WinkingSkull.com

A study aid for must-know anatomy

Register for WinkingSkull.com PLUS!

Your study aid for must-know anatomy

Gain a solid foundation in human anatomy with WinkingSkull.com, a study aid that is ideal for supplementing course study and for exam preparation. This user-friendly website features more than 200 stunning images derived from ***Atlas of Anatomy***.

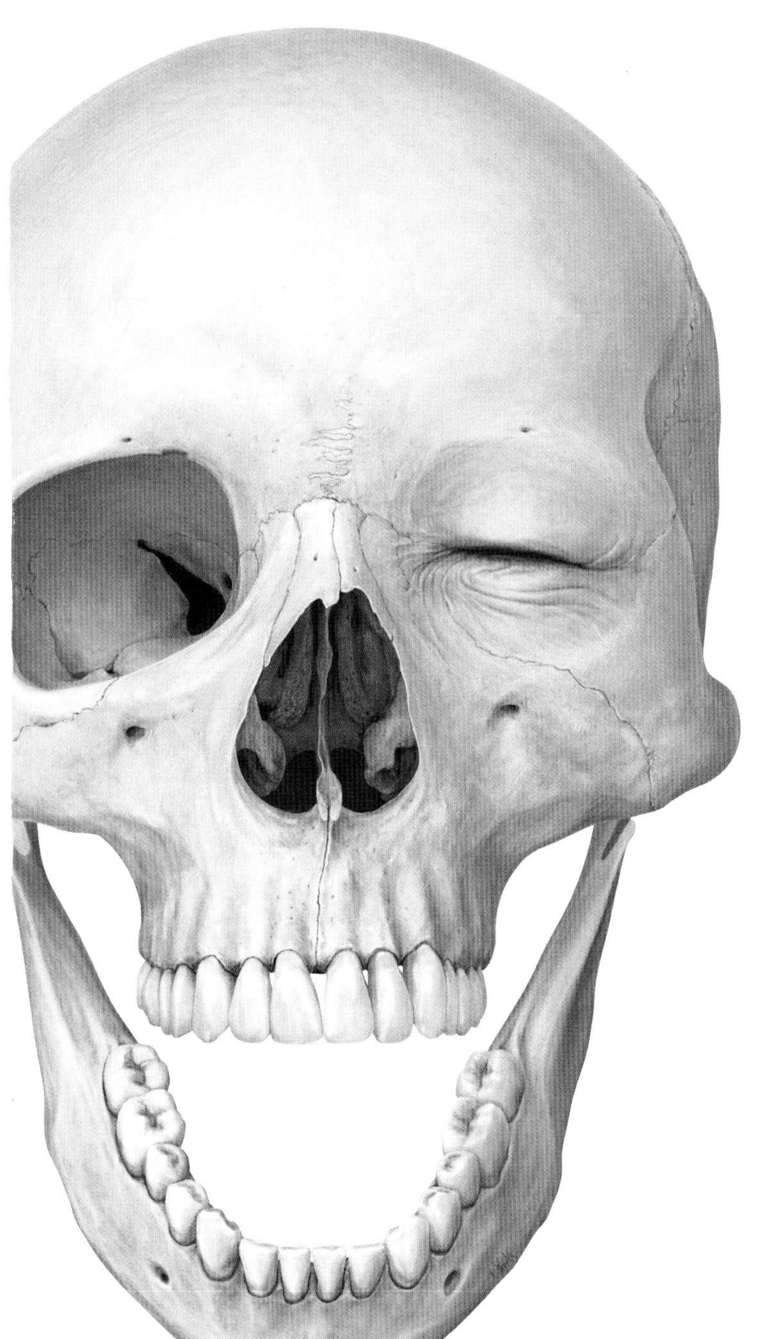

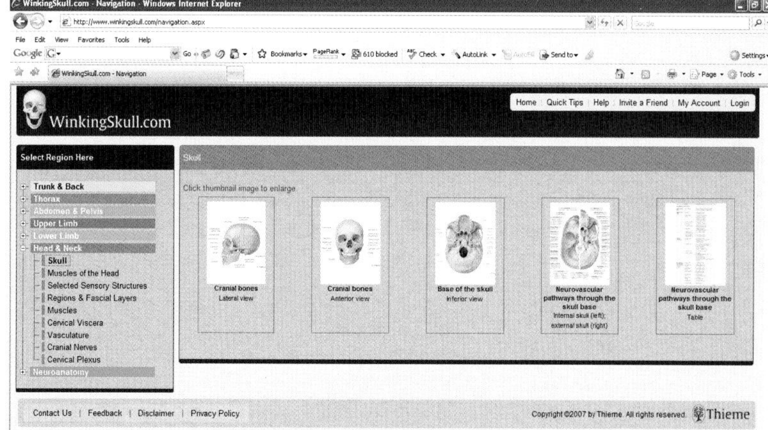
WinkingSkull.com
Home | Quick Tips | Help | Invite a Friend | My Account | Login
Select Region Here
Trunk & Back
Thorax
Abdomen & Pelvis
Upper Limb
Lower Limb
Head & Neck
Skull
Muscles of the Head
Selected Sensory Structures
Regions & Fascial Layers
Muscles
Cervical Viscera
Vasculature
Cranial Nerves
Cervical Plexus
Neuroanatomy
Skull
Click thumbnail image to enlarge
Cranial bones Lateral view
Cranial bones Anterior view
Base of the skull Inferior view
Contact Us | Feedback | Disclaimer | Privacy Policy
Thieme

FEATURES

- Must-know concepts for the study of anatomy
- An intuitive design that simplifies navigation
- Stunning, full-color illustrations—art of the 21st century!
- Timed tests to assess comprehension
- Test scores that are instantly available for viewing

Buyers of *Atlas of Anatomy* gain exclusive access to additional clinical content that builds on the highly practical scope of the book to prepare students for the clinical setting. This exclusive material includes:

- MRIs
- CT scans
- Sectional anatomy with explanatory schematics

Scratch the panel below to reveal the unique access code that will enable you to register for WinkingSkull.com PLUS. Log on to www.WinkingSkull.com to get started.

NOTE: This product cannot be returned if panel is scratched.

Atlas of Anatomy

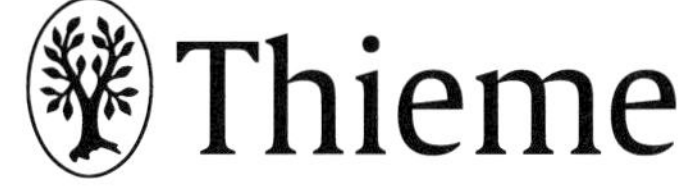
Thieme

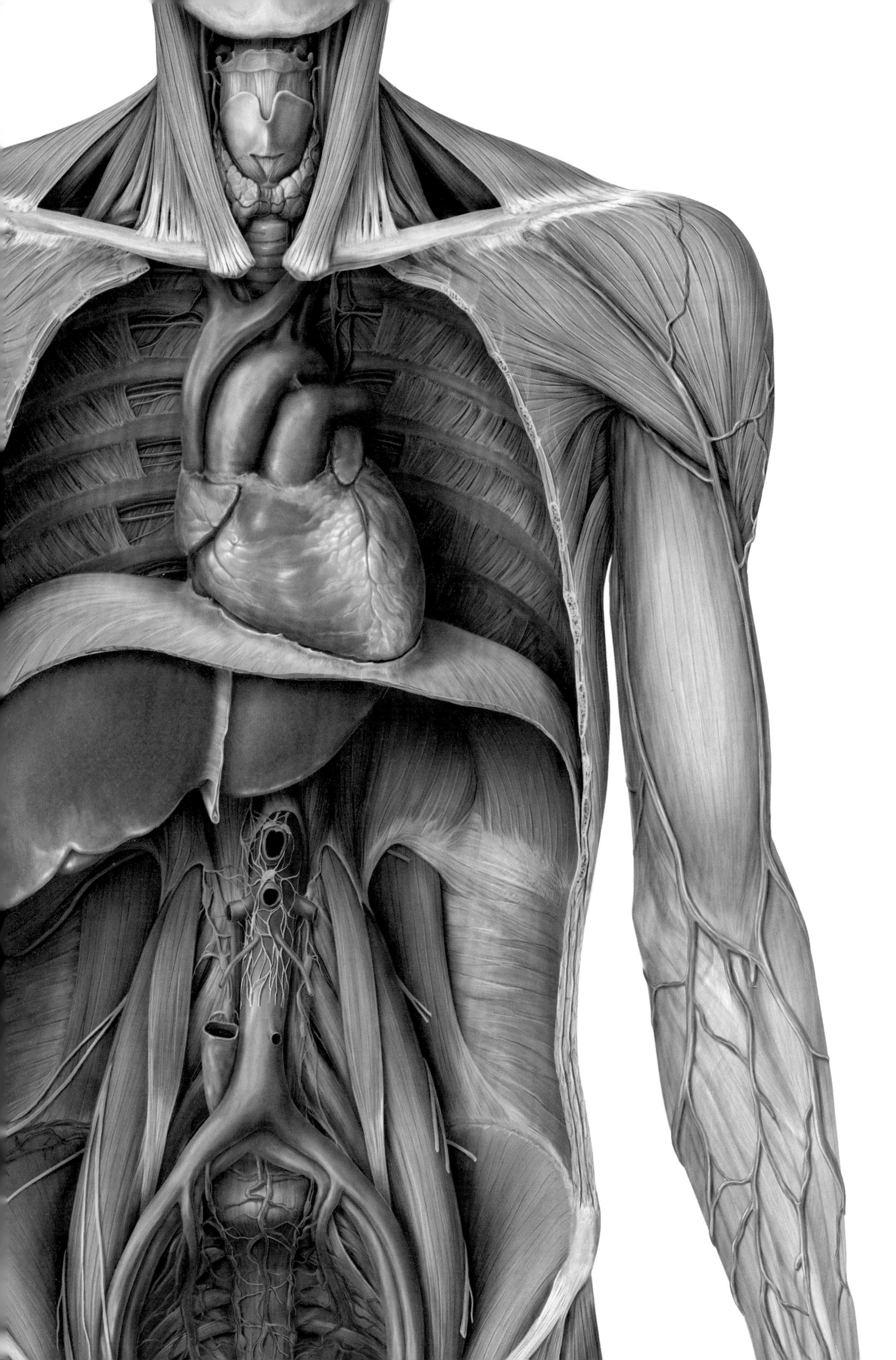

Atlas of Anatomy

Edited by
Anne M. Gilroy
Brian R. MacPherson
Lawrence M. Ross

Based on the work of
Michael Schuenke
Erik Schulte
Udo Schumacher

Consulting Editors
Jonas Broman
Anna Josephson

Illustrations by
Markus Voll
Karl Wesker

Thieme
New York · Stuttgart

Thieme Medical Publishers, Inc.
333 Seventh Avenue
New York, New York 10001

Based on the work of Michael Schuenke, MD, PhD,
Erik Schulte, MD, and Udo Schumacher, MD

Anne M. Gilroy, MA
Dept. of Cell Biology and Dept. of Surgery
University of Massachusetts Medical School
55 Lake Avenue North
Worcester, MA 01655-0333

Brian R. MacPherson, PhD
Department of Anatomy and Neurobiology
MN225 Chandler Medical Center
University of Kentucky College of Medicine
Lexington, KY 40536-0298

Lawrence M. Ross, MD, PhD
Department of Neurobiology and Anatomy
University of Texas Medical School at Houston
6431 Fannin, Suite 7.046
Houston, TX 77030

Michael Schuenke, MD, PhD
Institute of Anatomy
Christian Albrecht University Kiel
Olshausenstrasse 40
D-24098 Kiel

Erik Schulte, MD
Department of Anatomy and Cell Biology
Johannes Gutenberg University
Saarstrasse 19-21
D-55099 Mainz

Udo Schumacher, MD, FRCPath, CBiol, FIBiol, DSc
Institute of Anatomy II: Experimental Morphology
Center for Experimental Medicine
University Medical Center Hamburg-Eppendorf
Martinistrasse 52
D-20246 Hamburg

ISBN 978-1-60406-099-7

Developmental Editor: Bridget N. Queenan
Editorial Director, Educational Products: Cathrin Weinstein, MD
Senior Production Editor: Adelaide Elsie Starbecker
Director of Sales: Ross Lumpkin
National Sales Manager: James Nunn
Vice President, Production and Electronic Publishing: Anne T. Vinnicombe
Vice President, International Marketing and Sales: Cornelia Schulze
Chief Financial Officer: Peter van Woerden
President: Brian D. Scanlan

Consulting Editors
Jonas Broman, PhD
Anna Josephson, MD, PhD
Department of Neuroscience
Karolinska Institutet
S-17177 Stockholm

Illustrators
Markus Voll
Karl Wesker

Compositor: ICC Macmillan, Inc., Beverly, MA
Printer: Appl, Wemding, Germany

Library of Congress Cataloging-in-Publication Data is available from the publisher.

References: Detailed references are available from the publisher upon request.

Dedication

To my father, Francis Gilroy, whose dedication to medicine has been a greater inspiration to me than he has ever realized; to my students who lovingly tolerate, and sometimes share, my passion for human anatomy; and most of all to my sons, Colin & Bryan, whose love and support I treasure beyond all else.

To my friend and mentor, Dr. Ken McFadden of the Division of Anatomy at the University of Alberta, who ensured I received the training in gross anatomy instruction required to be successful, and to the thousands of professional students who I have taught over the past 30 years honing these skills. However, none of the success I've enjoyed during my time in academia would have been possible without the constant support, participation and encouragement of my wife, Cynthia Long.

To my wife, Irene; to the children, Chip, Jennifer, Jocelyn & Barry, Tricia, Scott, Katie & Snapper, and Trey; and to my students who have taught me so well.

Foreword

This Atlas of Anatomy is, in my opinion, the finest single volume atlas of human anatomy that has ever been created. Two factors make it so: the images and the way they have been organized.

The artists, Markus Voll and Karl Wesker, have created a new standard of excellence in anatomical art. Their graceful use of transparency and their sensitive representation of light and shadow give the reader an accurate three-dimensional understanding of every structure.

The authors have organized the images so that they give just the flow of information a student needs to build up a clear mental image of the human body. Each two-page spread is a self-contained lesson that unobtrusively shows the hand of an experienced and thoughtful teacher. I wish I could have held this book in my hands when I was a student; I envy any student who does so now.

Robert B. Acland
Louisville, KY
March 2008

Acknowledgments

We would like to thank the authors of the original award-winning Anatomy Series Michael Schuenke, Erik Schulte, and Udo Schumacher for their work over the course of many years.

We cordially thank the members of the Advisory Board for their contributions.

- Bruce M. Carlson, MD, PhD
  University of Michigan
  Ann Arbor, Michigan
- Derek Bryant (Class of 2011)
  University of Toronto Medical School
  Burlington, Ontario
- Peter Cole, MD
  Glamorum Healing Centre
  Orangeville, Ontario
- Michael Droller, MD
  The Mount Sinai Medical Center
  New York, New York
- Anthony Firth, PhD
  Imperial College London
  London
- Mark H. Hankin, PhD
  University of Toledo, College of Medicine
  Toledo, Ohio
- Katharine Hudson (Class of 2010)
  McGill Medical School
  Montreal, Quebec
- Christopher Lee (Class of 2010)
  Harvard Medical School
  Cambridge, Massachusetts
- Francis Liuzzi, PhD
  Lake Erie College of Osteopathic Medicine
  Bradenton, Florida
- Graham Louw, PhD
  University of Cape Town Medical School
  University of Cape Town
- Estomih Mtui, MD
  Weill Cornell Medical College
  New York, New York
- Srinivas Murthy, MD
  Harvard Medical School
  Boston, Massachusetts
- Jeff Rihn, MD
  The Rothman Institute
  Philadelphia, Pennsylvania
- Lawrence Rizzolo, PhD
  Yale University
  New Haven, Connecticut
- Mikel Snow, PhD
  University of Southern California
  Los Angeles, California
- Kelly Wright (Class of 2010)
  Wayne State University School of Medicine
  Detroit, Michigan

We gratefully acknowledge the contribution of the student translators from the Karolinska Institute in Stockholm, Sweden: Christoffer Brynte, Mårten Fällman, Jacob Lannerbro, and Hannah Sjöstedt.

Preface

Each of us was amazed and impressed with the extraordinary detail, accuracy, and beauty of the material that was created for the Thieme Atlas of Anatomy by authors Michael Schuenke, Erik Schulte, and Udo Schumacher and artists Markus Voll and Karl Wesker. We felt these atlases and their pedagogical concepts were one of the most significant additions to anatomical education in the past 50 years. It was our intent to use this exceptional material as the cornerstone of our effort to create a concise single volume Atlas of Anatomy for the curious and eager health science student.

Our challenge was first to select from this extensive collection those images that are most instructive and illustrative of current dissection approaches. Along the way, however, we realized that creating a single volume atlas was much more than choosing images: each image had to convey a significant amount of detail while the appeal and labeling needed to be clean and soothing to the eye. Therefore, hundreds of illustrations were drawn new or modified to fit the approach of this new atlas. In addition, key schematic diagrams and simplified summary-form tables were added wherever needed. Dozens of applicable radiographic images and important clinical correlates have been added where appropriate. Additionally, surface anatomy illustrations are accompanied by questions designed to direct the student's attention to anatomic detail that is most relevant in conducting the physical exam. Elements from each of these features are arranged in a regional format to facilitate common dissection approaches. Within each region the various components are examined systemically, followed by topographical images to tie the systems within the region together. In all of this, a clinical perspective on the anatomical structures is taken. The unique two facing pages "spread" format focuses the user to the area/topic being explored.

We hope these efforts, the results of close to 100 combined years of experience teaching the discipline of anatomy to bright, enthusiastic students, has resulted in a comprehensive, easy-to-use resource and reference.

We would like to thank our colleagues at Thieme Publishers who so professionally facilitated this effort. We cannot thank enough, Cathrin E. Schulz, MD, Editorial Director Educational Products, who so graciously reminded us of deadlines, while always being available to troubleshoot problems. More importantly, she encouraged, helped, and complimented our efforts.

We also wish to extend very special thanks and appreciation to Bridget Queenan, Developmental Editor, who edited and developed the manuscript with an outstanding talent for visualization and intuitive flow of information. We are very grateful to her for catching many details along the way while always patiently responding to requests for artwork and labeling changes.

Cordial thanks to Elsie Starbecker, Senior Production Editor, who with great care and speed produced this atlas with its over 2,200 illustrations. Finally thanks to Rebecca McTavish, Developmental Editor, for joining the team in the correction phase. Their hard work has made the Atlas of Anatomy a reality.

Anne M. Gilroy
Brian R. MacPherson
Lawrence M. Ross

March 2008,
Worcester, MA, Lexington, KY, and Houston, TX

Table of Contents

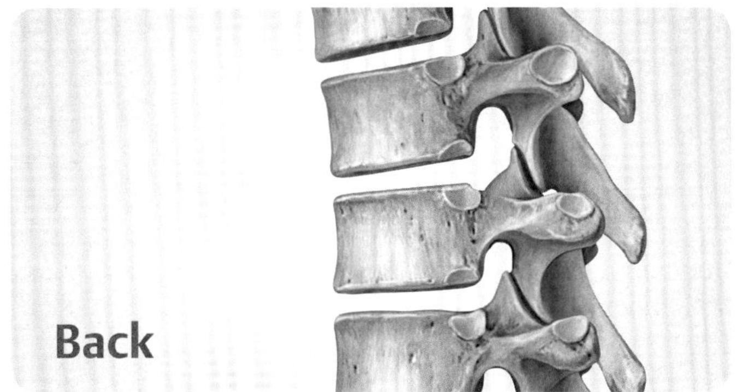
Back

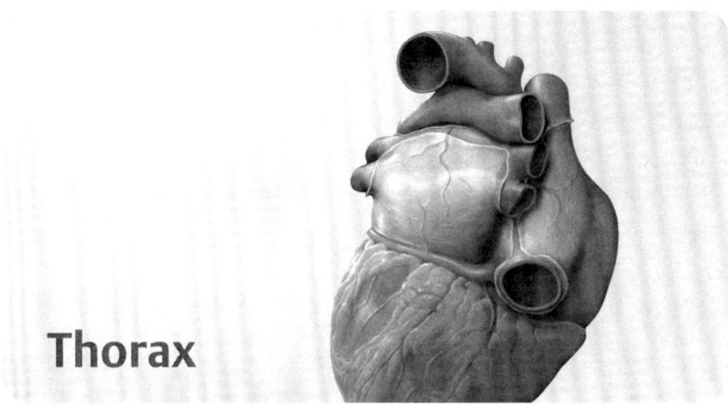
Thorax

1 Bones, Ligaments & Joints

Columna Vertebralis: Overview 2
Columna Vertebrales: Elements 4
Vertebrae Cervicale 6
Vertebrae Thoracicae and Lumbales 8
Os Sacrum and Os Coccygis 10
Discus Invertebralis 12
Articulationes Columnae Vertebralis: Overview 14
Joints of Columna Vertebralis: Craniovertebral Region 16
Vertebral Ligaments: Overview & Cervical Spine 18
Vertebral Ligaments: Thoracolumbar Spine 20

2 Muscles

Muscles of the Back: Overview 22
Intrinsic Muscles of the Cervical Spine 24
Intrinsic Muscles of the Back 26
Muscle Facts (I) 28
Muscle Facts (II) 30
Muscle Facts (III) 32

3 Neurovasculature

Arteries & Veins of the Back 34
Nerves of the Back 36
Neurovascular Topography of the Back 38

4 Surface Anatomy

Surface Anatomy 40

5 Thoracic Wall

Thoracic Skeleton 44
Sternum & Ribs 46
Joints of the Thoracic Cage 48
Thoracic Wall Muscle Facts 50
Diaphragm 52
Neurovasculature of the Diaphragm 54
Arteries & Veins of the Thoracic Wall 56
Nerves of the Thoracic Wall 58
Neurovascular Topography of the Thoracic Wall 60
Female Breast 62
Lymphatics of the Female Breast 64

6 Thoracic Cavity

Divisions of the Thoracic Cavity 66
Arteries of the Thoracic Cavity 68
Veins of the Thoracic Cavity 70
Lymphatics of the Thoracic Cavity 72
Nerves of the Thoracic Cavity 74

7 Mediastinum

Mediastinum: Overview 76
Mediastinum: Structures 78
Thymus & Pericardium 80
Heart in Situ 82
Heart: Surfaces & Chambers 84
Heart: Valves 86
Arteries & Veins of the Heart 88
Conduction & Innervation of the Heart 90
Heart: Radiology 92
Pre- & Postnatal Circulation 94
Esophagus 96
Neurovasculature of the Esophagus 98
Lymphatics of the Mediastinum 100

8 Pleural Cavity

Pleural Cavity 102
Lungs in Situ 104
Lung: Radiology 106
Bronchopulmonary Segments of the Lungs 108
Trachea & Bronchial Tree 110
Respiratory Mechanics 112
Pulmonary Arteries & Veins 114
Neurovasculature of the Tracheobronchial Tree 116
Lymphatics of the Pleural Cavity 118

9 Surface Anatomy

Surface Anatomy 120

Abdomen & Pelvis

10 Bones, Ligaments & Joints

Pelvic Girdle 124
Male & Female Pelvis 126
Pelvic Ligaments 128

11 Abdominal Wall

Muscles of the Abdominal Wall 130
Regio Inguinalis & Canalis Inguinalis 132
Abdominal Wall & Inguinal Hernias 134
Regio Perinealis 136
Abdominal Wall Muscle Facts 138
Pelvic Floor Muscle Facts 140

12 Spaces

Divisions of the Abdominopelvic Cavity 142
Cavitas Peritonealis & Greater Sac 144
Bursa Omentalis 146
Mesenterium & Posterior Wall 148
Contents of the Pelvis 150
Peritoneal Relationships 152
Pelvis & Perineum 154
Transverse Sections 156

13 Internal Organs

Gaster 158
Duodenum 160
Jejunum & Ileum 162
Cecum, Appendix & Colon 164
Rectum & Canalis Anulis 166
Hepar: Overview 168
Hepar: Segments & Lobes 170
Vesica Biliaris & Bile Ducts 172
Pancreas & Lien 174
Renes & Glandulae Suprarenales: Overview 176
Renes & Glandulae Suprarenales: Features 178
Ureter 180
Vesica Urinaria 182
Vesica Urinaria & Urethra 184

14 Reproductive Organs

Overview of the Genital Organs 186
Uterus & Ovaries 188
Vagina 190
Female External Genitalia 192
Neurovasculature of the Female Genitalia 194
Penis, Scrotum & Funiculus Spermaticus 196
Testis & Epididymis 198
Male Accessory Sex Glands 200
Neurovasculature of the Male Genitalia 202
Development of the Genitalia 204

15 Arteries & Veins

Arteries of the Abdomen 206
Aorta Abdominalis & Arteriae Renales 208
Truncus Coeliacus 210
Arteriae Mesenterica Superior & Inferior 212
Veins of the Abdomen 214
Vena Cava Inferior & Venae Renales 216
Vena Portae Hepatis 218
Venae Mesenterica Superior & Inferior 220
Arteries & Veins of the Pelvis 222
Arteries & Veins of the Rectum & Genitalia 224

16 Lymphatics

Lymph Nodes of the Abdomen & Pelvis 226
Lymph Nodes of the Posterior Abdominal Wall 228
Lymph Nodes of the Anterior Abdominal Organs 230
Lymph Nodes of the Intestines 232
Lymph Nodes of the Genitalia 234

17 Nerves

Plexus Autonomicus 236
Innervation of the Abdominal Organs 238
Innervation of the Intestines 240
Innervation of the Pelvis 242
Autonomic Innervation: Overview 244
Autonomic Innervation: Urinary & Genital Organs 246

18 Surface Anatomy

Surface Anatomy 248

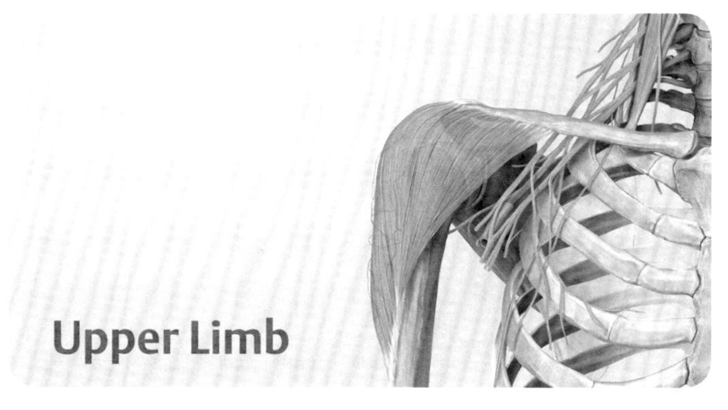
Upper Limb

19 Shoulder & Arm

Bones of the Upper Limb 252
Clavicula & Scapula 254
Humerus 256
Joints of the Shoulder 258
Joints of the Shoulder: Articulatio Humeri 260
Subacromial Space & Bursae 262
Anterior Muscles of the Shoulder & Arm (I) 264
Anterior Muscles of the Shoulder & Arm (II) 266
Posterior Muscles of the Shoulder & Arm (I) 268
Posterior Muscles of the Shoulder & Arm (II) 270
Muscle Facts (I) 272
Muscle Facts (II) 274
Muscle Facts (III) 276
Muscle Facts (IV) 278

20 Elbow & Forearm

Radius & Ulna 280
Articulatio Cubiti 282
Ligaments of Articulatio Cubiti 284
Radioulnar Joints 286
Muscles of the Forearm (I) 288
Muscles of the Forearm (II) 290
Muscle Facts (I) 292
Muscle Facts (II) 294
Muscle Facts (III) 296

21 Wrist & Hand

Bones of the Wrist & Hand 298
Joints of the Wrist & Hand 300
Ligaments of the Wrist & Hand 302
Ligaments of the Fingers 304
Muscles of the Hand: Superficial & Middle Layers 306
Muscles of the Hand: Middle & Deep Layers 308
Dorsum of the Hand 310
Muscle Facts (I) 312
Muscle Facts (II) 314

22 Neurovasculature

Arteries of the Upper Limb 316
Veins & Lymphatics of the Upper Limb 318
Nerves of Plexus Brachialis 320
Supraclavicular Branches & Fasciculus Posterior 322
Fasciculus Posterior: N. Axillaris & N. Radialis 324
Fasciculus Medialis & Fasciculus Lateralis 326
N. Medianus & N. Ulnaris 328
Superficial Veins & Nerves of the Upper Limb 330
Posterior Shoulder & Axilla 332
Anterior Shoulder 334
Topography of the Axilla 336
Topography of the Brachial & Cubital Regions 338
Topography of the Forearm 340
Topography of the Carpal Region 342
Topography of the Palm of the Hand 344
Topography of the Dorsum of the Hand 346
Transverse Sections 348

23 Surface Anatomy

Surface Anatomy (I) 350
Surface Anatomy (II) 352

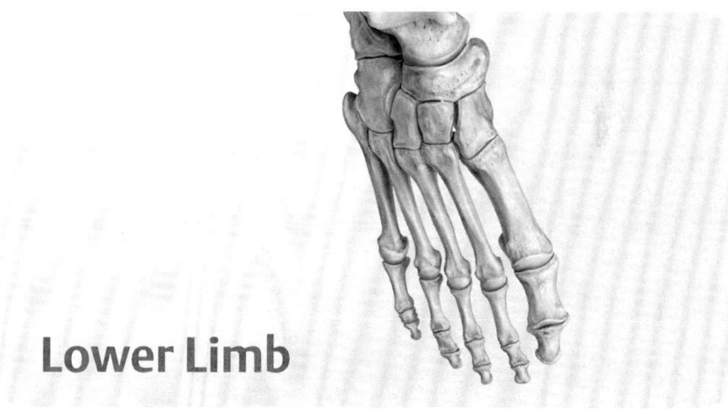
Lower Limb

24 Hip & Thigh

Bones of the Lower Limb 356
Pelvic Girdle & Os Coxae 358
Femur 360
Articulatio Coxae: Overview 362
Articulatio Coxae: Ligaments & Capsule 364
Anterior Muscles of the Thigh, Hip & Regio Glutealis (I) 366
Anterior Muscles of the Thigh, Hip & Regio Glutealis (II) 368
Posterior Muscles of the Thigh, Hip & Regio Glutealis (I) 370
Posterior Muscles of the Thigh, Hip & Regio Glutealis (II) 372
Muscle Facts (I) 374
Muscle Facts (II) 376
Muscle Facts (III) 378

25 Knee & Leg

Tibia & Fibula 380
Articulatio Genus: Overview 382
Articulatio Genus: Capsule, Ligaments & Bursae 384
Articulatio Genus: Ligaments & Menisci 386
Ligamenta Cruciata 388
Articulatio Genus Cavitas Articularis 390
Muscles of the Leg: Anterior & Lateral Views 392

Muscles of the Leg: Posterior View 394
Muscle Facts (I) 396
Muscle Facts (II) 398

26 Ankle & Foot

Ossa Pedis 400
Articulationes Pedis (I) 402
Articulationes Pedis (II) 404
Articulationes Pedis (III) 406
Ligaments of the Ankle & Foot 408
Plantar Vault & Arches of the Foot 410
Muscles of the Sole of the Foot 412
Muscles & Tendon Sheaths of the Foot 414
Muscle Facts (I) 416
Muscle Facts (II) 418

27 Neurovasculature

Arteries of the Lower Limb 420
Veins & Lymphatics of the Lower Limb 422
Plexus Lumbosacralis 424
Nerves of Plexus Lumbalis 426
Nerves of Plexus Lumbalis: N. Obturatoris & N. Femoralis 428
Nerves of Plexus Sacralis 430
Nerves of Plexus Sacralis: N. Ischiadicus 432
Superficial Nerves & Vessels of the Lower Limb 434
Topography of Regio Inguinalis 436
Topography of Regio Glutealis 438
Topography of the Anterior & Posterior Thigh 440
Topography of the Posterior & Medial Leg 442
Topography of the Lateral & Anterior Leg 444
Topography of Planta Pedis 446
Transverse Sections of the Thigh & Leg 448

28 Surface Anatomy

Surface Anatomy 450

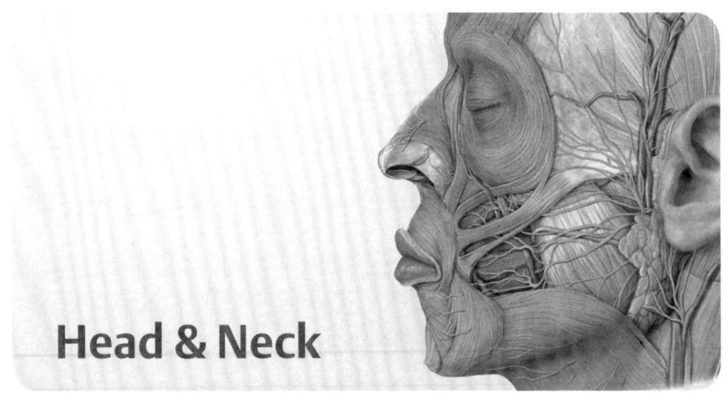
Head & Neck

29 Bones of the Head

Anterior & Lateral Skull 454
Posterior Skull & Calvaria 456
Base of the Skull 458
Os Ethmoidale & Os Sphenoidale 460

30 Muscles of the Skull & Face

Muscles of Facial Expression & of Mastication 462
Muscle Origins & Insertions on the Skull 464
Muscle Facts (I) 466
Muscle Facts (II) 468

31 Cranial Nerves

Cranial Nerves: Overview 470
CN I & II: N. Olfactorius & N. Opticus 472
CN III, IV & VI:
N. Oculomotorius, N. Trochlearis & N. Abducens 474
CN V: N. Trigeminus 476
CN VII: N. Facialis 478
CN VIII: N. Vestibulocochlearis 480
CN IX: N. Glossopharyngeus 482
CN X: N. Vagus 484
CN XI & XII: N. Accessorius & N. Hypoglossus 486

32 Neurovasculature of the Skull & Face

Innervation of the Face 488
Arteries of the Head & Neck 490
A. Carotis Externa:
Anterior, Medial & Posterior Branches 492
A. Carotis Externa: Terminal Branches 494
Veins of the Head & Neck 496
Topography of the Superficial Face 498
Topography of the Parotid Region & Fossa Temporalis 500
Topography of Fossa Infratemporalis 502
Topography of Fossa Pterygopalatina 504

33 Orbit & Eye

Bones of the Orbita 506
Muscles of the Orbita 508
Neurovasculature of the Orbita 510

Topography of the Orbita 512
Orbita & Eyelid 514
Eyeball (Bulbus Oculi) 516
Cornea, Iris & Lens 518

34 Nasal Cavity & Nose

Bones of the Nasal Cavity (Cavitas Nasi) 520
Paranasal Air Sinuses (Sinus Paranasales) 522
Neurovasculature of the Nasal Cavity 524

35 Temporal Bone & Ear

Os Temporale 526
External Ear (Auris Externa) & Auditory Canal 528
Middle Ear (Auris Media):
Tympanic Cavity (Cavitas Tympani) 530
Middle Ear: Ossicular Chain & Tympanic Membrane 532
Arteries of the Middle Ear 534
Inner Ear (Auris Interna) 536

36 Oral Cavity & Pharynx

Bones of the Oral Cavity (Cavitas Oris) 538
Articulatio Temporomandibularis 540
Teeth (Dentes) 542
Muscles of the Oral Cavity 544
Innervation of the Oral Cavity 546
Tongue (Lingua) 548
Topography of the Oral Cavity & Salivary Glands 550
Tonsils & Pharynx 552
Pharyngeal Muscles 554
Neurovasculature of the Pharynx 556

37 Neck

Bones & Ligaments of the Neck 558
Overview & Superficial Muscles of the Neck 560
Suprahyoid & Infrahyoid Muscles of the Neck 562
Deep Muscles of the Neck 564
Arteries & Veins of the Neck 566
Innervation of the Neck 568
Larynx: Cartilage & Structure 570
Larynx: Muscles & Levels 572
Neurovasculature of the Larynx, Thyroid & Parathyroids ... 574
Topography of the Neck: Regions & Fascia 576
Topography of the Anterior Cervical Region 578
Topography of the Anterior & Lateral Cervical Regions 580
Topography of the Lateral Cervical Region 582
Topography of the Posterior Cervical Region 584
Lymphatics of the Neck 586

38 Surface Anatomy

Surface Anatomy 588

Neuroanatomy

39 Brain & Spinal Cord

Nervous System: Overview 592
Telencephalon 594
Telencephalon & Diencephalon 596
Diencephalon, Brainstem & Cerebellum 598
Medulla Spinalis 600
Meninges 602
Ventricles & CSF Spaces 604

40 Blood Vessels of the Brain & Spinal Cord

Sinus Durae Matris & Veins of the Brain 606
Arteries of the Brain 608
Arteries & Veins of the Spinal Cord 610

41 Functional Systems

Circuitry 612
Sensory & Motor Pathways 614
Sensory Systems (I) 616
Sensory Systems (II) 618
Sensory Systems (III) 620

42 Autonomic Nervous System

Autonomic Nervous System 622

Appendix

Answers to Surface Anatomy Questions 626

Index 628

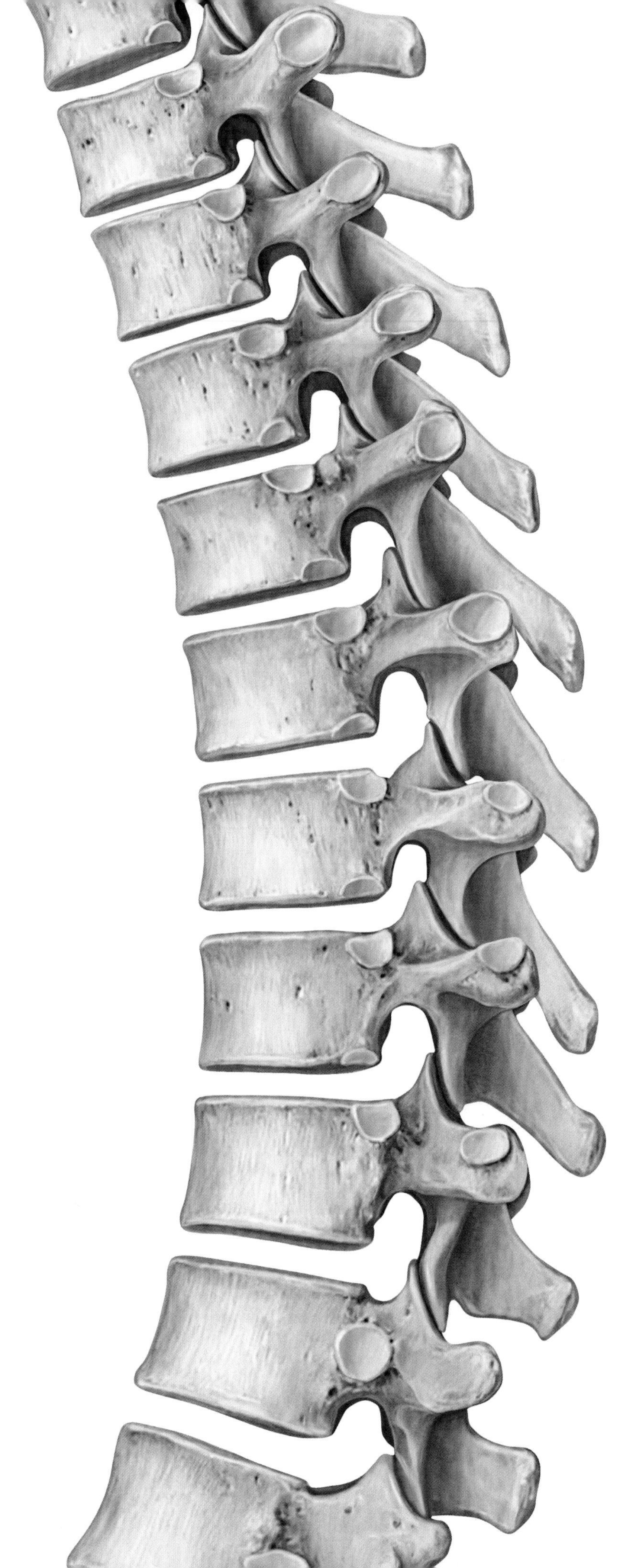

Back

1 Bones, Ligaments & Joints

Columna Vertebralis: Overview 2
Columna Vertebrales: Elements 4
Vertebrae Cervicales 6
Vertebrae Thoracicae and Lumbales 8
Os Sacrum and Os Coccygis 10
Discus Intervertebralis 12
Articulationes Columnae Vertebralis: Overview 14
Joints of Columna Vertebralis: Craniovertebral Region 16
Vertebral Ligaments: Overview & Cervical Spine 18
Vertebral Ligaments: Thoracolumbar Spine 20

2 Muscles

Muscles of the Back: Overview 22
Intrinsic Muscles of the Cervical Spine 24
Intrinsic Muscles of the Back 26
Muscle Facts (I) 28
Muscle Facts (II) 30
Muscle Facts (III) 32

3 Neurovasculature

Arteries & Veins of the Back 34
Nerves of the Back 36
Neurovascular Topography of the Back 38

4 Surface Anatomy

Surface Anatomy 40

Columna Vertebralis: Overview

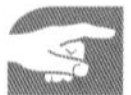

Columna vertebralis (spine) is divided into four regions: the cervical, thoracic, lumbar, and sacral spines. Both the cervical and lumbar spines demonstrate lordosis (inward curvature); the thoracic and sacral spines demonstrate kyphosis (outward curvature).

Fig. 1.1 **Columna vertebralis**
Left lateral view.

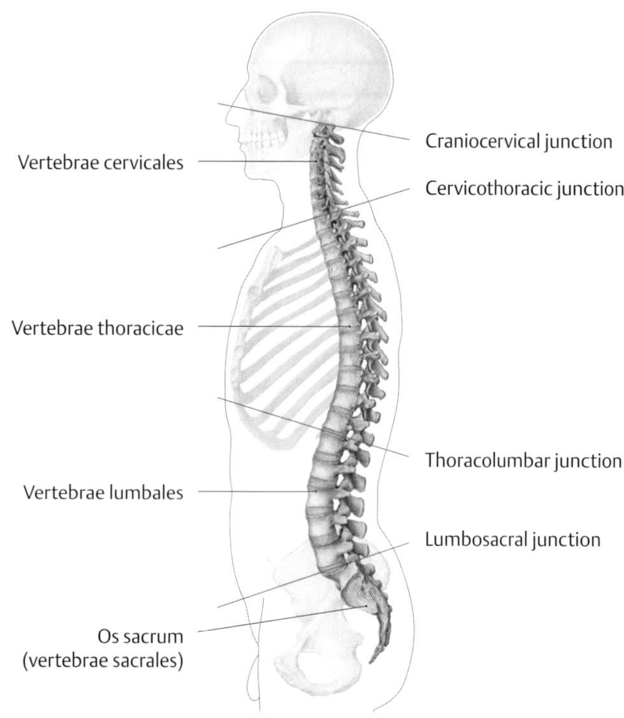

Vertebrae cervicales
Craniocervical junction
Cervicothoracic junction
Vertebrae thoracicae
Thoracolumbar junction
Vertebrae lumbales
Lumbosacral junction
Os sacrum
(vertebrae sacrales)

A Regions of the spine.

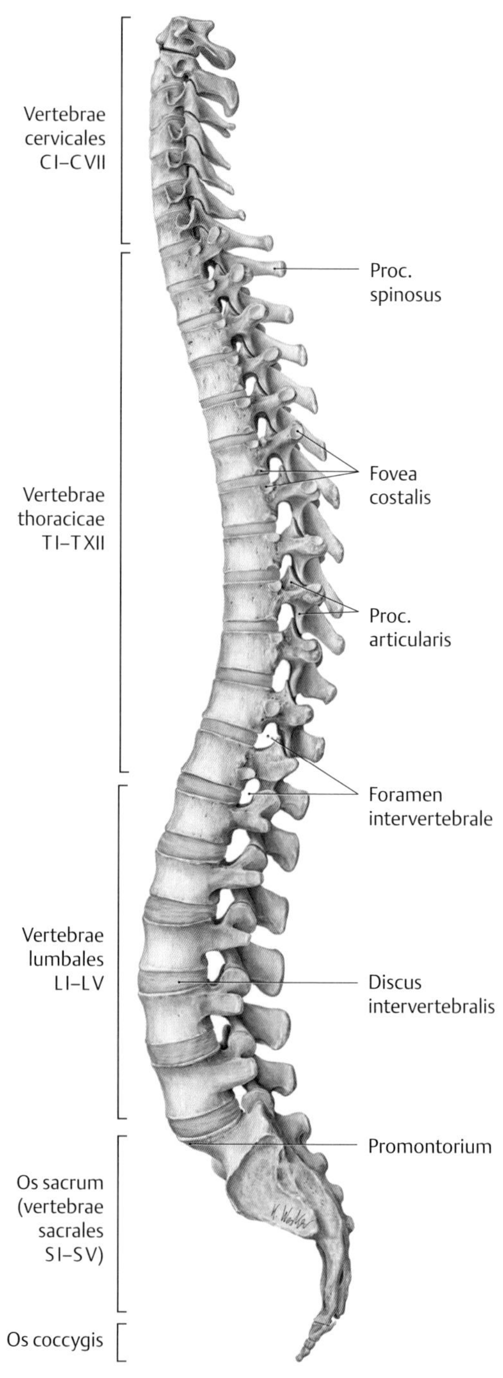

Vertebrae
cervicales
CI–CVII
Proc.
spinosus
Fovea
costalis
Vertebrae
thoracicae
TI–TXII
Proc.
articularis
Foramen
intervertebrale
Vertebrae
lumbales
LI–LV
Discus
intervertebralis
Promontorium
Os sacrum
(vertebrae
sacrales
SI–SV)
Os coccygis

B Bony vertebral column.

Clinical

Spinal development

The characteristic curvatures of the adult spine appear over the course of postnatal development, being only partially present in a newborn. The newborn has a "kyphotic" spinal curvature (**A**); lumbar lordosis develops later and becomes stable at puberty (**C**).

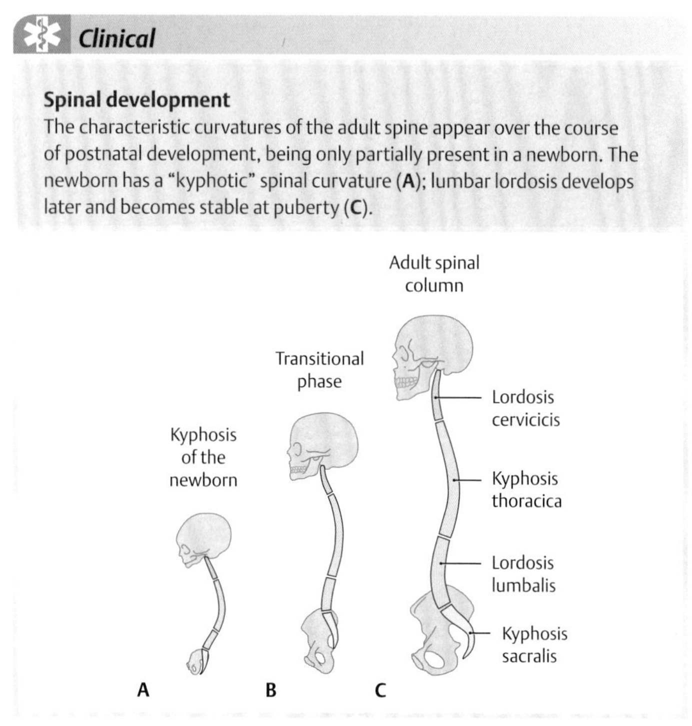

Adult spinal
column
Transitional
phase
Kyphosis
of the
newborn
Lordosis
cervicicis
Kyphosis
thoracica
Lordosis
lumbalis
Kyphosis
sacralis
A
B
C

Fig. 1.2 **Normal anatomical position of the spine**
Left lateral view.

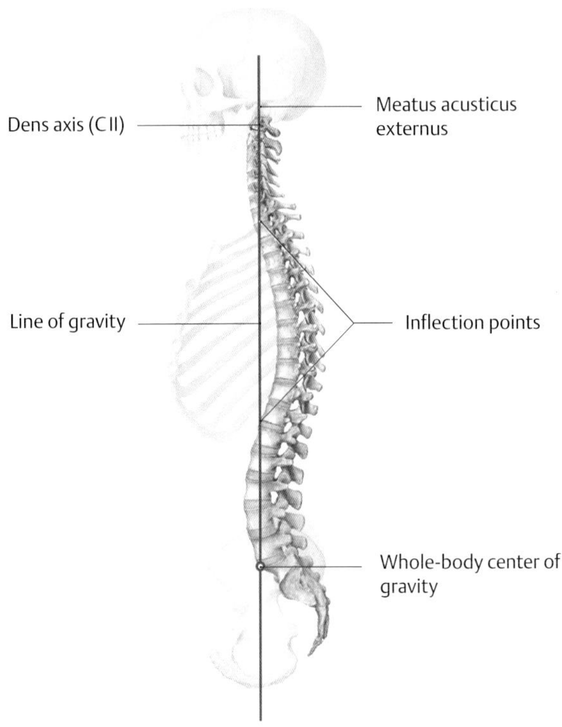
Dens axis (C II)
Meatus acusticus externus
Line of gravity
Inflection points
Whole-body center of gravity

A Line of gravity. The line of gravity passes through certain anatomical landmarks, including the inflection points at the cervicothoracic and thoracolumbar junctions. It continues through the center of gravity (anterior to the sacral promontory) before passing through the hip joint, knee, and ankle.

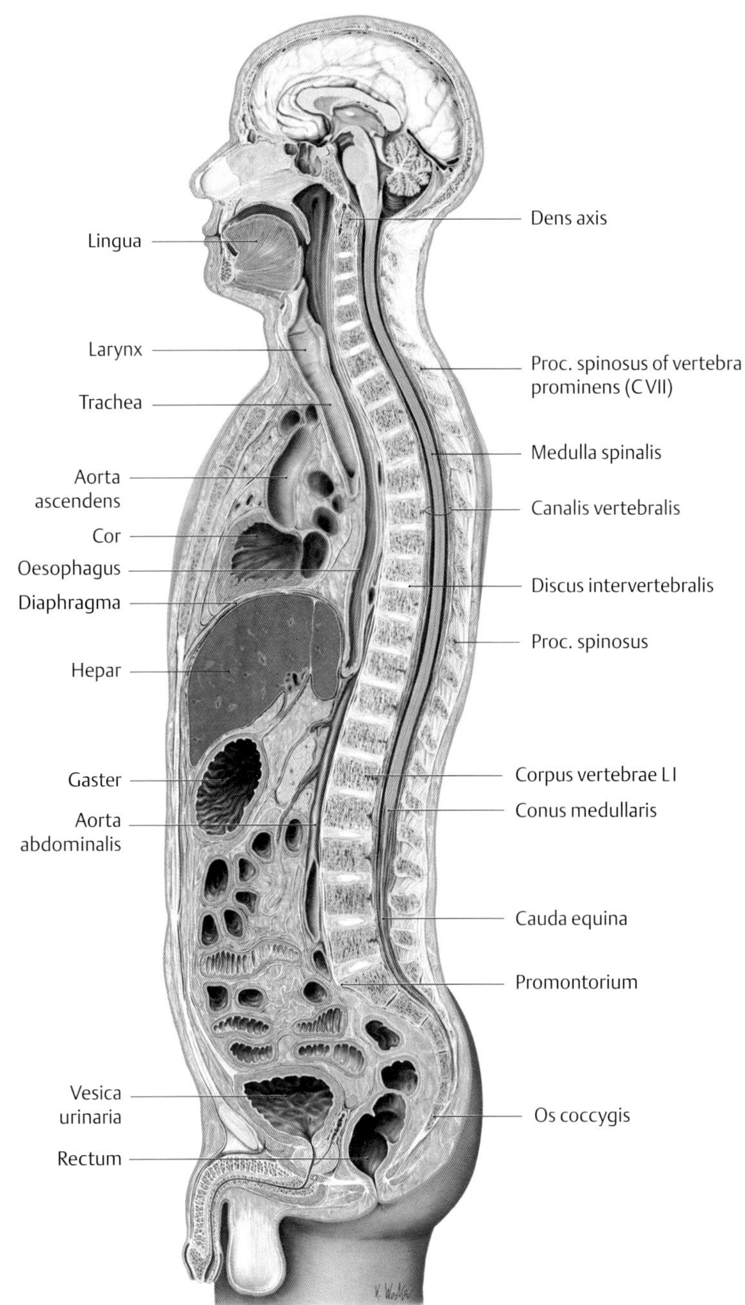
Lingua
Larynx
Trachea
Aorta ascendens
Cor
Oesophagus
Diaphragma
Hepar
Gaster
Aorta abdominalis
Vesica urinaria
Rectum
Dens axis
Proc. spinosus of vertebra prominens (C VII)
Medulla spinalis
Canalis vertebralis
Discus intervertebralis
Proc. spinosus
Corpus vertebrae L I
Conus medullaris
Cauda equina
Promontorium
Os coccygis

B Midsagittal section through an adult male.

Columna Vertebrales: Elements

Fig. 1.3 Bones of columna vertebrales

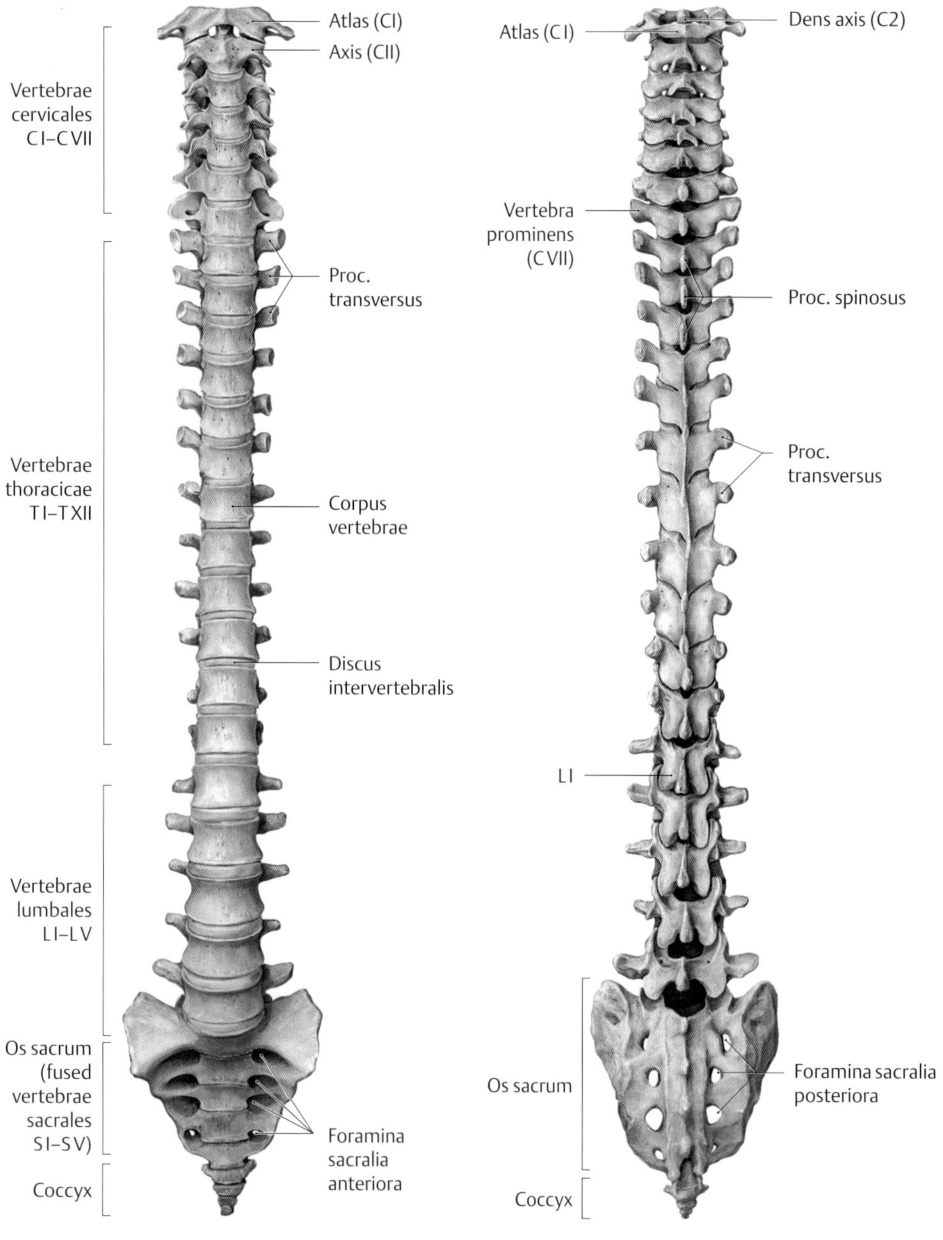
Atlas (CI)
Axis (CII)
Vertebrae cervicales CI–CVII
Proc. transversus
Vertebrae thoracicae TI–TXII
Corpus vertebrae
Discus intervertebralis
Vertebrae lumbales LI–LV
Os sacrum (fused vertebrae sacrales SI–SV)
Foramina sacralia anteriora
Coccyx
Atlas (CI)
Dens axis (C2)
Vertebra prominens (CVII)
Proc. spinosus
Proc. transversus
LI
Os sacrum
Foramina sacralia posteriora
Coccyx

A Anterior view.

B Posterior view.

Fig. 1.4 Palpable processus spinosus as landmarks

Posterior view. The easily palpated processus spinosus provide important landmarks during physical examination.

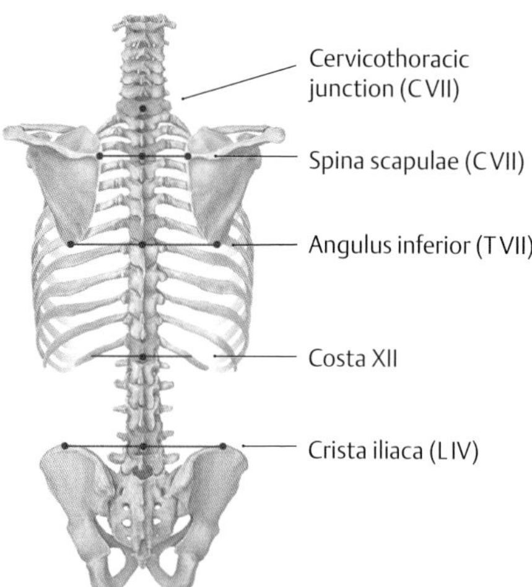
Cervicothoracic junction (CVII)
Spina scapulae (CVII)
Angulus inferior (TVII)
Costa XII
Crista iliaca (LIV)

Fig. 1.5 Structural elements of a vertebra

Left posterosuperior view. With the exception of the atlas (C I) and axis (C II), all vertebrae consist of the same structural elements.

Fig. 1.6 Typical vertebrae

Superior view.

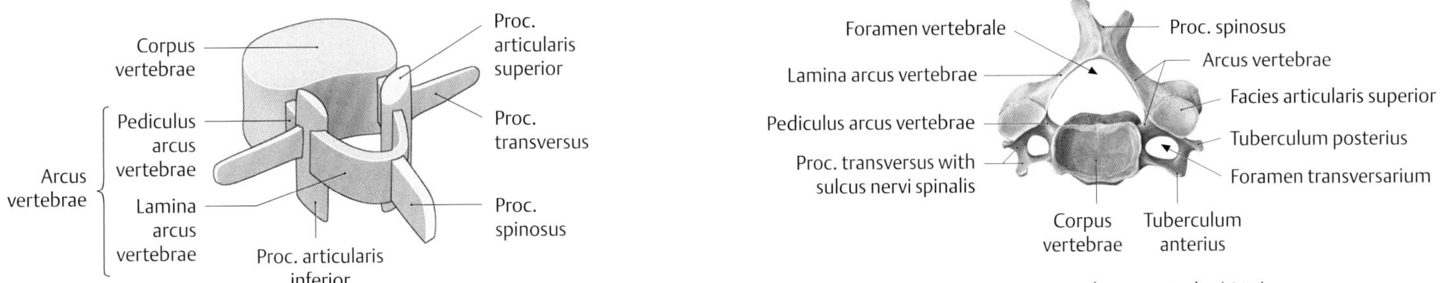

Corpus vertebrae
Proc. articularis superior
Pediculus arcus vertebrae
Proc. transversus
Arcus vertebrae
Lamina arcus vertebrae
Proc. spinosus
Proc. articularis inferior
Foramen vertebrale
Proc. spinosus
Lamina arcus vertebrae
Arcus vertebrae
Facies articularis superior
Pediculus arcus vertebrae
Tuberculum posterius
Proc. transversus with sulcus nervi spinalis
Foramen transversarium
Corpus vertebrae
Tuberculum anterius

A Vertebra cervicalis (C IV).

Fovea costalis
Proc. spinosus
Lamina arcus vertebrae
Proc. transversus
Pediculus arcus vertebrae
Facies articularis superior
Facies costalis inferior
Facies costalis superior
Corpus vertebrae

B Vertebra thoracalis (T VI).

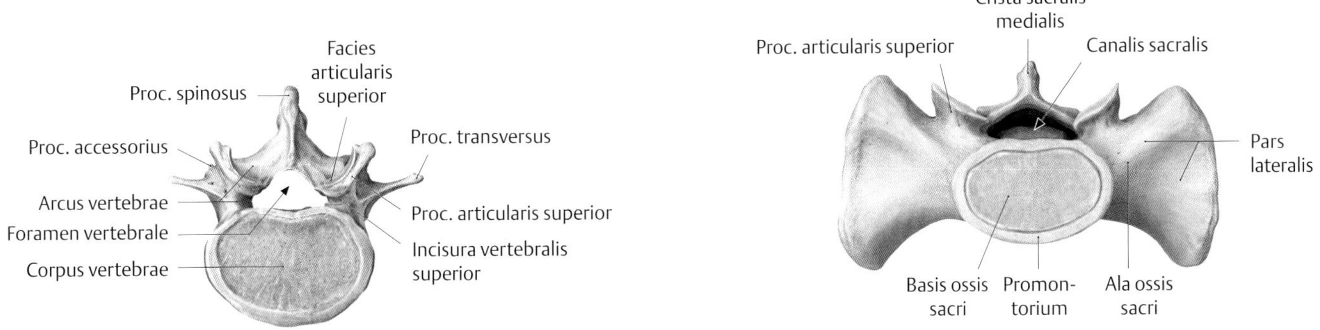

Proc. spinosus
Facies articularis superior
Proc. accessorius
Proc. transversus
Arcus vertebrae
Foramen vertebrale
Proc. articularis superior
Corpus vertebrae
Incisura vertebralis superior
Crista sacralis medialis
Proc. articularis superior
Canalis sacralis
Pars lateralis
Basis ossis sacri
Promon-torium
Ala ossis sacri

C Vertebra lumbalis (L IV).

D Os sacrum.

Table 1.1 Structural elements of vertebrae

Vertebrae	Body	Vertebral foramen	Transverse processes	Articular processes	Spinous process
Vertebrae cervicales C III*–C VII	Small (kidney-shaped)	Large (triangular)	Small (may be absent in C VII); tuberculum anterius and posterius enclose foramen transversum	Superoposteriorly and inferoanteriorly; oblique facets: most nearly horizontal	Short (C III–C V); bifid (C III–C VI); long (C VII)
Vertebrae thoracicae T I–T XII	Medium (heart-shaped); includes costal facets	Small (circular)	Large and strong; length decreases T I–T XII; costal facets (T I–T X)	Posteriorly (slightly laterally) and anteriorly (slightly medially); facets in coronal plane	Long, sloping postero-inferiorly; tip extends to level of vertebral body below
Vertebrae lumbales L I–L V	Large (kidney-shaped)	Medium (triangular)	Long and slender; proc. accessorius on posterior surface	Posteromedially (or medially) and anterolaterally (or laterally); facets nearly in sagittal plane; proc. mammilaris on posterior surface of each processus articularis superior	Short and broad
Vertebrae sacrales (os sacrum) S I–S V (fused)	Decreases from base to apex	Canalis sacralis	Fused to rudimentary rib (ribs, see pp. 44–47)	Superoposteriorly (SI) superior surface of lateral sacrumauricular surface	Crista sacralis mediana

*C I (atlas) and C II (axis) are considered atypical (see pp. 6–7).

Vertebrae Cervicales

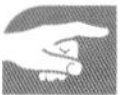

The seven vertebrae of the cervical spine differ most conspicuously from the common vertebral morphology. They are specialized to bear the weight of the head and allow the neck to move in all directions. C I and C II are known as the atlas and axis, respectively. C VII is called the vertebra prominens for its long, palpable spinous process.

Fig. 1.7 Cervical spine

Left lateral view.

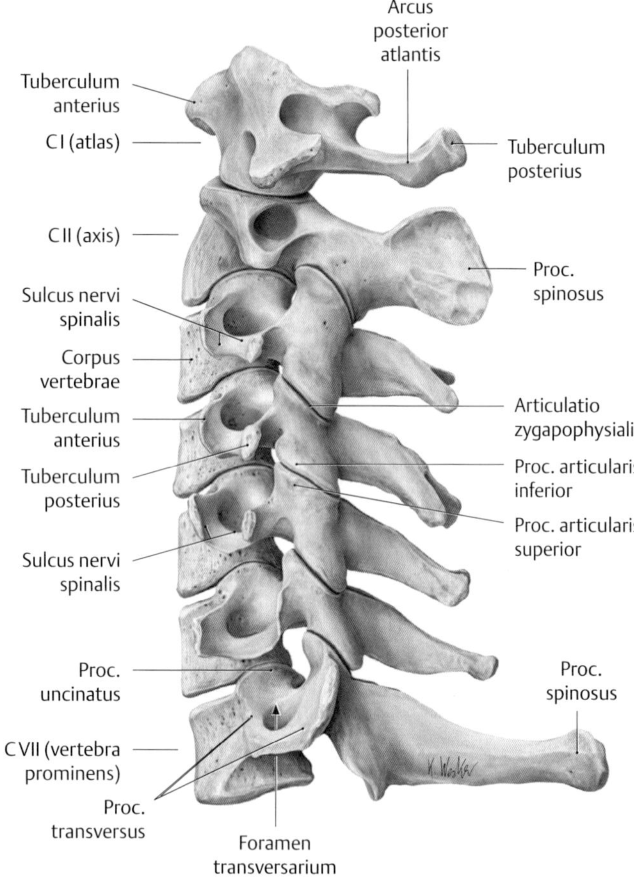
Arcus posterior atlantis
Tuberculum anterius
C I (atlas)
Tuberculum posterius
C II (axis)
Proc. spinosus
Sulcus nervi spinalis
Corpus vertebrae
Articulatio zygapophysialis
Tuberculum anterius
Tuberculum posterius
Proc. articularis inferior
Proc. articularis superior
Sulcus nervi spinalis
Proc. uncinatus
Proc. spinosus
C VII (vertebra prominens)
Proc. transversus
Foramen transversarium

A Bones of the cervical spine, left lateral view.

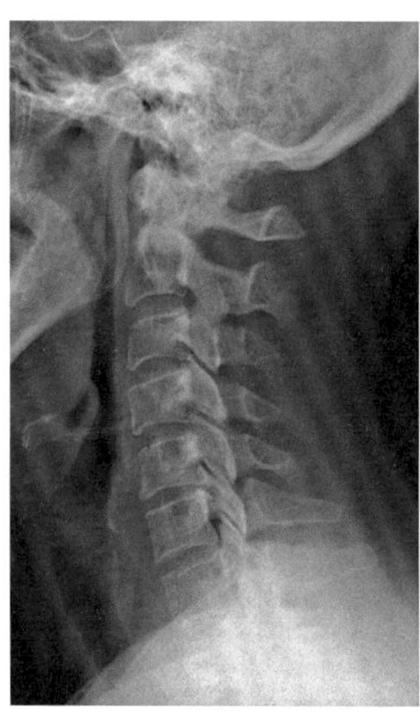

B Radiograph of the cervical spine, left lateral view.

Fig. 1.8 Atlas (C I)

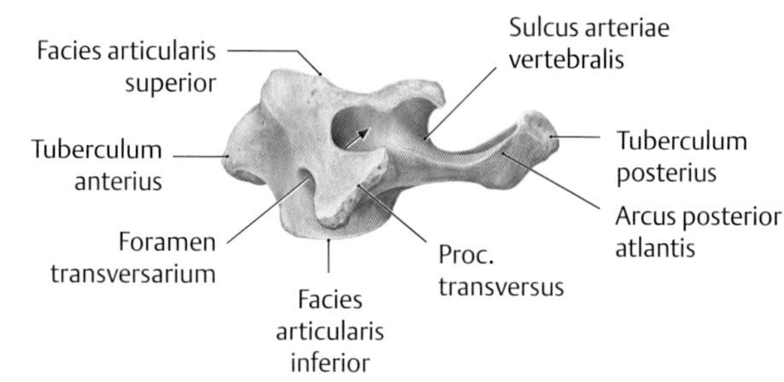
Facies articularis superior
Sulcus arteriae vertebralis
Tuberculum anterius
Tuberculum posterius
Arcus posterior atlantis
Foramen transversarium
Proc. transversus
Facies articularis inferior

A Left lateral view.

Fig. 1.9 Axis (C II)

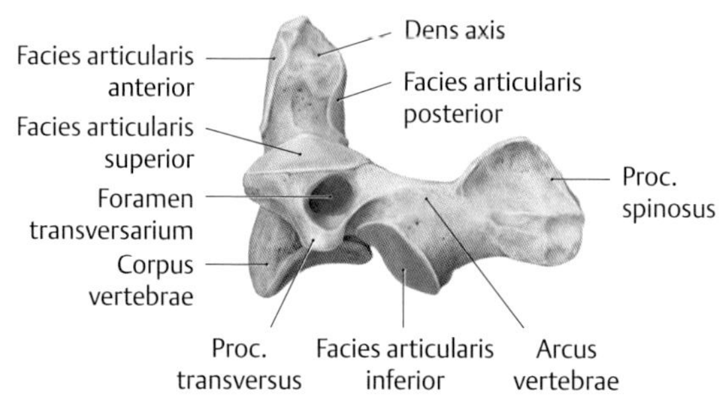
Dens axis
Facies articularis anterior
Facies articularis posterior
Facies articularis superior
Foramen transversarium
Proc. spinosus
Corpus vertebrae
Proc. transversus
Facies articularis inferior
Arcus vertebrae

A Left lateral view.

Fig. 1.10 Typical cervical vertebra (C IV)

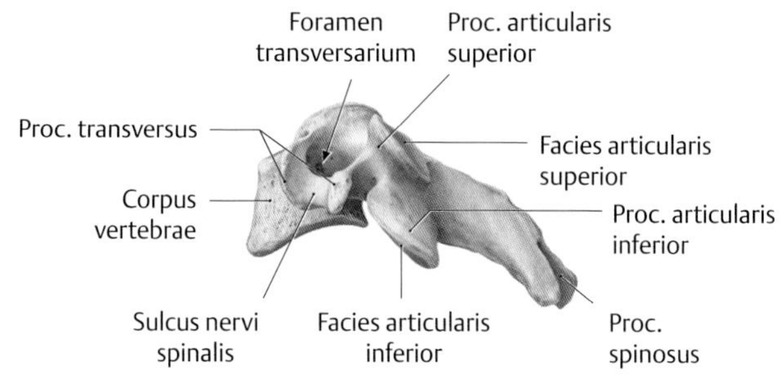
Foramen transversarium
Proc. articularis superior
Proc. transversus
Facies articularis superior
Corpus vertebrae
Proc. articularis inferior
Sulcus nervi spinalis
Facies articularis inferior
Proc. spinosus

A Left lateral view.

Clinical

Injuries in the cervical spine

The cervical spine is prone to hyperextension injuries, such as "whiplash," which can occur when the head extends back much farther than it normally would. The most common injuries of the cervical spine are fractures of the dens of the axis, traumatic spondylolisthesis (ventral slippage of a vertebral body), and atlas fractures. Patient prognosis is largely dependent on the spinal level of the injuries (see p. 600).

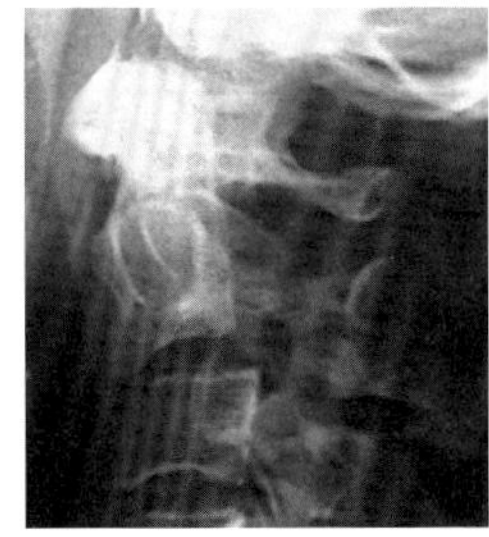

This patient hit the dashboard of his car while not wearing a seat belt. The resulting hyperextension caused the traumatic spondylolisthesis of C II (axis) with fracture of arcus vertebrae of C II, as well as tearing of the ligaments between C II and C III. This injury is often referred to as "hangman's fracture."

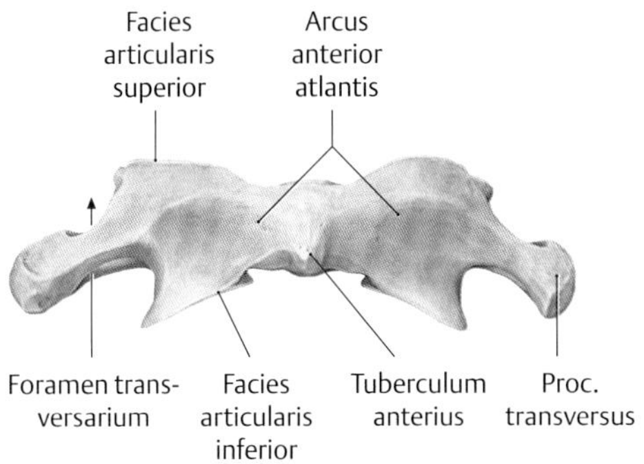
Facies articularis superior
Arcus anterior atlantis
Foramen transversarium
Facies articularis inferior
Tuberculum anterius
Proc. transversus

B Anterior view.

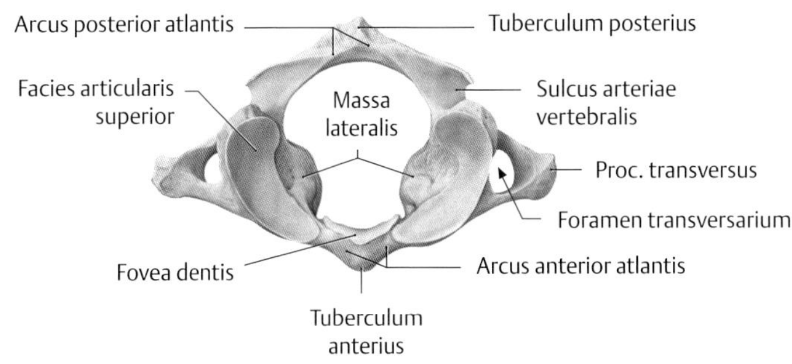
Arcus posterior atlantis
Tuberculum posterius
Facies articularis superior
Massa lateralis
Sulcus arteriae vertebralis
Proc. transversus
Foramen transversarium
Fovea dentis
Arcus anterior atlantis
Tuberculum anterius

C Superior view.

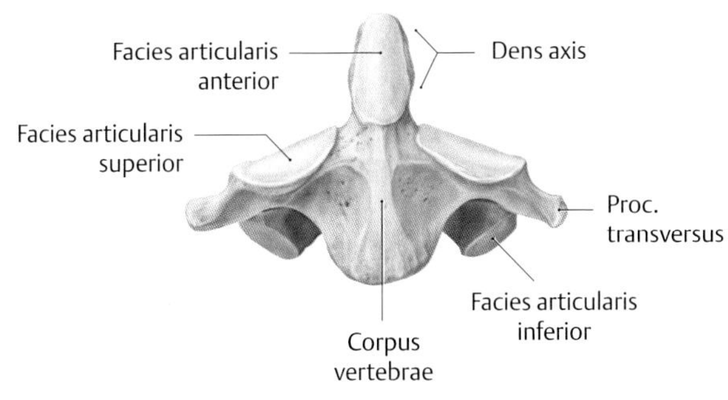
Facies articularis anterior
Dens axis
Facies articularis superior
Proc. transversus
Facies articularis inferior
Corpus vertebrae

B Anterior view.

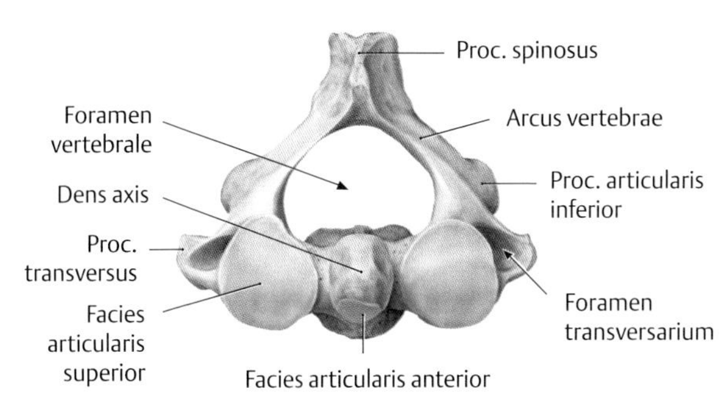
Proc. spinosus
Foramen vertebrale
Arcus vertebrae
Dens axis
Proc. articularis inferior
Proc. transversus
Facies articularis superior
Foramen transversarium
Facies articularis anterior

C Superior view.

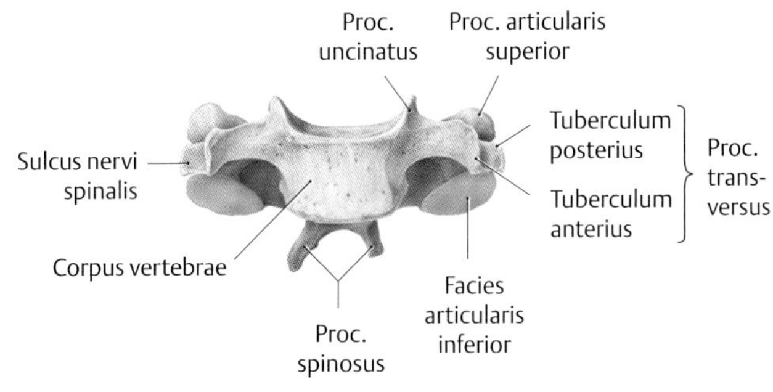
Proc. uncinatus
Proc. articularis superior
Tuberculum posterius
Proc. transversus
Tuberculum anterius
Sulcus nervi spinalis
Corpus vertebrae
Facies articularis inferior
Proc. spinosus

B Anterior view.

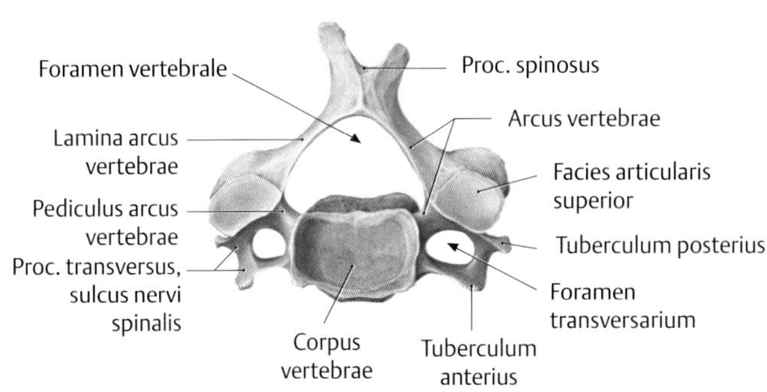
Foramen vertebrale
Proc. spinosus
Arcus vertebrae
Lamina arcus vertebrae
Facies articularis superior
Pediculus arcus vertebrae
Tuberculum posterius
Proc. transversus, sulcus nervi spinalis
Foramen transversarium
Corpus vertebrae
Tuberculum anterius

C Superior view.

Vertebrae Thoracicae and Lumbales

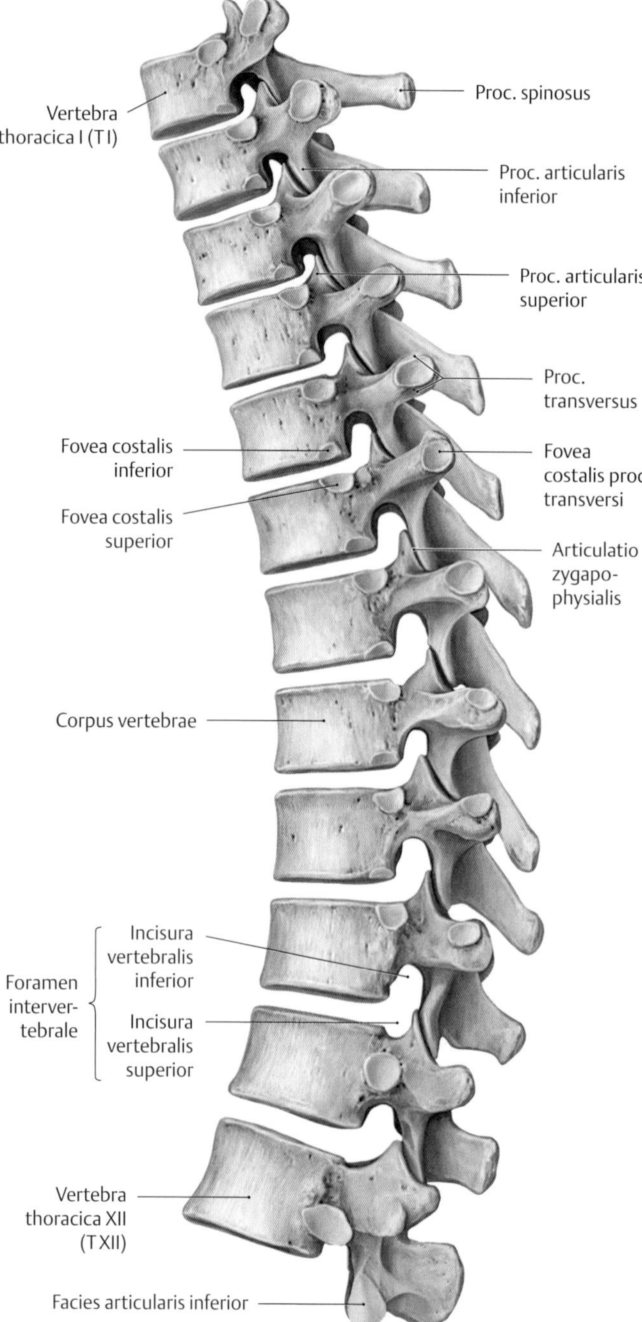

Proc. spinosus
Vertebra thoracica I (T I)
Proc. articularis inferior
Proc. articularis superior
Proc. transversus
Fovea costalis inferior
Fovea costalis proc. transversi
Fovea costalis superior
Articulatio zygapophysialis
Corpus vertebrae
Foramen intervertebrale
Incisura vertebralis inferior
Incisura vertebralis superior
Vertebra thoracica XII (T XII)
Facies articularis inferior

Fig. 1.11 **Thoracic spine**
Left lateral view.

Fig. 1.12 **Typical vertebra thoracalis (T VI)**

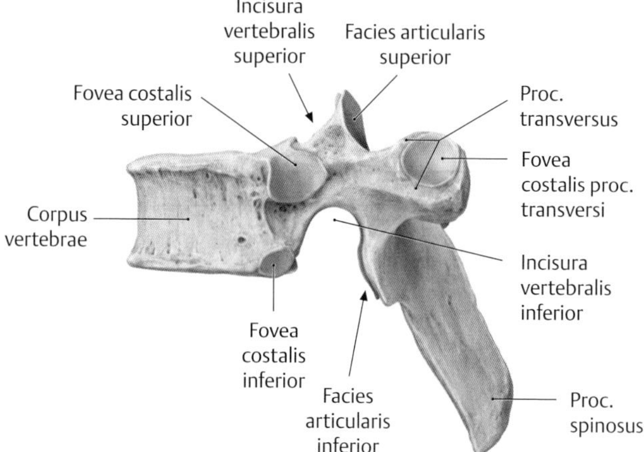

Incisura vertebralis superior
Facies articularis superior
Fovea costalis superior
Proc. transversus
Fovea costalis proc. transversi
Corpus vertebrae
Incisura vertebralis inferior
Fovea costalis inferior
Facies articularis inferior
Proc. spinosus

A Left lateral view.

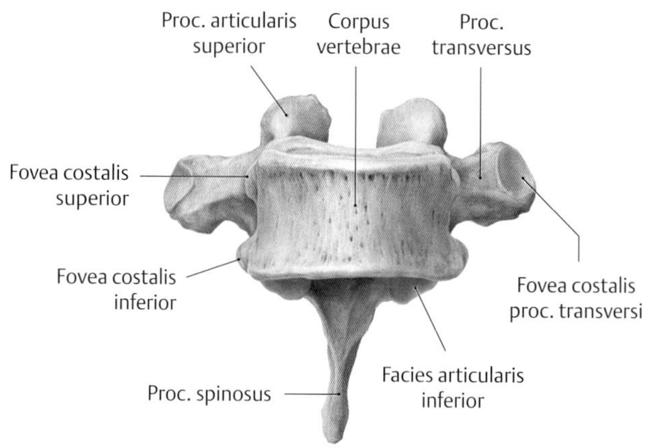

Proc. articularis superior
Corpus vertebrae
Proc. transversus
Fovea costalis superior
Fovea costalis inferior
Fovea costalis proc. transversi
Facies articularis inferior
Proc. spinosus

B Anterior view.

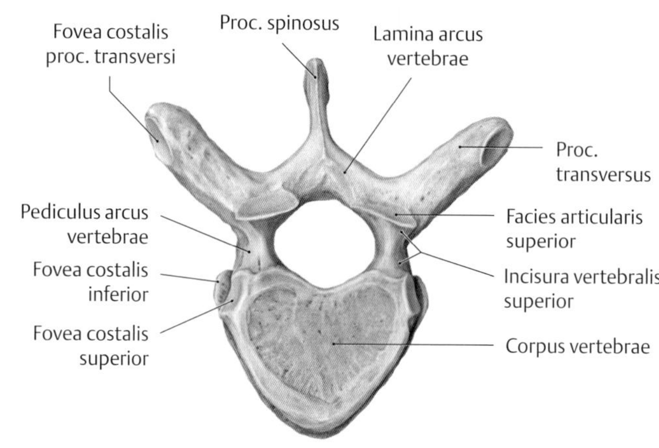

Fovea costalis proc. transversi
Proc. spinosus
Lamina arcus vertebrae
Proc. transversus
Pediculus arcus vertebrae
Facies articularis superior
Fovea costalis inferior
Incisura vertebralis superior
Fovea costalis superior
Corpus vertebrae

C Superior view.

Fig. 1.13 Lumbar spine

Left lateral view.

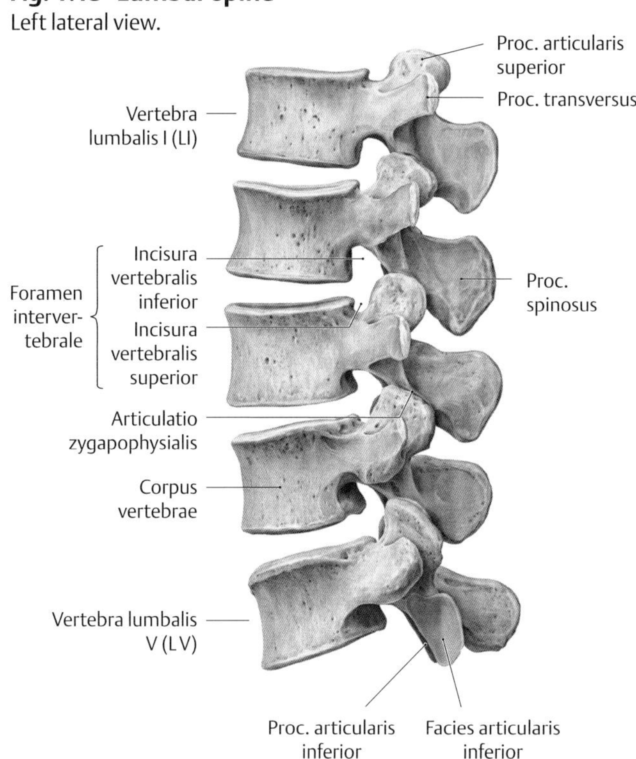
Proc. articularis superior
Proc. transversus
Vertebra lumbalis I (LI)
Foramen interver-tebrale
Incisura vertebralis inferior
Incisura vertebralis superior
Proc. spinosus
Articulatio zygapophysialis
Corpus vertebrae
Vertebra lumbalis V (LV)
Proc. articularis inferior
Facies articularis inferior

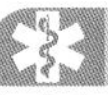

Clinical

Osteoporosis

The spine is the structure most affected by degenerative diseases of the skeleton, such as arthrosis and osteoporosis. In osteoporosis, more bone material gets reabsorbed than built up, resulting in a loss of bone mass. Symptoms include compression fractures and resulting back pain.

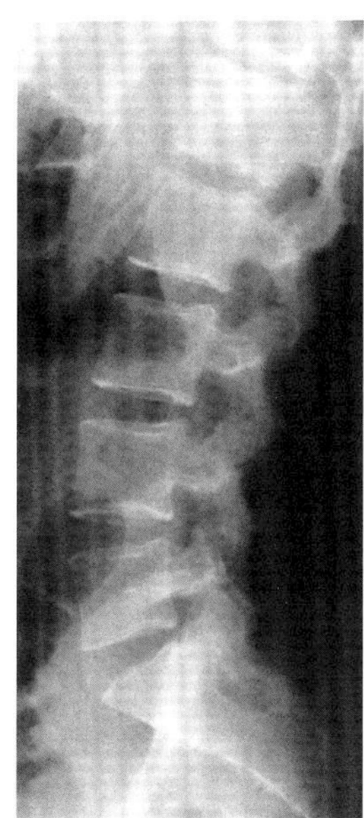

A Radiograph of a normal lumbar spine, left lateral view.

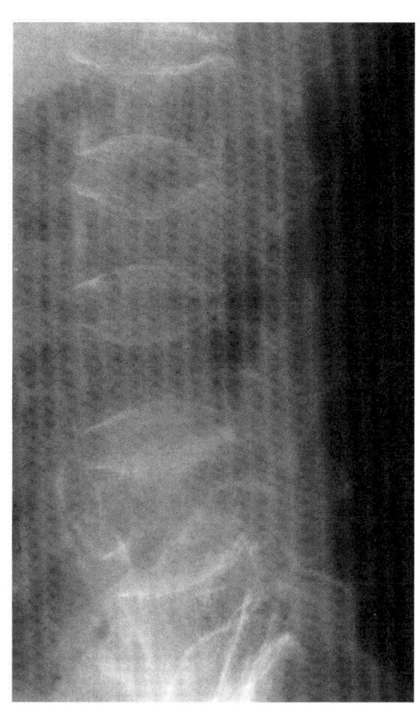

B Radiograph of an osteoporotic spine. Corpus vertebrae are decreased in density, and the internal trabecular structure is coarse. Lower and upper end plates are fractured.

Fig. 1.14 Typical vertebra lumbalis (LIV)

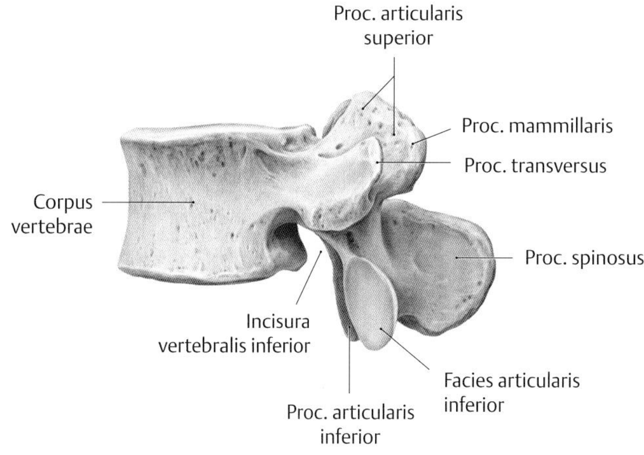
Proc. articularis superior
Proc. mammillaris
Proc. transversus
Corpus vertebrae
Proc. spinosus
Incisura vertebralis inferior
Facies articularis inferior
Proc. articularis inferior

A Left lateral view.

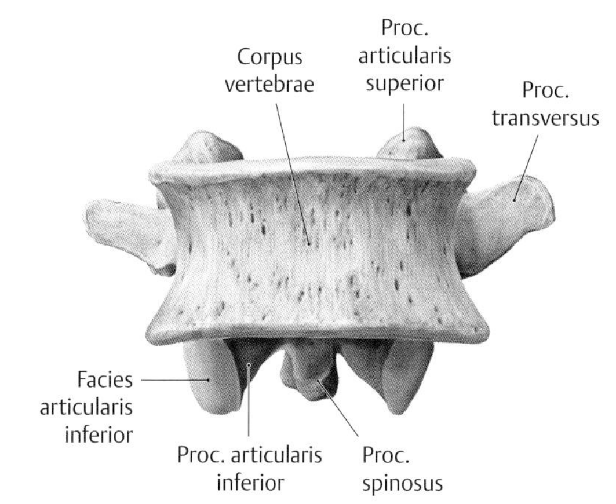
Corpus vertebrae
Proc. articularis superior
Proc. transversus
Facies articularis inferior
Proc. articularis inferior
Proc. spinosus

B Anterior view.

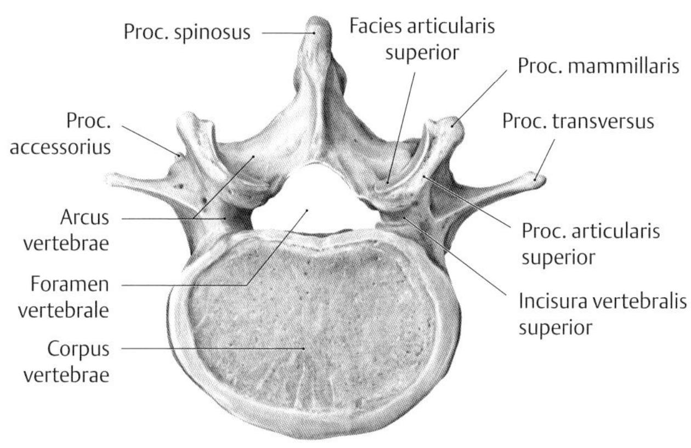
Proc. spinosus
Facies articularis superior
Proc. mammillaris
Proc. accessorius
Proc. transversus
Arcus vertebrae
Proc. articularis superior
Foramen vertebrale
Incisura vertebralis superior
Corpus vertebrae

C Superior view.

Os Sacrum and Os Coccygis

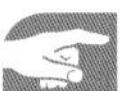

The sacrum is formed from five postnatally fused sacral vertebrae. The base of the sacrum articulates with the fifth lumbar vertebra (L V), and the apex articulates with the coccyx, a series of three or four rudimentary vertebrae.

Fig. 1.15 Os sacrum and os coccygis

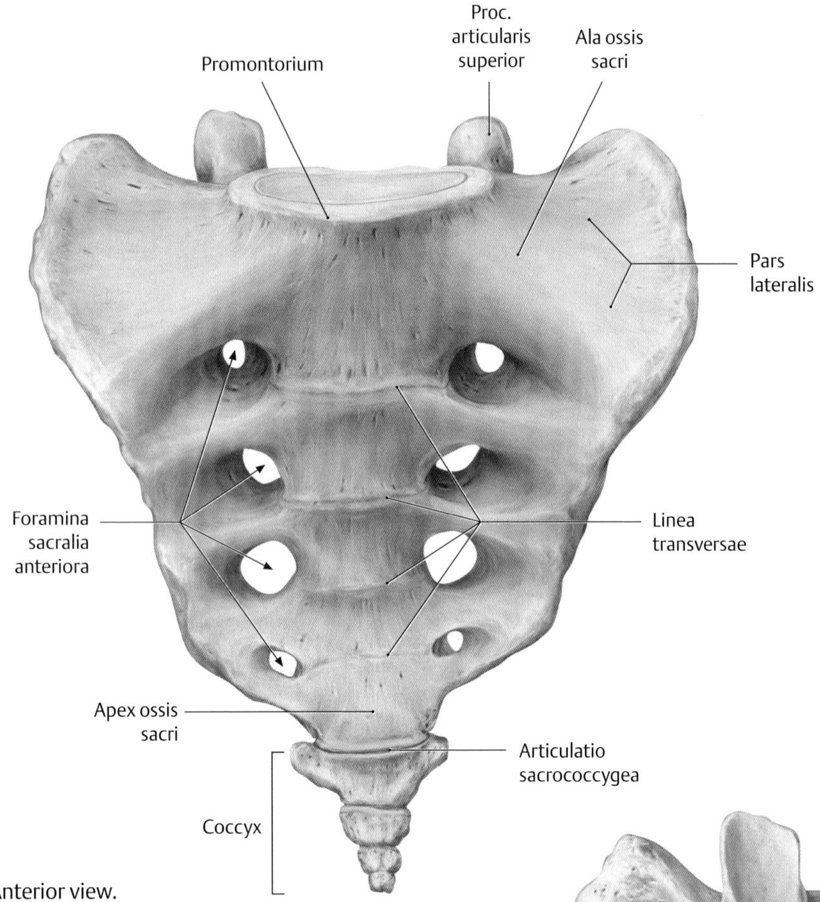

Promontorium
Proc. articularis superior
Ala ossis sacri
Pars lateralis
Foramina sacralia anteriora
Linea transversae
Apex ossis sacri
Articulatio sacrococcygea
Coccyx

A Anterior view.

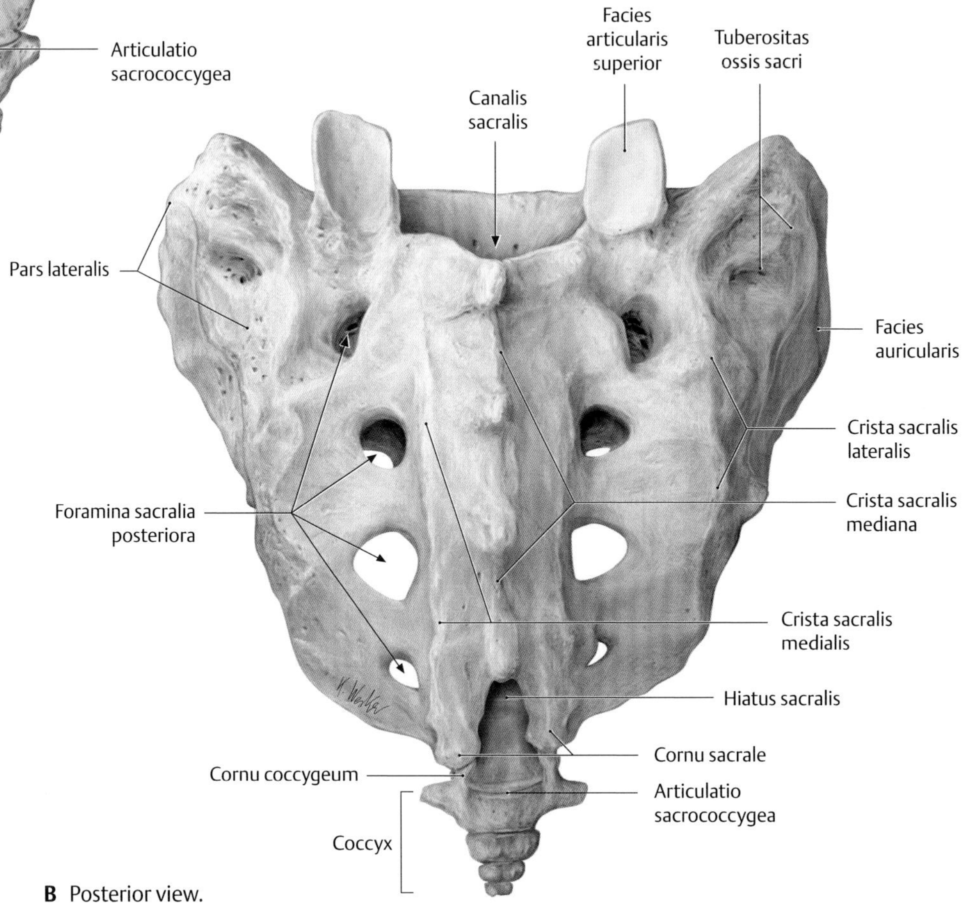

Canalis sacralis
Facies articularis superior
Tuberositas ossis sacri
Pars lateralis
Facies auricularis
Crista sacralis lateralis
Foramina sacralia posteriora
Crista sacralis mediana
Crista sacralis medialis
Hiatus sacralis
Cornu sacrale
Cornu coccygeum
Articulatio sacrococcygea
Coccyx

B Posterior view.

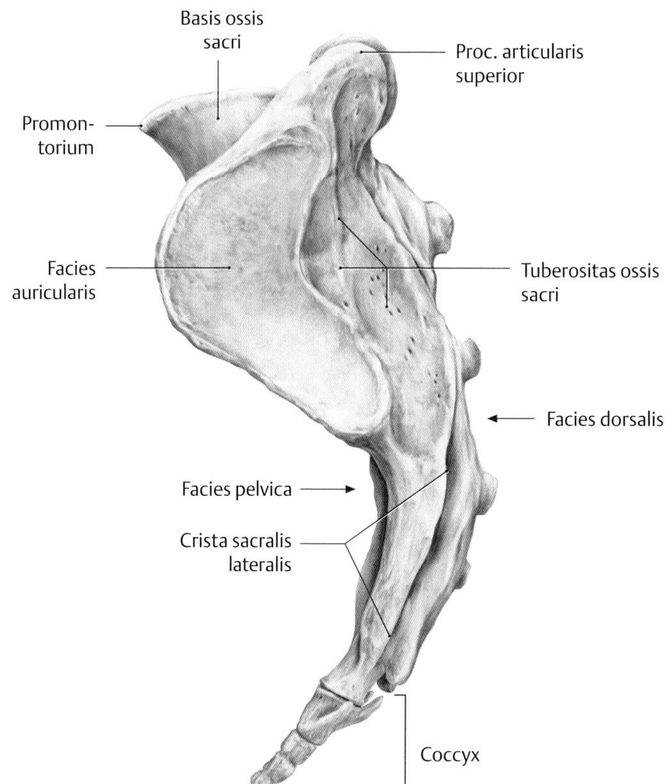
Basis ossis sacri
Proc. articularis superior
Promontorium
Facies auricularis
Tuberositas ossis sacri
Facies dorsalis
Facies pelvica
Crista sacralis lateralis
Coccyx

C Left lateral view.

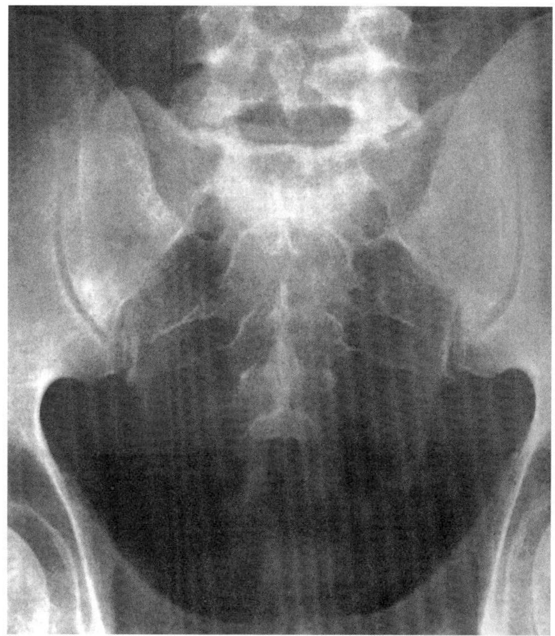

D Radiograph of sacrum, anteroposterior view.

Fig. 1.16 Os sacrum

Superior view.

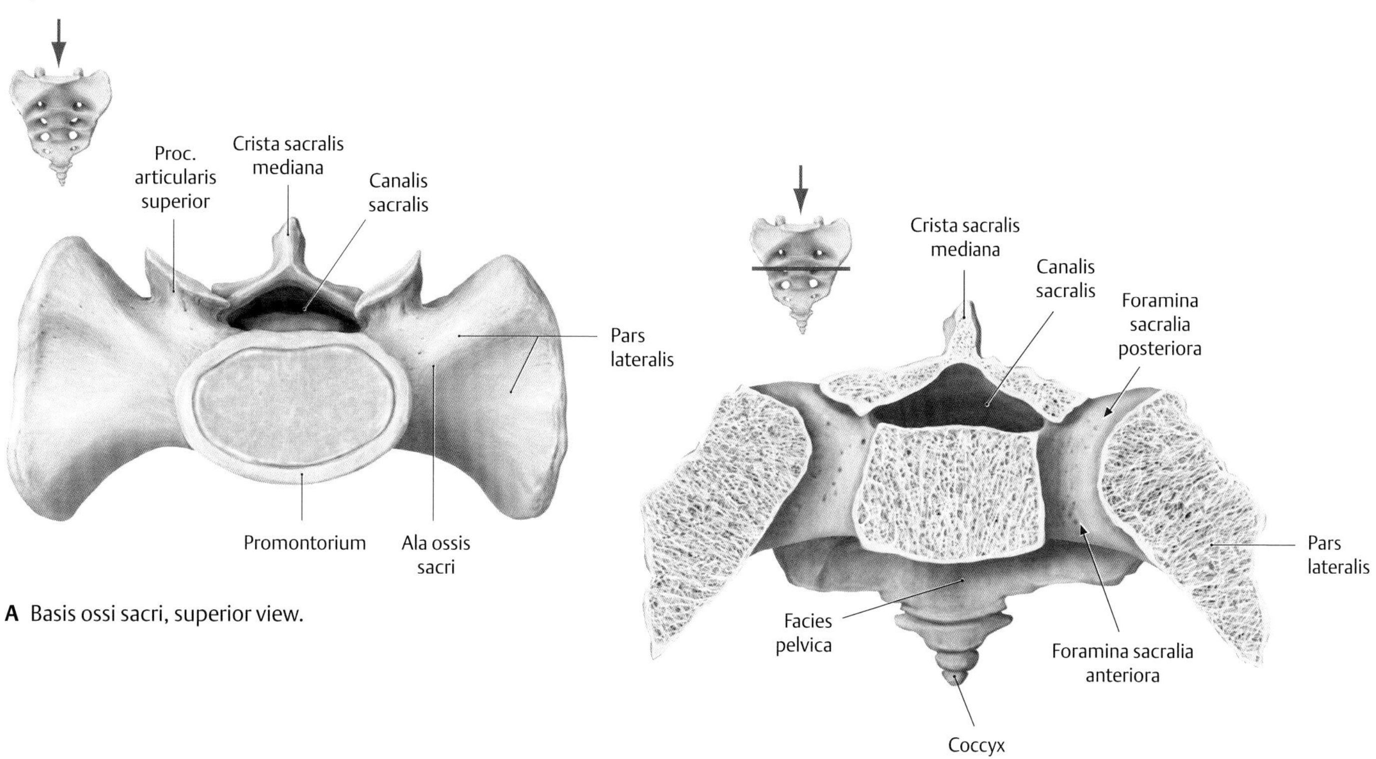
Proc. articularis superior
Crista sacralis mediana
Canalis sacralis
Pars lateralis
Promontorium
Ala ossis sacri
Crista sacralis mediana
Canalis sacralis
Foramina sacralia posteriora
Pars lateralis
Facies pelvica
Foramina sacralia anteriora
Coccyx

A Basis ossi sacri, superior view.

B Transverse section through second sacral vertebra demonstrating foramina sacralia anteriora and posteriora, superior view.

Discus Intervertebralis

Fig. 1.17 **Discus intervertebralis in columna vertebralis**
Sagittal section of T XI–T XII, left lateral view. The discus intervertebralis occupy the spaces between vertebrae (intervertebral joints, see p. 14).

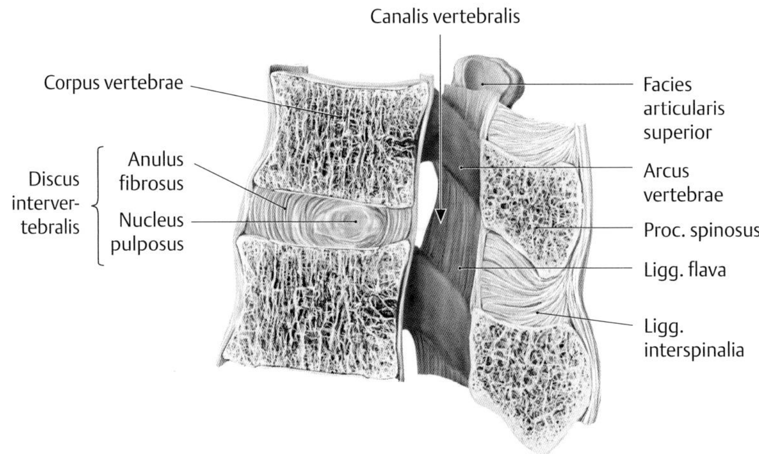

Canalis vertebralis
Corpus vertebrae
Discus interver-tebralis
Anulus fibrosus
Nucleus pulposus
Facies articularis superior
Arcus vertebrae
Proc. spinosus
Ligg. flava
Ligg. interspinalia

Fig. 1.18 **Structure of discus intervertebralis**
Anterosuperior view with the anterior half of the disk and the right half of the end plate removed. The intervertebral disk consists of an external fibrous ring (anulus fibrosus) and a gelatinous core (nucleus pulposus).

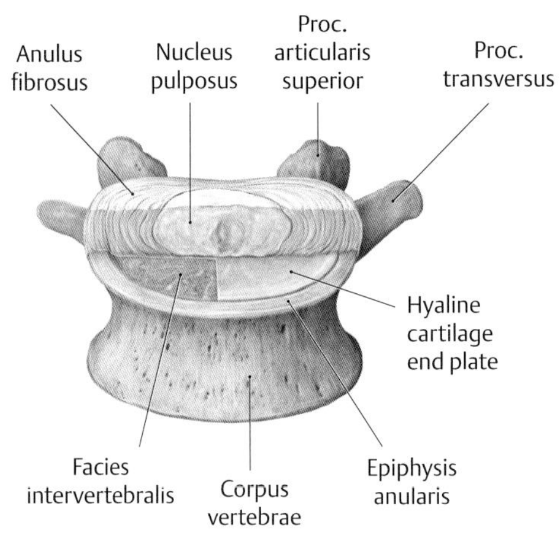

Anulus fibrosus
Nucleus pulposus
Proc. articularis superior
Proc. transversus
Hyaline cartilage end plate
Facies intervertebralis
Corpus vertebrae
Epiphysis anularis

Fig. 1.19 **Relation of discus intervertebralis to canalis vertebralis**
Fourth lumbar vertebra, superior view.

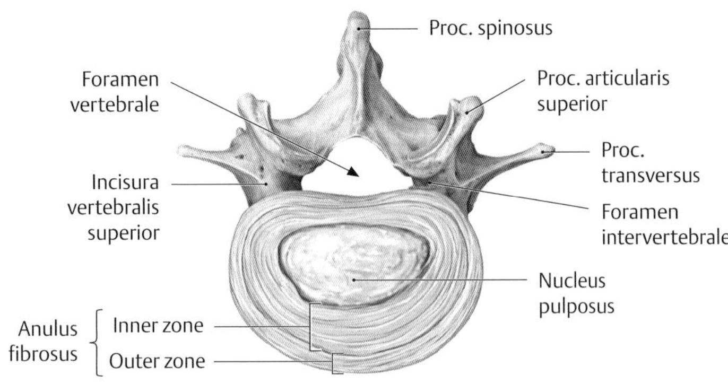

Proc. spinosus
Foramen vertebrale
Proc. articularis superior
Proc. transversus
Incisura vertebralis superior
Foramen intervertebrale
Nucleus pulposus
Anulus fibrosus
Inner zone
Outer zone

Fig. 1.20 **Outer zone of the anulus fibrosus**
Anterior view of L III–L IV with intervertebral disk.

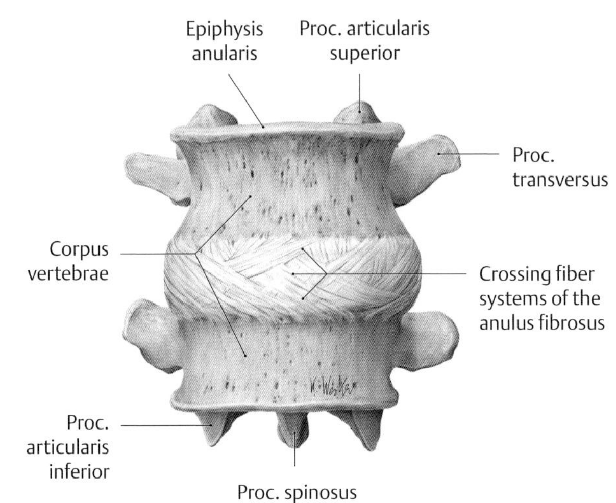

Epiphysis anularis
Proc. articularis superior
Proc. transversus
Corpus vertebrae
Crossing fiber systems of the anulus fibrosus
Proc. articularis inferior
Proc. spinosus

Clinical

Disk herniation, hernia disci intervertebralis, in the lumbar spine

As the stress resistance of the anulus fibrosus declines with age, the tissue of the nucleus pulposus may protrude through weak spots under loading. If the fibrous ring of the anulus ruptures completely, the herniated material may compress the contents of the intervertebral foramen (nerve roots and blood vessels). These patients often suffer from severe local back pain. Pain is also felt in the associated dermatome (see p. 600). When the motor part of the spinal nerve is affected, the muscles served by that spinal nerve will show weakening. It is an important diagnostic step to test the muscles innervated by a nerve from a certain spinal segment, as well as the sensitivity in the specific dermatome. Example: The first sacral nerve root (S1) innervates the gastrocnemius and soleus muscles; thus, standing or walking on toes can be affected (see p. 398).

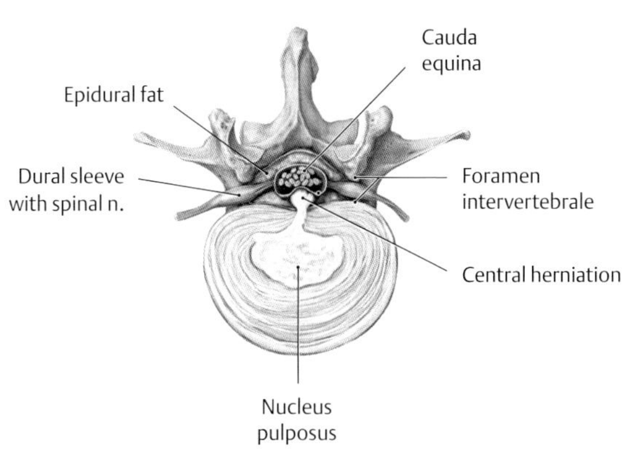
Cauda equina
Epidural fat
Dural sleeve with spinal n.
Foramen intervertebrale
Central herniation
Nucleus pulposus

A Superior view.

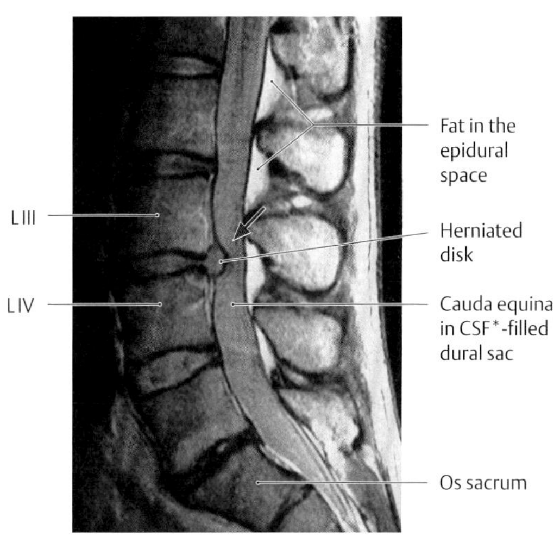
L III
L IV
Fat in the epidural space
Herniated disk
Cauda equina in CSF*-filled dural sac
Os sacrum

B Midsagittal T2-weighted MRI (magnetic resonance image).

Posterior herniation (A, B) In the MRI, a conspicuously herniated disk at the level of L III–L IV protrudes posteriorly (transligamentous herniation). The dural sac is deeply indented at that level. *CSF (cerebrospinal fluid).

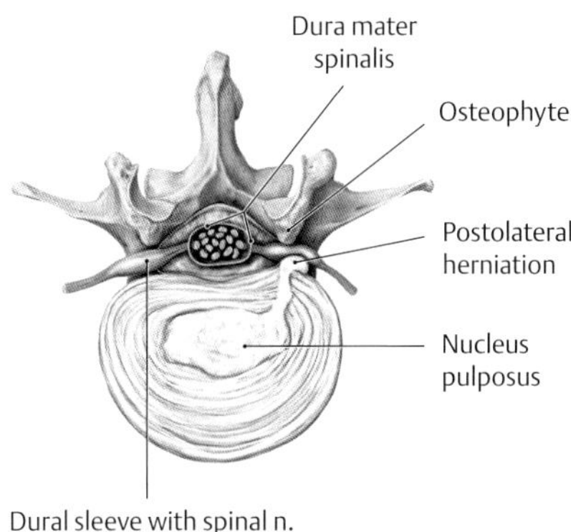
Dura mater spinalis
Osteophyte
Postolateral herniation
Nucleus pulposus
Dural sleeve with spinal n.

C Superior view.

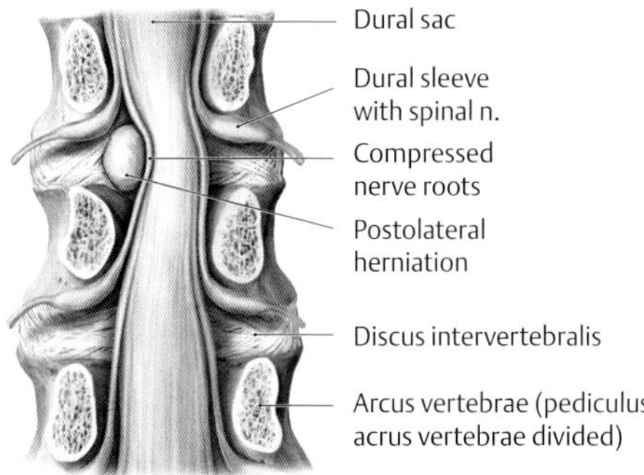
Dural sac
Dural sleeve with spinal n.
Compressed nerve roots
Postolateral herniation
Discus intervertebralis
Arcus vertebrae (pediculus acrus vertebrae divided)

D Posterior view, arcus vertebrae removed.

Posterolateral herniation (C, D) A posterolateral herniation may compress the spinal nerve as it passes through the intervertebral foramen. If more medially positioned, the herniation may spare the nerve at that level, but impact nerves at inferior levels.

Articulationes Columnae Vertebralis: Overview

Table 1.2 Joints of the vertebral column

Craniovertebral joints		
①	Articulationes atlantooccipitales	Occiput–C I
②	Articulationes atlantoaxiales	C I–C II
Joints of the vertebral bodies		
③	Articulationes uncovertebrales	C III–C VII
④	Articulationes intervertebrales	C I–S I
Joints of the vertebral arch		
⑤	Articulationes zygapophyseales	C I–S I

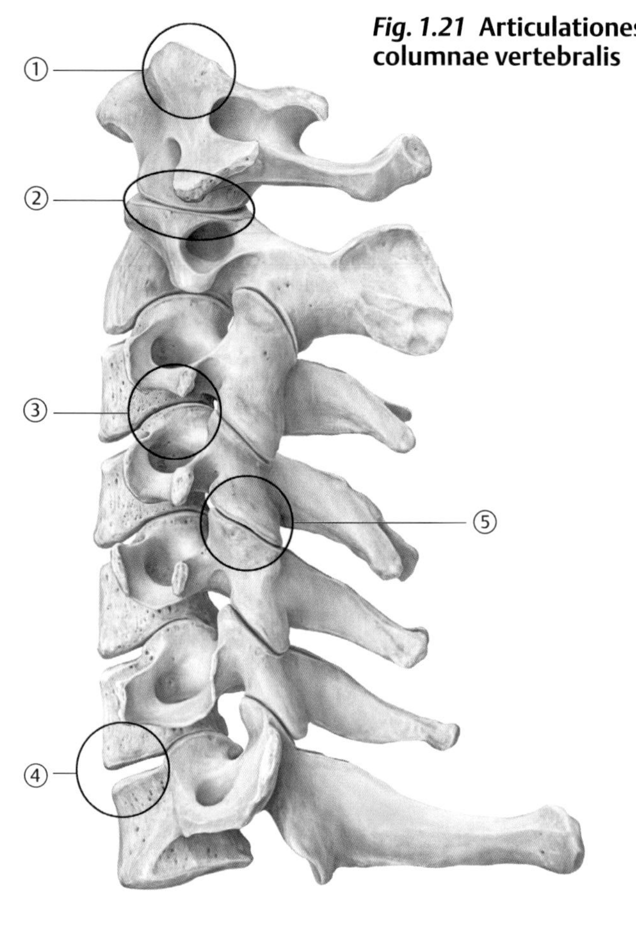
①
②
③
④
⑤

Fig. 1.21 **Articulationes columnae vertebralis**

Fig. 1.22 **Articulationes zygapophysiales (intervertebral facet)**

The orientation of articulationes zygapophysiales differs between the spinal regions, influencing the degree and direction of movement.

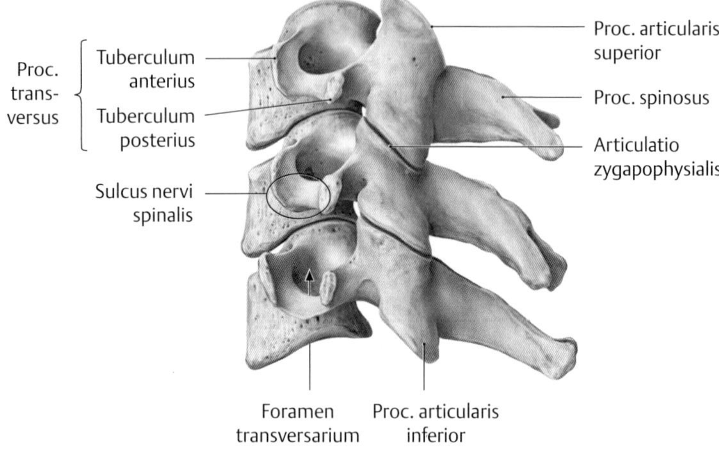
Proc. trans-versus
Tuberculum anterius
Tuberculum posterius
Sulcus nervi spinalis
Proc. articularis superior
Proc. spinosus
Articulatio zygapophysialis
Foramen transversarium
Proc. articularis inferior

A Cervical region, left lateral view. Articulationes zygapophysiales lie 45 degrees from the horizontal.

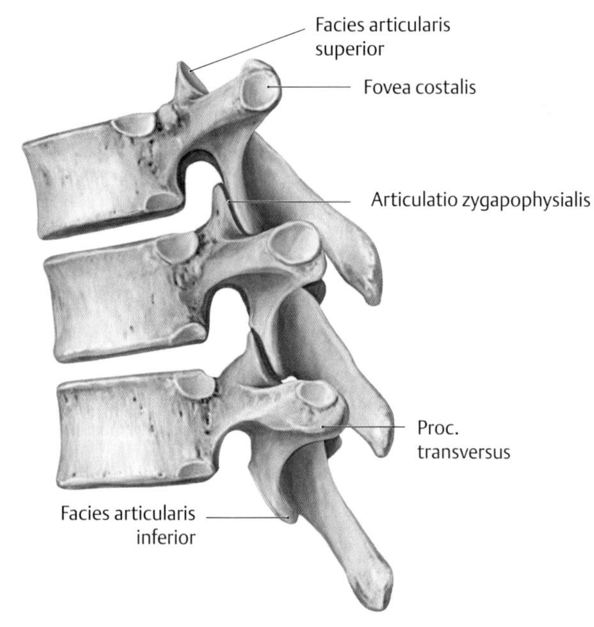
Facies articularis superior
Fovea costalis
Articulatio zygapophysialis
Proc. transversus
Facies articularis inferior

B Thoracic region, left lateral view. The joints lie in the coronal plane.

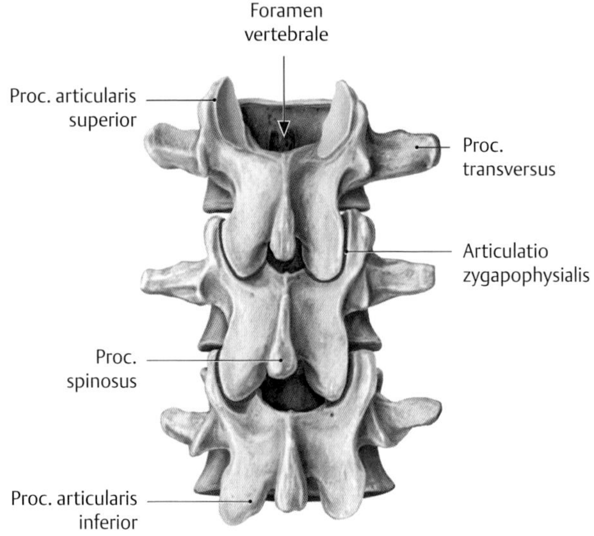
Foramen vertebrale
Proc. articularis superior
Proc. transversus
Articulatio zygapophysialis
Proc. spinosus
Proc. articularis inferior

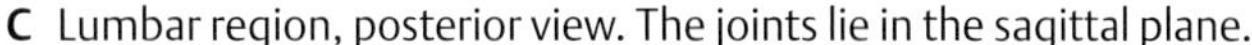

C Lumbar region, posterior view. The joints lie in the sagittal plane.

Fig. 1.23 Articulationes uncovertebrales

Anterior view. Articulationes uncovertebrales form during childhood between processus uncinatus of C III–C VI and corpus vertebrae immediately superior. The joints may result from fissures in the cartilage of the disks that assume an articular character. If the fissures become complete tears, the risk of pulposus herniation is increased (see p. 13).

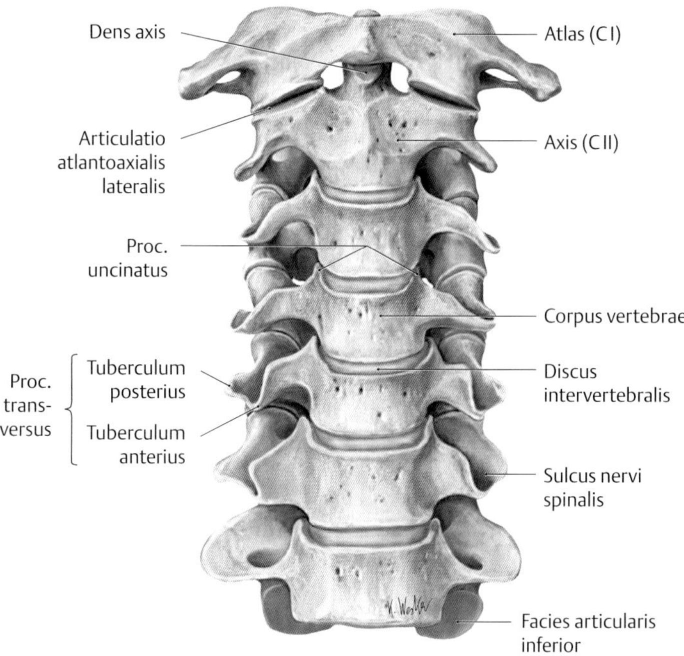
Dens axis
Atlas (C I)
Articulatio atlantoaxialis lateralis
Axis (C II)
Proc. uncinatus
Corpus vertebrae
Proc. trans-versus
Tuberculum posterius
Tuberculum anterius
Discus intervertebralis
Sulcus nervi spinalis
Facies articularis inferior

A Articulationes uncovertebrales in the cervical spine of an 18-year-old man, anterior view.

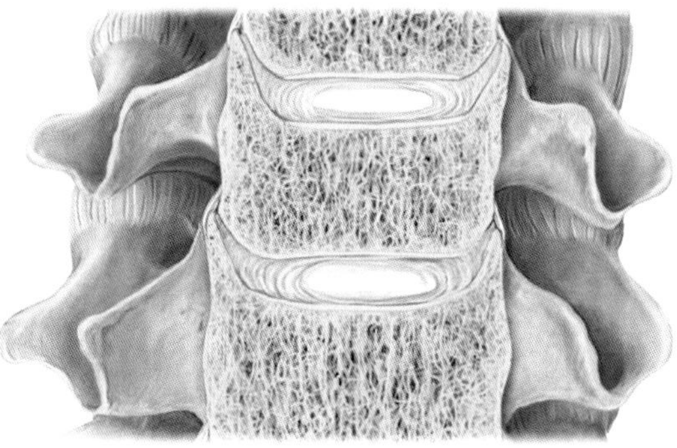

B Articulationes uncovertebrales (enlarged), anterior view of coronal section.

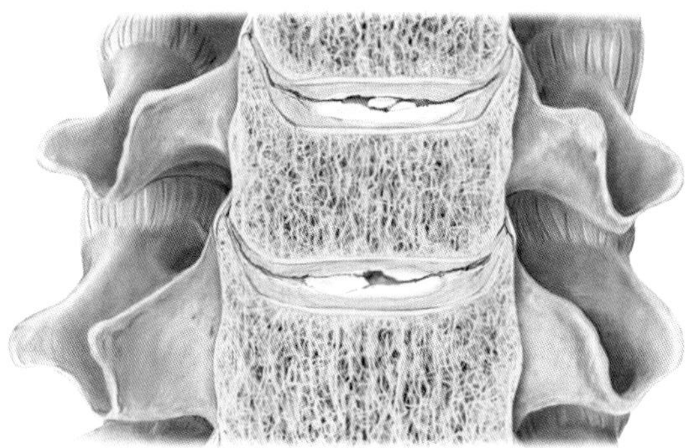

C Split discus intervertebralis, anterior view of coronal section.

Clinical

Proximity of nervus spinalis and arteria vertebralis to the processus uncinatus

Nervus spinalis and arteria vertebralis pass through the foramen transversarium and foramina intervertebrale, respectively. Bony outgrowths (osteophytes) resulting from uncovertebral arthrosis may compress both the nerve and the artery and can lead to chronic pain in the neck.

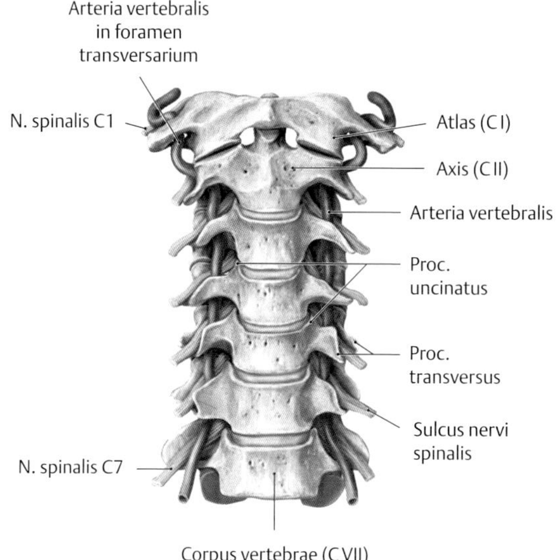
Arteria vertebralis in foramen transversarium
N. spinalis C1
Atlas (C I)
Axis (C II)
Arteria vertebralis
Proc. uncinatus
Proc. transversus
Sulcus nervi spinalis
N. spinalis C7
Corpus vertebrae (C VII)

A Cervical spine, anterior view.

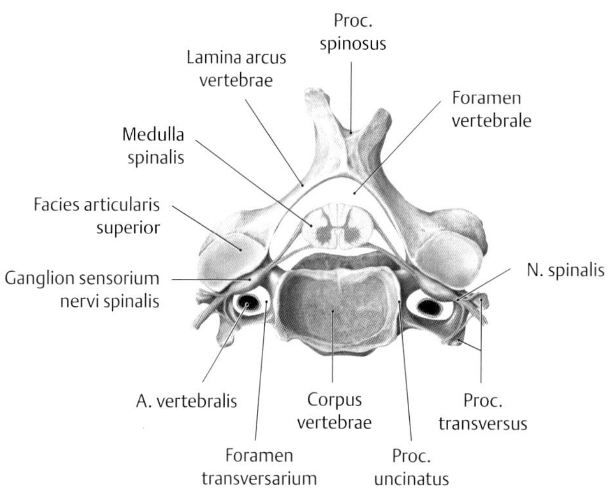
Proc. spinosus
Lamina arcus vertebrae
Foramen vertebrale
Medulla spinalis
Facies articularis superior
Ganglion sensorium nervi spinalis
N. spinalis
A. vertebralis
Corpus vertebrae
Proc. transversus
Foramen transversarium
Proc. uncinatus

B Fourth cervical vertebra, superior view.

Joints of Columna Vertebralis: Craniovertebral Region

Fig. 1.24 Craniovertebral joints

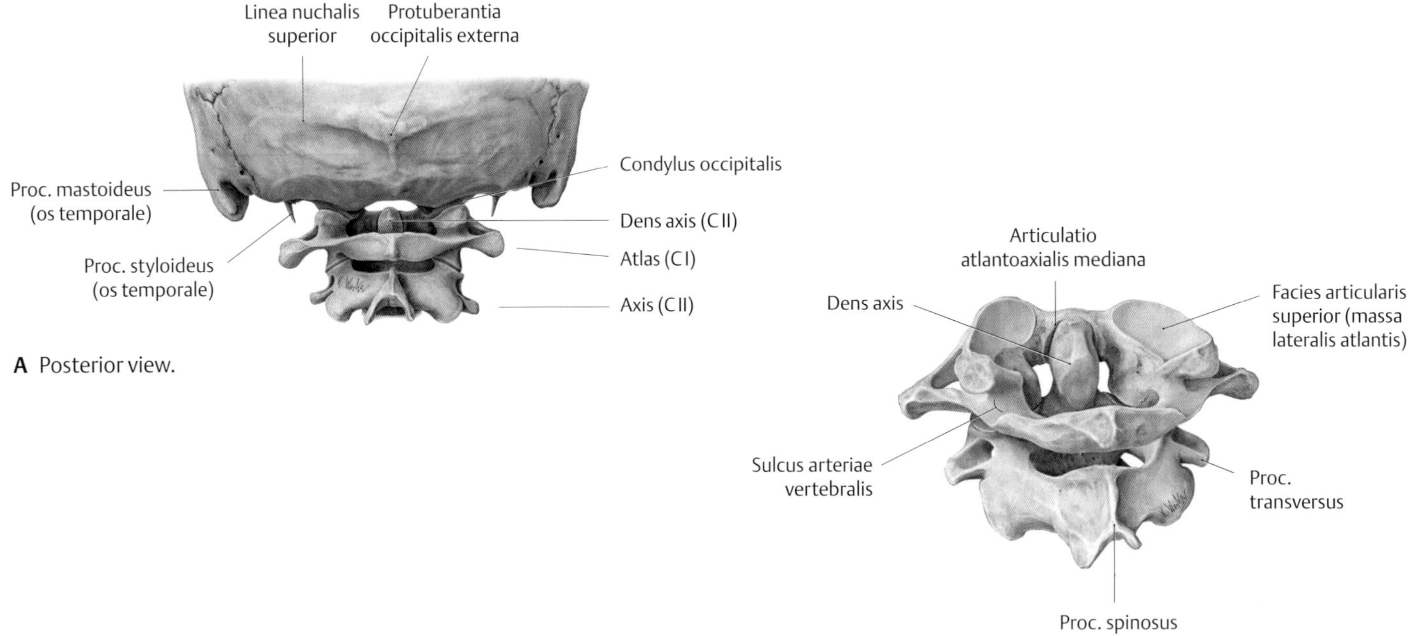
Linea nuchalis superior
Protuberantia occipitalis externa
Condylus occipitalis
Proc. mastoideus (os temporale)
Dens axis (C II)
Atlas (C I)
Proc. styloideus (os temporale)
Axis (C II)
Articulatio atlantoaxialis mediana
Dens axis
Facies articularis superior (massa lateralis atlantis)
Sulcus arteriae vertebralis
Proc. transversus
Proc. spinosus

A Posterior view.

B Atlas (C I) and axis (C II), posterosuperior view.

Fig. 1.25 Dissection of the craniovertebral joint ligaments

Posterior view.

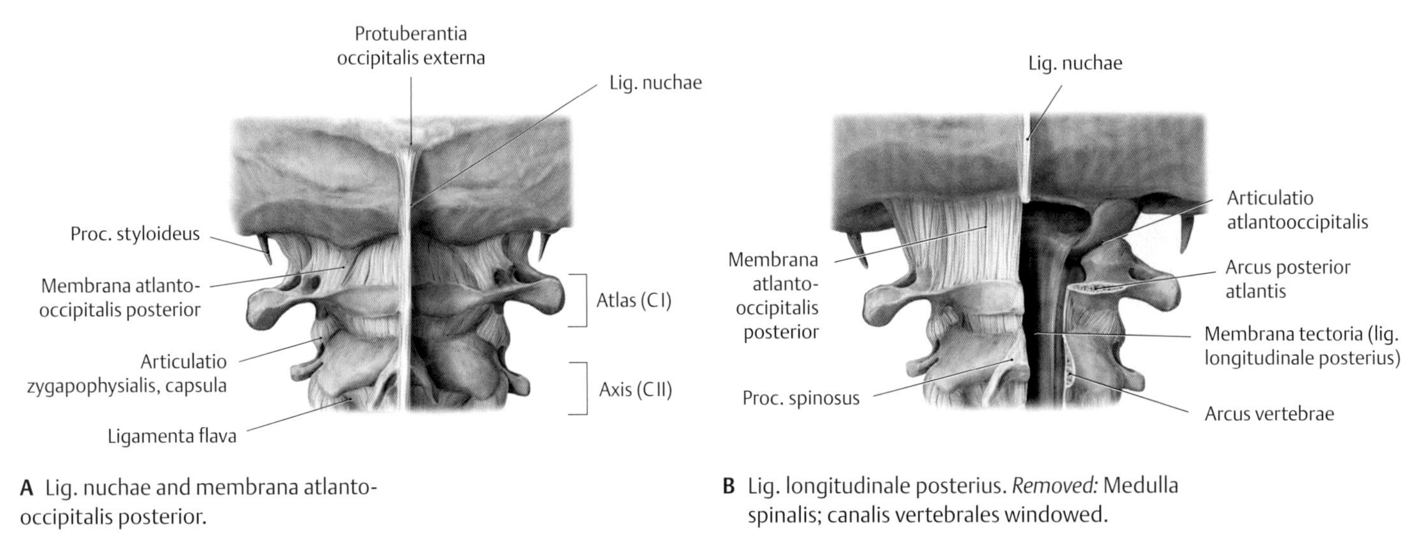
Protuberantia occipitalis externa
Lig. nuchae
Proc. styloideus
Membrana atlanto-occipitalis posterior
Atlas (C I)
Articulatio zygapophysialis, capsula
Axis (C II)
Ligamenta flava
Lig. nuchae
Articulatio atlantooccipitalis
Membrana atlanto-occipitalis posterior
Arcus posterior atlantis
Membrana tectoria (lig. longitudinale posterius)
Proc. spinosus
Arcus vertebrae

A Lig. nuchae and membrana atlanto-occipitalis posterior.

B Lig. longitudinale posterius. *Removed:* Medulla spinalis; canalis vertebrales windowed.

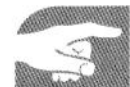

The atlanto-occipital joints are the two articulations between the convex condylus occipitalis of the occipital bone and the slightly concave facies articularis superior of the atlas (C I). The atlanto-axial joints are the two lateral and one medial articulations between the atlas (C I) and axis (C II).

Fig. 1.26 Ligaments of the craniovertebral joints

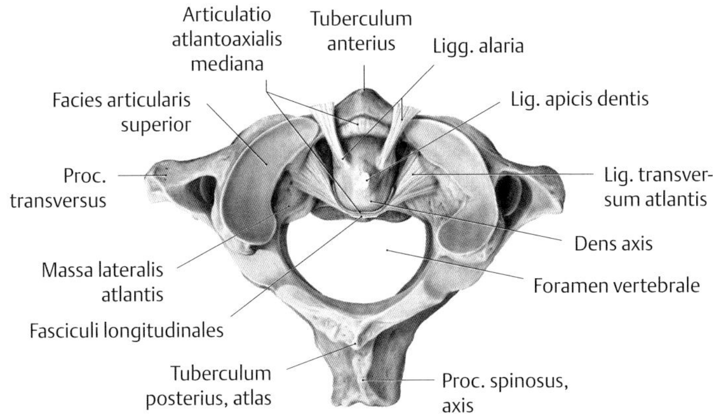
Articulatio atlantoaxialis mediana
Tuberculum anterius
Ligg. alaria
Facies articularis superior
Lig. apicis dentis
Proc. transversus
Lig. transversum atlantis
Dens axis
Massa lateralis atlantis
Foramen vertebrale
Fasciculi longitudinales
Tuberculum posterius, atlas
Proc. spinosus, axis

A Ligaments of articulatio atlantoaxialis mediana, superior view. Fovea dentis of the atlas is hidden by the joint capsule.

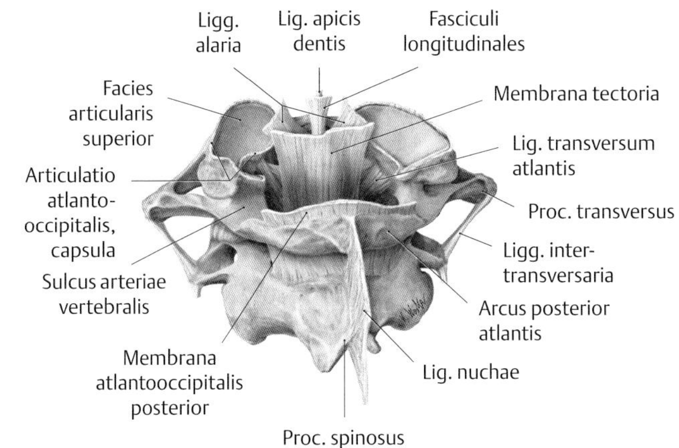
Ligg. alaria
Lig. apicis dentis
Fasciculi longitudinales
Facies articularis superior
Membrana tectoria
Lig. transversum atlantis
Articulatio atlanto-occipitalis, capsula
Proc. transversus
Ligg. inter-transversaria
Sulcus arteriae vertebralis
Arcus posterior atlantis
Membrana atlantooccipitalis posterior
Lig. nuchae
Proc. spinosus

B Ligaments of the craniovertebral joints, posterosuperior view. Dens axis is hidden by membrana tectoria.

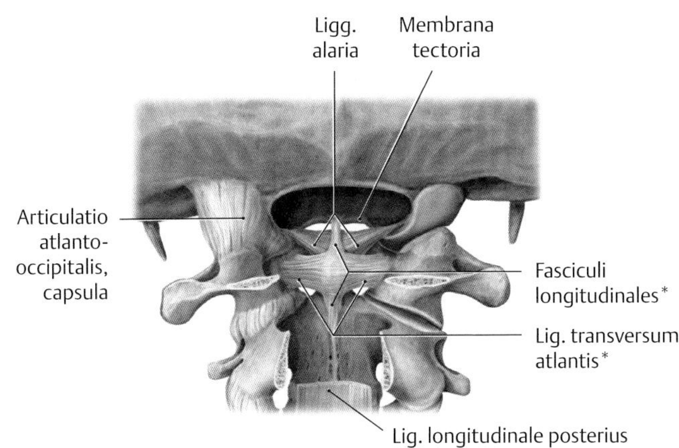
Ligg. alaria
Membrana tectoria
Articulatio atlanto-occipitalis, capsula
Fasciculi longitudinales*
Lig. transversum atlantis*
Lig. longitudinale posterius

C Lig. cruciforme atlantis (*). *Removed:* Membrana tectoria.

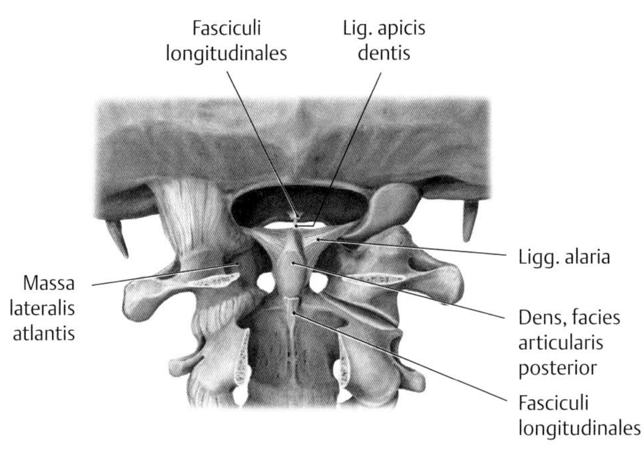
Fasciculi longitudinales
Lig. apicis dentis
Ligg. alaria
Massa lateralis atlantis
Dens, facies articularis posterior
Fasciculi longitudinales

D Ligg. alaria and lig. apicis dentis. *Removed:* Lig. transversum atlantis, fasciculi longitudinales.

Vertebral Ligaments: Overview & Cervical Spine

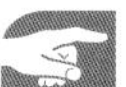

The ligaments of the spinal column bind the vertebrae and enable the spine to withstand high mechanical loads and shearing stresses and limit the range of motion. The ligaments are subdivided into vertebral body ligaments and vertebral arch ligaments.

Fig. 1.27 **Vertebral ligaments**
Viewed obliquely from the left posterior view.

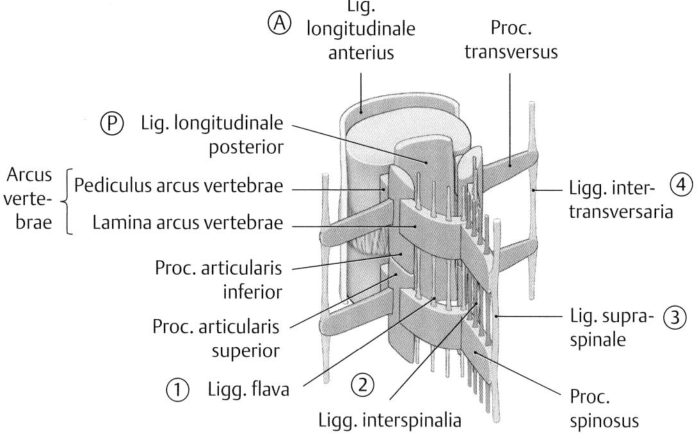
Ⓐ Lig. longitudinale anterius
Proc. transversus
Ⓟ Lig. longitudinale posterior
Arcus vertebrae
Pediculus arcus vertebrae
Lamina arcus vertebrae
Ligg. inter-transversaria ④
Proc. articularis inferior
Proc. articularis superior
Lig. supra-spinale ③
① Ligg. flava
②
Ligg. interspinalia
Proc. spinosus

Table 1.3 **Vertebral ligaments**		
Ligament		**Location**
Vertebral body ligaments		
Ⓐ	Lig. longitudinale anterius	Along anterior surface of vertebral body
Ⓟ	Lig. longitudinale posterius	Along posterior surface of vertebral body
Vertebral arch ligaments		
①	Lig. flava	Between laminae
②	Ligg. interspinosi	Between procc. spinosi
③	Ligg. supraspinosi	Along posterior ridge of procc. spinosi
④	Ligg. intertransversarii	Between procc. transversi
Lig. nuchae*		Between external protuberancia occipitalis and proc. spinosus of C VII

*Corresponds to a lig. supraspinosum that is broadened superiorly.

Fig. 1.28 **Ligamentum longitudinale anterius**
Lig. longitudinale anterius. Anterior view with base of skull removed.

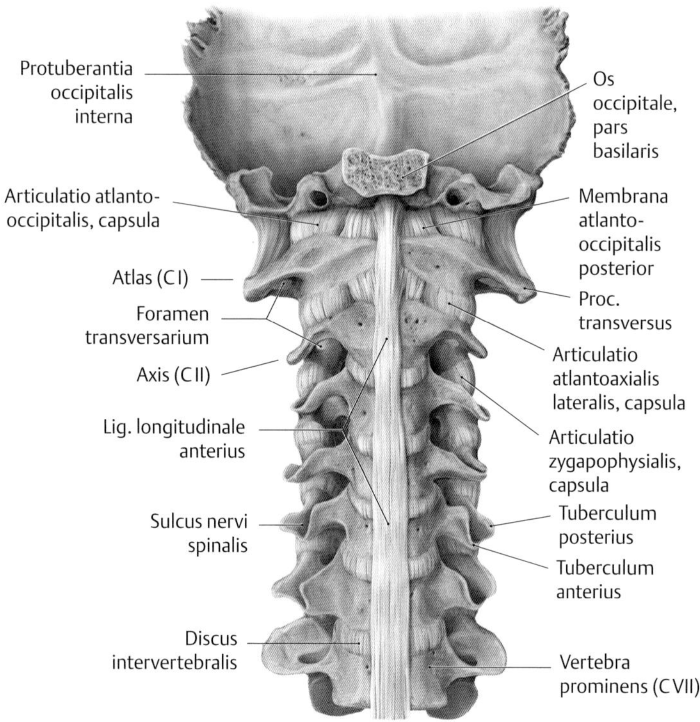
Protuberantia occipitalis interna
Os occipitale, pars basilaris
Articulatio atlanto-occipitalis, capsula
Membrana atlanto-occipitalis posterior
Atlas (C I)
Proc. transversus
Foramen transversarium
Articulatio atlantoaxialis lateralis, capsula
Axis (C II)
Lig. longitudinale anterius
Articulatio zygapophysialis, capsula
Sulcus nervi spinalis
Tuberculum posterius
Tuberculum anterius
Discus intervertebralis
Vertebra prominens (C VII)

Fig. 1.29 **Ligamentum longitudinale posterius**
Posterior view with canalis vertebralis windowed and medulla spinalis removed. The membrana tectoria is a broadened expansion of lig. longitudinale posterius.

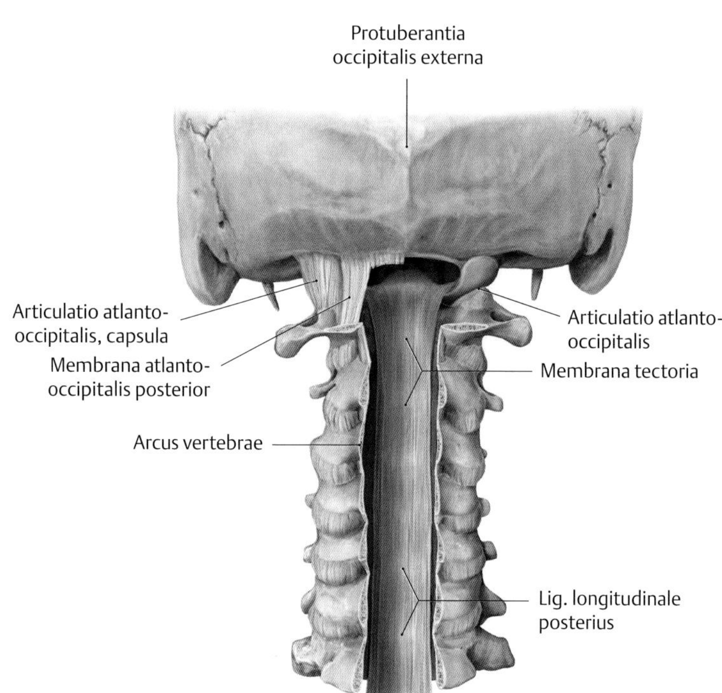
Protuberantia occipitalis externa
Articulatio atlanto-occipitalis, capsula
Articulatio atlanto-occipitalis
Membrana atlanto-occipitalis posterior
Membrana tectoria
Arcus vertebrae
Lig. longitudinale posterius

Fig. 1.30 Ligaments of the cervical spine

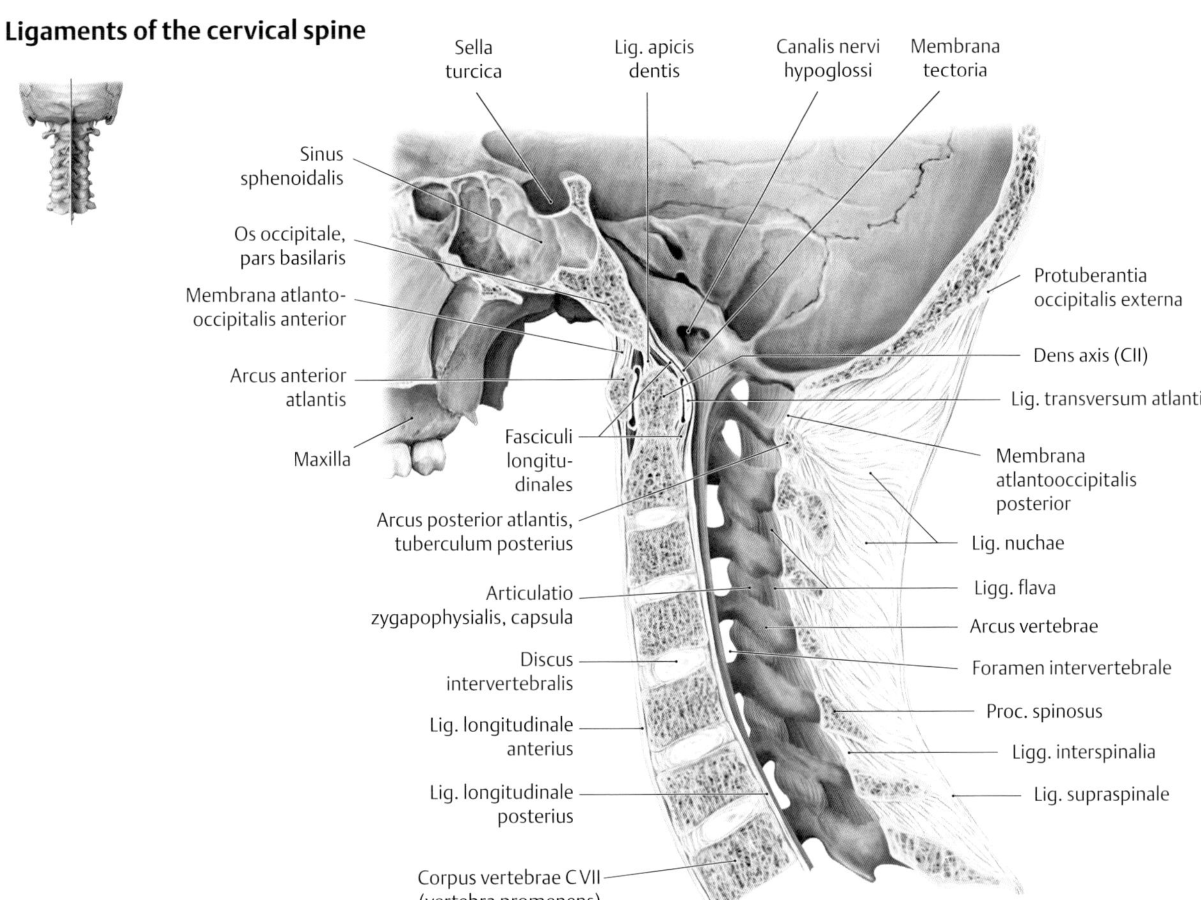
Sella turcica
Lig. apicis dentis
Canalis nervi hypoglossi
Membrana tectoria
Sinus sphenoidalis
Os occipitale, pars basilaris
Membrana atlanto-occipitalis anterior
Arcus anterior atlantis
Maxilla
Fasciculi longitu-dinales
Arcus posterior atlantis, tuberculum posterius
Articulatio zygapophysialis, capsula
Discus intervertebralis
Lig. longitudinale anterius
Lig. longitudinale posterius
Corpus vertebrae C VII (vertebra promenens)
Protuberantia occipitalis externa
Dens axis (CII)
Lig. transversum atlantis
Membrana atlantooccipitalis posterior
Lig. nuchae
Ligg. flava
Arcus vertebrae
Foramen intervertebrale
Proc. spinosus
Ligg. interspinalia
Lig. supraspinale

A Midsagittal section, left lateral view. Lig. nuchae is the broadened, sagittally oriented part of lig. supraspinale that extends from vertebra prominens (C VII) to protuberantia occipitalis externa.

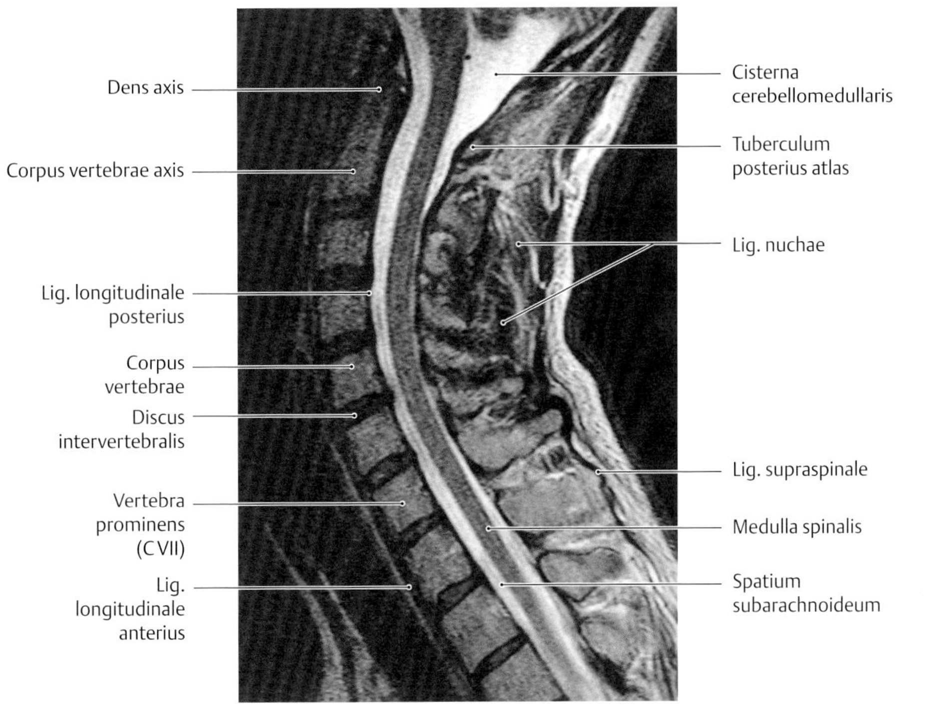
Dens axis
Corpus vertebrae axis
Lig. longitudinale posterius
Corpus vertebrae
Discus intervertebralis
Vertebra prominens (C VII)
Lig. longitudinale anterius
Cisterna cerebellomedullaris
Tuberculum posterius atlas
Lig. nuchae
Lig. supraspinale
Medulla spinalis
Spatium subarachnoideum

B Midsagittal T2-weighted MRI, left lateral view.

Vertebral Ligaments: Thoracolumbar Spine

Fig. 1.31 **Ligaments of the vertebral column: Thoracolumbar junction**
Left lateral view of T XI–L III, with T XI–T XII sectioned in the midsagittal plane.

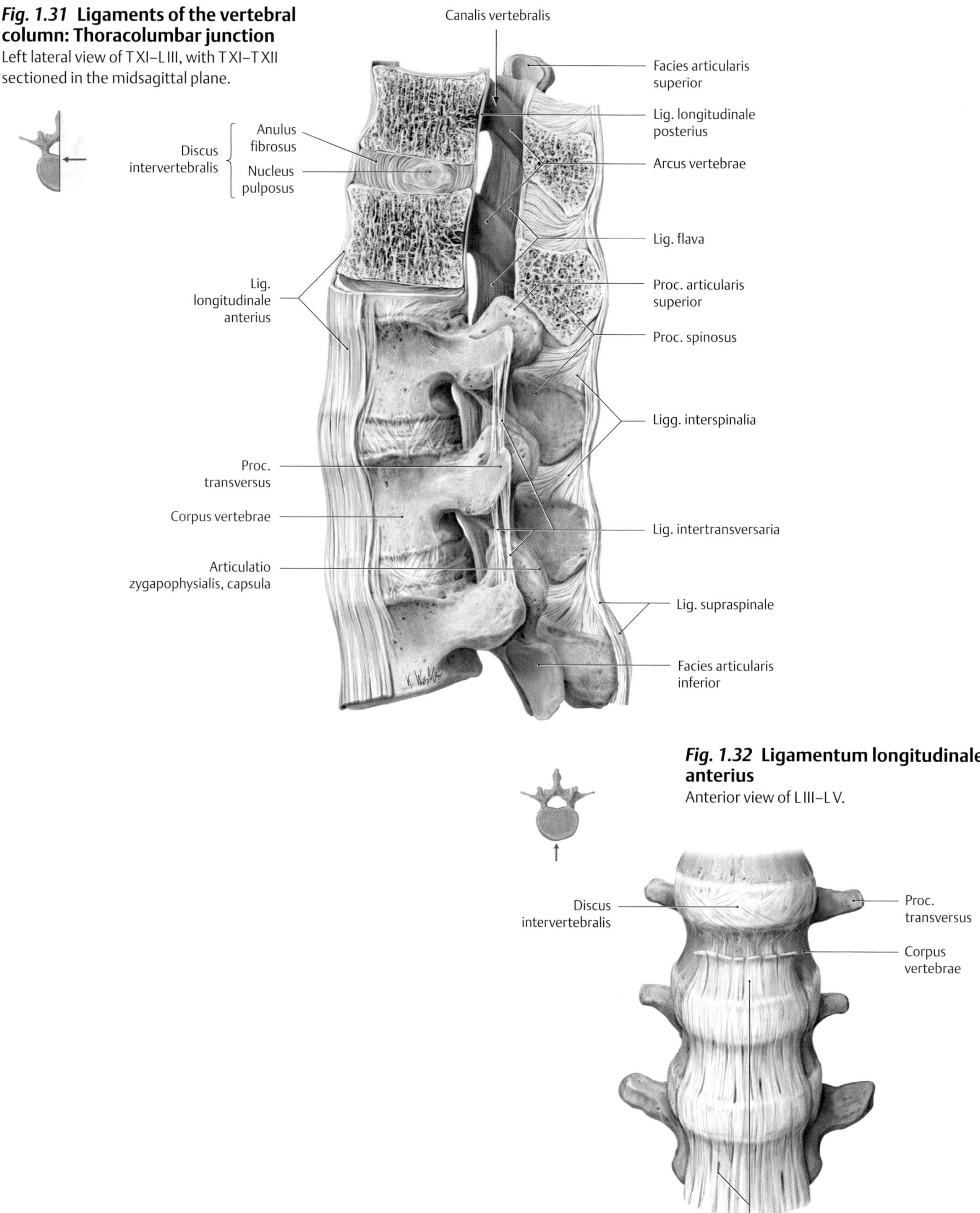
Canalis vertebralis
Facies articularis superior
Lig. longitudinale posterius
Arcus vertebrae
Discus intervertebralis
Anulus fibrosus
Nucleus pulposus
Lig. flava
Proc. articularis superior
Lig. longitudinale anterius
Proc. spinosus
Ligg. interspinalia
Proc. transversus
Corpus vertebrae
Lig. intertransversaria
Articulatio zygapophysialis, capsula
Lig. supraspinale
Facies articularis inferior
Discus intervertebralis
Proc. transversus
Corpus vertebrae
Lig. longitudinale anterius

Fig. 1.32 **Ligamentum longitudinale anterius**
Anterior view of L III–L V.

Fig. 1.33 Ligamentum flavum and ligamenta intertransversaria

Anterior view of opened canalis vertebralis at level of L II–L V. *Removed:* corpus vertebrae L II–L IV.

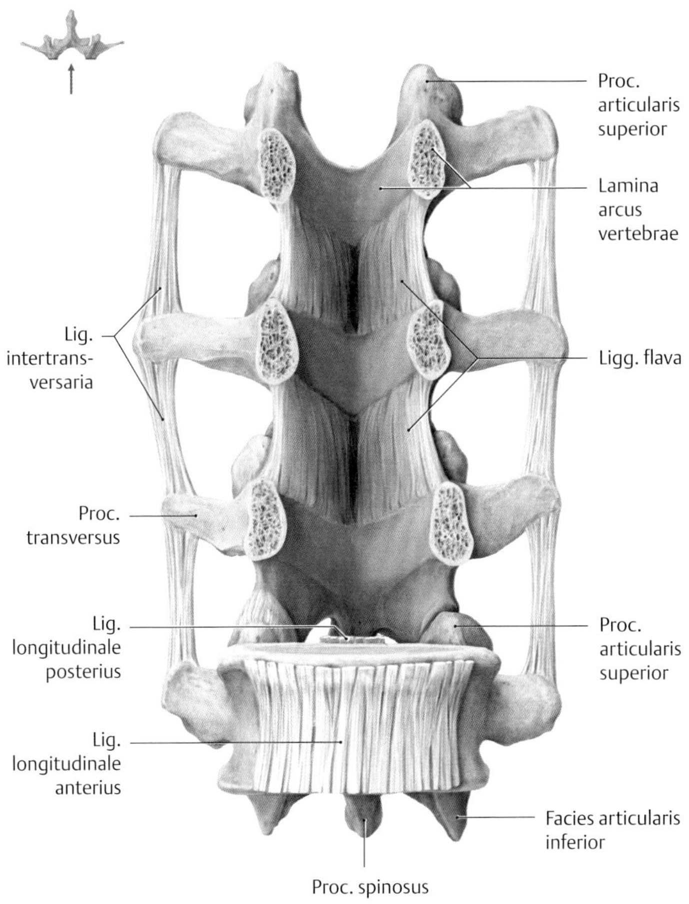
Proc. articularis superior
Lamina arcus vertebrae
Lig. intertrans-versaria
Ligg. flava
Proc. transversus
Lig. longitudinale posterius
Proc. articularis superior
Lig. longitudinale anterius
Facies articularis inferior
Proc. spinosus

Fig. 1.34 Ligamentum longitudinale posterius

Posterior view of opened canalis vertebralis at level of L II–L V. *Removed:* L II–L IV arcus vertebrae at pedicular level.

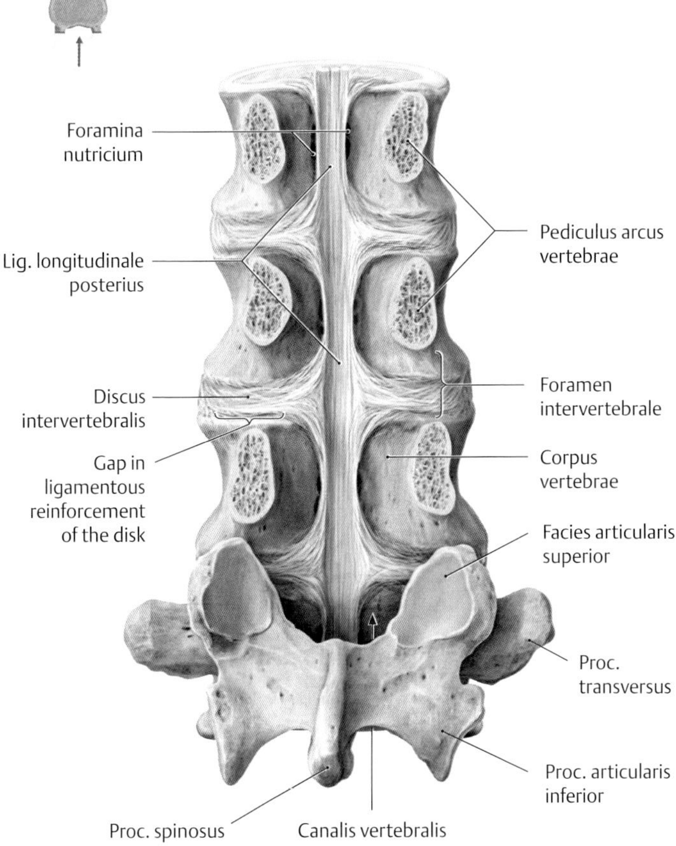
Foramina nutricium
Lig. longitudinale posterius
Pediculus arcus vertebrae
Discus intervertebralis
Foramen intervertebrale
Gap in ligamentous reinforcement of the disk
Corpus vertebrae
Facies articularis superior
Proc. transversus
Proc. articularis inferior
Proc. spinosus
Canalis vertebralis

Muscles of the Back: Overview

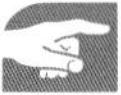

The muscles of the back are divided into two groups, the extrinsic and the intrinsic muscles, which are separated by lamina superficialis, fascia thoracolumbalis. The superficial extrinsic muscles are considered muscles of the upper limb that have migrated to the back; these muscles are discussed in Unit 4.

Fig. 2.1 **Superficial (extrinsic) muscles of the back**
Posterior view. *Removed:* M. trapezius and m. latissimus dorsi (right). *Revealed:* Fascia thoracolumbalis. *Note:* Lamina superficialis of the thoracolumbar fascia is reinforced by the aponeurotic origin of the latissimus dorsi.

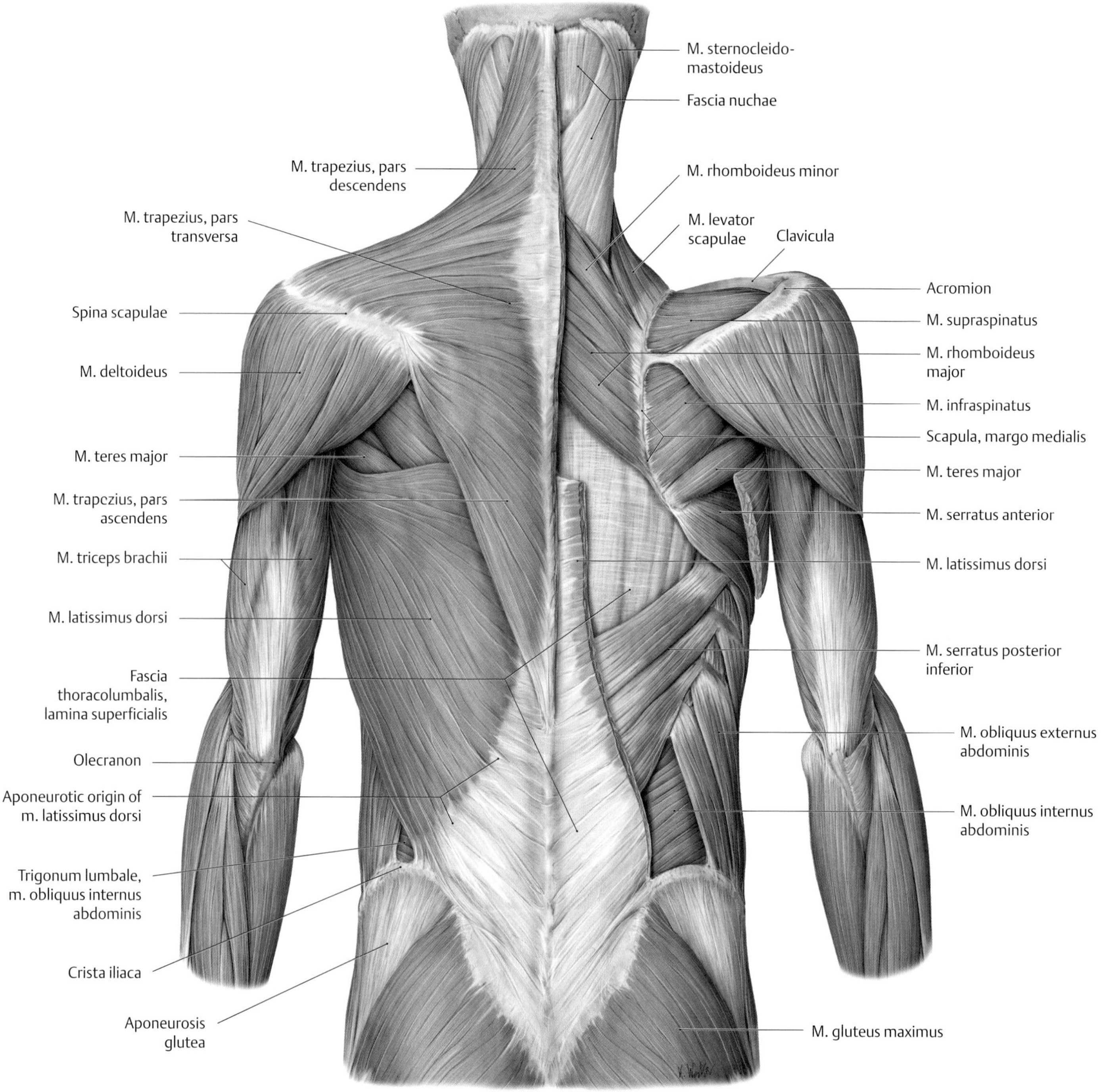

M. trapezius, pars descendens
M. trapezius, pars transversa
Spina scapulae
M. deltoideus
M. teres major
M. trapezius, pars ascendens
M. triceps brachii
M. latissimus dorsi
Fascia thoracolumbalis, lamina superficialis
Olecranon
Aponeurotic origin of m. latissimus dorsi
Trigonum lumbale, m. obliquus internus abdominis
Crista iliaca
Aponeurosis glutea
M. sternocleidomastoideus
Fascia nuchae
M. rhomboideus minor
M. levator scapulae
Clavicula
Acromion
M. supraspinatus
M. rhomboideus major
M. infraspinatus
Scapula, margo medialis
M. teres major
M. serratus anterior
M. latissimus dorsi
M. serratus posterior inferior
M. obliquus externus abdominis
M. obliquus internus abdominis
M. gluteus maximus

Fig. 2.2 Fascia thoracolumbalis

Transverse section, superior view. The intrinsic back muscles are sequestered in an osseofibrous canal, formed by fascia thoracolumbalis, archus, and processus spinosus and processus transversus of associated vertebrae. Fascia thoracolumbalis consists of a superficial layer, lamina superficialis, and a deep layer, lamina profunda, that unite at the lateral margin of the intrinsic back muscles. In the neck, the superficial layer blends with the fascia nuchae (deep layer), becoming continuous with fascia cervicalis (prevertebral layer).

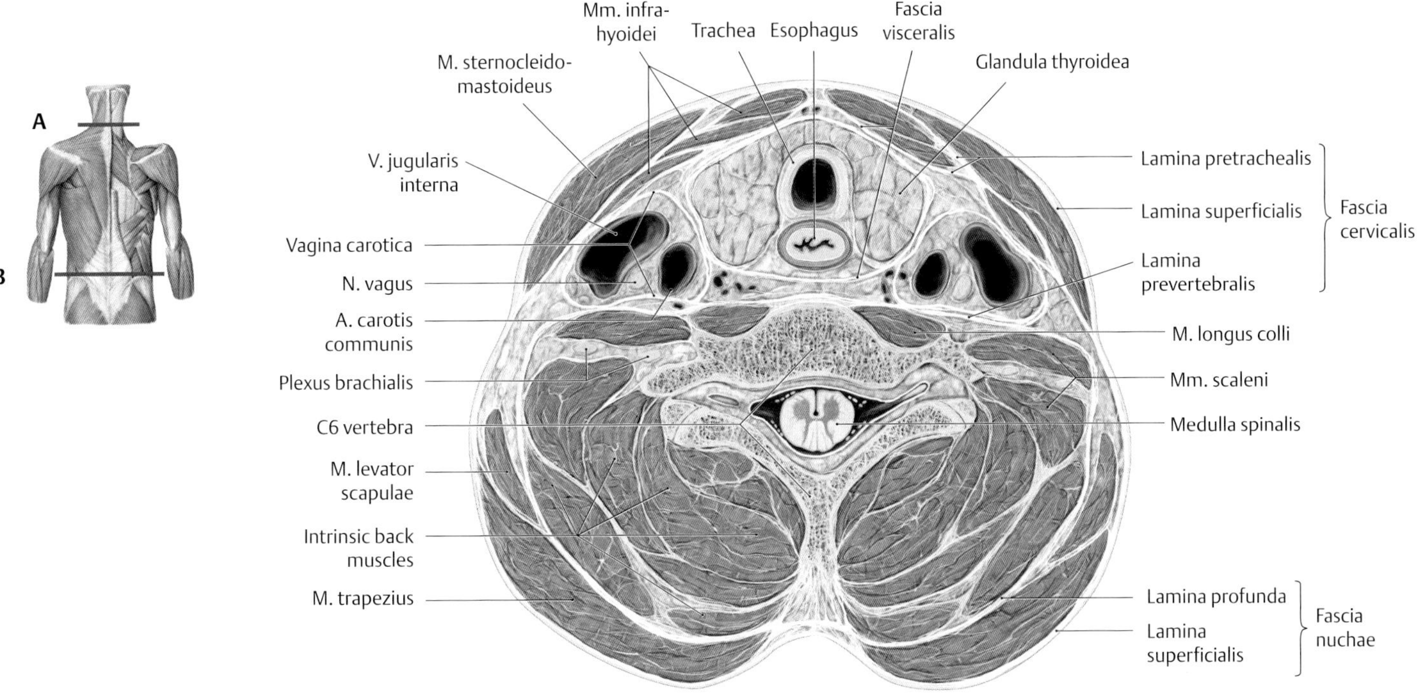
A
B
Mm. infra-hyoidei
Trachea
Esophagus
Fascia visceralis
M. sternocleido-mastoideus
Glandula thyroidea
V. jugularis interna
Lamina pretrachealis
Lamina superficialis
Fascia cervicalis
Vagina carotica
Lamina prevertebralis
N. vagus
A. carotis communis
M. longus colli
Plexus brachialis
Mm. scaleni
C6 vertebra
Medulla spinalis
M. levator scapulae
Intrinsic back muscles
M. trapezius
Lamina profunda
Lamina superficialis
Fascia nuchae

A Transverse section at level of CVI vertebra, superior view.

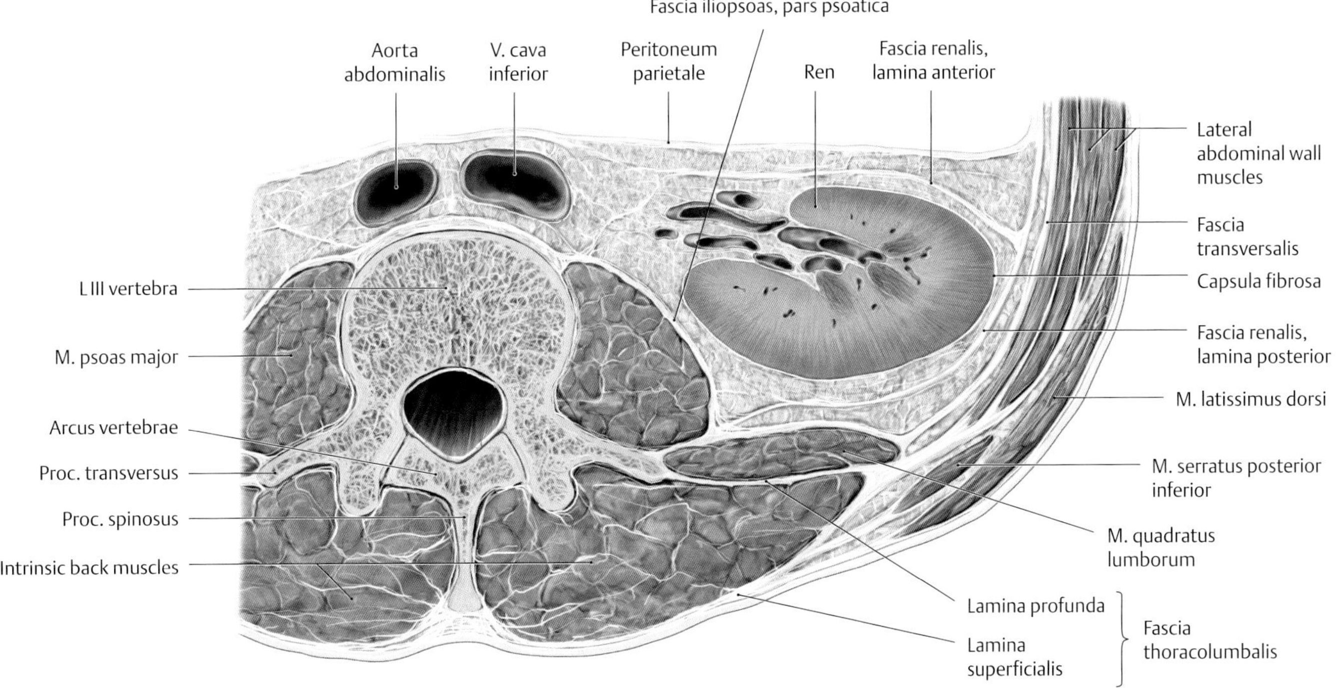
Fascia iliopsoas, pars psoatica
Aorta abdominalis
V. cava inferior
Peritoneum parietale
Ren
Fascia renalis, lamina anterior
Lateral abdominal wall muscles
Fascia transversalis
L III vertebra
Capsula fibrosa
M. psoas major
Fascia renalis, lamina posterior
M. latissimus dorsi
Arcus vertebrae
Proc. transversus
M. serratus posterior inferior
Proc. spinosus
M. quadratus lumborum
Intrinsic back muscles
Lamina profunda
Lamina superficialis
Fascia thoracolumbalis

B Transverse section at level of LIII, superior view.
Removed: Cauda equina and anterior trunk wall.

Intrinsic Muscles of the Cervical Spine

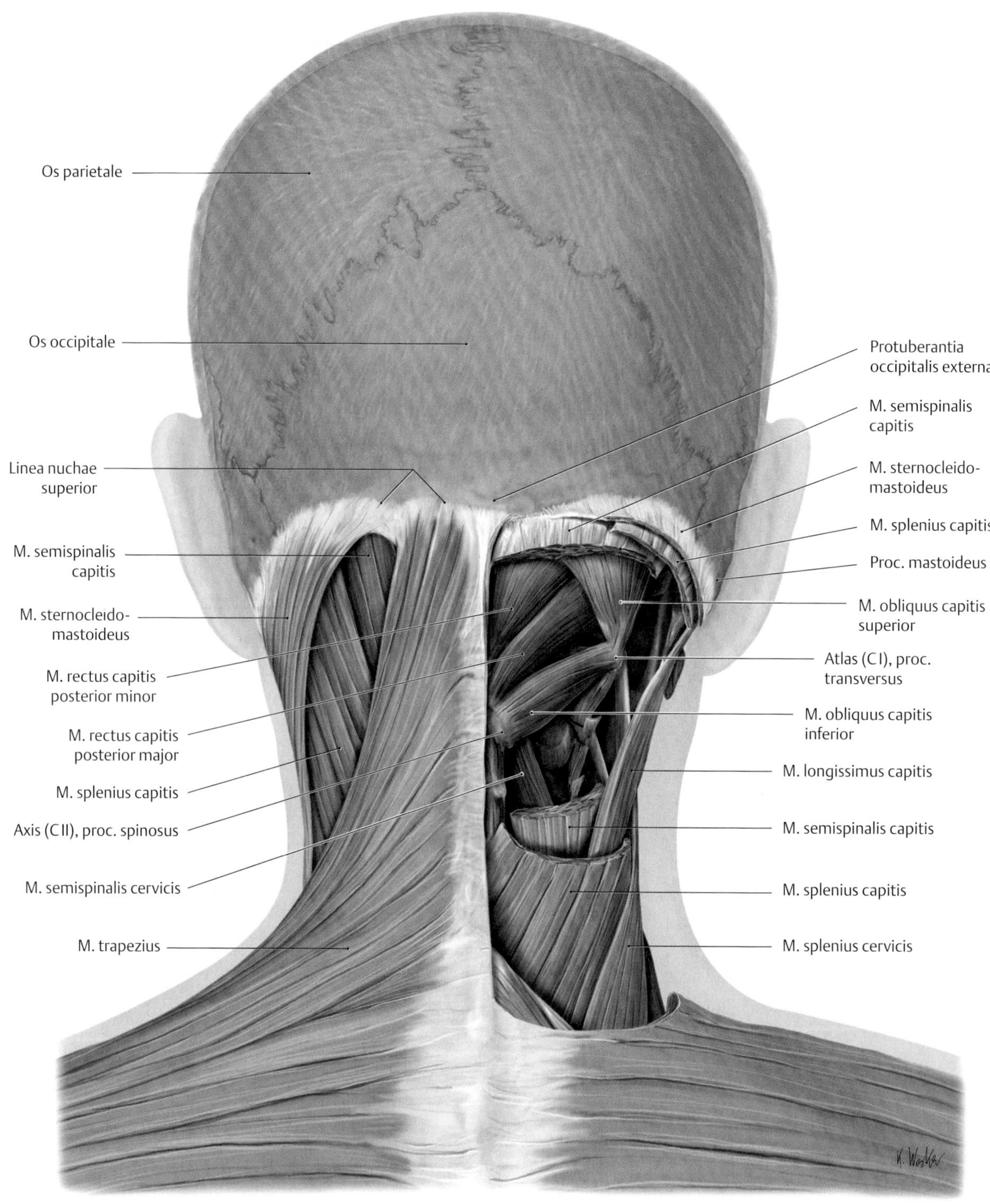
Os parietale
Os occipitale
Linea nuchae superior
M. semispinalis capitis
M. sternocleido-mastoideus
M. rectus capitis posterior minor
M. rectus capitis posterior major
M. splenius capitis
Axis (C II), proc. spinosus
M. semispinalis cervicis
M. trapezius
Protuberantia occipitalis externa
M. semispinalis capitis
M. sternocleido-mastoideus
M. splenius capitis
Proc. mastoideus
M. obliquus capitis superior
Atlas (C I), proc. transversus
M. obliquus capitis inferior
M. longissimus capitis
M. semispinalis capitis
M. splenius capitis
M. splenius cervicis

Fig. 2.3 **Muscles in the nuchal region**
Posterior view. *Removed:* M. trapezius, m. sternocleidomastoid, m. splenius, and m. semispinalis (right). *Revealed:* Musculi cervicis (right).

Fig. 2.4 **Short nuchal muscles**
Posterior view. See Fig. 2.6.

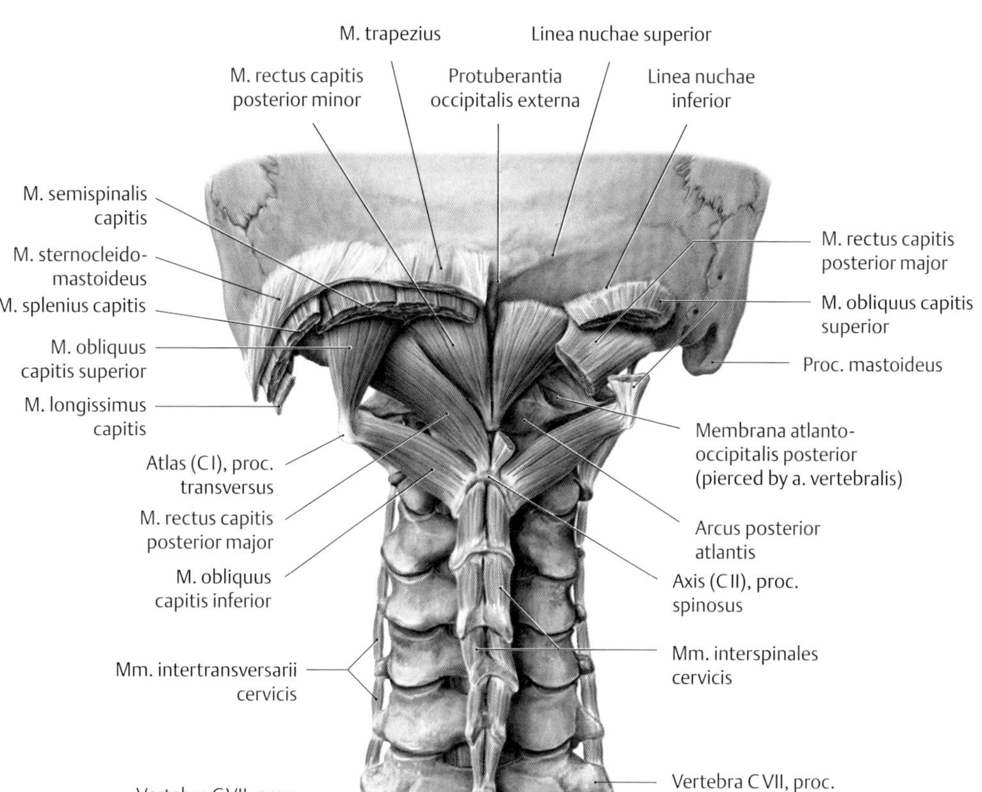
M. trapezius
Linea nuchae superior
M. rectus capitis posterior minor
Protuberantia occipitalis externa
Linea nuchae inferior
M. semispinalis capitis
M. sternocleido-mastoideus
M. splenius capitis
M. obliquus capitis superior
M. longissimus capitis
Atlas (C I), proc. transversus
M. rectus capitis posterior major
M. obliquus capitis inferior
Mm. intertransversarii cervicis
Vertebra C VII, proc. spinosus
M. rectus capitis posterior major
M. obliquus capitis superior
Proc. mastoideus
Membrana atlanto-occipitalis posterior (pierced by a. vertebralis)
Arcus posterior atlantis
Axis (C II), proc. spinosus
Mm. interspinales cervicis
Vertebra C VII, proc. transversus

A Course of the short nuchal muscles.

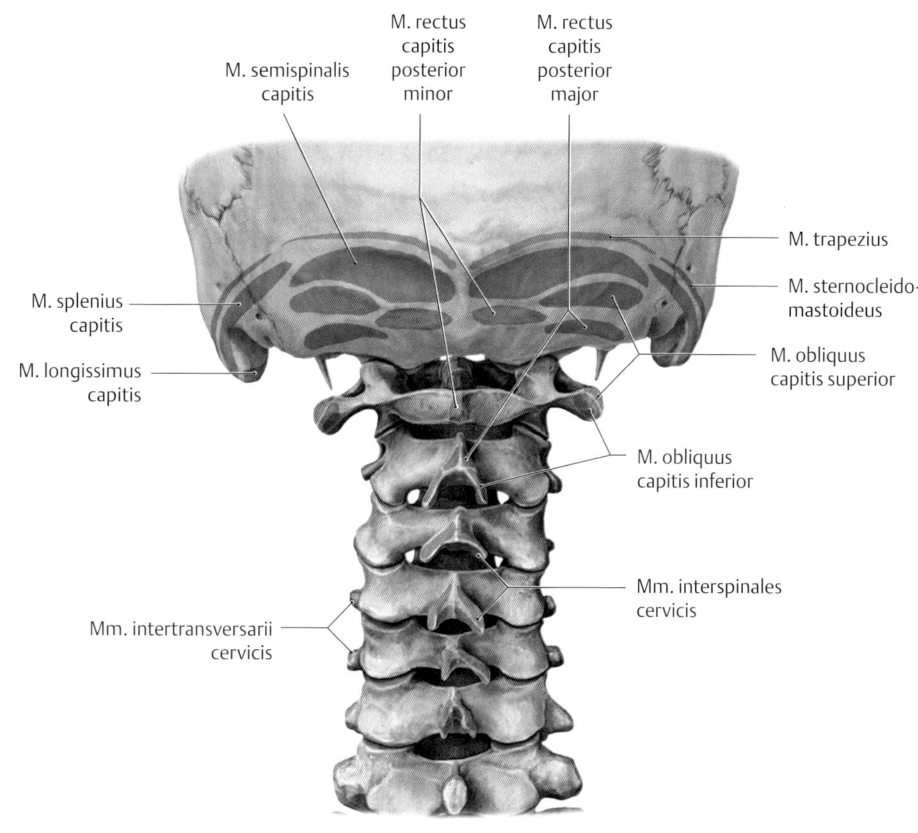
M. semispinalis capitis
M. rectus capitis posterior minor
M. rectus capitis posterior major
M. trapezius
M. sternocleido-mastoideus
M. splenius capitis
M. longissimus capitis
M. obliquus capitis superior
M. obliquus capitis inferior
Mm. interspinales cervicis
Mm. intertransversarii cervicis

B Origins (red) and insertions (blue) in the suboccipital region.

Intrinsic Muscles of the Back

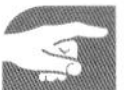

The extrinsic muscles of the back (m. trapezius, m. latissimus dorsi, m. levator scapulae, and m. rhomboideae) are discussed in Unit 4. M. serratus posterior, considered an intermediate extrinsic back muscle, has been included with the superficial intrinsic muscles in this unit.

Fig. 2.5 **Intrinsic muscles of the back**

Posterior view. Sequential dissection of fascia thoracolumbalis, superficial intrinsic muscles, intermediate intrinsic muscles, and deep intrinsic muscles of the back.

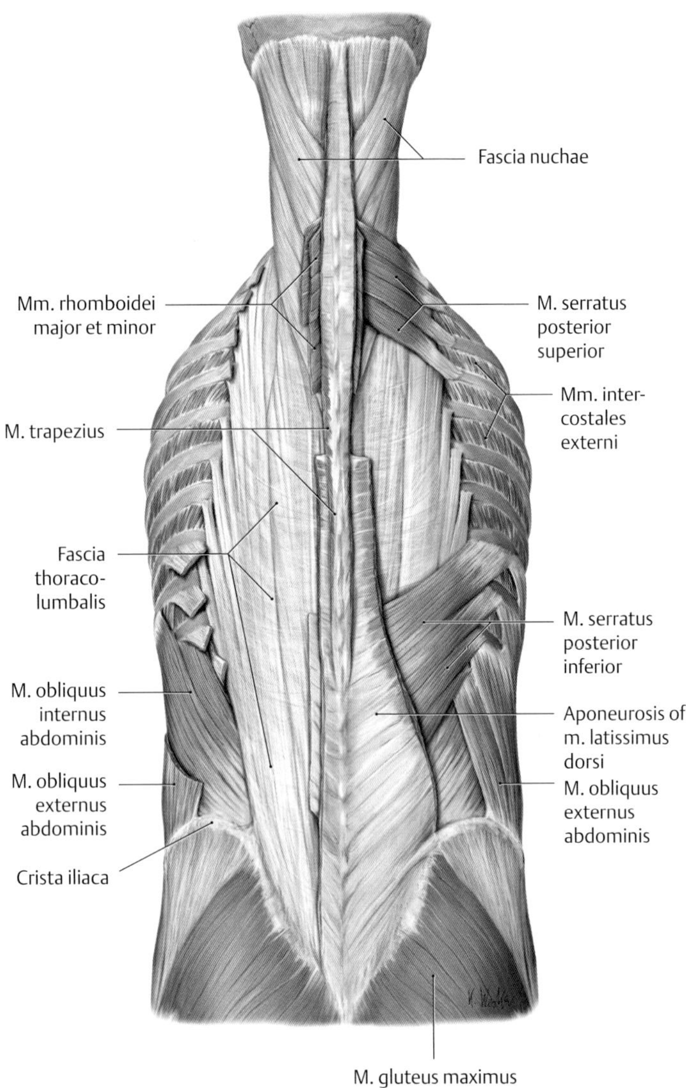
Fascia nuchae
Mm. rhomboidei major et minor
M. serratus posterior superior
Mm. inter-costales externi
M. trapezius
Fascia thoraco-lumbalis
M. serratus posterior inferior
M. obliquus internus abdominis
Aponeurosis of m. latissimus dorsi
M. obliquus externus abdominis
M. obliquus externus abdominis
Crista iliaca
M. gluteus maximus

A Fascia thoracolumbalis. *Removed:* Shoulder girdles and extrinsic back muscles (except m. serratus posterior and aponeurotic origin of m. latissimus dorsi). *Revealed:* Lamina superficialis fascia thoracolumbalis.

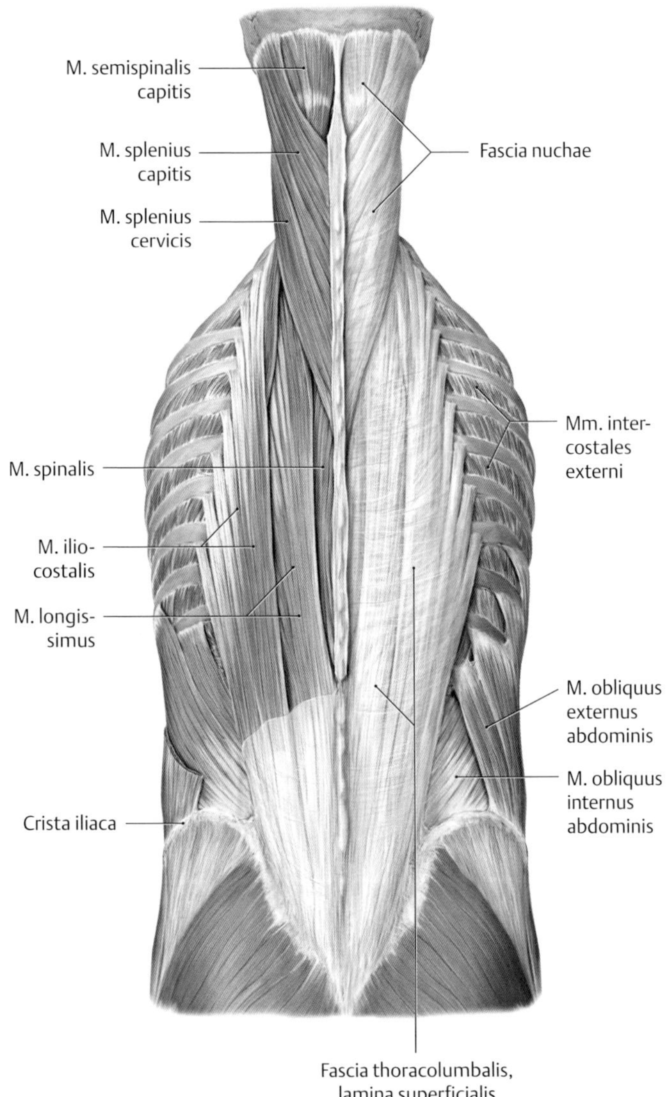
M. semispinalis capitis
M. splenius capitis
Fascia nuchae
M. splenius cervicis
Mm. inter-costales externi
M. spinalis
M. ilio-costalis
M. longis-simus
M. obliquus externus abdominis
M. obliquus internus abdominis
Crista iliaca
Fascia thoracolumbalis, lamina superficialis

B Superficial and intermediate intrinsic back muscles. *Removed:* Fascia thoracolumbalis (left). *Revealed:* M. erector spinae and m. splenius.

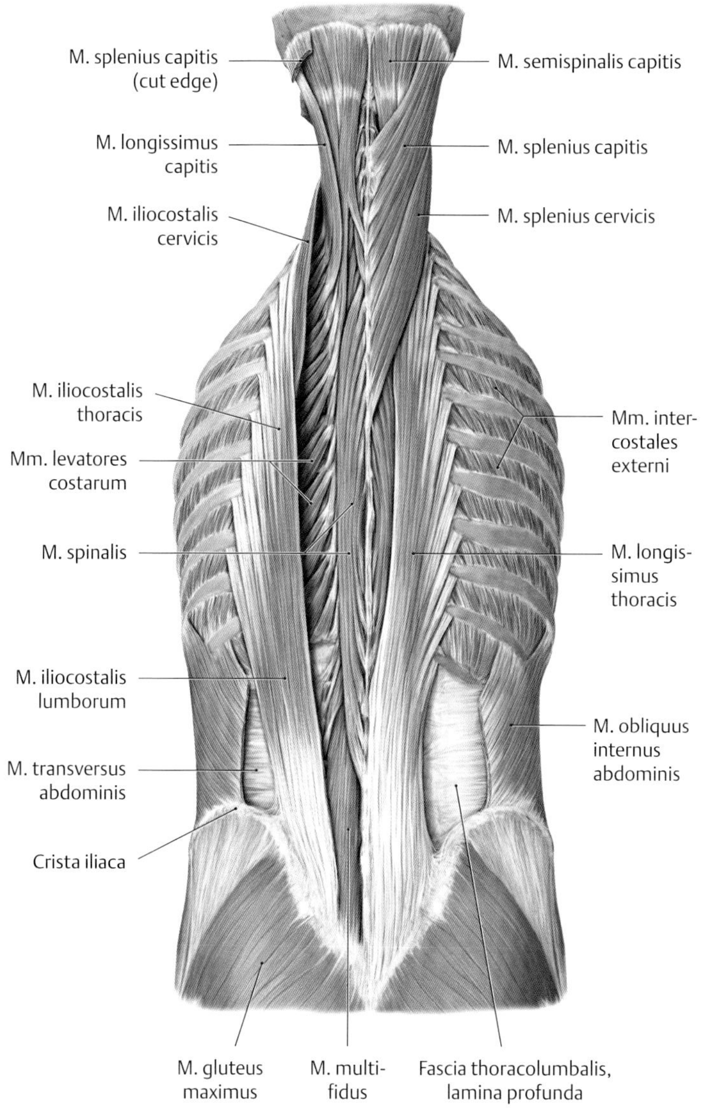
M. splenius capitis (cut edge)
M. semispinalis capitis
M. longissimus capitis
M. splenius capitis
M. iliocostalis cervicis
M. splenius cervicis
M. iliocostalis thoracis
Mm. intercostales externi
Mm. levatores costarum
M. spinalis
M. longissimus thoracis
M. iliocostalis lumborum
M. obliquus internus abdominis
M. transversus abdominis
Crista iliaca
M. gluteus maximus
M. multifidus
Fascia thoracolumbalis, lamina profunda

C Intermediate and deep intrinsic back muscles. *Removed:* M. longissimus thoracis and cervicis, m. splenius muscles (left); m. iliocostalis (right). *Note:* Lamina profunda of fascia thoracolumbalis gives origin to the internal oblique and transversus abdominus. *Revealed:* Deep muscles of the back.

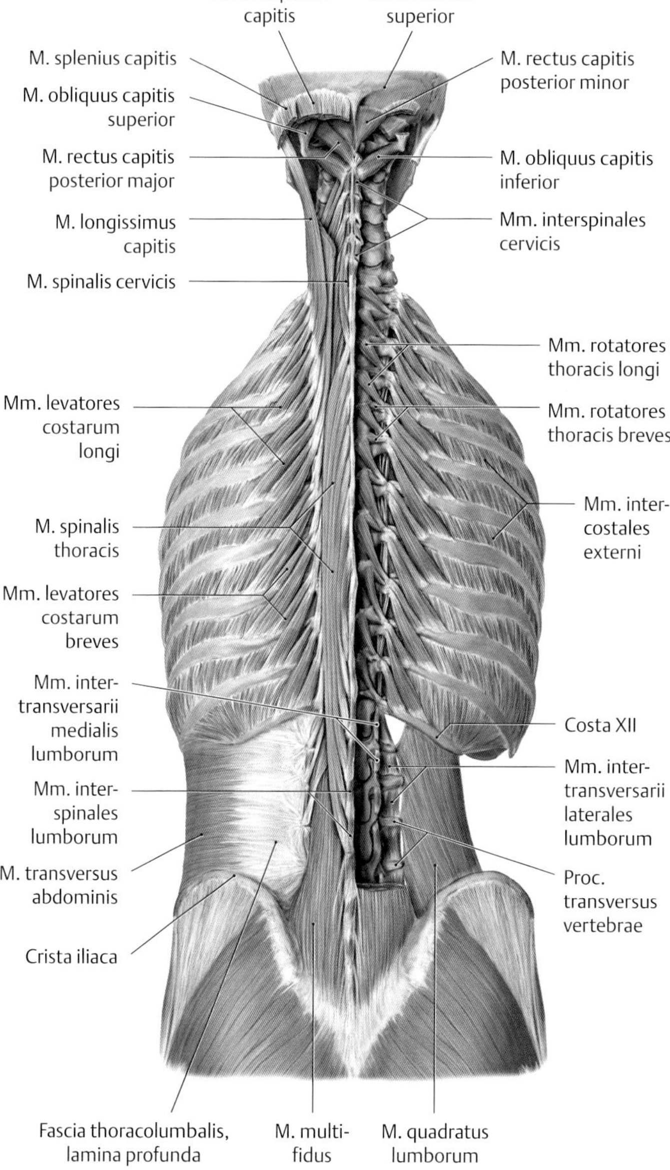
M. semispinalis capitis
Linea nuchae superior
M. splenius capitis
M. rectus capitis posterior minor
M. obliquus capitis superior
M. rectus capitis posterior major
M. obliquus capitis inferior
M. longissimus capitis
Mm. interspinales cervicis
M. spinalis cervicis
Mm. rotatores thoracis longi
Mm. levatores costarum longi
Mm. rotatores thoracis breves
Mm. intercostales externi
M. spinalis thoracis
Mm. levatores costarum breves
Mm. intertransversarii medialis lumborum
Costa XII
Mm. intertransversarii laterales lumborum
Mm. interspinales lumborum
M. transversus abdominis
Proc. transversus vertebrae
Crista iliaca
Fascia thoracolumbalis, lamina profunda
M. multifidus
M. quadratus lumborum

D Deep intrinsic back muscles. *Removed:* Superficial and intermediate intrinsic back muscles (all); deep fascial layer and m. multifidus (right). *Revealed:* M. intertransversarii and m. quadratus lumborum (right).

Muscle Facts (I)

Fig. 2.6 Short nuchal and craniovertebral joint muscles

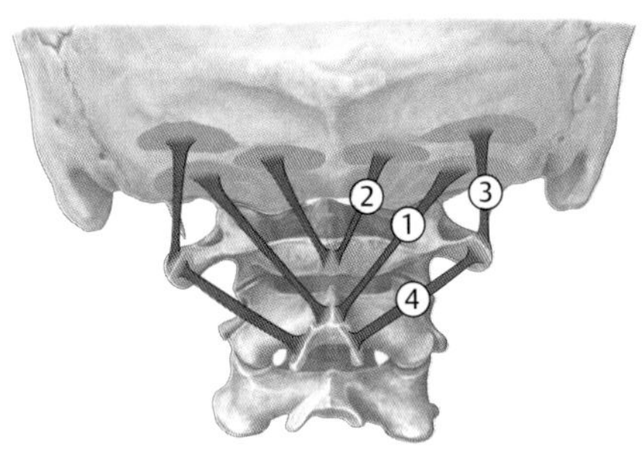

2
1
3
4

A Posterior view.

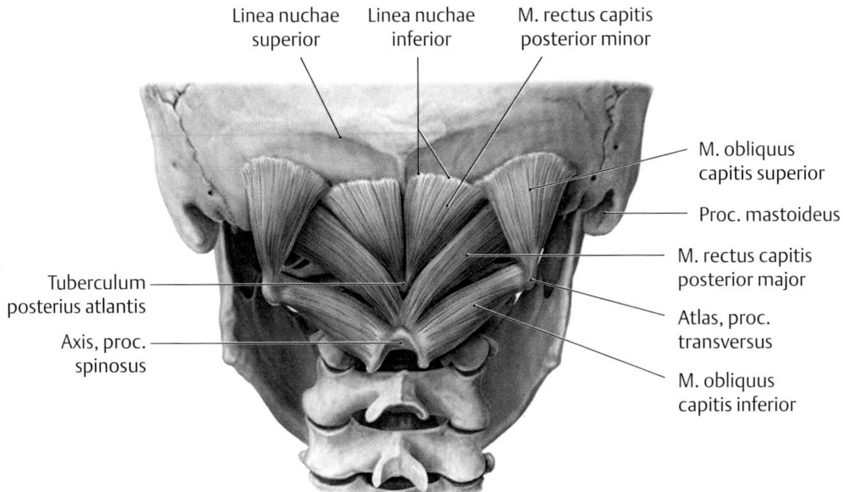

Linea nuchae superior
Linea nuchae inferior
M. rectus capitis posterior minor
M. obliquus capitis superior
Proc. mastoideus
M. rectus capitis posterior major
Tuberculum posterius atlantis
Atlas, proc. transversus
Axis, proc. spinosus
M. obliquus capitis inferior

B Suboccipital muscles, posterior view.

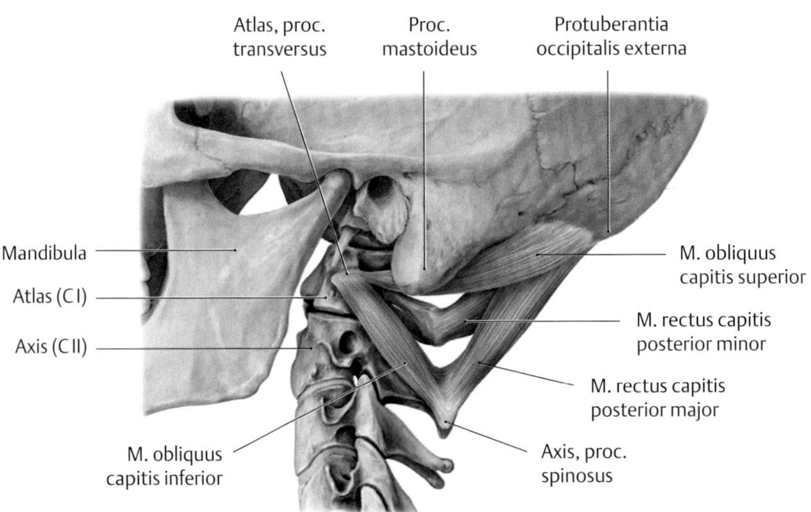

Atlas, proc. transversus
Proc. mastoideus
Protuberantia occipitalis externa
Mandibula
M. obliquus capitis superior
Atlas (C I)
Axis (C II)
M. rectus capitis posterior minor
M. rectus capitis posterior major
M. obliquus capitis inferior
Axis, proc. spinosus

C Suboccipital muscles, left lateral view.

Table 2.1 **Short nuchal and craniovertebral joint muscles**

Muscle		Origin	Insertion	Innervation	Action
M. rectus capitis posterior	① M. rectus capitis posterior major	C II (proc. spinosus)	Os occipitale (linea nuchalis inferior, middle third)	C1 (Ramus dorsalis = N. suboccipitalis)	*Bilateral:* Extends head *Unilateral:* Rotates head to same side
	② M. rectus capitis posterior minor	C I (tuberculum posterius)	Os occipitale (linea nuchalis inferior, inner third)		
M. obliquus capitis	③ M. obliquus capitis superior	C I (proc. transversus)	Os occipitale (linea nuchalis inferior, middle third; above m. rectus capitis posterior major)		*Bilateral:* Extends head *Unilateral:* Tilts head to same side; rotates to opposite side
	④ M. obliquus capitis inferior	C II (proc. spinosus)	C I (proc. transversus)		*Bilateral:* Extends head *Unilateral:* Rotates head to same side

Fig. 2.7 Prevertebral muscles

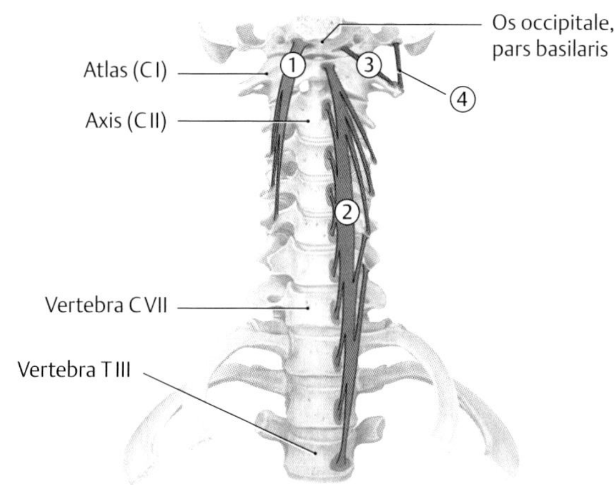
Os occipitale, pars basilaris
Atlas (C I)
Axis (C II)
Vertebra C VII
Vertebra T III
①
②
③
④

A Anterior view.

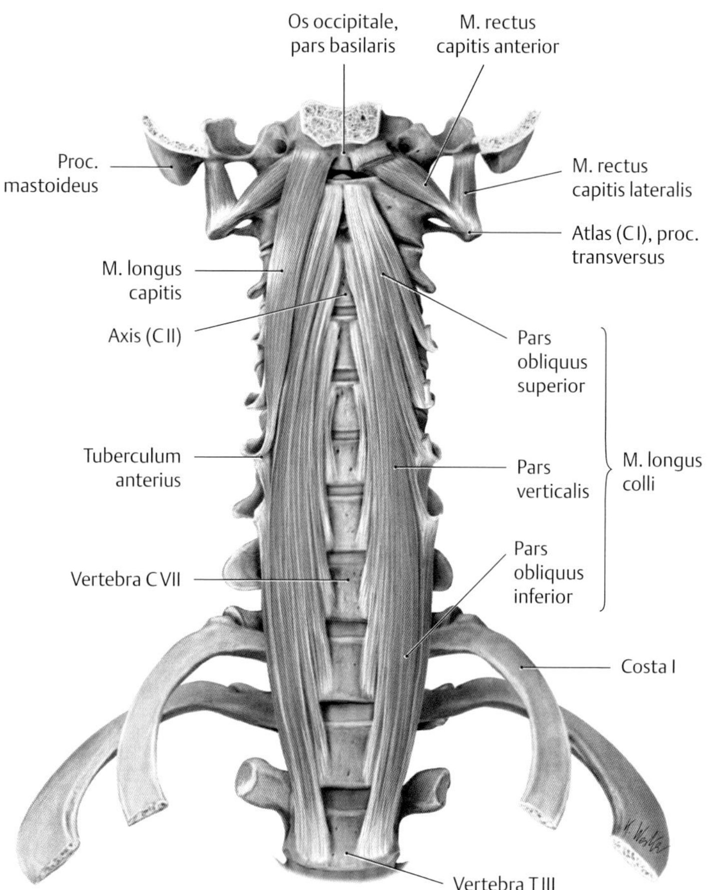
Os occipitale, pars basilaris
M. rectus capitis anterior
Proc. mastoideus
M. rectus capitis lateralis
Atlas (C I), proc. transversus
M. longus capitis
Axis (C II)
Pars obliquus superior
Tuberculum anterius
Pars verticalis
M. longus colli
Pars obliquus inferior
Vertebra C VII
Costa I
Vertebra T III

B Prevertebral muscles, anterior view. *Removed:* Longus capitis (left); cervical viscera.

Table 2.2 Prevertebral muscles

Muscle		Origin	Insertion	Innervation	Action
① M. longus capitis		C III–C VI (procc. transversi, tuberculi anteriores)	Os occipitale (pars basilaris)	Direct branches from plexus cervicalis (C1–C3)	*Bilateral:* Flexes head *Unilateral:* Tilts and slightly rotates head to same side
② M. longus colli (cervicis)	Pars verticalis (medial)	C V–T III (pars anterior of corpus vertebrae)	C II–C IV (pars anterior of corpus vertebrae)	Direct branches from plexus cervicalis (C2–C6)	*Bilateral:* Flexes cervical spine *Unilateral:* Tilts and rotates cervical spine to same side
	Pars obliquus superior	C III–C V (procc. transversi, tuberculi anteriores)	C I (procc. transversi, tuberculi anteriores)		
	Pars obliquus inferior	T I–T III (pars anterior of corpus vertebrae)	C V–C VI (procc. transversi, tuberculi anteriores)		
M. rectus capitis	③ M. rectus capitis anterior	C I (lateral mass)	Os occipitale (pars basilaris)	C1 (r. ventralis)	*Bilateral:* Flexion at articulatio atlantooccipitalis *Unilateral:* Lateral flexion at articulatio atlantooccipitalis
	④ M. rectus capitis lateralis	C I (proc. transversus)	Os occipitale (pars basilaris, lateral to condylus occipitalis)		

Muscle Facts (II)

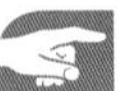

The intrinsic back muscles are divided into superficial, intermediate, and deep layers. M. serratus posterior are extrinsic back muscles, innervated by the ventral rami of intercostal nerves, not the dorsal rami, which innervate the intrinsic back muscles. They are included here as they are encountered in dissection of the back musculature.

Table 2.3 Superficial intrinsic back muscles

Muscle		Origin	Insertion	Innervation	Action
M. serratus posterior	① M. serratus posterior superior	Lig. nuchae; C VII–T III (procc. spinosi)	Costa II–IV (superior borders)	2nd–5th Nn. intercostales	Elevates ribs
	② M. serratus posterior inferior	T XI–L II (procc. spinosi)	Costa VIII–XII (inferior borders, near anguli)	Nn. spinales T9–T12 (r. ventralis)	Depresses ribs
Mm. splenii	③ M. splenius capitis	Ligamentum nuchae; C VII–T III (procc. spinosi)	Os occipitale (lateral linae nuchalis superior; proc. mastoideus)	Nn. spinales C1–C6 (r. dorsalis, lateral branches)	*Bilateral:* Extends cervical spine and head *Unilateral:* Flexes and rotates head to the same side
	④ M. splenius cervicis	T III–T VI (procc. spinosi)	C I–C II (procc. transversi)		

Fig. 2.8 **Superficial intrinsic back muscles (schematic)**
Right side, posterior view.

Fig. 2.9 **Intermediate intrinsic back muscles (schematic)**
Right side, posterior view. These muscles are collectively known as the erector spinae.

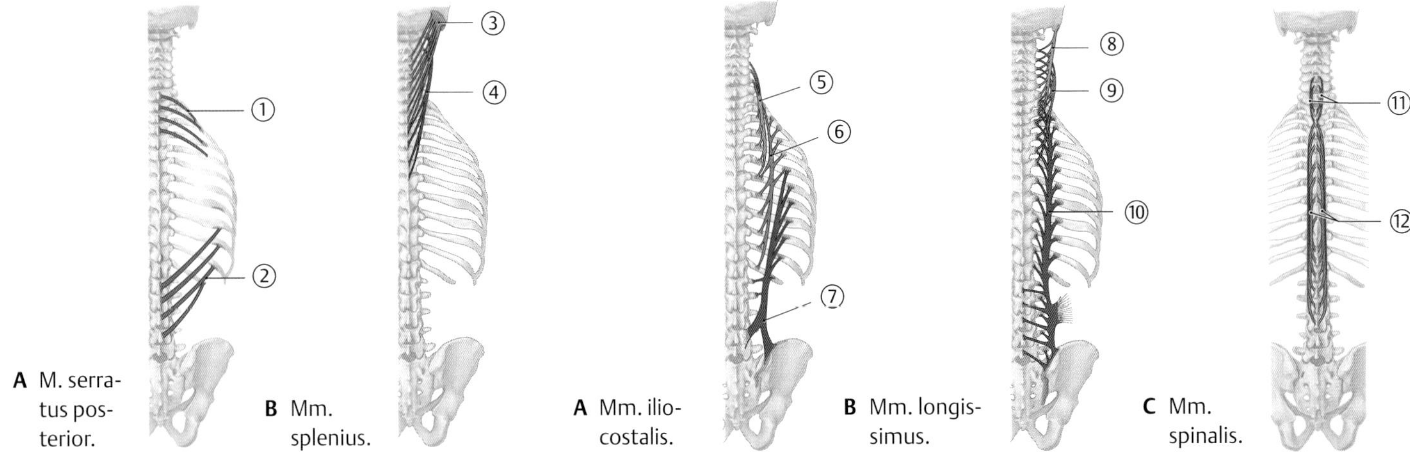
①
②
③
④
⑤
⑥
⑦
⑧
⑨
⑩
⑪
⑫

A M. serratus posterior. **B** Mm. splenius.

A Mm. iliocostalis. **B** Mm. longissimus. **C** Mm. spinalis.

Table 2.4 Intermediate intrinsic back muscles

Muscle		Origin	Insertion	Innervation	Action
Mm. iliocostales	⑤ M. iliocostalis cervicis	Costa III–VII	C IV–C VI (procc. transversi)	Nn. spinales C8–L1 (r. dorsalis, lateral branches)	*Bilateral:* Extends spine *Unilateral:* Bends spine laterally to same side
	⑥ M. iliocostalis thoracis	Costa VII–XII	Costa I–VI		
	⑦ M. illiocostalis lumborum	Os sacrum; crista iliaca; fascia thoracolumbalis	Costa VI–XII; fascia thoracolumbalis (deep layer); upper vertebrae lumbales (procc. transversi)		
Mm. longissimi	⑧ M. longissimus capitis	T I–T III (procc. transversi); C IV–C VII (procc. transversi and articulares)	Os temporale (proc. mastoideus)	Nn. spinales C1–L5 (r. dorsalis, lateral branches)	*Bilateral:* Extends head *Unilateral:* Flexes and rotates head to same side
	⑨ M. longissimus cervicis	T I–T VI (procc. transversi)	C II–C V (procc. transversi)		*Bilateral:* Extends spine *Unilateral:* Bends spine laterally to same side
	⑩ M. longissimus thoracis	Os sacrum; crista iliaca; vertebrae lumbales (procc. spinosi); lower vertebrae thoracicae (procc. transversi)	Costa II–XII; vertebrae lumbales (procc. costalis); vertebrae thoracicae (procc. transversi)		
Mm. spinales	⑪ M. spinalis cervicis	C V–T II (procc. spinosi)	C II–C V (procc. spinosi)	Nn. spinales (r. dorsalis)	*Bilateral:* Extends cervical and thoracic spine *Unilateral:* Bends cervical and thoracic spine to same side
	⑫ M. spinalis thoracis	T X–L III (procc. spinosi, lateral surfaces)	T II–T VIII (procc. spinosi, lateral surfaces)		

Fig. 2.10 **Superficial and intermediate intrinsic back muscles**
Posterior view.

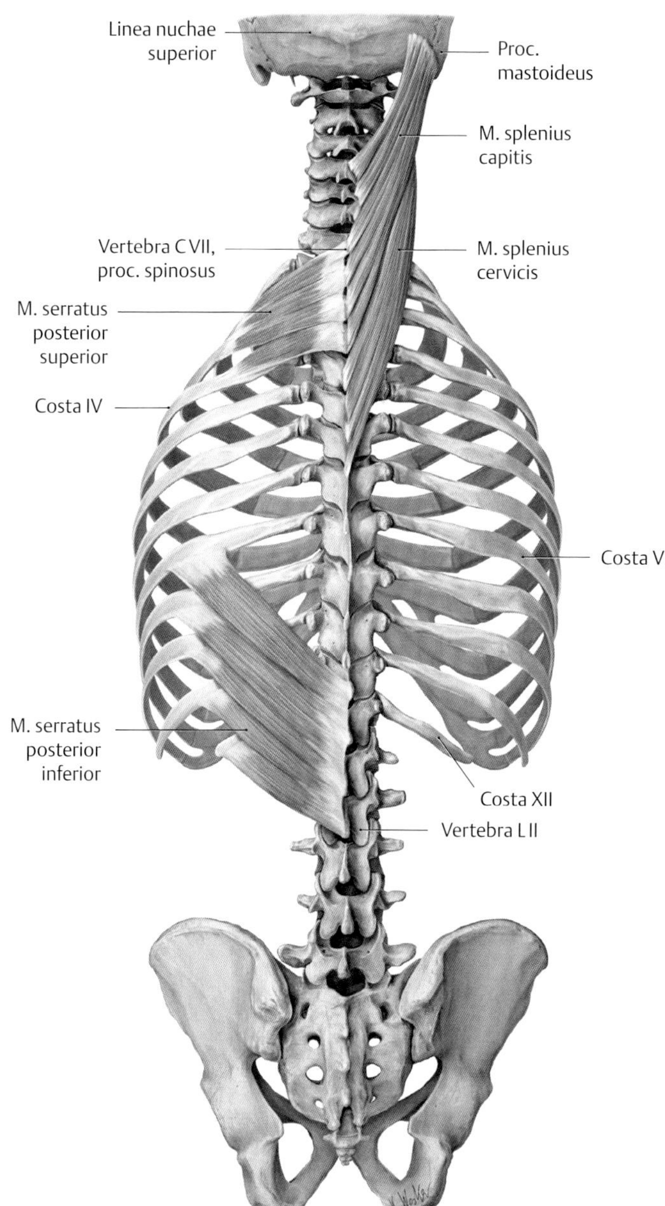
Linea nuchae superior
Proc. mastoideus
M. splenius capitis
Vertebra C VII, proc. spinosus
M. splenius cervicis
M. serratus posterior superior
Costa IV
Costa VIII
M. serratus posterior inferior
Costa XII
Vertebra L II

A M. splenius and m. serratus posterior.

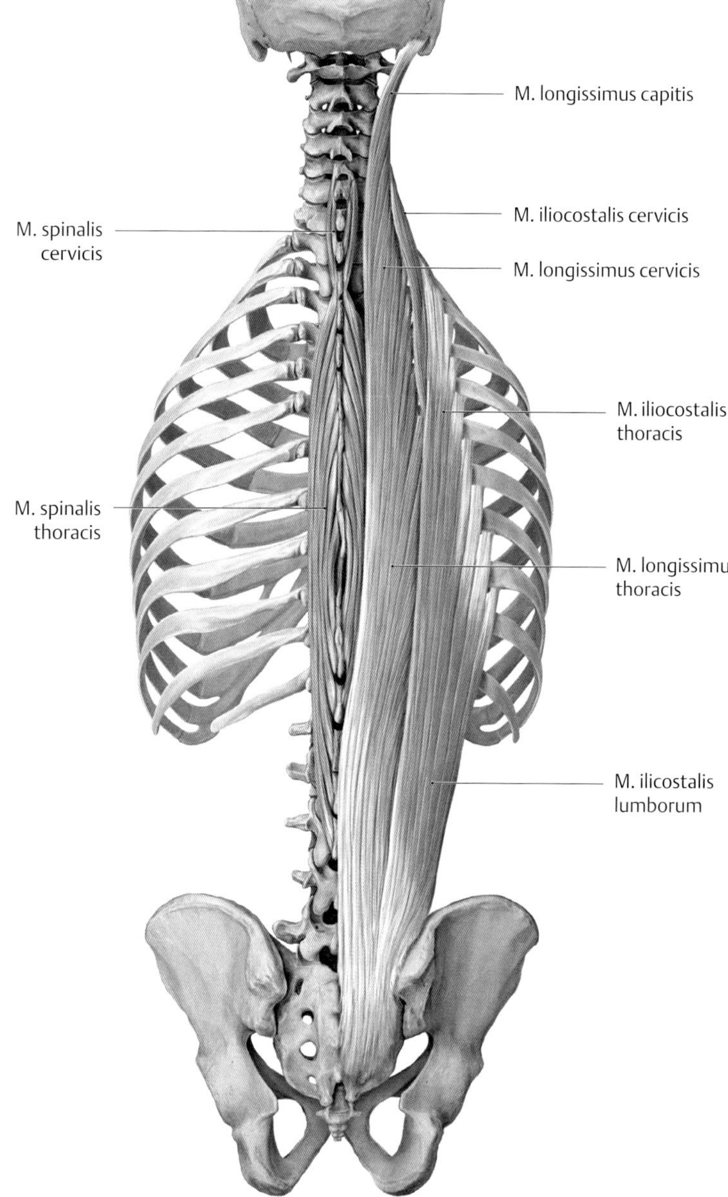
M. longissimus capitis
M. iliocostalis cervicis
M. spinalis cervicis
M. longissimus cervicis
M. iliocostalis thoracis
M. spinalis thoracis
M. longissimus thoracis
M. ilicostalis lumborum

B M. erector spinae: m. iliocostalis, longissimus, and spinalis.

Muscle Facts (III)

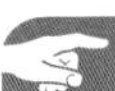

The deep intrinsic back muscles are divided into two groups: transversospinal and deep segmental muscles. The transversospinalis muscles pass between the transverse and spinous processes of the vertebrae.

Table 2.5 Transversospinalis muscles

Muscle		Origin	Insertion	Innervation	Action
Mm. rotatores	① Mm. rotatores breves	TI–TXII (between procc. transversi and spinosi of adjacent vertebrae)		Nn. spinales (r. dorsalis)	*Bilateral:* Extends thoracic spine *Unilateral:* Rotates spine to opposite side
	② Mm. rotatores longi	TI–TXII (between procc. transversi and spinosi, skipping one vertebra)			
Mm. multifidi ③		CII–sacrum (procc. transversi and spinosi, skipping two to four vertebrae)			*Bilateral:* Extends spine *Unilateral:* Flexes spine to same side, rotates to opposite side
Mm. semispinales	④ M. semispinalis capitis	CIV–TVII (procc. transversi and articulares)	Os occipitale (between linae nuchalis superior and inferior)		*Bilateral:* Extends thoracic and cervical spines and head (stabilizes articulationes craniovertebrales) *Unilateral:* Bends head, cervical and thoracic spines to same side, rotates to opposite side
	⑤ M. semispinalis cervicis	TI–TVI (procc. transversi)	CII–CV (procc. spinosi)		
	⑥ M. semispinalis thoracis	TVI–TXII (procc. transversi)	CVI–TIV (procc. spinosi)		

Fig. 2.11 Transversospinalis muscles (schematic)
Posterior view.

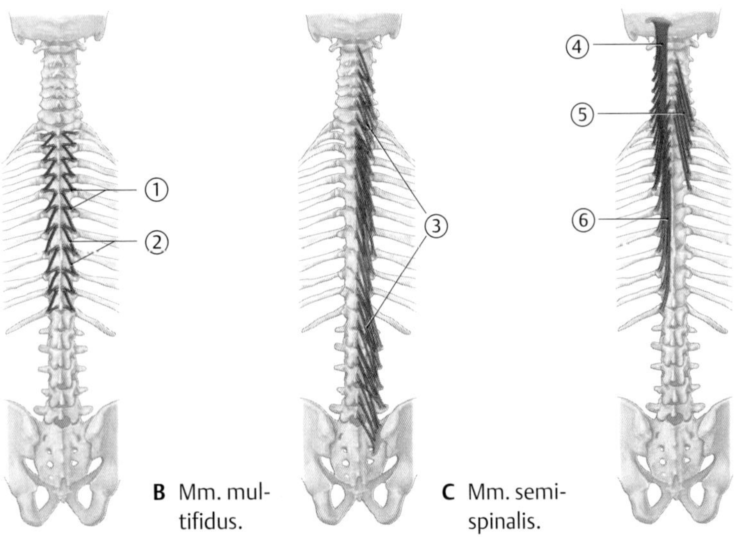

①
②
③
④
⑤
⑥

A Mm. rotatores. **B** Mm. multifidus. **C** Mm. semispinalis.

Fig. 2.12 Deep segmental muscles (schematic)
Posterior view.

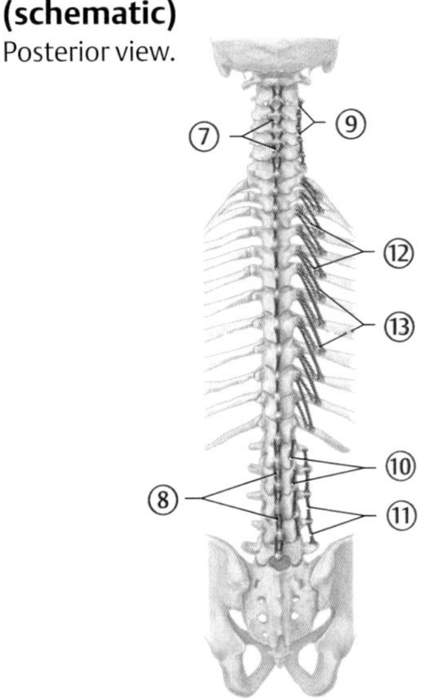

⑦
⑨
⑫
⑬
⑩
⑧
⑪

Table 2.6 Deep segmental back muscles

Muscle		Origin	Insertion	Innervation	Action
Mm. interspinales*	⑦ Mm. interspinales cervicis	CI–CVII (between procc. spinosi of adjacent vertebrae)		Nn. spinales (r.dorsalis)	Extends cervical and lumbar spines
	⑧ Mm. interspinales lumborum	LI–LV (between procc. spinosi of adjacent vertebrae)			
Mm. intertransversarii*	Mm. intertransversarii anterior cervicis	CII–CVII (between tuberculi anteriores of adjacent vertebrae)		Nn. spinales (r. ventralis)	*Bilateral:* Stabilizes and extends the cervical and lumbar spines *Unilateral:* Bends the cervical and lumbar spines laterally to same side
	⑨ Mm. intertransversarii posterior cervicis	CII–CVII (between tuberculi posteriores of adjacent vertebrae)		Nn. spinales (r. dorsalis)	
	⑩ Mm. intertransversarii mediales lumborum	LI–LV (between procc. mammilarii of adjacent vertebrae)			
	⑪ Mm. intertransversarii laterales lumborum	LI–LV (between procc. transversi of adjacent vertebrae)			
Mm. levatores costarum	⑫ Mm. levatores costarum breves	CVII–TXI (procc. transversi)	Angulus costae of next lower rib		*Bilateral:* Extends thoracic spine *Unilateral:* Bends thoracic spine to same side, rotates to opposite side
	⑬ Mm. levatores costarum longi		Angulus costae of rib two vertebrae below		

*Both the mm. interspinales and mm. intertransversarii traverse the entire spine; only their clinically relevant components have been included.

Fig. 2.13 Deep intrinsic back muscles

Posterior view.

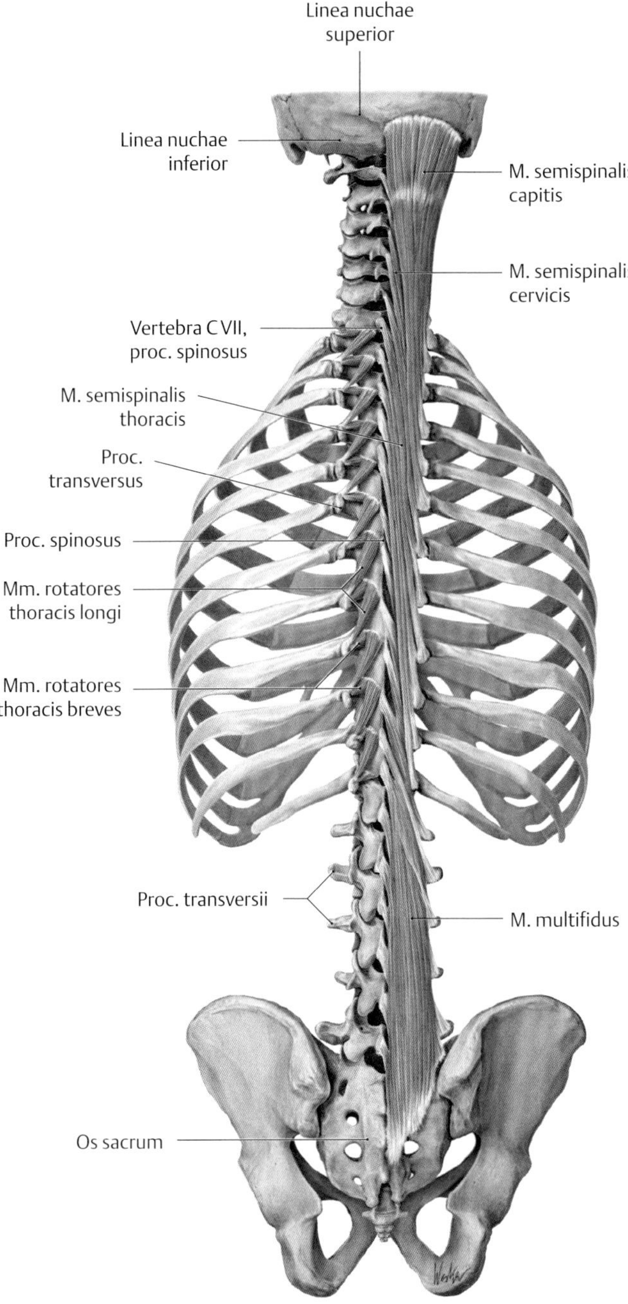
Linea nuchae superior
Linea nuchae inferior
M. semispinalis capitis
M. semispinalis cervicis
Vertebra C VII, proc. spinosus
M. semispinalis thoracis
Proc. transversus
Proc. spinosus
Mm. rotatores thoracis longi
Mm. rotatores thoracis breves
Proc. transversii
M. multifidus
Os sacrum

A Transversospinalis muscles: Mm. rotatores, mm. multifidus, and mm. semispinalis.

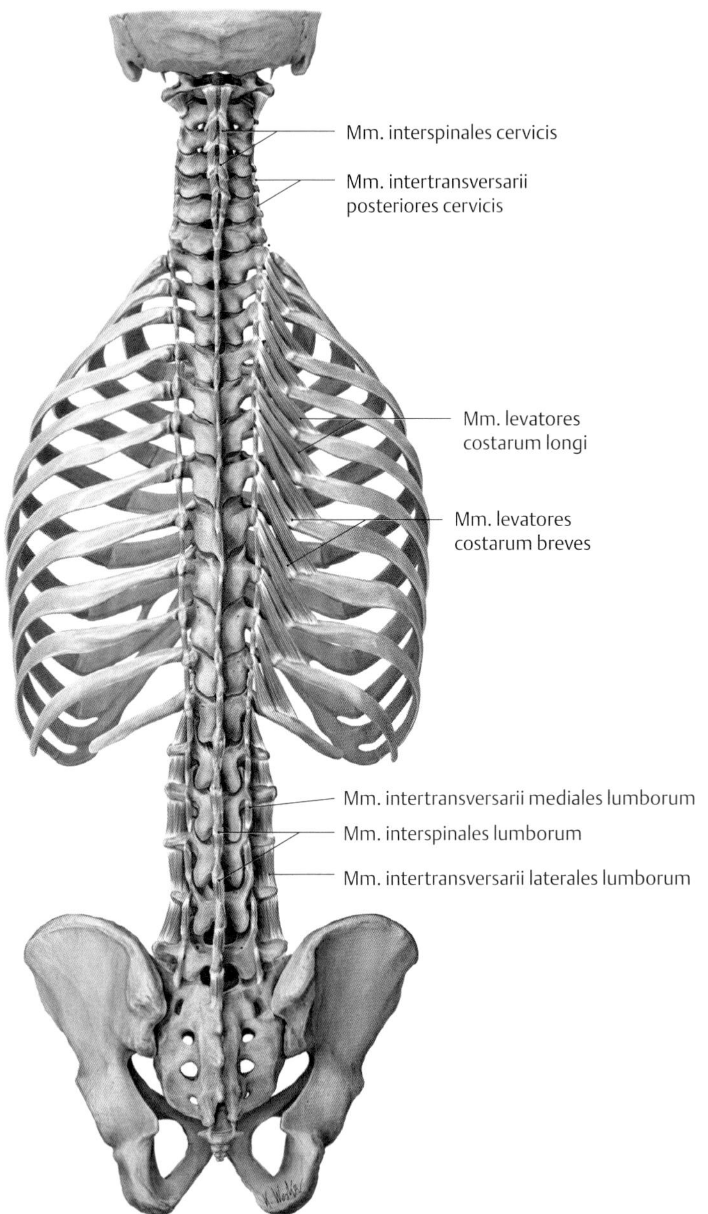
Mm. interspinales cervicis
Mm. intertransversarii posteriores cervicis
Mm. levatores costarum longi
Mm. levatores costarum breves
Mm. intertransversarii mediales lumborum
Mm. interspinales lumborum
Mm. intertransversarii laterales lumborum

B Deep segmental muscles: Mm. interspinales, mm. intertransversarii, and mm. levatores costarum.

Arteries & Veins of the Back

Fig. 3.1 Arteries of the back

The structures of the back are supplied by branches of a. intercostalis posterior, which arise from aorta thoracica or directly from a. subclavia.

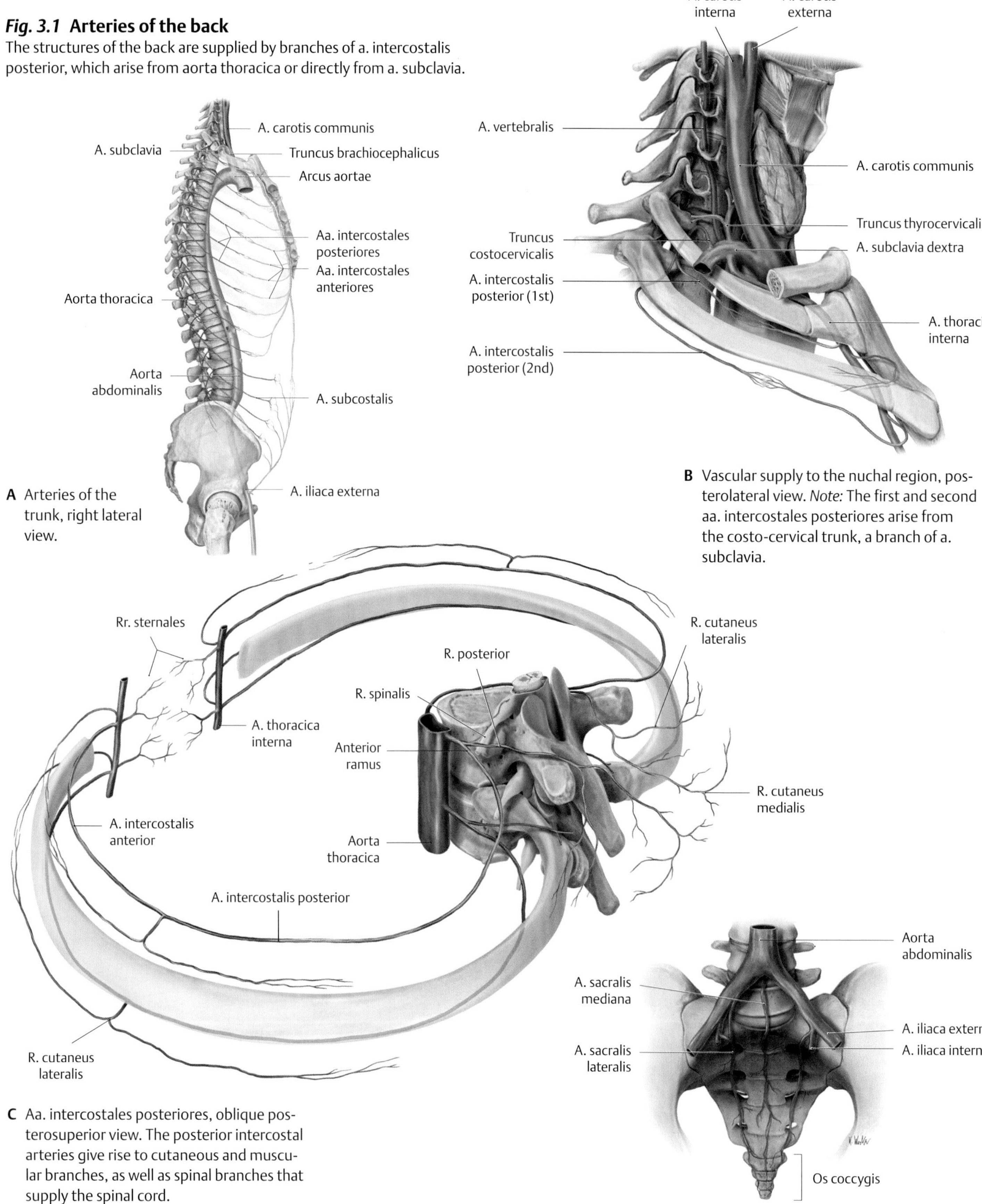

A. carotis communis
A. subclavia
Truncus brachiocephalicus
Arcus aortae
Aa. intercostales posteriores
Aa. intercostales anteriores
Aorta thoracica
Aorta abdominalis
A. subcostalis
A. iliaca externa
A. carotis interna
A. carotis externa
A. vertebralis
A. carotis communis
Truncus thyrocervicalis
Truncus costocervicalis
A. subclavia dextra
A. intercostalis posterior (1st)
A. thoracica interna
A. intercostalis posterior (2nd)
Rr. sternales
R. cutaneus lateralis
R. posterior
R. spinalis
A. thoracica interna
Anterior ramus
R. cutaneus medialis
A. intercostalis anterior
Aorta thoracica
A. intercostalis posterior
R. cutaneus lateralis
Aorta abdominalis
A. sacralis mediana
A. iliaca externa
A. iliaca interna
A. sacralis lateralis
Os coccygis

A Arteries of the trunk, right lateral view.

B Vascular supply to the nuchal region, posterolateral view. *Note:* The first and second aa. intercostales posteriores arise from the costo-cervical trunk, a branch of a. subclavia.

C Aa. intercostales posteriores, oblique posterosuperior view. The posterior intercostal arteries give rise to cutaneous and muscular branches, as well as spinal branches that supply the spinal cord.

D Vascular supply to the sacrum, anterior view.

Fig. 3.2 Veins of the back

The veins of the back drain into v. azygos via vv. intercostales superiores, vv. hemiazygos, and vv. lumbales ascendens. The interior of the spinal column is drained by plexus venosus vertebralis that runs the length of the spine.

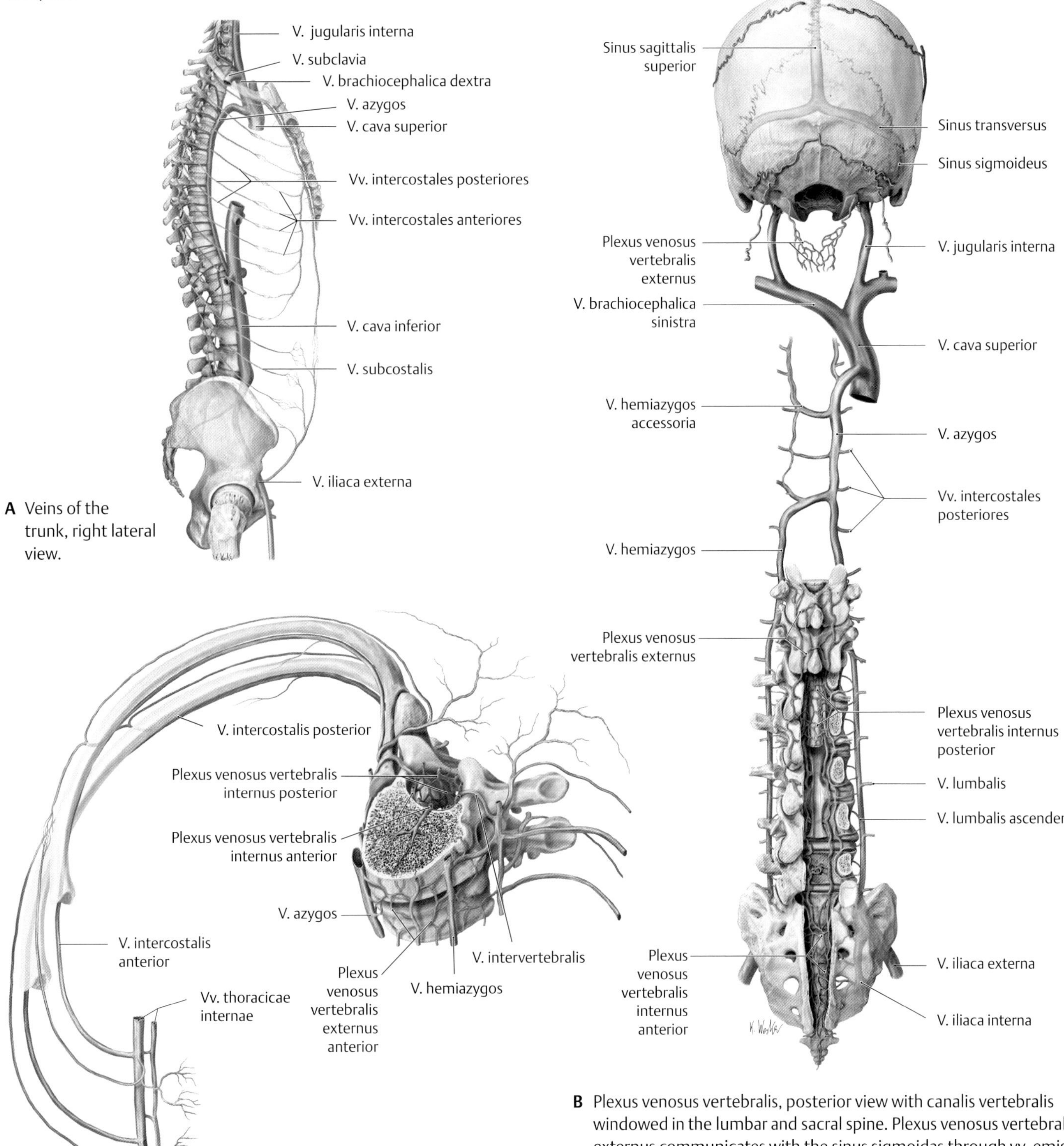
V. jugularis interna
V. subclavia
V. brachiocephalica dextra
V. azygos
V. cava superior
Vv. intercostales posteriores
Vv. intercostales anteriores
V. cava inferior
V. subcostalis
V. iliaca externa
Sinus sagittalis superior
Sinus transversus
Sinus sigmoideus
Plexus venosus vertebralis externus
V. jugularis interna
V. brachiocephalica sinistra
V. cava superior
V. hemiazygos accessoria
V. azygos
Vv. intercostales posteriores
V. hemiazygos
Plexus venosus vertebralis externus
Plexus venosus vertebralis internus posterior
V. lumbalis
V. lumbalis ascendens
Plexus venosus vertebralis internus anterior
V. iliaca externa
V. iliaca interna
V. intercostalis posterior
Plexus venosus vertebralis internus posterior
Plexus venosus vertebralis internus anterior
V. azygos
V. intercostalis anterior
V. intervertebralis
Plexus venosus vertebralis externus anterior
V. hemiazygos
Vv. thoracicae internae

A Veins of the trunk, right lateral view.

B Plexus venosus vertebralis, posterior view with canalis vertebralis windowed in the lumbar and sacral spine. Plexus venosus vertebralis externus communicates with the sinus sigmoidas through vv. emissariae in the skull. Plexus venosus vertebralis externus is divided into an anterior and a posterior portion that run along the exterior of the spinal column. Plexus venosus vertebralis internus anterior and posterior run in the foramen vertebrale and drain the spinal cord.

C Vv. intercostalis and plexus venosus vertebralis anterior, anterosuperior view. The intercostal veins follow a similar course as the intercostal nerves and arteries (see pp. 34, 36). *Note:* Plexus venosus vertebralis externus anterior can be seen communicating with v. azygos.

Nerves of the Back

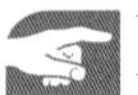

The back receives its innervation from branches of nn. spinales. The *posterior* rami of the spinal nerves supply most of the intrinsic muscles of the back. The extrinsic muscles of the back are supplied by the *anterior* rami of the spinal nerves.

Fig. 3.3 Nerves of the back

The anterior rami of n. spinalis T1–T11 form nn. intercostales, which course along the ribs and give rise to lateral and anterior cutaneous branches, rami cutaneri.

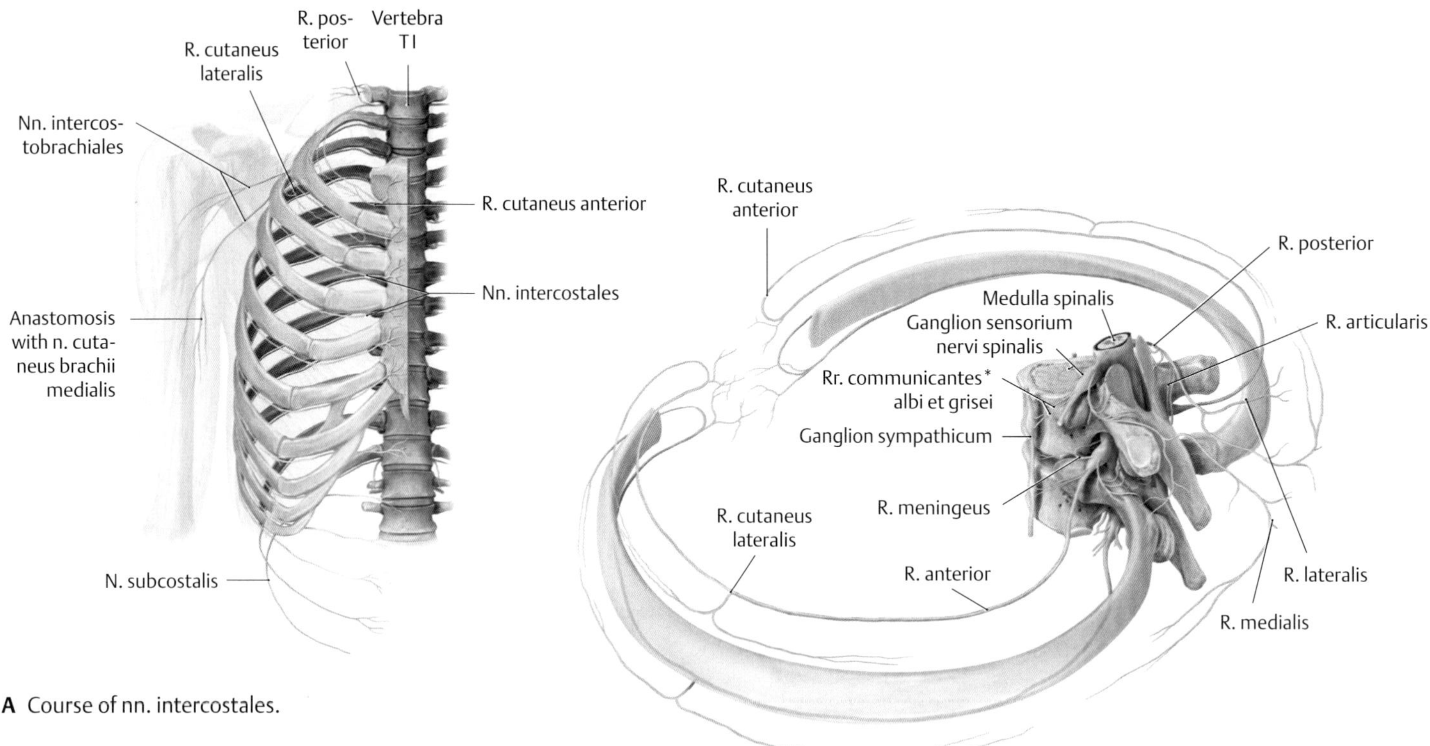
R. posterior
Vertebra T1
R. cutaneus lateralis
Nn. intercostobrachiales
R. cutaneus anterior
Nn. intercostales
Anastomosis with n. cutaneus brachii medialis
N. subcostalis
R. cutaneus anterior
R. posterior
Medulla spinalis
Ganglion sensorium nervi spinalis
R. articularis
Rr. communicantes* albi et grisei
Ganglion sympathicum
R. meningeus
R. cutaneus lateralis
R. anterior
R. lateralis
R. medialis

A Course of nn. intercostales.

B Nn. intercostales branches, superior view. Rami posteriores of nn. spinales give rise to muscular and cutaneous branches, as well as articular branches to the zygapophyseal joints. Rami anteriores of nn. spinales T1–T11 produce nn. intercostales (T12 produces n. subcostalis).

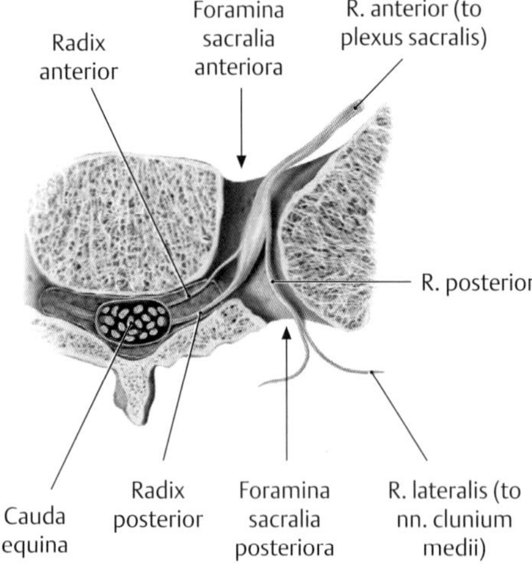
Radix anterior
Foramina sacralia anteriora
R. anterior (to plexus sacralis)
R. posterior
Cauda equina
Radix posterior
Foramina sacralia posteriora
R. lateralis (to nn. clunium medii)

C Nn. spinales branches in the sacral foramina. Superior view of transverse section through right half of sacrum.

Table 3.1 Branches of a spinal nerve

Branches			Territory
R. meningeus			Spinal meninges; ligaments of spinal column
R. dorsalis	Medial branches	Articular branch	Articulationes zygapophyseales
		Muscular branch	Intrinsic back muscles
		Cutaneous branch	Skin of posterior head, neck, back, and buttocks
	Lateral branches	Cutaneous branch	
		Muscular branch	Intrinsic back muscles
R. ventralis	Lateral cutaneous branches		Skin of lateral chest wall
	Anterior cutaneous branches		Skin of anterior chest wall

*The white and gray rami communicans carry pre- and postganglionic fibers between the sympathetic trunk and spinal nerve. They are shown on p. 622.

Fig. 3.4 **Nerves of the nuchal region**

Right side, posterior view. Like the back, the nuchal region receives most of its motor and sensory innervation from rami *posteriores* of nn. spinales. Rami posteriores of C1–C3 have specific names: n. suboccipital (C1), n. occipitalis major (C2), and n. occipitalis tertius (C3). N. occipitalis minor and n. auricularis major arise from the rami *anteriores* of the C1–C4 spinal nerves and innervate the skin of the anterolateral head and neck. Rami anteriores of C1–C4 also give rise to the *ansa cervicalis,* which innervates mm. infrahyoidales (see p. 562).

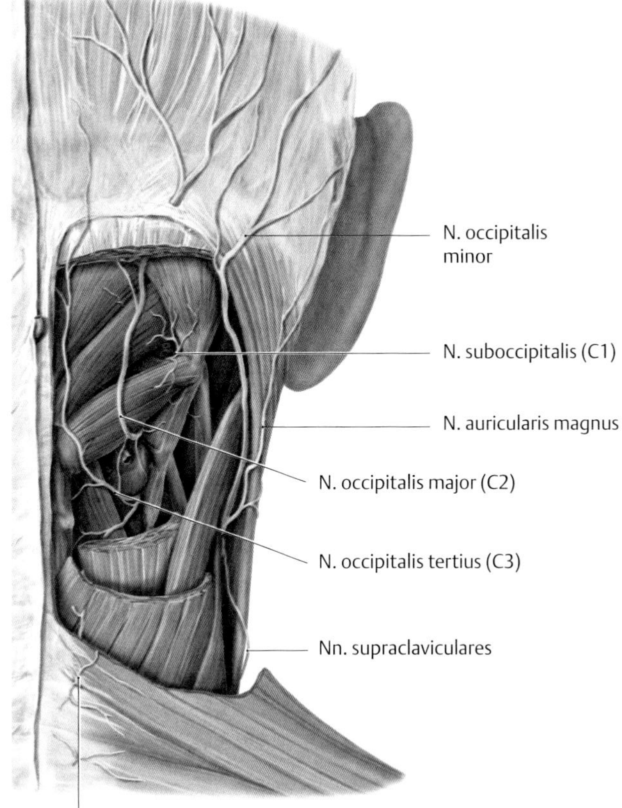
N. occipitalis minor
N. suboccipitalis (C1)
N. auricularis magnus
N. occipitalis major (C2)
N. occipitalis tertius (C3)
Nn. supraclaviculares
N. spinalis (C5), r. posterior

Fig. 3.5 **Cutaneous innervation of the back**

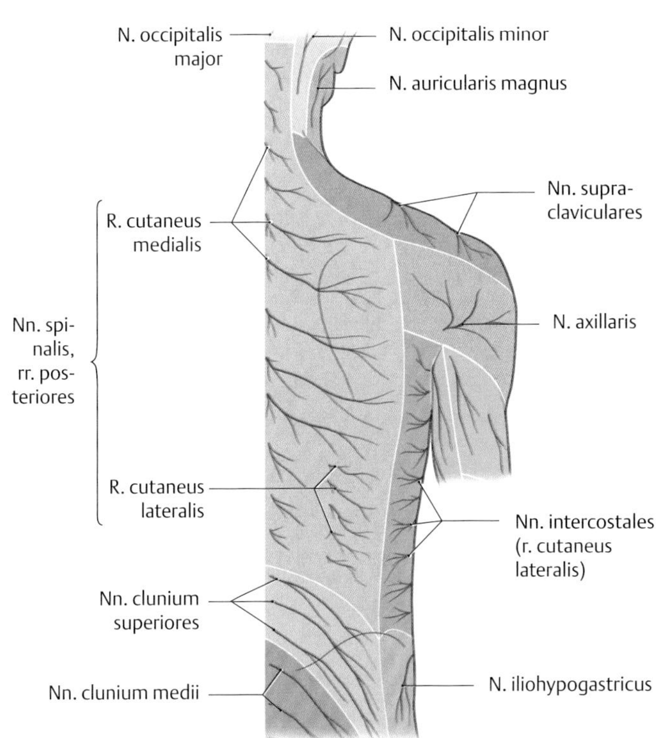
N. occipitalis major
N. occipitalis minor
N. auricularis magnus
R. cutaneus medialis
Nn. supra-claviculares
Nn. spi-nalis, rr. pos-teriores
N. axillaris
R. cutaneus lateralis
Nn. intercostales (r. cutaneus lateralis)
Nn. clunium superiores
Nn. clunium medii
N. iliohypogastricus

A Peripheral sensory cutaneous innervation of the back.

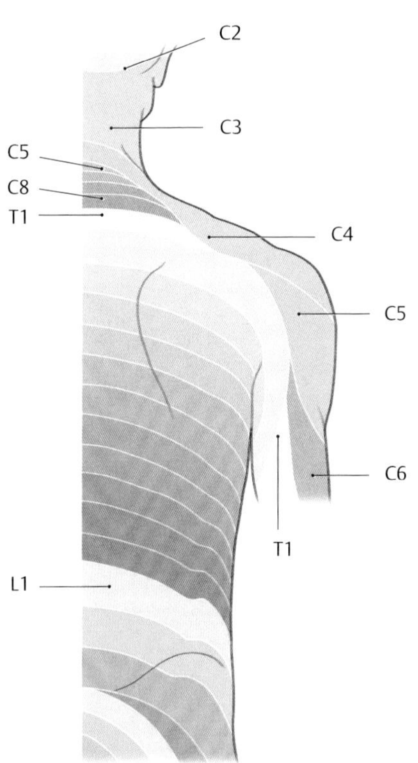
C2
C3
C5
C8
T1
C4
C5
C6
T1
L1

B Dermatomes: Segmental (radicular) cutaneous innervation of the back. *Note*: Ramus posterior of C1 is purely motor; there is consequently no C1 dermatome.

Neurovascular Topography of the Back

Fig. 3.6 Neurovasculature of the nuchal region
Posterior view. *Removed:* M. trapezius, m. sternocleidomastoid, m. splenius capitis, and m. semispinalis capitis. *Revealed:* Suboccipital region. See p. 60 for the course of the intercostal vessels.

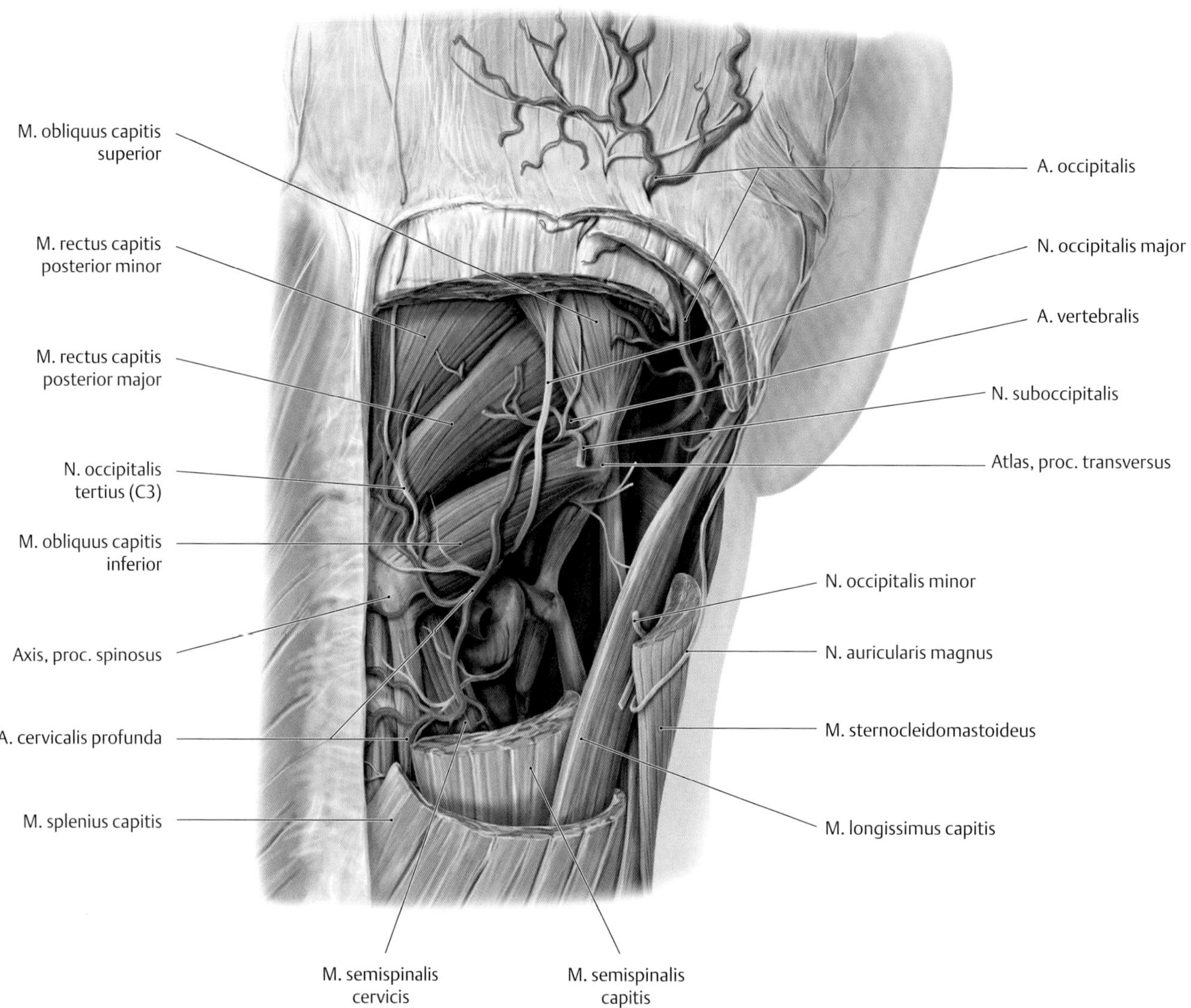
M. obliquus capitis superior
M. rectus capitis posterior minor
M. rectus capitis posterior major
N. occipitalis tertius (C3)
M. obliquus capitis inferior
Axis, proc. spinosus
A. cervicalis profunda
M. splenius capitis
A. occipitalis
N. occipitalis major
A. vertebralis
N. suboccipitalis
Atlas, proc. transversus
N. occipitalis minor
N. auricularis magnus
M. sternocleidomastoideus
M. longissimus capitis
M. semispinalis cervicis
M. semispinalis capitis

Fig. 3.7 **Neurovasculature of the back**
Posterior view. *Removed:* Muscle fascia (except fascia thoracolumbalis, lamina superficialis); m. latissimus dorsi (right). *Reflected:* M. trapezius (right). *Revealed:* A. transversa cervicis in the deep scapular region.

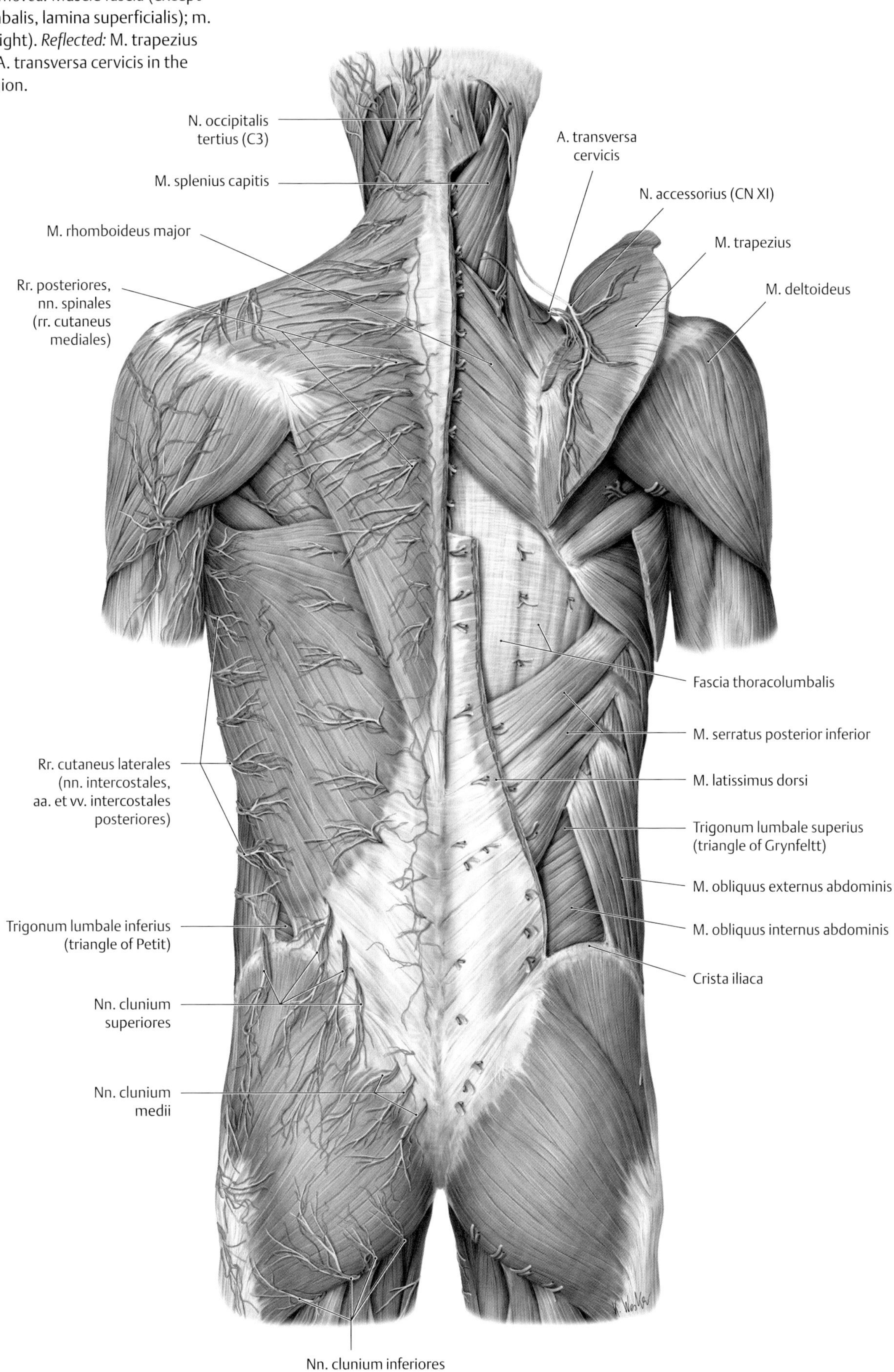
N. occipitalis tertius (C3)
M. splenius capitis
M. rhomboideus major
Rr. posteriores, nn. spinales (rr. cutaneus mediales)
A. transversa cervicis
N. accessorius (CN XI)
M. trapezius
M. deltoideus
Fascia thoracolumbalis
M. serratus posterior inferior
M. latissimus dorsi
Rr. cutaneus laterales (nn. intercostales, aa. et vv. intercostales posteriores)
Trigonum lumbale superius (triangle of Grynfeltt)
M. obliquus externus abdominis
M. obliquus internus abdominis
Trigonum lumbale inferius (triangle of Petit)
Crista iliaca
Nn. clunium superiores
Nn. clunium medii
Nn. clunium inferiores

Surface Anatomy

Fig. 4.1 Palpable structures in the back

Posterior view.

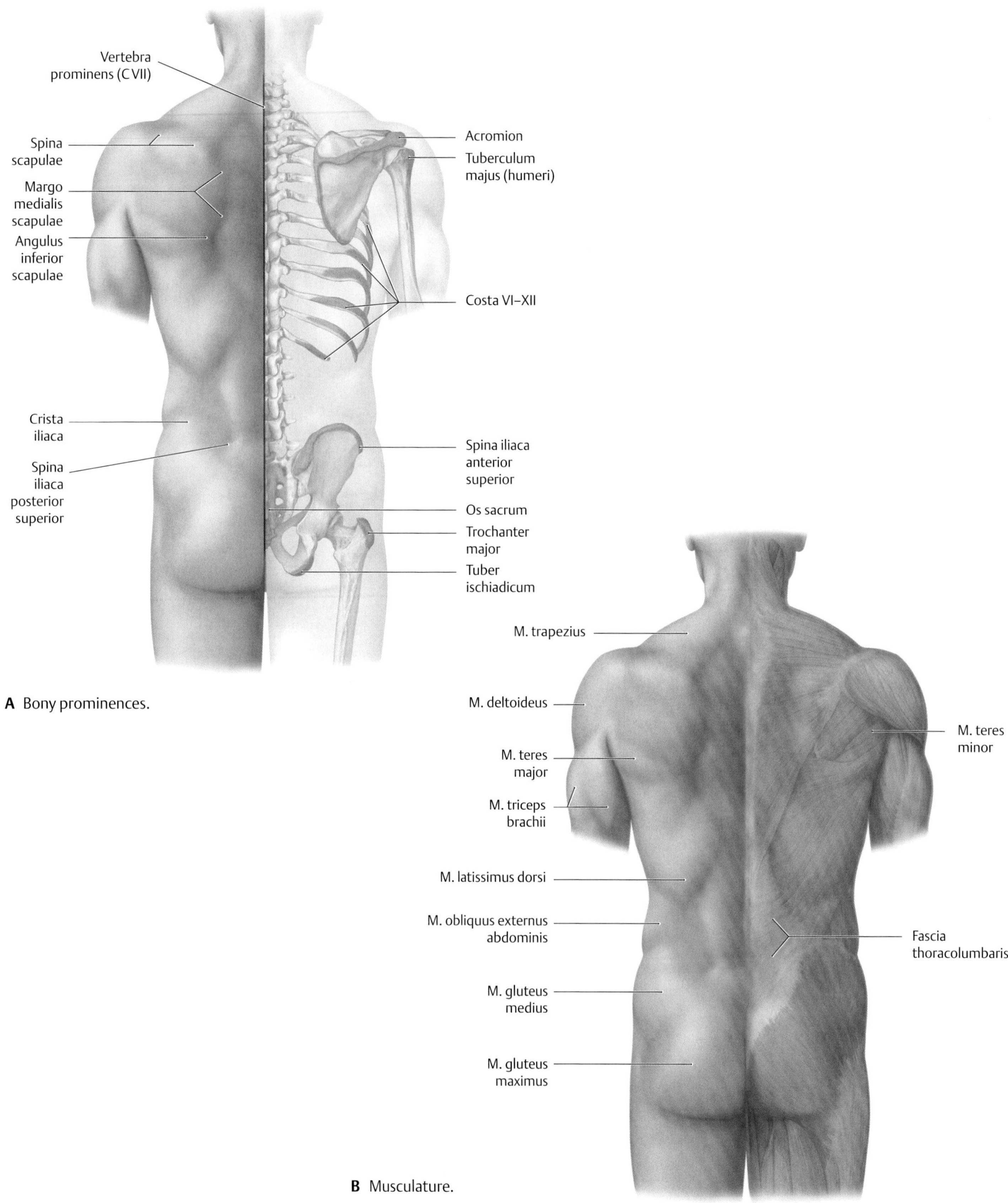

Vertebra prominens (C VII)
Spina scapulae
Margo medialis scapulae
Angulus inferior scapulae
Crista iliaca
Spina iliaca posterior superior
Acromion
Tuberculum majus (humeri)
Costa VI–XII
Spina iliaca anterior superior
Os sacrum
Trochanter major
Tuber ischiadicum
M. trapezius
M. deltoideus
M. teres major
M. triceps brachii
M. latissimus dorsi
M. obliquus externus abdominis
M. gluteus medius
M. gluteus maximus
M. teres minor
Fascia thoracolumbaris

A Bony prominences.

B Musculature.

Fig. 4.2 **Surface anatomy of the back**
Posterior view.

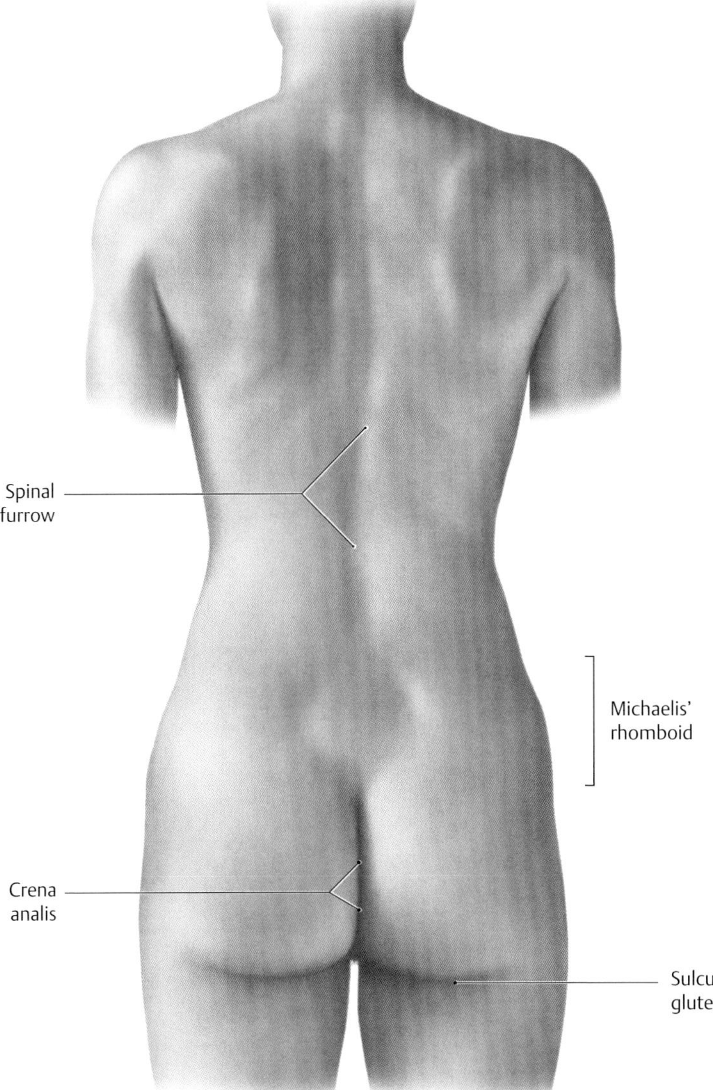
Spinal furrow
Michaelis' rhomboid
Crena analis
Sulcus gluteus

A Female back.

Q1: Michaelis' rhomboid can be used as an indicator of the width of the female pelvis. What are its boundaries?

Q2: The limb girdles are reliable indicators of specific vertebral levels. What level corresponds to the angulus interior of the scapula? What level corresponds to the crista iliaca?

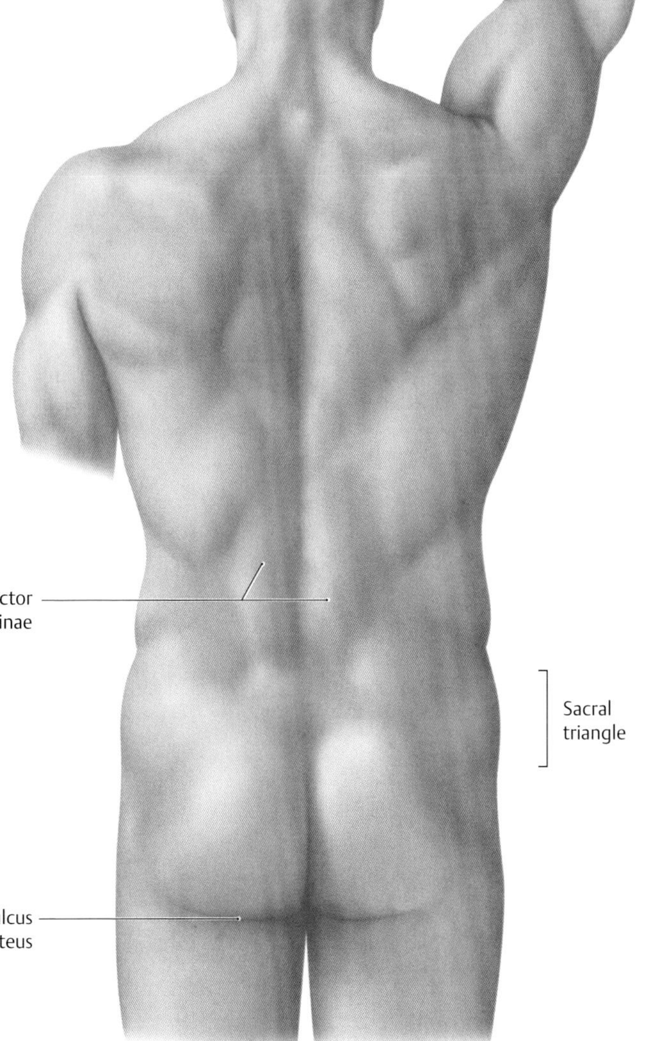
M. erector spinae
Sacral triangle
Sulcus gluteus

B Male back.

See answers beginning on p. 626.

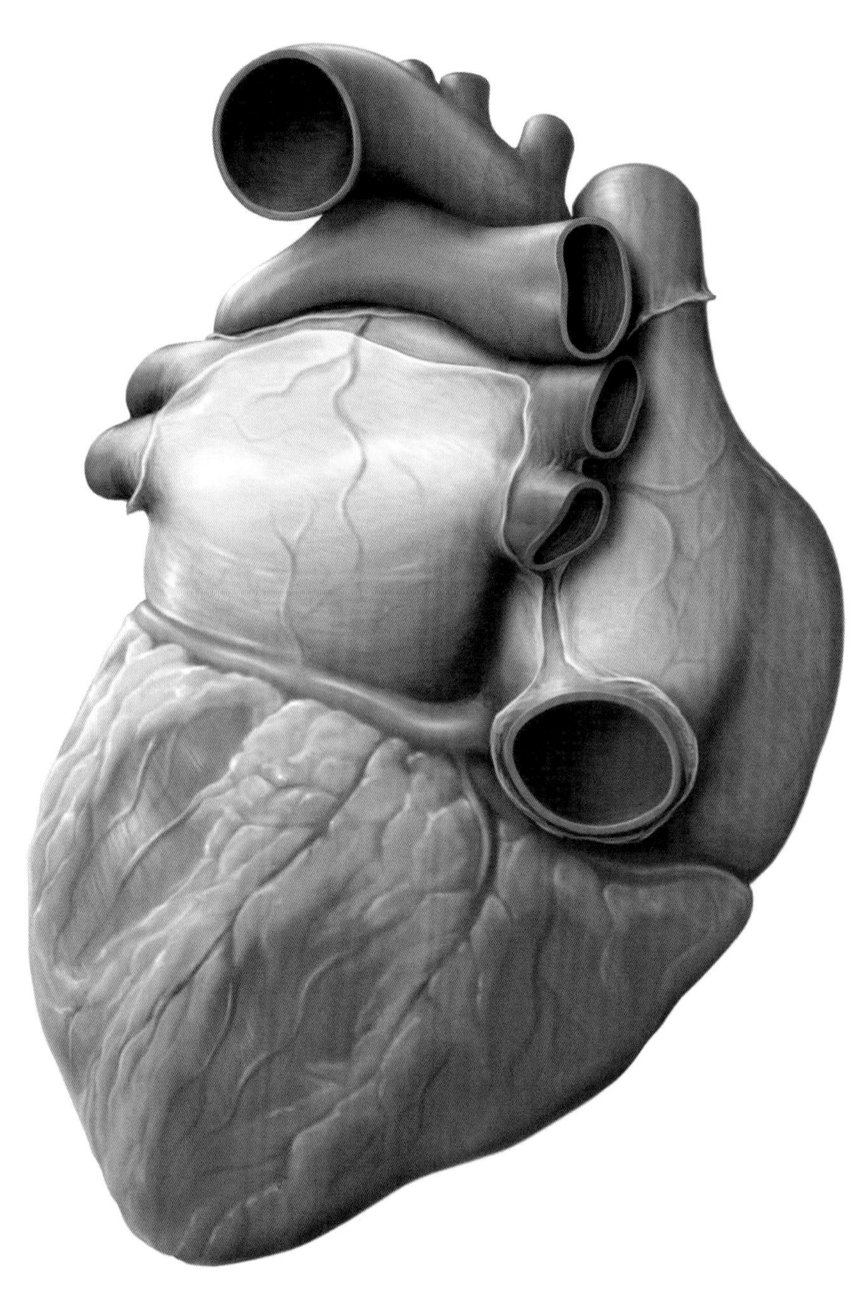

Thorax

5 Thoracic Wall

Thoracic Skeleton 44
Sternum & Ribs 46
Joints of the Thoracic Cage 48
Thoracic Wall Muscle Facts 50
Diaphragm 52
Neurovasculature of the Diaphragm 54
Arteries & Veins of the Thoracic Wall 56
Nerves of the Thoracic Wall 58
Neurovascular Topography of the Thoracic Wall 60
Female Breast 62
Lymphatics of the Female Breast 64

6 Thoracic Cavity

Divisions of the Thoracic Cavity 66
Arteries of the Thoracic Cavity 68
Veins of the Thoracic Cavity 70
Lymphatics of the Thoracic Cavity 72
Nerves of the Thoracic Cavity 74

7 Mediastinum

Mediastinum: Overview 76
Mediastinum: Structures 78
Thymus & Pericardium 80
Heart in Situ 82
Heart: Surfaces & Chambers 84
Heart: Valves 86
Arteries & Veins of the Heart 88
Conduction & Innervation of the Heart 90
Heart: Radiology 92
Pre- & Postnatal Circulation 94
Esophagus 96
Neurovasculature of the Esophagus 98
Lymphatics of the Mediastinum 100

8 Pleural Cavity

Pleural Cavity 102
Lungs in Situ 104
Lung: Radiology 106
Bronchopulmonary Segments of the Lungs 108
Trachea & Bronchial Tree 110
Respiratory Mechanics 112
Pulmonary Arteries & Veins 114
Neurovasculature of the Tracheobronchial Tree 116
Lymphatics of the Pleural Cavity 118

9 Surface Anatomy

Surface Anatomy 120

Thoracic Skeleton

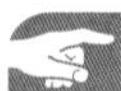

The thoracic skeleton consists of 12 vertebrae thoracicae (p. 8), 12 pairs of ribs with costal cartilages, and the sternum. In addition to participating in respiratory movements, it provides a measure of protection to vital organs. The female thorax is generally narrower and shorter than the male equivalent.

Fig. 5.1 Thoracic skeleton

Incisura clavicularis
Apertura thoracis superior
Incisura jugularis
Manubrium sterni
Angulus sterni
Corpus sterni
Proc. xiphoideus
Sternum
Cartilagines costales
Arcus costalis
Apertura thoracis inferior

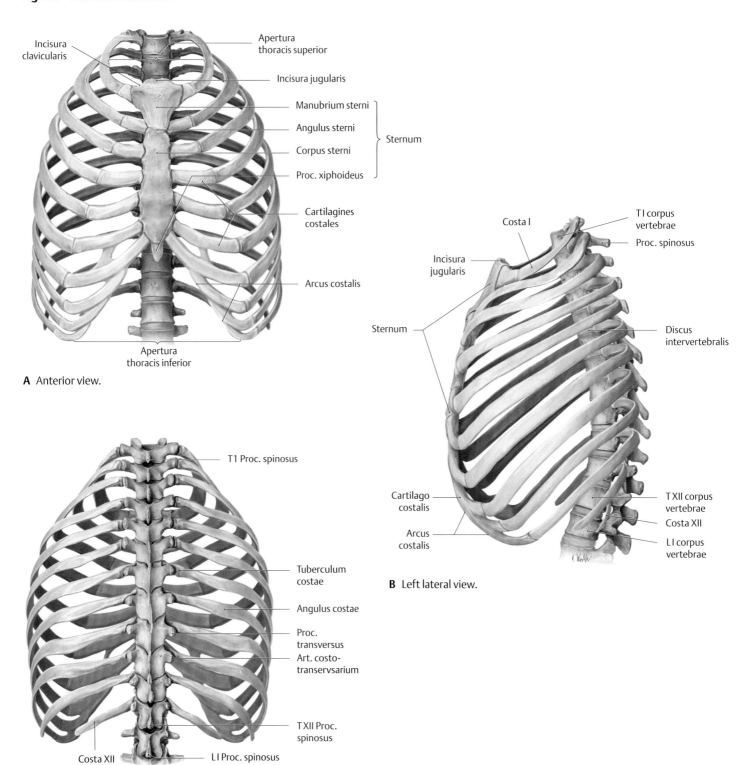

A Anterior view.

Costa I
T I corpus vertebrae
Proc. spinosus
Incisura jugularis
Sternum
Discus intervertebralis
Cartilago costalis
Arcus costalis
T XII corpus vertebrae
Costa XII
L I corpus vertebrae

B Left lateral view.

T1 Proc. spinosus
Tuberculum costae
Angulus costae
Proc. transversus
Art. costo-transervsarium
T XII Proc. spinosus
Costa XII
L I Proc. spinosus

C Posterior view.

Fig. 5.2 **Structure of a thoracic segment**
Superior view of 6th rib pair.

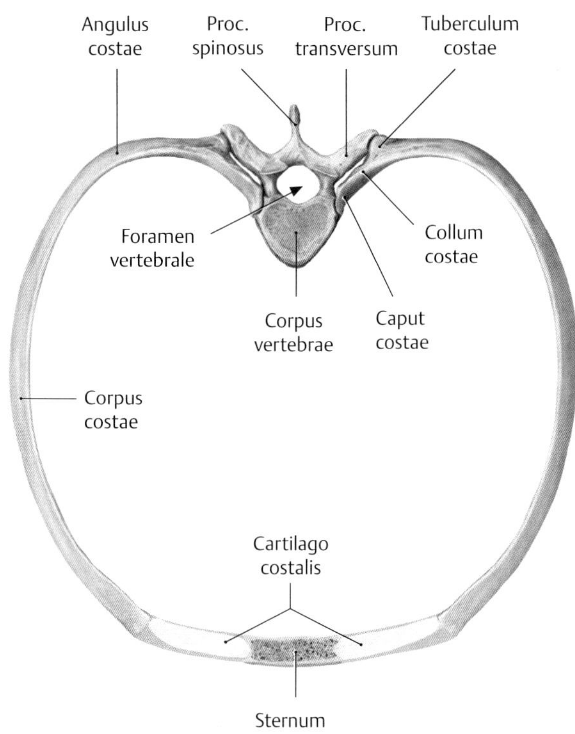
Angulus costae
Proc. spinosus
Proc. transversum
Tuberculum costae
Foramen vertebrale
Collum costae
Corpus vertebrae
Caput costae
Corpus costae
Cartilago costalis
Sternum

Table 5.1	**Elements of a thoracic segment**	
Vertebra		
Rib	Bony part (costal bone)	Caput costae
		Collum costae
		Tuberculum costae
		Corpus costae (including angulus costae)
	Costal part (cartilago costalis)	
Sternum (articulates with cartilago costalis of costae verae only; see Fig. 5.3)		

Fig. 5.3 **Types of ribs**
Left lateral view.

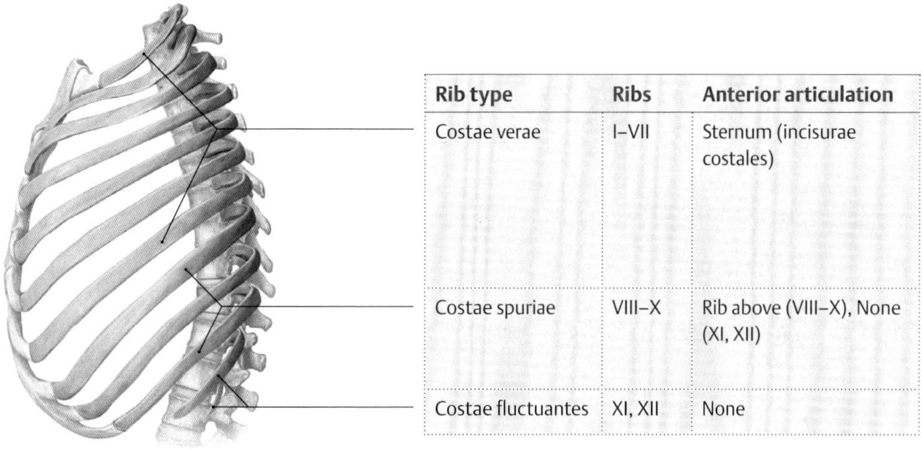

Rib type	Ribs	Anterior articulation
Costae verae	I–VII	Sternum (incisurae costales)
Costae spuriae	VIII–X	Rib above (VIII–X), None (XI, XII)
Costae fluctuantes	XI, XII	None

Sternum & Ribs

Fig. 5.4 **Sternum**

The sternum is a bladelike bone consisting of manubrium sterni, corpus sterni, and processus xiphoideus. The junction of the manubrium and corpus (angulus sterni) is typically elevated and marks the articulation of the second rib. The angulus sterni is an important landmark for internal structures.

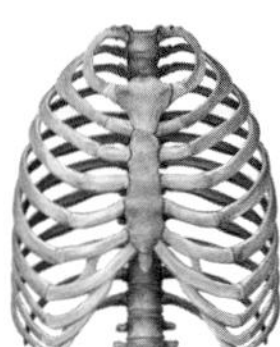

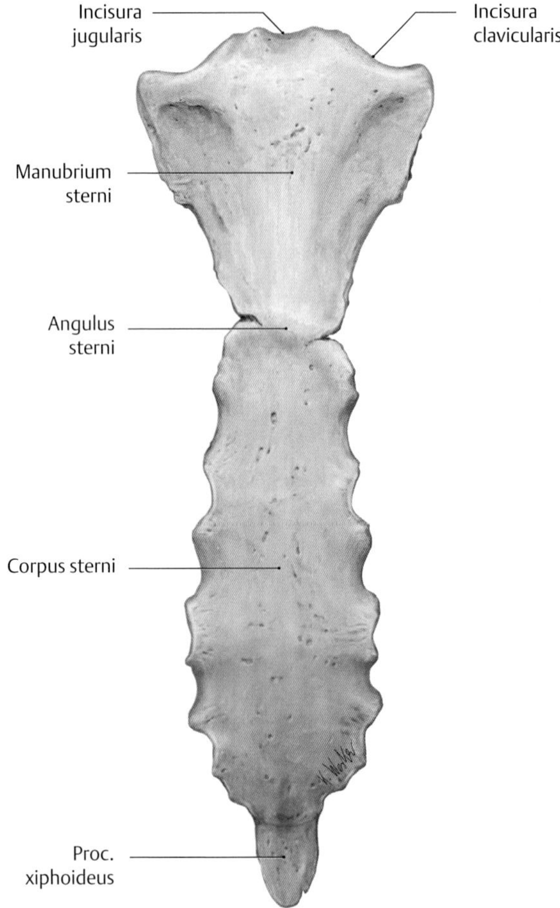
Incisura jugularis
Incisura clavicularis
Manubrium sterni
Angulus sterni
Corpus sterni
Proc. xiphoideus

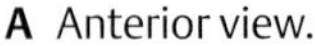

A Anterior view.

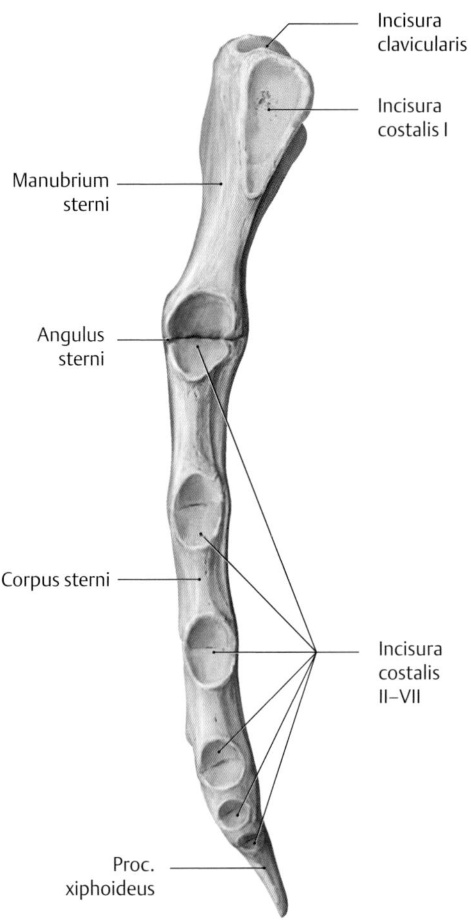
Incisura clavicularis
Incisura costalis I
Manubrium sterni
Angulus sterni
Corpus sterni
Incisura costalis II–VII
Proc. xiphoideus

B Left lateral view. The incisurae costales are sites of articulation with the costal cartilage of the true ribs (see Fig. 5.3).

Fig. 5.5 Costae

Right ribs, superior view. See pp. 258–259 for joints of the shoulder.

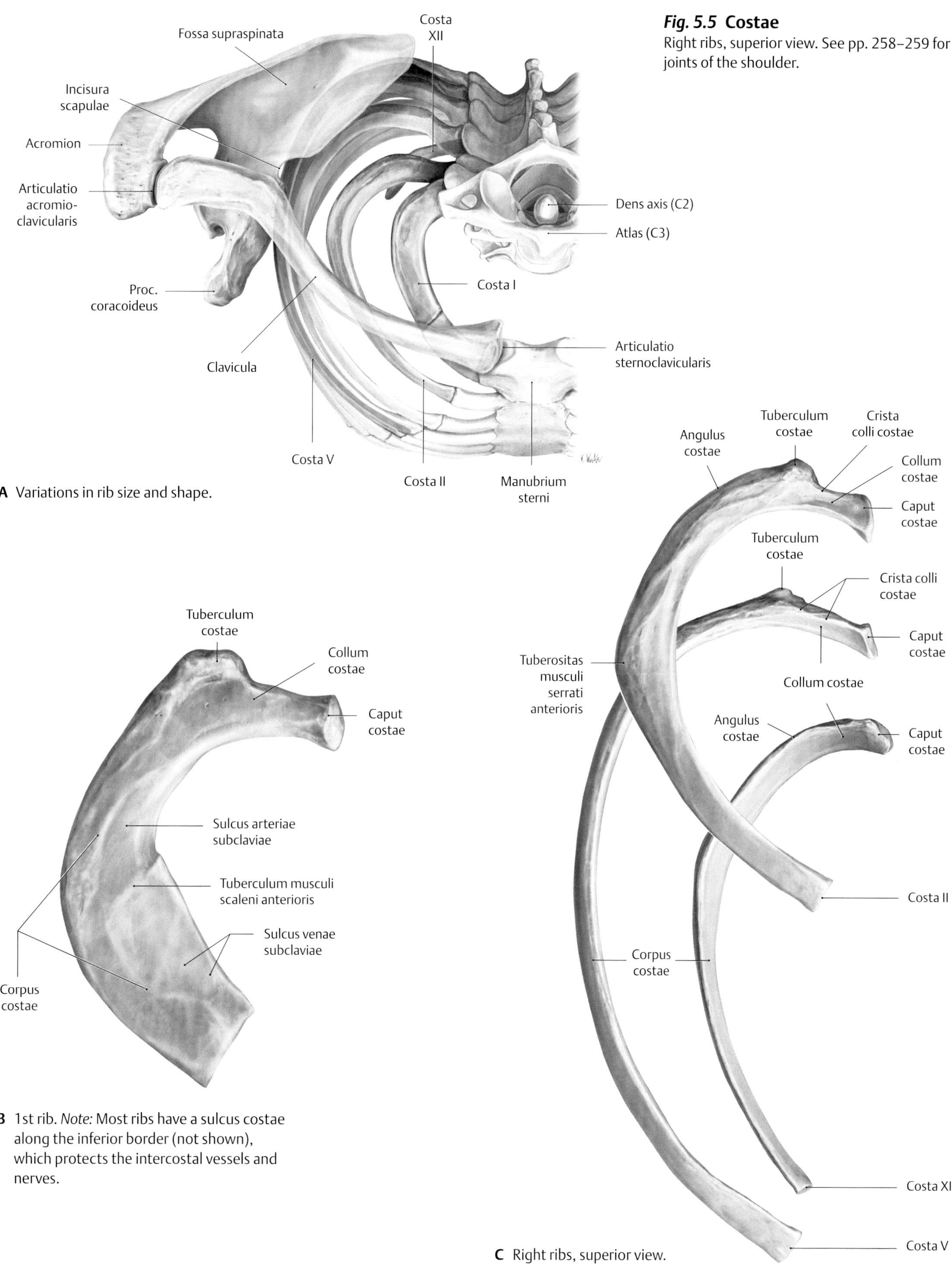

Fossa supraspinata
Costa XII
Incisura scapulae
Acromion
Articulatio acromio-clavicularis
Dens axis (C2)
Atlas (C3)
Costa I
Proc. coracoideus
Articulatio sternoclavicularis
Clavicula
Costa V
Costa II
Manubrium sterni
Tuberculum costae
Crista colli costae
Angulus costae
Collum costae
Caput costae
Tuberculum costae
Crista colli costae
Caput costae
Collum costae
Tuberositas musculi serrati anterioris
Angulus costae
Caput costae
Tuberculum costae
Collum costae
Caput costae
Sulcus arteriae subclaviae
Tuberculum musculi scaleni anterioris
Sulcus venae subclaviae
Corpus costae
Costa II
Corpus costae
Costa XI
Costa V

A Variations in rib size and shape.

B 1st rib. *Note:* Most ribs have a sulcus costae along the inferior border (not shown), which protects the intercostal vessels and nerves.

C Right ribs, superior view.

Joints of the Thoracic Cage

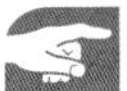

The diaphragma is the chief muscle for quiet respiration (see p. 52). The muscles of the thoracic wall (see p. 50) contribute to deep (forced) inspiration.

Fig. 5.6 **Rib cage movement**

Full inspiration (red); full expiration (blue). In deep inspiration, there is an increase in transverse and sagittal thoracic diameters, as well as the infrasternal angle. The descent of the diaphragm further increases the volume of the thoracic cavity.

Inspiration

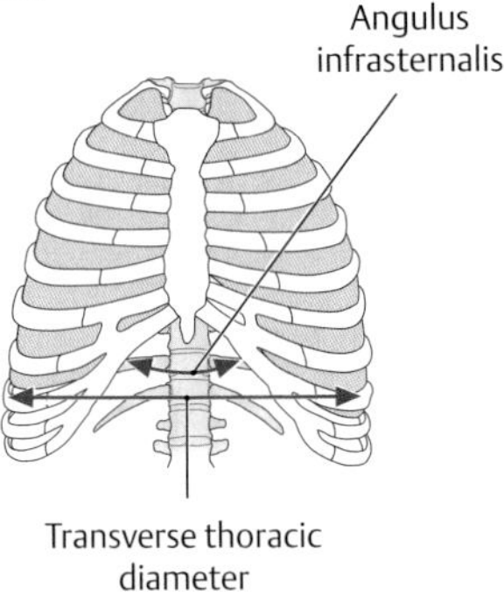
Angulus infrasternalis
Transverse thoracic diameter

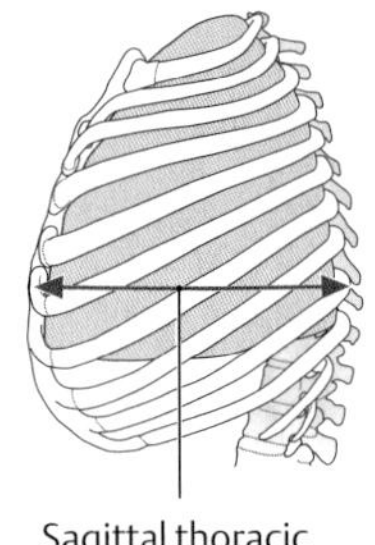
Sagittal thoracic diameter

Expiration

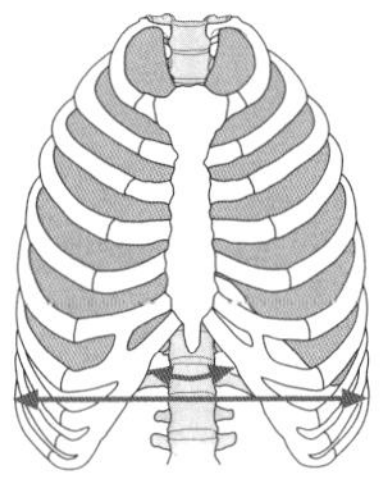

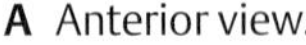

A Anterior view.

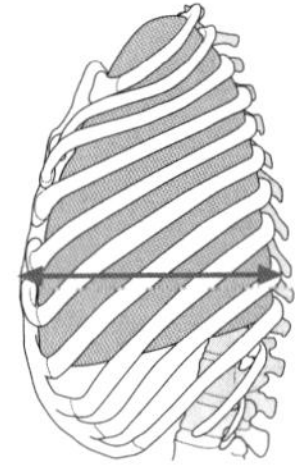

B Left lateral view.

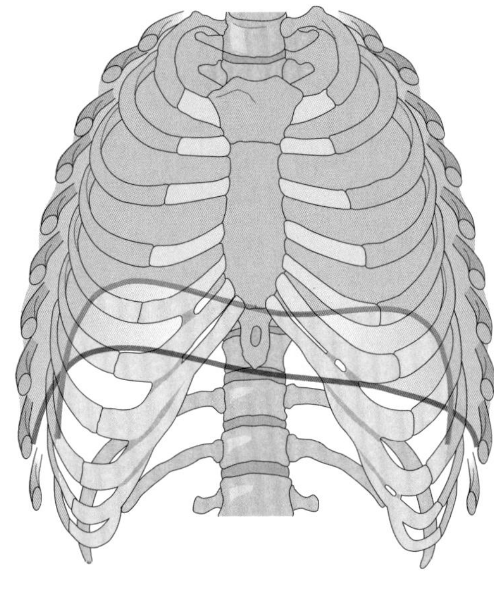

C Position of diaphragm during respiration.

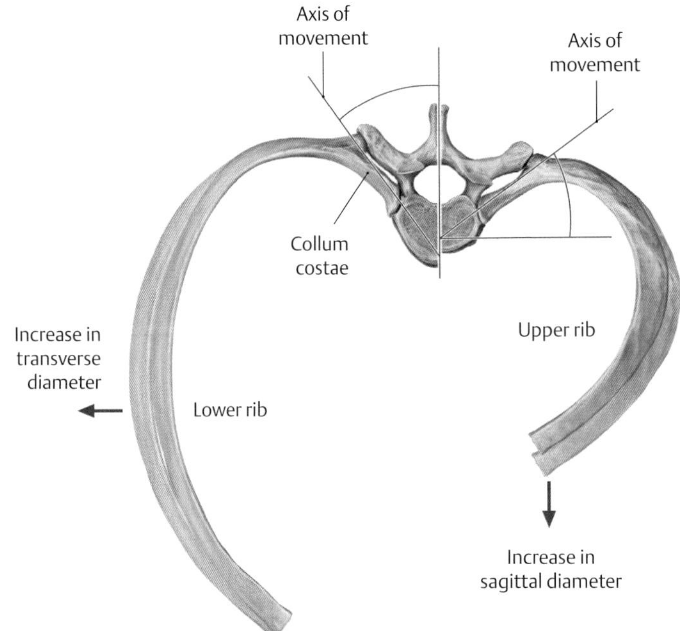
Axis of movement
Axis of movement
Collum costae
Upper rib
Increase in transverse diameter
Lower rib
Increase in sagittal diameter

D Axes of rib movement, superior view.

Fig. 5.7 Sternocostal joints

Anterior view with right half of sternum sectioned frontally. True joints are generally found only at ribs 2 to 5; ribs 1, 6, and 7 attach to the sternum by synchondroses.

Fig. 5.8 Costovertebral joints

Two synovial joints make up the costovertebral articulation of each rib. The costal tubercle of each rib articulates with the costal facet of its accompanying vertebra (**A**). The head of most ribs articulates with the vertebra of its own number and the vertebra immediately superior. Ribs 1, 11, and 12 typically articulate only with their own vertebrae.

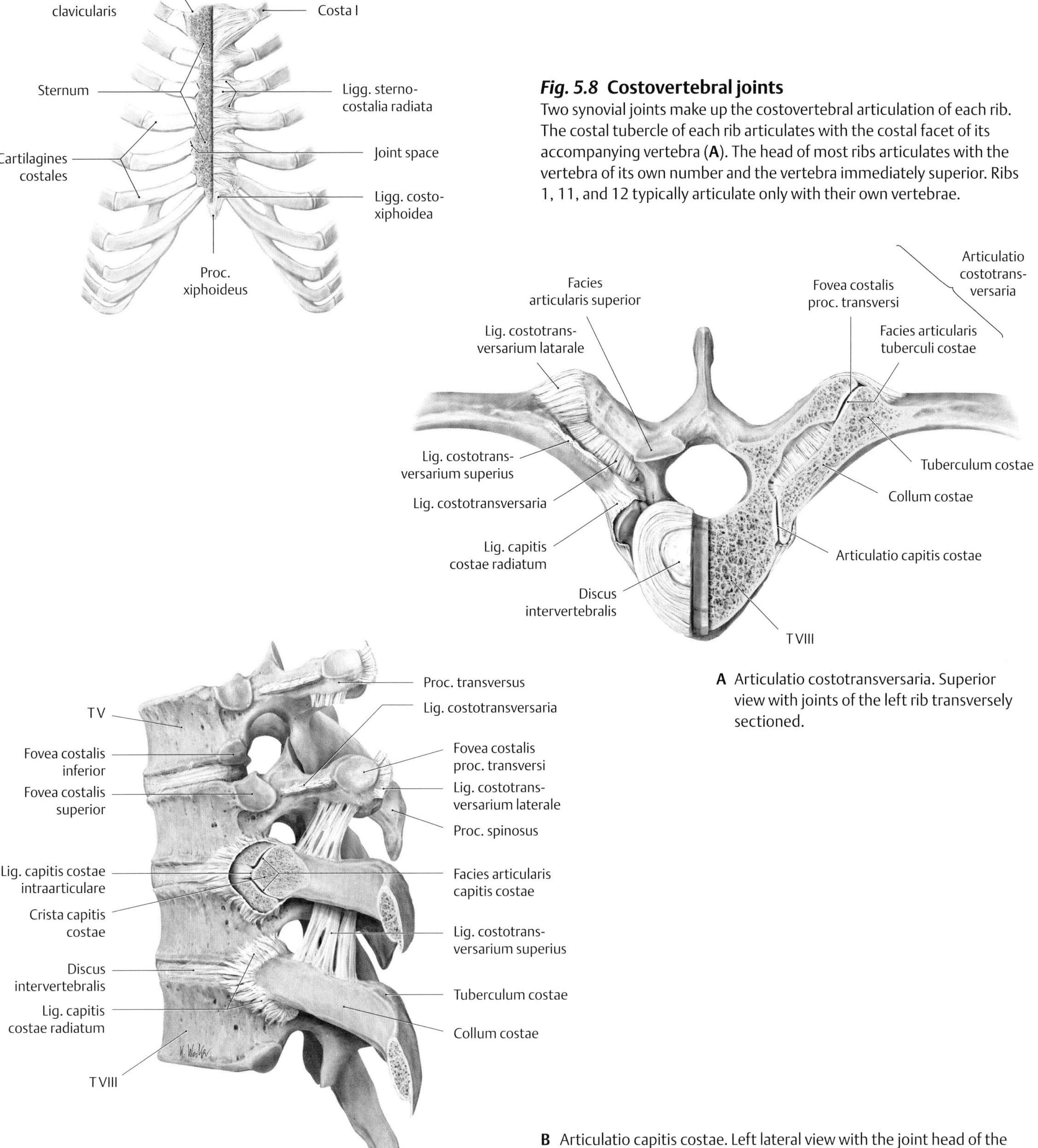

Incisura clavicularis
Costa I
Sternum
Ligg. sterno-costalia radiata
Cartilagines costales
Joint space
Ligg. costo-xiphoidea
Proc. xiphoideus
Articulatio costotrans-versaria
Facies articularis superior
Fovea costalis proc. transversi
Lig. costotrans-versarium latarale
Facies articularis tuberculi costae
Tuberculum costae
Lig. costotrans-versarium superius
Collum costae
Lig. costotransversaria
Lig. capitis costae radiatum
Articulatio capitis costae
Discus intervertebralis
T VIII
Proc. transversus
T V
Lig. costotransversaria
Fovea costalis inferior
Fovea costalis proc. transversi
Fovea costalis superior
Lig. costotrans-versarium laterale
Proc. spinosus
Lig. capitis costae intraarticulare
Facies articularis capitis costae
Crista capitis costae
Lig. costotrans-versarium superius
Discus intervertebralis
Tuberculum costae
Lig. capitis costae radiatum
Collum costae
T VIII

A Articulatio costotransversaria. Superior view with joints of the left rib transversely sectioned.

B Articulatio capitis costae. Left lateral view with the joint head of the 7th rib opened.

Thoracic Wall Muscle Facts

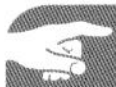

The muscles of the thoracic wall are primarily responsible for chest respiration, although other muscles aid in *deep* inspiration: m. pectoralis major and m. serratus anterior are discussed with the shoulder (see pp. 264–267), and m. serratus posterior is discussed with the back (see p. 30).

Fig. 5.9 Muscles of the thoracic wall

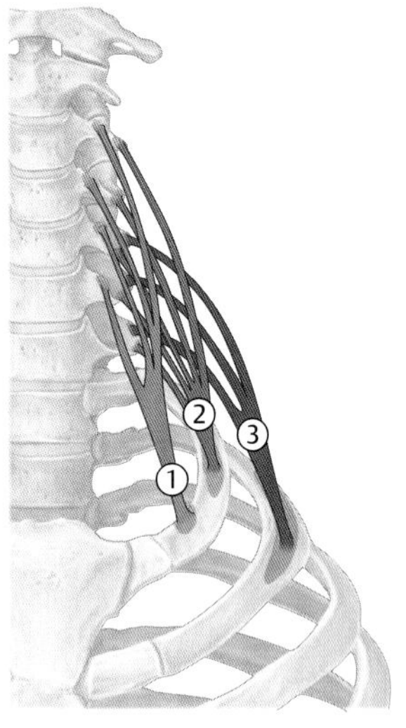

①
②
③

A Mm. scaleni, anterior view.

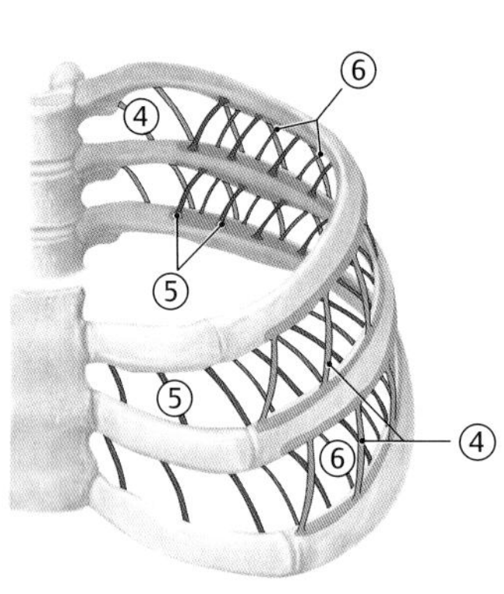

⑥
④
⑤
⑤
⑥
④

B Mm. intercostales, anterior view.

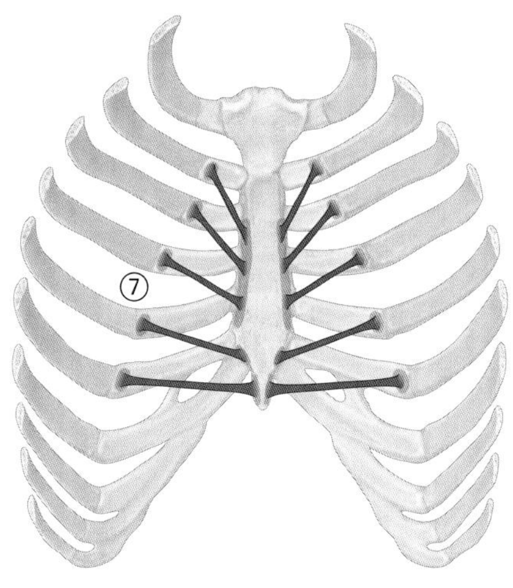

⑦

C M. transversus thoracis, posterior view.

Table 5.2 Muscles of the thoracic wall

Muscle		Origin	Insertion	Innervation	Action
Mm. scaleni	① M. scalenus anterior	Vertebrae CIII–CVI (proc. transversus, tuberculum anterius)	Costa I (Tuberculum m. scaleni anterioris)	Direct branches from cervical and brachial plexus (C3–C6)	*With ribs mobile*: Raises upper ribs (inspiration) *With ribs fixed*: Bends cervical spine to same side (unilateral); flexes neck (bilateral)
	② M. scalenus medius	Vertebrae CIV–CVI (proc. transversus, tuberculum posterius)	Costa I (posterior to sulcus arteriae subclaviae)		
	③ M. scalenus posterior		Costa II (outer surface)		
Mm. intercostales	④ M. intercostalis externus	Lower margin of rib to upper margin of next lower rib (courses obliquely forward and downward from tuberculum costae to chondro-osseous junction)		Nn. intercostales I–XI	Raises ribs (inspiration); supports intercostal spaces; stabilizes chest wall
	⑤ M. intercostalis internus	Lower margin of rib to lower margin of next lower rib (courses obliquely forward and upward from angulus costae to sternum)			Lowers ribs (expiration); supports intercostal spaces, stabilizes chest wall
	⑥ M. intercostalis intimus				
Mm. subcostales		Lower margin of lower ribs to inner surface of ribs two to three ribs below		Variable lower nn. intercostales	Raises ribs (inspiration)
⑦ M. transversus thoracis		Sternum and proc. xiphoideus (inner surface)	Costae II–VI (cartilago costalis, inner surface)	Nn. intercostales II–VII	Weakly lowers ribs (expiration)

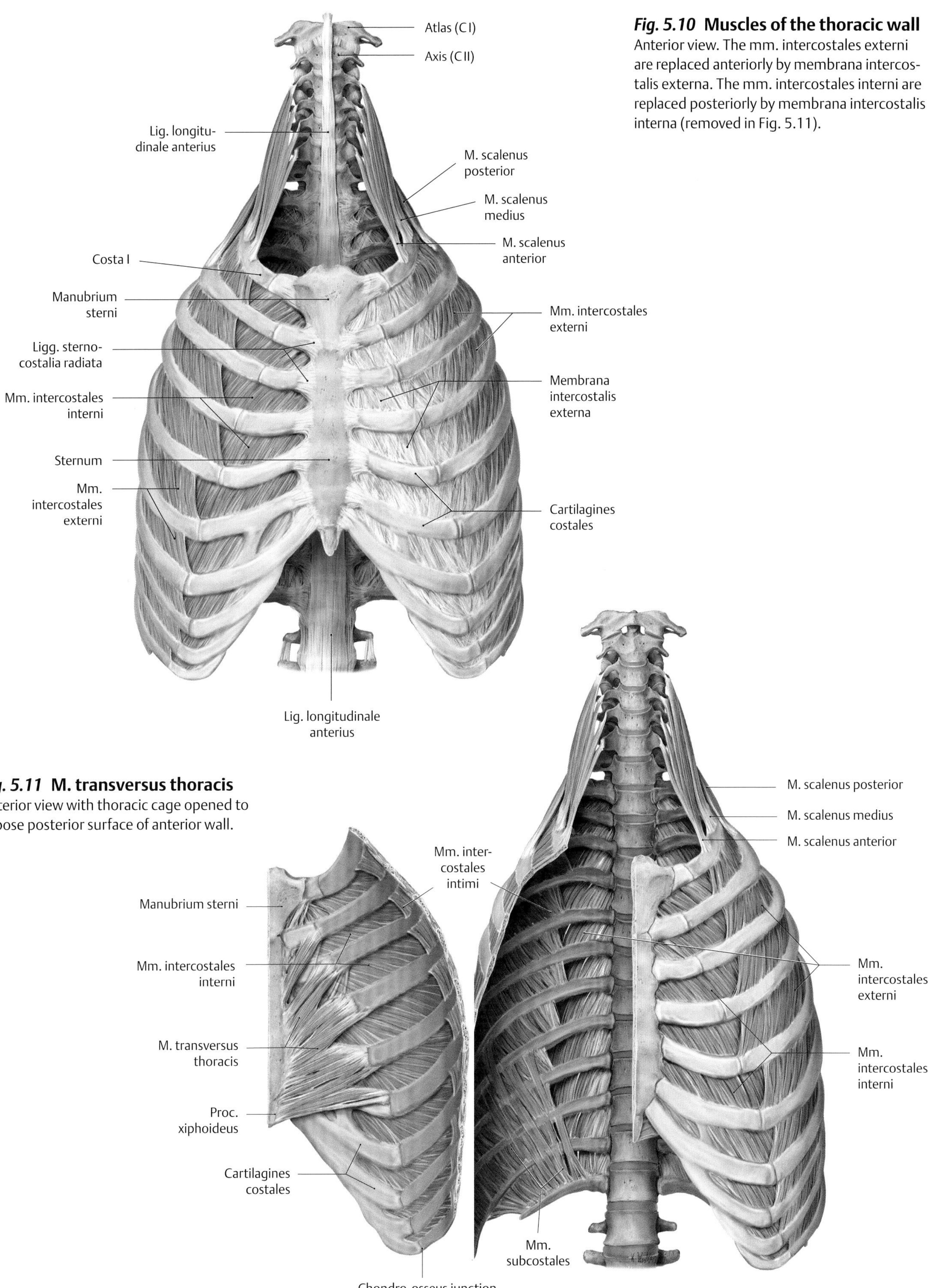
Atlas (C I)
Axis (C II)
Lig. longitu-
dinale anterius
M. scalenus
posterior
M. scalenus
medius
M. scalenus
anterior
Costa I
Manubrium
sterni
Mm. intercostales
externi
Ligg. sterno-
costalia radiata
Membrana
intercostalis
externa
Mm. intercostales
interni
Sternum
Mm.
intercostales
externi
Cartilagines
costales
Lig. longitudinale
anterius
M. scalenus posterior
M. scalenus medius
M. scalenus anterior
Mm. inter-
costales
intimi
Manubrium sterni
Mm. intercostales
interni
Mm.
intercostales
externi
M. transversus
thoracis
Mm.
intercostales
interni
Proc.
xiphoideus
Cartilagines
costales
Mm.
subcostales
Chondro-osseus junction

Fig. 5.10 **Muscles of the thoracic wall**
Anterior view. The mm. intercostales externi are replaced anteriorly by membrana intercostalis externa. The mm. intercostales interni are replaced posteriorly by membrana intercostalis interna (removed in Fig. 5.11).

Fig. 5.11 **M. transversus thoracis**
Anterior view with thoracic cage opened to expose posterior surface of anterior wall.

Diaphragm

Fig. 5.12 Diaphragma
The diaphragma, which separates the thorax from the abdomen, has two asymmetric domes and three apertures (for the aorta, vena cava, and esophagus; see Fig. 5.13B).

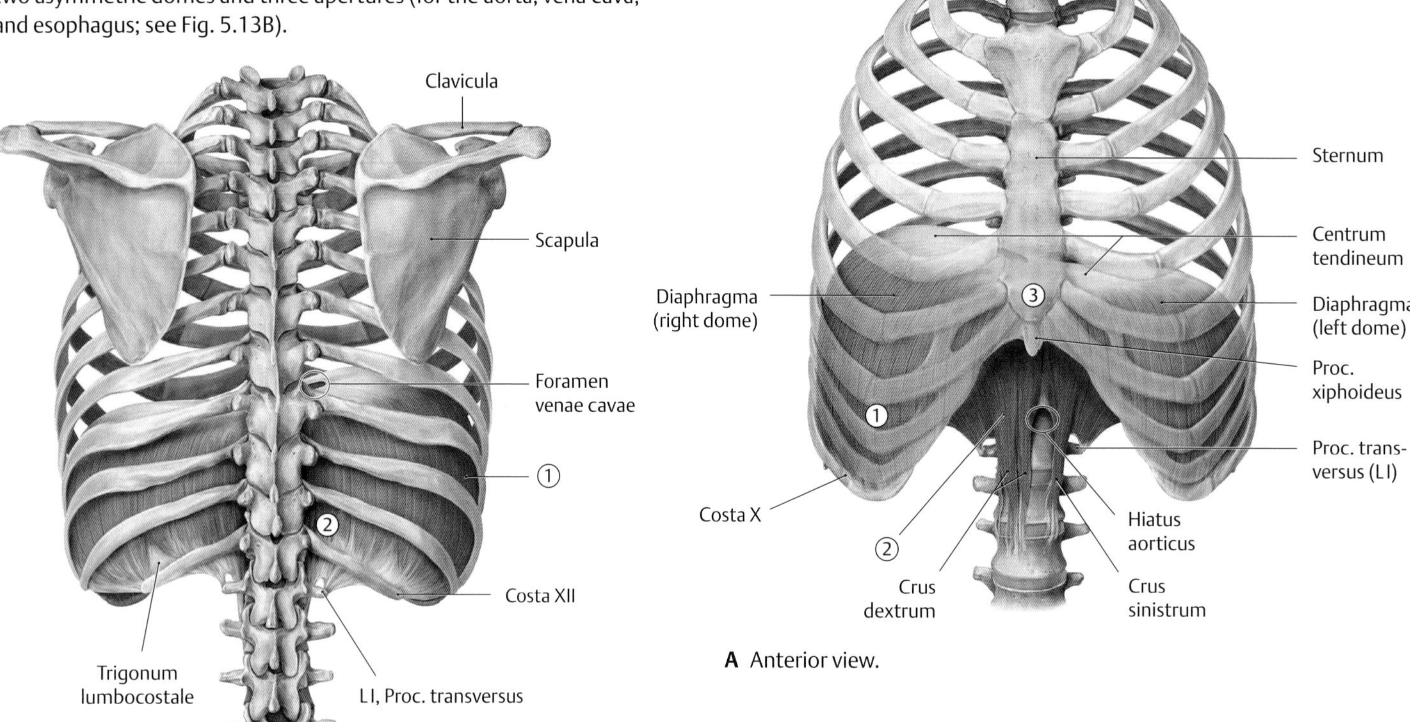

Clavicula
Scapula
Foramen venae cavae
①
②
Costa XII
Trigonum lumbocostale
L I, Proc. transversus
Sternum
Centrum tendineum
Diaphragma (right dome)
③
Diaphragma (left dome)
Proc. xiphoideus
①
Proc. transversus (L I)
Costa X
②
Hiatus aorticus
Crus dextrum
Crus sinistrum

A Anterior view.

B Posterior view.

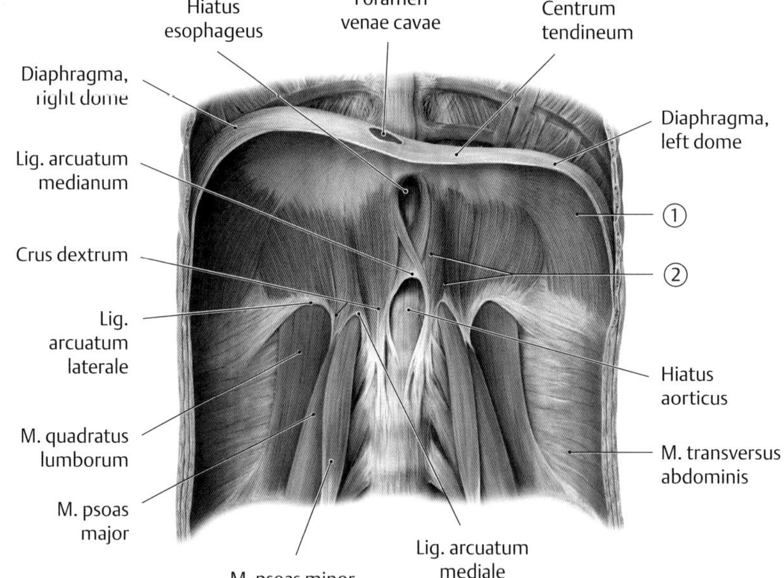

Hiatus esophageus
Foramen venae cavae
Centrum tendineum
Diaphragma, right dome
Diaphragma, left dome
Lig. arcuatum medianum
①
Crus dextrum
②
Lig. arcuatum laterale
Hiatus aorticus
M. quadratus lumborum
M. transversus abdominis
M. psoas major
M. psoas minor
Lig. arcuatum mediale

C Coronal section with diaphragma in intermediate position.

Table 5.3 Diaphragm

Muscle		Origin	Insertion	Innervation	Action
Diaphragma	① Pars costalis diaphragmatis	Costae VII–XII (inner surface; lower margin of arcus costalis)	Centrum tendineum	N. phrenicus (C3–C5, plexus cervicalis)	Principal muscle of respiration (diaphragmatic and thoracic breathing); aids in compressing abdominal viscera (abdominal press)
	② Pars lumbalis diaphragmatis	Medial part: corpus vertebrae LI–LIII, disci intervertebrales, and lig. longitudinale anterius as right and left crura			
		Lateral parts: lig. arcuatum mediale and lig. arcuatum laterale			
	③ Pars sternalis diaphragmatis	Processus xiphoideus (posterior surface)			

Fig. 5.13 Diaphragma in situ

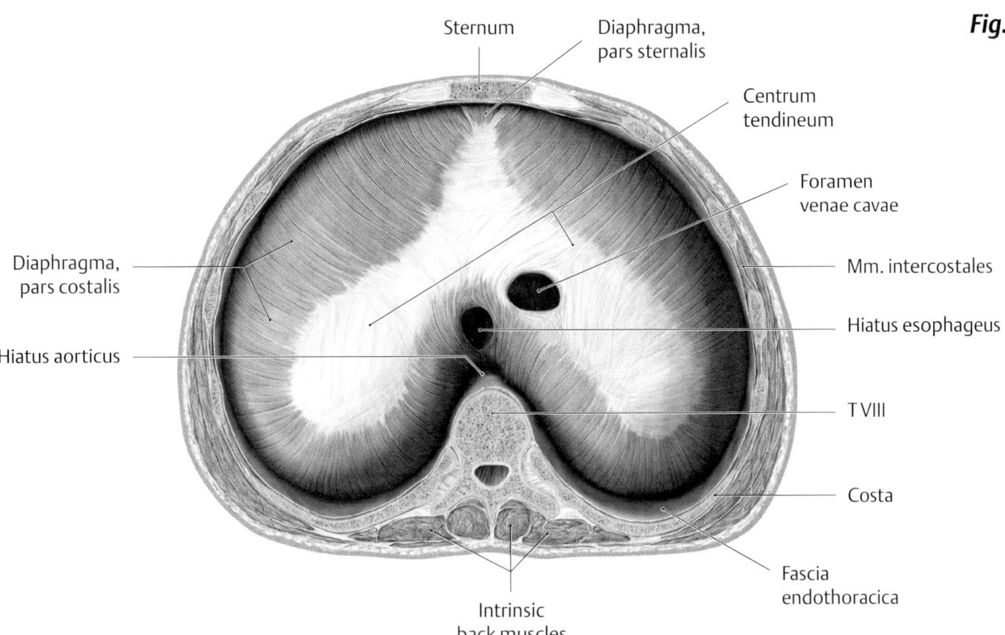
Sternum
Diaphragma, pars sternalis
Centrum tendineum
Foramen venae cavae
Diaphragma, pars costalis
Mm. intercostales
Hiatus esophageus
Hiatus aorticus
T VIII
Costa
Fascia endothoracica
Intrinsic back muscles

A Superior view.

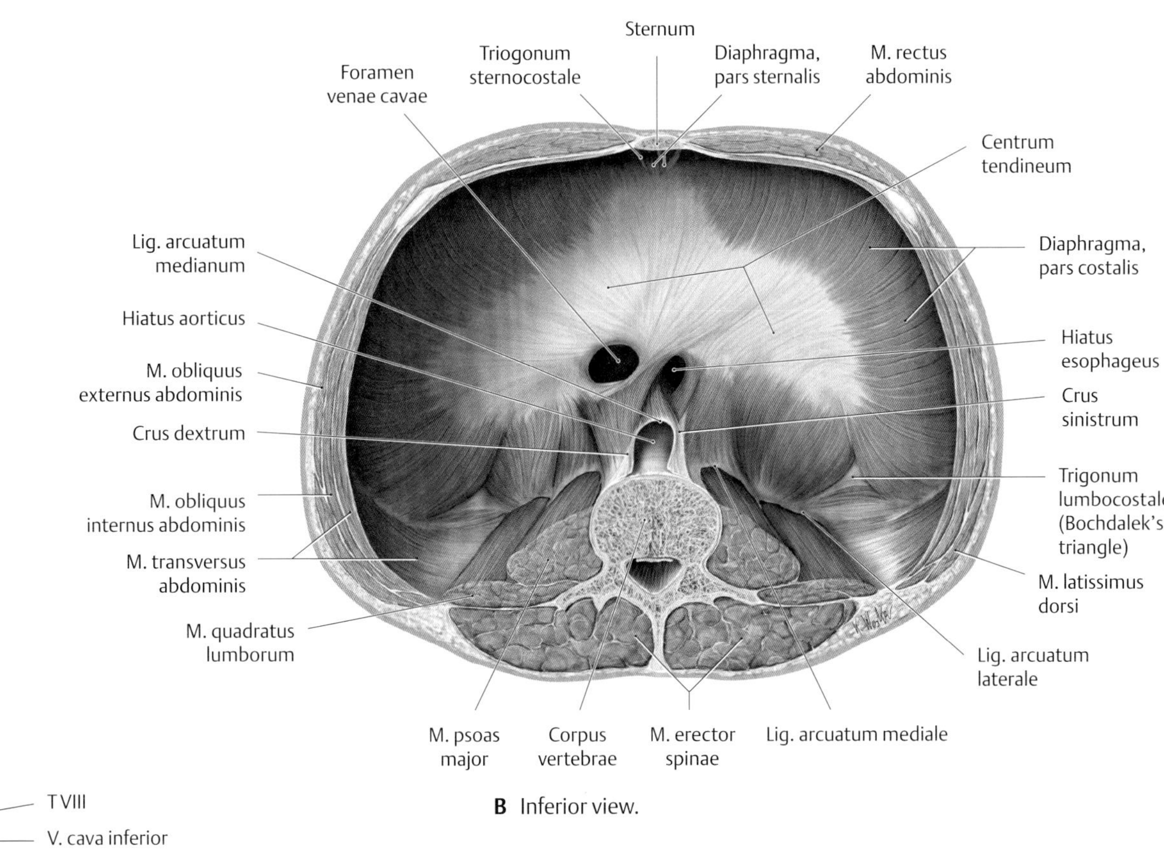
Sternum
Foramen venae cavae
Triogonum sternocostale
Diaphragma, pars sternalis
M. rectus abdominis
Centrum tendineum
Lig. arcuatum medianum
Diaphragma, pars costalis
Hiatus aorticus
Hiatus esophageus
M. obliquus externus abdominis
Crus sinistrum
Crus dextrum
Trigonum lumbocostale (Bochdalek's triangle)
M. obliquus internus abdominis
M. transversus abdominis
M. latissimus dorsi
M. quadratus lumborum
Lig. arcuatum laterale
M. psoas major
Corpus vertebrae
M. erector spinae
Lig. arcuatum mediale

B Inferior view.

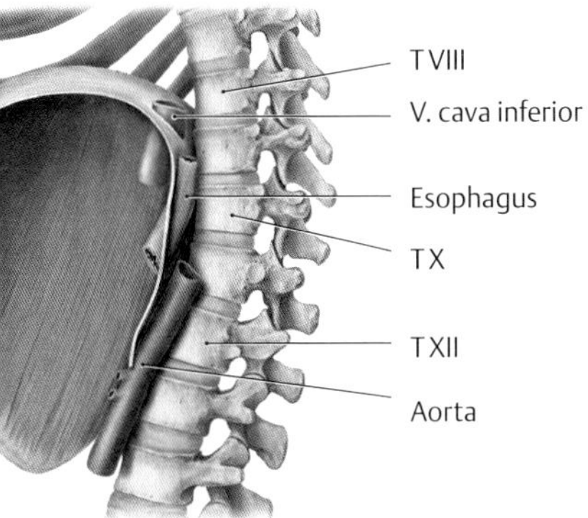
T VIII
V. cava inferior
Esophagus
T X
T XII
Aorta

C Diaphragmatic apertures, left lateral view.

Neurovasculature of the Diaphragm

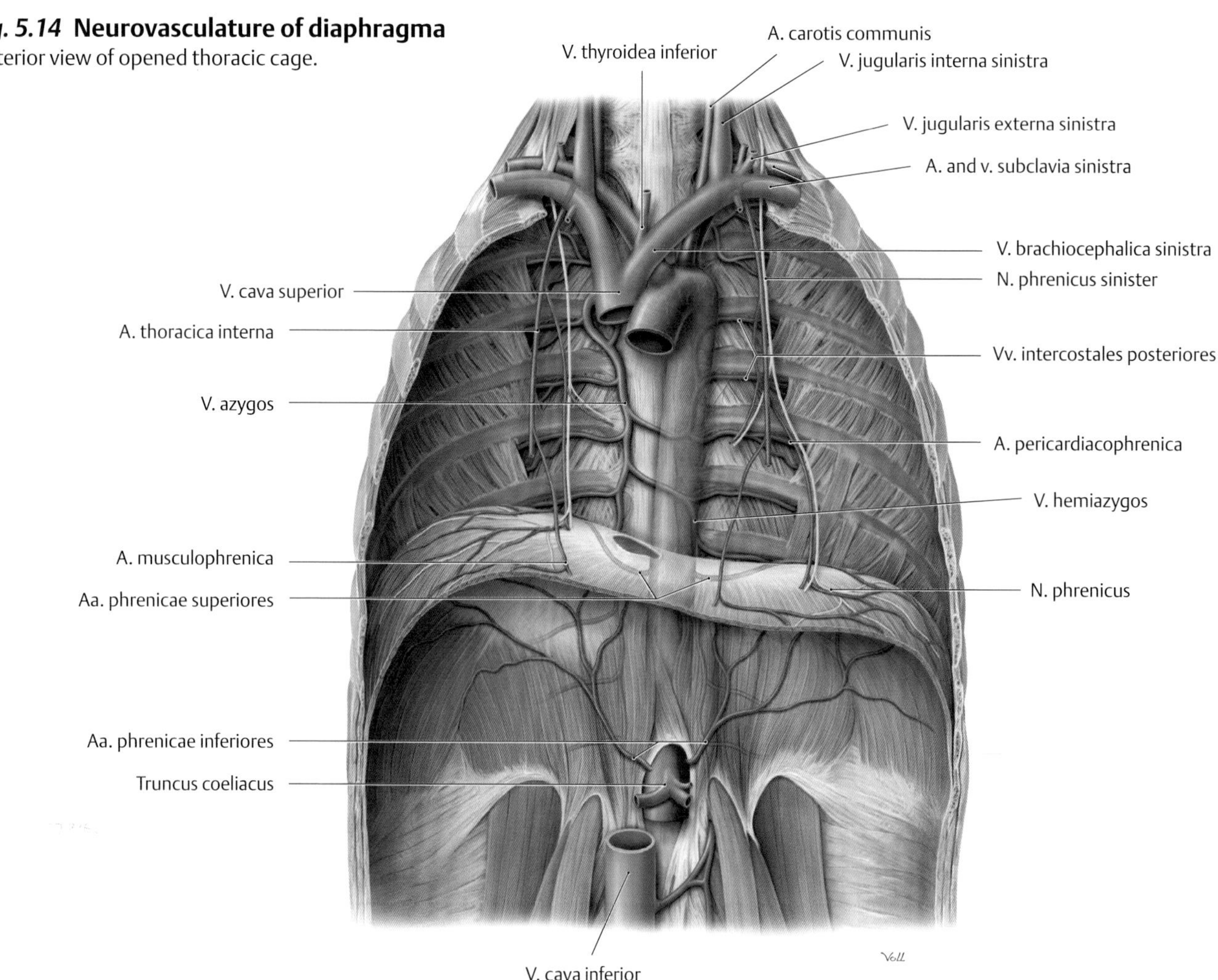
V. thyroidea inferior
A. carotis communis
V. jugularis interna sinistra
V. jugularis externa sinistra
A. and v. subclavia sinistra
V. brachiocephalica sinistra
N. phrenicus sinister
V. cava superior
A. thoracica interna
Vv. intercostales posteriores
V. azygos
A. pericardiacophrenica
V. hemiazygos
A. musculophrenica
Aa. phrenicae superiores
N. phrenicus
Aa. phrenicae inferiores
Truncus coeliacus
V. cava inferior

Fig. 5.14 **Neurovasculature of diaphragma**
Anterior view of opened thoracic cage.

Fig. 5.15 **Innervation of the diaphragm**
Anterior view. The n. phrenicus lies on the lateral surface of the fibrous pericardium together with the pericardiacophrenic arteries and veins. *Note*: The n. phrenicus also innervates the pericardium.

C3
C4
C5
M. scalenus anterior
N. phrenicus sinister
Costa
Mm. intercostales
To pleura parietalis, pars mediastinalis
Rr. pericardiaci
To pleura parietalis, pars diaphragmatica
Nn. intercostales
Diaphragma

— Efferent fibers — Afferent fibers

Table 5.4 Blood vessels of the diaphragm

Artery	Origin	Vein	Drainage
A. phrenica inferior (chief blood supply)	Aorta abdominalis; occasionally from truncus coeliacus	Vv. intercostales posteriores	Right side: V. azygos ; Left side: V. hemiazygos
Aa. phrenicae superiores	Aorta thoracica	Vv. phrenicae superiores	
A. pericardiacophrenica	A. thoracica interna	V. intercostalis superior dextra	
A. musculophrenica			

Fig. 5.16 Arteries and nerves of diaphragma

Note: The margins of diaphragma receive sensory innervation from the lowest intercostal nerves.

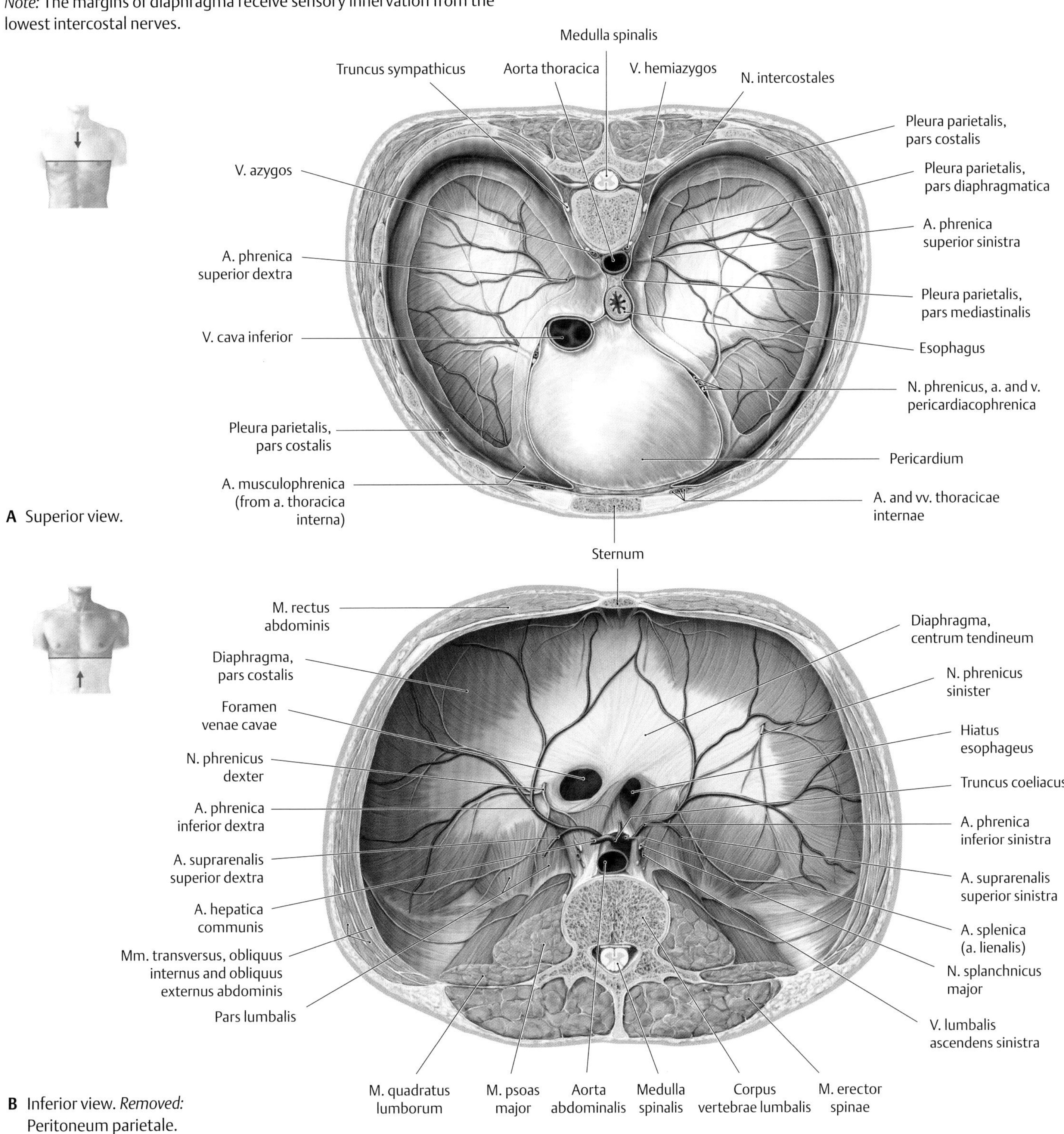

Medulla spinalis
Truncus sympathicus
Aorta thoracica
V. hemiazygos
N. intercostales
Pleura parietalis, pars costalis
V. azygos
Pleura parietalis, pars diaphragmatica
A. phrenica superior sinistra
A. phrenica superior dextra
Pleura parietalis, pars mediastinalis
V. cava inferior
Esophagus
N. phrenicus, a. and v. pericardiacophrenica
Pleura parietalis, pars costalis
Pericardium
A. musculophrenica (from a. thoracica interna)
A. and vv. thoracicae internae
Sternum
M. rectus abdominis
Diaphragma, centrum tendineum
Diaphragma, pars costalis
N. phrenicus sinister
Foramen venae cavae
Hiatus esophageus
N. phrenicus dexter
Truncus coeliacus
A. phrenica inferior dextra
A. phrenica inferior sinistra
A. suprarenalis superior dextra
A. suprarenalis superior sinistra
A. hepatica communis
A. splenica (a. lienalis)
Mm. transversus, obliquus internus and obliquus externus abdominis
N. splanchnicus major
Pars lumbalis
V. lumbalis ascendens sinistra
M. quadratus lumborum
M. psoas major
Aorta abdominalis
Medulla spinalis
Corpus vertebrae lumbalis
M. erector spinae

A Superior view.

B Inferior view. *Removed:* Peritoneum parietale.

Arteries & Veins of the Thoracic Wall

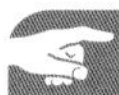

Aa. intercostales posteriores anostomose with aa. intercostales anteriores to supply the structures of the thoracic wall. Aa. intercostales posteriores branch from aorta thoracica, with the exception of the 1st and 2nd, which arise from a. intercostalis suprema (a branch of truncus costocervicalis).

Table 5.5 Arteries of the thoracic wall

Origin	Branch
A. subclavia and a. axillaris	A. thoracica superior
	A. thoracica lateralis
	A. thoracoacromialis
	Aa. intercostales posteriores (1st and 2nd; see p. 34)
Aorta thoracica	Aa. intercostales posteriores (3rd through 12th)
A. thoracica interna	Aa. intercostales anteriores
	A. musculophrenica
	A. epigastrica superior

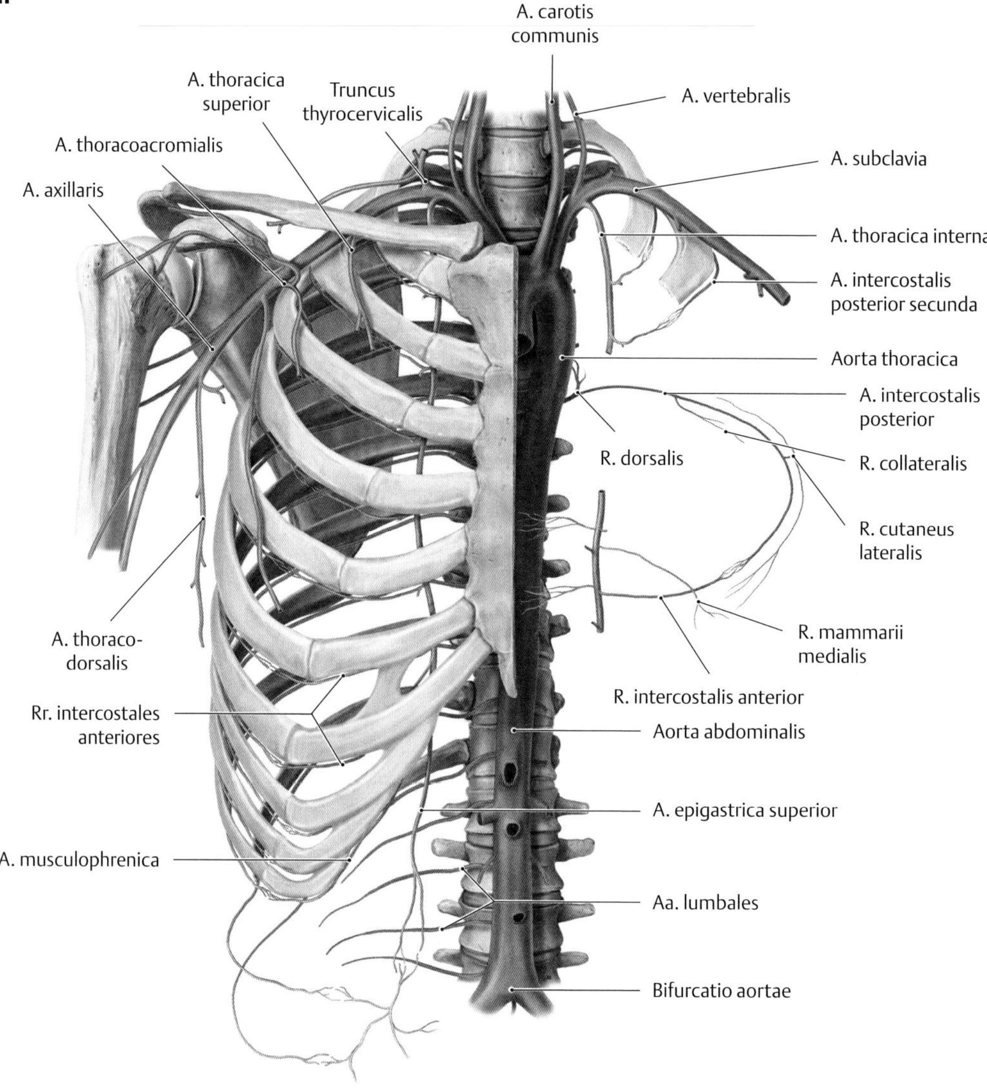

A. carotis communis
A. thoracica superior
Truncus thyrocervicalis
A. vertebralis
A. thoracoacromialis
A. subclavia
A. axillaris
A. thoracica interna
A. intercostalis posterior secunda
Aorta thoracica
A. intercostalis posterior
R. dorsalis
R. collateralis
R. cutaneus lateralis
A. thoraco-dorsalis
R. mammarii medialis
R. intercostalis anterior
Rr. intercostales anteriores
Aorta abdominalis
A. epigastrica superior
A. musculophrenica
Aa. lumbales
Bifurcatio aortae

Fig. 5.17 **Arteries of the thoracic wall**
Anterior view.

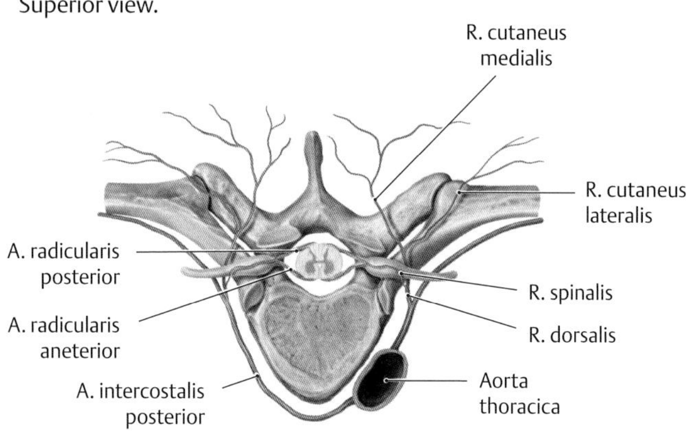

R. cutaneus medialis
R. cutaneus lateralis
A. radicularis posterior
R. spinalis
A. radicularis aneterior
R. dorsalis
A. intercostalis posterior
Aorta thoracica

Fig. 5.18 **Branches of aa. intercostales posteriores**
Superior view.

Table 5.6 Branches of the intercostal arteries

Artery	Branches		Supplies
Aa. intercostales posteriores	Ramus dorsalis	Rami spinales	Spinal cord
		Ramus cutaneus medialis	Posterior thoracic wall
		Ramus cutaneus lateralis	
	Ramus collateralis		Lateral thoracic wall
AA. intercostales anteriores	Ramus cutaneus lateralis*		Anterior thoracic wall

*The rami mammarii laterales from ramus cutaneus lateralis supplies the breast along with rami mammari mediales from a thoracic interna.

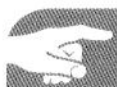

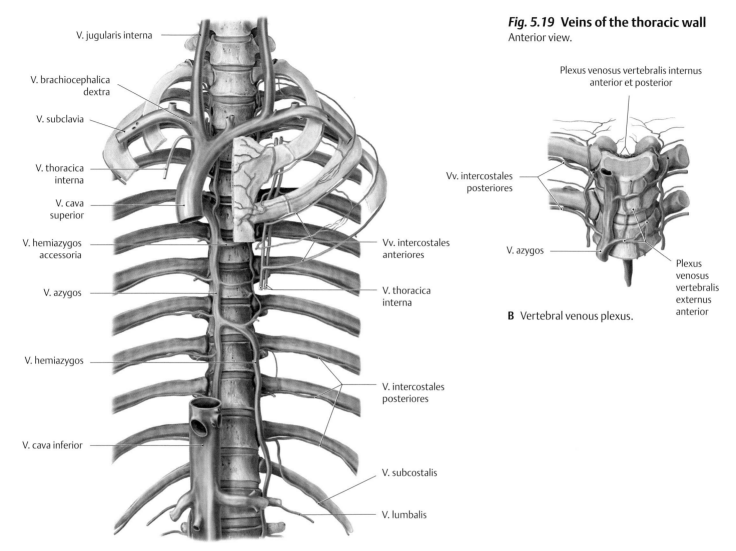

The vv. intercostales drain primarily into the azygos system, but also into v. thoracica interna. This blood ultimately returns to the heart via v. cava superior. The vv. intercostales follow a similar course to their arterial counterparts. However, the veins of the vertebral column form an external vertebral venous plexus that traverses the entire length of the spine (see p. 35).

V. jugularis interna
V. brachiocephalica dextra
V. subclavia
V. thoracica interna
V. cava superior
V. hemiazygos accessoria
V. azygos
V. hemiazygos
V. cava inferior
Vv. intercostales anteriores
V. thoracica interna
V. intercostales posteriores
V. subcostalis
V. lumbalis

A Anterior view with rib cage opened.

Fig. 5.19 Veins of the thoracic wall

Anterior view.

Plexus venosus vertebralis internus anterior et posterior
Vv. intercostales posteriores
V. azygos
Plexus venosus vertebralis externus anterior

B Vertebral venous plexus.

Fig. 5.20 Superficial veins

Anterior view. The vv. thoracoepigastricae are a potential superficial collateral venous drainage route in the event of superior or inferior vena cava obstruction.

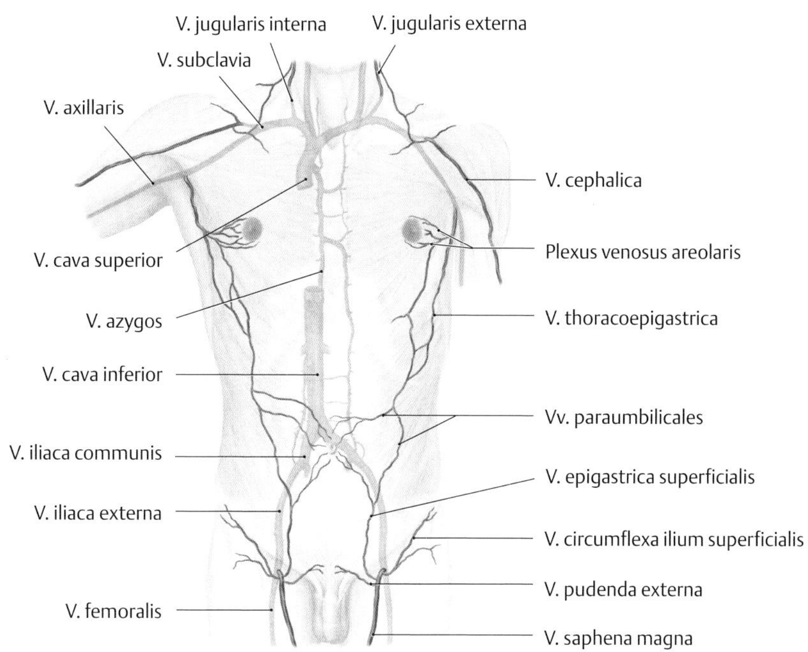
V. jugularis interna
V. jugularis externa
V. subclavia
V. axillaris
V. cephalica
Plexus venosus areolaris
V. cava superior
V. azygos
V. thoracoepigastrica
V. cava inferior
Vv. paraumbilicales
V. iliaca communis
V. epigastrica superficialis
V. iliaca externa
V. circumflexa ilium superficialis
V. pudenda externa
V. femoralis
V. saphena magna

Nerves of the Thoracic Wall

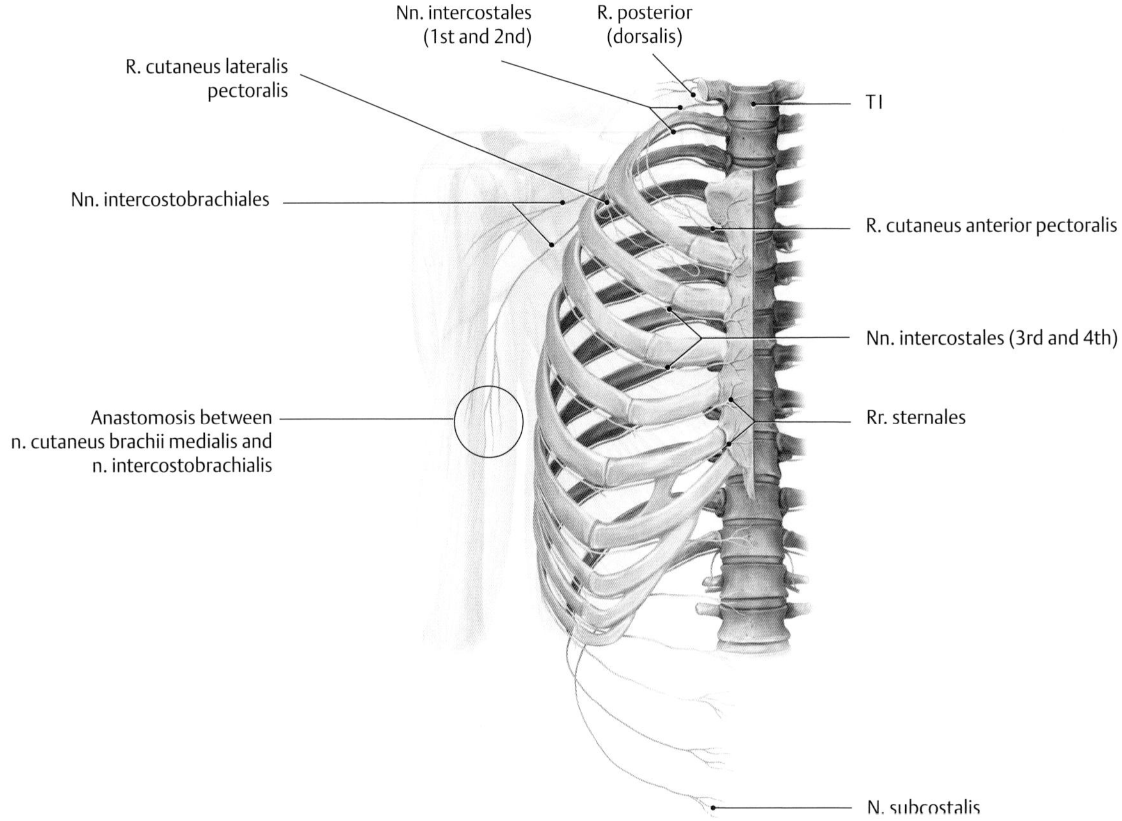
Nn. intercostales
(1st and 2nd)
R. posterior
(dorsalis)
R. cutaneus lateralis
pectoralis
T I
Nn. intercostobrachiales
R. cutaneus anterior pectoralis
Nn. intercostales (3rd and 4th)
Anastomosis between
n. cutaneus brachii medialis and
n. intercostobrachialis
Rr. sternales
N. subcostalis

Fig. 5.21 **Nn. intercostales**
Anterior view. The 1st rib has been removed to reveal the 1st and 2nd intercostal nerves.

Fig. 5.22 **Thoracic wall: Peripheral sensory cutaneous innervation**

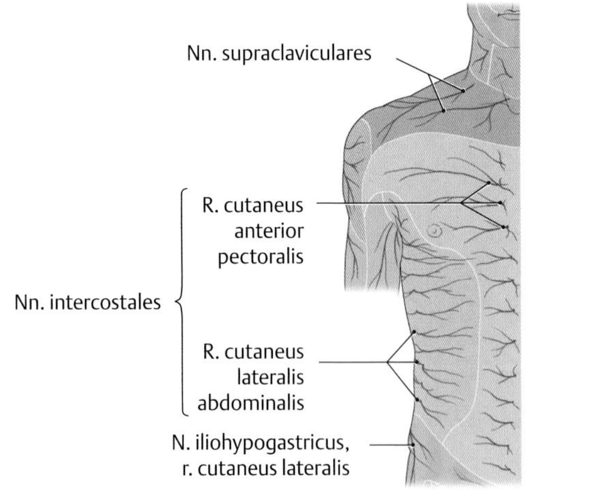
Nn. supraclaviculares
R. cutaneus
anterior
pectoralis
Nn. intercostales
R. cutaneus
lateralis
abdominalis
N. iliohypogastricus,
r. cutaneus lateralis

A Anterior view.

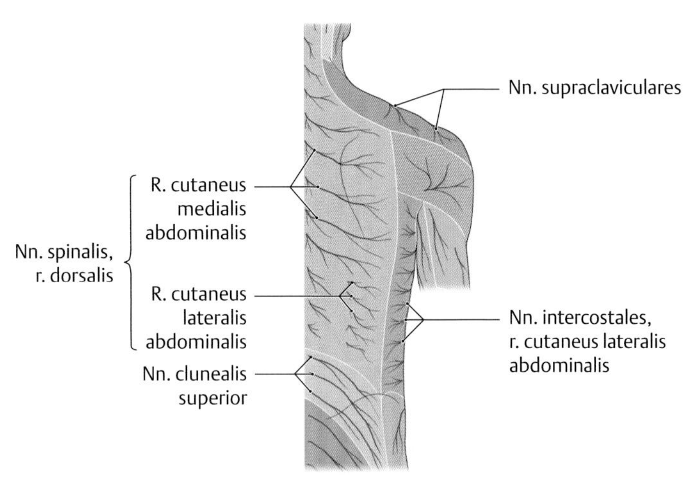
Nn. supraclaviculares
R. cutaneus
medialis
abdominalis
Nn. spinalis,
r. dorsalis
R. cutaneus
lateralis
abdominalis
Nn. intercostales,
r. cutaneus lateralis
abdominalis
Nn. clunealis
superior

B Posterior view.

Fig. 5.23 Spinal nerve branches

Superior view. Formed by the union of the posterior (sensory) and anterior (motor) roots, the at-most 1 cm-long n. spinales courses through the intervertebral foramen and exits the vertebral canal. Its ramus posterior innervates the skin and intrinsic muscles of the back; its ramus anterior forms the nn. intercostales. See p. 36 for more details.

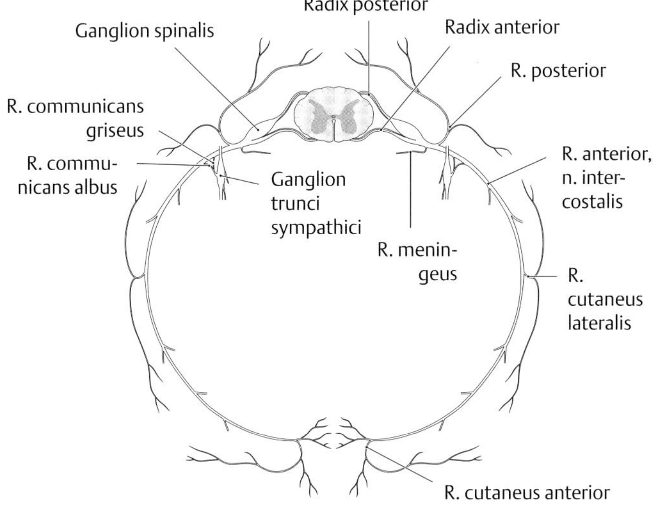
Radix posterior
Ganglion spinalis
Radix anterior
R. posterior
R. communicans griseus
R. communicans albus
Ganglion trunci sympathici
R. anterior, n. intercostalis
R. meningeus
R. cutaneus lateralis
R. cutaneus anterior

Fig. 5.24 Course of nn. intercostales

Coronal section, anterior view.

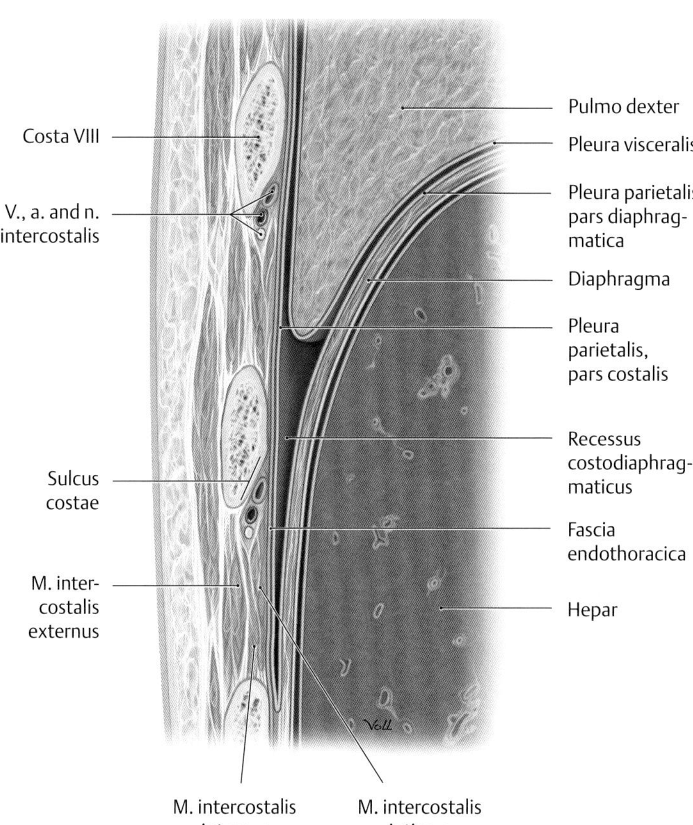
Pulmo dexter
Costa VIII
Pleura visceralis
V., a. and n. intercostalis
Pleura parietalis, pars diaphragmatica
Diaphragma
Pleura parietalis, pars costalis
Recessus costodiaphragmaticus
Sulcus costae
Fascia endothoracica
M. intercostalis externus
Hepar
M. intercostalis internus
M. intercostalis intimus

Fig. 5.25 Thoracic wall: Dermatomes

Landmarks: T4 generally includes the nipple; T6 innervates the skin over processus xiphoideus.

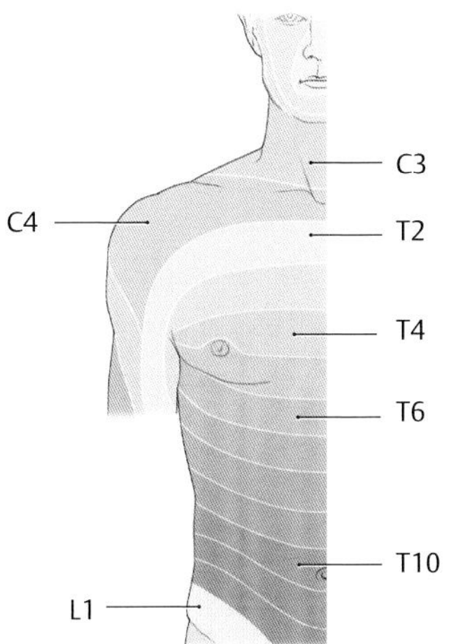
C3
C4
T2
T4
T6
T10
L1

A Anterior view.

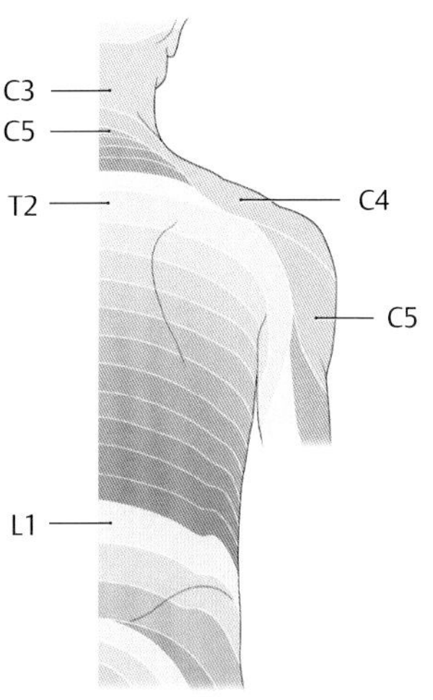
C3
C5
T2
C4
C5
L1

B Posterior view.

Neurovascular Topography of the Thoracic Wall

Fig. 5.26 **Anterior structures**
Anterior view (see pp. 34–39 for neurovasculature of the back).

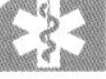

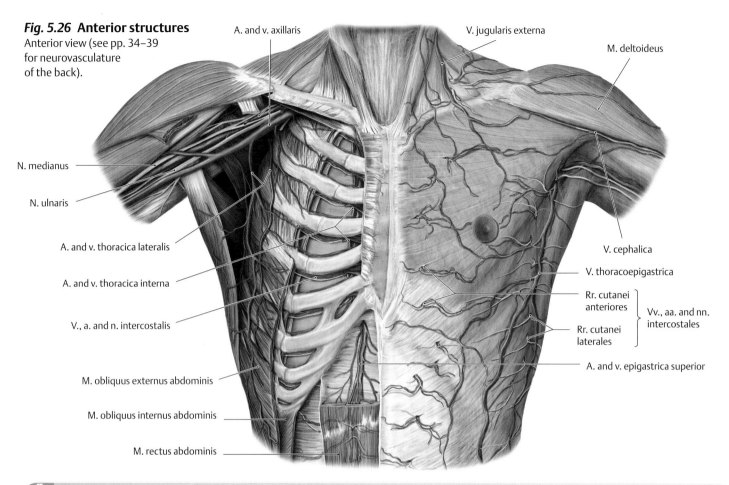
A. and v. axillaris
V. jugularis externa
M. deltoideus
N. medianus
N. ulnaris
A. and v. thoracica lateralis
A. and v. thoracica interna
V., a. and n. intercostalis
M. obliquus externus abdominis
M. obliquus internus abdominis
M. rectus abdominis
V. cephalica
V. thoracoepigastrica
Rr. cutanei anteriores
Rr. cutanei laterales
Vv., aa. and nn. intercostales
A. and v. epigastrica superior

Clinical

Insertion of a chest tube

Abnormal fluid collection in the pleural space (e.g., pleural effusion due to bronchial carcinoma) may necessitate the insertion of a chest tube. Generally, the optimal puncture site in a sitting patient is at the level of the 7th or 8th intercostal space on the posterior axillary line. The drain should always be introduced at the upper margin of a rib to avoid injuring the intercostal vein, artery, and nerve. See p. 113 for details on collapsed lungs.

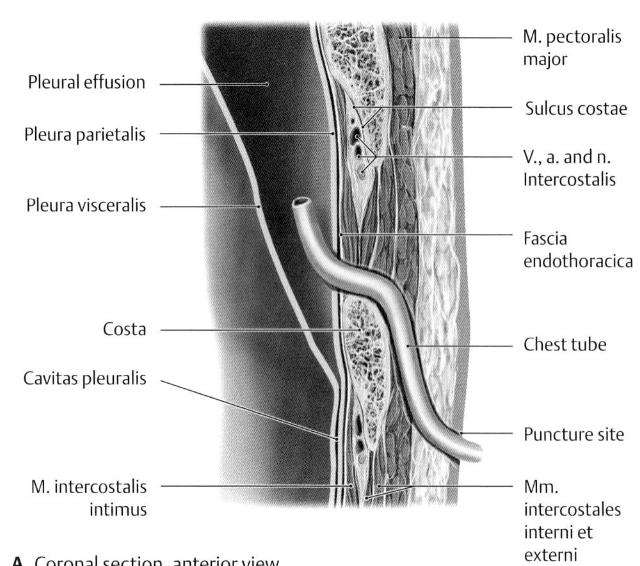
Pleural effusion
Pleura parietalis
Pleura visceralis
Costa
Cavitas pleuralis
M. intercostalis intimus
M. pectoralis major
Sulcus costae
V., a. and n. Intercostalis
Fascia endothoracica
Chest tube
Puncture site
Mm. intercostales interni et externi

A Coronal section, anterior view.

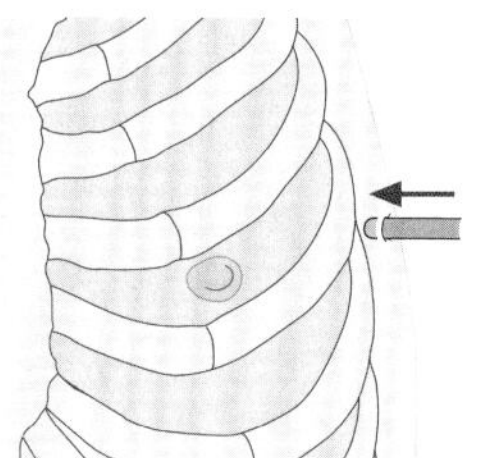

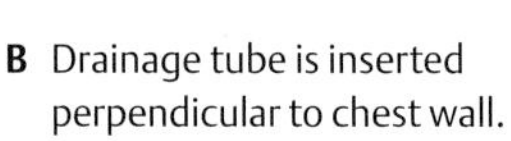

B Drainage tube is inserted perpendicular to chest wall.

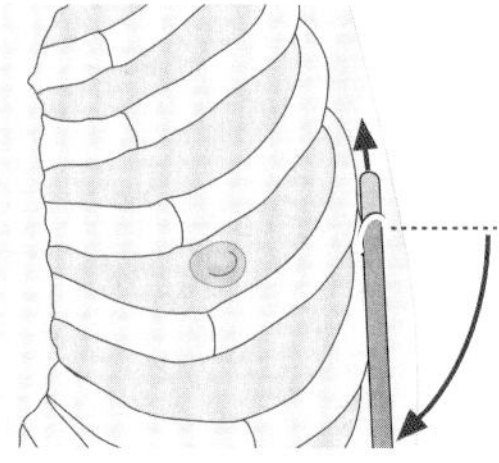

C At ribs, the tube is angled and advanced parallel to the chest wall in the subcutaneous plane.

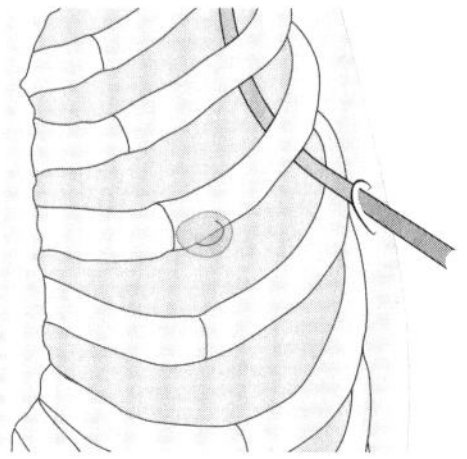

D At the superior margin of the rib, the tube is passed through the intercostal muscles and advanced into the pleural cavity.

Fig. 5.27 **Intercostal structures in cross section**
Transverse section, anterosuperior view.

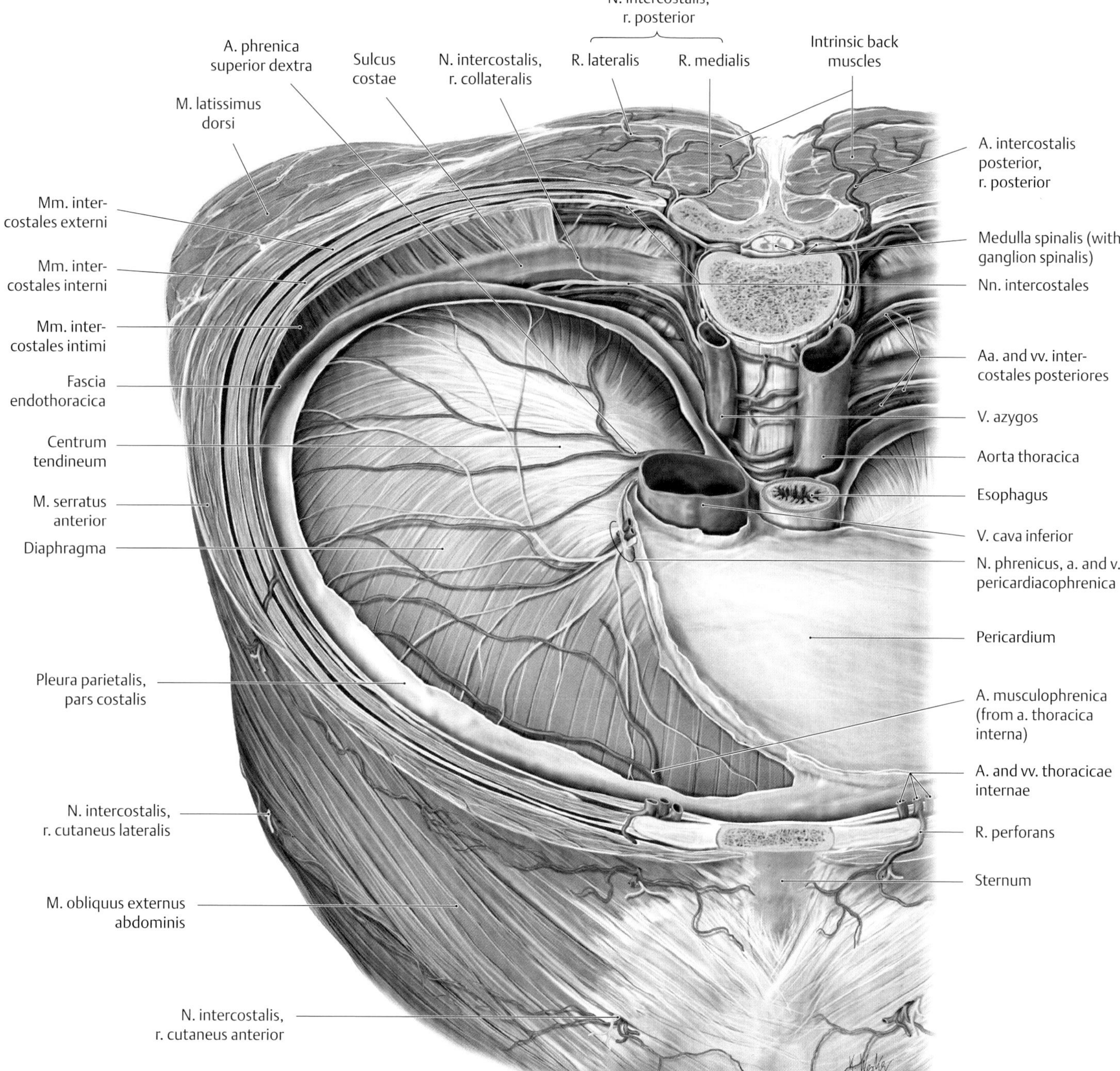
N. intercostalis, r. posterior
R. lateralis
R. medialis
A. phrenica superior dextra
Sulcus costae
N. intercostalis, r. collateralis
Intrinsic back muscles
M. latissimus dorsi
A. intercostalis posterior, r. posterior
Mm. intercostales externi
Medulla spinalis (with ganglion spinalis)
Mm. intercostales interni
Nn. intercostales
Mm. intercostales intimi
Aa. and vv. intercostales posteriores
Fascia endothoracica
V. azygos
Centrum tendineum
Aorta thoracica
M. serratus anterior
Esophagus
V. cava inferior
Diaphragma
N. phrenicus, a. and v. pericardiacophrenica
Pericardium
Pleura parietalis, pars costalis
A. musculophrenica (from a. thoracica interna)
A. and vv. thoracicae internae
N. intercostalis, r. cutaneus lateralis
R. perforans
Sternum
M. obliquus externus abdominis
N. intercostalis, r. cutaneus anterior

Female Breast

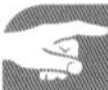

The female breast, a modified sweat gland in the subcutaneous tissue layer, consists of glandular tissue, fibrous stroma, and fat. The breast extends from the 2nd to the 6th rib and is loosely attached to the pectoral, axillary, and superficial abdominal fascia by connective tissue. The breast is additionally supported by suspensory ligaments. An extension of the breast tissue into the axilla, the axillary tail, is often present.

Fig. 5.28 Female breast
Right breast, anterior view.

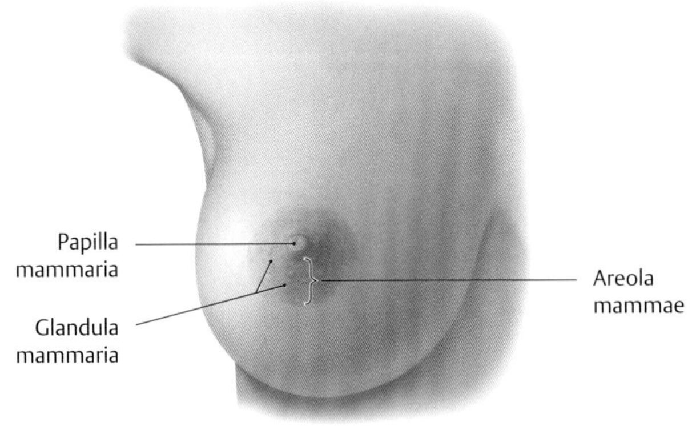
Papilla mammaria
Glandula mammaria
Areola mammae

Fig. 5.29 Mammary ridges
Rudimentary mammary glands form in both sexes along the mammary ridges. Occasionally, these may persist in humans to form accessory nipples (*polythelia*), although only the thoracic pair normally remains.

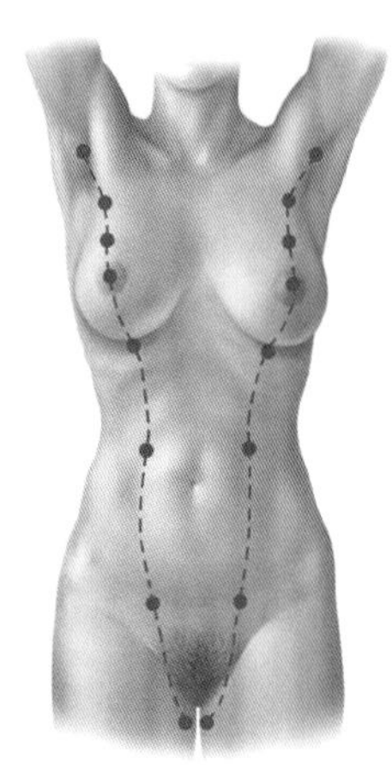

Fig. 5.30 Blood supply to the breast

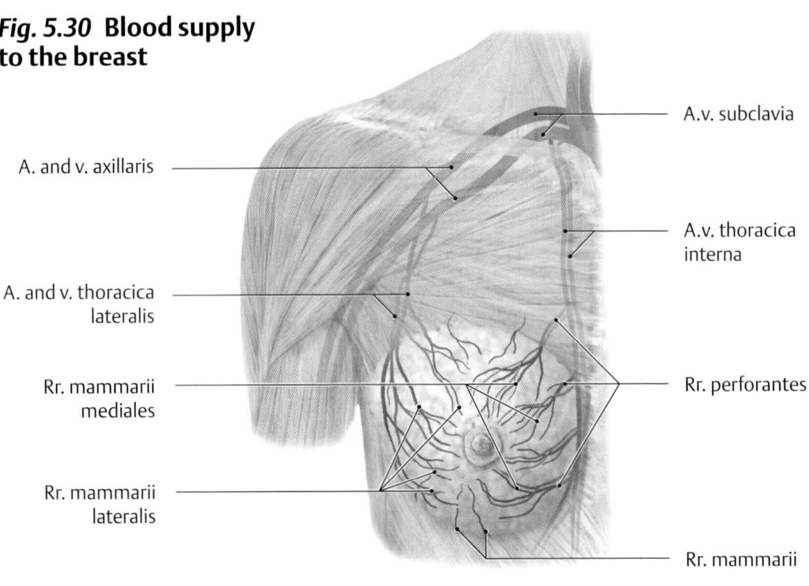
A.v. subclavia
A. and v. axillaris
A.v. thoracica interna
A. and v. thoracica lateralis
Rr. mammarii mediales
Rr. perforantes
Rr. mammarii lateralis
Rr. mammarii

Fig. 5.31 Sensory innervation of the breast

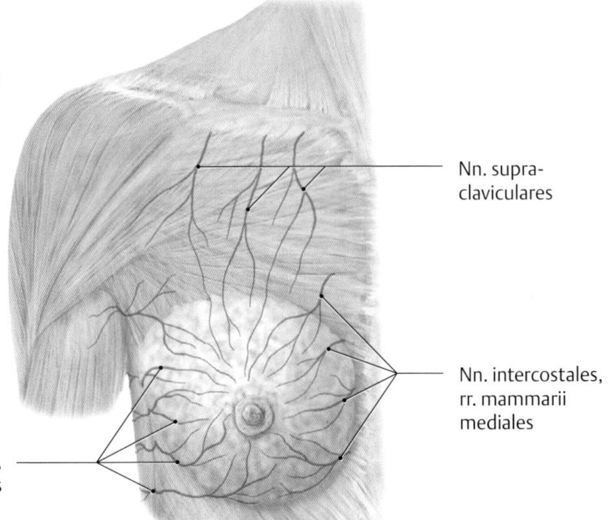
Nn. supra-claviculares
Nn. intercostales, rr. mammarii mediales
Nn. intercostales, rr. mammarii lateralis

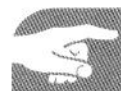

The glandular tissue is composed of 10 to 20 individual lobes, each with its own ductus lactiferi. The gland ducts open on the elevated papilla mammaria at the center of the pigmented areola mammae. Just proximal to the duct opening is a dilated portion called the sinus lactiferi. Areolar elevations are the openings of the areolar glands (sebaceous). The glands and lactiferous ducts are surrounded by firm, fibrofatty tissue with a rich blood supply.

Fig. 5.32 Structures of the breast

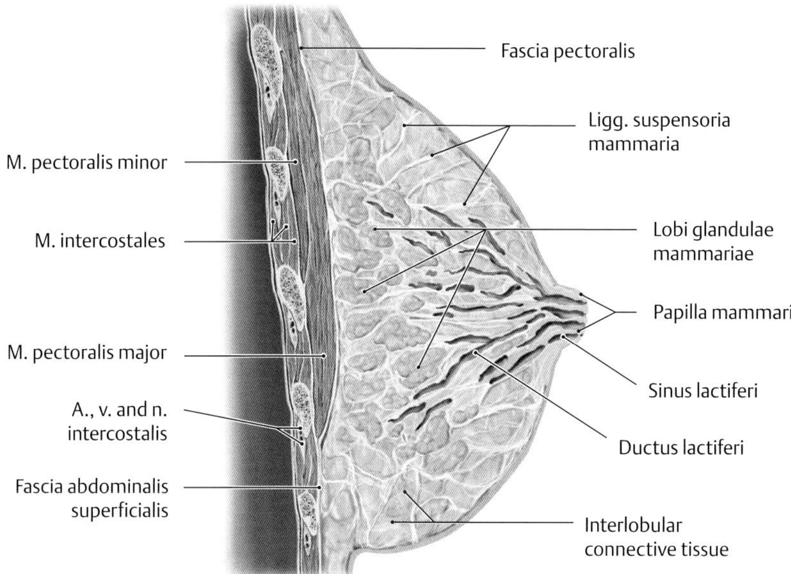
Fascia pectoralis
Ligg. suspensoria mammaria
M. pectoralis minor
M. intercostales
Lobi glandulae mammariae
Papilla mammari
M. pectoralis major
Sinus lactiferi
A., v. and n. intercostalis
Ductus lactiferi
Fascia abdominalis superficialis
Interlobular connective tissue

A Sagittal section along midclavicular line.

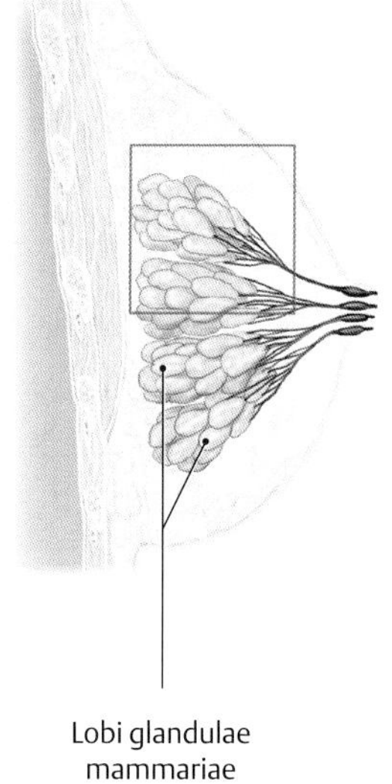
Lobi glandulae mammariae

B Duct system and portions of a lobe, sagittal section. In the nonlactating breast (shown here), the lobules contain clusters of rudimentary acini.

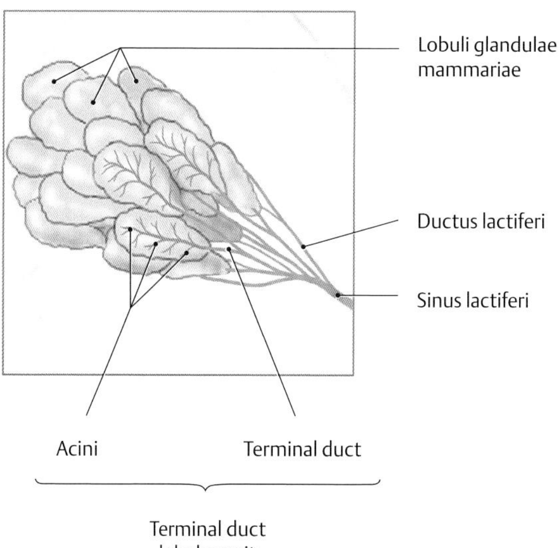
Lobuli glandulae mammariae
Ductus lactiferi
Sinus lactiferi
Acini
Terminal duct
Terminal duct lobular unit

C Terminal duct lobular unit (TDLU). The clustered acini composing the lobule empty into a terminal ductule; these structures are collectively known as the TDLU.

Lymphatics of the Female Breast

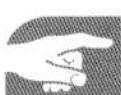

The lymphatic vessels of the breast (not shown) are divided into three systems: superficial, subcutaneous, and deep. These drain primarily into the nll. axillares, which are classified based on their relationship to the pectoralis minor (Table 5.7). The medial portion of the breast is drained by nll. parasternales, which are associated with the internal thoracic vessels.

Fig. 5.33 **Axillary lymph nodes**

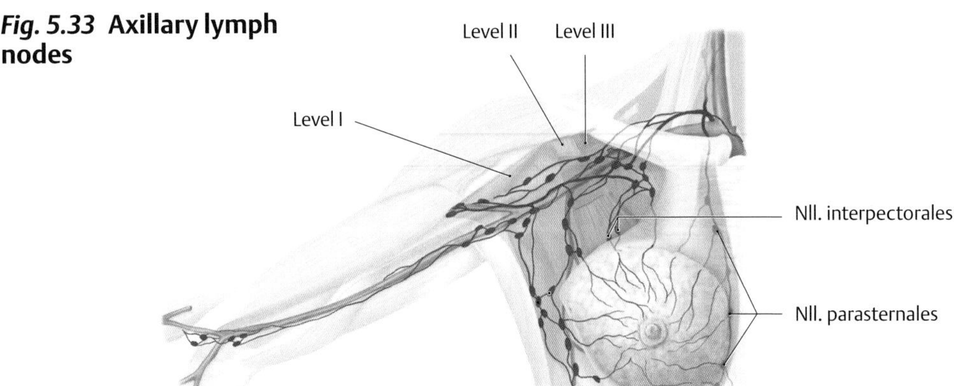
Level II
Level III
Level I
Nll. interpectorales
Nll. parasternales

A Lymphatic drainage of the breast.

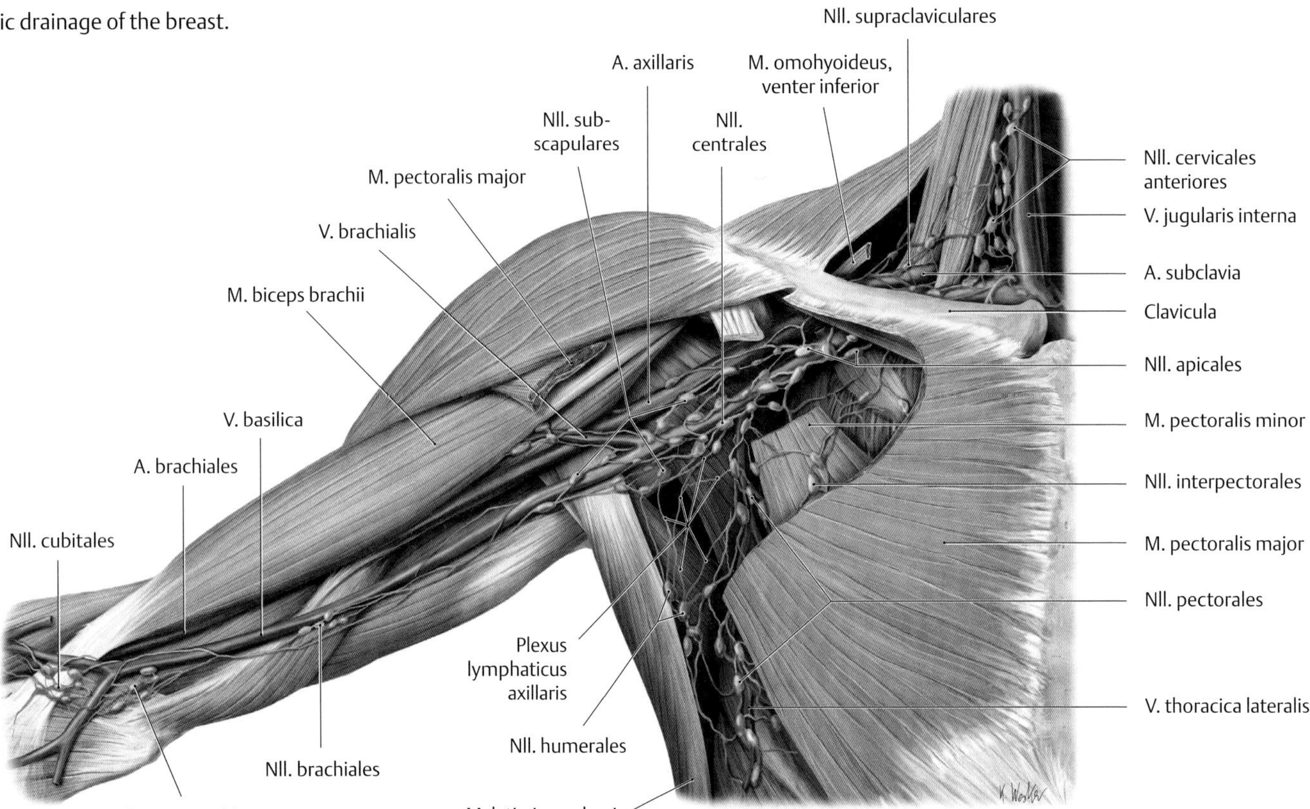
Nll. supraclaviculares
A. axillaris
M. omohyoideus, venter inferior
Nll. sub-scapulares
Nll. centrales
M. pectoralis major
V. brachialis
M. biceps brachii
V. basilica
A. brachiales
Nll. cubitales
Nll. cervicales anteriores
V. jugularis interna
A. subclavia
Clavicula
Nll. apicales
M. pectoralis minor
Nll. interpectorales
M. pectoralis major
Nll. pectorales
V. thoracica lateralis
Plexus lymphaticus axillaris
Nll. humerales
Nll. brachiales
Nll. supratrochleares
M. latissimus dorsi

B Anterior view.

Table 5.7 **Levels of axillary lymph nodes**

Level		Position	Lymph nodes (Nll.)
I	Lower axillary group	Lateral to m. pectoralis minor	Nll. pectorales/anteriores
			Nll. subscapulares/posteriores
			Nll. humerales/laterales
			Nll. centrales
II	Middle axillary group	Along m. pectoralis minor	Nll. interpectorales
III	Upper infraclavicular group	Medial to m. pectoralis minor	Nll. apicales

Clinical

Breast cancer

Stem cells in the intralobular connective tissue give rise to tremendous cell growth, necessary for duct system proliferation and acini differentiation. This makes the terminal duct lobular unit (TDLU) the most common site of origin of malignant breast tumors.

Lobuli glandulae mammariae
Ductus lactiferi
Sinus lactiferi
Acini
Terminal duct
Terminal duct lobular unit

A Terminal duct lobular unit.

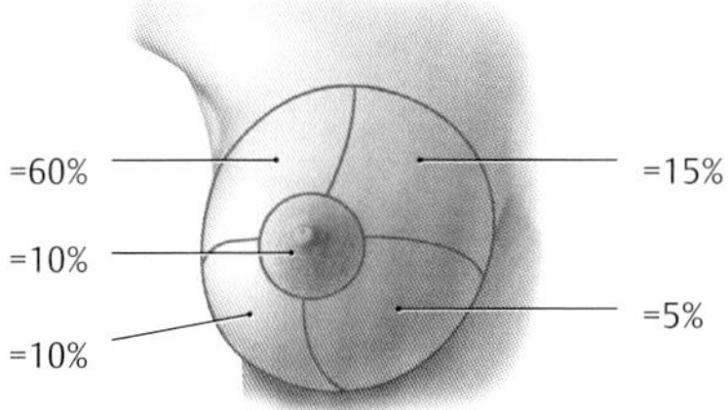
≈60%
≈10%
≈10%
≈15%
≈5%

B Origin of malignant tumors by quadrant.

Tumors originating in the breast spread via the lymphatic vessels. The deep system of lymphatic drainage (level III) is of particular importance, although the parasternal lymph nodes provide a route by which tumor cells may spread across the midline. The survival rate in breast cancer correlates most strongly with the number of lymph nodes involved at the axillary nodal level. Metastatic involvement is gauged through scintigraphic mapping with radiolabeled colloids (technetium [Tc] 99m sulfur microcolloid). The downstream sentinel node is the first to receive lymphatic drainage from the tumor and is therefore the first to be visualized with radiolabeling. Once identified, it can then be removed (via *sentinel lymphadenectomy*) and histologically examined for tumor cells. This method is 98% accurate in predicting the level of axillary nodal involvement.

Metastatic involvement	5-year survival rate
Level I	65%
Level II	31%
Level III	~0%

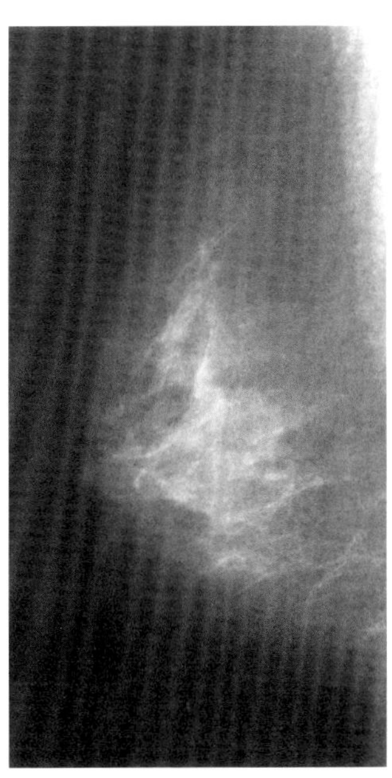

C Normal mammogram.

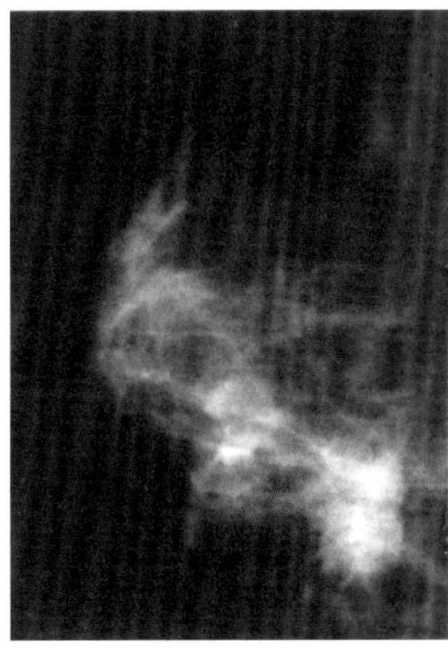

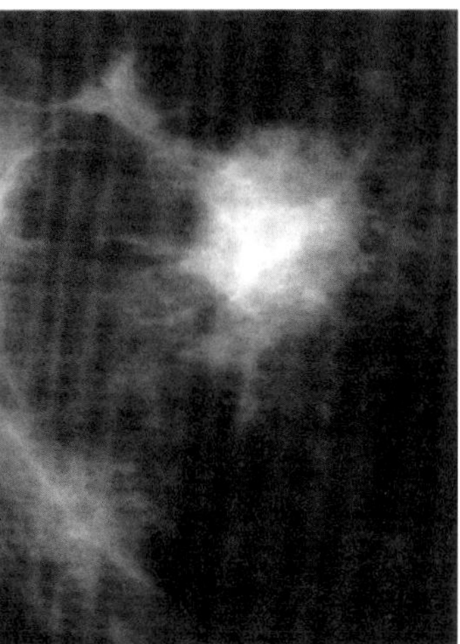

D Mammogram of invasive ductal carcinoma. The large lesion has changed the architecture of the neighboring breast tissue.

Divisions of the Thoracic Cavity

The thoracic cavity is divided into three large spaces: the mediastinum (p. 76) and the two pleural cavities (p. 102).

Fig. 6.1 Thoracic cavity
Coronal section, anterior view.

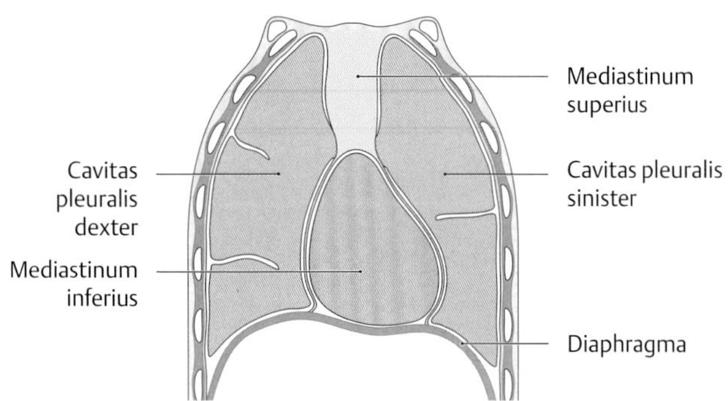
Mediastinum superius
Cavitas pleuralis dexter
Cavitas pleuralis sinister
Mediastinum inferius
Diaphragma

A Divisions of the thoracic cavity.

Table 6.1 Major structures of the thoracic cavity

Mediastinum	Mediastinum superius		Thymus, great vessels, trachea, esophagus, and ductus thoracicus
	Mediastinum inferius	Mediastinum anterius	Thymus
		Mediastinum medium	Cor, pericardium, and roots of great vessels
		Mediastinum posterius	Aorta thoracica, ductus thoracicus, esophagus, and azygos venous system
Cavitas pleuralis	Cavitas pleuralis dexter		Pulmo dexter
	Cavitas pleuralis sinister		Pulmo sinister

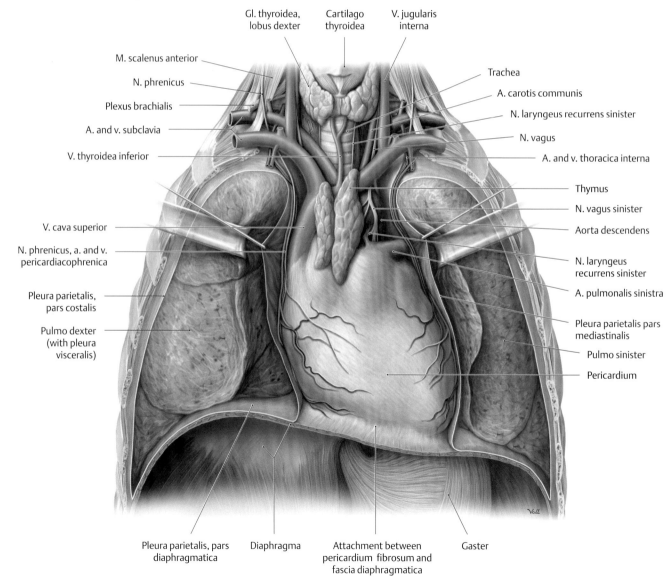

Gl. thyroidea, lobus dexter
Cartilago thyroidea
V. jugularis interna
M. scalenus anterior
N. phrenicus
Plexus brachialis
A. and v. subclavia
V. thyroidea inferior
Trachea
A. carotis communis
N. laryngeus recurrens sinister
N. vagus
A. and v. thoracica interna
Thymus
N. vagus sinister
Aorta descendens
V. cava superior
N. phrenicus, a. and v. pericardiacophrenica
N. laryngeus recurrens sinister
A. pulmonalis sinistra
Pleura parietalis, pars costalis
Pleura parietalis pars mediastinalis
Pulmo dexter (with pleura visceralis)
Pulmo sinister
Pericardium
Pleura parietalis, pars diaphragmatica
Diaphragma
Attachment between pericardium fibrosum and fascia diaphragmatica
Gaster

B Opened thoracic cavity. *Removed:* Thoracic wall; connective tissue of anterior mediastinum.

Fig. 6.2 Divisions of the mediastinum

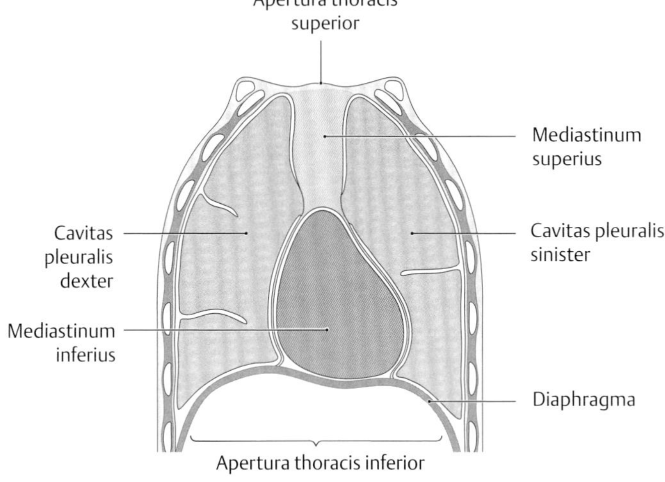
Apertura thoracis superior
Mediastinum superius
Cavitas pleuralis dexter
Cavitas pleuralis sinister
Mediastinum inferius
Diaphragma
Apertura thoracis inferior

A Anterior view (coronal section).

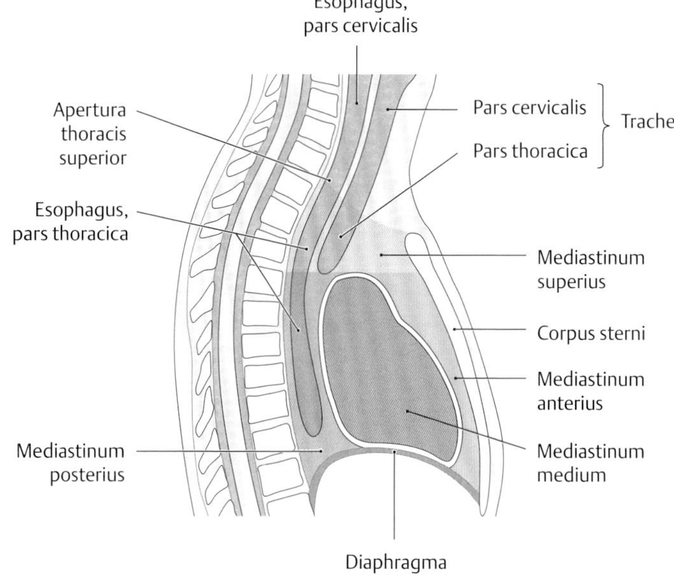
Esophagus, pars cervicalis
Apertura thoracis superior
Pars cervicalis
Pars thoracica
Trachea
Esophagus, pars thoracica
Mediastinum superius
Corpus sterni
Mediastinum anterius
Mediastinum posterius
Mediastinum medium
Diaphragma

B Lateral view (midsagittal section).

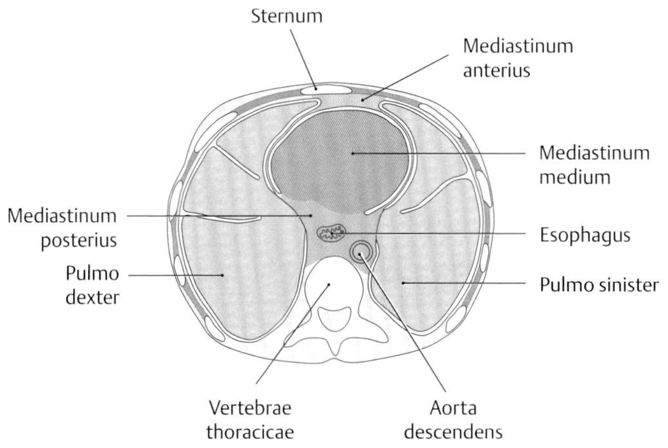
Sternum
Mediastinum anterius
Mediastinum medium
Mediastinum posterius
Esophagus
Pulmo dexter
Pulmo sinister
Vertebrae thoracicae
Aorta descendens

C Inferior view (transverse section).

Fig. 6.3 Transverse sections of the thorax

Computed tomography (CT) scan of thorax, inferior view.

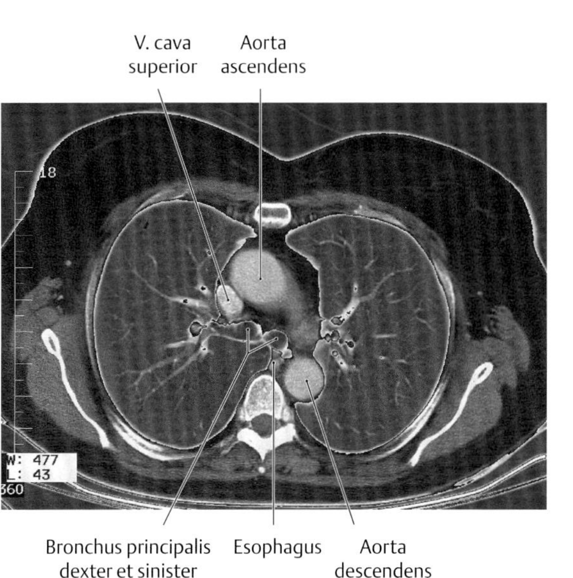
V. cava superior
Aorta ascendens
18
W: 477
L: 43
360
Bronchus principalis dexter et sinister
Esophagus
Aorta descendens

A Mediastinum superius.

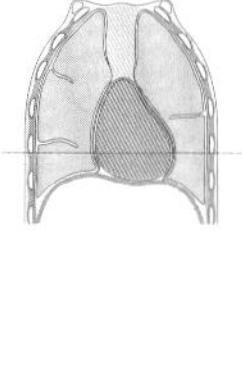

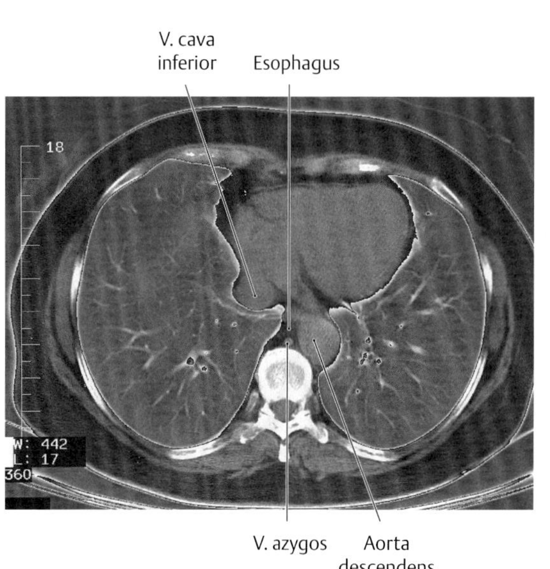
V. cava inferior
Esophagus
18
W: 442
L: 17
360
V. azygos
Aorta descendens

B Mediastinum inferius.

Arteries of the Thoracic Cavity

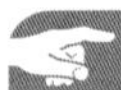

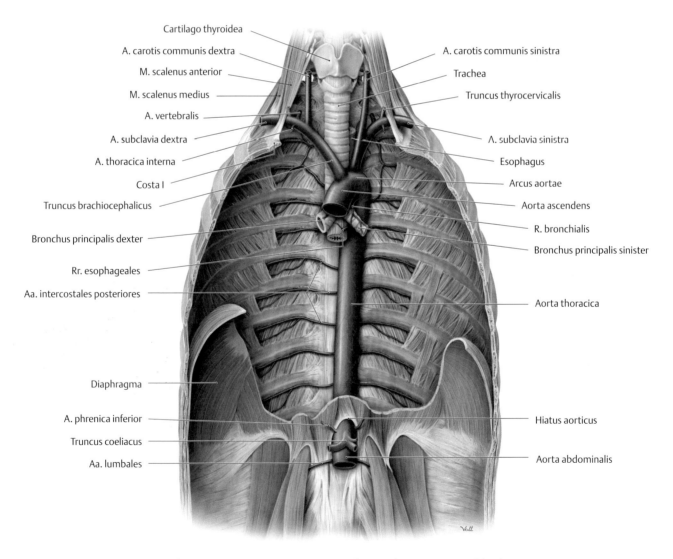

The arcus aortae has three major branches: truncus brachiocephalicus, a. carotis communis sinistra, and a. subclavia sinistra. After arcus aortae, the aorta begins its descent, becoming aorta thoracica at the level of angulus sterni and aorta abdominalis once it passes through hiatus aorticus in the diaphragm.

Fig. 6.4 Thoracic aorta

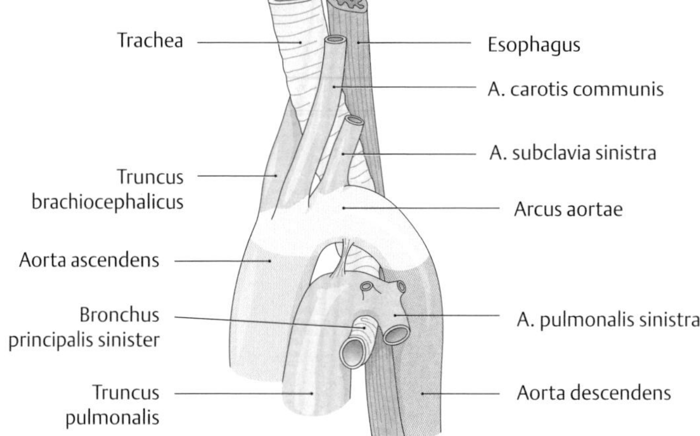
Trachea
Esophagus
A. carotis communis
A. subclavia sinistra
Truncus brachiocephalicus
Arcus aortae
Aorta ascendens
Bronchus principalis sinister
A. pulmonalis sinistra
Truncus pulmonalis
Aorta descendens

A Parts of the aorta, left lateral view. *Note:* The arcus aortae begins and ends at the level of angulus sterni (see p. 46).

Cartilago thyroidea
A. carotis communis dextra
M. scalenus anterior
M. scalenus medius
A. vertebralis
A. subclavia dextra
A. thoracica interna
Costa I
Truncus brachiocephalicus
Bronchus principalis dexter
Rr. esophageales
Aa. intercostales posteriores
Diaphragma
A. phrenica inferior
Truncus coeliacus
Aa. lumbales
A. carotis communis sinistra
Trachea
Truncus thyrocervicalis
A. subclavia sinistra
Esophagus
Arcus aortae
Aorta ascendens
R. bronchialis
Bronchus principalis sinister
Aorta thoracica
Hiatus aorticus
Aorta abdominalis

B Aorta thoracica in situ, anterior view. *Removed:* Heart, lungs, portions of diaphragma.

Table 6.2	Branches of the thoracic aorta		
The thoracic organs are supplied by direct branches from aorta thoracica, as well as indirect branches from aa. subclaviae.			
Branches			**Region supplied**
Truncus brachiocephalicus	A. subclavia dextra		See a. subclavia sinistra
	A. carotis communis dextra		Head and neck
A. carotis communis sinistra			
A. subclavia sinistra	A. vertebralis		
	A. thoracica interna	Aa. intercostales anteriores	Anterior chest wall
		Rr. thymici	Thymus
		Rr. mediastinales	Mediastinum posterius
		A. pericardiacophrenica	Pericardium, diaphragma
	Truncus thyrocervicalis	A. thyroida inferior	Esophagus, trachea, gl. thyroida
	Truncus costocervicalis	A. intercostalis suprema	Chest wall
Aorta thoracica, pars descendens	Visceral branches		Cor, pericardium, bronchi, trachea, esophagus
	Parietal branches	Aa. intercostales posteriores	Posterior chest wall
		Aa. phrenicae superiores	Diaphragma

Clinical

Aortic dissection

A tear in the inner wall (intima) of the aorta allows blood to separate the layers of the aortic wall, creating a "false lumen" and potentially resulting in life-threatening aortic rupture. Symptoms are dyspnea (shortness of breath) and sudden onset of excruciating pain. Acute aortic dissections occur most often in the ascending aorta and generally require surgery. More distal aortic dissections may be treated conservatively, provided there are no complications (e.g., obstruction of blood supply to the organs, in which case a stent may be inserted to restore perfusion). Aortic dissections occurring at the base of a coronary artery may cause myocardial infarction.

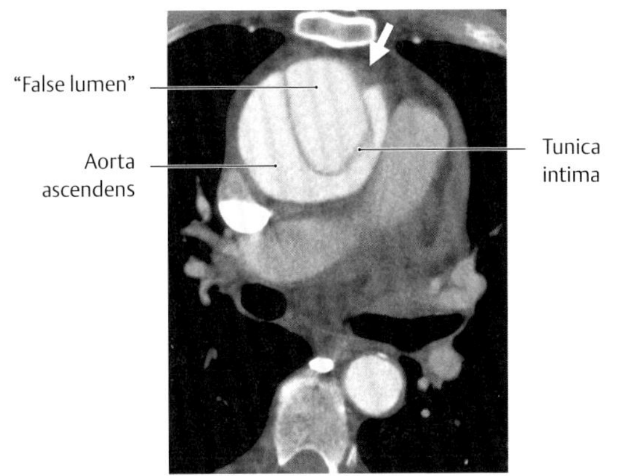
"False lumen"
Aorta ascendens
Tunica intima

A Aortic dissection. Parts of the intima are still attached to the connective tissue in the wall of the aorta (*arrow*).

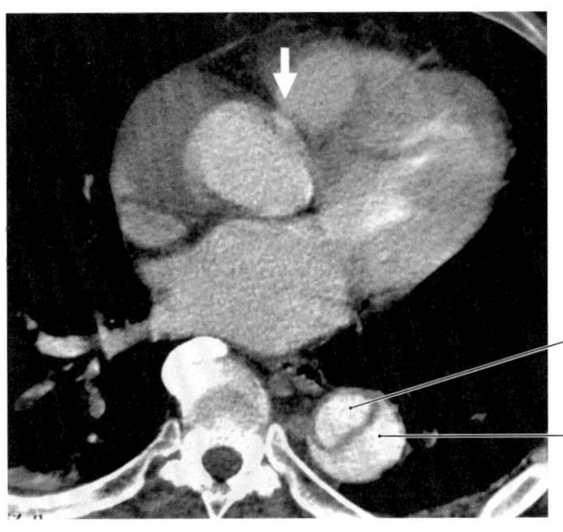
"False lumen"
Aorta descendens

B The flow in the coronary arteries is intact (*arrow*).

Veins of the Thoracic Cavity

The v. cava superior is formed by the union of the two vv. brachiocephalicae at the level of the T II–T III junction. It receives blood drained by the azygos system (v. cava inferior has no tributaries in the thorax).

Fig. 6.5 V. cava superior and azygos system

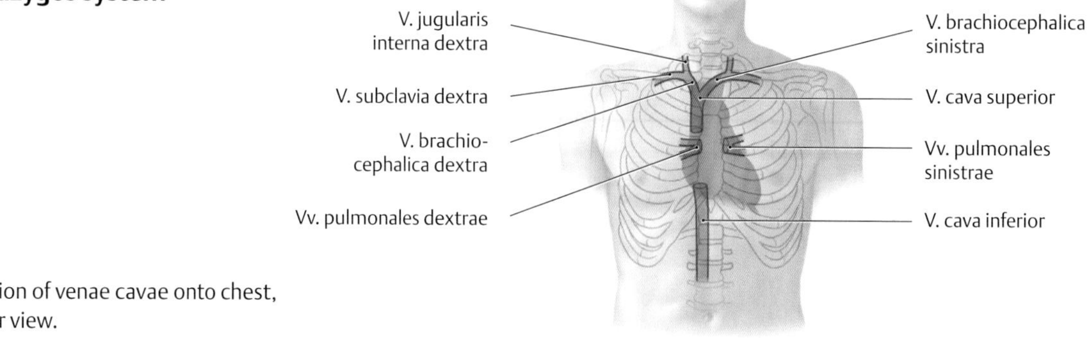
V. jugularis interna dextra
V. subclavia dextra
V. brachio-cephalica dextra
Vv. pulmonales dextrae
V. brachiocephalica sinistra
V. cava superior
Vv. pulmonales sinistrae
V. cava inferior

A Projection of venae cavae onto chest, anterior view.

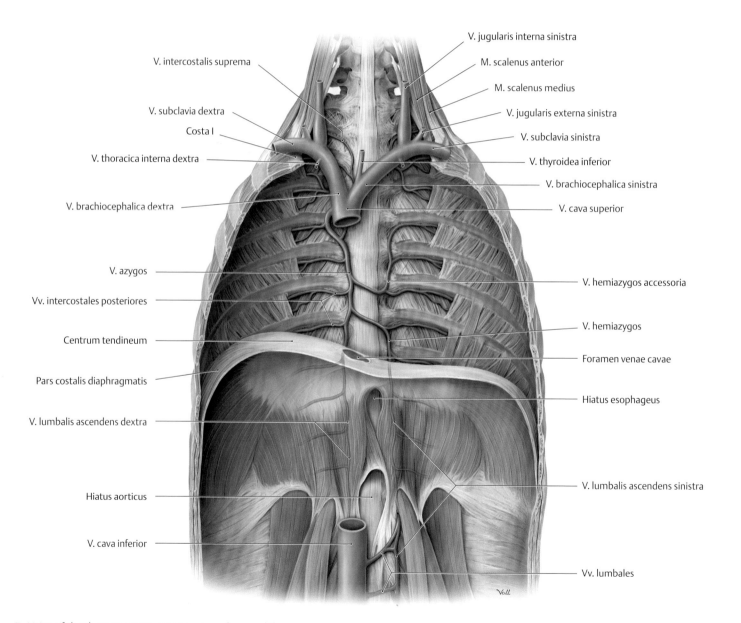

V. intercostalis suprema
V. subclavia dextra
Costa I
V. thoracica interna dextra
V. brachiocephalica dextra
V. azygos
Vv. intercostales posteriores
Centrum tendineum
Pars costalis diaphragmatis
V. lumbalis ascendens dextra
Hiatus aorticus
V. cava inferior
V. jugularis interna sinistra
M. scalenus anterior
M. scalenus medius
V. jugularis externa sinistra
V. subclavia sinistra
V. thyroidea inferior
V. brachiocephalica sinistra
V. cava superior
V. hemiazygos accessoria
V. hemiazygos
Foramen venae cavae
Hiatus esophageus
V. lumbalis ascendens sinistra
Vv. lumbales

B Veins of the thoracic cavity, anterior view of opened thorax.

Table 6.3 Thoracic tributaries of the superior vena cava

Major vein	Tributaries		Region drained
Vv. brachiocephalicae	V. thyroidea inferior		Esophagus, trachea, gl. thyroidea
	V. jugularis interna		Head, neck, upper limb
	V. jugularis externa		
	V. subclavia		
	V. intercostalis suprema		
	Vv. pericardiacae		
	V. intercostalis superior sinistra		
Azygos system (left side: v. hemiazygos and v. hemiazygos accessoria; right side: v. azygos)	Visceral branches		Trachea, bronchi, esophagus
	Parietal branches	Vv. intercostales posteriores	Inner chest wall and diaphragm
		Vv. phrenicae superiores	
		V. intercostalis superior dextra	
Vv. thoracicae internae	Vv. thymicae		Thymus
	Vv. mediastinales		Mediastinum posterius
	Vv. intercostales anteriores		Anterior chest wall
	Vv. pericardiacophrenicae		Pericardium
	Vv. musculophrenicae		Diaphragma

Note: Structures of the mediastinum superius may also drain directly to vv. brachiocephalicae via vv. tracheales, vv. esophageales and vv. mediastinales.

***Fig. 6.6* Azygos system**
Anterior view.

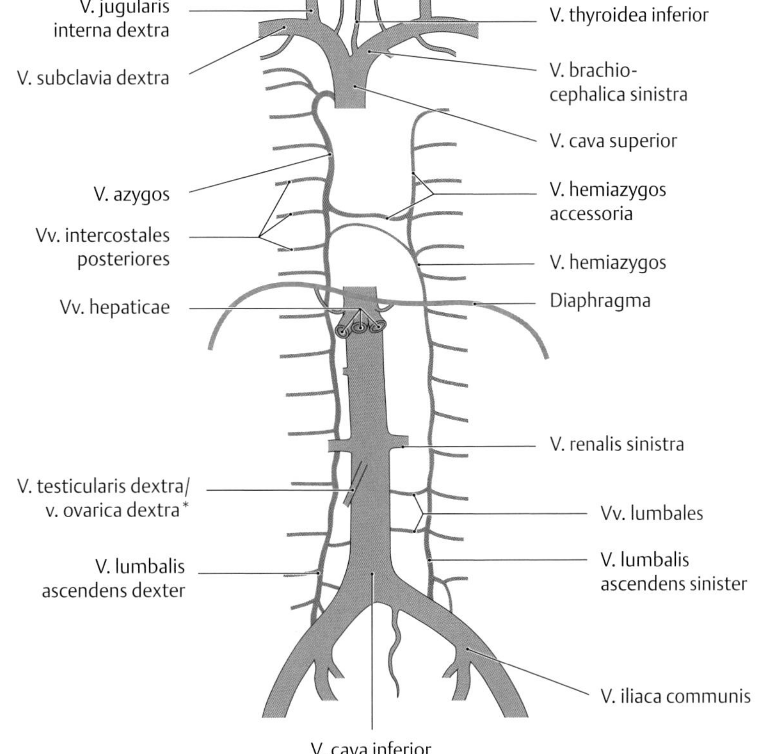
V. jugularis interna dextra
V. subclavia dextra
V. azygos
Vv. intercostales posteriores
Vv. hepaticae
V. testicularis dextra/ v. ovarica dextra*
V. lumbalis ascendens dexter
V. cava inferior
V. thyroidea inferior
V. brachio-cephalica sinistra
V. cava superior
V. hemiazygos accessoria
V. hemiazygos
Diaphragma
V. renalis sinistra
Vv. lumbales
V. lumbalis ascendens sinister
V. iliaca communis

*V. testicularis/ovarica sin. arises from v. renalis sin.

Lymphatics of the Thoracic Cavity

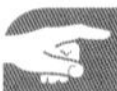

The body's chief lymph vessel is ductus thoracicus. Beginning in the abdomen at the level of L I as the *cisterna chyli*, the ductus thoracicus empties into the junction of v. jugularis interna sinistra and v. subclavia sinistra. The ductus lymphaticus dexter drains to the junction of v. jugularis interna dextra and v. subclavia dextra.

Fig. 6.7 **Lymphatic trunks in the thorax**
Anterior view of opened thorax.

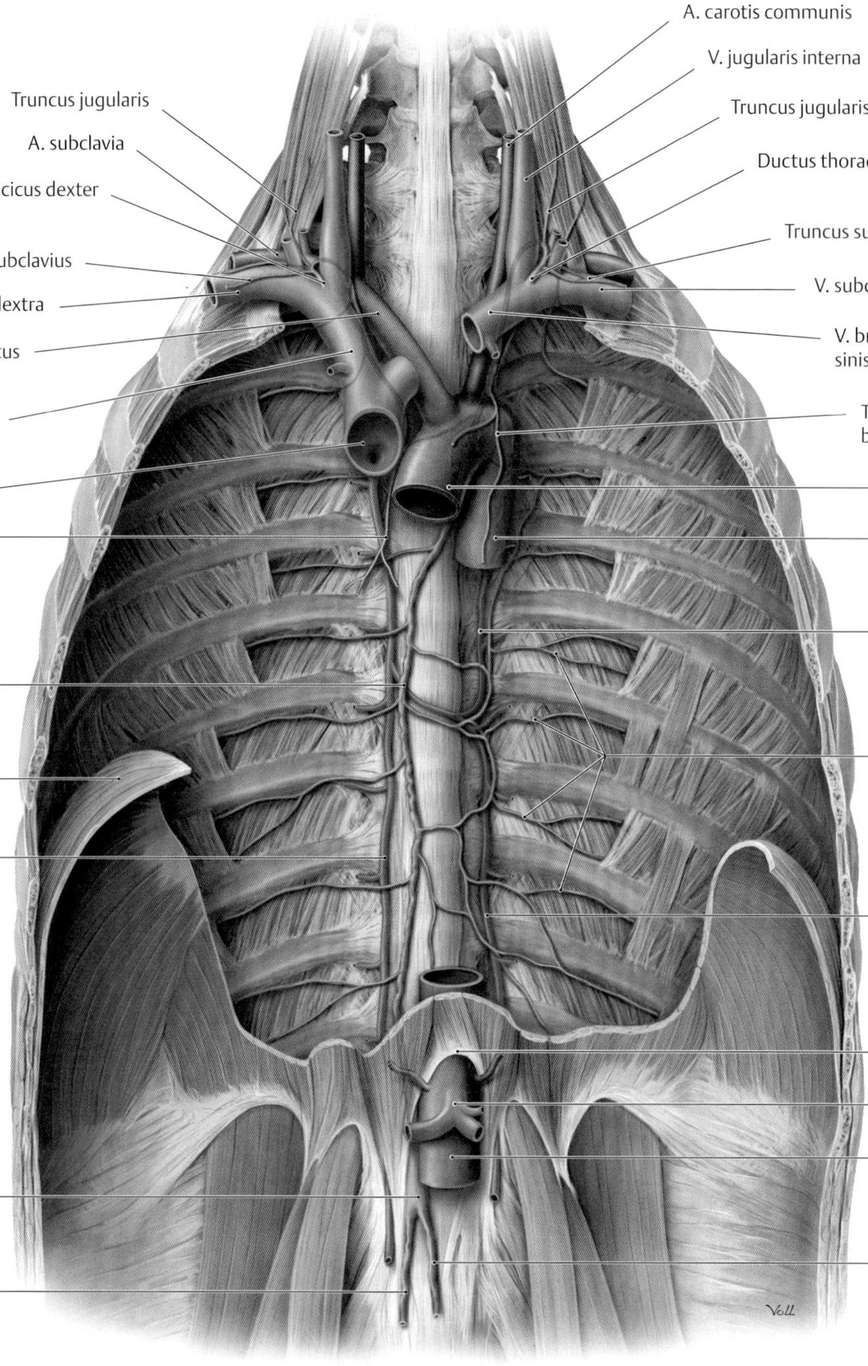

Truncus jugularis
A. subclavia
Ductus thoracicus dexter
Truncus subclavius
V. subclavia dextra
Truncus brachiocephalicus
V. brachiocephalica dextra
V. cava superior
Truncus bronchomediastinalis
Ductus thoracicus
Diaphragma
V. azygos
Cisterna chyli
Truncus lumbalis dexter
A. carotis communis
V. jugularis interna
Truncus jugularis
Ductus thoracicus
Truncus subclavius
V. subclavia sinistra
V. brachiocephalica sinistra
Truncus bronchomediastinalis
Aorta ascendens
Aorta thoracica
V. hemiazygos accessoria
Intercostal lymphatics
V. hemiazygos
Hiatus aorticus
Truncus coeliacus
Aorta abdominalis
Truncus lumbalis sinister
Voll

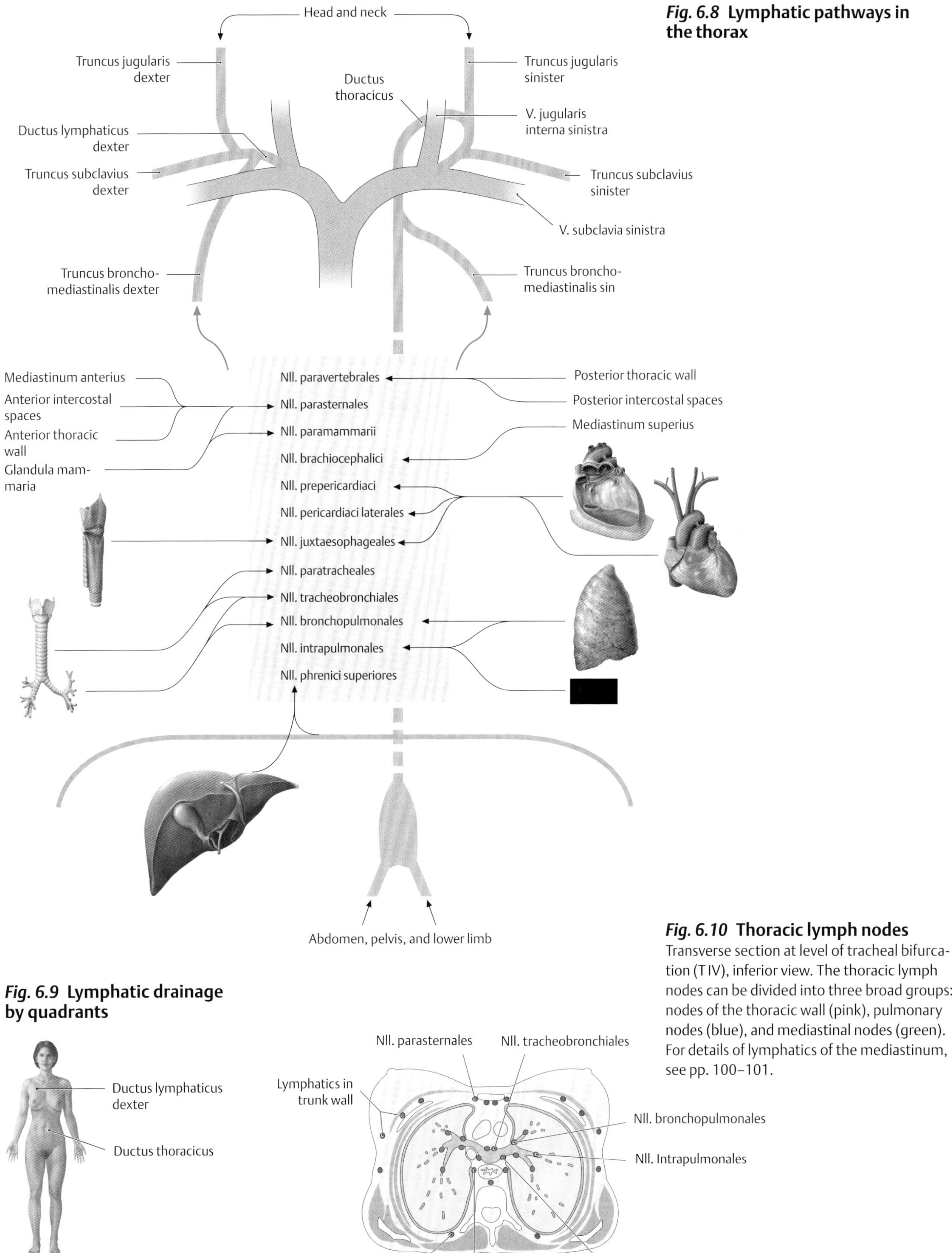
Head and neck
Truncus jugularis dexter
Ductus thoracicus
Truncus jugularis sinister
V. jugularis interna sinistra
Ductus lymphaticus dexter
Truncus subclavius dexter
Truncus subclavius sinister
V. subclavia sinistra
Truncus broncho-mediastinalis dexter
Truncus broncho-mediastinalis sin
Mediastinum anterius
Anterior intercostal spaces
Anterior thoracic wall
Glandula mammaria
Nll. paravertebrales
Nll. parasternales
Nll. paramammarii
Nll. brachiocephalici
Nll. prepericardiaci
Nll. pericardiaci laterales
Nll. juxtaesophageales
Nll. paratracheales
Nll. tracheobronchiales
Nll. bronchopulmonales
Nll. intrapulmonales
Nll. phrenici superiores
Posterior thoracic wall
Posterior intercostal spaces
Mediastinum superius
Abdomen, pelvis, and lower limb
Ductus lymphaticus dexter
Ductus thoracicus
Nll. parasternales
Nll. tracheobronchiales
Lymphatics in trunk wall
Nll. bronchopulmonales
Nll. Intrapulmonales
Nll. intercostales
Nll. juxtaesophageales
Nll. paratracheales

Fig. 6.8 **Lymphatic pathways in the thorax**

Fig. 6.9 **Lymphatic drainage by quadrants**

Fig. 6.10 **Thoracic lymph nodes**
Transverse section at level of tracheal bifurcation (T IV), inferior view. The thoracic lymph nodes can be divided into three broad groups: nodes of the thoracic wall (pink), pulmonary nodes (blue), and mediastinal nodes (green). For details of lymphatics of the mediastinum, see pp. 100–101.

Nerves of the Thoracic Cavity

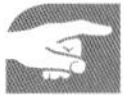

Thoracic innervation is mostly autonomic, arising from the paravertebral sympathetic trunks and parasympathetic vagus nerves. There are two exceptions: the phrenic nerves innervate the pericardium and diaphragm (p. 54), and the intercostal nerves innervate the thoracic wall (p. 58).

Fig. 6.11 **Nerves in the thorax**
Anterior view of opened thorax.

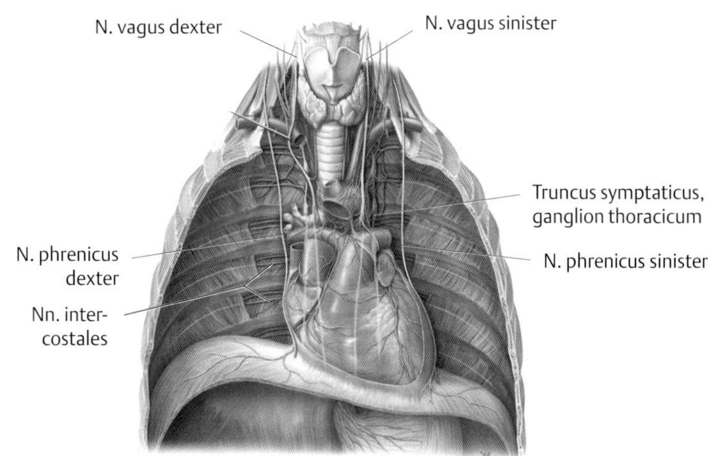
N. vagus dexter
N. vagus sinister
Truncus symptaticus, ganglion thoracicum
N. phrenicus dexter
N. phrenicus sinister
Nn. intercostales

A Thoracic innervation.

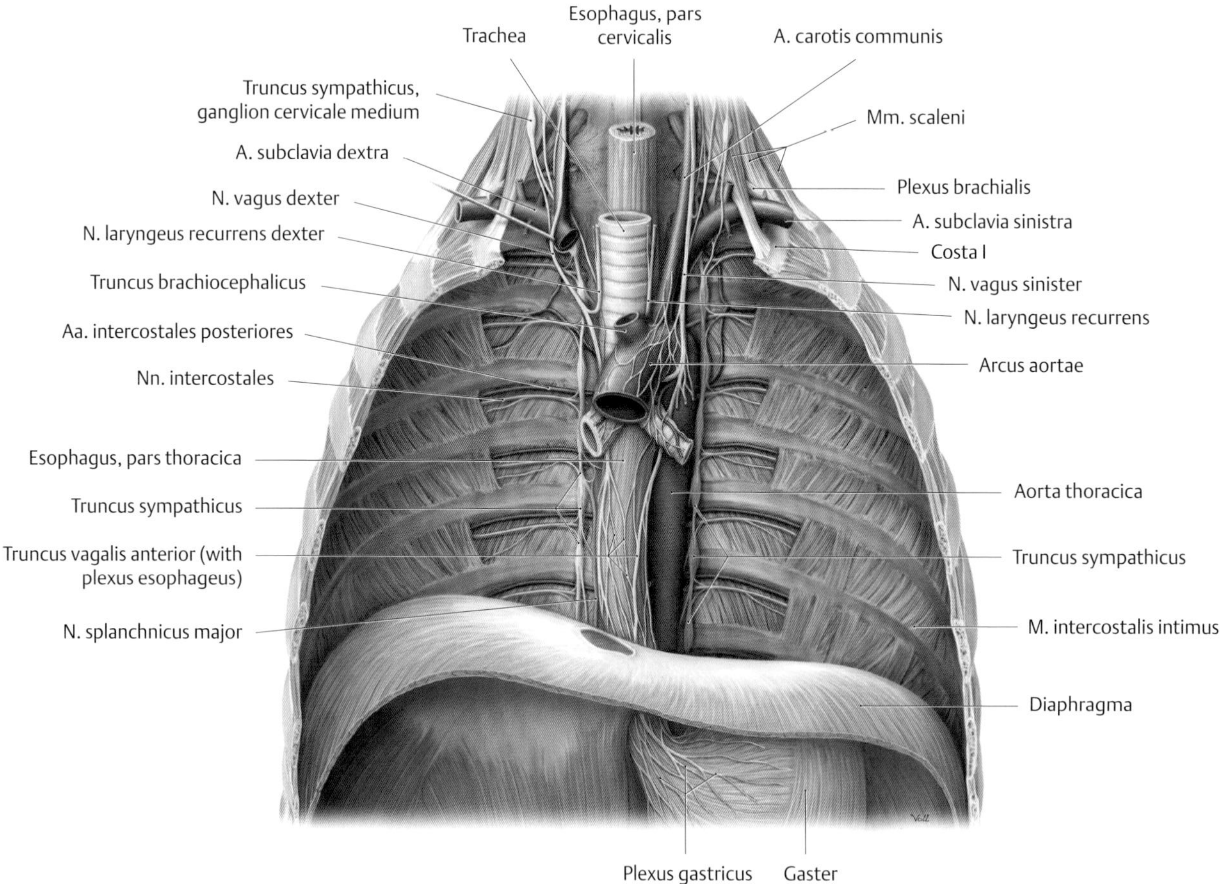
Trachea
Esophagus, pars cervicalis
A. carotis communis
Truncus sympathicus, ganglion cervicale medium
Mm. scaleni
A. subclavia dextra
Plexus brachialis
N. vagus dexter
A. subclavia sinistra
N. laryngeus recurrens dexter
Costa I
Truncus brachiocephalicus
N. vagus sinister
N. laryngeus recurrens
Aa. intercostales posteriores
Arcus aortae
Nn. intercostales
Esophagus, pars thoracica
Aorta thoracica
Truncus sympathicus
Truncus vagalis anterior (with plexus esophageus)
Truncus sympathicus
M. intercostalis intimus
N. splanchnicus major
Diaphragma
Plexus gastricus anterior
Gaster

B Nerves of the thorax in situ. *Note:* The recurrent laryngeal nerves have been slightly anteriorly retracted; normally, they occupy the groove between the trachea and the esophagus, making them vulnerable during thyroid gland surgery.

The autonomic nervous system innervates smooth muscle, cardiac muscle, and glands. It is subdivided into the sympathetic (red) and parasympathetic (blue) nervous systems, which together regulates blood flow, secretions, and organ function.

Fig. 6.12 Sympathetic and parasympathetic nervous systems in the thorax

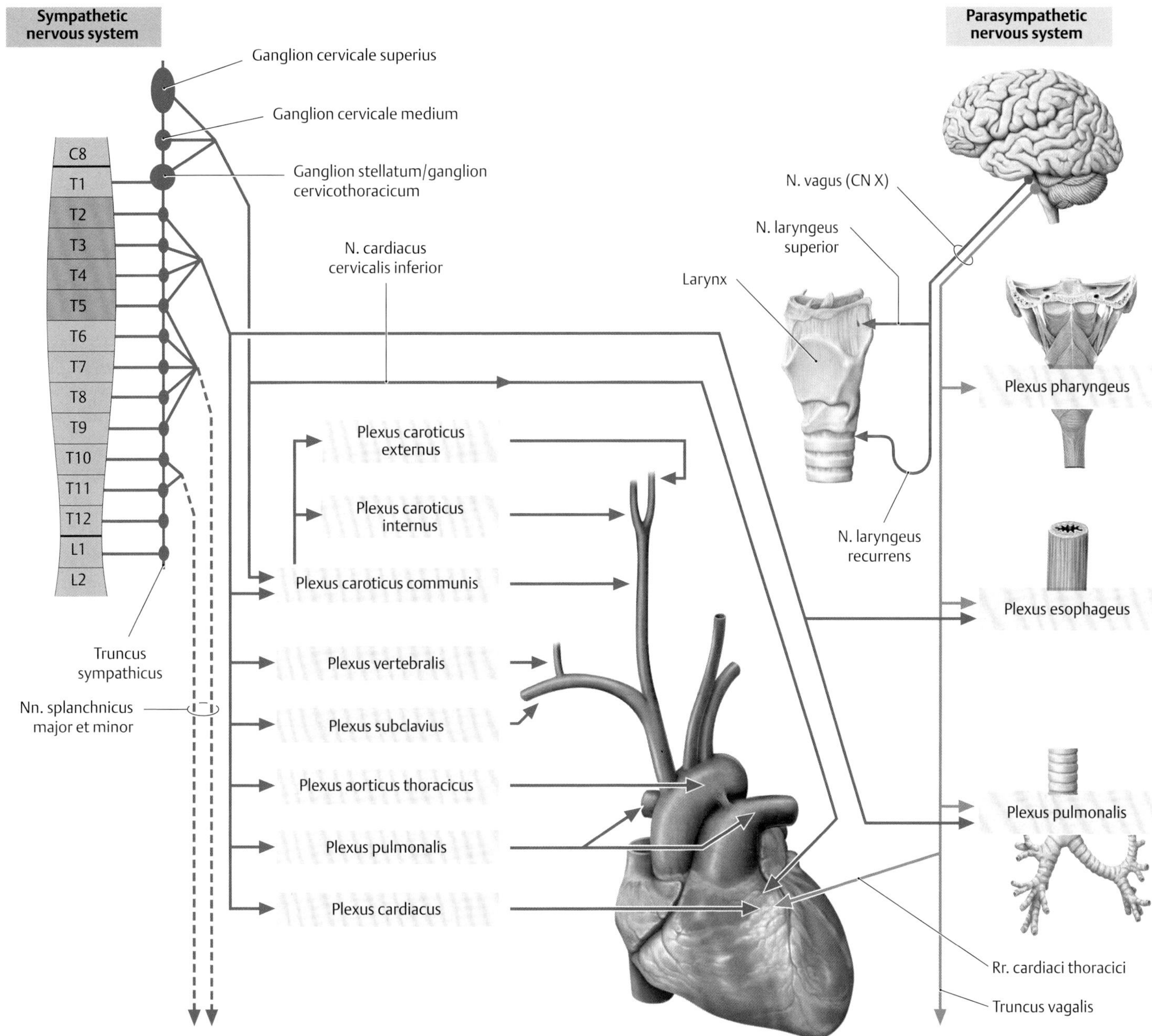
Sympathetic nervous system
Parasympathetic nervous system
Ganglion cervicale superius
Ganglion cervicale medium
Ganglion stellatum/ganglion cervicothoracicum
C8
T1
T2
T3
T4
T5
T6
T7
T8
T9
T10
T11
T12
L1
L2
N. cardiacus cervicalis inferior
Truncus sympathicus
Nn. splanchnicus major et minor
Plexus caroticus externus
Plexus caroticus internus
Plexus caroticus communis
Plexus vertebralis
Plexus subclavius
Plexus aorticus thoracicus
Plexus pulmonalis
Plexus cardiacus
N. vagus (CN X)
N. laryngeus superior
Larynx
N. laryngeus recurrens
Plexus pharyngeus
Plexus esophageus
Plexus pulmonalis
Rr. cardiaci thoracici
Truncus vagalis

Table 6.4 Peripheral sympathetic nervous system

Origin of presynaptic fibers*	Ganglion cells	Course of postsynaptic fibers	Target
Spinal cord	Truncus sympathicus	Follow nn. intercostales	Blood vessels and glands in chest wall
		Accompany intrathoracic aa.	Visceral targets
		Gather in n. splanchnicus major and n. splanchnicus minor	Abdomen

*The axons of presynaptic neurons exit the spinal cord via the anterior roots and synapse with *post*synaptic neurons in the sympathetic ganglia.

Table 6.5 Peripheral parasympathetic nervous system

Origin of presynaptic fibers	Course of presynaptic motor axons*		Target
Brainstem	N. vagus (CN X)	Rr. cardiaci	Plexus cardiacus
		Rr. esophagei	Plexus esophageus
		Rr. tracheales	Trachea
		Rr. bronchiales	Plexus pulmonalis (bronchi, pulmonary vessels)

*The ganglion cells of the parasympathetic nervous system are scattered in microscopic groups in their target organs. The n. vagus thus carries the *pre*synaptic motor axons to these targets.
CN = cranial nerve.

Mediastinum: Overview

The mediastinum is the space in the thorax between the pleural sacs of the lungs. It is divided into two parts: superior and inferior. The inferior mediastinum is further divided into anterior, middle, and posterior portions.

Fig. 7.1 Divisions of the mediastinum

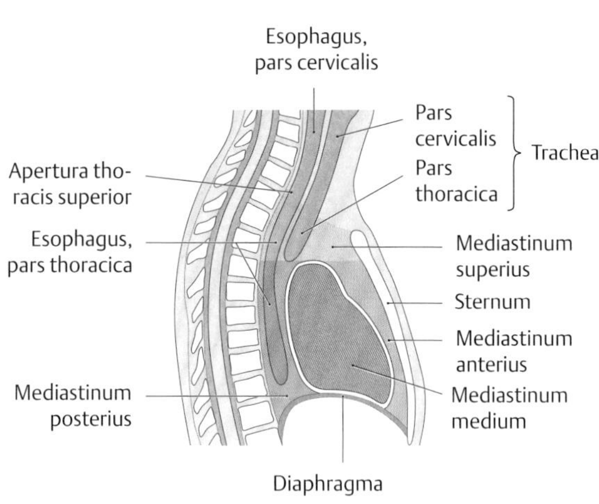
Esophagus, pars cervicalis
Pars cervicalis
Pars thoracica
Trachea
Apertura thoracis superior
Esophagus, pars thoracica
Mediastinum superius
Sternum
Mediastinum anterius
Mediastinum posterius
Mediastinum medium
Diaphragma

A Schematic.

Table 7.1 Contents of the mediastinum

	Mediastinum superius	Mediastinum inferius		
		Mediastinum anterius	*Mediastinum medium*	*Mediastinum posterius*
Organs	• Thymus • Trachea • Esophagus • Ductus thoracicus	• Thymus (in children, see Fig. 7.5)	• Heart • Pericardium	• Esophagus
Arteries	• Arcus aortae • Truncus brachiocephalicus • A. carotis communis sinistra • A. subclavia sinistra	• Smaller vessels	• Aorta ascendens • Truncus pulmonalis and aa. pulmonales • Aa. and vv. pericardiacophrenicae	• Aorta thoracica and branches • Ductus thoracicus
Veins and lymph vessels	• V. cava superior • Vv. brachiocephalicae • Ductus thoracicus	• Smaller vessels, lymphatics, and lymph nodes	• V. cava superior • V. azygos • Vv. pulmonales • Aa. and vv. pericardiacophrenicae	• V. azygos • V. hemiazygos • Ductus thoracicus
Nerves	• Nn. vagi • N. laryngeus recurrens sinister • Cardiac nerves • Nn. phrenici	• None	• Nn. phrenici	• Nn. vagi

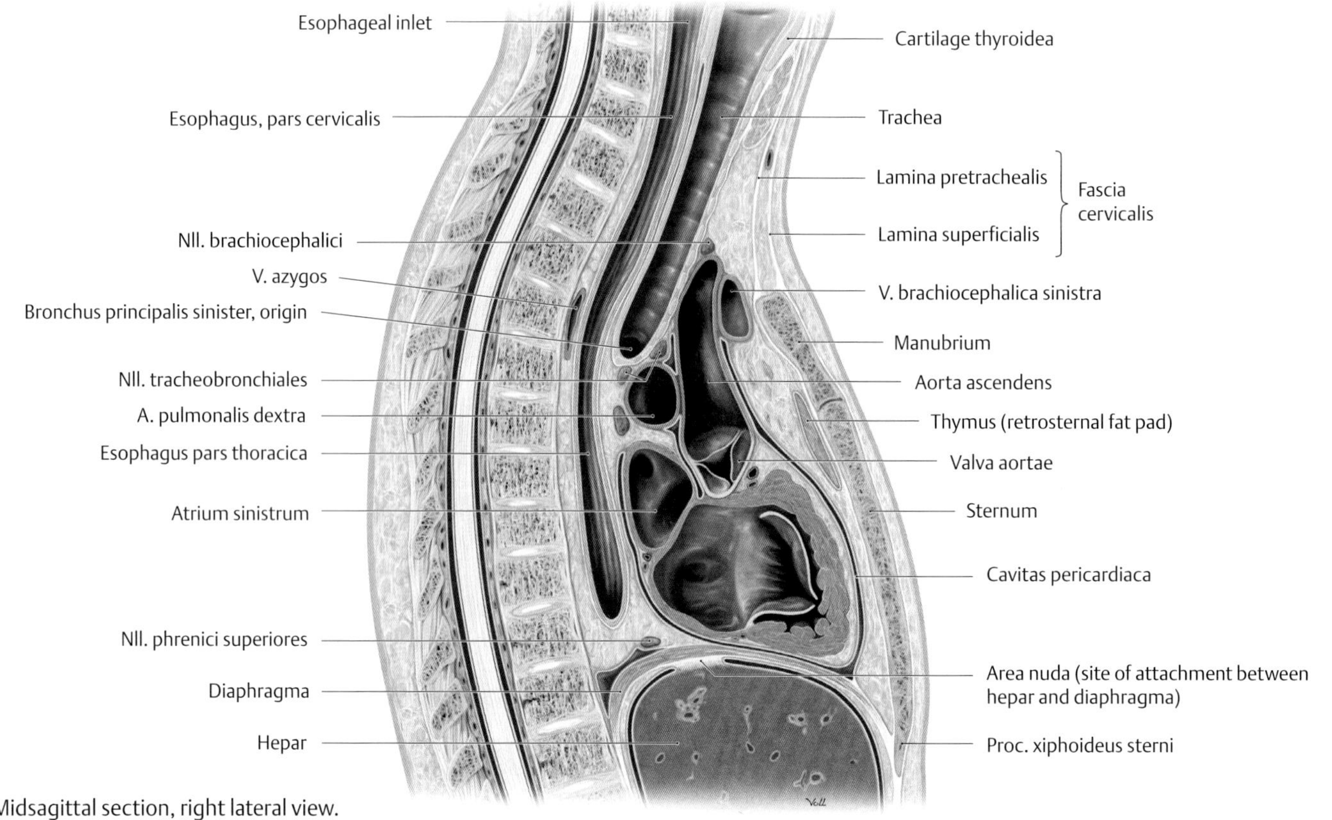
Esophageal inlet
Esophagus, pars cervicalis
Nll. brachiocephalici
V. azygos
Bronchus principalis sinister, origin
Nll. tracheobronchiales
A. pulmonalis dextra
Esophagus pars thoracica
Atrium sinistrum
Nll. phrenici superiores
Diaphragma
Hepar
Cartilage thyroidea
Trachea
Lamina pretrachealis
Lamina superficialis
Fascia cervicalis
V. brachiocephalica sinistra
Manubrium
Aorta ascendens
Thymus (retrosternal fat pad)
Valva aortae
Sternum
Cavitas pericardiaca
Area nuda (site of attachment between hepar and diaphragma)
Proc. xiphoideus sterni

B Midsagittal section, right lateral view.

Fig. 7.2 Contents of the mediastinum

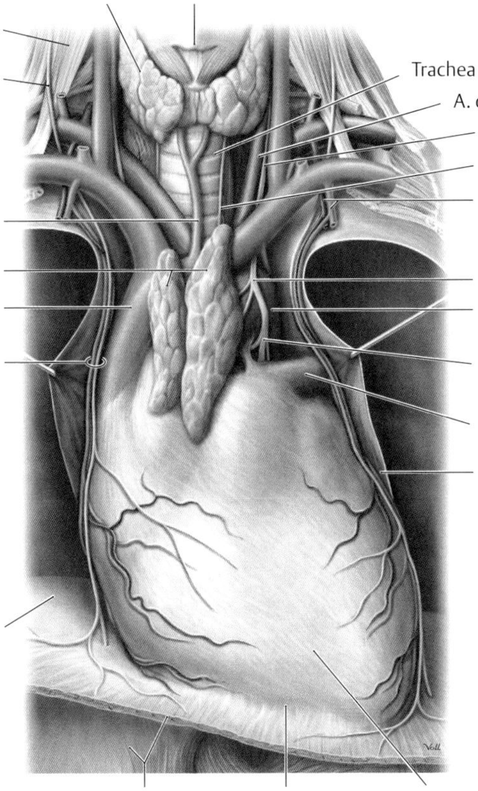

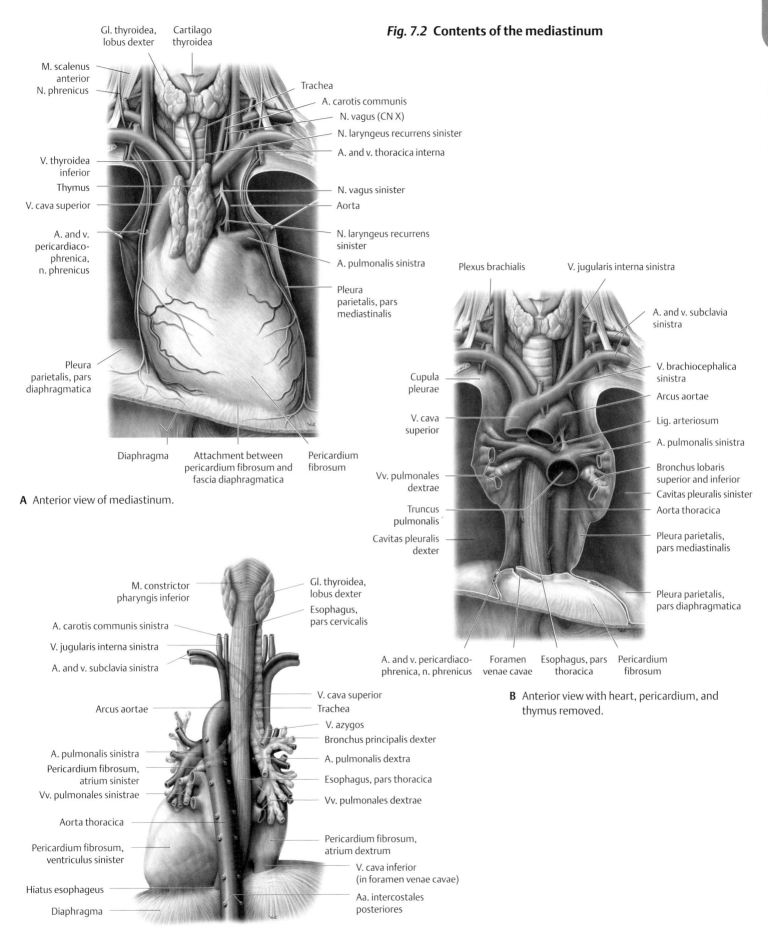

Gl. thyroidea, lobus dexter
Cartilago thyroidea
M. scalenus anterior
N. phrenicus
Trachea
A. carotis communis
N. vagus (CN X)
N. laryngeus recurrens sinister
A. and v. thoracica interna
V. thyroidea inferior
Thymus
V. cava superior
N. vagus sinister
Aorta
A. and v. pericardiaco-phrenica, n. phrenicus
N. laryngeus recurrens sinister
A. pulmonalis sinistra
Pleura parietalis, pars mediastinalis
Pleura parietalis, pars diaphragmatica
Diaphragma
Attachment between pericardium fibrosum and fascia diaphragmatica
Pericardium fibrosum

A Anterior view of mediastinum.

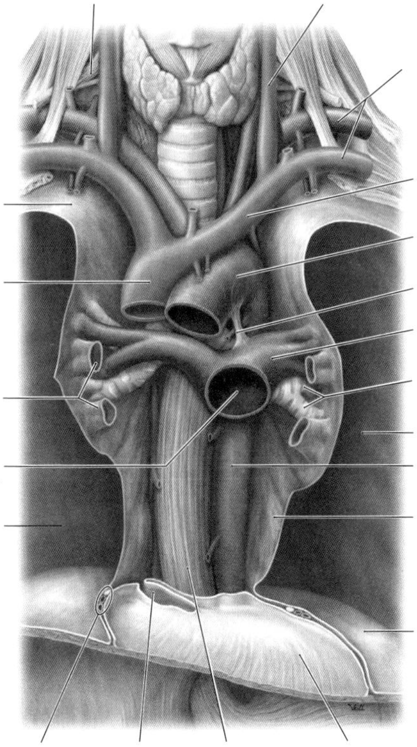

Plexus brachialis
V. jugularis interna sinistra
A. and v. subclavia sinistra
Cupula pleurae
V. brachiocephalica sinistra
Arcus aortae
V. cava superior
Lig. arteriosum
A. pulmonalis sinistra
Bronchus lobaris superior and inferior
Vv. pulmonales dextrae
Cavitas pleuralis sinister
Truncus pulmonalis
Aorta thoracica
Cavitas pleuralis dexter
Pleura parietalis, pars mediastinalis
Pleura parietalis, pars diaphragmatica
A. and v. pericardiaco-phrenica, n. phrenicus
Foramen venae cavae
Esophagus, pars thoracica
Pericardium fibrosum

B Anterior view with heart, pericardium, and thymus removed.

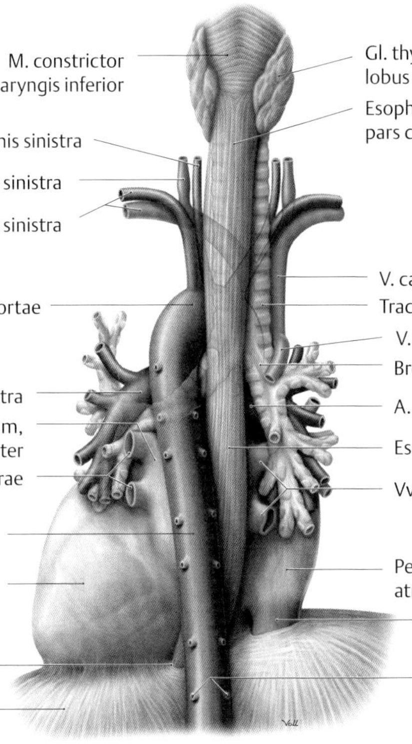

M. constrictor pharyngis inferior
Gl. thyroidea, lobus dexter
Esophagus, pars cervicalis
A. carotis communis sinistra
V. jugularis interna sinistra
A. and v. subclavia sinistra
V. cava superior
Arcus aortae
Trachea
V. azygos
Bronchus principalis dexter
A. pulmonalis sinistra
A. pulmonalis dextra
Pericardium fibrosum, atrium sinister
Esophagus, pars thoracica
Vv. pulmonales sinistrae
Vv. pulmonales dextrae
Aorta thoracica
Pericardium fibrosum, atrium dextrum
Pericardium fibrosum, ventriculus sinister
V. cava inferior (in foramen venae cavae)
Hiatus esophageus
Aa. intercostales posteriores
Diaphragma

C Posterior view.

Mediastinum: Structures

Fig. 7.3 Mediastinum

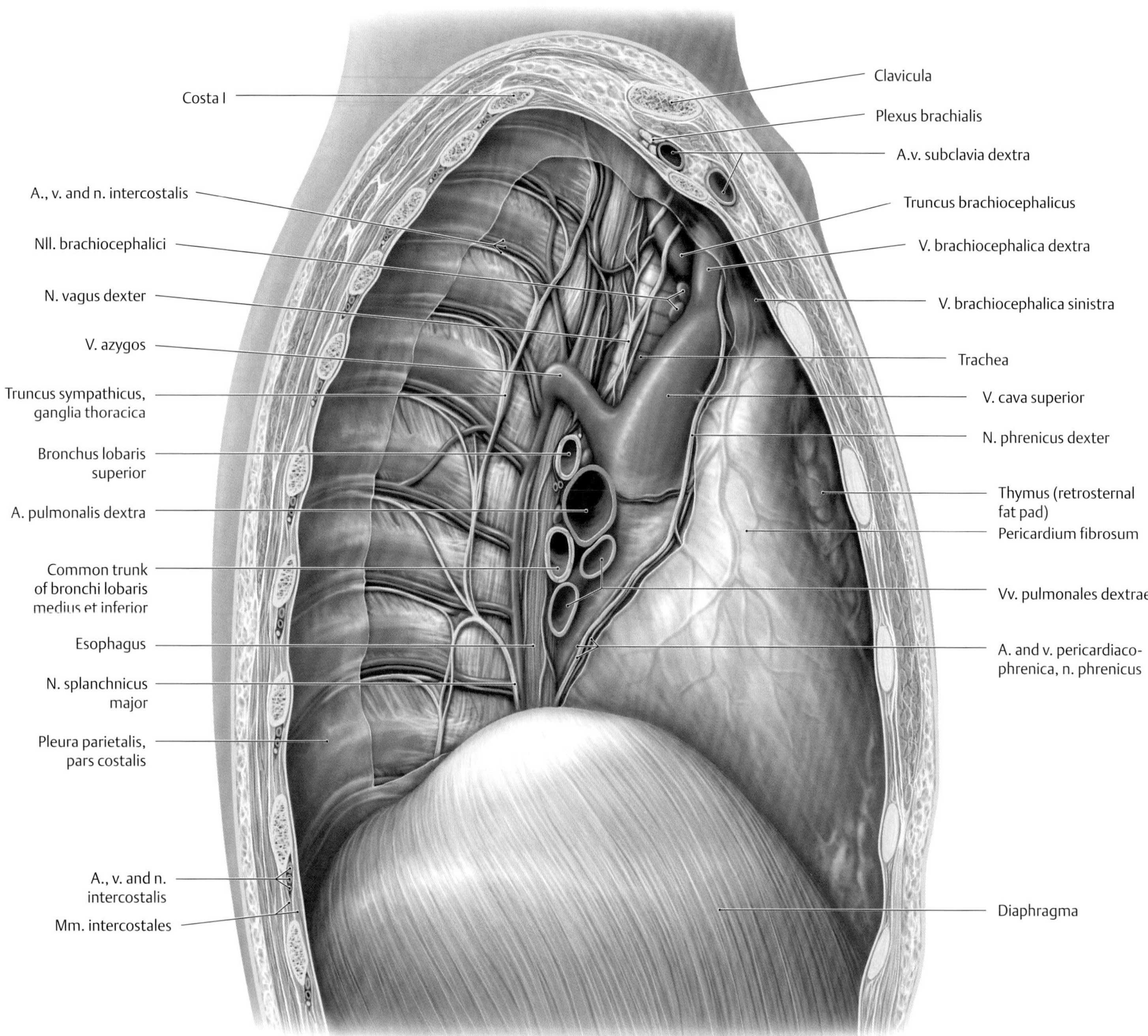

Costa I
A., v. and n. intercostalis
Nll. brachiocephalici
N. vagus dexter
V. azygos
Truncus sympathicus, ganglia thoracica
Bronchus lobaris superior
A. pulmonalis dextra
Common trunk of bronchi lobaris medius et inferior
Esophagus
N. splanchnicus major
Pleura parietalis, pars costalis
A., v. and n. intercostalis
Mm. intercostales
Clavicula
Plexus brachialis
A.v. subclavia dextra
Truncus brachiocephalicus
V. brachiocephalica dextra
V. brachiocephalica sinistra
Trachea
V. cava superior
N. phrenicus dexter
Thymus (retrosternal fat pad)
Pericardium fibrosum
Vv. pulmonales dextrae
A. and v. pericardiaco-phrenica, n. phrenicus
Diaphragma

A Right lateral view, parasagittal section. Note the many structures passing between the superior and inferior (middle and posterior) mediastinum.

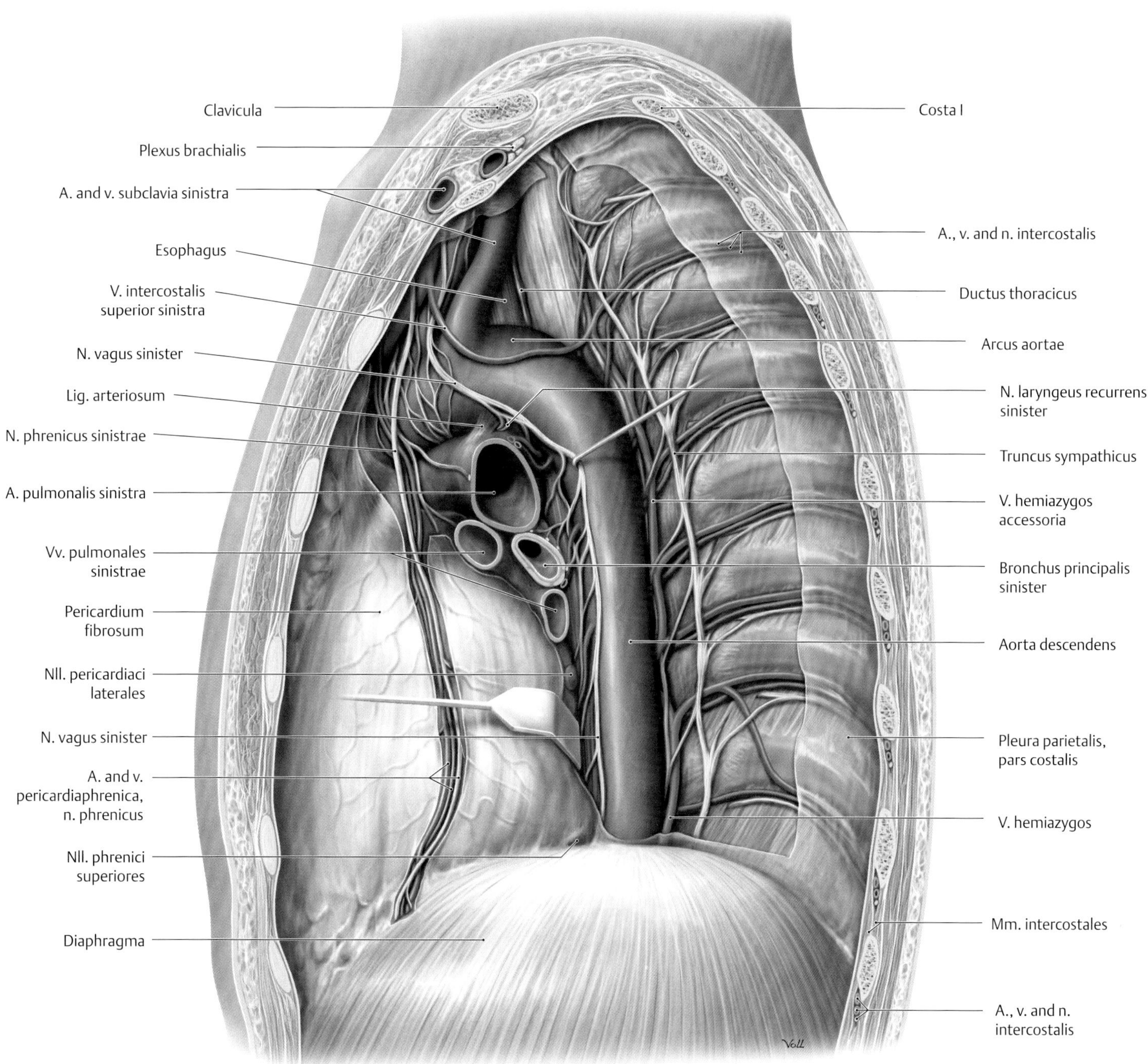
Clavicula
Plexus brachialis
A. and v. subclavia sinistra
Esophagus
V. intercostalis superior sinistra
N. vagus sinister
Lig. arteriosum
N. phrenicus sinistrae
A. pulmonalis sinistra
Vv. pulmonales sinistrae
Pericardium fibrosum
Nll. pericardiaci laterales
N. vagus sinister
A. and v. pericardiaphrenica, n. phrenicus
Nll. phrenici superiores
Diaphragma
Costa I
A., v. and n. intercostalis
Ductus thoracicus
Arcus aortae
N. laryngeus recurrens sinister
Truncus sympathicus
V. hemiazygos accessoria
Bronchus principalis sinister
Aorta descendens
Pleura parietalis, pars costalis
V. hemiazygos
Mm. intercostales
A., v. and n. intercostalis

B Left lateral view, parasagittal section. *Removed:* Left lung and pleura parietale. *Revealed:* Posterior mediastinal structures.

Thymus & Pericardium

Fig. 7.4 Thymus and pericardium in situ
Anterior view of coronal section. The thymus lies in the superior mediastinum.

V. jugularis interna
Gl. thyroidea
V. thyroidea inferior
N. laryngeus recurrens sinister
N. vagus (CN X)
A. and v. subclavia
N. phrenicus
A. and v. thoracica interna
V. cava superior
Thymus
A. and v. pericardiacophrenica, n. phrenicus
Pulmo dexter
Pleura parietalis, pars diaphragmatica
Pleura parietalis, pars mediastinalis
Pericardium fibrosum

Fig. 7.5 Thymus
Anterior view of opened thorax of a 2-year-old child. The thymus is well developed at this age, extending inferiorly into the anterior mediastinum (compare with Fig. 7.4). The thymus grows throughout childhood; at puberty, high levels of circulating sex hormones cause the thymus to atrophy.

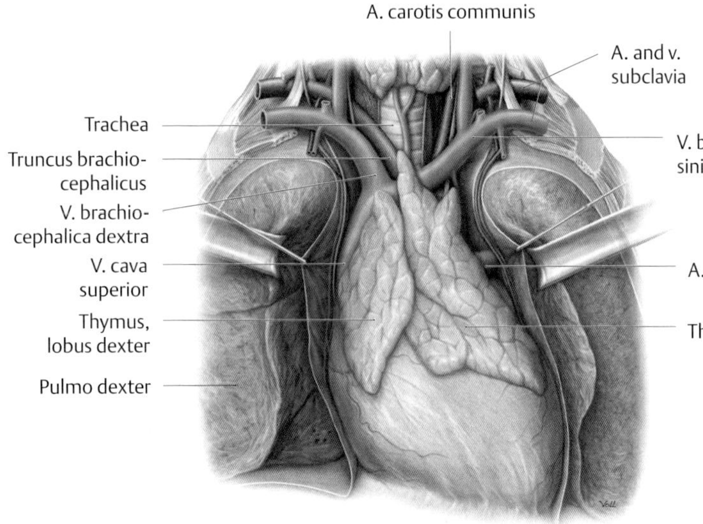
A. carotis communis
A. and v. subclavia
Trachea
Truncus brachio-cephalicus
V. brachio-cephalica dextra
V. cava superior
Thymus, lobus dexter
Pulmo dexter
V. brachiocephalica sinistra
A. pulmonalis sinistra
Thymus, lobus sin

Fig. 7.6 Pericardium
Anterior view of opened thorax with flaps of pericardium fibrosum reflected.

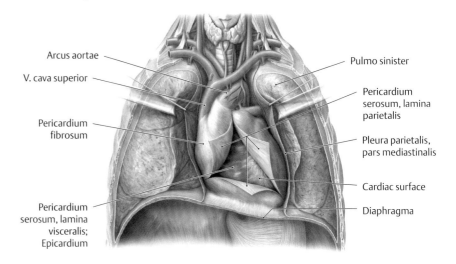

Arcus aortae
V. cava superior
Pericardium fibrosum
Pericardium serosum, lamina visceralis; Epicardium
Pulmo sinister
Pericardium serosum, lamina parietalis
Pleura parietalis, pars mediastinalis
Cardiac surface
Diaphragma

Fig. 7.7 Reflections of pericardium serosum

Anterior view. The lamina parietalis and lamina visceralis (epicardium) of the pericardium serosum are continuous with one another around the great vessels of the heart. The passage between the arterial- and venous-associated reflections is the sinus transversus pericardii (see **B**).

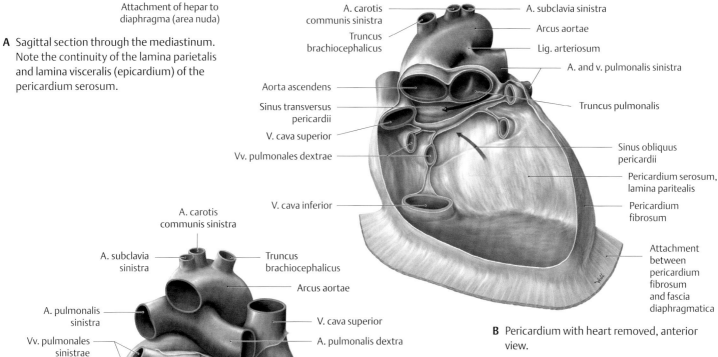

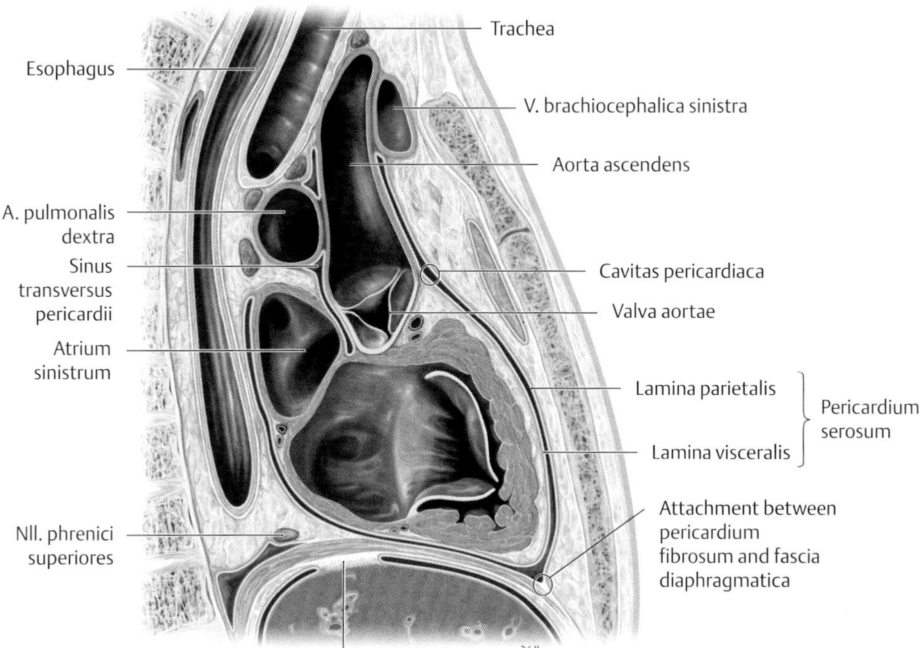
Trachea
Esophagus
V. brachiocephalica sinistra
Aorta ascendens
A. pulmonalis dextra
Sinus transversus pericardii
Cavitas pericardiaca
Valva aortae
Atrium sinistrum
Lamina parietalis
Lamina visceralis
Pericardium serosum
Attachment between pericardium fibrosum and fascia diaphragmatica
Nll. phrenici superiores
Attachment of hepar to diaphragma (area nuda)

A Sagittal section through the mediastinum. Note the continuity of the lamina parietalis and lamina visceralis (epicardium) of the pericardium serosum.

A. carotis communis sinistra
A. subclavia sinistra
Arcus aortae
Truncus brachiocephalicus
Lig. arteriosum
A. and v. pulmonalis sinistra
Aorta ascendens
Truncus pulmonalis
Sinus transversus pericardii
V. cava superior
Sinus obliquus pericardii
Vv. pulmonales dextrae
Pericardium serosum, lamina paritealis
V. cava inferior
Pericardium fibrosum
Attachment between pericardium fibrosum and fascia diaphragmatica

B Pericardium with heart removed, anterior view.

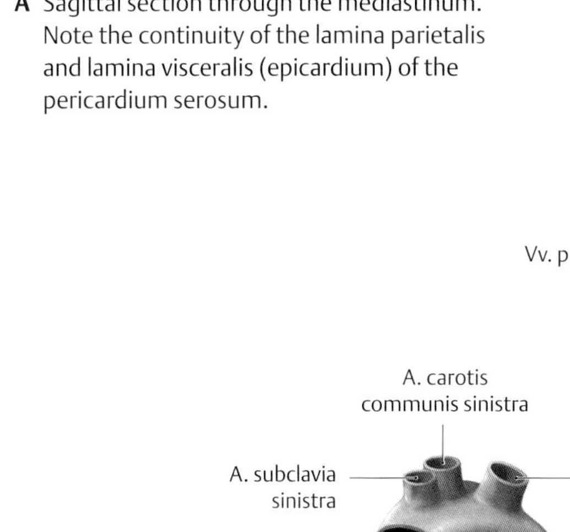
A. carotis communis sinistra
A. subclavia sinistra
Truncus brachiocephalicus
Arcus aortae
A. pulmonalis sinistra
V. cava superior
Vv. pulmonales sinistrae
A. pulmonalis dextra
Auricula sinistra
Vv. pulmonales dextrae
Atrium sinistrum
Atrium dextrum
Ventriculus sinister
Pericardium serosum, lamina visceralis
Reflected edge (continuous with pericardium serosum, lamina parietalis)
Sinus coronarius
V. cava inferior

C Heart removed from pericardium fibrosum, posterior view. Note the reflection of the epicardium (cut edges).

Heart in Situ

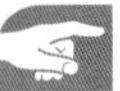

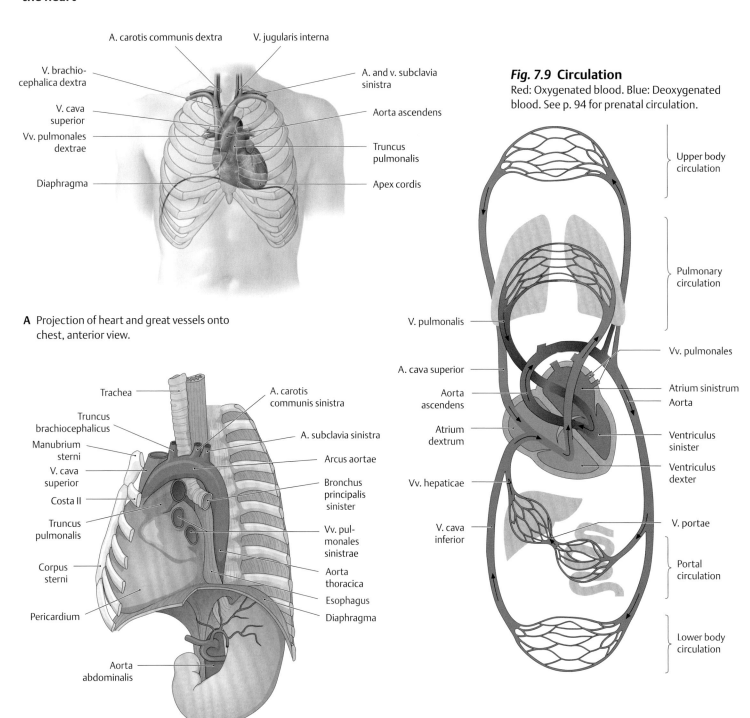

The heart is located posterior to the sternum in the middle portion of the inferior mediastinum. The heart projects into the left side of the thoracic cavity.

Fig. 7.8 Topographical relations of the heart

A. carotis communis dextra
V. jugularis interna
V. brachio-cephalica dextra
A. and v. subclavia sinistra
V. cava superior
Aorta ascendens
Vv. pulmonales dextrae
Truncus pulmonalis
Diaphragma
Apex cordis

A Projection of heart and great vessels onto chest, anterior view.

Trachea
A. carotis communis sinistra
Truncus brachiocephalicus
Manubrium sterni
A. subclavia sinistra
V. cava superior
Arcus aortae
Costa II
Bronchus principalis sinister
Truncus pulmonalis
Vv. pulmonales sinistrae
Corpus sterni
Aorta thoracica
Esophagus
Pericardium
Diaphragma
Aorta abdominalis

B Left lateral view.

Fig. 7.9 Circulation

Red: Oxygenated blood. Blue: Deoxygenated blood. See p. 94 for prenatal circulation.

Upper body circulation
Pulmonary circulation
V. pulmonalis
Vv. pulmonales
A. cava superior
Atrium sinistrum
Aorta ascendens
Aorta
Atrium dextrum
Ventriculus sinister
Ventriculus dexter
Vv. hepaticae
V. portae
V. cava inferior
Portal circulation
Lower body circulation

Fig. 7.10 **Heart in situ**
Anterior view.

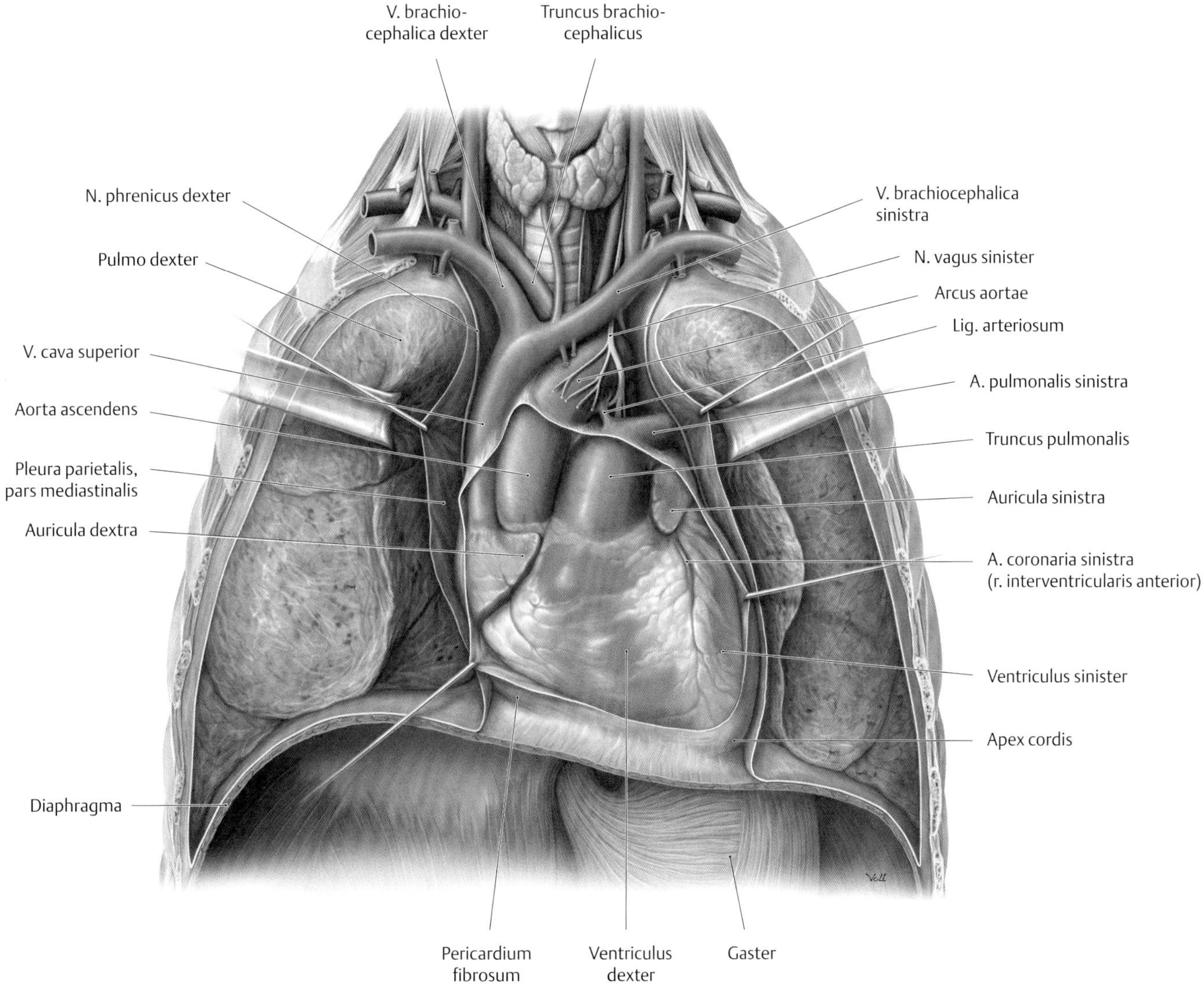
V. brachio-
cephalica dexter
Truncus brachio-
cephalicus
N. phrenicus dexter
Pulmo dexter
V. cava superior
Aorta ascendens
Pleura parietalis,
pars mediastinalis
Auricula dextra
Diaphragma
V. brachiocephalica
sinistra
N. vagus sinister
Arcus aortae
Lig. arteriosum
A. pulmonalis sinistra
Truncus pulmonalis
Auricula sinistra
A. coronaria sinistra
(r. interventricularis anterior)
Ventriculus sinister
Apex cordis
Pericardium
fibrosum
Ventriculus
dexter
Gaster

Heart: Surfaces & Chambers

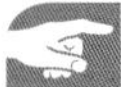

Note the reflection of lamina visceralis (epicardium) to become lamina parietalis of the pericardium serosum.

Fig. 7.11 **Surfaces of the heart**
The heart has three surfaces: anterior (facies sternocostalis), posterior (basis cordis), and inferior (facies diaphragmatica).

A. subclavia sinistra
A. carotis communis sinistra
Arcus aortae
Lig. arteriosum
Truncus brachio-cephalicus
A. pulmonalis sinistra
A. pulmonalis dextra
Vv. pulmonales sinistrae
V. cava superior
Truncus pulmonalis
Aorta ascendens
Auricula sinistra
Auricula dextra
Atrium dextrum
Pericardium (reflected edge)
Sulcus coronarius
Sulcus inter-ventricularis anterior
Ventriculus dexter
Ventriculus sinister
V. cava inferior
Apex cordis

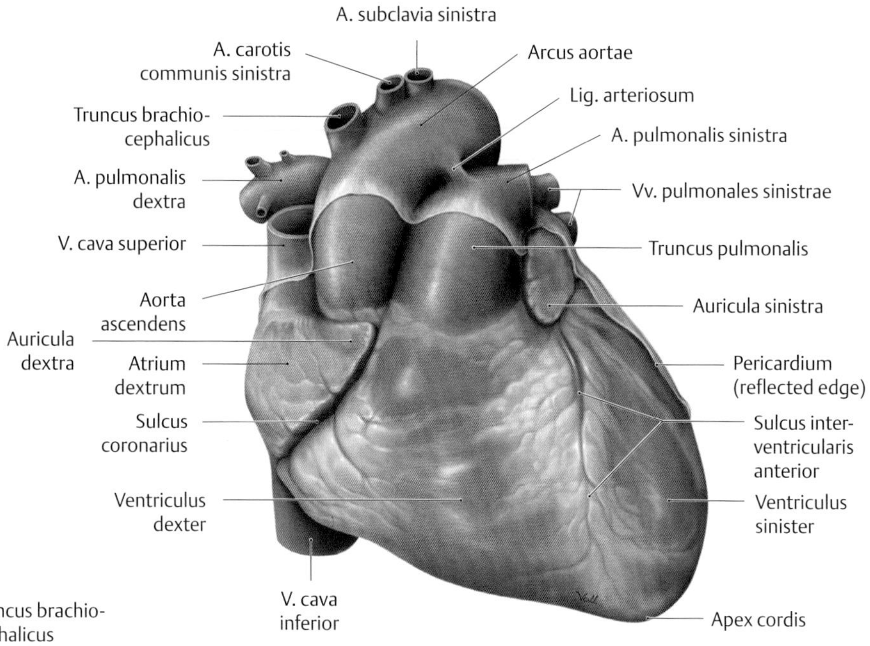

A Anterior surface (facies sternocostalis).

A. carotis communis sinistra
A. subclavia sinistra
Truncus brachio-cephalicus
Arcus aortae
A. pulmonalis sinistra
V. cava superior
Vv. pulmonales sinistrae
A. pulmonalis dextra
Auricula sinistra
Vv. pulmonales dextrae
Atrium sinistrum
Atrium dextrum
Ventriculus sinister
Pericardium (reflected edge)
Sinus coronarius
V. cava inferior

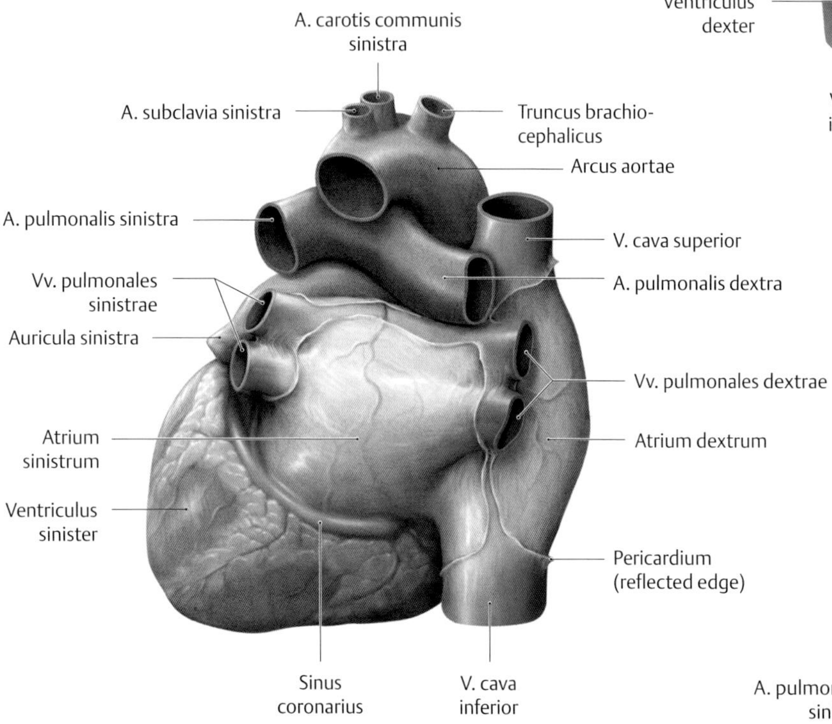

B Posterior surface (basis cordis).

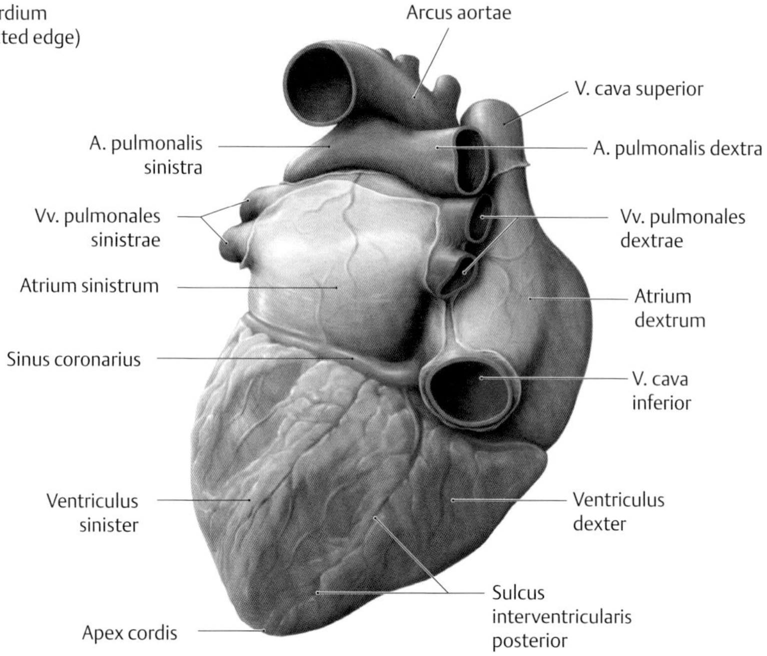

Arcus aortae
V. cava superior
A. pulmonalis sinistra
A. pulmonalis dextra
Vv. pulmonales sinistrae
Vv. pulmonales dextrae
Atrium sinistrum
Atrium dextrum
Sinus coronarius
V. cava inferior
Ventriculus sinister
Ventriculus dexter
Sulcus interventricularis posterior
Apex cordis

C Inferior surface (facies diaphragmatica).

Fig. 7.12 Chambers of the heart

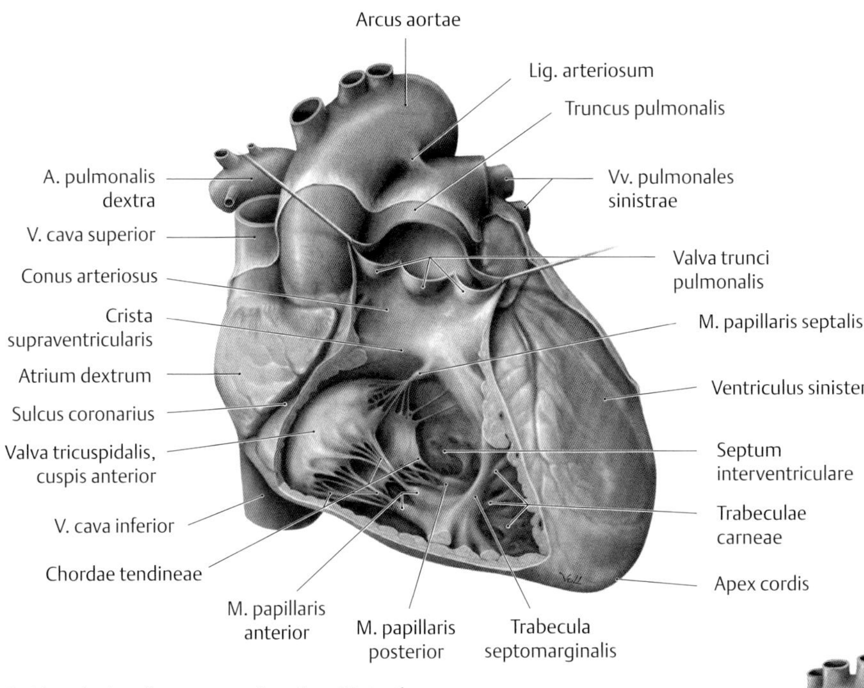
Arcus aortae
Lig. arteriosum
Truncus pulmonalis
A. pulmonalis dextra
Vv. pulmonales sinistrae
V. cava superior
Conus arteriosus
Valva trunci pulmonalis
Crista supraventricularis
M. papillaris septalis
Atrium dextrum
Ventriculus sinister
Sulcus coronarius
Valva tricuspidalis, cuspis anterior
Septum interventriculare
V. cava inferior
Trabeculae carneae
Chordae tendineae
Apex cordis
M. papillaris anterior
M. papillaris posterior
Trabecula septomarginalis

A Ventriculus dexter, anterior view. Note the crista supraventricularis, which marks the adult boundary between the embryonic ventricle and the bulbus cordis (now conus arteriosus).

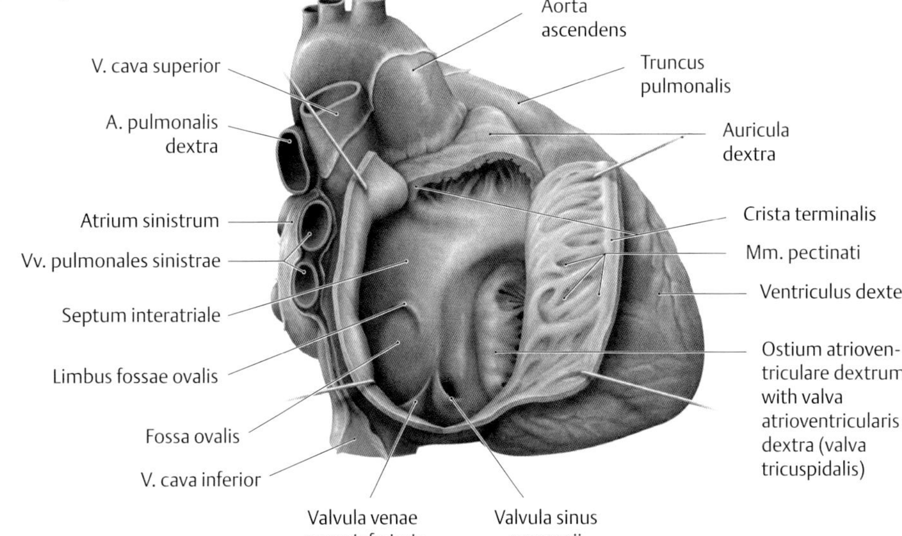
Aorta ascendens
V. cava superior
Truncus pulmonalis
A. pulmonalis dextra
Auricula dextra
Atrium sinistrum
Crista terminalis
Vv. pulmonales sinistrae
Mm. pectinati
Ventriculus dexter
Septum interatriale
Limbus fossae ovalis
Ostium atrioventriculare dextrum with valva atrioventricularis dextra (valva tricuspidalis)
Fossa ovalis
V. cava inferior
Valvula venae cavae inferioris
Valvula sinus coronarii

B Atrium dextrum, right lateral view.

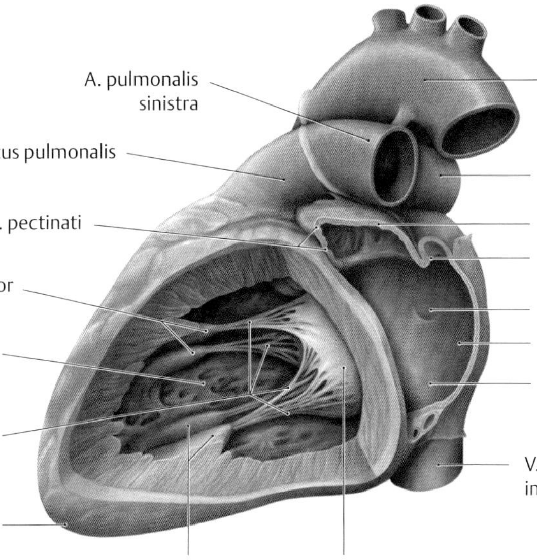

A. pulmonalis sinistra
Arcus aortae
Truncus pulmonalis
A. pulmonalis dextra
Mm. pectinati
Auricula sinistra
V. pulmonalis sinistra superior
M. papillaris anterior
Valvula foraminis ovalis
Atrium sinistrum
Trabeculae carneae of septum interventriculare
Septum interatriale
Chordae tendineae
V. cava inferior
Apex cordis
M. papillaris posterior
Valva mitralis

C Atrium sinister and ventriculus sinister, left lateral view. Note the irregular trabeculae carneae characteristic of the ventricular wall.

Heart: Valves

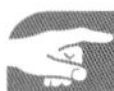

The cardiac valves are divided into two groups: semilunar and atrioventricular. The two semilunar valves (valva aortae and valva trunci pulmonalis) located at the base of the two great arteries of the heart regulate passage of blood from the ventricles to the aorta and truncus pulmonalis. The two valva atrioventricularis (sinistra and dextra) lie at the interface between the atria and ventricles.

***Fig. 7.13* Cardiac valves**
Plane of cardiac valves, superior view. *Removed:* Atria and great arteries.

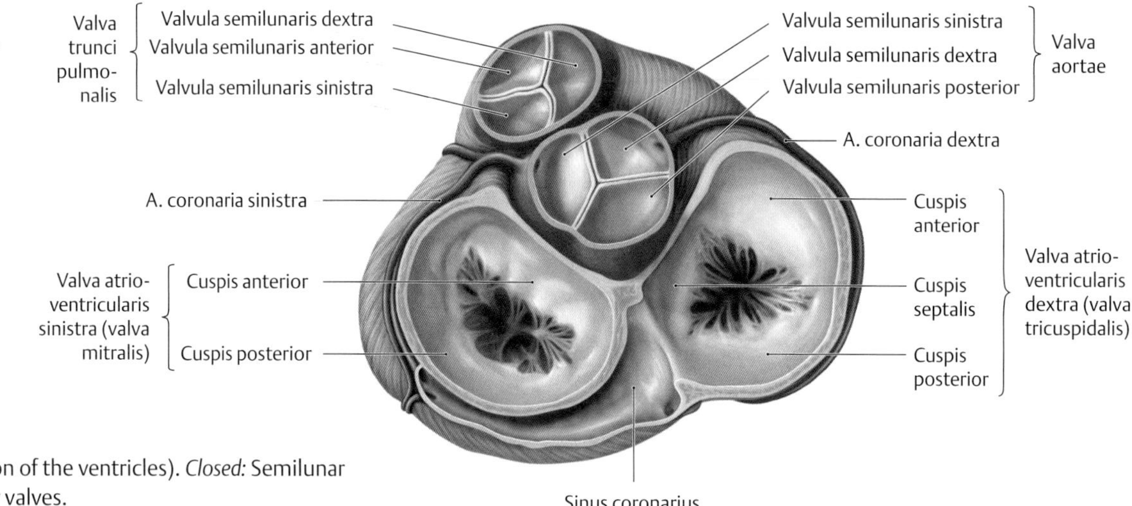
Valva trunci pulmonalis
Valvula semilunaris dextra
Valvula semilunaris anterior
Valvula semilunaris sinistra
Valvula semilunaris sinistra
Valvula semilunaris dextra
Valvula semilunaris posterior
Valva aortae
A. coronaria dextra
A. coronaria sinistra
Valva atrioventricularis sinistra (valva mitralis)
Cuspis anterior
Cuspis posterior
Cuspis anterior
Cuspis septalis
Cuspis posterior
Valva atrioventricularis dextra (valva tricuspidalis)
Sinus coronarius

A Ventricular diastole (relaxation of the ventricles). *Closed:* Semilunar valves. *Open:* Atrioventricular valves.

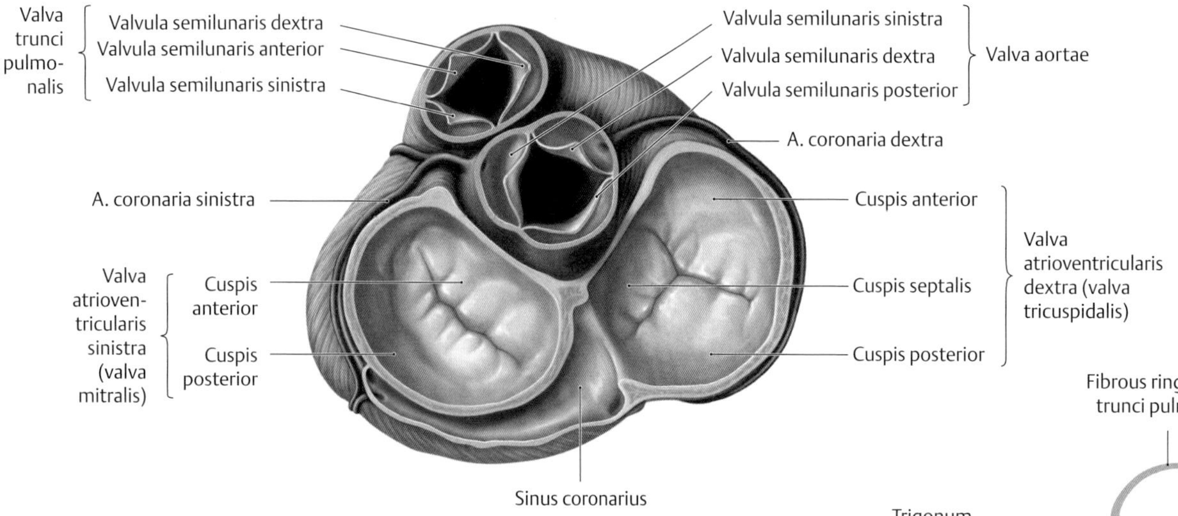

Valva trunci pulmonalis
Valvula semilunaris dextra
Valvula semilunaris anterior
Valvula semilunaris sinistra
Valvula semilunaris sinistra
Valvula semilunaris dextra
Valvula semilunaris posterior
Valva aortae
A. coronaria dextra
A. coronaria sinistra
Valva atrioventricularis sinistra (valva mitralis)
Cuspis anterior
Cuspis posterior
Cuspis anterior
Cuspis septalis
Cuspis posterior
Valva atrioventricularis dextra (valva tricuspidalis)
Sinus coronarius

B Ventricular systole (contraction of the ventricles). *Closed:* Valvae atrioventriculares. *Open:* Valva aortae and valva trunci pulmonalis.

Fibrous ring of valva trunci pulmonalis
Trigonum fibrosum sinister
Tendo infundibuli
Fibrous ring of valva aortae
Trigonum fibrosum dextrum
Anulus fibrosus sinister
Opening for the bundle of His
Anulus fibrosus dexter

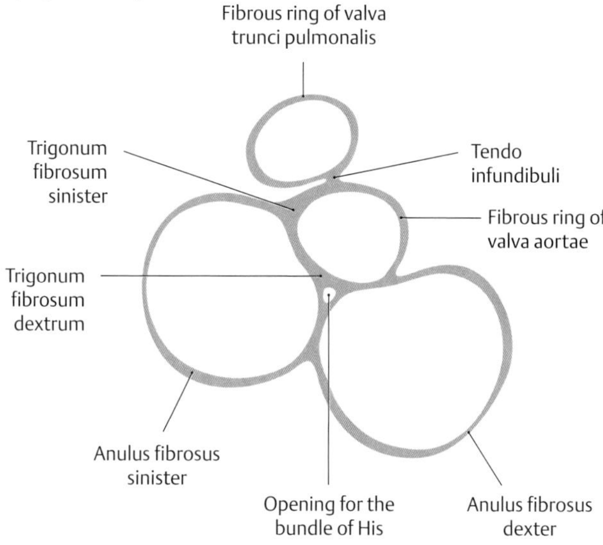

C Cardiac skeleton. The cardiac skeleton is formed by dense fibrous connective tissue. The anuli fibrosi (rings) and intervening trigonum fibrosum dextrum and sinister separate the atria from the ventricles. This provides mechanical stability, electrical insulation (see p. 90 for cardiac conduction system), and an attachment point for the cardiac muscles and valve cusps.

Fig. 7.14 Semilunar valves

Valves have been longitudinally sectioned and opened.

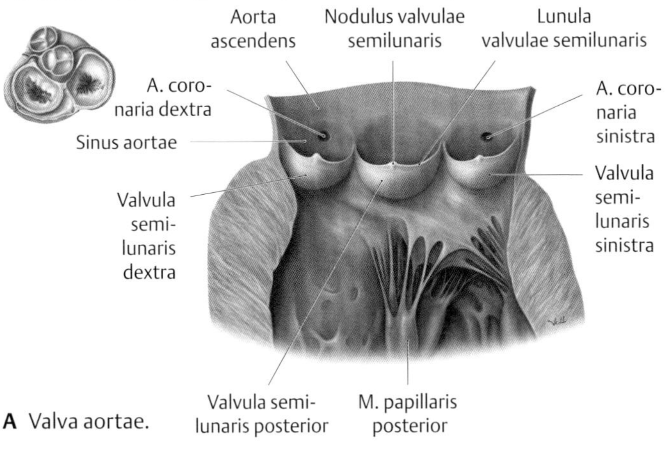
Aorta ascendens
Nodulus valvulae semilunaris
Lunula valvulae semilunaris
A. coronaria dextra
A. coronaria sinistra
Sinus aortae
Valvula semilunaris sinistra
Valvula semilunaris dextra
Valvula semilunaris posterior
M. papillaris posterior

A Valva aortae.

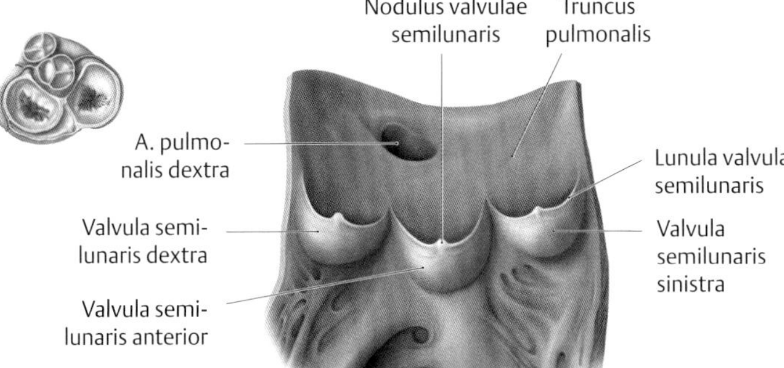
Nodulus valvulae semilunaris
Truncus pulmonalis
A. pulmonalis dextra
Lunula valvulae semilunaris
Valvula semilunaris dextra
Valvula semilunaris sinistra
Valvula semilunaris anterior

B Valva trunci pulmonalis.

Fig. 7.15 Atrioventricular valves

Anterior view during ventricular systole.

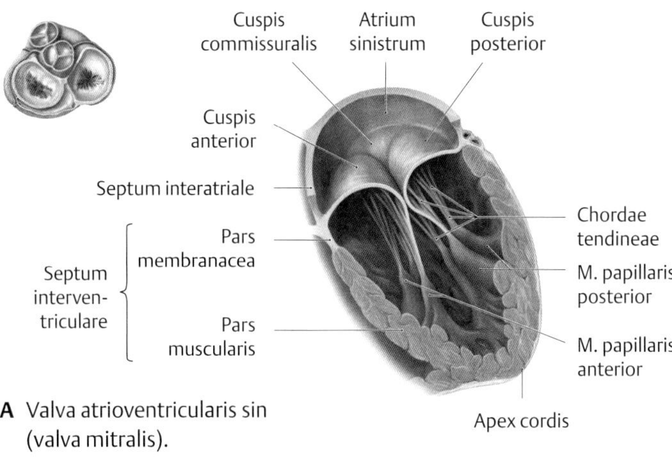
Cuspis commissuralis
Atrium sinistrum
Cuspis posterior
Cuspis anterior
Septum interatriale
Septum interventriculare
Pars membranacea
Pars muscularis
Chordae tendineae
M. papillaris posterior
M. papillaris anterior
Apex cordis

A Valva atrioventricularis sin (valva mitralis).

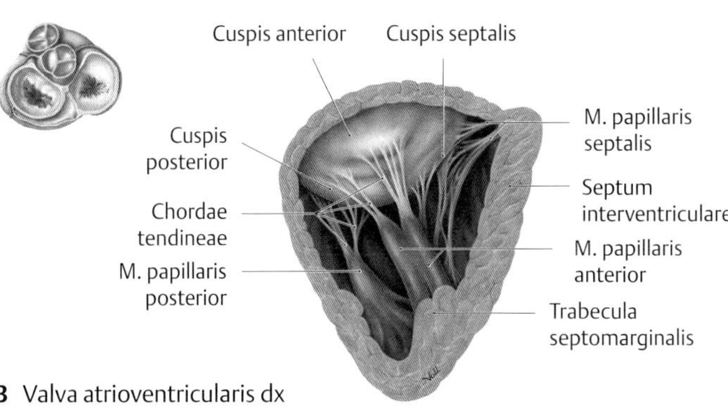
Cuspis anterior
Cuspis septalis
Cuspis posterior
M. papillaris septalis
Septum interventriculare
Chordae tendineae
M. papillaris anterior
M. papillaris posterior
Trabecula septomarginalis

B Valva atrioventricularis dx (valva tricuspidalis).

Clinical

Auscultation of the cardiac valves

Heart sounds, produced by closure of the semilunar and atrioventricular valves, are carried by the blood flowing through the valve. The resulting sounds are therefore best heard "downstream," at defined auscultation sites (dark circles). Valvular heart disease causes turbulent blood flow through the valve; this produces a murmur that may be detected in the colored regions.

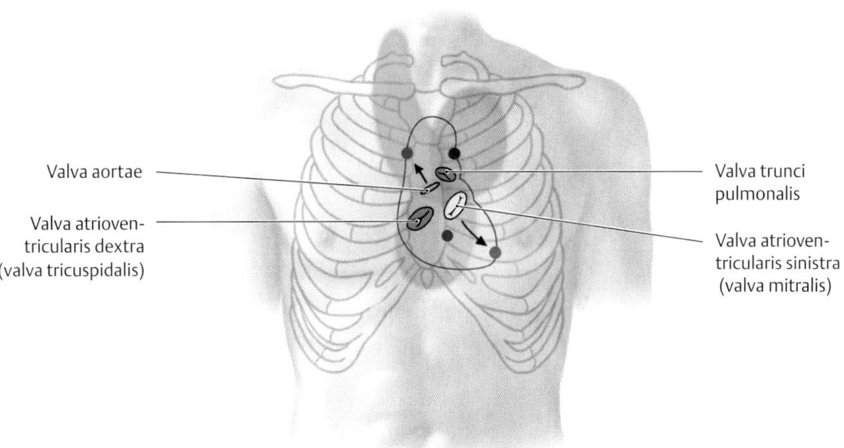
Valva aortae
Valva atrioventricularis dextra (valva tricuspidalis)
Valva trunci pulmonalis
Valva atrioventricularis sinistra (valva mitralis)

Table 7.2 Position and auscultation sites of cardiac valves

Valve	Anatomical projection	Auscultation site
Valva aortae	Left sternal border (at level of 3rd rib)	Right 2nd intercostal space (at sternal margin)
Valva trunci pulmonalis	Left sternal border (at level of 3rd costal cartilage)	Left 2nd intercostal space (at sternal margin)
Valva atrioventricularis sinistra (valva mitralis)	Left 4th/5th costal cartilage	Left 5th intercostal space (at midclavicular line) or apex cordis
Valva atrioventricular dextra (valva tricuspidalis)	Sternum (at level of 3rd costal cartilage)	Left 5th intercostal space (at sternal margin)

Arteries & Veins of the Heart

Fig. 7.16 Coronary arteries and cardiac veins

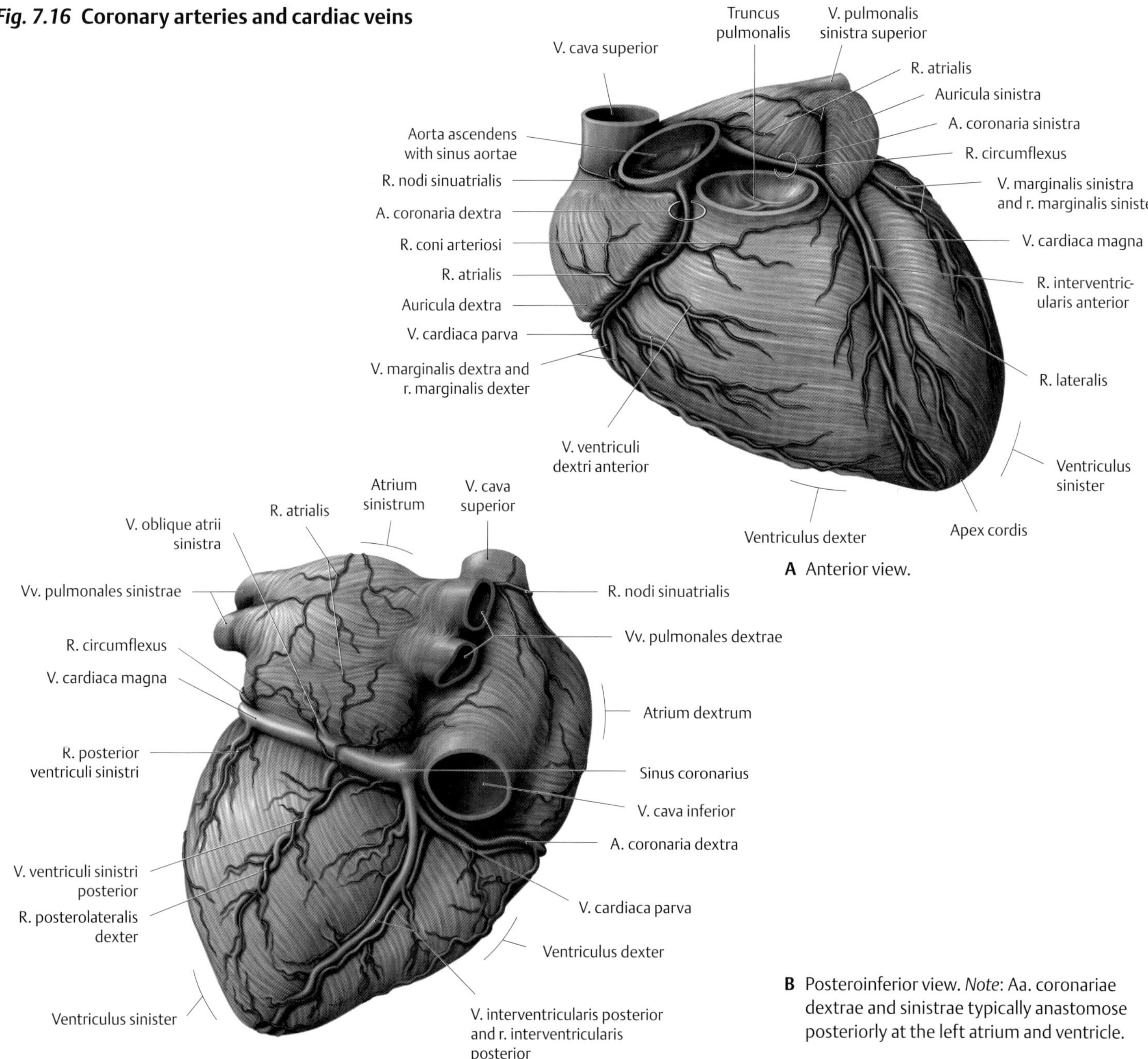

Truncus pulmonalis
V. pulmonalis sinistra superior
V. cava superior
R. atrialis
Auricula sinistra
A. coronaria sinistra
R. circumflexus
Aorta ascendens with sinus aortae
R. nodi sinuatrialis
V. marginalis sinistra and r. marginalis sinister
A. coronaria dextra
V. cardiaca magna
R. coni arteriosi
R. atrialis
R. interventricularis anterior
Auricula dextra
V. cardiaca parva
V. marginalis dextra and r. marginalis dexter
R. lateralis
V. ventriculi dextri anterior
Ventriculus sinister
Ventriculus dexter
Apex cordis
R. atrialis
Atrium sinistrum
V. cava superior
V. oblique atrii sinistra
Vv. pulmonales sinistrae
R. nodi sinuatrialis
Vv. pulmonales dextrae
R. circumflexus
V. cardiaca magna
Atrium dextrum
R. posterior ventriculi sinistri
Sinus coronarius
V. cava inferior
A. coronaria dextra
V. ventriculi sinistri posterior
R. posterolateralis dexter
V. cardiaca parva
Ventriculus dexter
Ventriculus sinister
V. interventricularis posterior and r. interventricularis posterior

A Anterior view.

B Posteroinferior view. *Note*: Aa. coronariae dextrae and sinistrae typically anastomose posteriorly at the left atrium and ventricle.

Table 7.3 Branches of the coronary arteries

A. coronaria sinistra	A. coronaria dextra
R. circumflexus • Rr. atriales • R. marginalis sinister • R. posterior ventriculi sinistra	R. nodi sinuatrialis R. coni arteriosi Rr. atriales R. marginalis dexter
R. interventricularis anterior (left anterior descending a., LAD) • R. coni arteriosi • R. lateralis • Rr. interventriculares septales	R. interventricularis posterior • Rr. interventriculares septales Rr. nodi atrioventricularis R. posterolateralis dexter

Table 7.4 Divisions of the cardiac veins

Vein	Tributaries	Drainage
Vv. cardiacae (cordis) anteriores (not shown)		Atrium dextrum
V. cardiaca (cordis) magna	V. interventricularis anterior	Sinus coronarius
	V. marginalis sinistra	
	V. obliqua atrii sinistra	
V. ventriculi sinistra posterior		
V. interventricularis posterior [v. cardiaca (cordis) media]		
Vv. cardiacae (cordis) minimae	Vv. ventricularis dextrae	
	V. marginalis dextra	

Fig. 7.17 Distribution of the coronary arteries

Anterior and posterior views of the heart, with superior views of transverse sections through the ventricles. The distribution of the coronary arteries differs from person to person. A. coronaria dextra and branches (green); a. coronaria sinistra and branches (red).

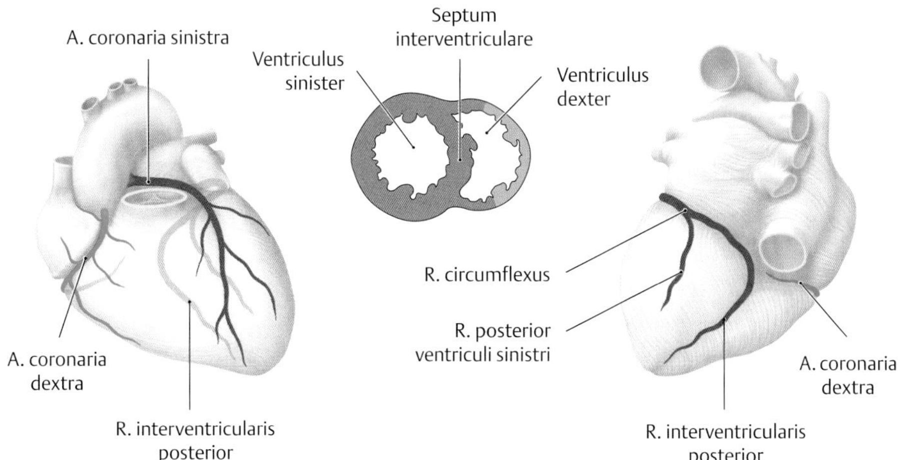
A. coronaria sinistra
Ventriculus sinister
Septum interventriculare
Ventriculus dexter
R. circumflexus
R. posterior ventriculi sinistri
A. coronaria dextra
R. interventricularis posterior
A. coronaria dextra
R. interventricularis posterior

A Left coronary dominance (~15%).

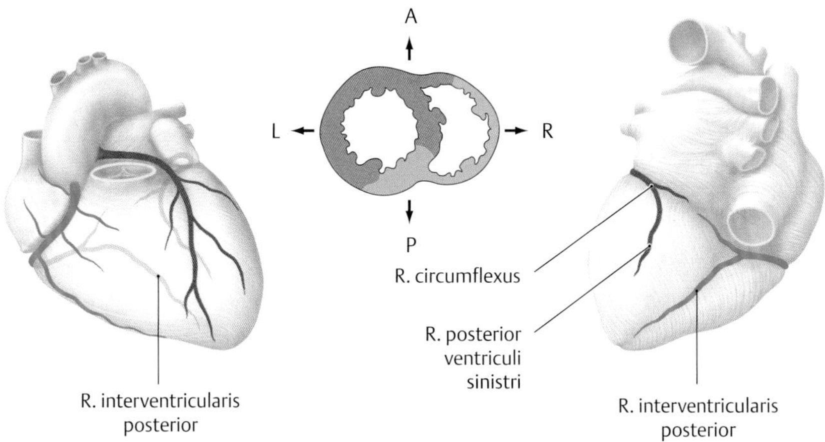
A
L
R
P
R. circumflexus
R. posterior ventriculi sinistri
R. interventricularis posterior
R. interventricularis posterior

B Balanced distribution (~70%).

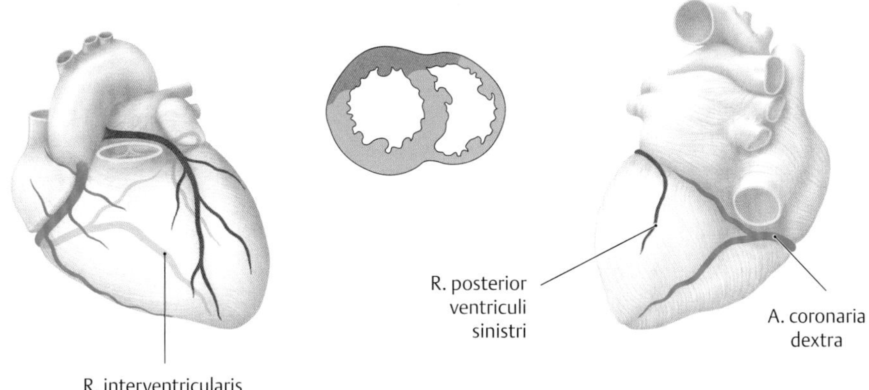
R. posterior ventriculi sinistri
A. coronaria dextra
R. interventricularis posterior

C Right coronary dominance (~15%).

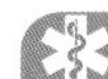

Clinical

Disturbed coronary blood flow

Although the coronary arteries are connected by structural anastomoses, they are end arteries from a functional standpoint. The most frequent cause of deficient blood flow is *atherosclerosis*, a narrowing of the coronary lumen due to plaque-like deposits on the vessel wall. When the decrease in luminal size (stenosis) reaches a critical point, coronary blood flow is restricted, causing chest pain (*angina pectoris*). Initially, this pain is induced by physical effort, but eventually it persists at rest, often radiating to characteristic sites (e.g., left arm, left side of head and neck). A myocardial infarction occurs when deficient blood supply causes myocardial tissue to die (necrosis). The location and extent of the infarction depends on the stenosed vessel (see **A–E**, after Heinecker).

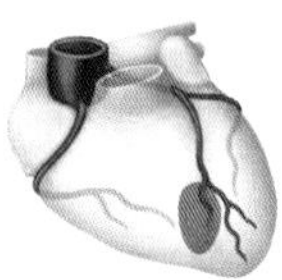

A Supra-apical anterior infarction.

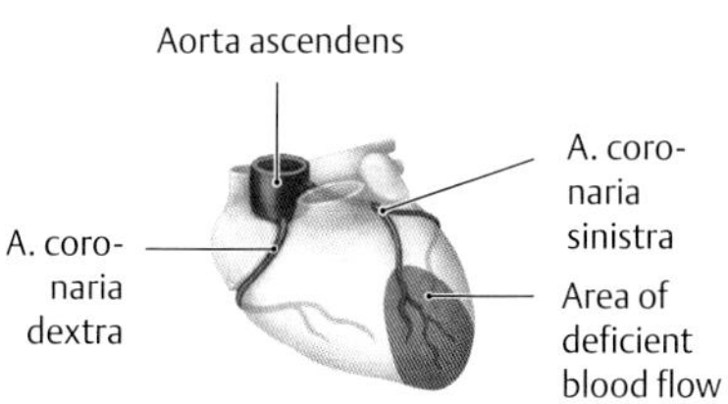
Aorta ascendens
A. coronaria dextra
A. coronaria sinistra
Area of deficient blood flow

B Apical anterior infarction.

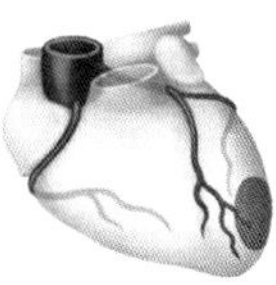

C Anterior lateral infarction.

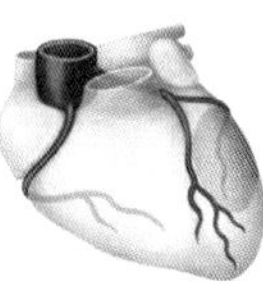

D Posterior lateral infarction.

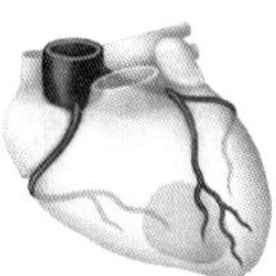

E Posterior infarction.

Conduction & Innervation of the Heart

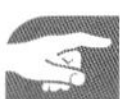

Contraction of cardiac muscle is modulated by the cardiac conduction system. This system of specialized myocardial cells generates and conducts excitatory impulses in the heart. The conduction system contains two nodes, both located in the atria: the nodus sinuatrialis (SA node), known as the pacemaker, and the nodus atrioventricularis (AV node).

Fig. 7.18 Cardiac conduction system

V. cava superior
Interatrial bundle
Nodus sinuatrialis
Anterior, middle and posterior internodal bundles
Nodus atrioventricularis
Crus dextrum
Fasciculus atrioventricularis
Crus sinistrum
Septum interventriculare

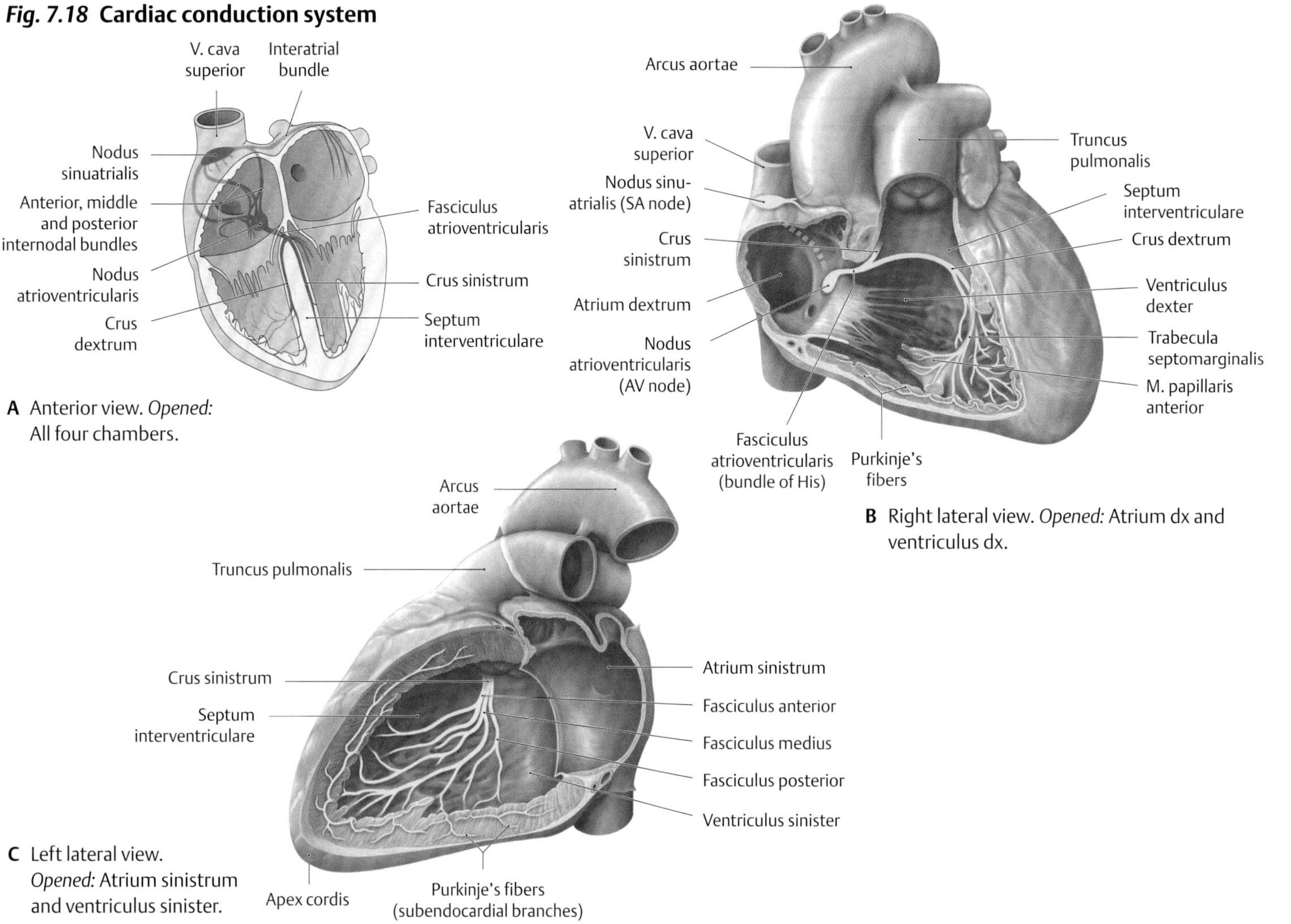

A Anterior view. *Opened:* All four chambers.

Arcus aortae
V. cava superior
Nodus sinuatrialis (SA node)
Crus sinistrum
Atrium dextrum
Nodus atrioventricularis (AV node)
Fasciculus atrioventricularis (bundle of His)
Purkinje's fibers
Truncus pulmonalis
Septum interventriculare
Crus dextrum
Ventriculus dexter
Trabecula septomarginalis
M. papillaris anterior

B Right lateral view. *Opened:* Atrium dx and ventriculus dx.

Arcus aortae
Truncus pulmonalis
Crus sinistrum
Septum interventriculare
Apex cordis
Purkinje's fibers (subendocardial branches)
Atrium sinistrum
Fasciculus anterior
Fasciculus medius
Fasciculus posterior
Ventriculus sinister

C Left lateral view. *Opened:* Atrium sinistrum and ventriculus sinister.

Clinical

Electrocardiogram (ECG)

The cardiac impulse (a physical dipole) travels across the heart and may be detected with electrodes. The use of three electrodes that separately record electrical activity of the heart along three axes or vectors (Einthoven limb leads) generates an electrocardiogram (ECG). The ECG graphs the cardiac cycle ("heartbeat"), reducing it to a series of waves, segments, and intervals. These ECG components can be used to determine whether cardiac impulses are normal or abnormal (e.g., myocardial infarction, chamber enlargement). *Note:* Although only three leads are required, a standard ECG examination includes at least two others (Goldberger, Wilson leads).

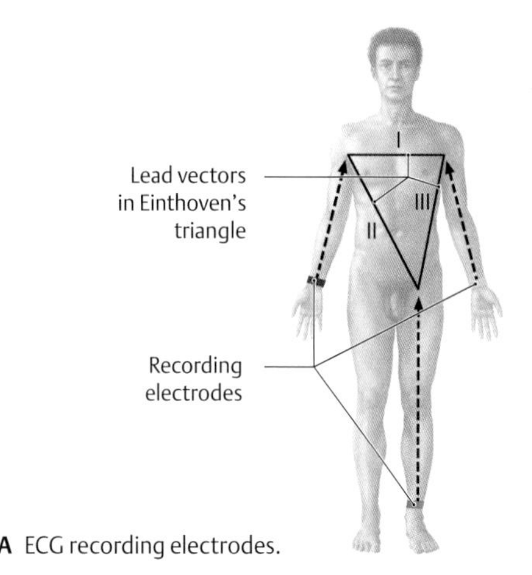
Lead vectors in Einthoven's triangle
I
II
III
Recording electrodes

A ECG recording electrodes.

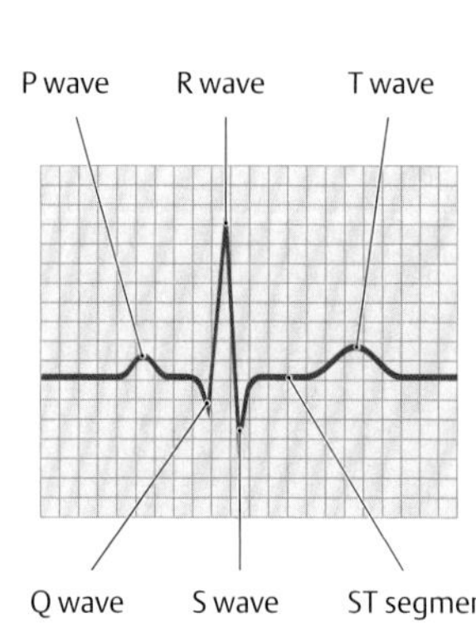
P wave
R wave
T wave
Q wave
S wave
ST segment

B ECG.

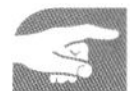

Sympathetic innervation: Presynaptic neurons from T1 to T6 spinal cord segments send fibers to synapse on postsynaptic neurons in the cervical and upper thoracic sympathetic ganglia. The three cervical nn. cardiaci and thoracic rr. cardiaci contribute to the cardiac plexus. Parasympathetic innervation: Presynaptic neurons and fibers reach the heart via rr. cardiaci, some of which also arise in the cervical region. They synapse on postsynaptic neurons near the SA node and along the coronary arteries.

Fig. 7.19 Autonomic innervation of the heart

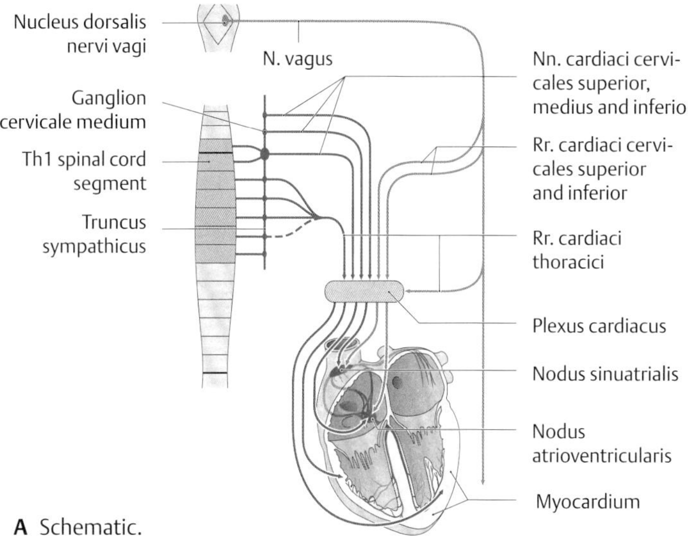
Nucleus dorsalis nervi vagi
N. vagus
Ganglion cervicale medium
Th1 spinal cord segment
Truncus sympathicus
Nn. cardiaci cervicales superior, medius and inferior
Rr. cardiaci cervicales superior and inferior
Rr. cardiaci thoracici
Plexus cardiacus
Nodus sinuatrialis
Nodus atrioventricularis
Myocardium

A Schematic.

Truncus sympathicus, ganglion cervicale inferius
Rr. cardiaci to plexus cardiacus
Plexus cardiacus
Nn. cardiaci cervicales
Arcus aortae, plexus aorticus thoracicus
A. pulmonalis and vv. pulmonales, plexus pulmonalis
Plexus cardiacus (along aa. coronariae)

B Autonomic plexuses of the heart, right lateral view. Note the continuity between the cardiac, aortic, and pulmonary plexuses.

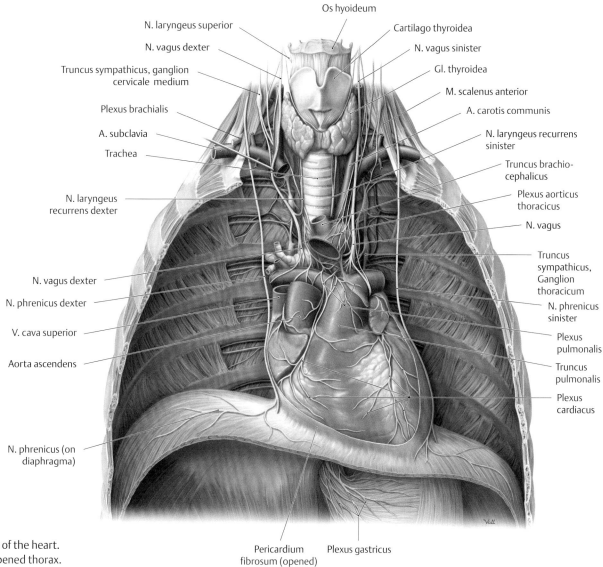

Os hyoideum
N. laryngeus superior
Cartilago thyroidea
N. vagus dexter
N. vagus sinister
Truncus sympathicus, ganglion cervicale medium
Gl. thyroidea
M. scalenus anterior
Plexus brachialis
A. carotis communis
A. subclavia
N. laryngeus recurrens sinister
Trachea
Truncus brachiocephalicus
N. laryngeus recurrens dexter
Plexus aorticus thoracicus
N. vagus
Truncus sympathicus, Ganglion thoracicum
N. vagus dexter
N. phrenicus dexter
N. phrenicus sinister
V. cava superior
Plexus pulmonalis
Aorta ascendens
Truncus pulmonalis
Plexus cardiacus
N. phrenicus (on diaphragma)
Pericardium fibrosum (opened)
Plexus gastricus

C Autonomic nerves of the heart. Anterior view of opened thorax.

Heart: Radiology

Table 7.5 Borders of the heart	
Border	**Defining structures**
Right cardiac border	Atrium dextrum
	V. cava superior
Apex cordis	Ventriculus sinister
Left cardiac border	Arcus aortae ("aortic knob")
	Truncus pulmonalis
	Atrium sinistrum
	Ventriculus sinister
Inferior cardiac border	Ventriculus sinister
	Ventriculus dexter

Fig. 7.20 Cardiac borders and configurations

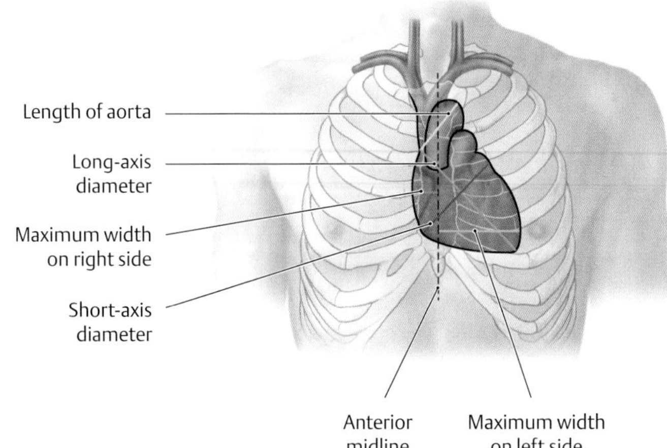

Length of aorta
Long-axis diameter
Maximum width on right side
Short-axis diameter
Anterior midline
Maximum width on left side

Fig. 7.21 Radiographic appearance of the heart

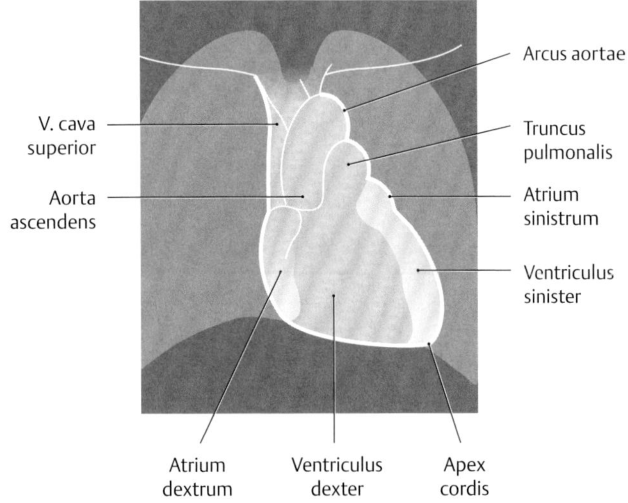

V. cava superior
Aorta ascendens
Arcus aortae
Truncus pulmonalis
Atrium sinistrum
Ventriculus sinister
Atrium dextrum
Ventriculus dexter
Apex cordis

A Anterior view.

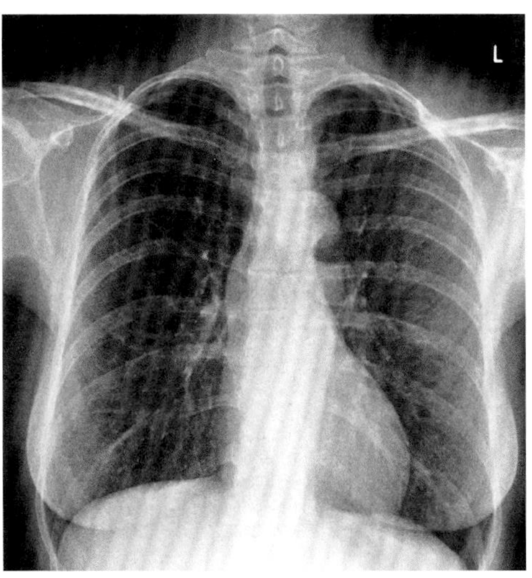

L

B Anteroposterior chest radiograph.

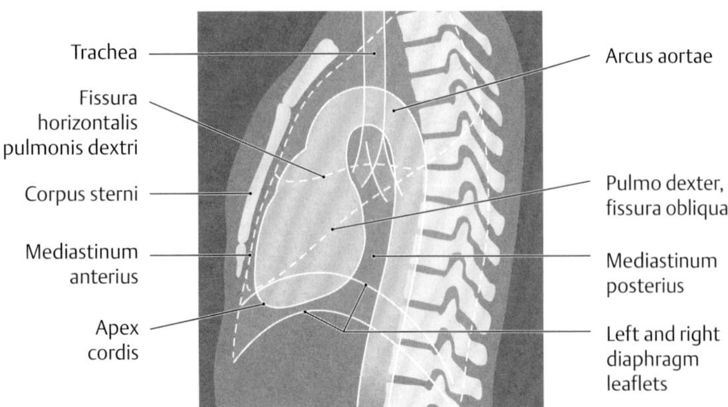

Trachea
Fissura horizontalis pulmonis dextri
Corpus sterni
Mediastinum anterius
Apex cordis
Arcus aortae
Pulmo dexter, fissura obliqua
Mediastinum posterius
Left and right diaphragm leaflets

C Lateral view. *Visible:* Diaphragma leaflets and lungs. The arcus aortae forms a sling over the left bronchus principalis. Note the narrowness of the anterior mediastinum relative to the posterior mediastinum.

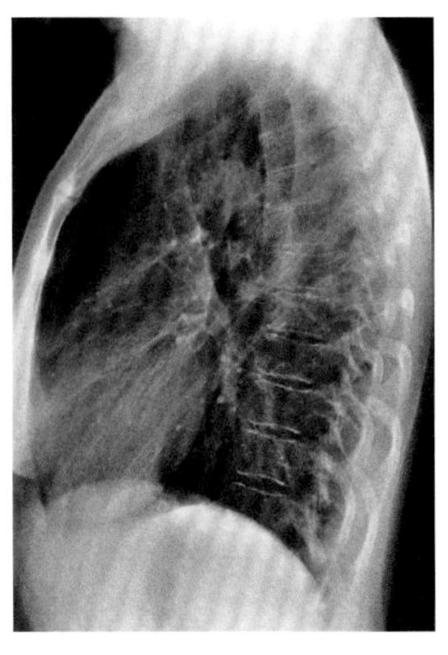

D Left lateral chest radiograph.

Fig. 7.22 Heart in transverse section

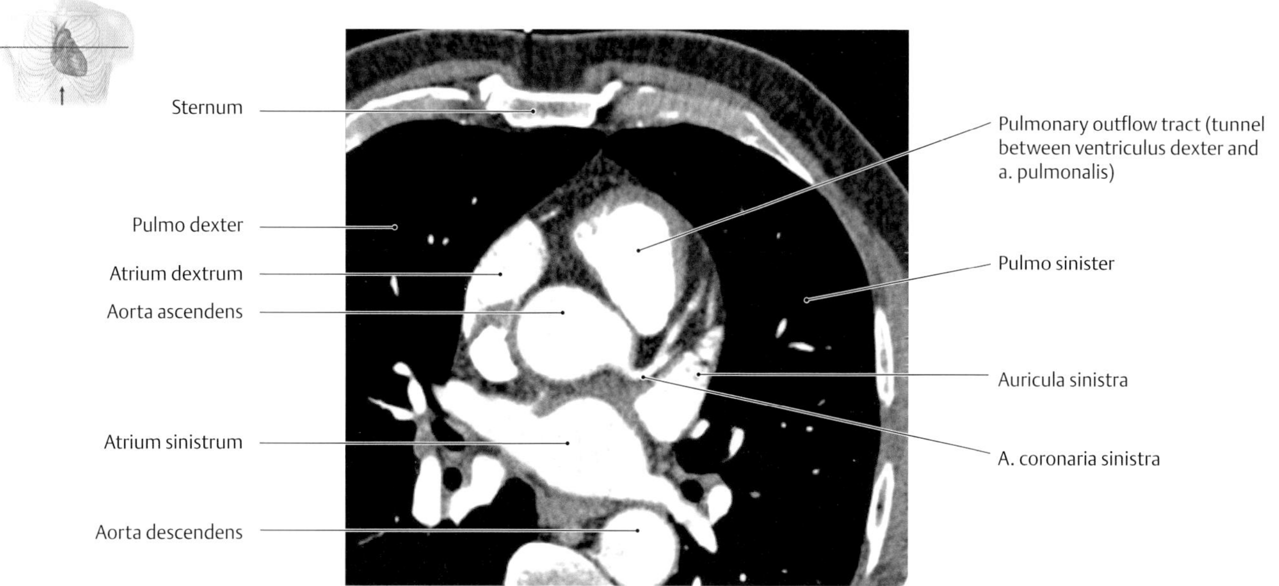
Sternum
Pulmo dexter
Atrium dextrum
Aorta ascendens
Atrium sinistrum
Aorta descendens
Pulmonary outflow tract (tunnel between ventriculus dexter and a. pulmonalis)
Pulmo sinister
Auricula sinistra
A. coronaria sinistra

A Heart in normal chest magnetic resonance imaging (MRI). The cardiac chambers are clearly displayed owing to the high signal intensity, and the lungs are not visualized.

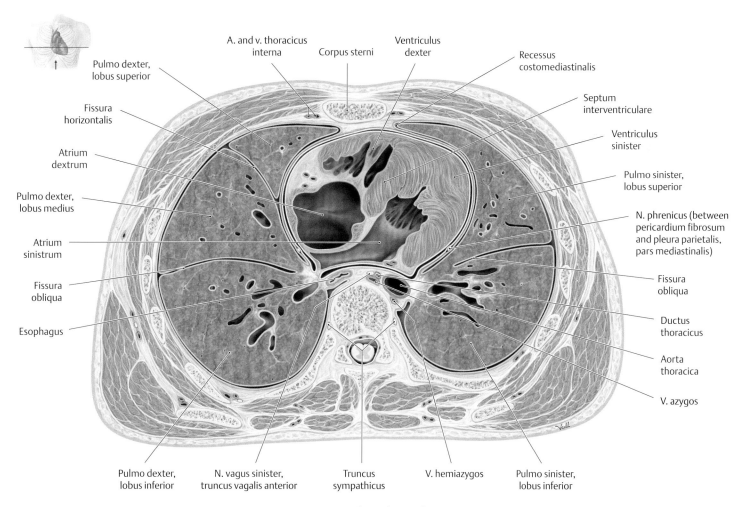

Pulmo dexter, lobus superior
A. and v. thoracicus interna
Corpus sterni
Ventriculus dexter
Recessus costomediastinalis
Fissura horizontalis
Septum interventriculare
Ventriculus sinister
Atrium dextrum
Pulmo sinister, lobus superior
Pulmo dexter, lobus medius
N. phrenicus (between pericardium fibrosum and pleura parietalis, pars mediastinalis)
Atrium sinistrum
Fissura obliqua
Fissura obliqua
Ductus thoracicus
Esophagus
Aorta thoracica
V. azygos
Pulmo dexter, lobus inferior
N. vagus sinister, truncus vagalis anterior
Truncus sympathicus
V. hemiazygos
Pulmo sinister, lobus inferior

B Transverse section through T8, inferior view.

Pre- & Postnatal Circulation

Fig. 7.23 Prenatal circulation
After Fritsch and Kühnel.

① Oxygenated and nutrient-rich fetal blood from the placenta passes to the fetus via the v. umbilicalis.

② Approximately half of this blood bypasses the liver (via ductus venosus) and enters v. cava inferior. The remainder enters v. portae to supply the liver with nutrients and oxygen.

③ Blood entering atrium dextrum from v. cava inferior bypasses ventriculus dx (as the lungs are not yet functioning) to enter atrium sinistrum via foramen ovale, a right-to-left shunt.

④ Blood from v. cava superior enters atrium dextrum, passes to ventriculus dexter, and moves into truncus pulmonalis. Most of this blood enters the aorta via the ductus arteriosus, a right-to-left shunt.

⑤ The partially oxygenated blood in the aorta returns to the placenta via the paired aa. umbilicales that arise from aa. iliacae interna.

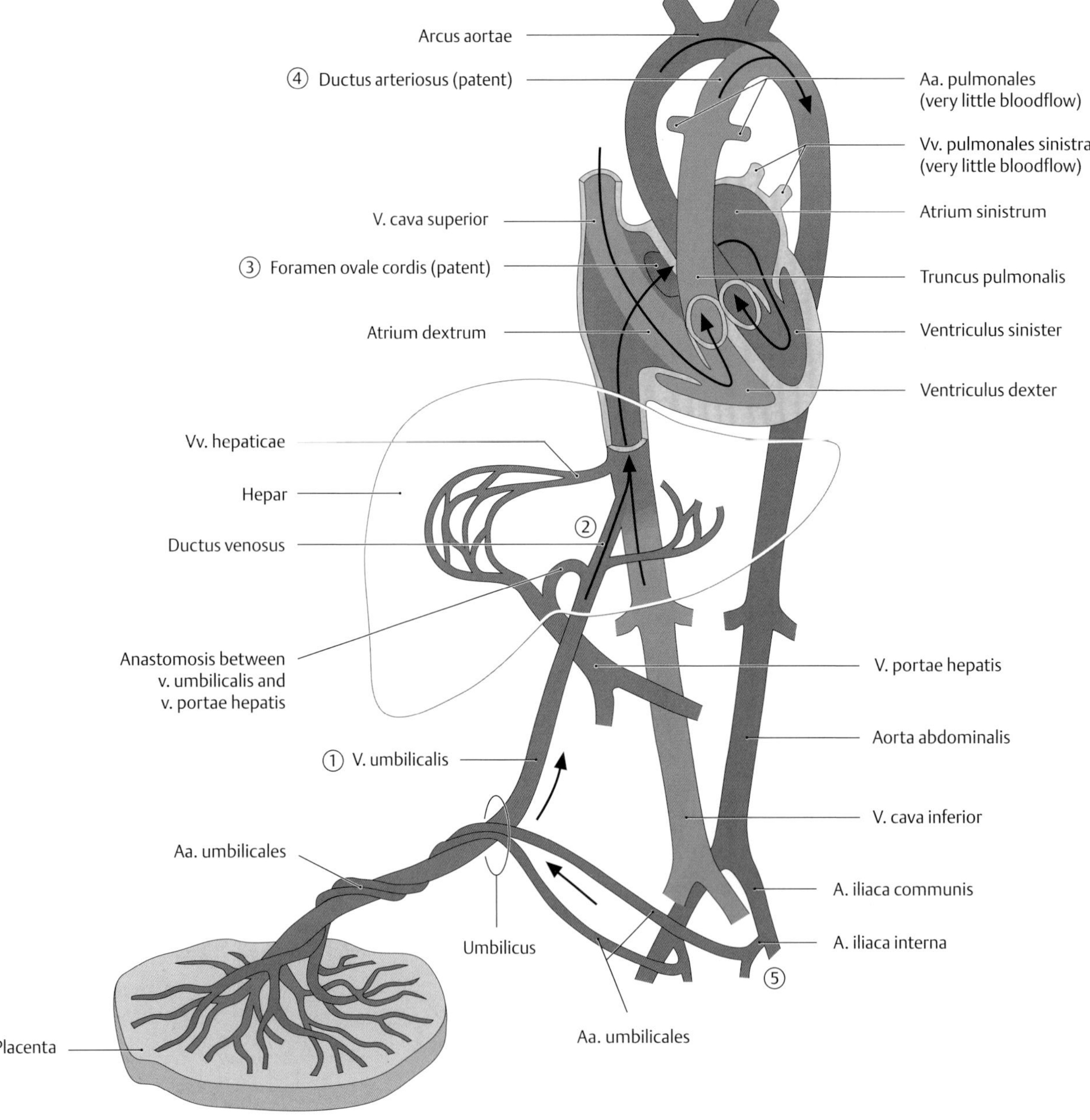

Arcus aortae
④ Ductus arteriosus (patent)
Aa. pulmonales (very little bloodflow)
Vv. pulmonales sinistrae (very little bloodflow)
V. cava superior
Atrium sinistrum
③ Foramen ovale cordis (patent)
Truncus pulmonalis
Atrium dextrum
Ventriculus sinister
Ventriculus dexter
Vv. hepaticae
Hepar
②
Ductus venosus
Anastomosis between v. umbilicalis and v. portae hepatis
V. portae hepatis
Aorta abdominalis
① V. umbilicalis
V. cava inferior
Aa. umbilicales
A. iliaca communis
Umbilicus
A. iliaca interna
⑤
Placenta
Aa. umbilicales

① As pulmonary respiration begins at birth, pulmonary blood pressure falls, causing blood from truncus pulmonalis to enter vv. pulmonales.

② The foramen ovale and ductus arteriosus close, eliminating the fetal right-to-left shunts. The pulmonary and systemic circulations in the heart are now separate.

③ As the infant is separated from the placenta, aa. umbilicales occlude (except for the proximal portions), along with v. umbilicalis and ductus venosus.

④ Blood to be metabolized now passes through the liver.

Fig. 7.24 **Postnatal circulation**
After Fritsch and Kühnel.

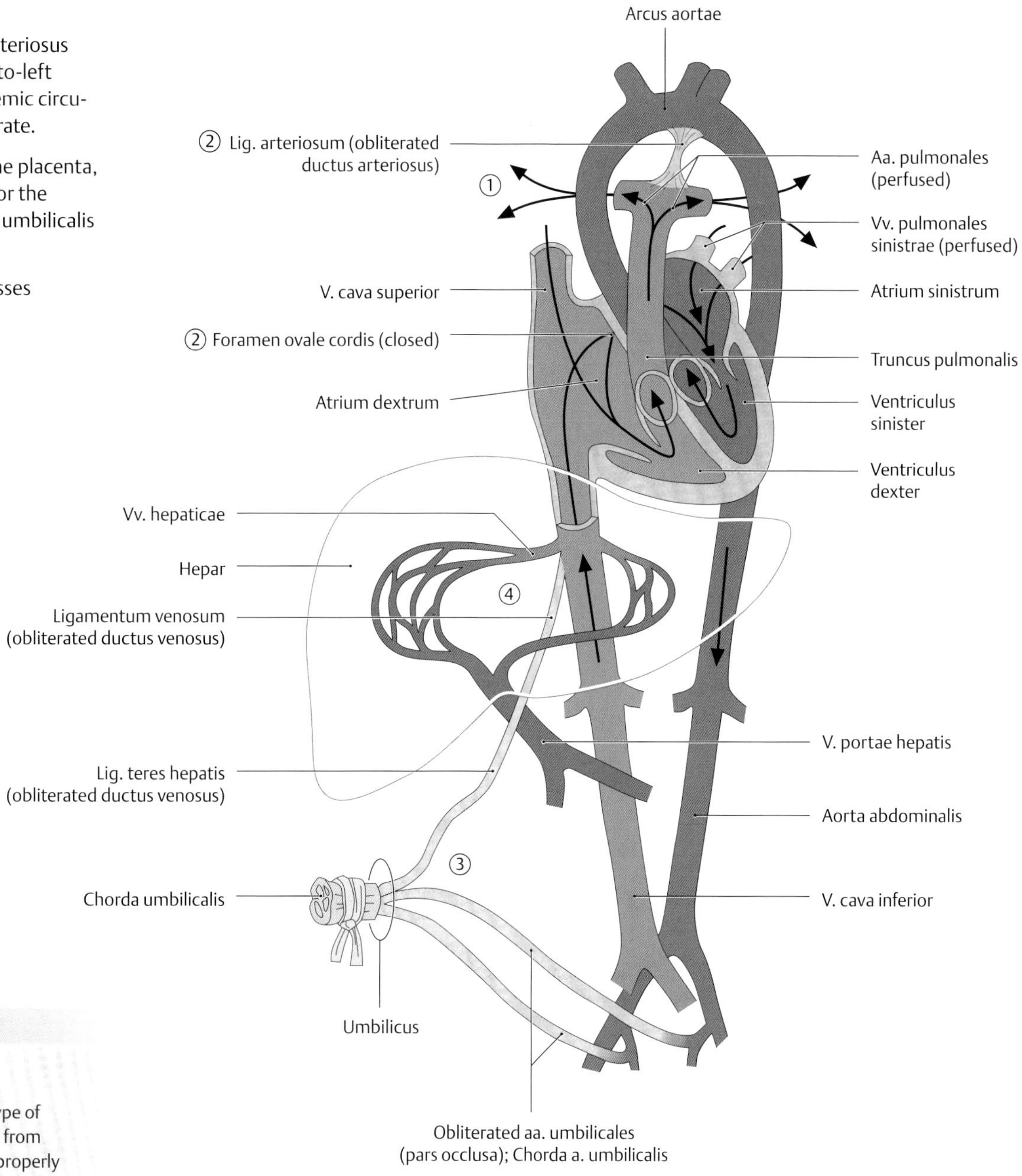

Arcus aortae
② Lig. arteriosum (obliterated ductus arteriosus)
①
Aa. pulmonales (perfused)
Vv. pulmonales sinistrae (perfused)
V. cava superior
Atrium sinistrum
② Foramen ovale cordis (closed)
Truncus pulmonalis
Atrium dextrum
Ventriculus sinister
Ventriculus dexter
Vv. hepaticae
Hepar
④
Ligamentum venosum (obliterated ductus venosus)
V. portae hepatis
Lig. teres hepatis (obliterated ductus venosus)
Aorta abdominalis
③
Chorda umbilicalis
V. cava inferior
Umbilicus
Obliterated aa. umbilicales (pars occlusa); Chorda a. umbilicalis

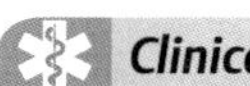 ***Clinical***

Septal defects
Septal defects, the most common type of congenital heart defect, allow blood from the left chambers of the heart to improperly pass into the right chambers during systole. Ventrical septal defect (VSD, shown below) is the most common form. Patent foramen ovale, the most prevalent form of *atrial* septal defect (ASD), results from improper closure of the fetal shunt.

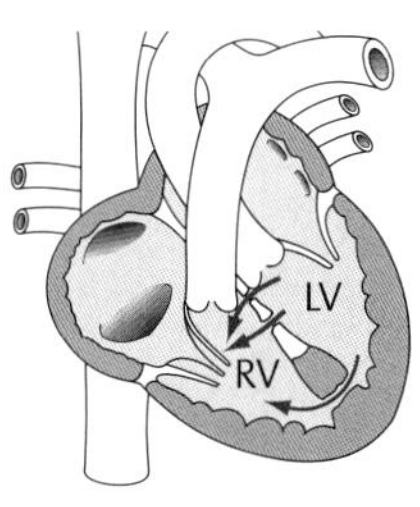
LV
RV

Table 7.6 **Derivatives of fetal circulatory structures**

Fetal structure	Adult remnant
Ductus arteriosus	Ligamentum arteriosum
Foramen ovale	Fossa ovalis
Ductus venosus	Ligamentum venosum
V. umbilicalis	Lig. teres hepatis
A. umbilicalis	Chorda a. umbilicalis

Esophagus

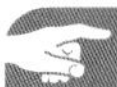

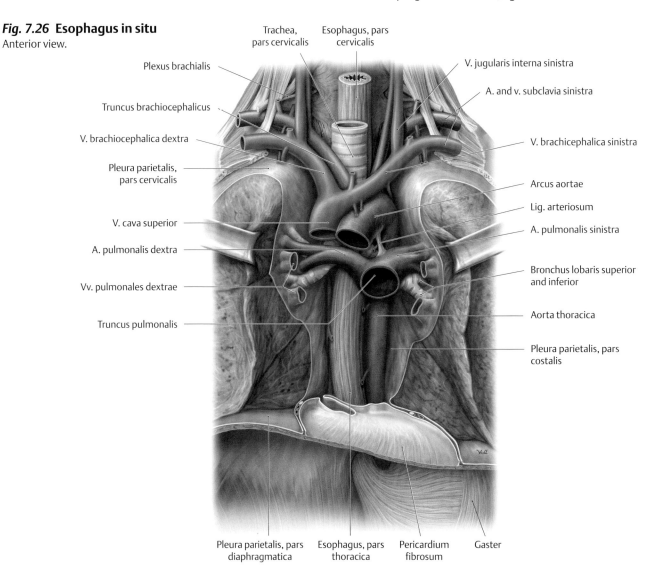

The esophagus is divided into three parts: cervical (C VI–T I), thoracic (T I to the esophageal hiatus of the diaphragm), and abdominal (the diaphragm to the cardiac orifice of the stomach). It descends slightly to the right of aorta thoracica and pierces diaphragma slightly to the left, just below processus xiphoideus.

Fig. 7.25 Esophagus: Location and constrictions

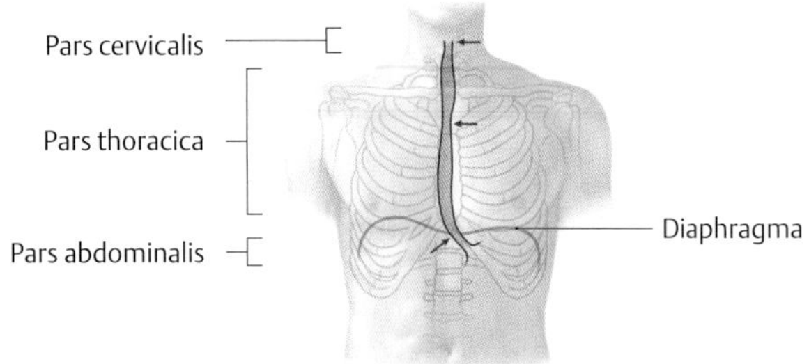
Pars cervicalis
Pars thoracica
Pars abdominalis
Diaphragma

A Projection of esophagus onto chest wall. Esophageal constrictions are indicated with arrows.

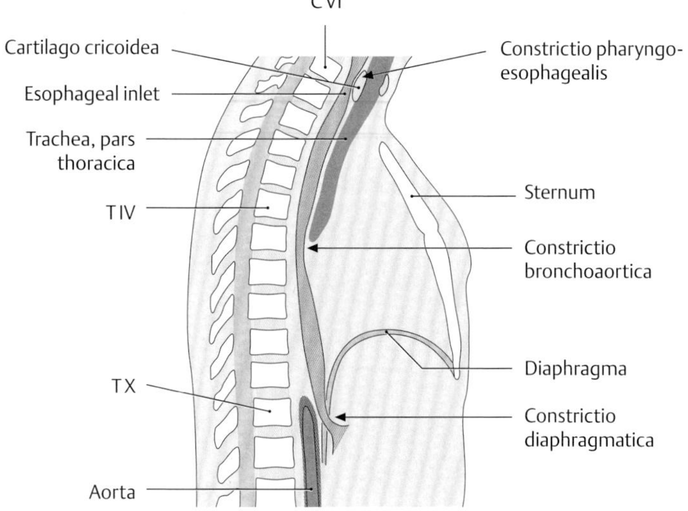
C VI
Cartilago cricoidea
Esophageal inlet
Trachea, pars thoracica
T IV
T X
Aorta
Constrictio pharyngo-esophagealis
Sternum
Constrictio bronchoaortica
Diaphragma
Constrictio diaphragmatica

B Esophageal constrictions, right lateral view.

Fig. 7.26 Esophagus in situ

Anterior view.

Trachea, pars cervicalis
Esophagus, pars cervicalis
Plexus brachialis
Truncus brachiocephalicus
V. brachiocephalica dextra
Pleura parietalis, pars cervicalis
V. cava superior
A. pulmonalis dextra
Vv. pulmonales dextrae
Truncus pulmonalis
V. jugularis interna sinistra
A. and v. subclavia sinistra
V. brachicephalica sinistra
Arcus aortae
Lig. arteriosum
A. pulmonalis sinistra
Bronchus lobaris superior and inferior
Aorta thoracica
Pleura parietalis, pars costalis
Pleura parietalis, pars diaphragmatica
Esophagus, pars thoracica
Pericardium fibrosum
Gaster

Fig. 7.27 **Structure of the esophagus**

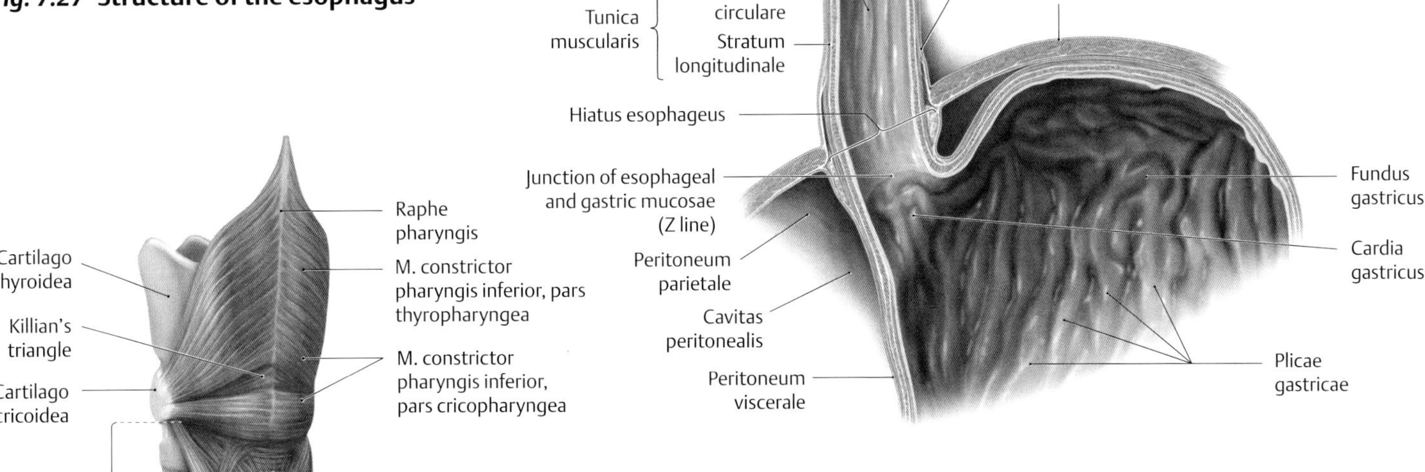

Raphe pharyngis
Cartilago thyroidea
M. constrictor pharyngis inferior, pars thyropharyngea
Killian's triangle
M. constrictor pharyngis inferior, pars cricopharyngea
Cartilago cricoidea
Tunica muscularis, stratum circulare
Trachea
Esophagus
Tunica muscularis, stratum longitudinale
Tunica muscularis, stratum circulare
Tela submucosa
Tunica mucosa
Tunica mucosa (longitudinal folds)
Pars mediastinalis
Pars diaphragmatica
Pleura parietalis
Tunica muscularis
Stratum circulare
Stratum longitudinale
Hiatus esophageus
Junction of esophageal and gastric mucosae (Z line)
Fundus gastricus
Cardia gastricus
Peritoneum parietale
Cavitas peritonealis
Peritoneum viscerale
Plicae gastricae

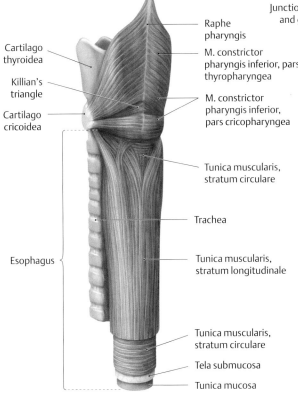

A Esophageal wall, oblique left posterior view. Pharynx (p. 552); trachea (p. 110).

B Esophagogastric junction, anterior view. A true sphincter is not identifiable at this junction; instead, the diaphragmatic muscle of the hiatus esophageus functions as a sphincter. The junction of esophageal and gastric mucosae is often referred to as the "Z line" because of its zigzag form.

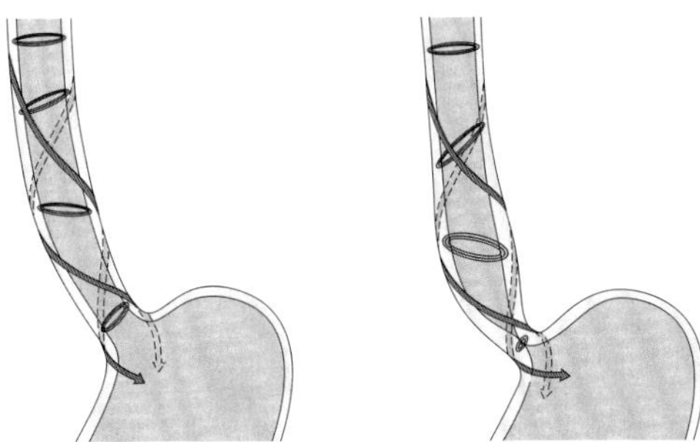

C Functional architecture of esophageal muscle.

Clinical

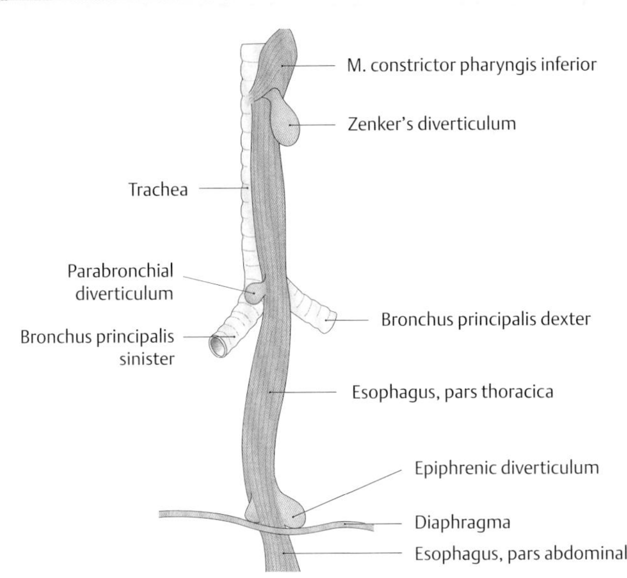

M. constrictor pharyngis inferior
Zenker's diverticulum
Trachea
Parabronchial diverticulum
Bronchus principalis dexter
Bronchus principalis sinister
Esophagus, pars thoracica
Epiphrenic diverticulum
Diaphragma
Esophagus, pars abdominalis

Esophageal diverticula

Diverticula (abnormal outpouchings or sacs) generally develop at weak spots in the esophageal wall. There are three main types of esophageal diverticula:

- Hypopharyngeal (pharyngo-esophageal) diverticula: Outpouchings occurring at the junction of the pharynx and the esophagus. These include Zenker's diverticula (70% of cases).
- "True" traction diverticula: Protrusion of all wall layers, not typically occurring at characteristic weak spots. However, they generally result from an inflammatory process (e.g., lymphangitis) and are thus common at sites where the esophagus closely approaches the bronchi and bronchial lymph nodes (thoracic or parabronchial diverticula).
- "False" pulsion diverticula: Herniations of the mucosa and submucosa through weak spots in the muscular coat due to a rise in esophageal pressure (e.g., during normal swallowing). These include parahiatal and epiphrenic diverticula occurring above the esophageal aperture of the diaphragm (10% of cases).

Neurovasculature of the Esophagus

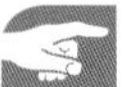

Sympathetic innervation: Presynaptic fibers arise from the T2–T6 spinal cord segments. Postsynaptic fibers arise from the truncus sympaticus to join the plexus esophageus. Parasympathetic innervation: Presynaptic fibers arise from the dorsal vagal nucleus and travel in the nn. vagi to form the extensive plexus esophageus. *Note:* The postsynaptic neurons are in the wall of the esophagus. Fibers to the cervical portion of the esophagus travel in the n. laryngeus recurrens.

Fig. 7.28 **Autonomic innervation of the esophagus**

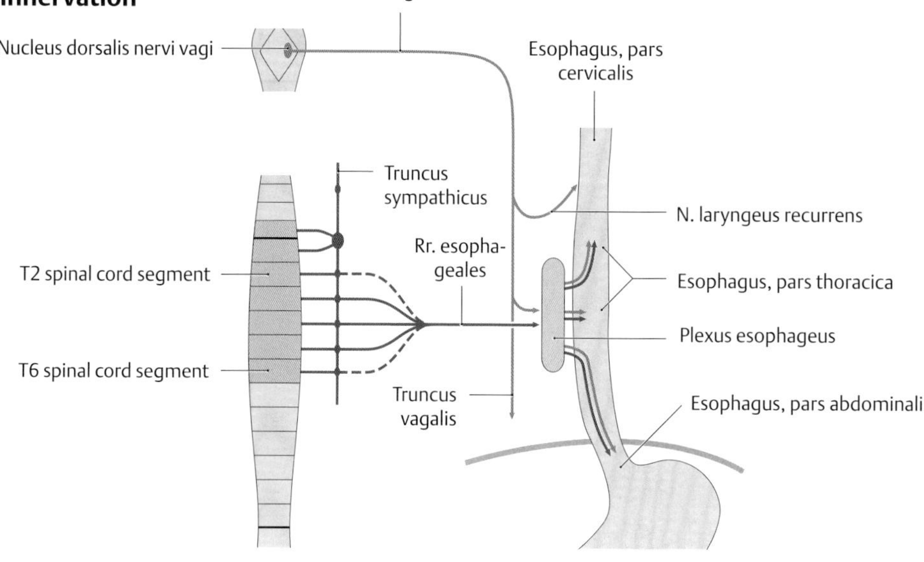
N.vagus
Nucleus dorsalis nervi vagi
Esophagus, pars cervicalis
Truncus sympathicus
N. laryngeus recurrens
Rr. esophageales
T2 spinal cord segment
Esophagus, pars thoracica
Plexus esophageus
T6 spinal cord segment
Truncus vagalis
Esophagus, pars abdominalis

Fig. 7.29 **Esophageal plexus**

The left and right n. vagus initially descend on the left and right sides of the esophagus. As they begin to contribute to the plexus esophageus, they shift to anterior and posterior positions, respectively. As the nn. vagi continue into the abdomen, they are named the truncus vagalis anterior and posterior.

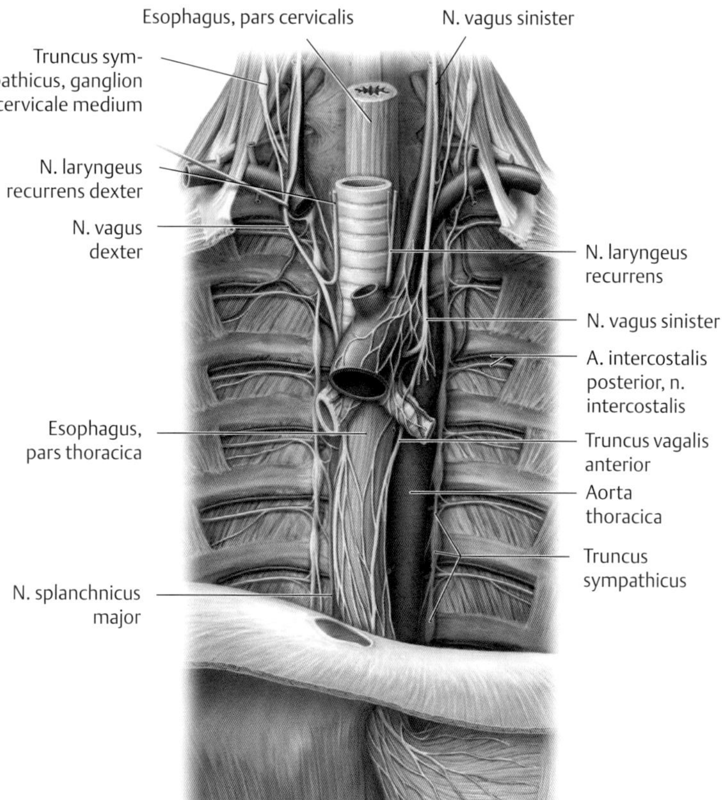
Esophagus, pars cervicalis
N. vagus sinister
Truncus sympathicus, ganglion cervicale medium
N. laryngeus recurrens dexter
N. vagus dexter
N. laryngeus recurrens
N. vagus sinister
A. intercostalis posterior, n. intercostalis
Esophagus, pars thoracica
Truncus vagalis anterior
Aorta thoracica
Truncus sympathicus
N. splanchnicus major

A Plexus esophageus in situ. Anterior view.

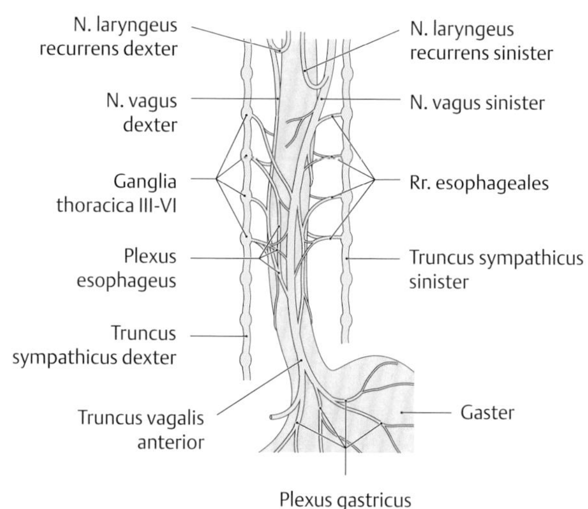
N. laryngeus recurrens dexter
N. laryngeus recurrens sinister
N. vagus dexter
N. vagus sinister
Ganglia thoracica III-VI
Rr. esophageales
Plexus esophageus
Truncus sympathicus sinister
Truncus sympathicus dexter
Truncus vagalis anterior
Gaster
Plexus gastricus anterior

B Anterior view. Note the postsynaptic sympathetic contribution to the plexus esophageus.

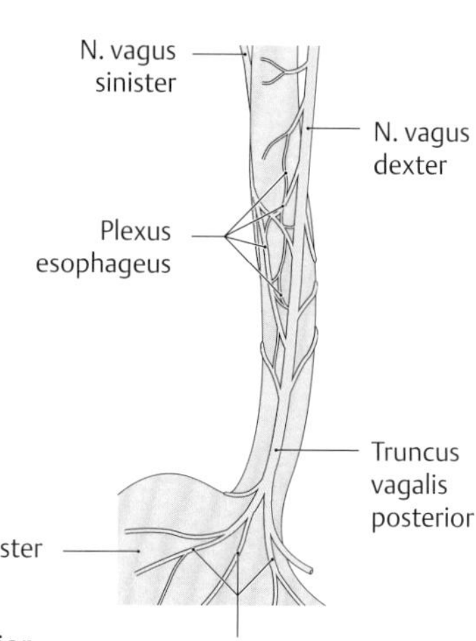
N. vagus sinister
N. vagus dexter
Plexus esophageus
Truncus vagalis posterior
Gaster
Plexus gastricus posterior

C Posterior view.

Fig. 7.30 Esophageal arteries
Anterior view.

A. carotis communis sinistra
A. thyroidea inferior
M. scalenus anterior
Truncus thyrocervicalis
Rr. esophageales
A. thoracica interna
A. subclavia sinistra
A. vertebralis
Trachea
Arcus aortae
Bronchus principalis sinister
Rr. esophageales (from aorta thoracica)
Aa. intercostales posteriores
Aorta thoracica
Diaphragma
Fundus gastricus
R. esophagealis
A. phrenica inferior sinistra
Truncus coeliacus
A. gastrica sinistra
A. hepatica communis
Aorta abdominalis

Fig. 7.31 Esophageal veins
Anterior view.

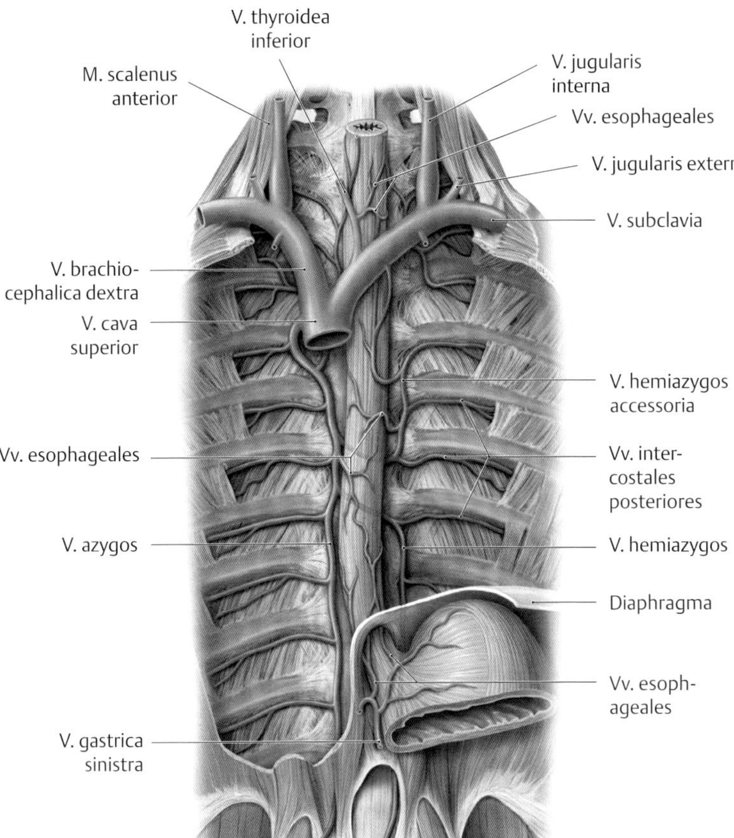
V. thyroidea inferior
M. scalenus anterior
V. jugularis interna
Vv. esophageales
V. jugularis externa
V. subclavia
V. brachio-cephalica dextra
V. cava superior
V. hemiazygos accessoria
Vv. esophageales
Vv. inter-costales posteriores
V. azygos
V. hemiazygos
Diaphragma
Vv. esoph-ageales
V. gastrica sinistra

Table 7.7	Blood vessels of the esophagus	
Part	**Origin of esophageal arteries**	**Drainage of esophageal veins**
Pars cervicalis	A. thyroida inferior	V. thyroida inferior
	Rarely direct branches from truncus thyro-cervicalis or a. carotis communis	V. brachiocephalica sinistra
Pars thoracica	Aorta (four or five aa. esophageales)	Upper left: V. hemiazygos accessoria or v. brachio-cephalica sinistra
		Lower left: V. hemiazygos
		Right side: V. azygos
Pars abdominalis	A. gastrica sinistra	V. gastrica sinistra

Lymphatics of the Mediastinum

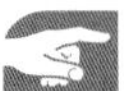

The nll. phrenici superiores drain lymph from the diaphragm, pericardium, lower esophagus, lung, and liver into the truncus bronchomediastinalis. The nll. phrenici inferiores, found in the abdomen, collect lymph from the diaphragm and lower lobes of the lung and convey it to the truncus lumbalis. *Note:* The pericardium may also drain superiorly to the nll. brachiocephalici.

Fig. 7.32 **Lymph nodes of the mediastinum and thoracic cavity**
Left anterior oblique view.

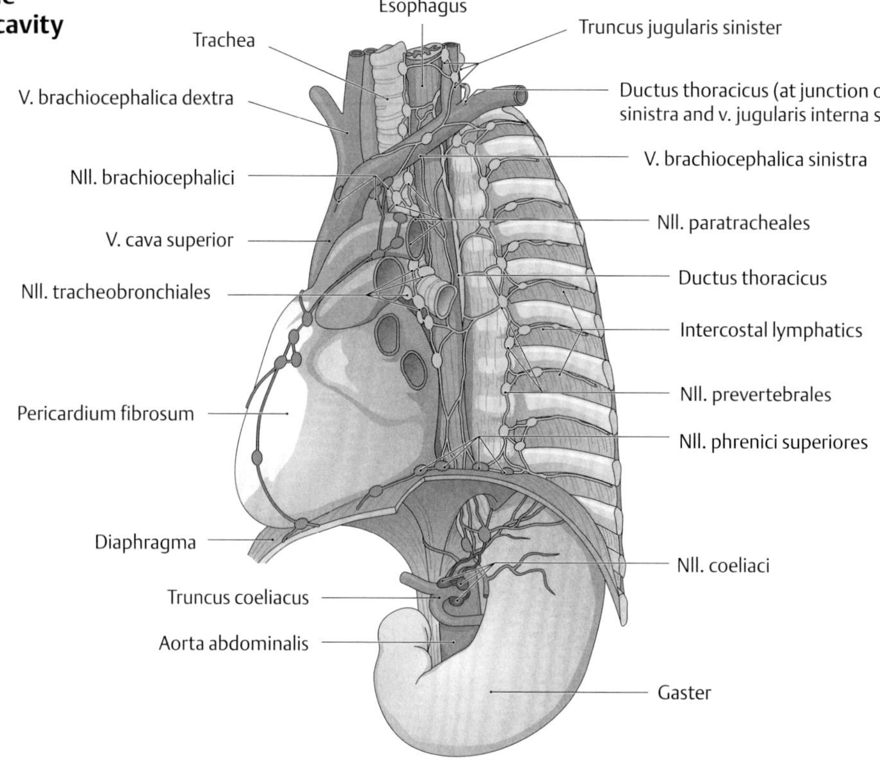
Esophagus
Trachea
Truncus jugularis sinister
V. brachiocephalica dextra
Ductus thoracicus (at junction of v. subclavia sinistra and v. jugularis interna sinistra)
V. brachiocephalica sinistra
Nll. brachiocephalici
Nll. paratracheales
V. cava superior
Ductus thoracicus
Nll. tracheobronchiales
Intercostal lymphatics
Nll. prevertebrales
Pericardium fibrosum
Nll. phrenici superiores
Diaphragma
Nll. coeliaci
Truncus coeliacus
Aorta abdominalis
Gaster

Fig. 7.33 **Lymphatic drainage of the heart**
A unique "crossed" drainage pattern exists in the heart: lymph from the left atrium and ventricle drains to the right venous junction, whereas lymph from the right atrium and ventricle drains to the left venous junction.

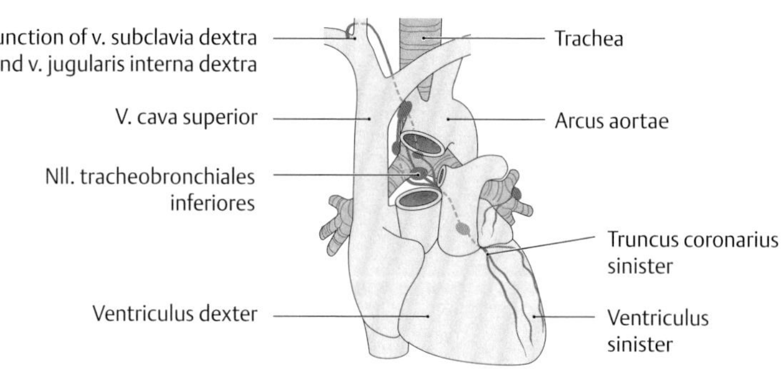
Junction of v. subclavia dextra and v. jugularis interna dextra
Trachea
V. cava superior
Arcus aortae
Nll. tracheobronchiales inferiores
Truncus coronarius sinister
Ventriculus dexter
Ventriculus sinister

A Lymphatic drainage of the left chambers, anterior view.

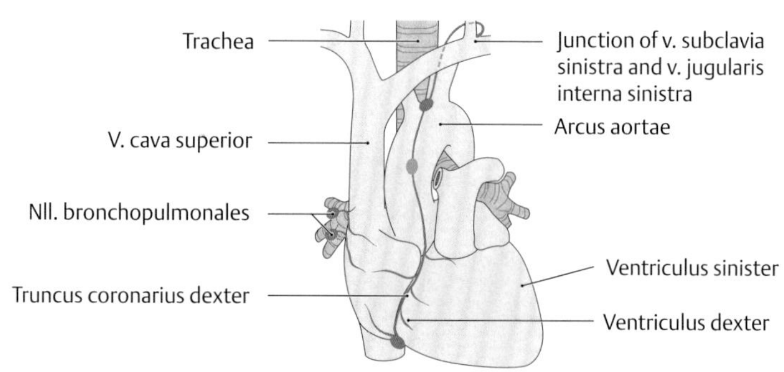
Trachea
Junction of v. subclavia sinistra and v. jugularis interna sinistra
Arcus aortae
V. cava superior
Nll. bronchopulmonales
Ventriculus sinister
Truncus coronarius dexter
Ventriculus dexter

B Lymphatic drainage of the right chambers, anterior view.

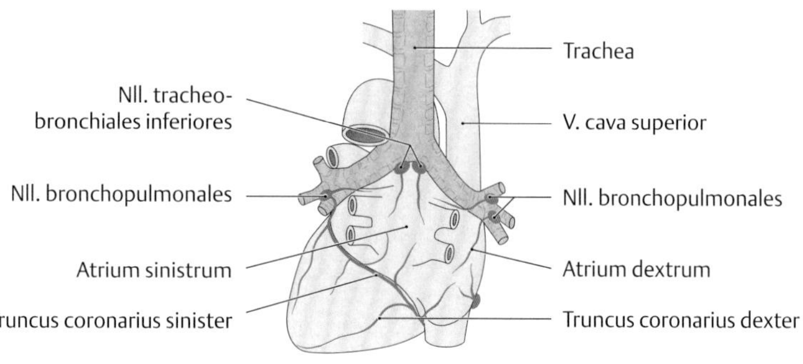
Trachea
Nll. tracheo-bronchiales inferiores
V. cava superior
Nll. bronchopulmonales
Nll. bronchopulmonales
Atrium sinistrum
Atrium dextrum
Truncus coronarius sinister
Truncus coronarius dexter

C Posterior view.

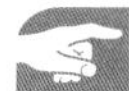

The nll. juxtaesophageales drain the esophagus. Lymphatic drainage of the cervical part of the esophagus is primarily cranial, to the nll. cervicales profundi and then to the truncus jugularis. The thoracic part of the esophagus drains to the trunci bronchomediastinales in two parts: the upper half drains cranially, and the lower half drains inferiorly via the nll. phrenici superiores. The nll. bronchopulmonales and paratracheales drain lymph from the lungs, bronchi, and trachea into the truncus bronchomediastinales (see p. 118).

Fig. 7.34 Mediastinal lymph nodes

Nll. juxta-esophageales
Esophagus
Trachea
Nll. paratracheales
Bronchus principalis dexter
Broncus principalis sinister
Nll. tracheo-bronchiales inferiores
Nll. juxtaesophageales
Diaphragma
Nll. phrenici-inferiores
Anulus lymphaticus cardiae (inconstant)
Gaster

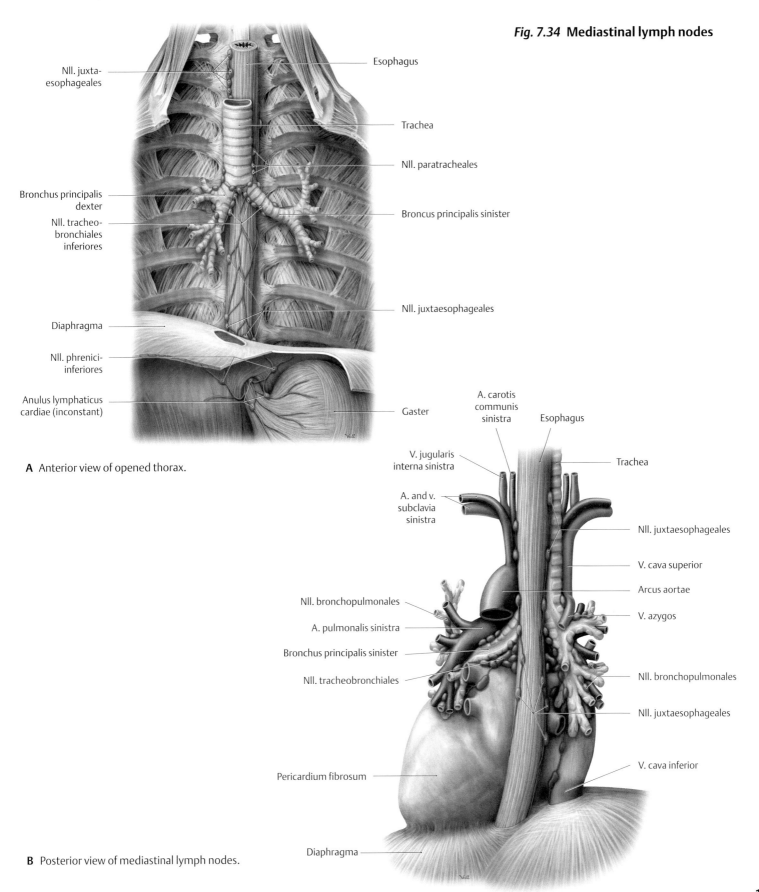

A Anterior view of opened thorax.

A. carotis communis sinistra
Esophagus
V. jugularis interna sinistra
Trachea
A. and v. subclavia sinistra
Nll. juxtaesophageales
V. cava superior
Arcus aortae
Nll. bronchopulmonales
V. azygos
A. pulmonalis sinistra
Bronchus principalis sinister
Nll. tracheobronchiales
Nll. bronchopulmonales
Nll. juxtaesophageales
V. cava inferior
Pericardium fibrosum
Diaphragma

B Posterior view of mediastinal lymph nodes.

Pleural Cavity

The paired pleural cavities (cavitas pleuralis) contain the left and right lungs. They are completely separated from each other by the mediastinum and are under negative atmospheric pressure (see respiratory mechanics, pp. 112–113).

Fig. 8.1 Pleural cavity

Pleural cavities and lungs projected onto thoracic skeleton.

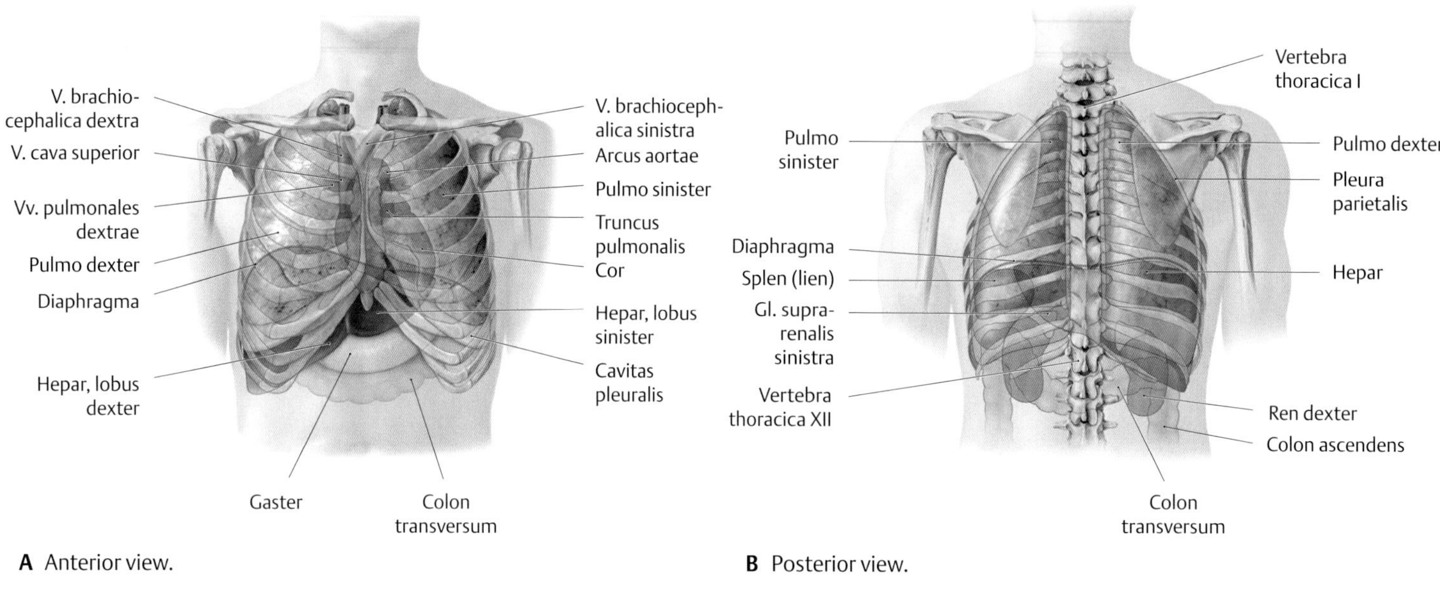

V. brachio-cephalica dextra
V. cava superior
Vv. pulmonales dextrae
Pulmo dexter
Diaphragma
Hepar, lobus dexter
Gaster
Colon transversum
V. brachioceph-alica sinistra
Arcus aortae
Pulmo sinister
Truncus pulmonalis
Cor
Hepar, lobus sinister
Cavitas pleuralis
Pulmo sinister
Diaphragma
Splen (lien)
Gl. supra-renalis sinistra
Vertebra thoracica XII
Vertebra thoracica I
Pulmo dexter
Pleura parietalis
Hepar
Ren dexter
Colon ascendens
Colon transversum

A Anterior view.

B Posterior view.

Fig. 8.2 Boundaries of the pleural cavities and lungs

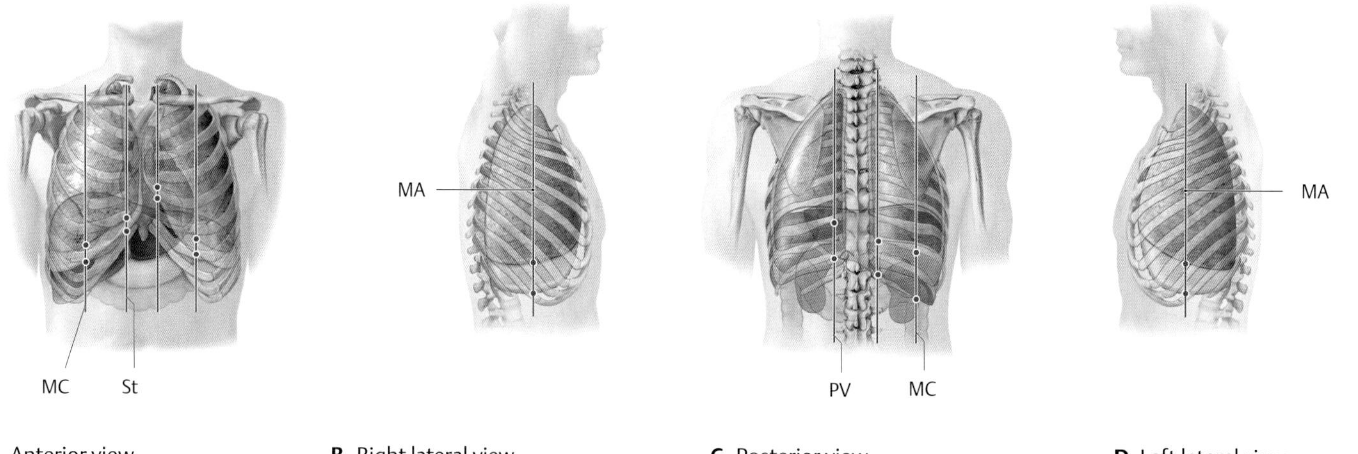

MC
St
MA
PV
MC
MA

A Anterior view.

B Right lateral view.

C Posterior view.

D Left lateral view.

Table 8.1 Pleural cavity boundaries and reference points

Reference line	Right pleura parietale	Pulmo dexter	Pulmo sinister	Left pleura parietale
Sternal line (St)	Costa VII	Costa VI	Costa IV	Costa IV
Midclavicular line (MC)	Cartilago costalis costa VIII	Costa VI	Costa VI	Costa VIII
Midaxillary line (MA)	Costa X	Costa VIII	Costa VIII	Costa X
Paravertebral line (PV)	Vertebra Th XII	Costa X	Costa X	Vertebra Th XII

Fig. 8.3 Pleura parietale

The pleural cavity is bounded by two serous layers. The pleura visceralis (pulmonalis) covers the lungs, and the pleura parietale lines the inner surface of the thoracic cavity. The four parts of the pleura parietale (pars costalis, pars diaphragmatica, pars mediastinalis, and cupula pleura) are continuous.

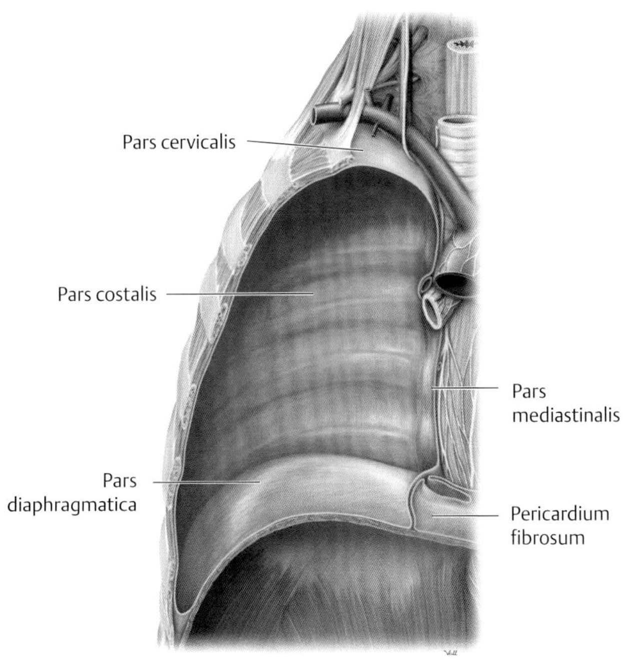

Pars cervicalis
Pars costalis
Pars mediastinalis
Pars diaphragmatica
Pericardium fibrosum

A Parts of the pleura parietale. *Opened:* Right pleural cavity, anterior view.

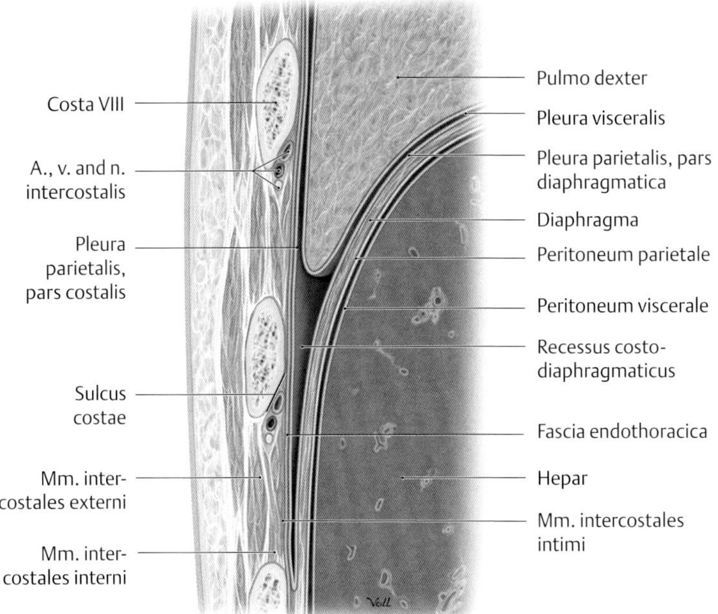

Costa VIII
A., v. and n. intercostalis
Pleura parietalis, pars costalis
Sulcus costae
Mm. intercostales externi
Mm. intercostales interni
Pulmo dexter
Pleura visceralis
Pleura parietalis, pars diaphragmatica
Diaphragma
Peritoneum parietale
Peritoneum viscerale
Recessus costodiaphragmaticus
Fascia endothoracica
Hepar
Mm. intercostales intimi

B Recessus costodiaphragmaticus, coronal section, anterior view. Reflection of the pars diaphragmatica onto the inner thoracic wall (becoming the pars costalis) forms the recessus costodiaphragmaticus.

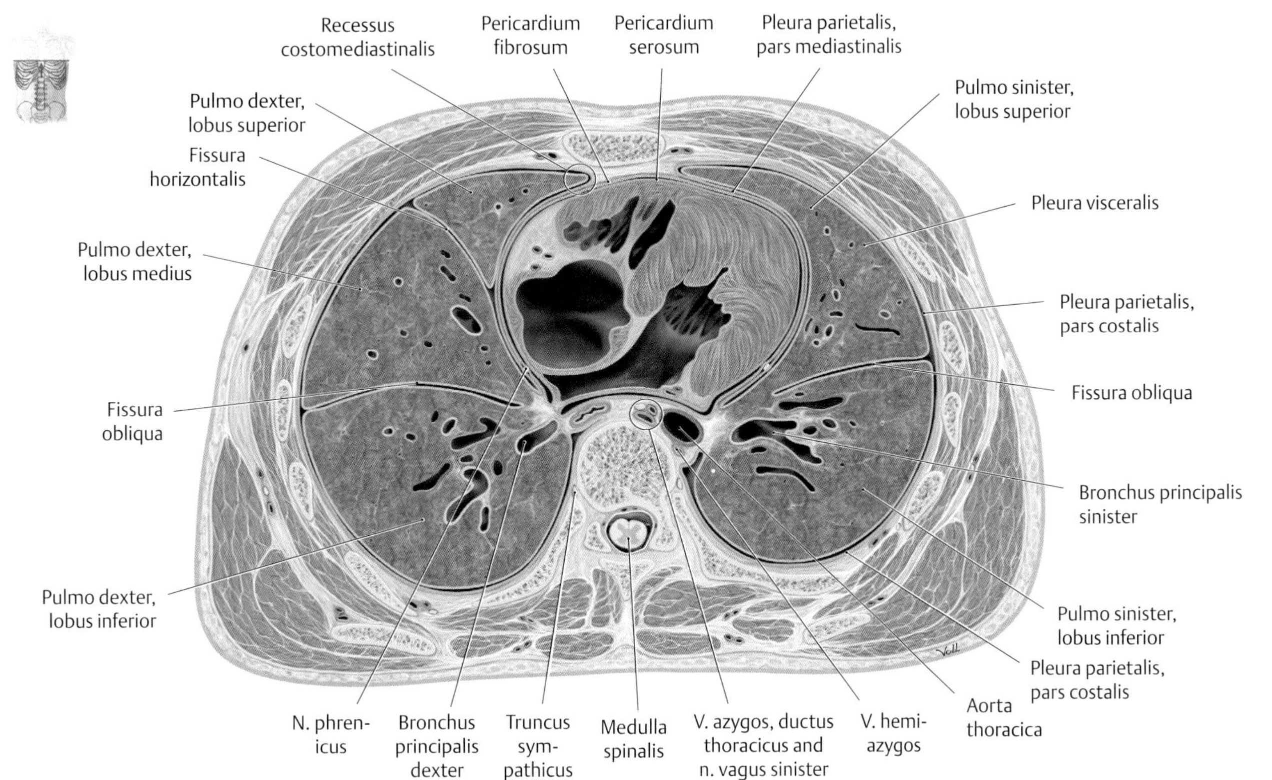

Recessus costomediastinalis
Pericardium fibrosum
Pericardium serosum
Pleura parietalis, pars mediastinalis
Pulmo dexter, lobus superior
Fissura horizontalis
Pulmo dexter, lobus medius
Fissura obliqua
Pulmo dexter, lobus inferior
Pulmo sinister, lobus superior
Pleura visceralis
Pleura parietalis, pars costalis
Fissura obliqua
Bronchus principalis sinister
Pulmo sinister, lobus inferior
Pleura parietalis, pars costalis
Aorta thoracica
N. phrenicus
Bronchus principalis dexter
Truncus sympathicus
Medulla spinalis
V. azygos, ductus thoracicus and n. vagus sinister
V. hemiazygos

C Transverse section, inferior view. Reflection of the pars costalis pleura parietalis onto the pericardium forms the recessus costomediastinalis.

Lungs in Situ

***Fig. 8.4* Lungs in situ**
The left and right lungs occupy the full volume of the pleural cavity. Note that the left lung is slightly smaller than the right due to the asymmetrical position of the heart.

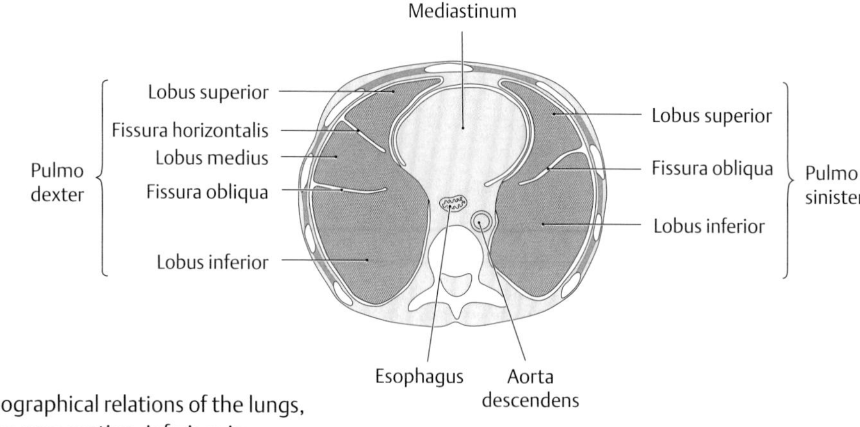
Mediastinum
Pulmo dexter
Lobus superior
Fissura horizontalis
Lobus medius
Fissura obliqua
Lobus inferior
Lobus superior
Fissura obliqua
Lobus inferior
Pulmo sinister
Esophagus
Aorta descendens

A Topographical relations of the lungs, transverse section, inferior view.

Truncus brachio-cephalicus
Cupula pleurae
Apex pulmonis
Pulmo dexter (lobus superior)
V. cava superior
A. pulmonalis dextra
Vv. pulmonales dextrae
Pulmo dexter (fissura horizontalis)
Truncus pulmonalis
Pulmo dexter (lobus medius)
Pulmo dexter (fissura obliqua)
Pulmo dexter (lobus inferior)
Recessus costo-diaphragmaticus
A. and v. subclavia sinistra
V. brachio-cephalica sinistra
Arcus aortae
A. pulmonalis sinistra
Bronchus lobaris superior and inferior
Pulmo sinister (lobus superior)
Aorta thoracica
Pleura parietalis, pars mediastinalis
Pulmo sinister (fissura obliqua)
Pleura parietalis, pars costalis
Pulmo sinister (lobus inferior)
Diaphragma
Pleura parietalis, pars diaphragmatica
Esophagus, pars thoracica
Pericardium fibrosum

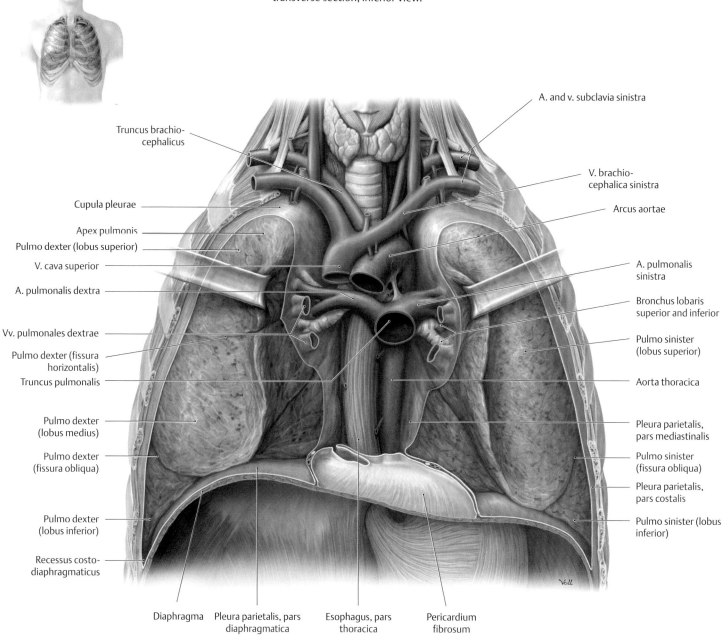

B Anterior view with lungs retracted.

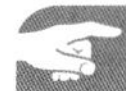

The fissura obliqua and fissura horizontalis divide the right lung into three lobi: superior, middle, and inferior. The fissura obliqua divides the left lung into two lobi: superior and inferior. The apex of each lung extends into the root of the neck. The hilum pulmonalis is the location at which the bronchi and neurovascular structures connect to the lung.

Fig. 8.5 Gross anatomy of the lungs

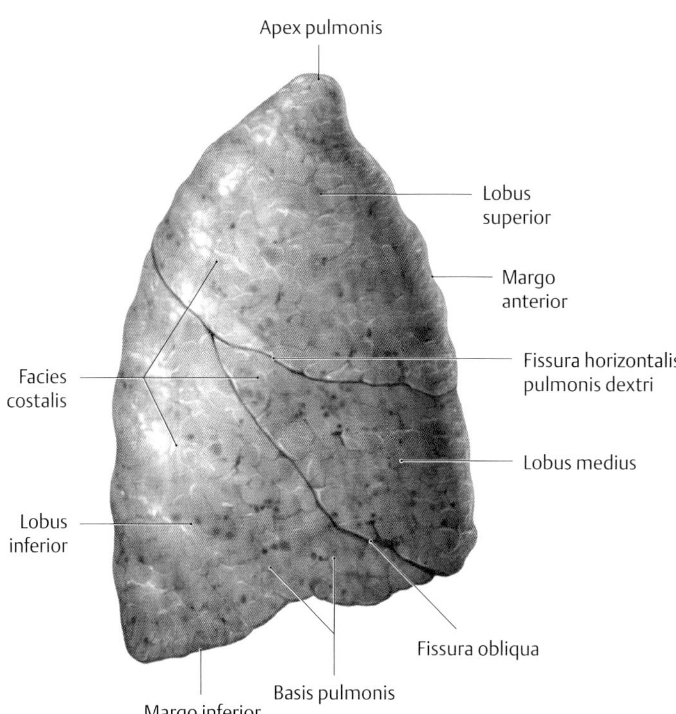
Apex pulmonis
Lobus superior
Margo anterior
Fissura horizontalis pulmonis dextri
Facies costalis
Lobus medius
Lobus inferior
Fissura obliqua
Basis pulmonis
Margo inferior

A Right lung, lateral view.

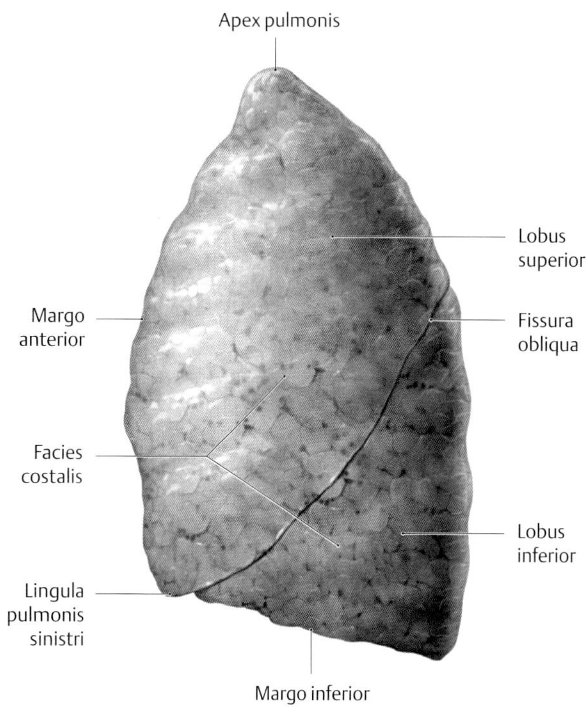
Apex pulmonis
Lobus superior
Margo anterior
Fissura obliqua
Facies costalis
Lobus inferior
Lingula pulmonis sinistri
Margo inferior

B Left lung, lateral view.

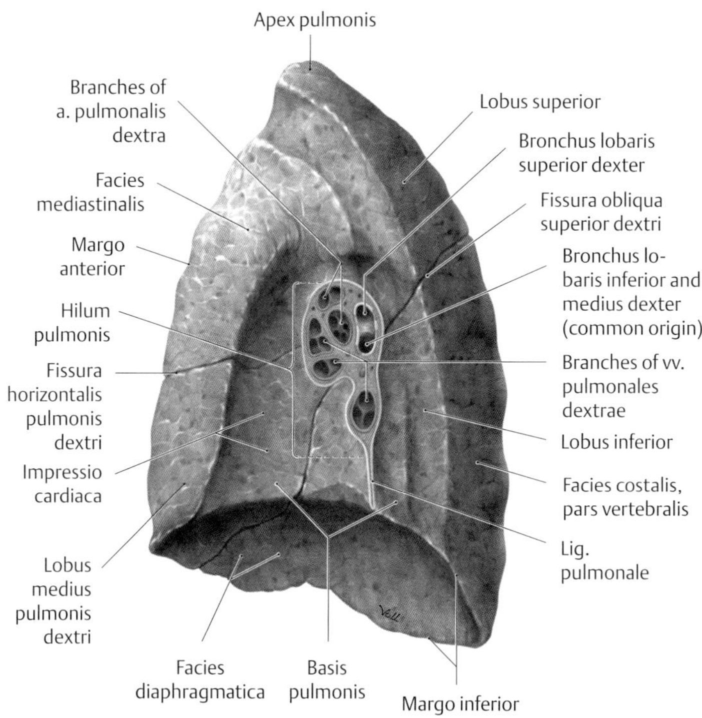
Apex pulmonis
Branches of a. pulmonalis dextra
Lobus superior
Bronchus lobaris superior dexter
Facies mediastinalis
Fissura obliqua superior dextri
Margo anterior
Bronchus lo-baris inferior and medius dexter (common origin)
Hilum pulmonis
Branches of vv. pulmonales dextrae
Fissura horizontalis pulmonis dextri
Lobus inferior
Impressio cardiaca
Facies costalis, pars vertebralis
Lig. pulmonale
Lobus medius pulmonis dextri
Facies diaphragmatica
Basis pulmonis
Margo inferior

C Right lung, medial view.

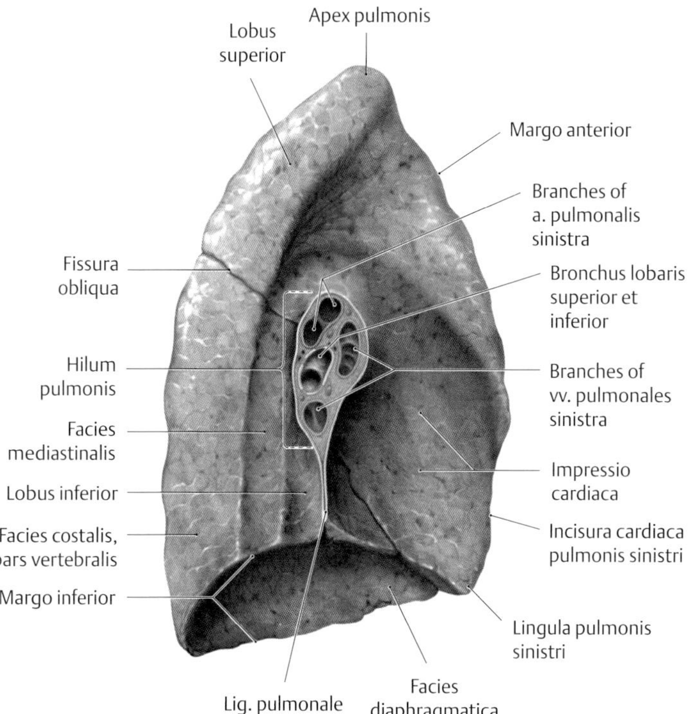
Lobus superior
Apex pulmonis
Margo anterior
Branches of a. pulmonalis sinistra
Fissura obliqua
Bronchus lobaris superior et inferior
Hilum pulmonis
Branches of vv. pulmonales sinistra
Facies mediastinalis
Impressio cardiaca
Lobus inferior
Incisura cardiaca pulmonis sinistri
Facies costalis, pars vertebralis
Margo inferior
Lingula pulmonis sinistri
Lig. pulmonale
Facies diaphragmatica

D Left lung, medial view.

Lung: Radiology

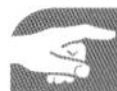

The regions of the lungs show varying degrees of lucency in chest radiographs. The perihilar region where the main bronchi and vessels enter and exit the lung is less radiolucent than the peripheral region, which contains small-caliber vascular branches and segmental bronchi. The perihilar lung region is also covered by the heart. These "shadows" appear as white or bright areas on the radiograph (radiographs are negatives: areas that are impermeable to light will appear bright).

Fig. 8.6 Radiographic appearance of the lungs

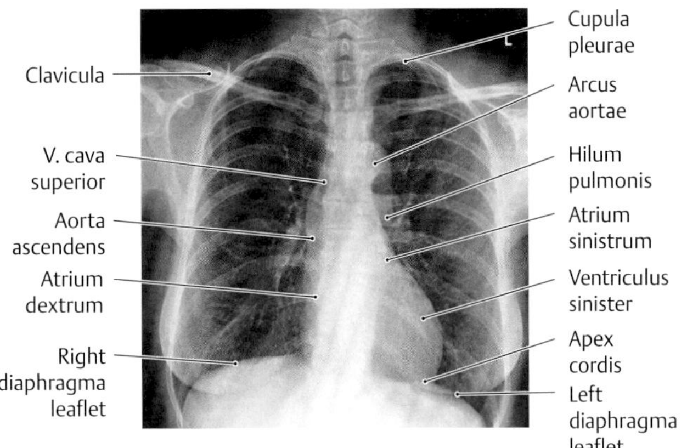
Clavicula
V. cava superior
Aorta ascendens
Atrium dextrum
Right diaphragma leaflet
Cupula pleurae
Arcus aortae
Hilum pulmonis
Atrium sinistrum
Ventriculus sinister
Apex cordis
Left diaphragma leaflet
L

A Normal anteroposterior chest radiograph.

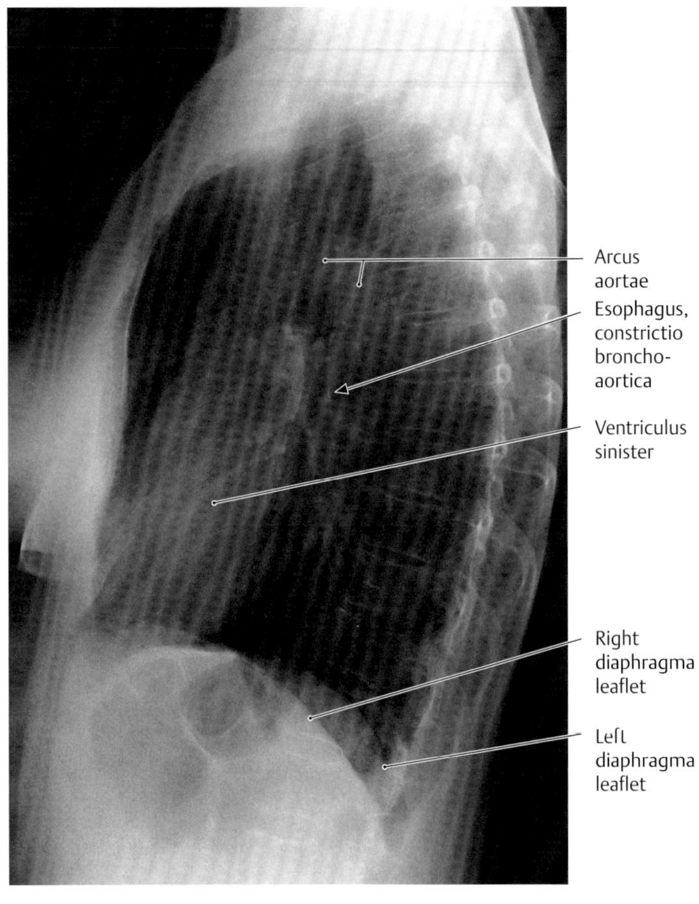
Arcus aortae
Esophagus, constrictio broncho-aortica
Ventriculus sinister
Right diaphragma leaflet
Left diaphragma leaflet

B Normal lateral chest radiograph.

Fig. 8.7 Opacity in lung diseases

Lateral and anterior views of the right and left lungs. Opacity (decreased radiolucency) may be observed in diseased lung areas. Increased opacity may be due to fluid infiltration (inflammation) or tissue proliferation (neoplasia). These opacities are easier to detect in the peripheral part of the lung, which is inherently more radiolucent. *Note:* Opacities that conform to segmental lung boundaries are almost invariably due to pulmonary inflammation.

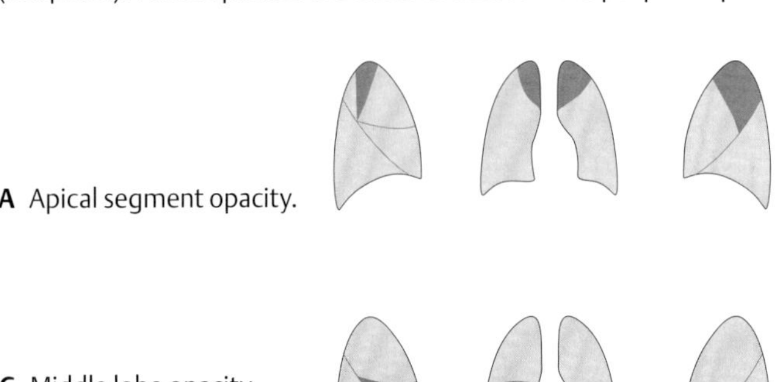

A Apical segment opacity.

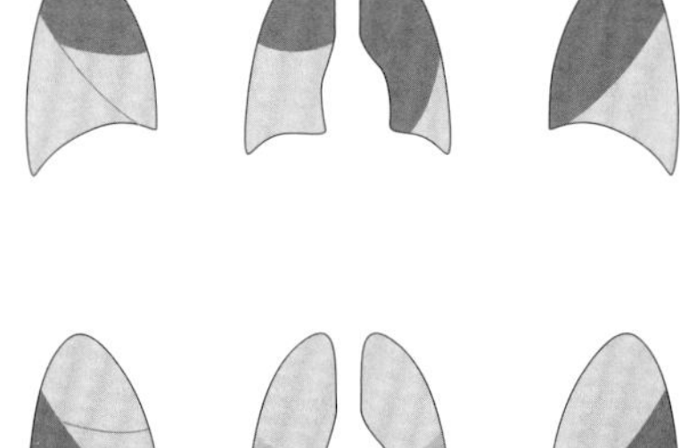

B Upper lobe opacity.

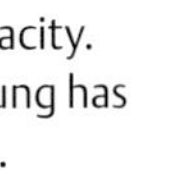

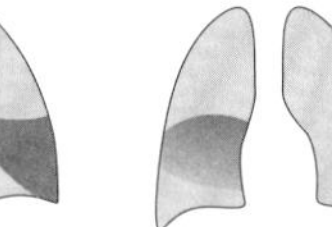

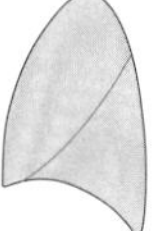

C Middle lobe opacity. *Note*: The left lung has no middle lobe.

D Lower lobe opacity.

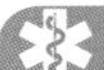 Clinical

Diseases of the lung

Increased opacity in the lungs does not necessarly correspond to segmental boundaries. Fluid accumulation in the lungs also creates characteristic "shadows" in pulmonary radiographs.

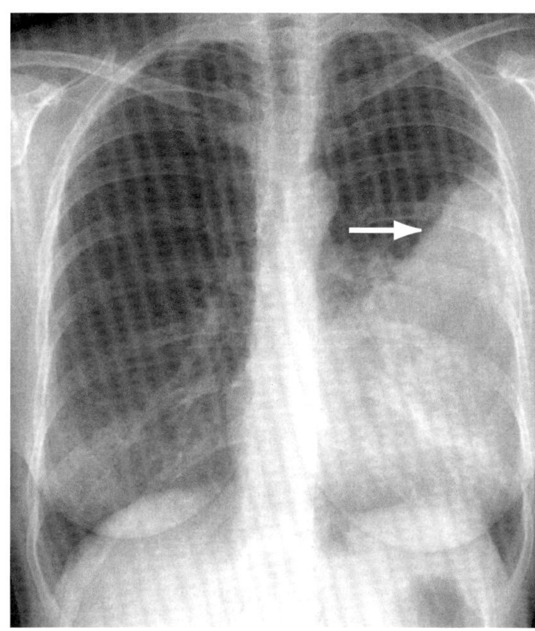

A Lingular pneumonia. The horizontal fissure can be seen (arrow). *Note*: The heart is much more difficult to visualize here due to increased opacity of segments IV and V.

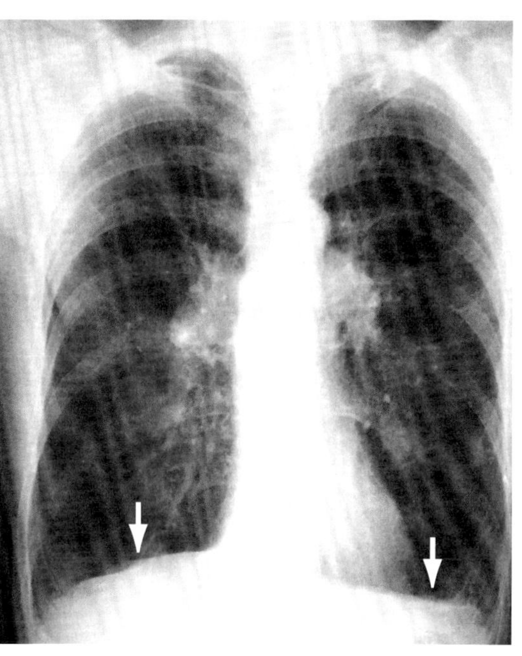

B Pulmonary emphysema. The chest radiograph reveals diaphragmatic depression (flattening of the domes of the diaphragm, arrows) with corresponding changes in the orientation of the cardiac shadow. The heart assumes a vertical orientation due to the low diaphragm (a lateral radiograph would reveal an increased retrosternal space). The central pulmonary arteries are dilated but taper dramatically at the segmental level.

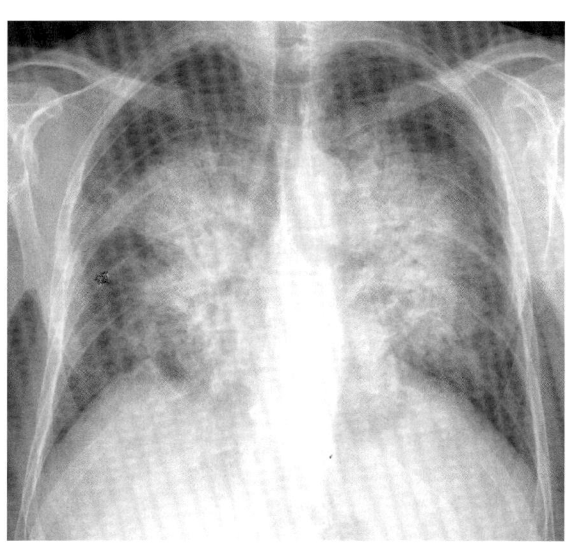

C Pulmonary edema complicating acute myocardial infarction. Dilation of vessels increases the number of visible vascular structures. This image shows a butterfly pattern of edema and bilateral pleural effusion.

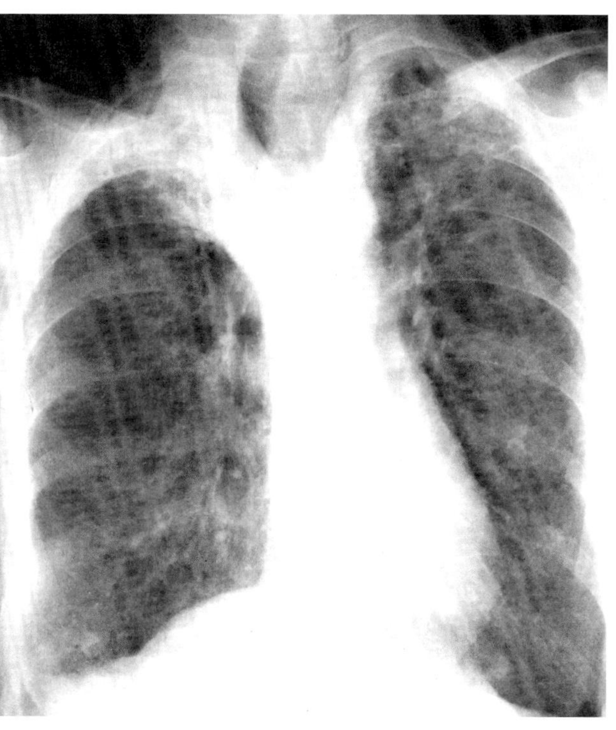

D Tuberculosis. Note the thickening of the pleura and the radiating fibrous bands. This image does not contain the small pulmonary nodules (tuberculomas) often found in the upper zones of the lung.

Bronchopulmonary Segments of the Lungs

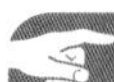

The lung lobes are subdivided into bronchopulmonary segments (segmenta bronchopulmonalia), each supplied by a tertiary (segmental) bronchus. *Note:* These subdivisions are not defined by surface boundaries but by origin.

Fig. 8.8 **Segmentation of the lung**
Anterior view. See pp. 110–111 for details of the trachea and bronchial tree.

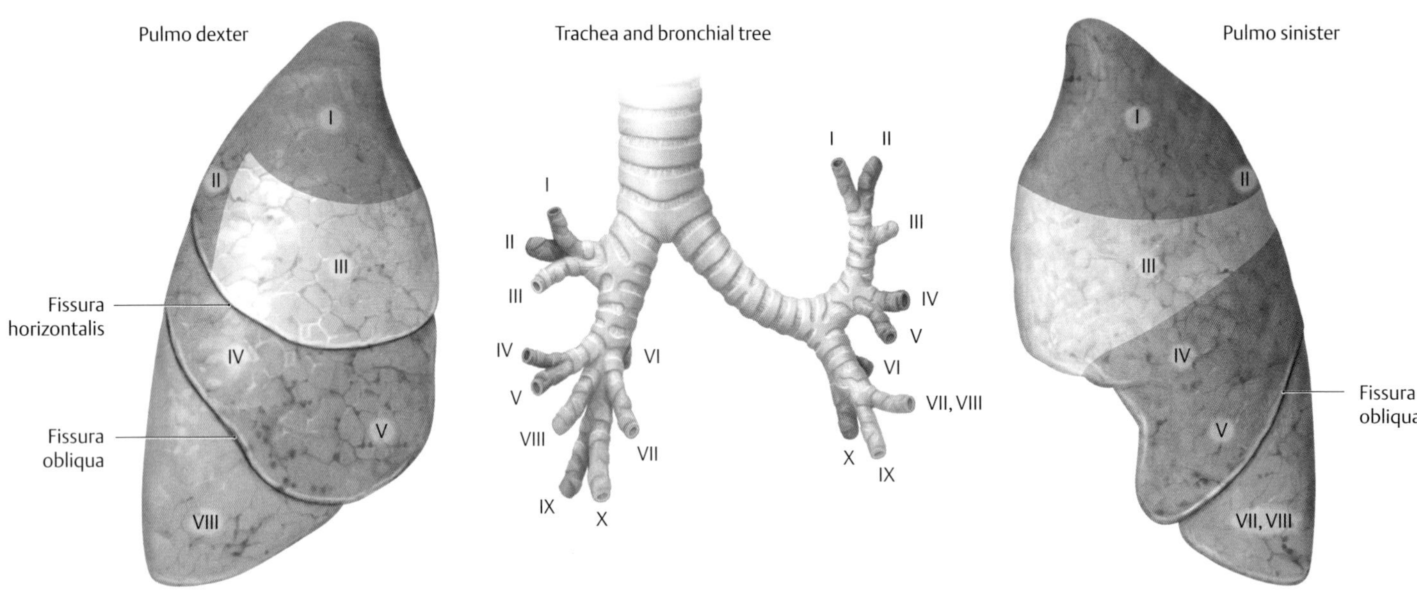
Pulmo dexter
I
II
III
Fissura horizontalis
IV
Fissura obliqua
V
VIII
Trachea and bronchial tree
I
II
III
IV
V
VI
VIII
VII
IX
X
I
II
III
IV
V
VI
VII, VIII
X
IX
Pulmo sinister
I
II
III
IV
Fissura obliqua
V
VII, VIII

Fig. 8.9 **Posteroanterior bronchogram**
Anterior view of right lung.

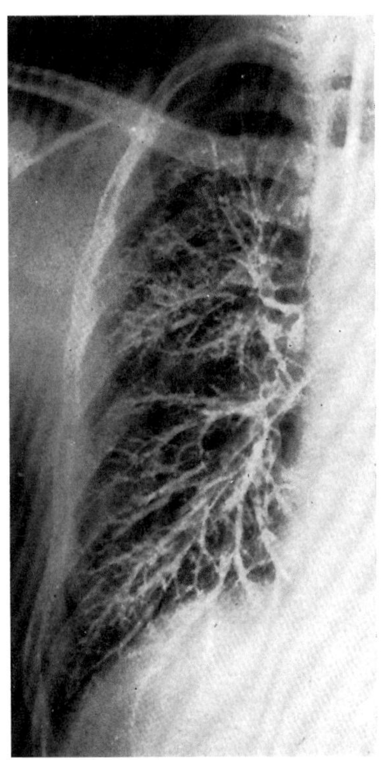

Table 8.2 **Segmental architecture of the lungs**

Each segment is supplied by a bronchus segmentalis of the same name (e.g., the bronchus segmentalis apicalis supplies the segmentum apicale). See pp. 110–111 for details of the trachea and bronchial tree.

	Pulmo dexter	Pulmo sinister	
	Lobus superior		
I	Segmentum apicale	Segmentum apicoposterius	I
II	Segmentum posterius		II
III	Segmentum anterius		III
	Lobus medius	**Lingula pulmonis sinistra**	
IV	Segmentum laterale	Segmentum lingulare superius	IV
V	Segmentum mediale	Segmentum lingulare inferius	V
	Inferior lobe		
VI	Segmentum superius		VI
VII	Segmentum basale mediale (cardiacum)		VII
VIII	Segmentum basale anterius		VIII
IX	Segmentum basale laterale		IX
X	Segmentum basale posterius		X

Fig. 8.10 Right lung: Bronchopulmonary segments

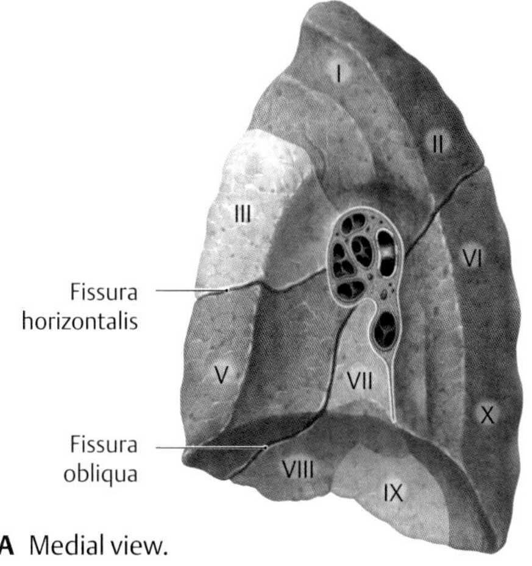

I
II
III
VI
Fissura horizontalis
V
VII
X
Fissura obliqua
VIII
IX

A Medial view.

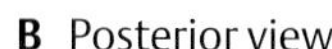

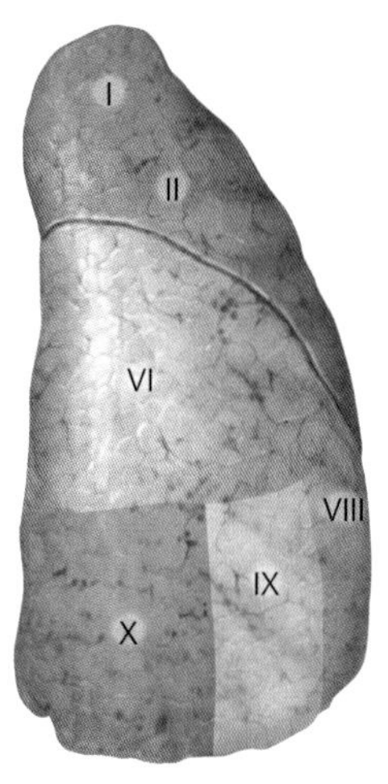

I
II
VI
VIII
IX
X

B Posterior view.

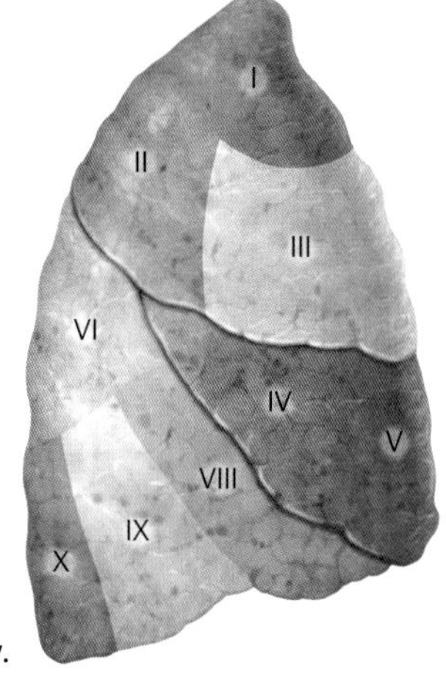

I
II
III
VI
IV
V
VIII
IX
X

C Lateral view.

Fig. 8.11 Left lung: Bronchopulmonary segments

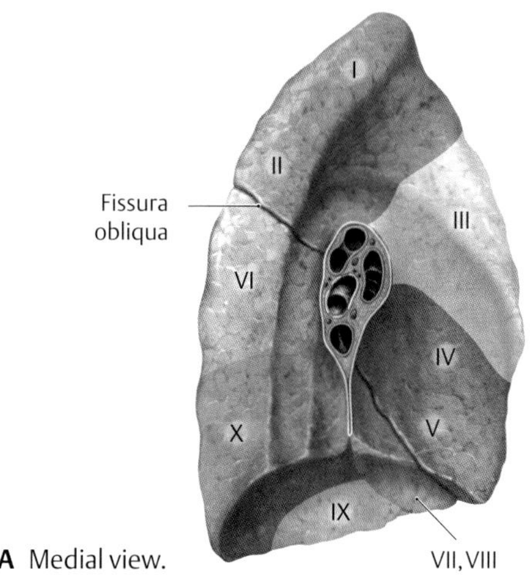

I
II
Fissura obliqua
III
VI
IV
X
V
IX
VII, VIII

A Medial view.

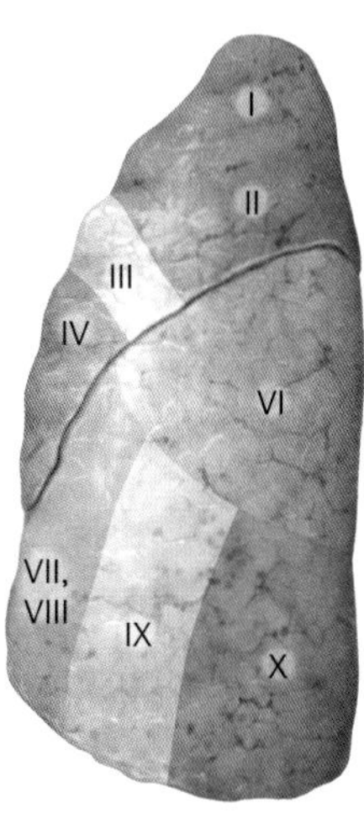

I
II
III
IV
VI
VII, VIII
IX
X

B Posterior view.

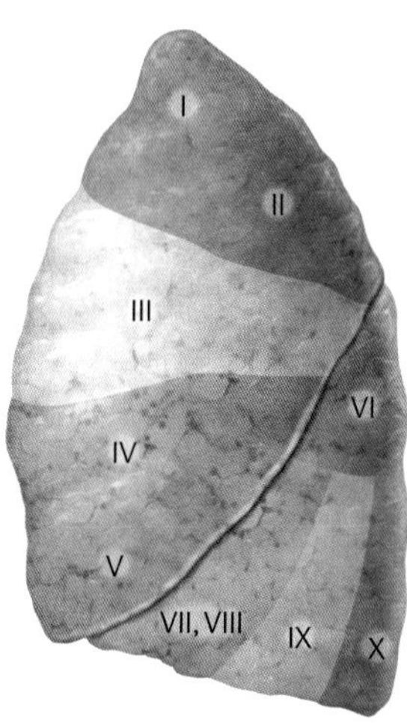

I
II
III
VI
IV
V
VII, VIII
IX
X

C Lateral view.

Clinical

Lung resections

Lung cancer, emphysema, or tuberculosis may necessitate the surgical removal of damaged portions of the lung. Surgeons exploit the anatomical subdivision of the lungs into lobes and segments when excising damaged tissue.

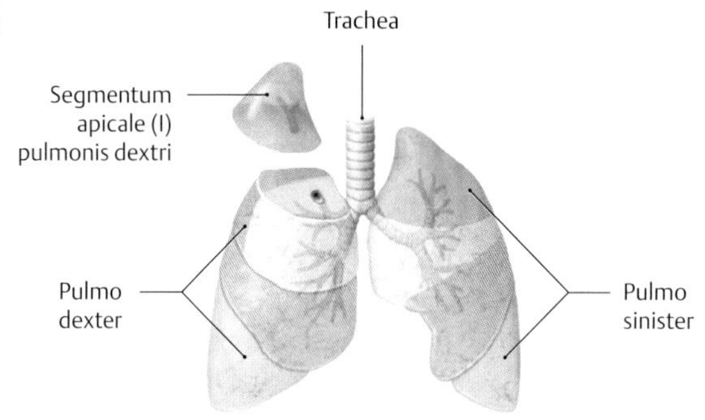

Trachea
Segmentum apicale (I) pulmonis dextri
Pulmo dexter
Pulmo sinister

A Segmentectomy (wedge resection): Removal of one or more segments.

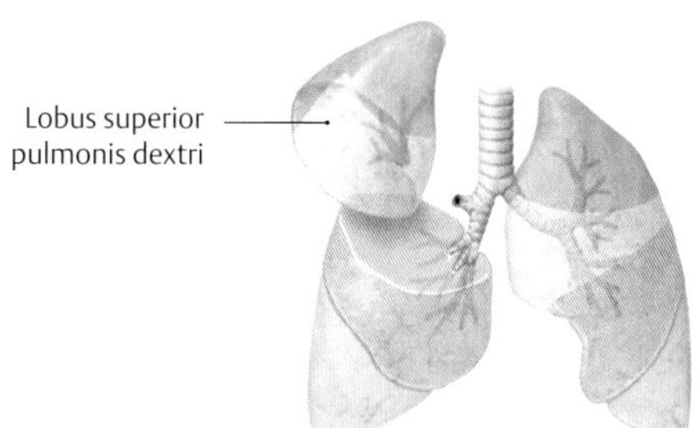

Lobus superior pulmonis dextri

B Lobectomy: Removal of lobe.

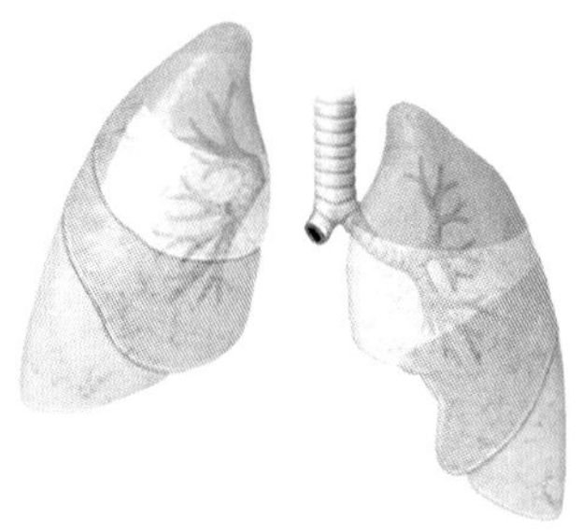

C Pneumonectomy: Removal of entire lung.

Trachea & Bronchial Tree

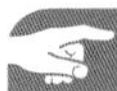

At or near the level of the angulus sterni, the lowest tracheal cartilage extends anteroposteriorly, forming the carina tracheae. The trachea bifurcates at the carina into the bronchi principales dexter and sinister. Each bronchus principalis gives off bronchi lobares to the corresponding lung.

Fig. 8.12 Trachea
See p. 574 for the structures of the thyroid.

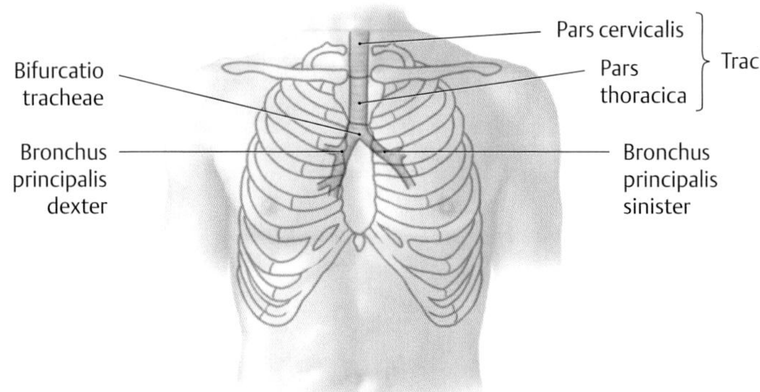
Bifurcatio tracheae
Bronchus principalis dexter
Pars cervicalis
Pars thoracica
Trachea
Bronchus principalis sinister

A Projection of trachea onto chest.

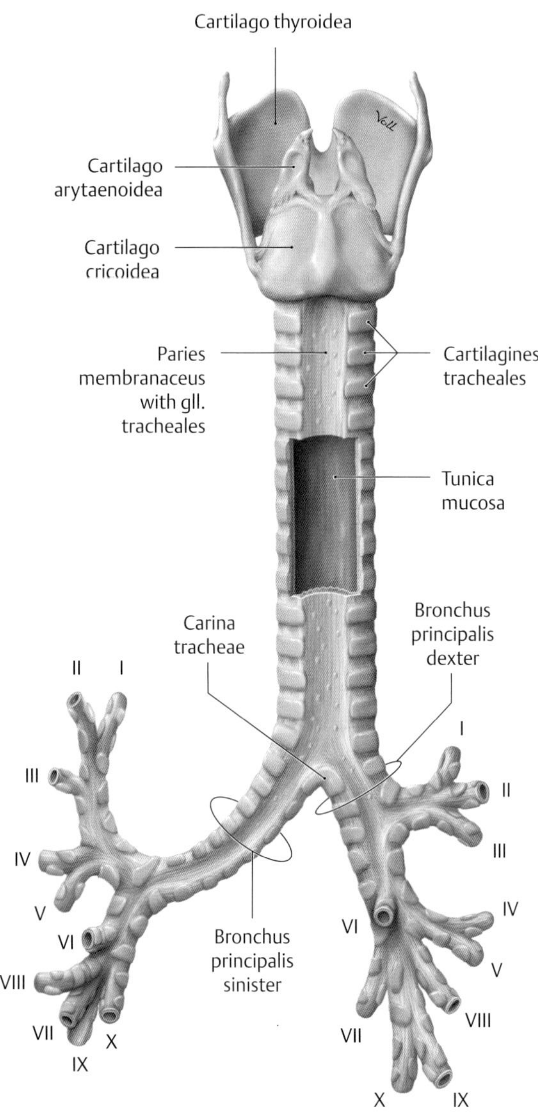
Cartilago thyroidea
Cartilago arytaenoidea
Cartilago cricoidea
Paries membranaceus with gll. tracheales
Cartilagines tracheales
Tunica mucosa
Carina tracheae
Bronchus principalis dexter
Bronchus principalis sinister
I
II
III
IV
V
VI
VII
VIII
IX
X

C Posterior view with opened posterior wall.

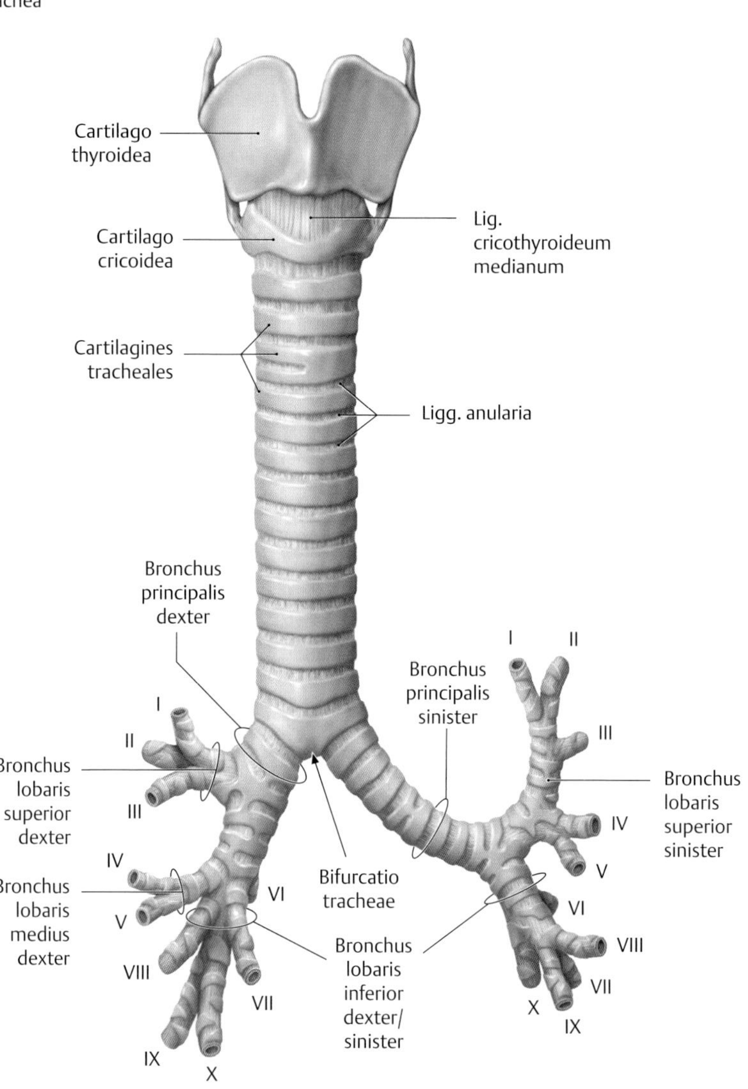
Cartilago thyroidea
Cartilago cricoidea
Lig. cricothyroideum medianum
Cartilagines tracheales
Ligg. anularia
Bronchus principalis dexter
Bronchus principalis sinister
Bronchus lobaris superior dexter
Bronchus lobaris medius dexter
Bifurcatio tracheae
Bronchus lobaris inferior dexter/ sinister
Bronchus lobaris superior sinister
I
II
III
IV
V
VI
VII
VIII
IX
X

B Anterior view.

Clinical

Foreign body aspiration

Toddlers are at particularly high risk of potentially fatal aspiration of foreign bodies. In general, foreign bodies are more likely to become lodged in the right bronchus principalis than the left: the left bronchus diverges more sharply at the tracheal bifurcation, while the right bronchus is relatively straight.

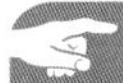

The conducting portion of the bronchial tree extends from the bifurcatio tracheae to the bronchiolus terminalis, inclusive. The respiratory portion consists of the bronchiolus respiratorius, ductuli alveolares, sacculi alveolares, and alveoli.

Fig. 8.13 Bronchial tree

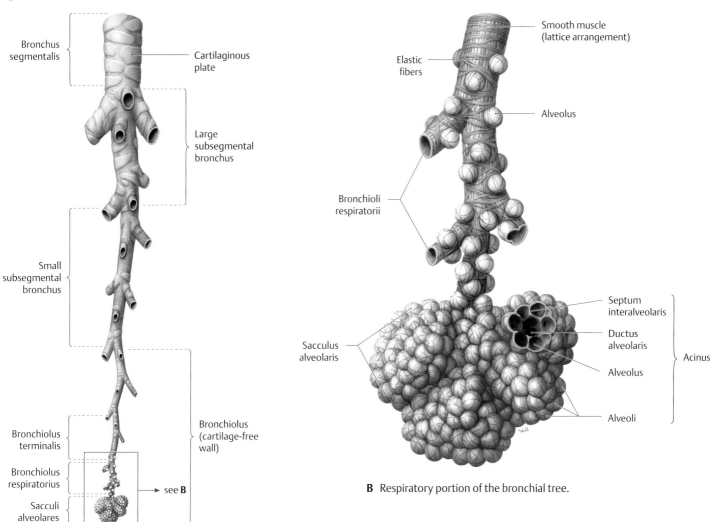

Bronchus segmentalis

Cartilaginous plate

Large subsegmental bronchus

Small subsegmental bronchus

Bronchiolus terminalis

Bronchiolus (cartilage-free wall)

Bronchiolus respiratorius

see **B**

Sacculi alveolares

A Divisions of the bronchial tree.

Smooth muscle (lattice arrangement)

Elastic fibers

Alveolus

Bronchioli respiratorii

Septum interalveolaris

Ductus alveolaris

Sacculus alveolaris

Acinus

Alveolus

Alveoli

B Respiratory portion of the bronchial tree.

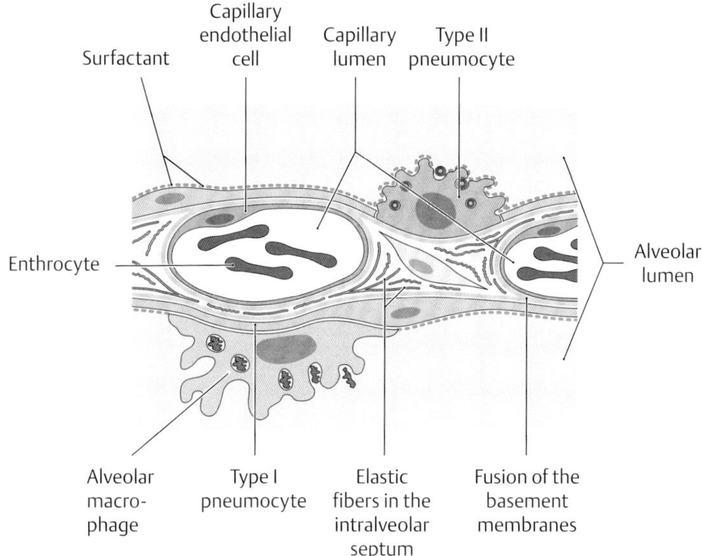
Capillary endothelial cell
Surfactant
Capillary lumen
Type II pneumocyte
Enthrocyte
Alveolar lumen
Alveolar macro-phage
Type I pneumocyte
Elastic fibers in the intralveolar septum
Fusion of the basement membranes

C Epithelial lining of the alveoli.

Clinical

Respiratory compromise

The most common cause of respiratory compromise at the bronchial level is asthma. Compromise at the alveolar level may result from increased diffusion distance, decreased aeration (emphysema), or fluid infiltration (e.g., pneumonia).

Diffusion distance: Gaseous exchange takes place between the alveolar and capillary lumens in the alveoli (see Fig. 8.13C). At these sites, the basement membranes of capillary endothelial cells are fused with those of type I alveolar epithelial cells, lowering the exchange distance to 0.5 μm. Diseases that increase this diffusion distance (e.g., edematous fluid collection or inflammation) result in compromised respiration.

Condition of alveoli: In diseases like emphysema, which occurs in chronic obstructive pulmonary disease (COPD), alveoli are destroyed or damaged. This reduces the surface area available for gaseous exchange.

Production of surfactant: Surfactant is a protein-phospholipid film that lowers the surface tension of the alveoli, making it easier for the lung to expand. The immature lungs of a preterm infant often fail to produce sufficient surfactant, leading to respiratory problems. Surfactant is produced and absorbed by alveolar epithelial cells (pneumocytes). Type I alveolar epithelial cells absorb surfactant; type II produce and distribute it.

Respiratory Mechanics

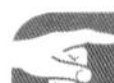

The mechanics of respiration are based on a rhythmic increase and decrease in thoracic volume, with an associated expansion and contraction of the lungs. *Inspiration* (red): Contraction of the diaphragm leaflets lowers the diaphragma into the inspiratory position, increasing the volume of the pleural cavity along the vertical axis. Contraction of the thoracic muscles (mm. intercostales externi, mm. scaleni, and m. serratus posterior) elevates the ribs, expanding the pleural cavity along the sagittal and transverse axes (Fig. 8.15A,B). Surface tension in the pleural space causes the pleura viscerale and parietale to adhere; thus, changes in thoracic volume alter the volume of the lungs. This is particularly evident in the pleural recesses: at functional residual capacity (resting position between inspiration and expiration), the lung does not fully occupy the pleural cavity. As the pleural cavity expands, a negative intrapleural pressure is generated. The air pressure differential results in an influx of air (inspiration). *Expiration* (blue): During passive expiration, the muscles of the thoracic cage relax and the diaphragma returns to its expiratory position. Contraction of the lungs increases the pulmonary pressure and expels air from the lungs. For forcible expiration, the mm. intercostalis interni (with the m. transversus thoracis and mm. subcostales) can actively lower the rib cage more rapidly and to a greater extent than through passive elastic recoil.

Fig. 8.14 **Respiratory changes in thoracic volume**
Inspiratory position (red); expiratory position (blue).

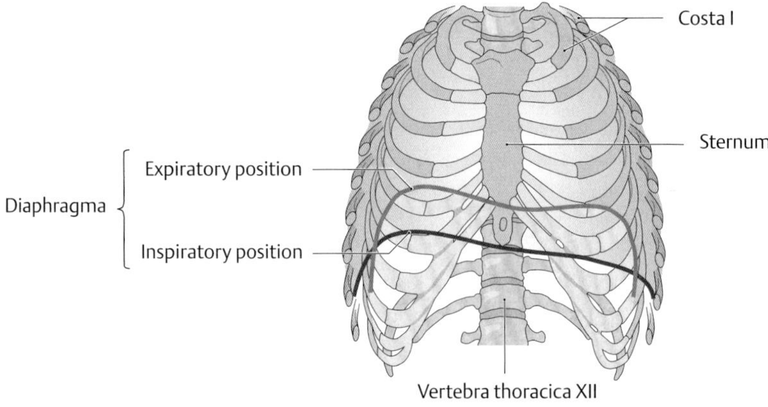
Costa I
Sternum
Diaphragma
Expiratory position
Inspiratory position
Vertebra thoracica XII

Fig. 8.15 **Inspiration: Pleural cavity expansion**

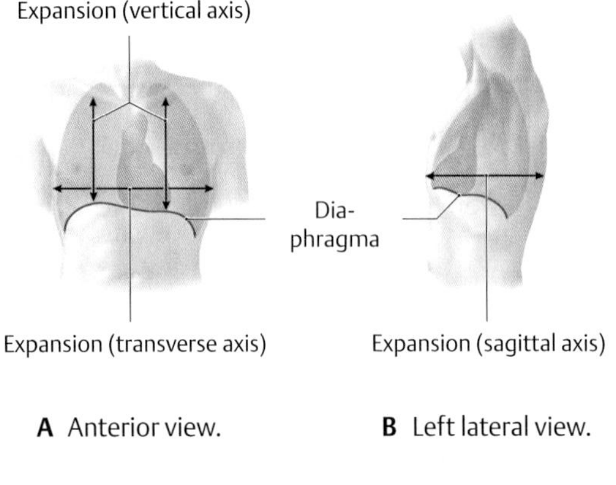
Expansion (vertical axis)
Dia-
phragma
Expansion (transverse axis)
Expansion (sagittal axis)

A Anterior view.

B Left lateral view.

Inspiration

Costa I

Apertura thoracica superior

Angulus infrasternalis

C Anterolateral view.

Fig. 8.16 **Expiration: Pleural cavity contraction**

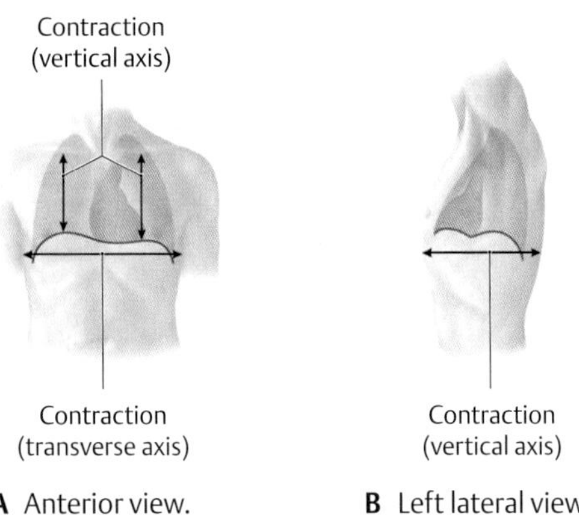
Contraction
(vertical axis)
Contraction
(transverse axis)
Contraction
(vertical axis)

A Anterior view.

B Left lateral view.

Expiration

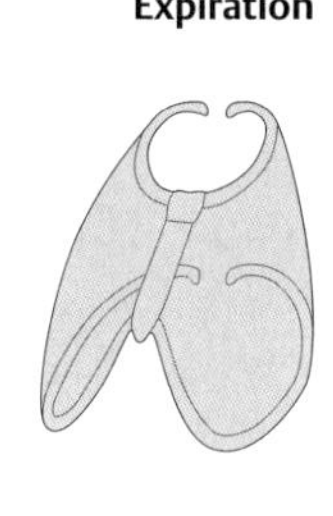

C Anterolateral view.

Fig. 8.17 **Respiratory changes in lung volume**

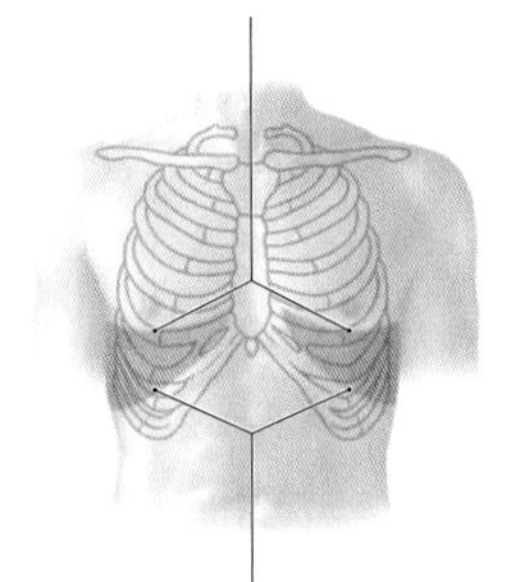
Inferior border of lung (full expiration)
Inferior border of lung (full inspiration)

Fig. 8.18 Inspiration: Lung expansion

Pulmo dexter (full inspiration)
Diaphragma
Recessus costodiaphragmaticus

Fig. 8.19 Expiration: Lung contraction

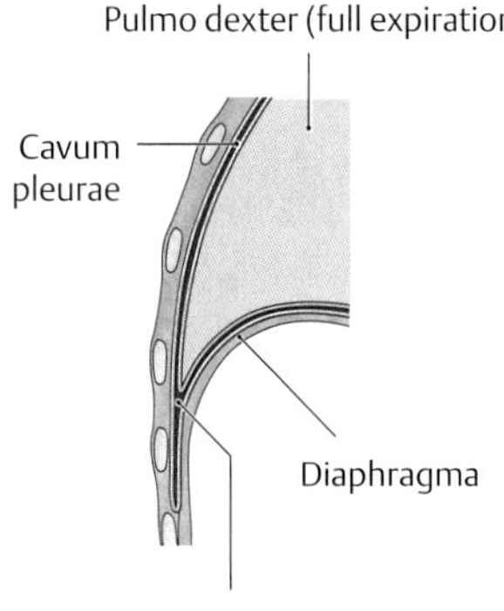
Pulmo dexter (full expiration)
Cavum pleurae
Diaphragma
Recessus costodiaphragmaticus

Fig. 8.20 Movements of the lung and bronchial tree

As the volume of the lung changes with the thoracic cavity, the entire bronchial tree moves within the lung. These structural movements are more pronounced in portions of the bronchial tree distant from the pulmonary hilum.

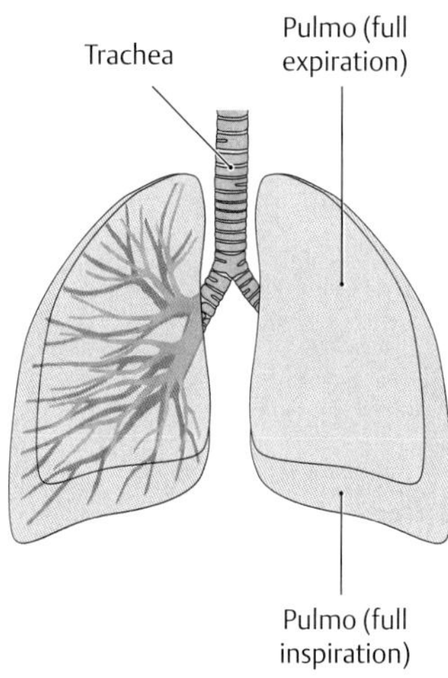
Trachea
Pulmo (full expiration)
Pulmo (full inspiration)

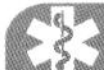

Clinical

Pneumothorax

The pleural space is normally sealed from the outside environment. Injury to the parietal pleura, visceral pleura, or lung allows air to enter the pleural cavity (pneumothorax). The lung collapses due to its inherent elasticity, and the patient's ability to breathe is compromised. The uninjured lung continues to function under normal pressure variations, resulting in "mediastinal flutter": the mediastinum shifts toward the normal side during inspiration and returns to the midline during expiration. Tension (valve) pneumothorax occurs when traumatically detached and displaced tissure covers the defect in the thoracic wall from the inside. This mobile flap allows air to enter, but not escape, the pleural cavity, causing a pressure buildup. The mediastinum shifts to the normal side, which may cause kinking of the great vessels and prevent the return of venous blood to the heart. Without treatment, tension pneumothorax is invariably fatal.

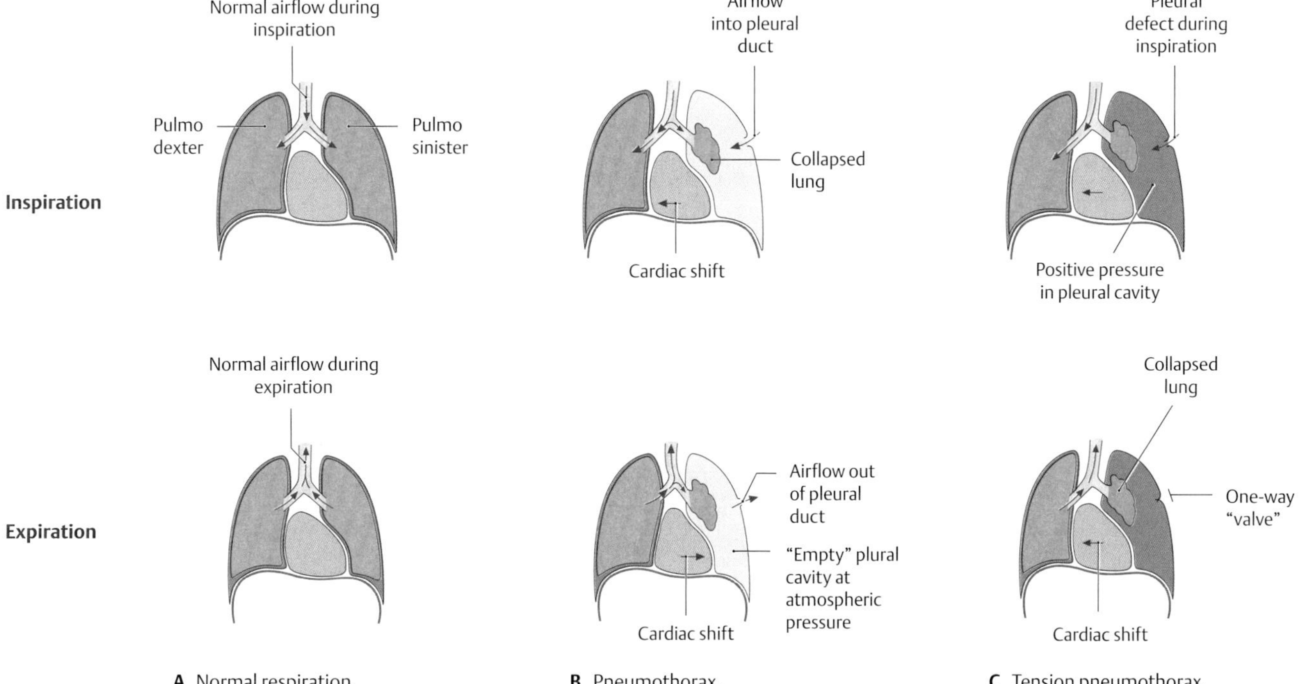
Inspiration
Expiration
Normal airflow during inspiration
Pulmo dexter
Pulmo sinister
Normal airflow during expiration
Airflow into pleural duct
Collapsed lung
Cardiac shift
Airflow out of pleural duct
"Empty" plural cavity at atmospheric pressure
Cardiac shift
Pleural defect during inspiration
Positive pressure in pleural cavity
Collapsed lung
One-way "valve"
Cardiac shift

A Normal respiration.

B Pneumothorax.

C Tension pneumothorax.

Pulmonary Arteries & Veins

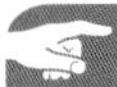

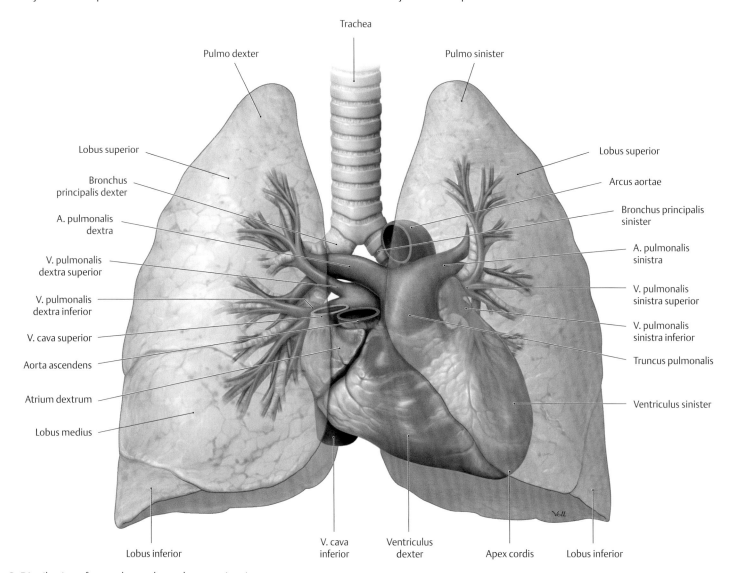

The truncus pulmonalis arises from the right ventriculus and divides into a left and right a. pulmonalis for each lung. The paired vv. pulmonales open into the left atrium on each side. The aa. pulmonales accompany and follow the branching of the bronchial tree, whereas the vv. pulmonales do not, being located at the margins of the pulmonary lobules.

Fig. 8.21 **Pulmonary arteries and veins**
Anterior view.

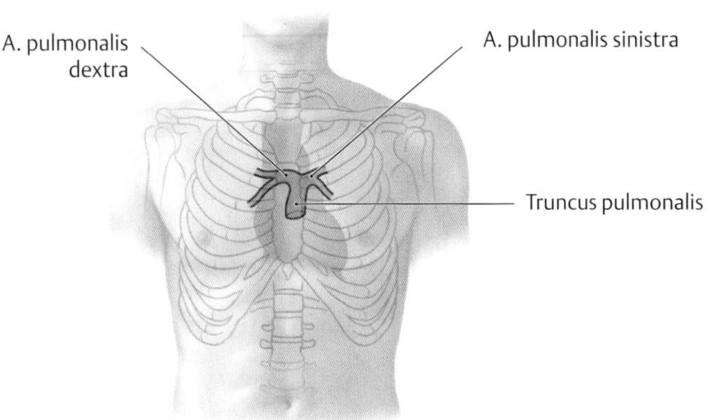
A. pulmonalis dextra
A. pulmonalis sinistra
Truncus pulmonalis

A Projection of aa. pulmonales on chest wall.

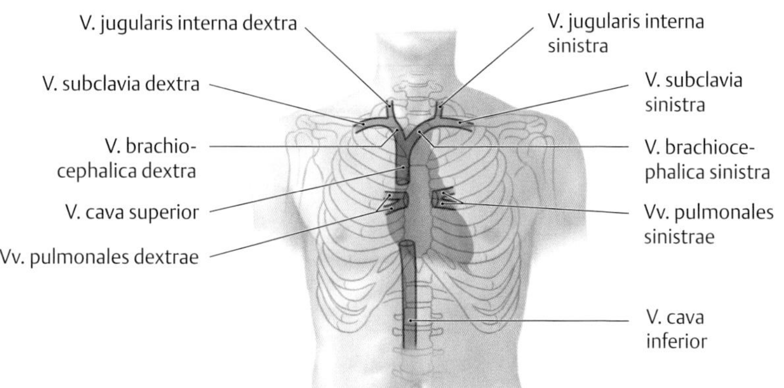
V. jugularis interna dextra
V. jugularis interna sinistra
V. subclavia dextra
V. subclavia sinistra
V. brachio-cephalica dextra
V. brachioce-phalica sinistra
V. cava superior
Vv. pulmonales sinistrae
Vv. pulmonales dextrae
V. cava inferior

B Projection of vv. pulmonales on chest wall.

Trachea
Pulmo dexter
Pulmo sinister
Lobus superior
Lobus superior
Arcus aortae
Bronchus principalis dexter
Bronchus principalis sinister
A. pulmonalis dextra
A. pulmonalis sinistra
V. pulmonalis dextra superior
V. pulmonalis sinistra superior
V. pulmonalis dextra inferior
V. pulmonalis sinistra inferior
V. cava superior
Truncus pulmonalis
Aorta ascendens
Atrium dextrum
Ventriculus sinister
Lobus medius
Lobus inferior
V. cava inferior
Ventriculus dexter
Apex cordis
Lobus inferior

C Distribution of aa. and vv. pulmonales, anterior view.

Fig. 8.22 Aa. pulmonales

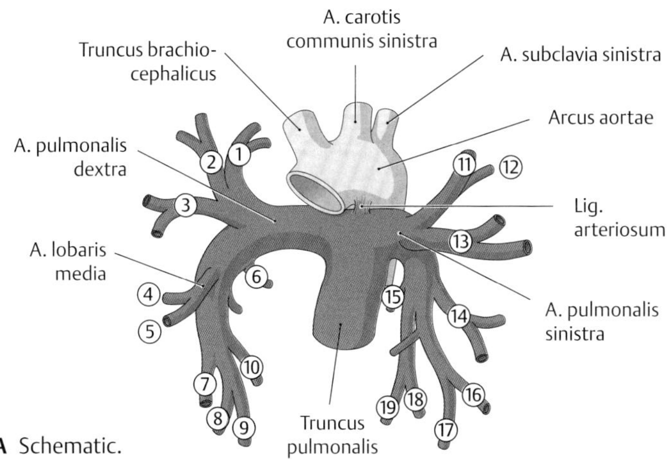
A. carotis communis sinistra
Truncus brachio-cephalicus
A. subclavia sinistra
Arcus aortae
A. pulmonalis dextra
Lig. arteriosum
A. lobaris media
A. pulmonalis sinistra
Truncus pulmonalis
1
2
3
4
5
6
7
8
9
10
11
12
13
14
15
16
17
18
19

A Schematic.

Table 8.3 Aa. pulmonales and their branches

A. pulmonales dextra			A. pulmonales sinistra
Aa. lobares superiores			
①	A. segmentalis apicalis		⑪
②	A. segmentalis posterior		⑫
③	A. segmentalis anterior		⑬
A. lobaris media			
④	A. segmentalis lateralis	A. lingularis	⑭
⑤	A. segmentalis medialis		
Aa. lobares inferiores			
⑥	A. segmentalis superior		⑮
⑦	A. segmentalis basalis anterior		⑯
⑧	A. segmentalis basalis lateralis		⑰
⑨	A. segmentalis basalis posterior		⑱
⑩	A. segmentalis basalis medialis		⑲

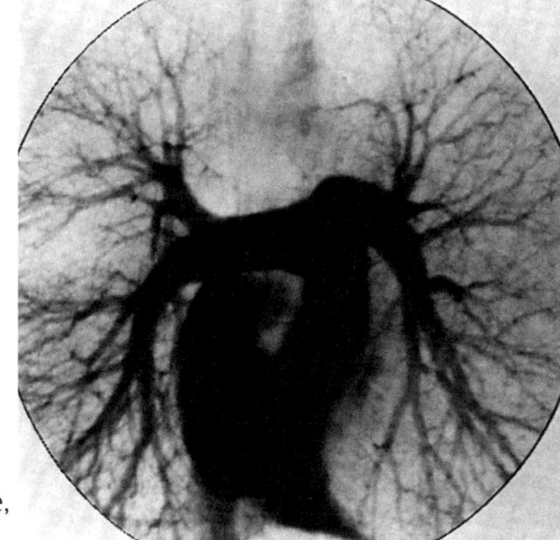

B Pulmonary arteriogram, arterial phase, anterior view.

Fig. 8.23 Vv. pulmonales

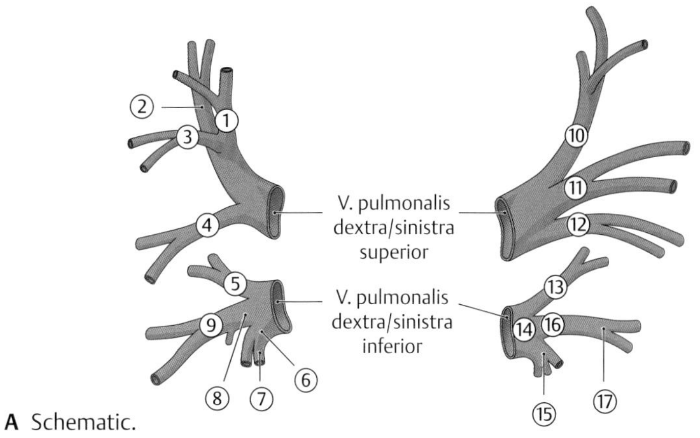
V. pulmonalis dextra/sinistra superior
V. pulmonalis dextra/sinistra inferior
1
2
3
4
5
6
7
8
9
10
11
12
13
14
15
16
17

A Schematic.

Table 8.4 Vv. pulmonales and their tributaries

Vv. pulmonales dextra			Vv. pulmonales sinistra
Vv. superiores			
①	V. apicalis	V. apicoposterior	⑩
②	V. posterior		
③	V. anterior	V. anterior	⑪
④	V. lobi medii	V. lingularis	⑫
Vv. inferiores			
⑤	V. superior		⑬
⑥	V. basalis communis		⑭
⑦	V. basalis inferior		⑮
⑧	V. basalis superior		⑯
⑨	V. basalis anterior		⑰

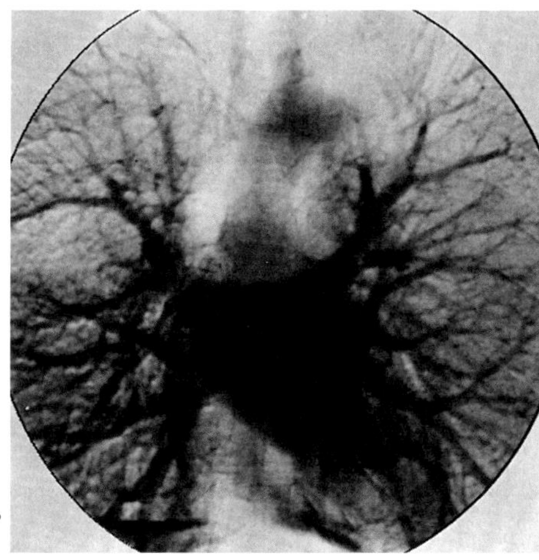

B Pulmonary arteriogram, venous phase, anterior view.

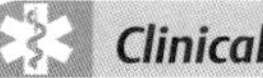

Clinical

Pulmonary embolism

Potentially life-threatening pulmonary embolism occurs when blood clots migrate through the venous system and become lodged in one of the arteries supplying the lungs. Symptoms include dyspnea (difficulty breathing) and tachycardia (increased heart rate). Most pulmonary emboli originate from stagnant blood in the veins of the lower limb and pelvis (venous thromboemboli). Causes include immobilization, disordered blood coagulation, and trauma. *Note:* A thromboembolus is a thrombus (blood clot) that has migrated (embolised).

Neurovasculature of the Tracheobronchial Tree

Fig. 8.24 **Pulmonary vasculature**
The pulmonary system is responsible for gaseous exchange within the lung. The branches of a. pulmonalis (shown in blue) carry *deoxygenated* blood and follow the bronchial tree. The branches of vv. pulmonales (red) are the only veins in the body carrying *oxygenated* blood, which they receive from the alveolar capillaries at the periphery of the lobulus.

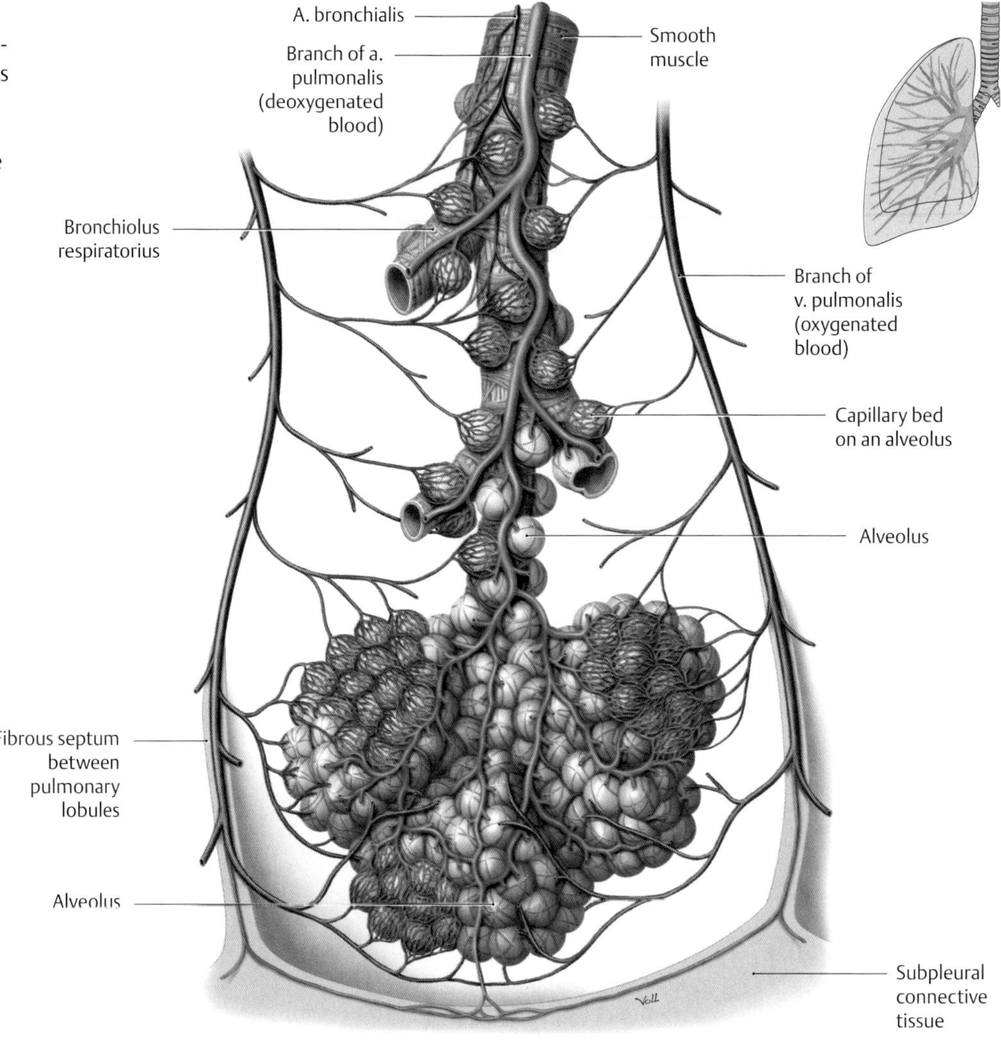
A. bronchialis
Branch of a. pulmonalis (deoxygenated blood)
Smooth muscle
Bronchiolus respiratorius
Branch of v. pulmonalis (oxygenated blood)
Capillary bed on an alveolus
Alveolus
Fibrous septum between pulmonary lobules
Alveolus
Subpleural connective tissue

Fig. 8.25 **Aa. bronchiales**
The bronchial tree receives its nutrients via the aa. bronchiales, found in the adventitia of the airways. Typically, there are one to three aa. bronchiales arising directly from the aorta. Origin from an a. intercostalis posterior may also occur.

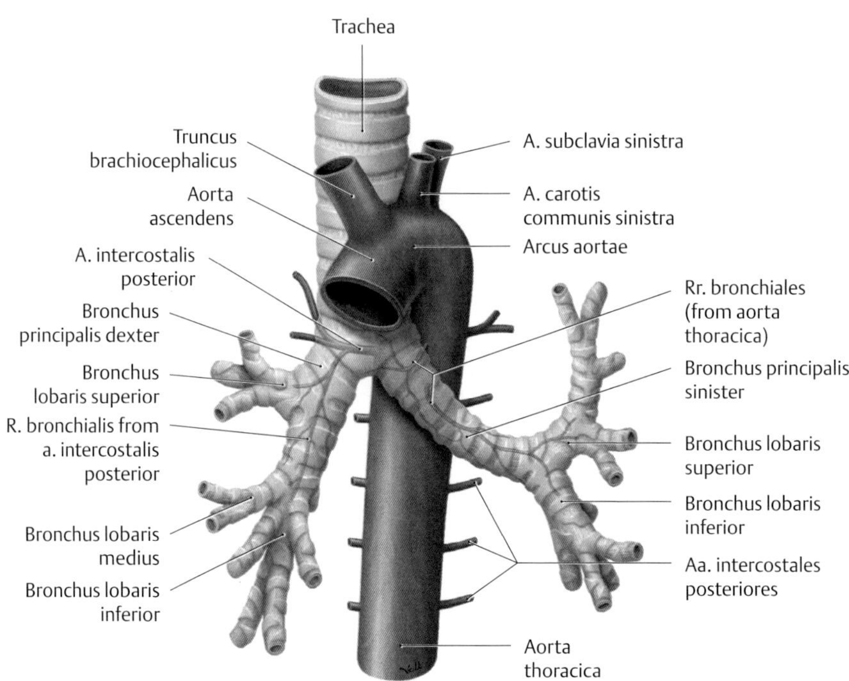
Trachea
Truncus brachiocephalicus
Aorta ascendens
A. intercostalis posterior
Bronchus principalis dexter
Bronchus lobaris superior
R. bronchialis from a. intercostalis posterior
Bronchus lobaris medius
Bronchus lobaris inferior
A. subclavia sinistra
A. carotis communis sinistra
Arcus aortae
Rr. bronchiales (from aorta thoracica)
Bronchus principalis sinister
Bronchus lobaris superior
Bronchus lobaris inferior
Aa. intercostales posteriores
Aorta thoracica

Fig. 8.26 Vv. bronchiales
Blood supplied by the aa. bronchiales is drained from the proximal tracheobronchial tree by the vv. bronchiales to the azygos system.

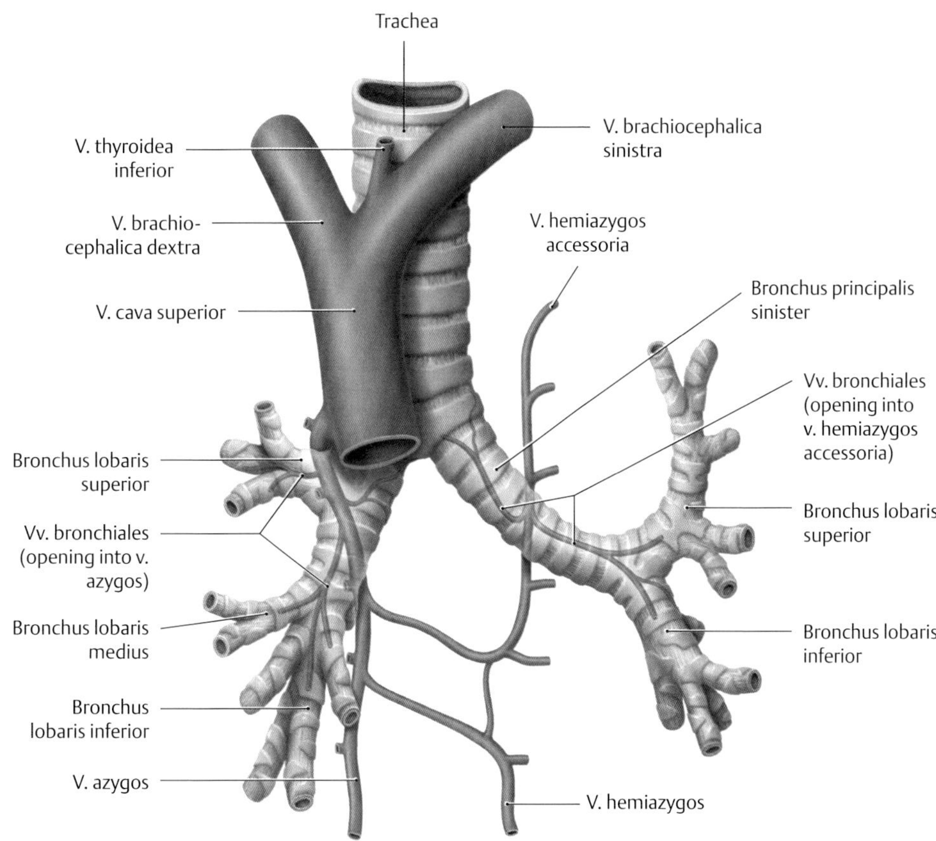
Trachea
V. thyroidea inferior
V. brachiocephalica sinistra
V. brachio-cephalica dextra
V. hemiazygos accessoria
V. cava superior
Bronchus principalis sinister
Vv. bronchiales (opening into v. hemiazygos accessoria)
Bronchus lobaris superior
Vv. bronchiales (opening into v. azygos)
Bronchus lobaris superior
Bronchus lobaris medius
Bronchus lobaris inferior
Bronchus lobaris inferior
V. azygos
V. hemiazygos

Fig. 8.27 Autonomic innervation of the tracheobronchial tree
Sympathetic innervation (red); parasympathetic innervation (blue).

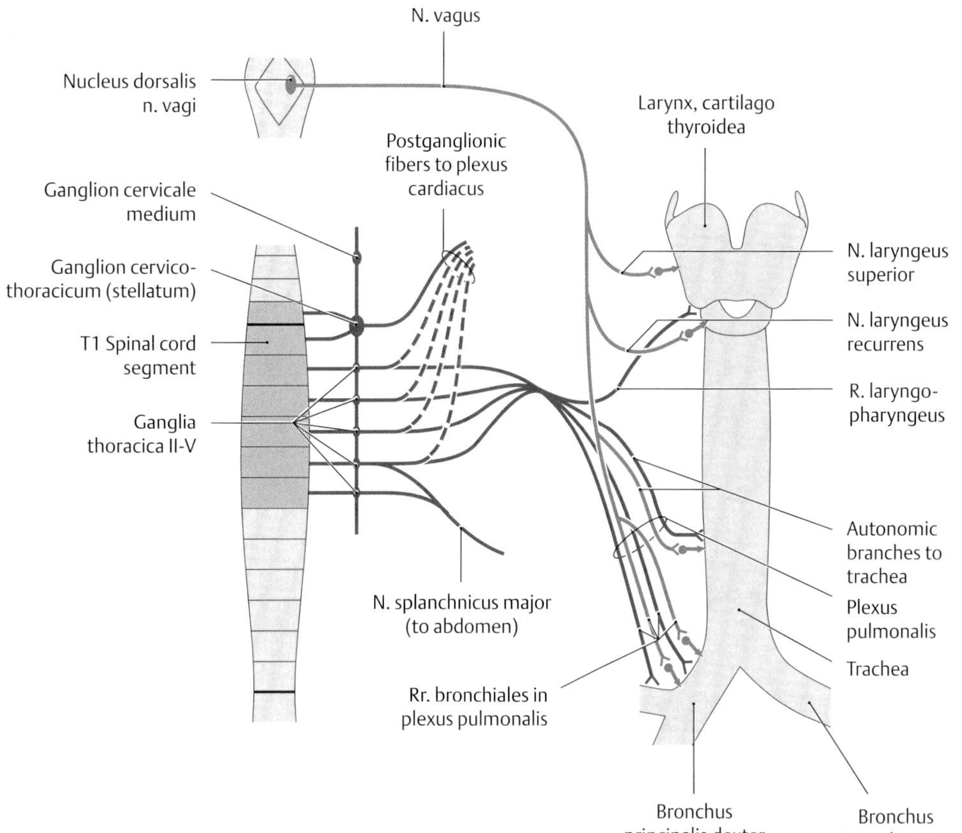
N. vagus
Nucleus dorsalis n. vagi
Larynx, cartilago thyroidea
Postganglionic fibers to plexus cardiacus
Ganglion cervicale medium
Ganglion cervico-thoracicum (stellatum)
N. laryngeus superior
N. laryngeus recurrens
T1 Spinal cord segment
R. laryngo-pharyngeus
Ganglia thoracica II-V
Autonomic branches to trachea
Plexus pulmonalis
N. splanchnicus major (to abdomen)
Trachea
Rr. bronchiales in plexus pulmonalis
Bronchus principalis dexter
Bronchus principalis sinister

Lymphatics of the Pleural Cavity

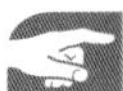

The lungs and bronchi are drained by two lymphatic drainage systems. The peribronchial network follows the bronchial tree, draining lymph from the bronchi and most of the lungs. The subpleural network collects lymph from the peripheral lung and pleura visceralis.

Fig. 8.28 **Lymphatic drainage of the pleural cavity**
Transverse section, inferior view.

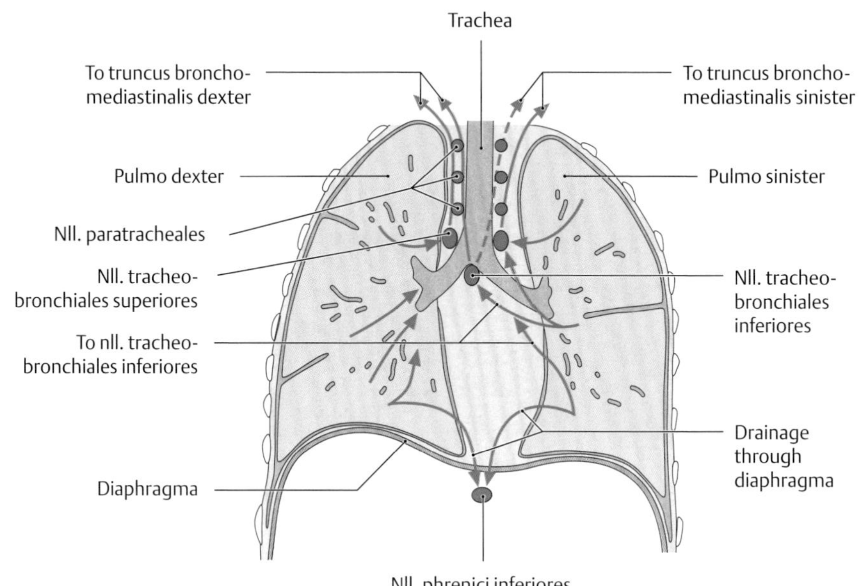
Trachea
To truncus broncho-mediastinalis dexter
To truncus broncho-mediastinalis sinister
Pulmo dexter
Pulmo sinister
Nll. paratracheales
Nll. tracheo-bronchiales superiores
Nll. tracheo-bronchiales inferiores
To nll. tracheo-bronchiales inferiores
Drainage through diaphragma
Diaphragma
Nll. phrenici inferiores

A Peribronchial network, coronal section. Nll. intrapulmonales along the bronchial tree drain lymph from the lungs into the nll. bronchopulmonales. Lymph then passes sequentially through the nll. tracheo-bronchiales inferiores and superiores, nll. paratracheales, truncus bronchomediastinalis, and finally to the ductus lymphaticus dexter or ductus thoracicus. *Note:* Significant amounts of lymph from the left lower lobe drain to the nll. tracheobronchiales superiores dextrae.

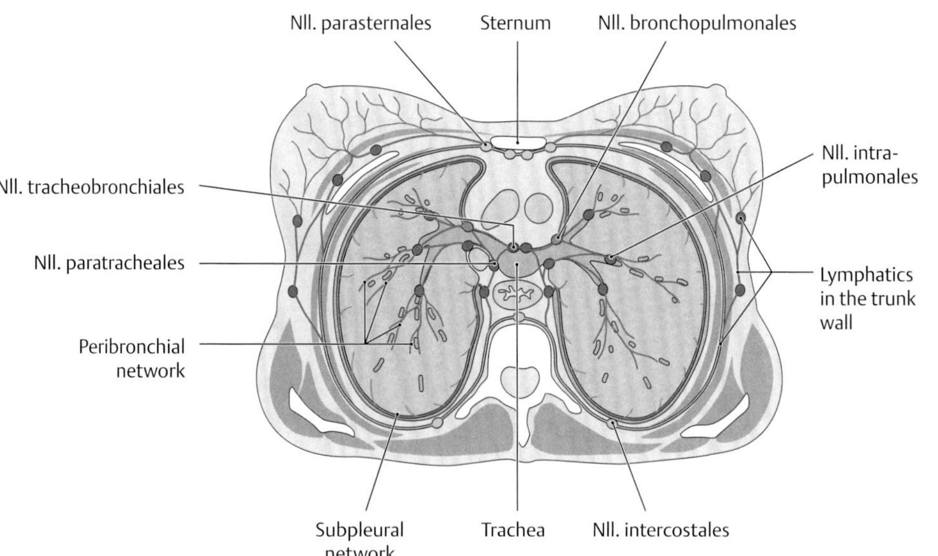
Nll. parasternales
Sternum
Nll. bronchopulmonales
Nll. intra-pulmonales
Nll. tracheobronchiales
Nll. paratracheales
Lymphatics in the trunk wall
Peribronchial network
Subpleural network
Trachea
Nll. intercostales

B Subpleural network, transverse section, superior view.

Fig. 8.29 **Lymph nodes of the pleural cavity**
Anterior view of pulmonary nodes.

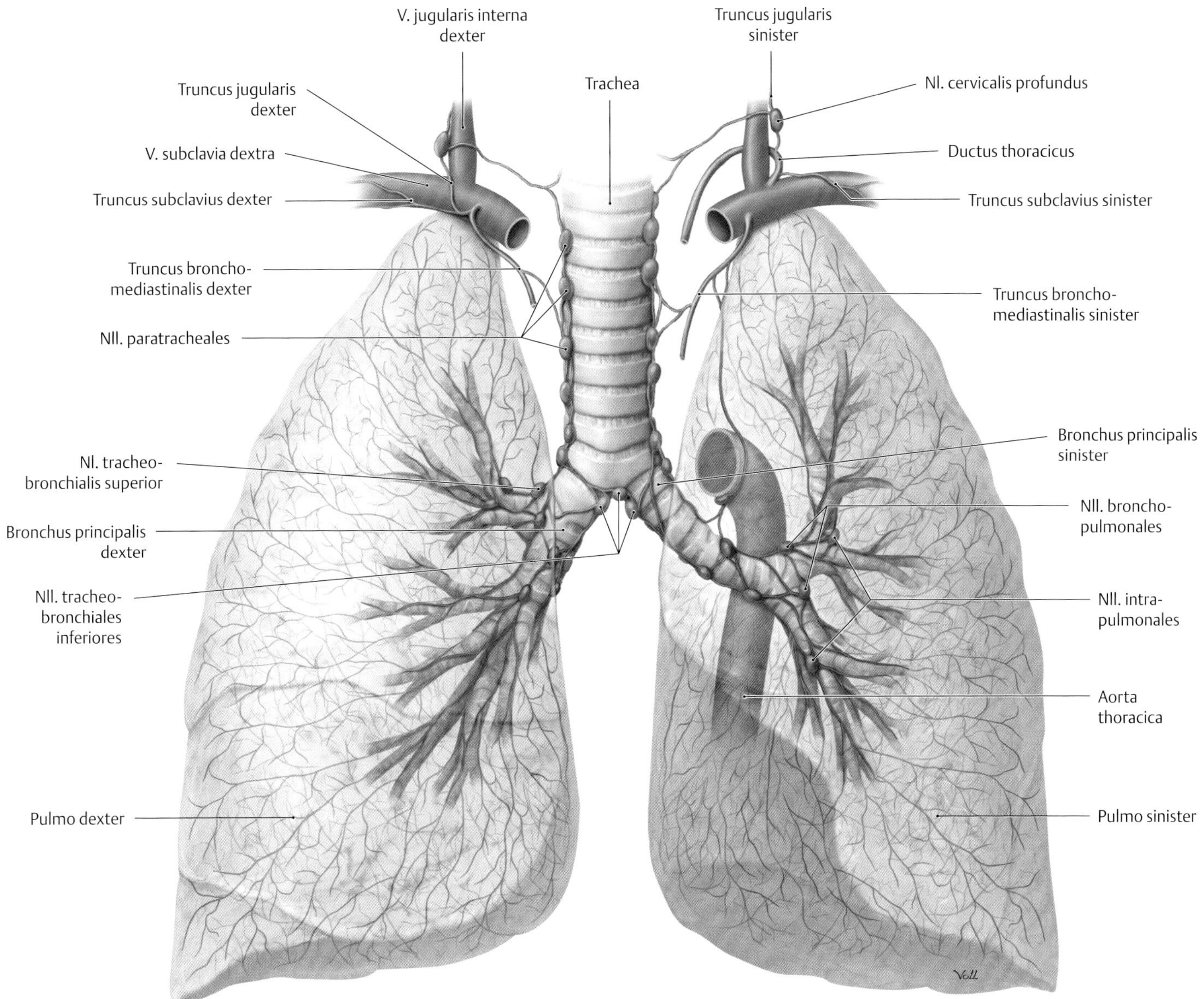
V. jugularis interna dexter
Truncus jugularis sinister
Truncus jugularis dexter
Trachea
Nl. cervicalis profundus
V. subclavia dextra
Ductus thoracicus
Truncus subclavius dexter
Truncus subclavius sinister
Truncus broncho-mediastinalis dexter
Truncus broncho-mediastinalis sinister
Nll. paratracheales
Bronchus principalis sinister
Nl. tracheo-bronchialis superior
Nll. broncho-pulmonales
Bronchus principalis dexter
Nll. tracheo-bronchiales inferiores
Nll. intra-pulmonales
Aorta thoracica
Pulmo dexter
Pulmo sinister

Surface Anatomy

Fig. 9.1 **Palpable structures in the thorax**
Anterior view. See pp. 40–41 for structures of the back.

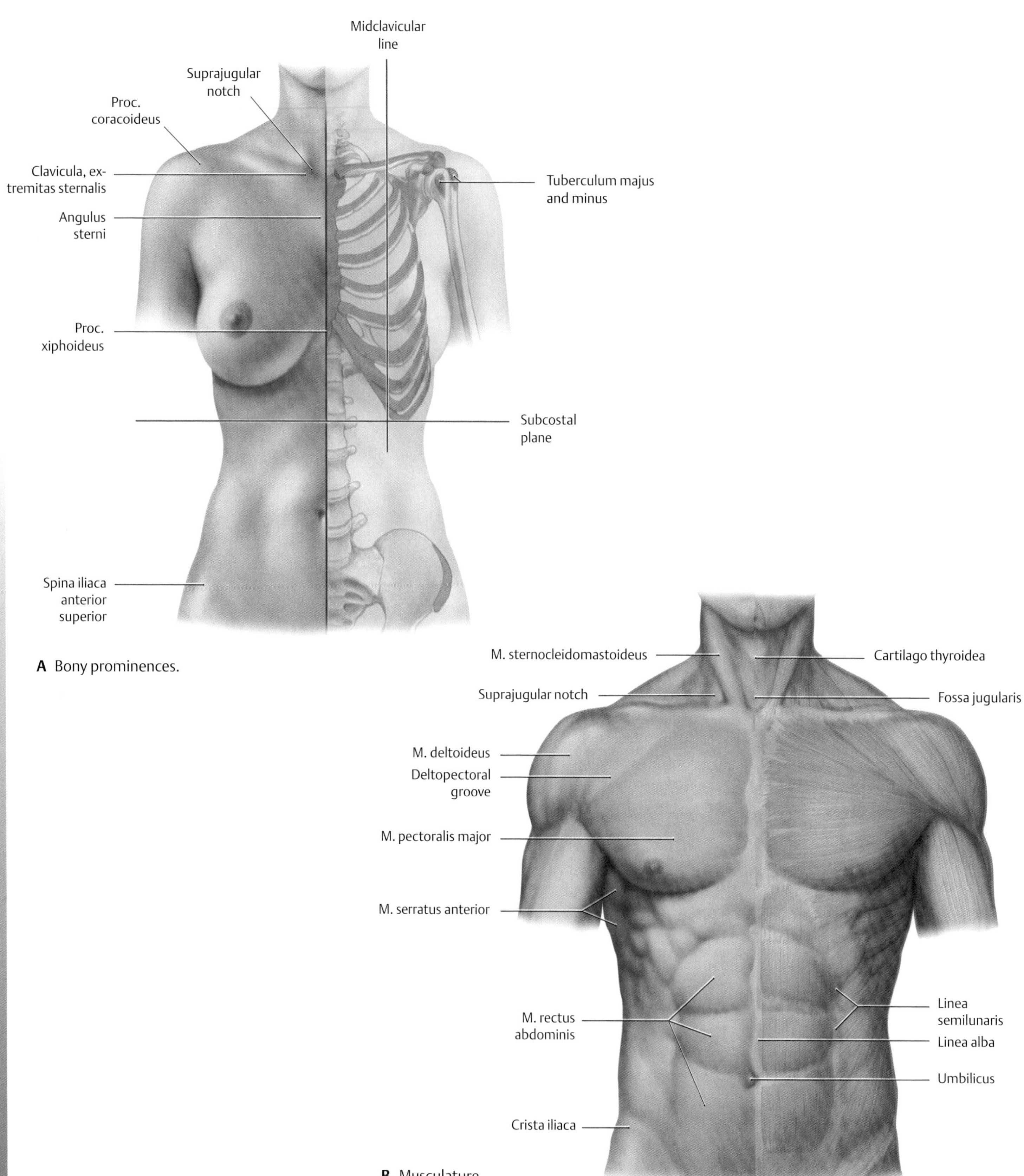
Midclavicular line
Suprajugular notch
Proc. coracoideus
Clavicula, extremitas sternalis
Tuberculum majus and minus
Angulus sterni
Proc. xiphoideus
Subcostal plane
Spina iliaca anterior superior
M. sternocleidomastoideus
Cartilago thyroidea
Suprajugular notch
Fossa jugularis
M. deltoideus
Deltopectoral groove
M. pectoralis major
M. serratus anterior
Linea semilunaris
M. rectus abdominis
Linea alba
Umbilicus
Crista iliaca

A Bony prominences.

B Musculature.

Fig. 9.2 **Surface anatomy of the thorax**
Anterior view. See pp. 40–41 for structures of the back.

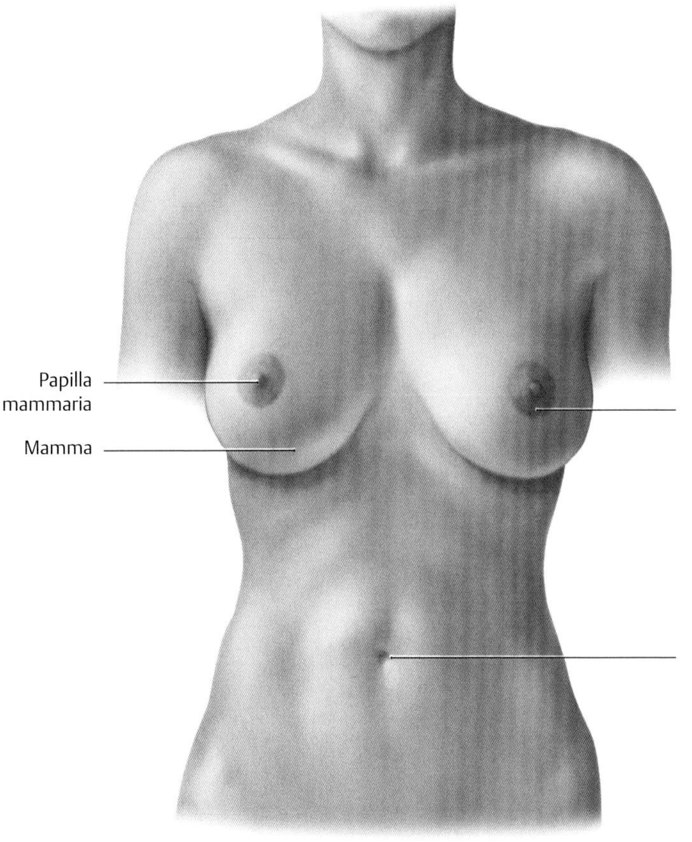
Papilla mammaria
Mamma
Areola mammae
Umbilicus

A Female thorax.

Q1: A female patient has given a history of detecting a "lump" during a self-examination. How would you proceed? Where would you palpate for lymph nodes?

Q2: You are presented with the anterior chest of your first hospital patient. How would you formulate a plan to optimally examine the four valves of the heart?

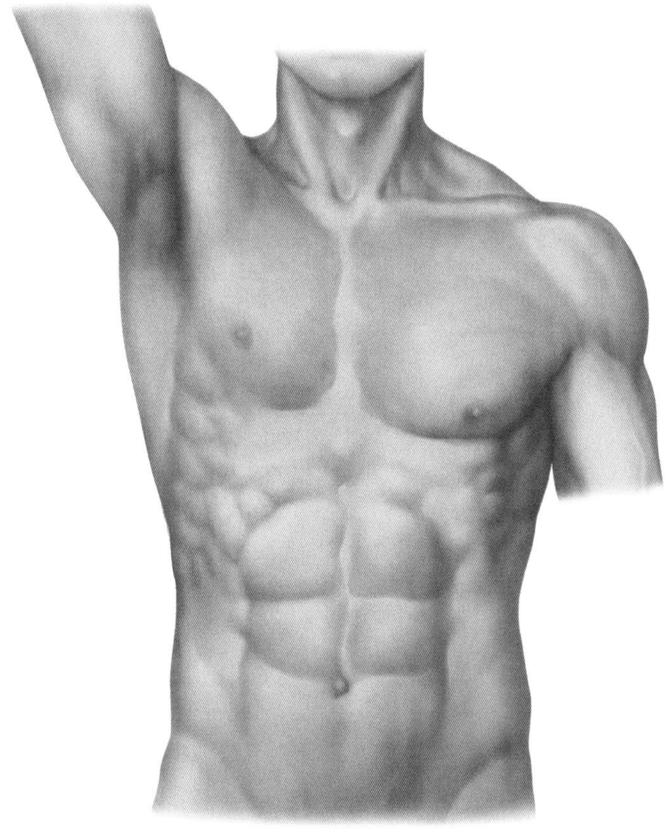

B Male thorax.

See answers beginning on p. 626.

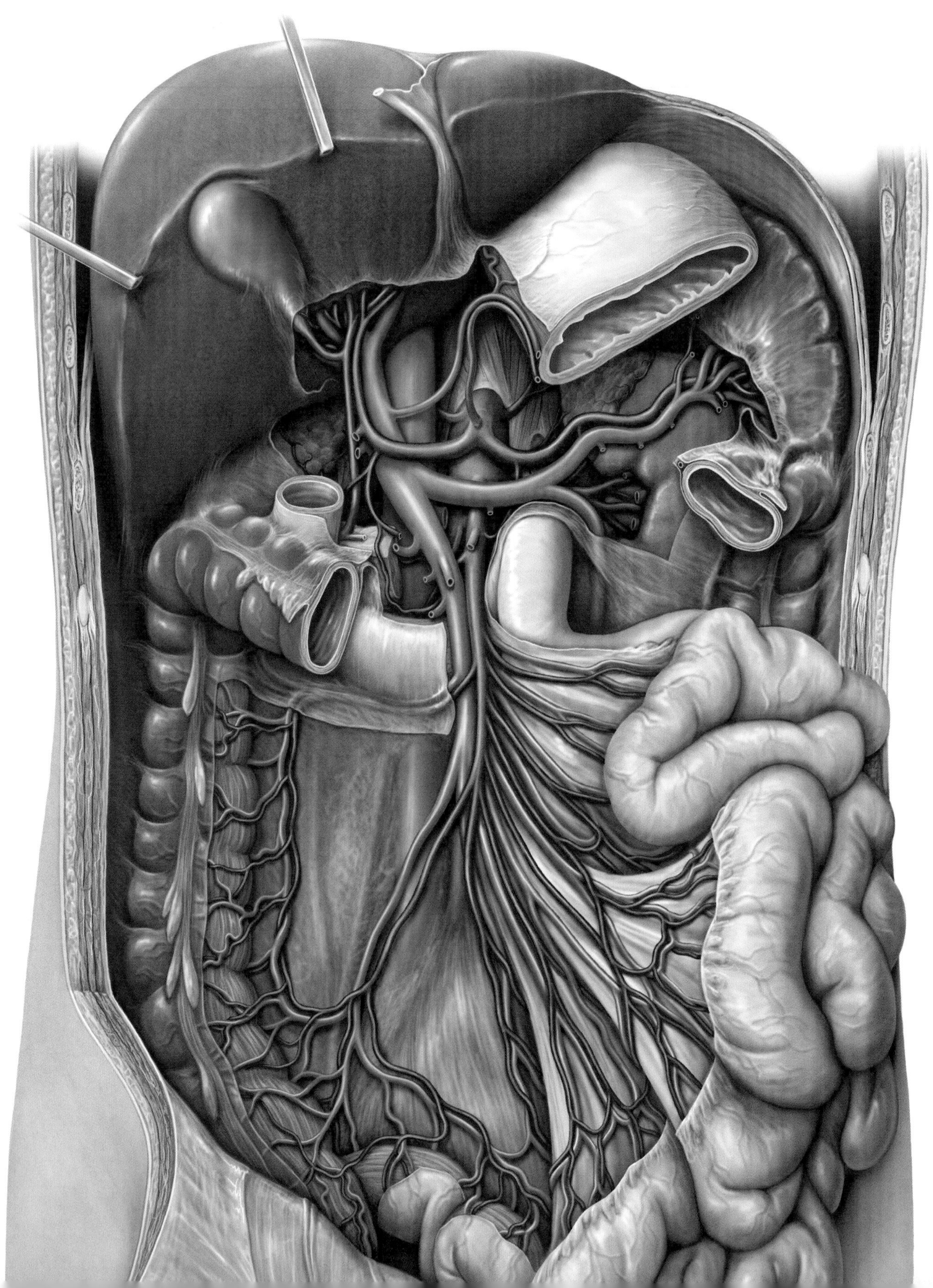

Abdomen & Pelvis

10 Bones, Ligaments & Joints

Pelvic Girdle . . . 124
Male & Female Pelvis . . . 126
Pelvic Ligaments . . . 128

11 Abdominal Wall

Muscles of the Abdominal Wall . . . 130
Regio Inguinalis & Canalis Inguinalis . . . 132
Abdominal Wall & Inguinal Hernias . . . 134
Regio Perinealis . . . 136
Abdominal Wall Muscle Facts . . . 138
Diaphragma Pelvis Muscle Facts . . . 140

12 Spaces

Divisions of the Abdominopelvic Cavity . . . 142
Cavitas Peritonealis & Greater Sac . . . 144
Bursa Omentalis . . . 146
Mesenterium & Posterior Wall . . . 148
Contents of the Pelvis . . . 150
Peritoneal Relationships . . . 152
Pelvis & Perineum . . . 154
Transverse Sections . . . 156

13 Internal Organs

Gaster . . . 158
Duodenum . . . 160
Jejunum & Ileum . . . 162
Cecum, Appendix & Colon . . . 164
Rectum & Canalis Analis . . . 166
Hepar: Overview . . . 168
Hepar: Segments & Lobes . . . 170
Vesica Biliaris & Bile Ducts . . . 172
Pancreas & Lien . . . 174
Renes & Glandulae Suprarenales: Overview . . . 176
Renes & Glandulae Suprarenales: Features . . . 178
Ureter . . . 180
Vesica Urinaria . . . 182
Vesica Urinaria & Urethra . . . 184

14 Reproductive Organs

Overview of the Genital Organs . . . 186
Uterus & Ovaries . . . 188
Vagina . . . 190
Female External Genitalia . . . 192
Neurovasculature of the Female Genitalia . . . 194
Penis, Scrotum & Funiculus Spermaticus . . . 196
Testis & Epididymis . . . 198
Male Accessory Sex Glands . . . 200
Neurovasculature of the Male Genitalia . . . 202
Development of the Genitalia . . . 204

15 Arteries & Veins

Arteries of the Abdomen . . . 206
Aorta Abdominalis & Arteriae Renales . . . 208
Truncus Coeliacus . . . 210
Arteriae Mesenterica Superior & Inferior . . . 212
Veins of the Abdomen . . . 214
Vena Cava Inferior & Venae Renales . . . 216
Vena Portae Hepatis . . . 218
Venae Mesenterica Superior & Inferior . . . 220
Arteries & Veins of the Pelvis . . . 222
Arteries & Veins of the Rectum & Genitalia . . . 224

16 Lymphatics

Lymph Nodes of the Abdomen & Pelvis . . . 226
Lymph Nodes of the Posterior Abdominal Wall . . . 228
Lymph Nodes of the Anterior Abdominal Organs . . . 230
Lymph Nodes of the Intestines . . . 232
Lymph Nodes of the Genitalia . . . 234

17 Nerves

Plexus Autonomicus . . . 236
Innervation of the Abdominal Organs . . . 238
Innervation of the Intestines . . . 240
Innervation of the Pelvis . . . 242
Autonomic Innervation: Overview . . . 244
Autonomic Innervation: Urinary & Genital Organs . . . 246

18 Surface Anatomy

Surface Anatomy . . . 248

Pelvic Girdle

Fig. 10.1 **Pelvic girdle**
Anterosuperior view. The pelvic girdle consists of the two os coxae and the sacrum (see p. 358).

Fig. 10.2 **Os coxae**
Os coxae dexter (male).

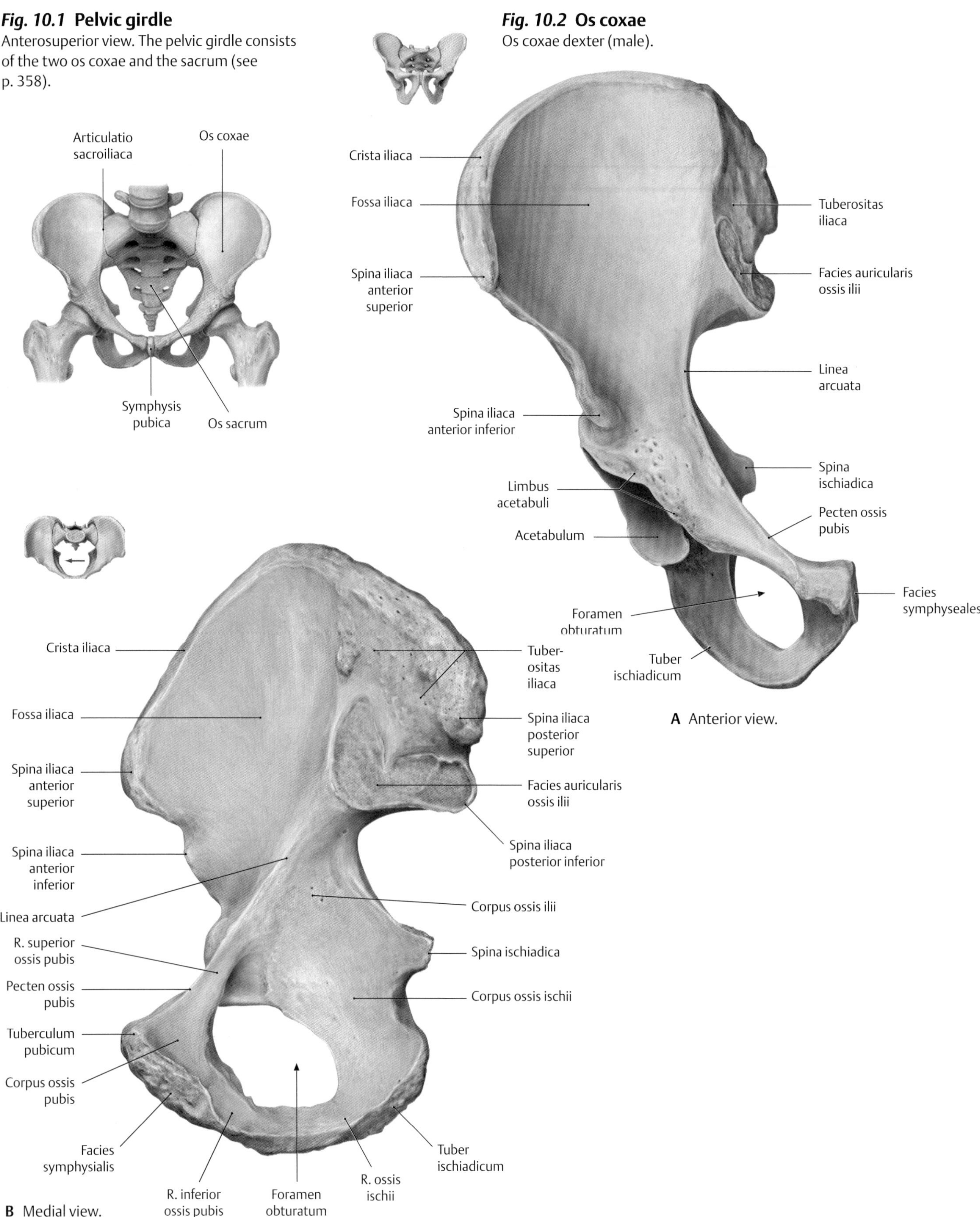
Articulatio sacroiliaca
Os coxae
Symphysis pubica
Os sacrum
Crista iliaca
Fossa iliaca
Tuberositas iliaca
Facies auricularis ossis ilii
Spina iliaca anterior superior
Linea arcuata
Spina iliaca anterior inferior
Spina ischiadica
Limbus acetabuli
Pecten ossis pubis
Acetabulum
Facies symphyseales
Foramen obturatum
Tuber ischiadicum
Crista iliaca
Tuber-ositas iliaca
Fossa iliaca
Spina iliaca posterior superior
Spina iliaca anterior superior
Facies auricularis ossis ilii
Spina iliaca posterior inferior
Spina iliaca anterior inferior
Linea arcuata
Corpus ossis ilii
R. superior ossis pubis
Spina ischiadica
Pecten ossis pubis
Corpus ossis ischii
Tuberculum pubicum
Corpus ossis pubis
Facies symphysialis
Tuber ischiadicum
R. ossis ischii
R. inferior ossis pubis
Foramen obturatum

A Anterior view.

B Medial view.

Fig. 10.3 Triradiate cartilage of os coxae

Os coxae dexter, lateral view. Os coxae consists of the os ilium, os ischii, and os pubis.

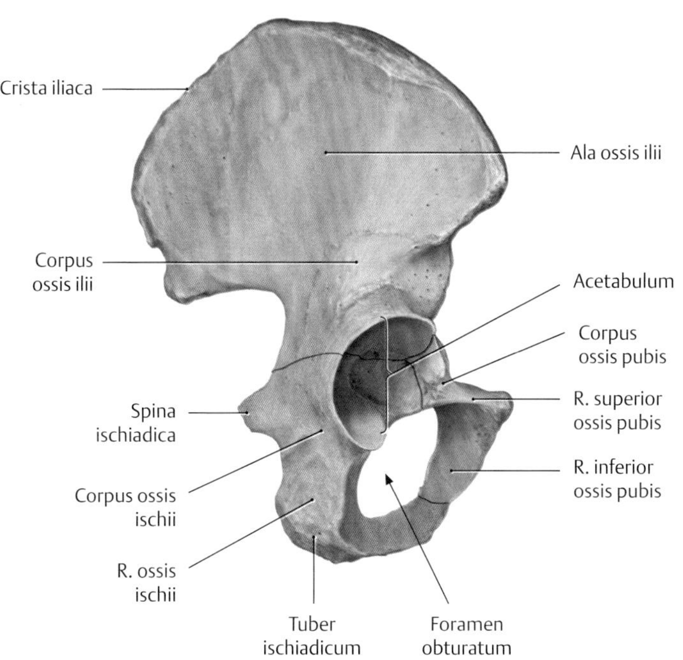
Crista iliaca
Ala ossis ilii
Corpus ossis ilii
Acetabulum
Corpus ossis pubis
Spina ischiadica
R. superior ossis pubis
R. inferior ossis pubis
Corpus ossis ischii
R. ossis ischii
Tuber ischiadicum
Foramen obturatum

A Junction of the triradiate cartilage.

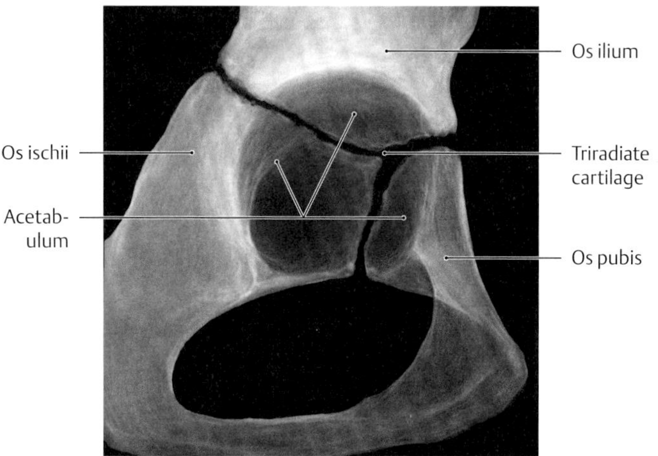
Os ilium
Os ischii
Triradiate cartilage
Acetabulum
Os pubis

B Radiograph of a child's acetabulum. Os coxae dexter, lateral view.

Fig. 10.4 Os coxae: Lateral view

Right hip bone (male).

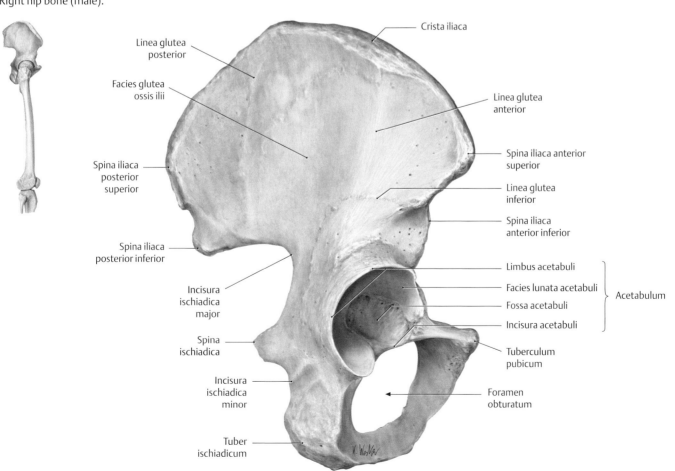

Crista iliaca
Linea glutea posterior
Facies glutea ossis ilii
Linea glutea anterior
Spina iliaca anterior superior
Spina iliaca posterior superior
Linea glutea inferior
Spina iliaca anterior inferior
Spina iliaca posterior inferior
Limbus acetabuli
Facies lunata acetabuli
Fossa acetabuli
Incisura acetabuli
Acetabulum
Incisura ischiadica major
Spina ischiadica
Tuberculum pubicum
Incisura ischiadica minor
Foramen obturatum
Tuber ischiadicum

Male & Female Pelvis

Fig. 10.5 Female pelvis

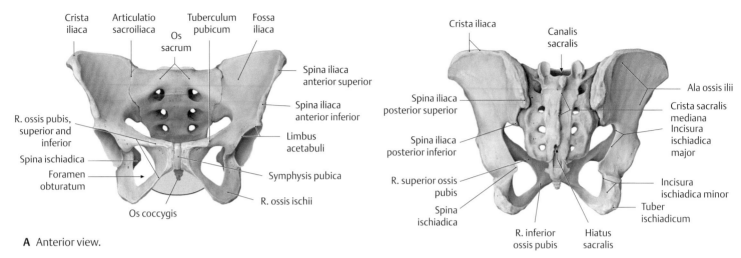

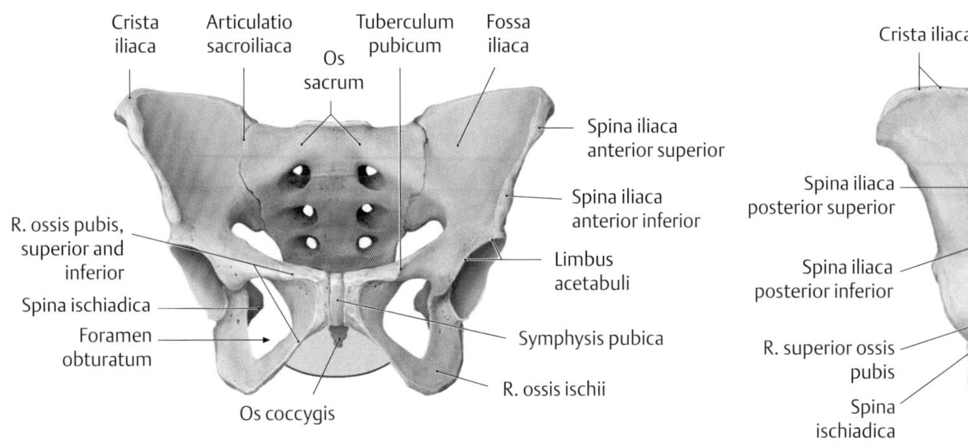
Crista iliaca
Articulatio sacroiliaca
Os sacrum
Tuberculum pubicum
Fossa iliaca
Spina iliaca anterior superior
Spina iliaca anterior inferior
R. ossis pubis, superior and inferior
Limbus acetabuli
Spina ischiadica
Foramen obturatum
Symphysis pubica
R. ossis ischii
Os coccygis
Crista iliaca
Canalis sacralis
Ala ossis ilii
Spina iliaca posterior superior
Crista sacralis mediana
Incisura ischiadica major
Spina iliaca posterior inferior
R. superior ossis pubis
Incisura ischiadica minor
Spina ischiadica
Tuber ischiadicum
R. inferior ossis pubis
Hiatus sacralis

A Anterior view.

B Posterior view.

Fig. 10.6 Male pelvis

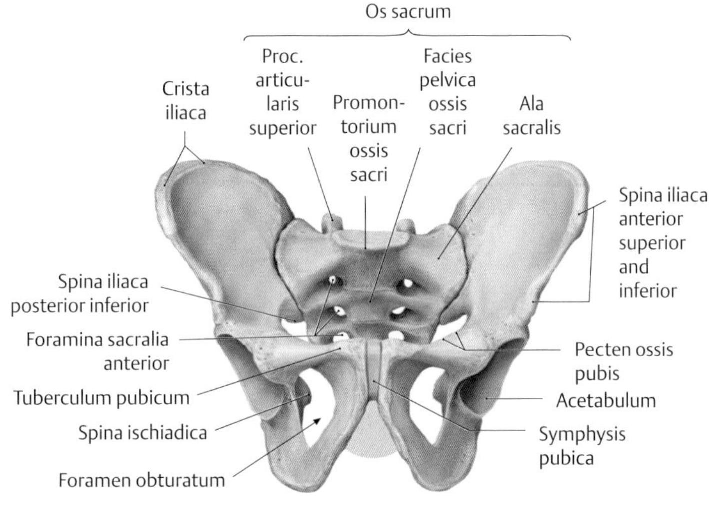
Os sacrum
Crista iliaca
Proc. articularis superior
Promontorium ossis sacri
Facies pelvica ossis sacri
Ala sacralis
Spina iliaca anterior superior and inferior
Spina iliaca posterior inferior
Foramina sacralia anterior
Pecten ossis pubis
Tuberculum pubicum
Acetabulum
Spina ischiadica
Symphysis pubica
Foramen obturatum

A Anterior view.

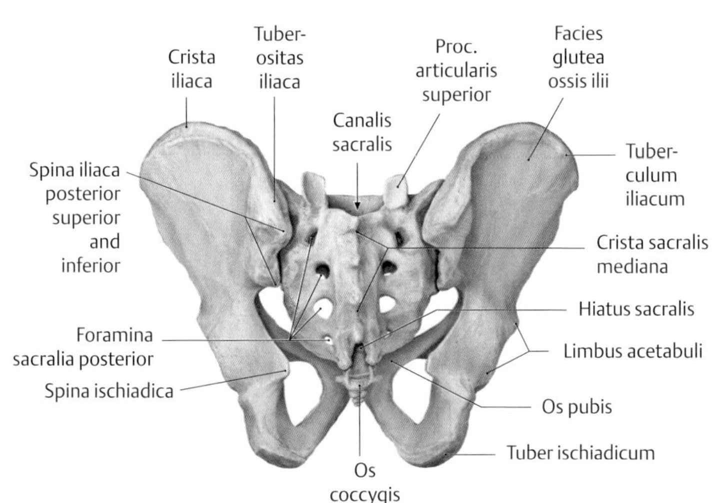
Crista iliaca
Tuberositas iliaca
Proc. articularis superior
Facies glutea ossis ilii
Canalis sacralis
Spina iliaca posterior superior and inferior
Tuberculum iliacum
Crista sacralis mediana
Hiatus sacralis
Foramina sacralia posterior
Limbus acetabuli
Spina ischiadica
Os pubis
Tuber ischiadicum
Os coccygis

B Posterior view.

Fig. 10.7 Female pelvis: Superior view

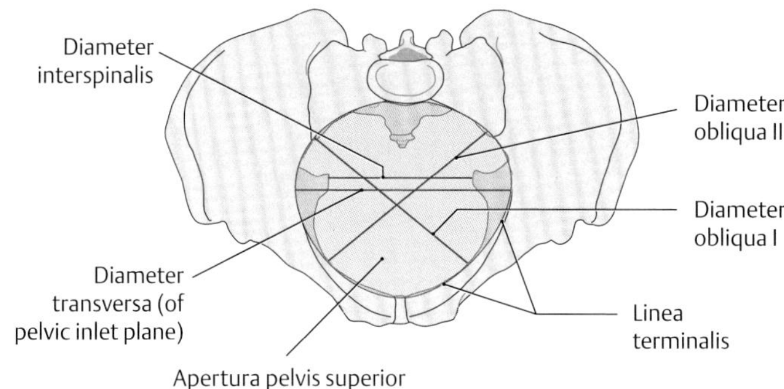
Diameter interspinalis
Diameter obliqua II
Diameter obliqua I
Diameter transversa (of pelvic inlet plane)
Linea terminalis
Apertura pelvis superior

A Pelvic measurements.

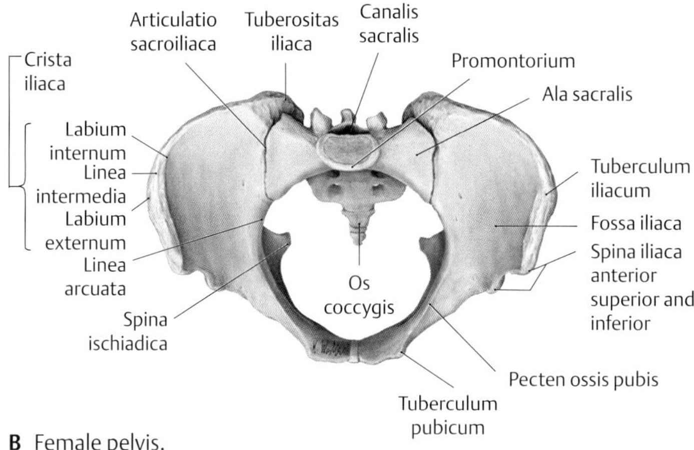
Crista iliaca
Labium internum
Linea intermedia
Labium externum
Linea arcuata
Spina ischiadica
Articulatio sacroiliaca
Tuberositas iliaca
Canalis sacralis
Promontorium
Ala sacralis
Tuberculum iliacum
Fossa iliaca
Spina iliaca anterior superior and inferior
Os coccygis
Pecten ossis pubis
Tuberculum pubicum

B Female pelvis.

Fig. 10.8 Male pelvis: Superior view

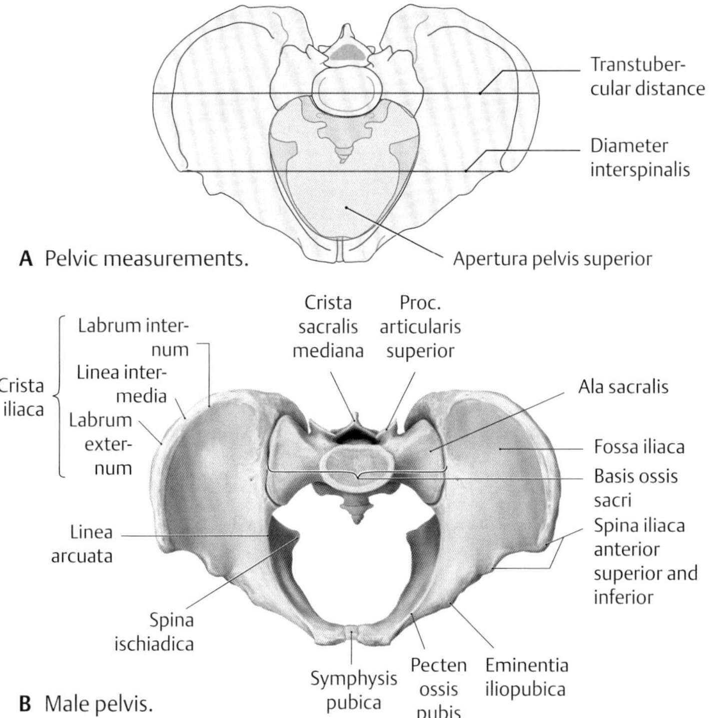
Transtuber-cular distance
Diameter interspinalis
Apertura pelvis superior
Crista iliaca
Labrum inter-num
Linea inter-media
Labrum exter-num
Crista sacralis mediana
Proc. articularis superior
Ala sacralis
Fossa iliaca
Basis ossis sacri
Spina iliaca anterior superior and inferior
Linea arcuata
Spina ischiadica
Symphysis pubica
Pecten ossis pubis
Eminentia iliopubica

A Pelvic measurements.

B Male pelvis.

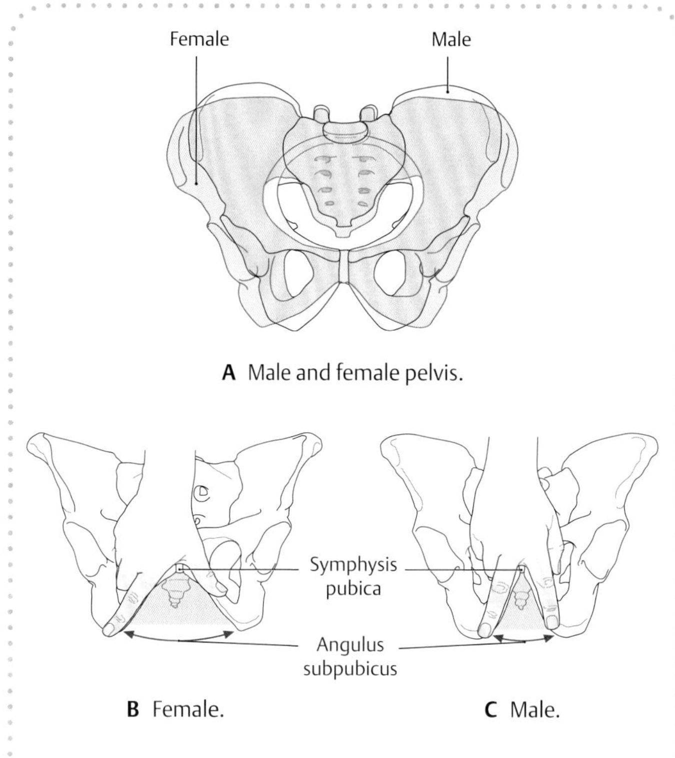
Female
Male
Symphysis pubica
Angulus subpubicus

A Male and female pelvis.

B Female.

C Male.

Table 10.1 Gender-specific features of the pelvis

Structure	Female	Male
Pelvis major	Wide and shallow	Narrow and deep
Aperatura pelvis superior	Transversely oval	Heart-shaped
Aperatura pelvis inferior	Roomy and round	Narrow and oblong
Tuber ischiadicum	Everted	Inverted
Cavitas pelvis	Roomy and shallow	Narrow and deep
Os sacrum	Short, wide, and flat	Long, narrow, and convex
Angulus subpubicus	90–100 degrees	70 degrees

Clinical

Childbirth

A non-optimal relation between the maternal pelvis and the fetal head may lead to complications during childbirth, potentially necessitating a caesarean section. Maternal causes include earlier pelvic trauma and innate malformations. Fetal causes include hydrocephalus (disturbed circulation of cerebrospinal fluid, leading to brain dilation and cranial expansion).

Pelvic Ligaments

Fig. 10.9 **Ligaments of the pelvis**
Male pelvis.

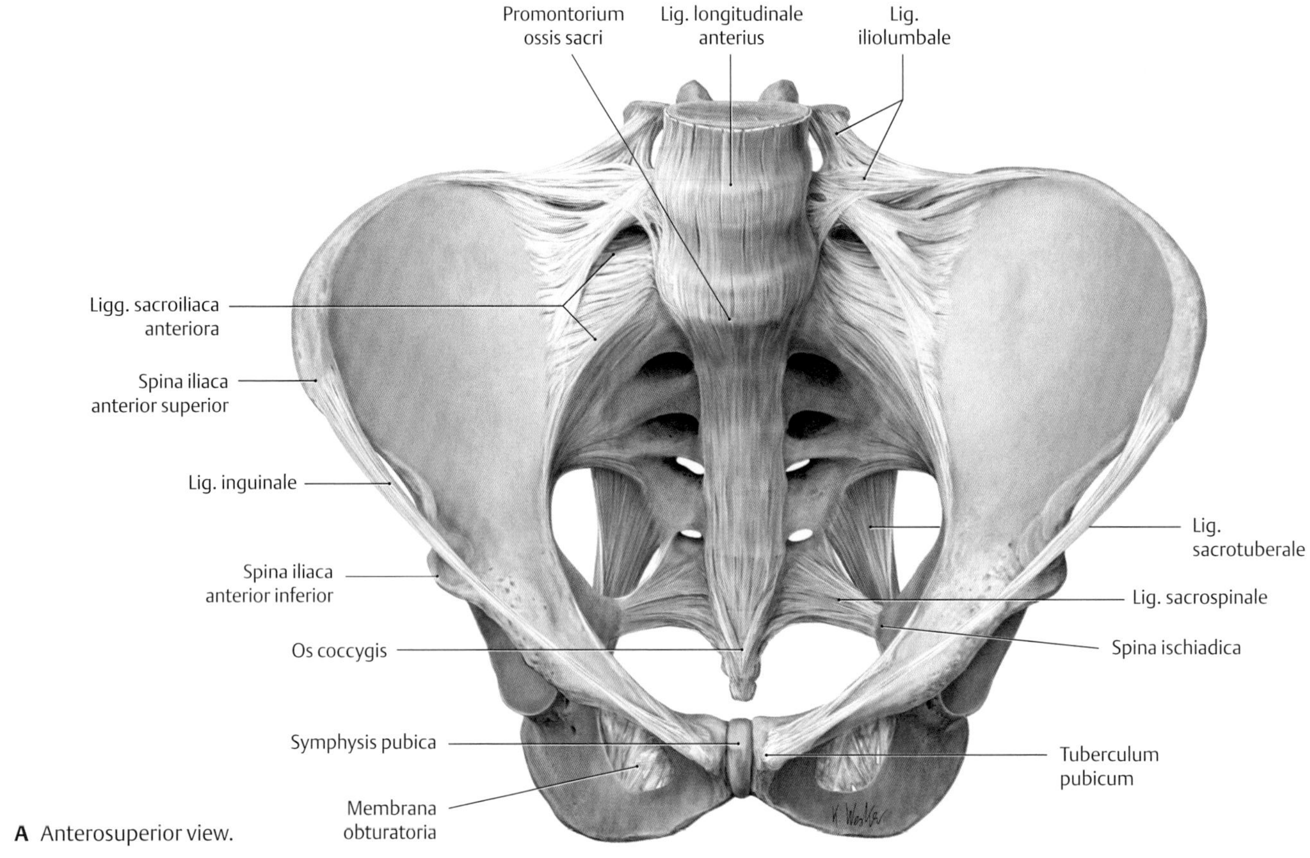

Promontorium ossis sacri
Lig. longitudinale anterius
Lig. iliolumbale
Ligg. sacroiliaca anteriora
Spina iliaca anterior superior
Lig. inguinale
Lig. sacrotuberale
Spina iliaca anterior inferior
Lig. sacrospinale
Spina ischiadica
Os coccygis
Symphysis pubica
Tuberculum pubicum
Membrana obturatoria

A Anterosuperior view.

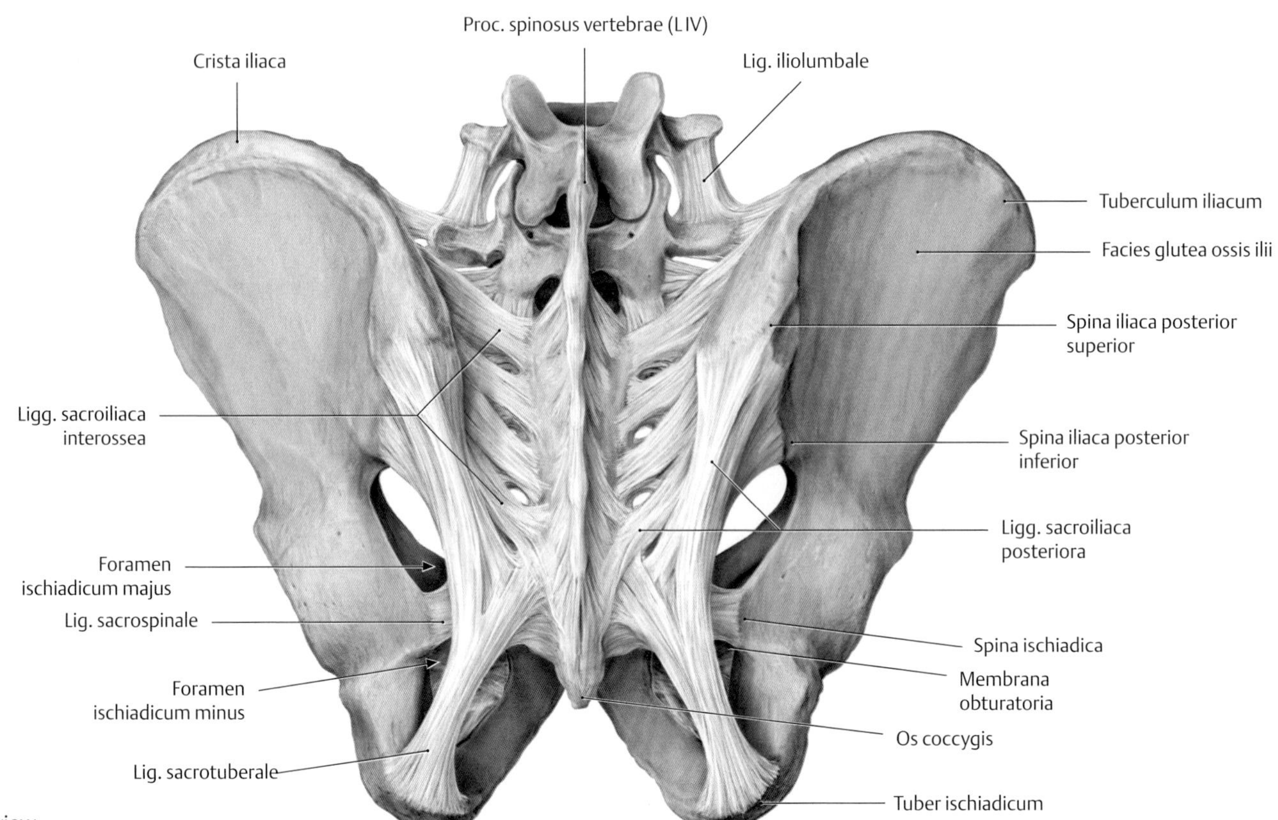

Proc. spinosus vertebrae (L IV)
Crista iliaca
Lig. iliolumbale
Tuberculum iliacum
Facies glutea ossis ilii
Spina iliaca posterior superior
Ligg. sacroiliaca interossea
Spina iliaca posterior inferior
Ligg. sacroiliaca posteriora
Foramen ischiadicum majus
Lig. sacrospinale
Spina ischiadica
Membrana obturatoria
Foramen ischiadicum minus
Os coccygis
Lig. sacrotuberale
Tuber ischiadicum

B Posterior view.

Fig. 10.10 Ligaments of art. sacroiliaca

Male pelvis.

Discus intervertebralis
Proc. spinosus vertebrae (LV)
Promontorium
Os sacrum
Spina iliaca anterior superior
Canalis sacralis
Ligg. sacroiliaca anteriora
Foramen ischiadicum majus
Linea arcuata
Lig. sacrospinale
Pecten ossis pubis
Hiatus sacralis
Spina ischiadica
Foramen ischiadicum minus
Os coccygis
Lig. sacrotuberale
Facies symphysialis
Membrana obturatoria
Tuber ischiadicum

A Right half of pelvis, medial view.

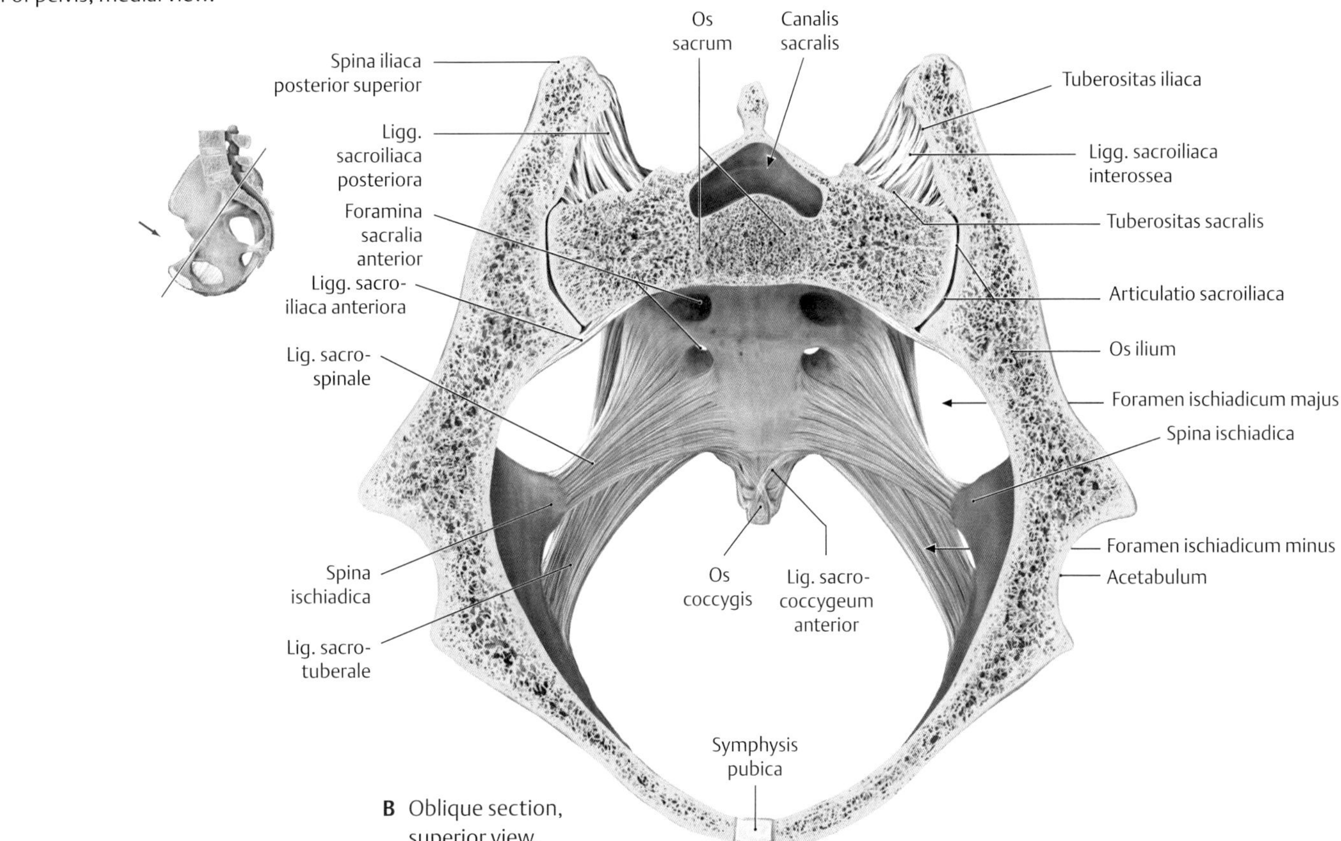
Os sacrum
Canalis sacralis
Spina iliaca posterior superior
Tuberositas iliaca
Ligg. sacroiliaca posteriora
Ligg. sacroiliaca interossea
Foramina sacralia anterior
Tuberositas sacralis
Ligg. sacroiliaca anteriora
Articulatio sacroiliaca
Os ilium
Lig. sacrospinale
Foramen ischiadicum majus
Spina ischiadica
Foramen ischiadicum minus
Acetabulum
Spina ischiadica
Os coccygis
Lig. sacrococcygeum anterior
Lig. sacrotuberale
Symphysis pubica

B Oblique section, superior view.

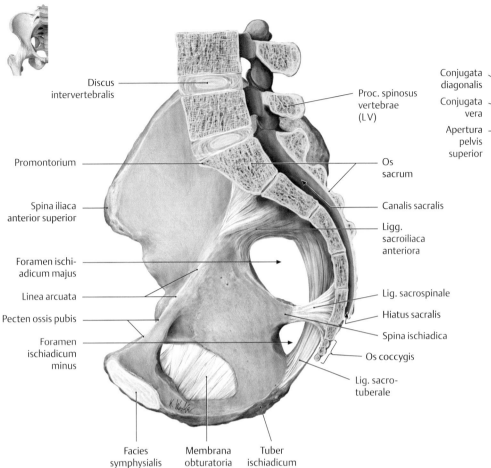

Fig. 10.11 Pelvic measurements

Right half of female pelvis, medial view. See Table 10.1.

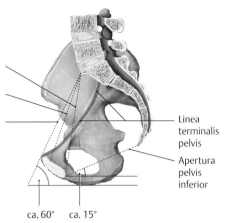

Conjugata diagonalis
Conjugata vera
Apertura pelvis superior
Linea terminalis pelvis
Apertura pelvis inferior
ca. 60°
ca. 15°

Muscles of the Abdominal Wall

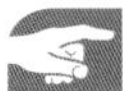

The anterolateral muscles of the abdominal wall consist of m. obliquus externus abdominis, m. obliquus internus abdominis and m. transversus abdominis. The posterior or deep abdominal wall muscles (notably the m. psoas major) are functionally hip muscles (see p. 138).

Fig. 11.1 **Muscles of the abdominal wall**

Right side, anterior view.

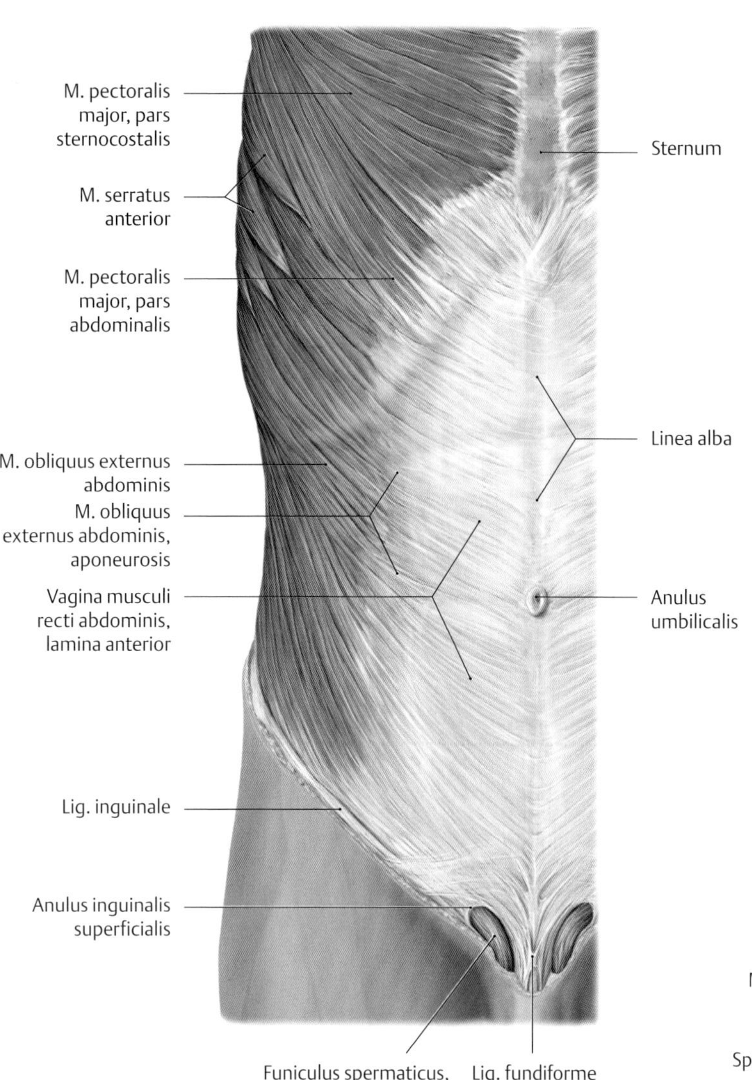

M. pectoralis major, pars sternocostalis
M. serratus anterior
M. pectoralis major, pars abdominalis
M. obliquus externus abdominis
M. obliquus externus abdominis, aponeurosis
Vagina musculi recti abdominis, lamina anterior
Lig. inguinale
Anulus inguinalis superficialis
Funiculus spermaticus, m. cremaster
Lig. fundiforme penis
Sternum
Linea alba
Anulus umbilicalis

A Superficial abdominal wall muscles.

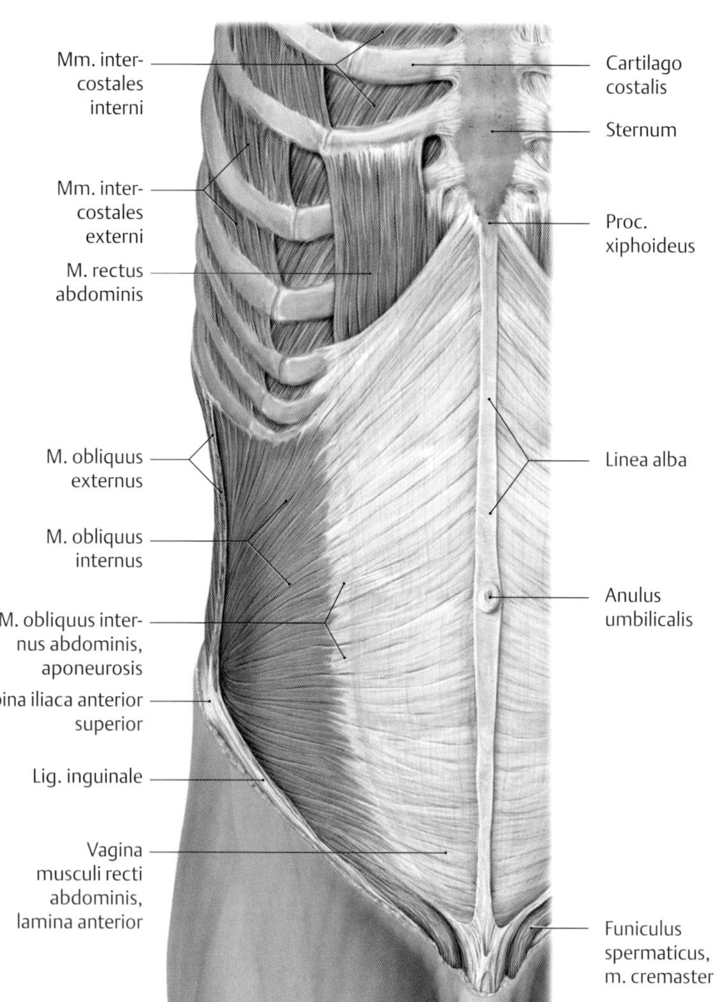

Mm. intercostales interni
Mm. intercostales externi
M. rectus abdominis
M. obliquus externus
M. obliquus internus
M. obliquus internus abdominis, aponeurosis
Spina iliaca anterior superior
Lig. inguinale
Vagina musculi recti abdominis, lamina anterior
Cartilago costalis
Sternum
Proc. xiphoideus
Linea alba
Anulus umbilicalis
Funiculus spermaticus, m. cremaster

B *Removed:* M. obliquus externus abdominis, m. pectoralis major, and m. serratus anterior.

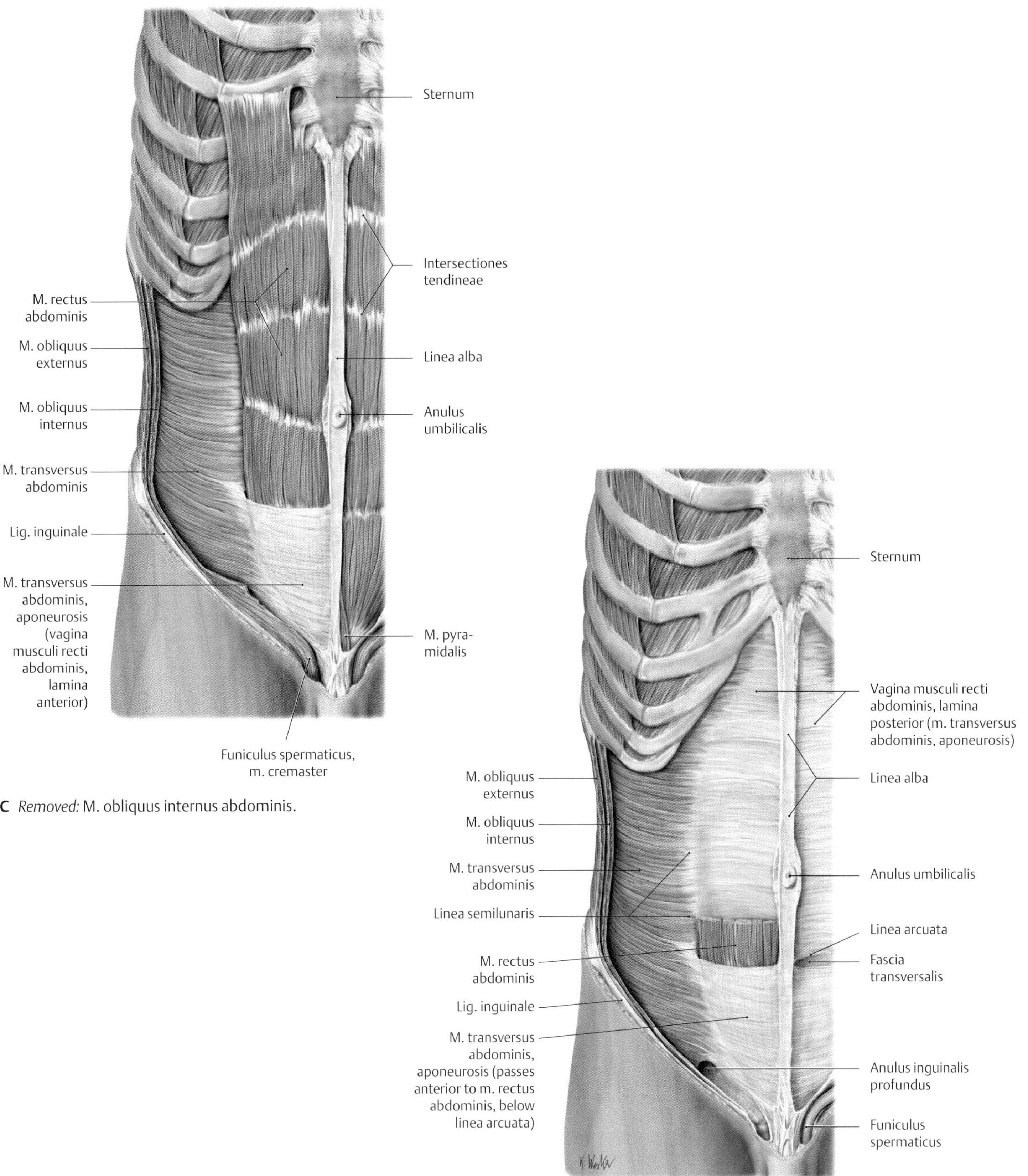

Sternum
Intersectiones tendineae
M. rectus abdominis
M. obliquus externus
Linea alba
M. obliquus internus
Anulus umbilicalis
M. transversus abdominis
Lig. inguinale
M. transversus abdominis, aponeurosis (vagina musculi recti abdominis, lamina anterior)
M. pyra-midalis
Funiculus spermaticus, m. cremaster
Sternum
Vagina musculi recti abdominis, lamina posterior (m. transversus abdominis, aponeurosis)
M. obliquus externus
Linea alba
M. obliquus internus
M. transversus abdominis
Anulus umbilicalis
Linea semilunaris
Linea arcuata
M. rectus abdominis
Fascia transversalis
Lig. inguinale
M. transversus abdominis, aponeurosis (passes anterior to m. rectus abdominis, below linea arcuata)
Anulus inguinalis profundus
Funiculus spermaticus

C *Removed:* M. obliquus internus abdominis.

D *Removed:* M. rectus abdominis.

Regio Inguinalis & Canalis Inguinalis

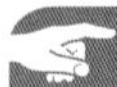

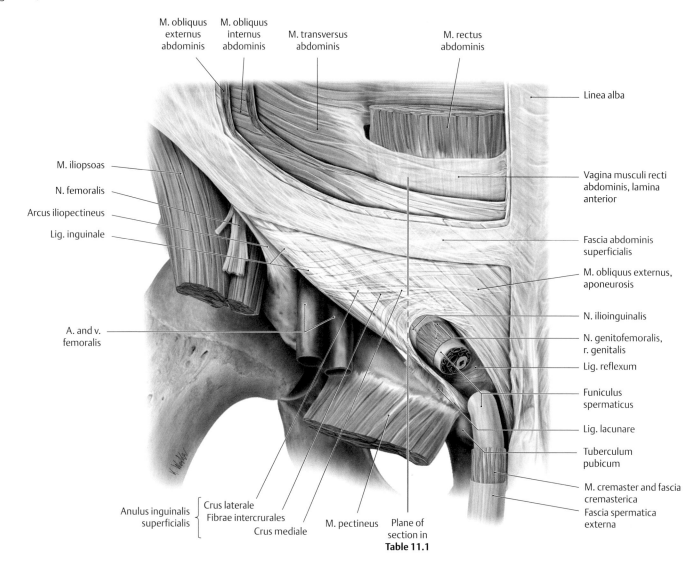

The regio inguinalis is the junction of the anterior abdominal wall and the anterior thigh. The canalis inguinalis is an important site for the passage of structures into and out of the abdominal cavity (e.g., components of funiculus spermaticus).

Fig. 11.2 **Inguinal region**
Right side, anterior view.

M. obliquus externus abdominis
M. obliquus internus abdominis
M. transversus abdominis
M. rectus abdominis
Linea alba
M. iliopsoas
N. femoralis
Arcus iliopectineus
Lig. inguinale
Vagina musculi recti abdominis, lamina anterior
Fascia abdominis superficialis
M. obliquus externus, aponeurosis
N. ilioinguinalis
A. and v. femoralis
N. genitofemoralis, r. genitalis
Lig. reflexum
Funiculus spermaticus
Lig. lacunare
Tuberculum pubicum
M. cremaster and fascia cremasterica
Fascia spermatica externa
Anulus inguinalis superficialis: Crus laterale, Fibrae intercrurales, Crus mediale
M. pectineus
Plane of section in **Table 11.1**

Table 11.1	Structures of the inguinal canal		
Structures			**Formed by**
Wall	Anterior wall	①	M. obliquus externus abdominis aponeurosis
	Roof	②	M. obliquus internus abdominis
		③	M. transversus abdominis
	Posterior wall	④	Fascia transversalis
		⑤	Peritoneum parietale
	Floor	⑥	Lig. inguinale (densely interwoven fibers of the lower m.obliquus externus abdominis aponeurosis and adjacent fascia lata of thigh)
Openings	Anulus inguinalis superficialis		Opening in m. obliquus externus abdominis aponeurosis; bounded by crus mediale and laterale; intercrural fibers, and reflected lig. inguinale
	Anulus inguinalis profundus		Outpouching of the fascia transversalis lateral to the plica umbilicalis lateralis (vasa epigastrica inferiora)
Sagittal section through plane in Fig. 11.2.			

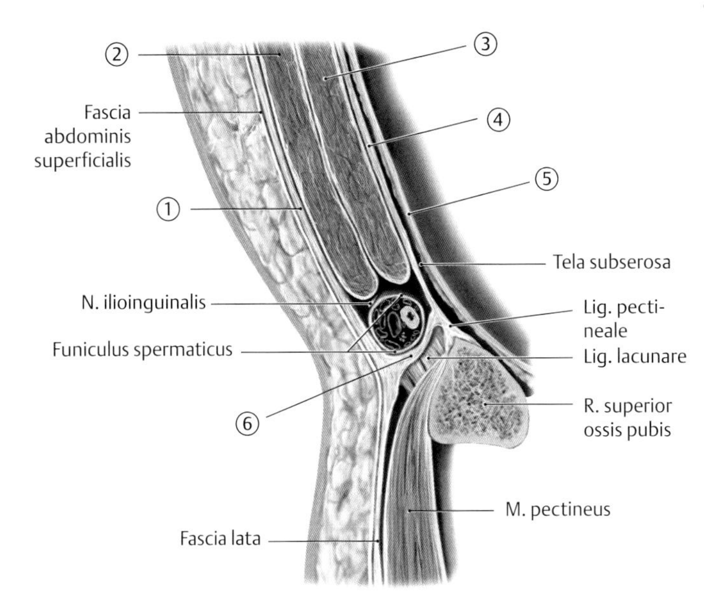

②
③
Fascia abdominis superficialis
④
⑤
①
Tela subserosa
N. ilioinguinalis
Lig. pectineale
Funiculus spermaticus
Lig. lacunare
R. superior ossis pubis
⑥
M. pectineus
Fascia lata

Fig. 11.3 Dissection of the regio inguinalis

Right side, anterior view.

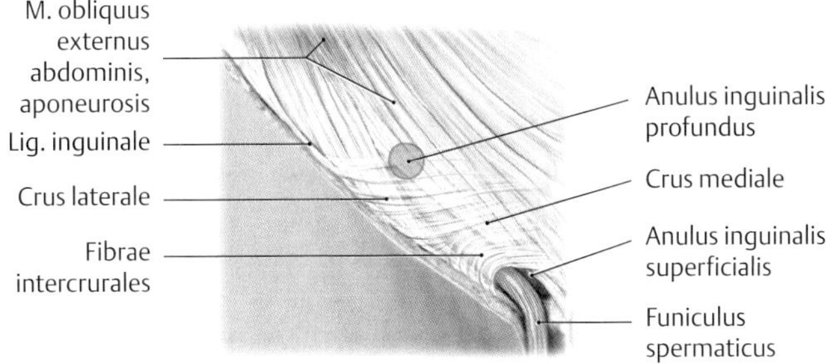

M. obliquus externus abdominis, aponeurosis
Lig. inguinale
Crus laterale
Fibrae intercrurales
Anulus inguinalis profundus
Crus mediale
Anulus inguinalis superficialis
Funiculus spermaticus

A Superficial layer.

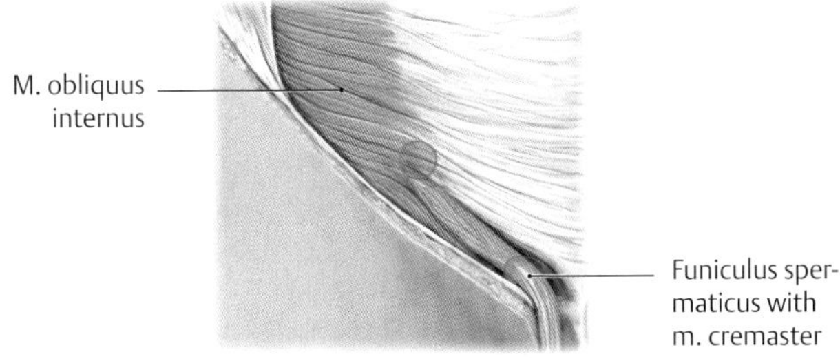

M. obliquus internus
Funiculus spermaticus with m. cremaster

B *Removed:* Aponeurosis of m. obliquus externus abdominis.

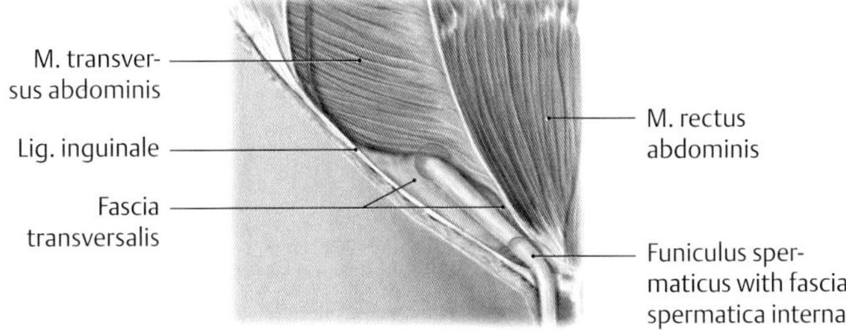

M. transversus abdominis
Lig. inguinale
Fascia transversalis
M. rectus abdominis
Funiculus spermaticus with fascia spermatica interna

C *Removed:* M. obliquus internus abdominis.

Fig. 11.4 Opening of canalis inguinalis

Right side, anterior view.

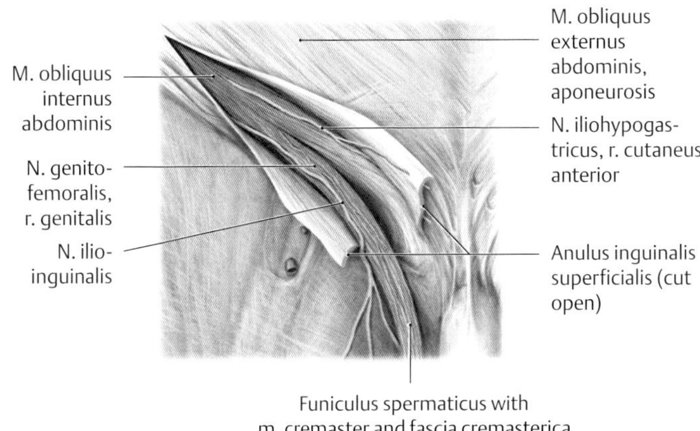

M. obliquus internus abdominis
N. genitofemoralis, r. genitalis
N. ilioinguinalis
M. obliquus externus abdominis, aponeurosis
N. iliohypogastricus, r. cutaneus anterior
Anulus inguinalis superficialis (cut open)
Funiculus spermaticus with m. cremaster and fascia cremasterica

A *Divided:* Aponeurosis of m. obliquus externus abdominis.

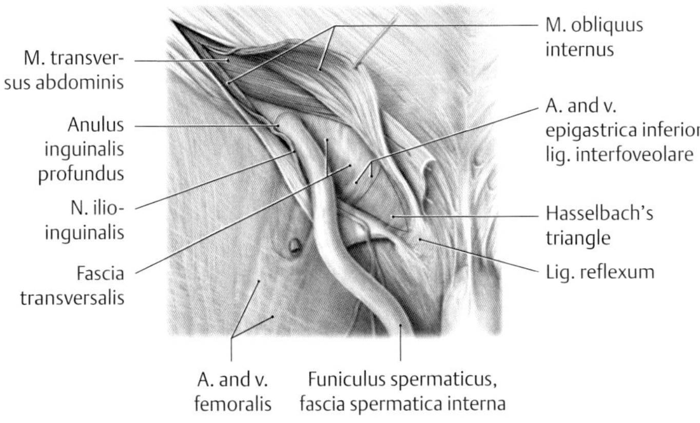

M. transversus abdominis
Anulus inguinalis profundus
N. ilioinguinalis
Fascia transversalis
M. obliquus internus
A. and v. epigastrica inferior, lig. interfoveolare
Hasselbach's triangle
Lig. reflexum
A. and v. femoralis
Funiculus spermaticus, fascia spermatica interna

B *Divided:* M. obliquus internus abdominis and m. cremaster.

The rectus sheath is created by fusion of the aponeuroses of m. transversus abdominis and mm. obliquus externus et infernus internus abdominis. The inferior edge of the posterior rectus sheath is called the linea arcuata.

Fig. 11.5 Abdominal wall and rectus sheath

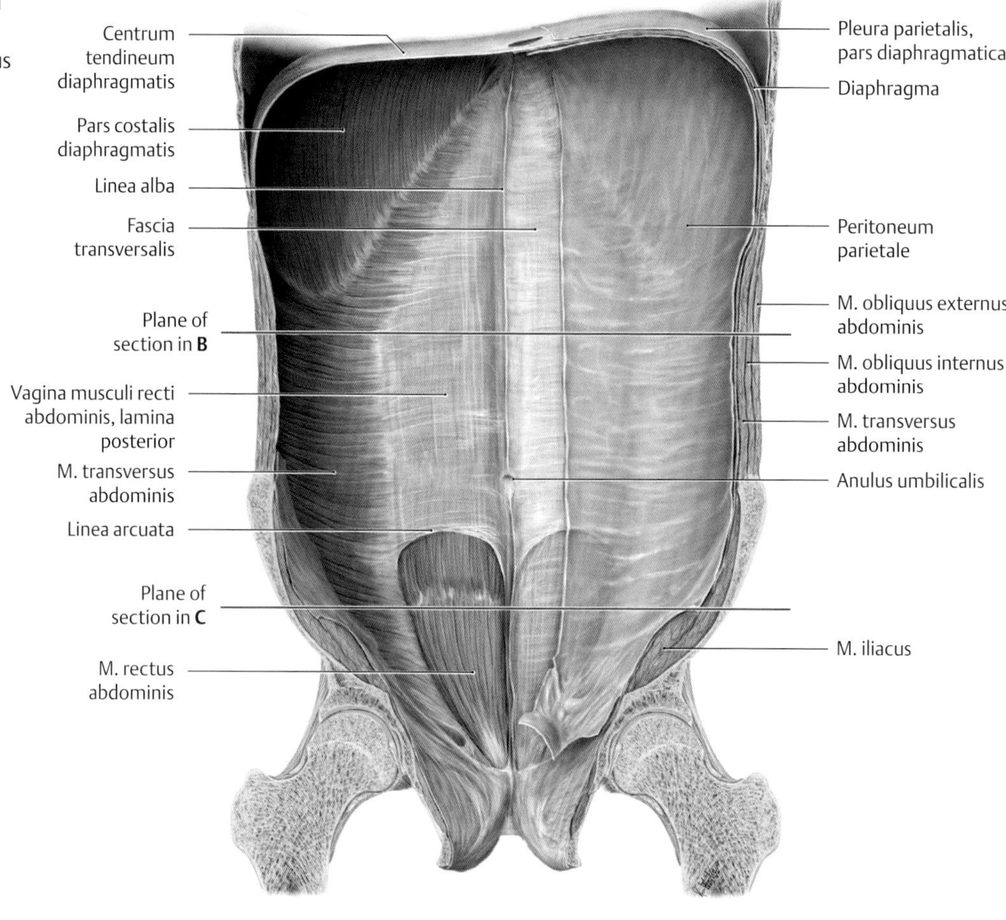

Centrum tendineum diaphragmatis
Pars costalis diaphragmatis
Linea alba
Fascia transversalis
Plane of section in **B**
Vagina musculi recti abdominis, lamina posterior
M. transversus abdominis
Linea arcuata
Plane of section in **C**
M. rectus abdominis
Pleura parietalis, pars diaphragmatica
Diaphragma
Peritoneum parietale
M. obliquus externus abdominis
M. obliquus internus abdominis
M. transversus abdominis
Anulus umbilicalis
M. iliacus

A Posterior (internal) view of the anterior abdominal wall.

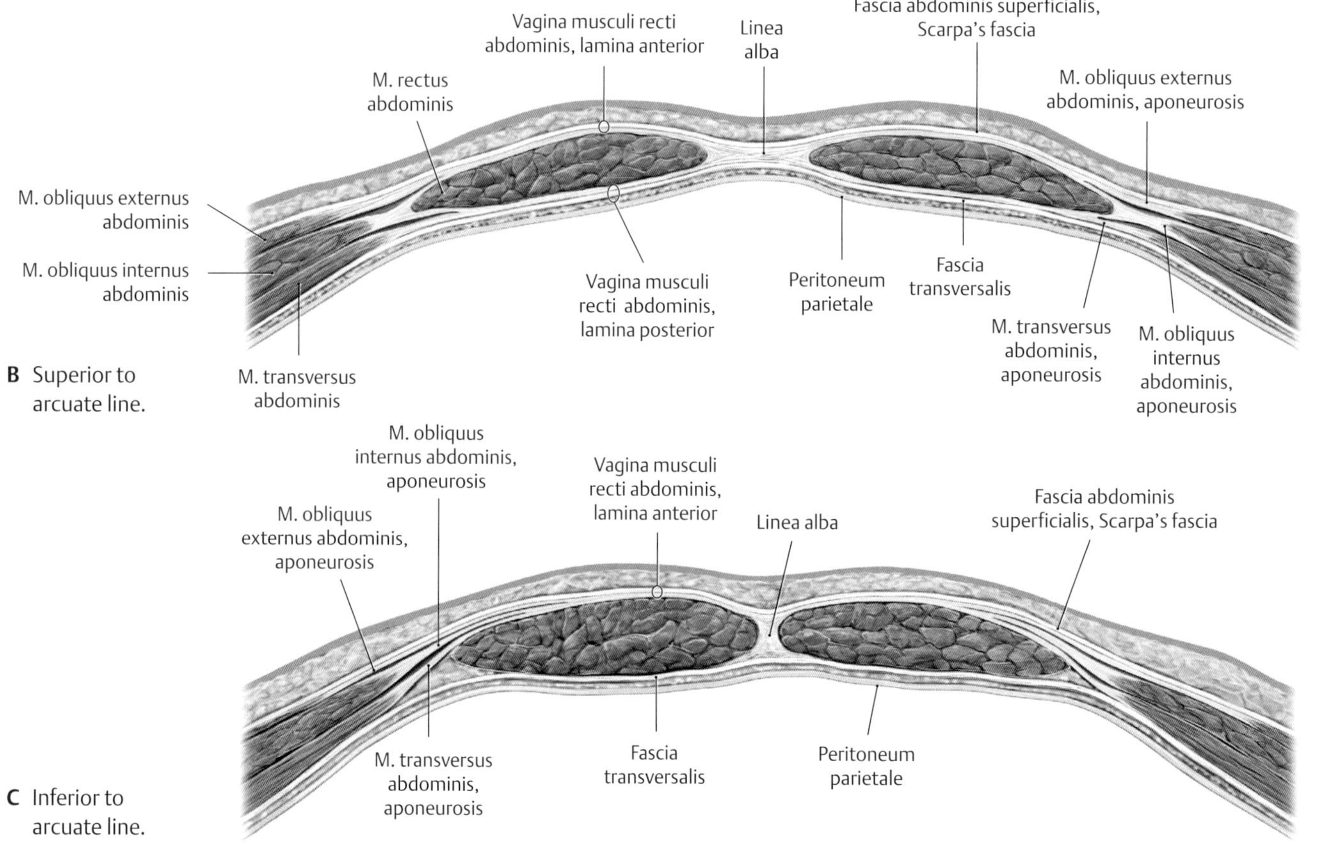

Vagina musculi recti abdominis, lamina anterior
Linea alba
Fascia abdominis superficialis, Scarpa's fascia
M. rectus abdominis
M. obliquus externus abdominis, aponeurosis
M. obliquus externus abdominis
M. obliquus internus abdominis
Vagina musculi recti abdominis, lamina posterior
Peritoneum parietale
Fascia transversalis
M. transversus abdominis, aponeurosis
M. obliquus internus abdominis, aponeurosis
M. transversus abdominis
M. obliquus internus abdominis, aponeurosis
M. obliquus externus abdominis, aponeurosis
Vagina musculi recti abdominis, lamina anterior
Linea alba
Fascia abdominis superficialis, Scarpa's fascia
M. transversus abdominis, aponeurosis
Fascia transversalis
Peritoneum parietale

B Superior to arcuate line.

C Inferior to arcuate line.

Fig. 11.6 **Abdominal wall: Internal surface anatomy**
Coronal section, posterior view. The three fossae of the anterior abdominal wall (*circled*) are sites of potential herniation.

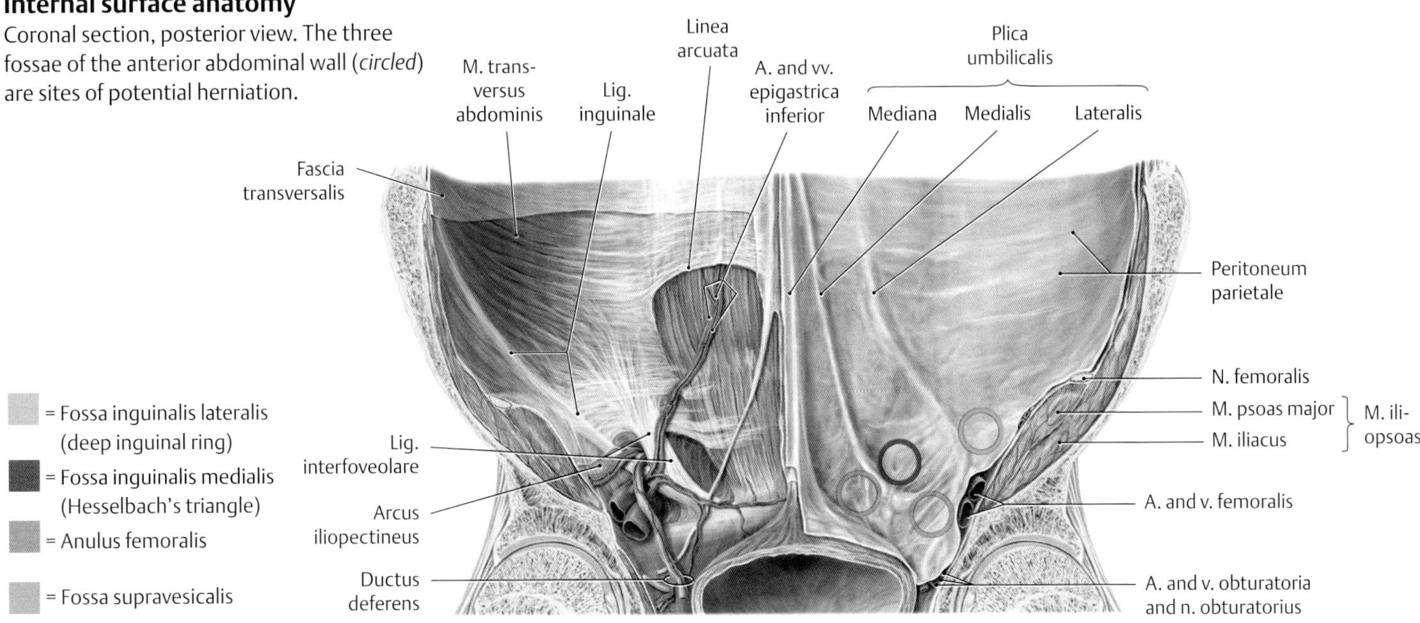

Linea arcuata
Plica umbilicalis
M. trans-versus abdominis
Lig. inguinale
A. and vv. epigastrica inferior
Mediana
Medialis
Lateralis
Fascia transversalis
Peritoneum parietale
N. femoralis
M. psoas major
M. iliacus
M. ili-opsoas
= Fossa inguinalis lateralis (deep inguinal ring)
= Fossa inguinalis medialis (Hesselbach's triangle)
= Anulus femoralis
= Fossa supravesicalis
Lig. interfoveolare
Arcus iliopectineus
Ductus deferens
A. and v. femoralis
A. and v. obturatoria and n. obturatorius

Clinical

Inguinal and femoral hernias

Indirect inguinal hernias occur in younger males and may be congenital or acquired; direct inguinal hernias are always acquired. Femoral hernias are acquired and more common in females.

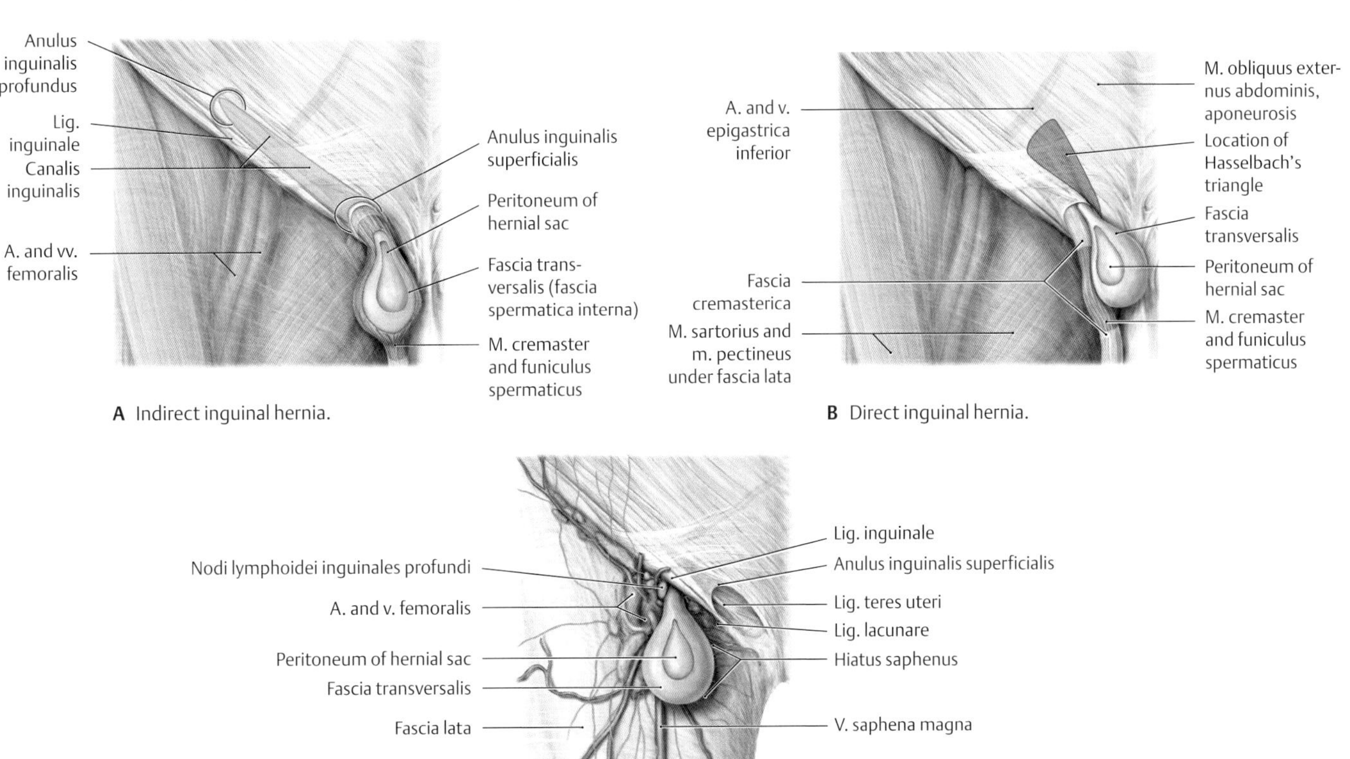

Anulus inguinalis profundus
Lig. inguinale
Canalis inguinalis
A. and vv. femoralis
Anulus inguinalis superficialis
Peritoneum of hernial sac
Fascia trans-versalis (fascia spermatica interna)
M. cremaster and funiculus spermaticus
A. and v. epigastrica inferior
Fascia cremasterica
M. sartorius and m. pectineus under fascia lata
M. obliquus exter-nus abdominis, aponeurosis
Location of Hasselbach's triangle
Fascia transversalis
Peritoneum of hernial sac
M. cremaster and funiculus spermaticus
Nodi lymphoidei inguinales profundi
A. and v. femoralis
Peritoneum of hernial sac
Fascia transversalis
Fascia lata
Lig. inguinale
Anulus inguinalis superficialis
Lig. teres uteri
Lig. lacunare
Hiatus saphenus
V. saphena magna

A Indirect inguinal hernia.

B Direct inguinal hernia.

C Femoral hernia.

Regio Perinealis

Fig. 11.7 Perineum and diaphragma pelvis: Female
Lithotomy position, caudal (inferior) view. See p. 192 for the external genitalia.

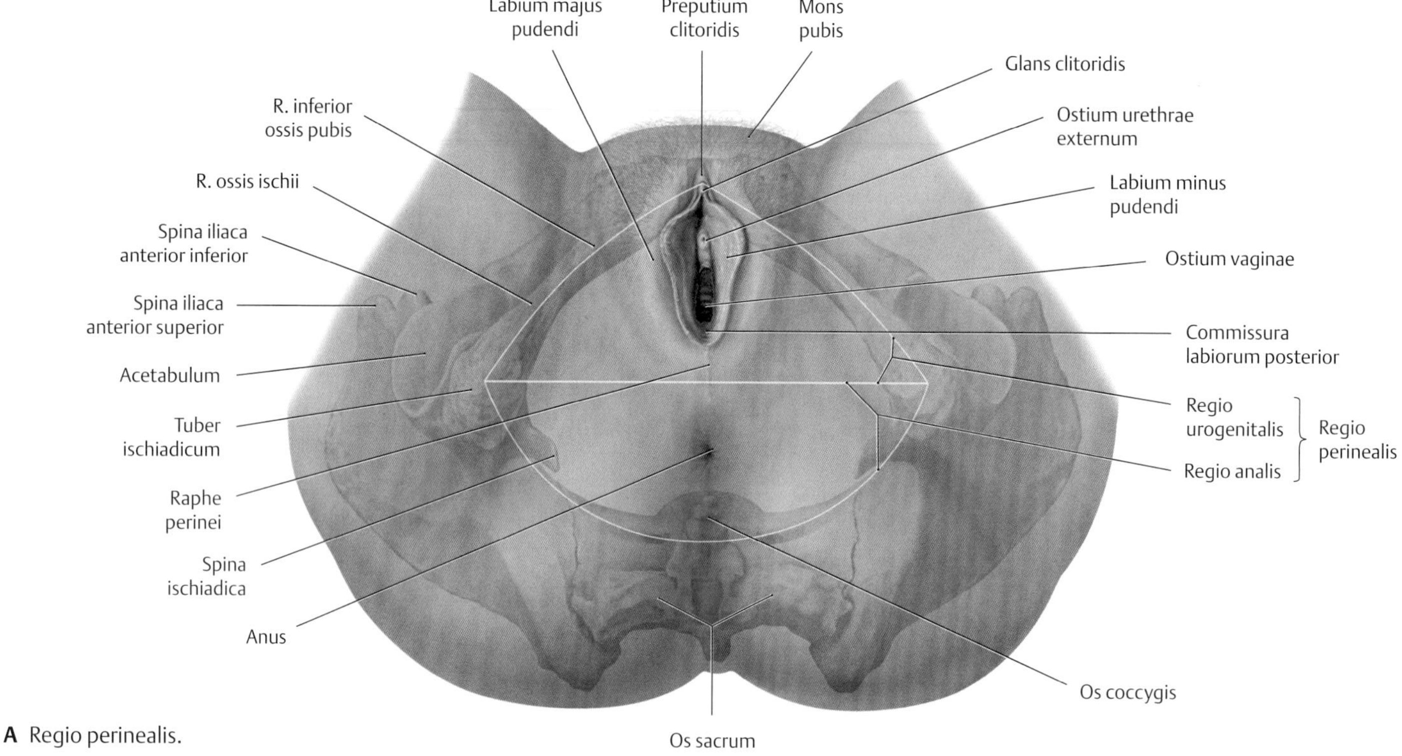
Labium majus pudendi
Preputium clitoridis
Mons pubis
Glans clitoridis
R. inferior ossis pubis
Ostium urethrae externum
R. ossis ischii
Labium minus pudendi
Spina iliaca anterior inferior
Ostium vaginae
Spina iliaca anterior superior
Commissura labiorum posterior
Acetabulum
Tuber ischiadicum
Regio urogenitalis
Regio analis
Regio perinealis
Raphe perinei
Spina ischiadica
Anus
Os coccygis
Os sacrum

A Regio perinealis.

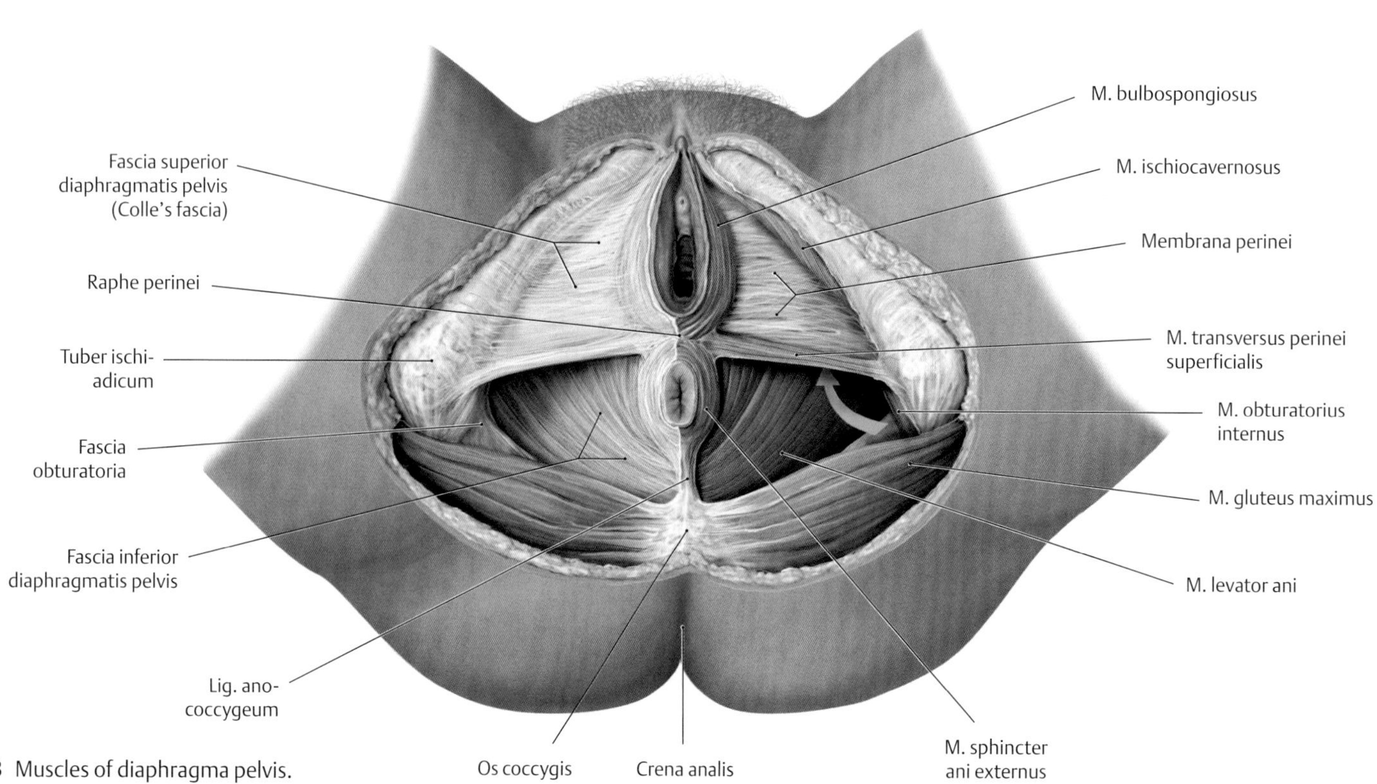
M. bulbospongiosus
Fascia superior diaphragmatis pelvis (Colle's fascia)
M. ischiocavernosus
Membrana perinei
Raphe perinei
Tuber ischiadicum
M. transversus perinei superficialis
M. obturatorius internus
Fascia obturatoria
M. gluteus maximus
Fascia inferior diaphragmatis pelvis
M. levator ani
Lig. anococcygeum
Os coccygis
Crena analis
M. sphincter ani externus

B Muscles of diaphragma pelvis.

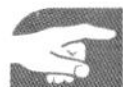

The bilateral boundaries of the perineum in both sexes are the symphysis pubica, r. ischiopubicus, tuber ischiadicum, lig. sacrotuberale, and the coccyx. The green arrows indicate the anterior recess of fossa ischioanalis, superior to the urogenital muscles.

Fig. 11.8 **Perineum and pelvic floor: Male**

Lithotomy position, caudal (inferior) view. See p. 196 for the genitalia.

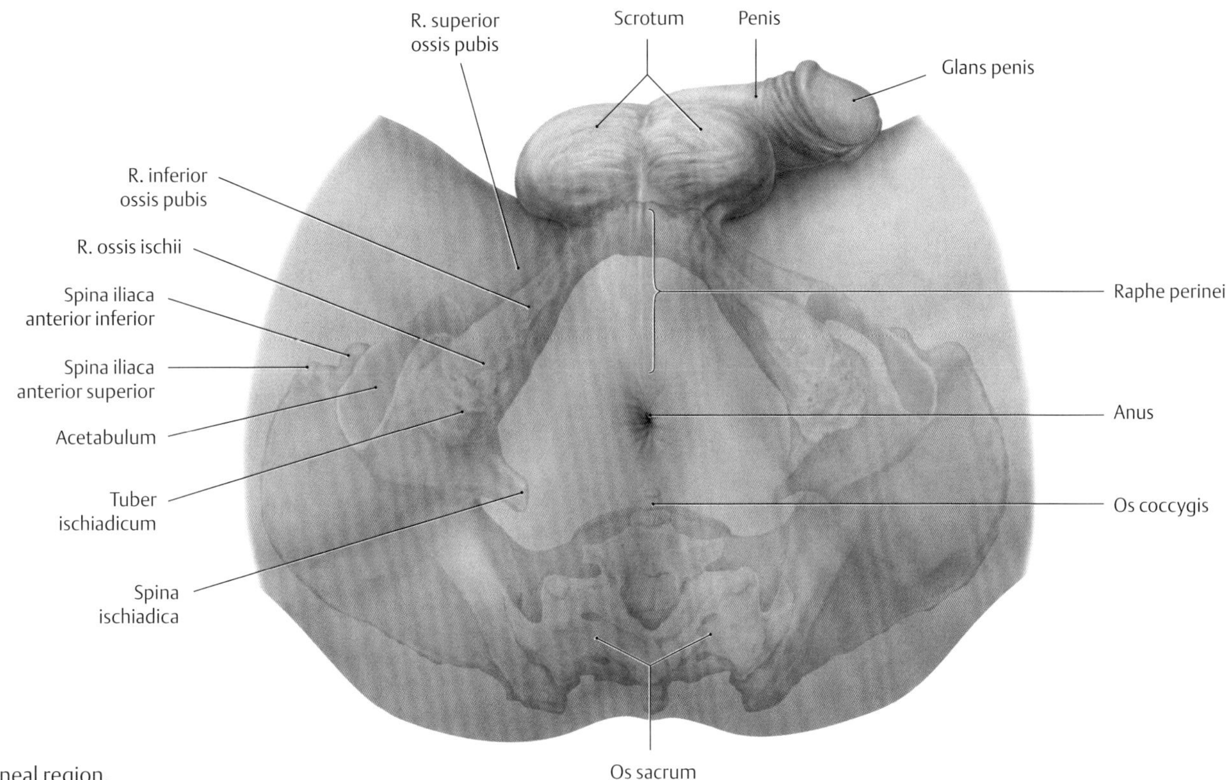

R. superior ossis pubis
Scrotum
Penis
Glans penis
R. inferior ossis pubis
R. ossis ischii
Spina iliaca anterior inferior
Spina iliaca anterior superior
Acetabulum
Tuber ischiadicum
Spina ischiadica
Raphe perinei
Anus
Os coccygis
Os sacrum

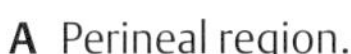

A Perineal region.

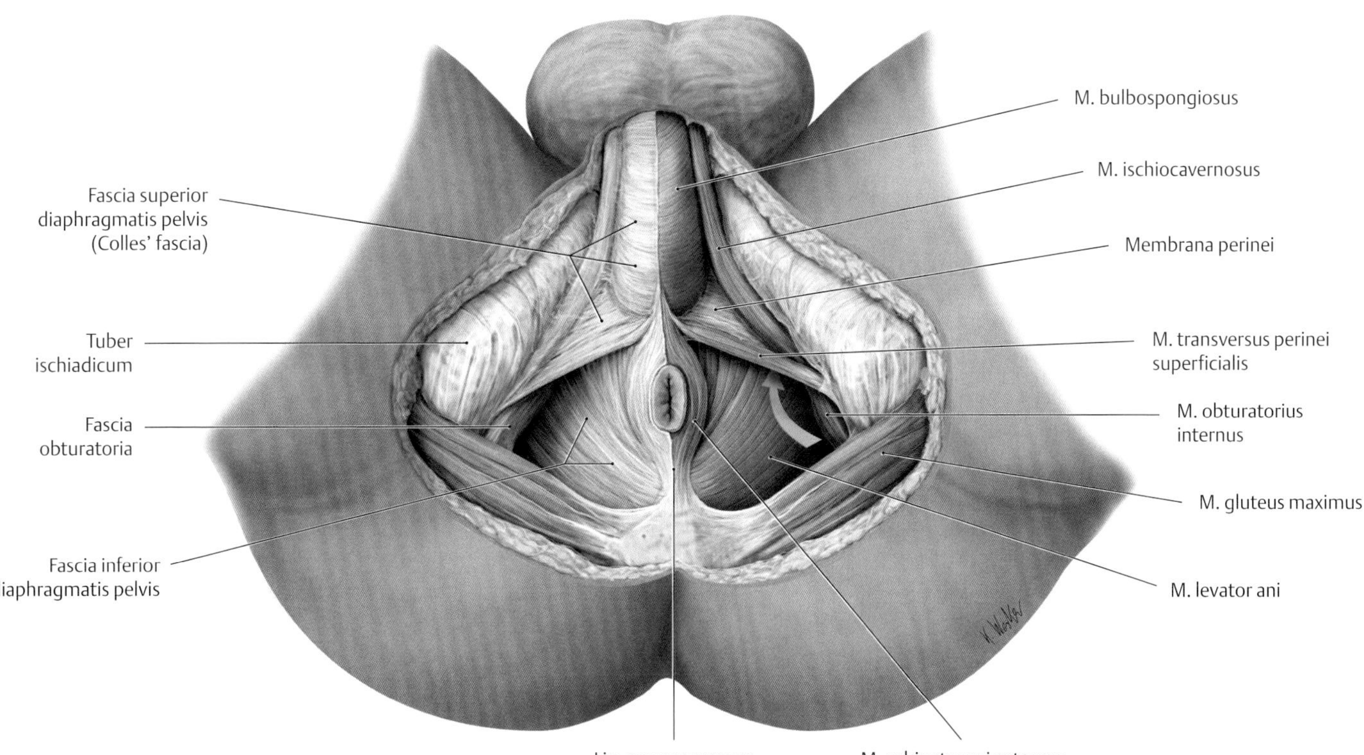

M. bulbospongiosus
M. ischiocavernosus
Membrana perinei
M. transversus perinei superficialis
M. obturatorius internus
M. gluteus maximus
M. levator ani
Fascia superior diaphragmatis pelvis (Colles' fascia)
Tuber ischiadicum
Fascia obturatoria
Fascia inferior diaphragmatis pelvis
Lig. anococcygeum
M. sphincter ani externus

B Muscles of the pelvic floor.

Abdominal Wall Muscle Facts

Fig. 11.9 Anterior muscles
Anterior view.

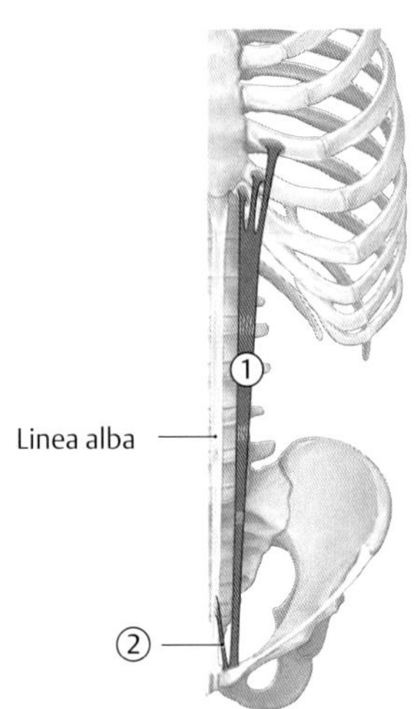

①
Linea alba
②

Fig. 11.10 Anterolateral muscles
Anterior view.

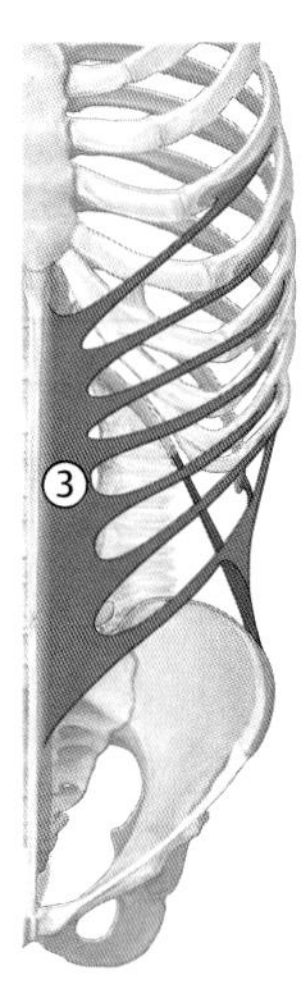

③

A M. obliquus externus abdominis.

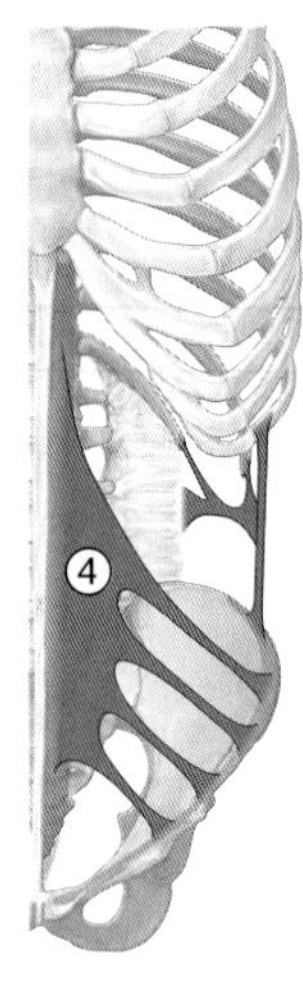

④

B M. obliquus internus abdominis.

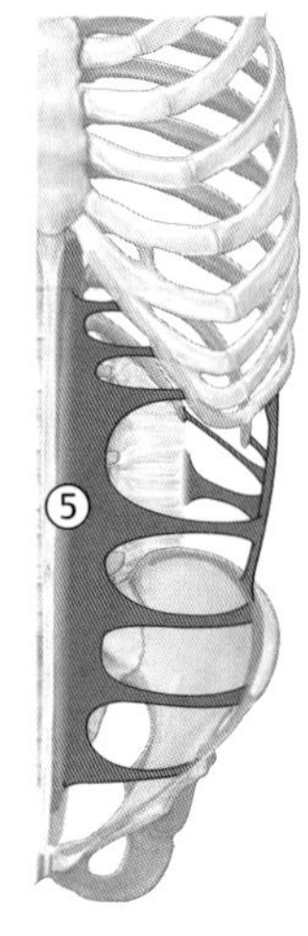

⑤

C M. transversus abdominis.

Fig. 11.11 Posterior muscles
Anterior view. M. psoas major and m. iliacus are together known as the m. iliopsoas.

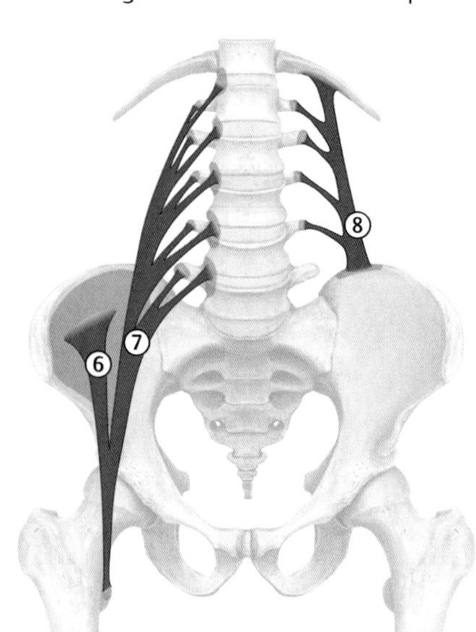

⑧
⑦
⑥

Table 11.2 Abdominal wall muscles

Muscle		Origin	Insertion	Innervation	Action
Anterior abdominal wall muscles					
① M. rectus abdominis		Os pubis (between tuberculum pubicum and symphyse)	Cartilago costalis of Costa V–VII, proc. xiphoideus of sternum	Nn. intercostales (T5–T12)	Flexes trunk, compresses abdomen, stabilizes pelvis
② M. pyramidalis		Os pubis (anterior to m. rectus abdominis)	Linea alba (runs within the vagina musculi recti abdominis)	N. subcostalis (12th N. intercostalis)	Tenses linea alba
Anterolateral abdominal wall muscles					
③ M. obliquus externus abdominis		Costa V–XII (outer surface)	Linea alba, tuberculum pubicum, anterior Sacra iliaca	Nn. intercostales (T7–T12)	*Unilateral:* Bends trunk to same side, rotates trunk to opposite side *Bilateral:* Flexes trunk, compresses abdomen, stabilizes pelvis
④ M. obliquus internus abdominis		Fascia thoracolumbalis (lamina profunda), crista iliaca (linea intermedia), spina iliaca anterior superior, fascia m. iliopsoas	Costa X–XII (lower borders), linea alba lamina anterior and posterior)	Nn. intercostales (T7–T12), N. ilio-hypogastricus, N. ilioinguinalis	
⑤ M. transversus abdominis		7th to 12th cartilago costalis (inner surfaces), fascia thoracolumbalis (lamina profunda), crista iliaca, spina iliaca anterior superior (labium internum), fascia M. iliopsoas	Linea alba, crista pubica		*Unilateral:* Rotates trunk to same side *Bilateral:* Compresses abdomen
Posterior abdominal wall muscles					
⑥ M. psoas major	Pars superficialis	T XII–L IV Corpus vertebrae and associated Discus intervertebralis (lateral surfaces)	Femur (trochanter minor), joint insertion as m. iliopsoas	Direct branches from plexus lumbalis (L2–L4)	Articulatio coxae: Flexion and external rotation lumbar spine (with femur fixed): *Unilateral:* Contraction bends trunk laterally *Bilateral:* Contraction raises trunk from supine position
	Pars profunda	L I–L V (Procc. costales)			
⑦ M. iliacus		Fossa iliaca		N. femoralis (L2–L4)	
⑧ M. quadratus lumborum		Crista iliaca and lig. iliolumbare (not shown)	Costa XII, L I–L IV corpus vertebrae (procc. transversi)	T12, L1–L4 Nn. spinales	*Unilateral:* Bends trunk to same side *Bilateral:* Bearing down and expiration, stabilizes Costa XII

Fig. 11.12 Anterior and posterior abdominal wall muscles
Anterior view.

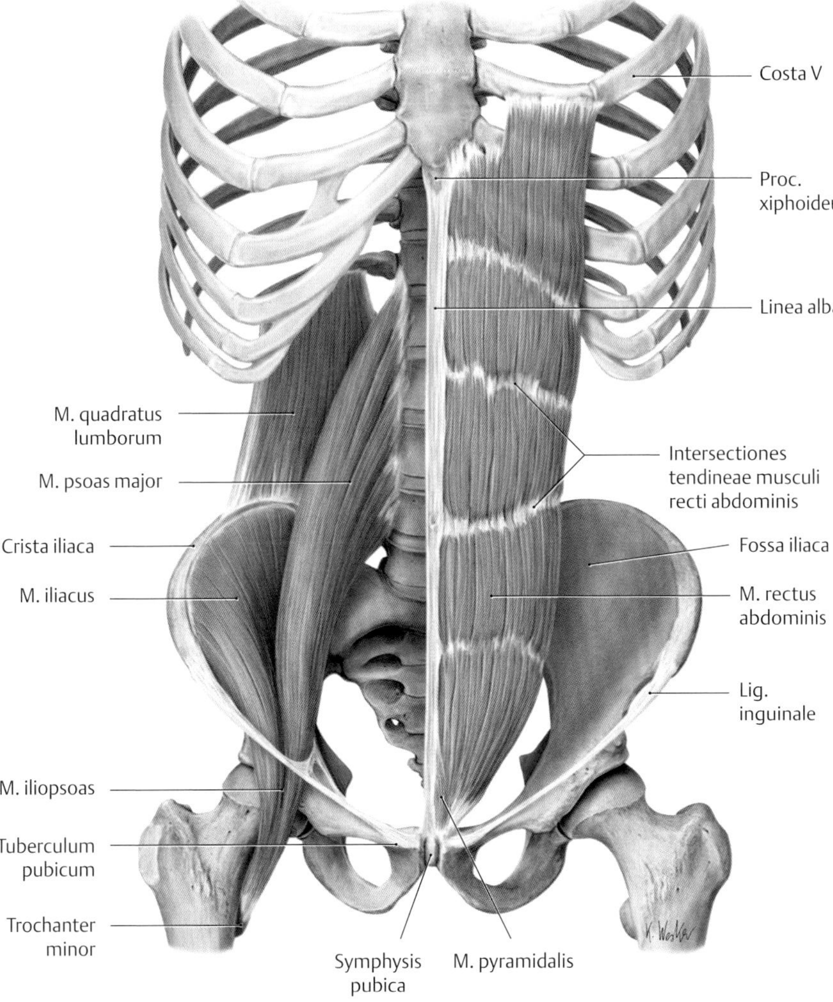
Costa V
Proc. xiphoideus
Linea alba
M. quadratus lumborum
M. psoas major
Intersectiones tendineae musculi recti abdominis
Crista iliaca
Fossa iliaca
M. iliacus
M. rectus abdominis
Lig. inguinale
M. iliopsoas
Tuberculum pubicum
Trochanter minor
Symphysis pubica
M. pyramidalis
A Anterior and posterior muscles.

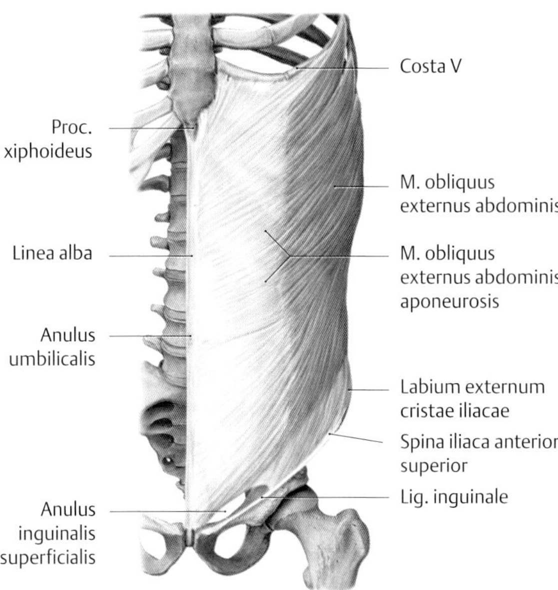
Costa V
Proc. xiphoideus
M. obliquus externus abdominis
Linea alba
M. obliquus externus abdominis, aponeurosis
Anulus umbilicalis
Labium externum cristae iliacae
Spina iliaca anterior superior
Lig. inguinale
Anulus inguinalis superficialis
B M. obliquus externus abdominis.

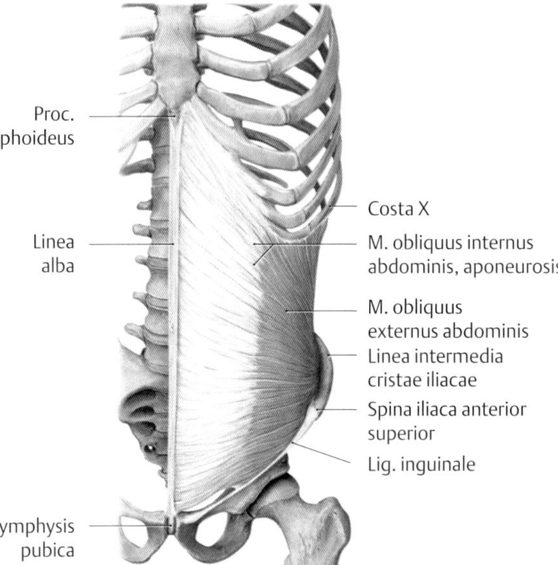
Proc. xiphoideus
Costa X
Linea alba
M. obliquus internus abdominis, aponeurosis
M. obliquus externus abdominis
Linea intermedia cristae iliacae
Spina iliaca anterior superior
Lig. inguinale
Symphysis pubica
C M. obliquus internus abdominis.

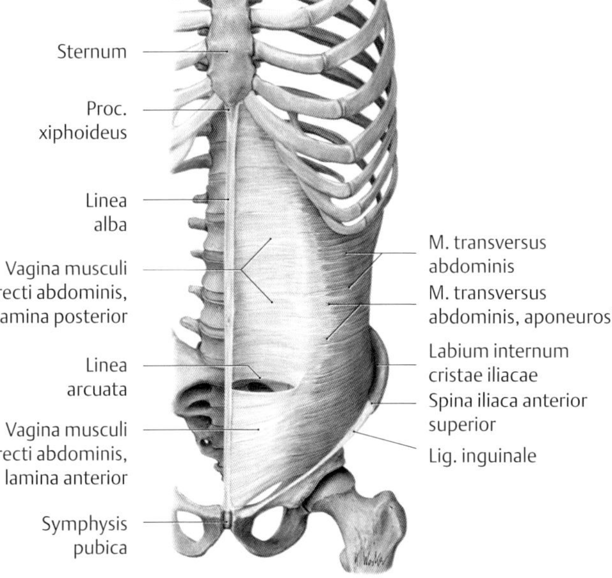
Sternum
Proc. xiphoideus
Linea alba
Vagina musculi recti abdominis, lamina posterior
M. transversus abdominis
M. transversus abdominis, aponeurosis
Linea arcuata
Labium internum cristae iliacae
Spina iliaca anterior superior
Vagina musculi recti abdominis, lamina anterior
Lig. inguinale
Symphysis pubica
D M. transversus abdominis.

Diaphragma Pelvis Muscle Facts

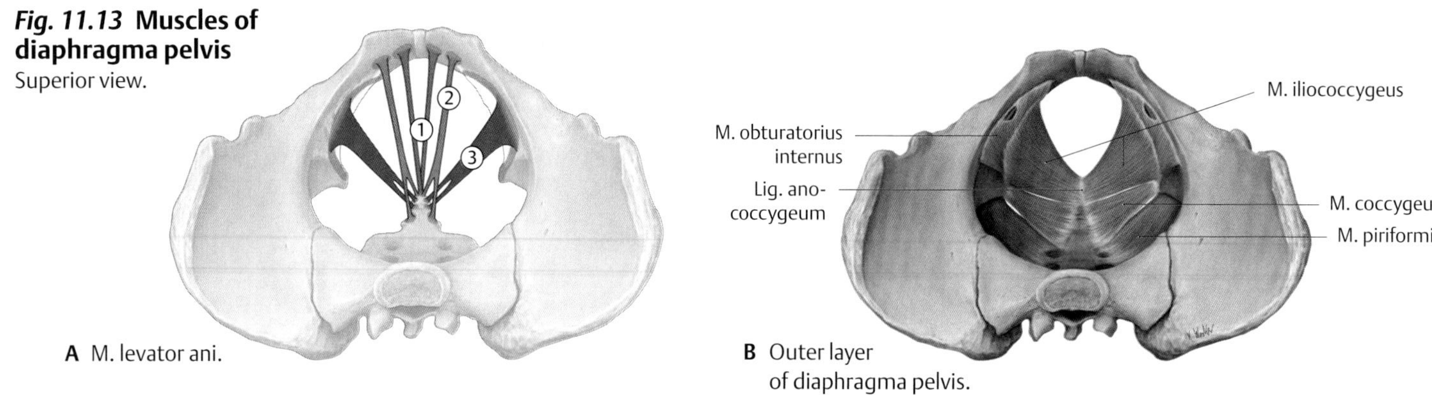

1
2
3
M. iliococcygeus
M. obturatorius internus
Lig. anococcygeum
M. coccygeus
M. piriformis

Fig. 11.13 **Muscles of diaphragma pelvis**
Superior view.

A M. levator ani.

B Outer layer of diaphragma pelvis.

Table 11.3 Muscles of the pelvic floor

Muscle		Origin	Insertion	Innervation	Action
Muscles of the pelvic diaphragm					
M. levator ani	① M. puborectalis	R. pubis superior (both sides of symphysis pubica)	Lig. anococcygeum	Direct branches of plexus sacralis (S4), inferior anal n.	Diaphragma pelvis: Supports pelvic viscera
	② M. pubococcygeus	Os pubis (lateral to origin of m.puborectalis)	Lig. anococcygeum, os coccygis		
	③ M. iliococcygeus	Internal fascia of m. obturatorius internus of m. levator ani (tendinous arch)			
M. coccygeus		Os sacrum (inferior end)	Spina ischiadicum	Direct branches from plexus sacralis (S4–S5)	Supports pelvic viscera, flexes os coccygis
Muscles of the pelvic wall (parietal muscles)					
M. piriformis*		Os sacrum (facies pelvica)	Femur (apex of trochanter major)	Direct branches from plexus sacralis (S1–S2)	Articulatio coxae: External rotation, stabilization, and abduction of flexed hip
M. obturatorius internus*		Membrane of m.obturatorius internus and bony boundaries (inner surface)	Femur (trochanter major, medial surface)	Direct branches from plexus sacralis (L5–S1)	Articulatio coxae: External rotation and abduction of flexed hip
Sphincter and erector muscles					
④ M. sphincter ani externus		Encircles anus (runs posteriorly from perineum to lig. anococcygeum)		N. pudendus (S2–S4)	Closes anus
⑤ M. sphincter urethrae externus		Encircles urethra (division of m. transversus perinei profundus)			Closes urethra
⑥ M. bulbospongiosus		Runs anteriorly from perineum to clitoris (females) or raphe penis (males)			Females: Compresses glandula vestibularis major Males: Assists in erection
⑦ M. ischiocavernosus		R. ischiadicus	Crus clitoridis or crus penis		Maintains erection by squeezing blood into corpus cavernosum of clitoris or penis

*The piriformis and obturator internus are considered muscles of the hip (see p. 374).
The female and male external genitalia are shown on pp. 194, 203.

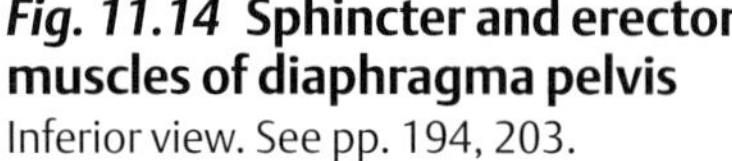
Fig. 11.14 **Sphincter and erector muscles of diaphragma pelvis**
Inferior view. See pp. 194, 203.

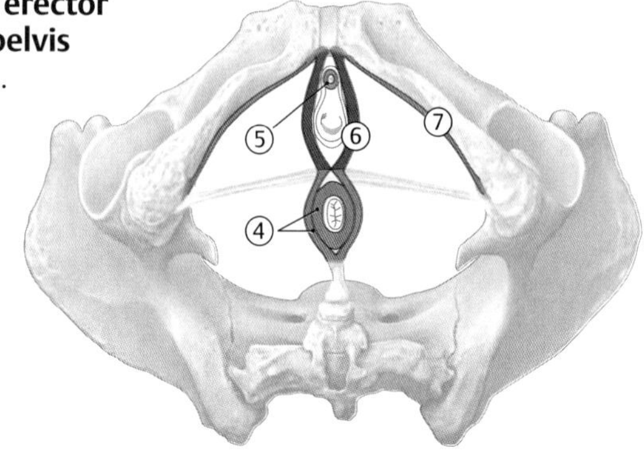

5
6
7
4

Fig. 11.15 **Diaphragma pelvis**
Female pelvis.

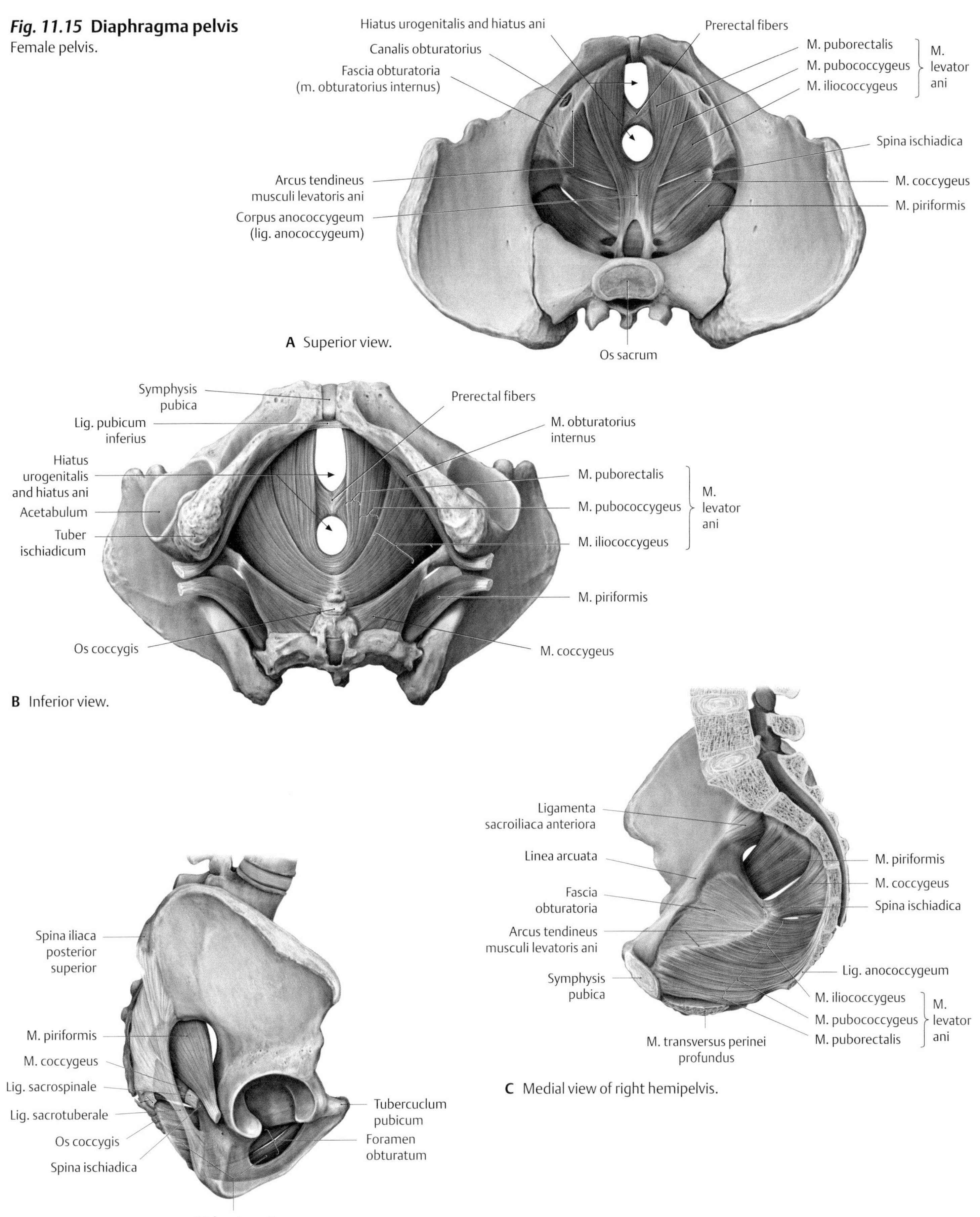
Hiatus urogenitalis and hiatus ani
Canalis obturatorius
Fascia obturatoria (m. obturatorius internus)
Arcus tendineus musculi levatoris ani
Corpus anococcygeum (lig. anococcygeum)
Prerectal fibers
M. puborectalis
M. pubococcygeus
M. iliococcygeus
M. levator ani
Spina ischiadica
M. coccygeus
M. piriformis
Os sacrum
Symphysis pubica
Lig. pubicum inferius
Hiatus urogenitalis and hiatus ani
Acetabulum
Tuber ischiadicum
Os coccygis
Prerectal fibers
M. obturatorius internus
M. puborectalis
M. pubococcygeus
M. iliococcygeus
M. levator ani
M. piriformis
M. coccygeus
Ligamenta sacroiliaca anteriora
Linea arcuata
Fascia obturatoria
Arcus tendineus musculi levatoris ani
Symphysis pubica
M. piriformis
M. coccygeus
Spina ischiadica
Lig. anococcygeum
M. iliococcygeus
M. pubococcygeus
M. puborectalis
M. levator ani
M. transversus perinei profundus
Spina iliaca posterior superior
M. piriformis
M. coccygeus
Lig. sacrospinale
Lig. sacrotuberale
Os coccygis
Spina ischiadica
M. levator ani
Tubercuclum pubicum
Foramen obturatum

A Superior view.

B Inferior view.

C Medial view of right hemipelvis.

D Right lateral view.

Divisions of the Abdominopelvic Cavity

***Fig. 12.1* Organ layers and quadrants**
Anterior view. The organs of the abdomen and pelvis can be classified by layer, by quadrant (using the umbilicus at L4), by level (upper and lower abdomen, and pelvis), or with respect to the presence of mesenterium (Table 12.1).

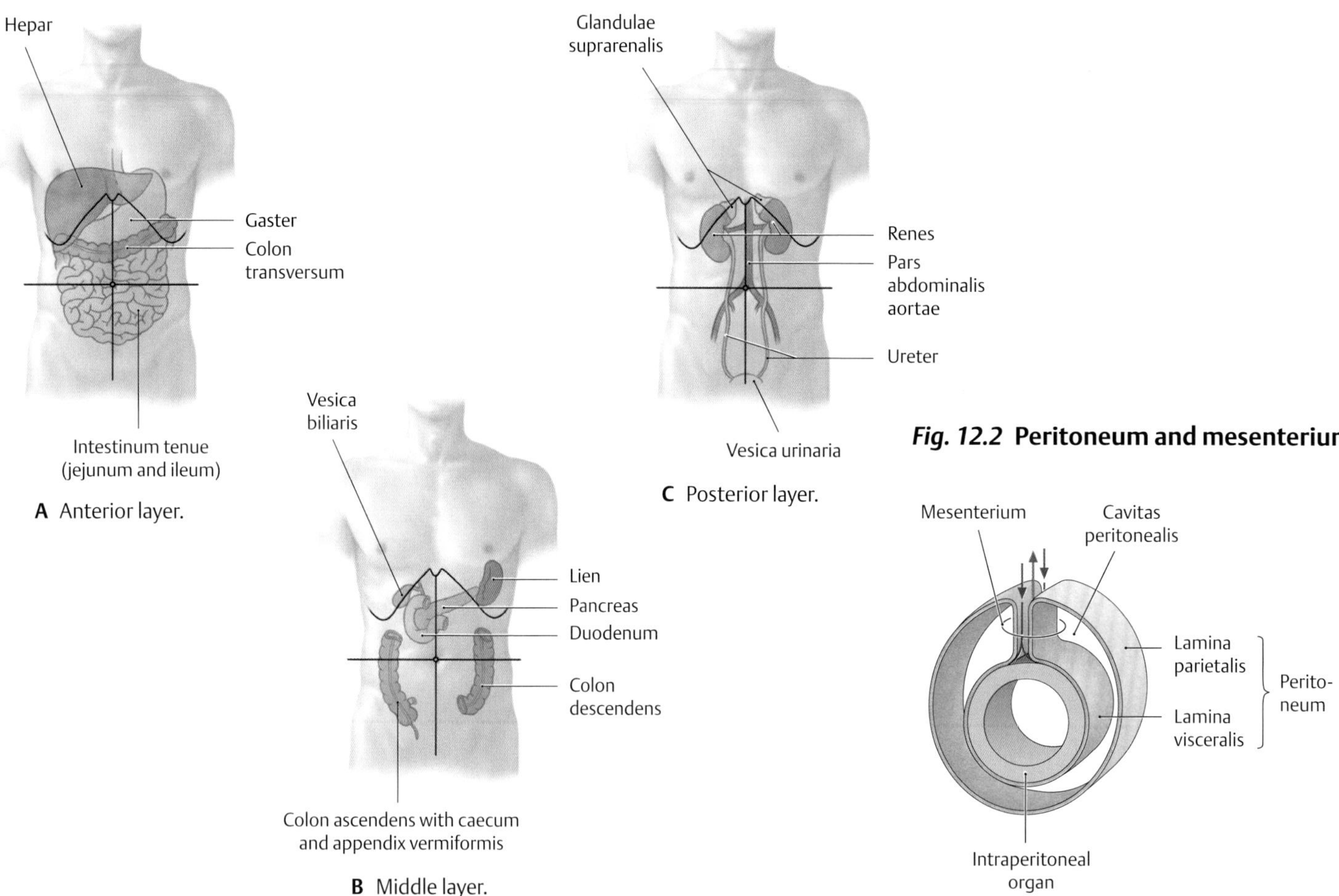
Hepar
Gaster
Colon transversum
Intestinum tenue (jejunum and ileum)
Vesica biliaris
Lien
Pancreas
Duodenum
Colon descendens
Colon ascendens with caecum and appendix vermiformis
Glandulae suprarenalis
Renes
Pars abdominalis aortae
Ureter
Vesica urinaria
Mesenterium
Cavitas peritonealis
Lamina parietalis
Lamina visceralis
Perito-neum
Intraperitoneal organ

A Anterior layer.

B Middle layer.

C Posterior layer.

***Fig. 12.2* Peritoneum and mesenterium**

Table 12.1 Organs of the abdomen and pelvis

Location		Organs		
Intraperitoneal organs: These organs have a mesenterium and are completely covered by the peritoneum.				
Cavitas peritonealis abdominalis		• Gaster • Intestinum tenue (jejunum, ileum, some of the pars superior of the duodenum) • Lien • Hepar		• Vesica biliaris • Caecum with appendix vermiformis (portions of variable size may be retroperitoneal) • Intestinum crassum (colon transversum and colon sigmoideum)
Cavitas peritonealis pelvis		• Uterus (fundus and corpus)	• Ovarium	• Tuba uterina
Extraperitoneal organs: These organs either have no mesenterium or lost it during development.				
Retroperitoneal	Primarily	• Ren	• Glandulae suprarenalis	• Cervix uteri
	Secondarily	• Duodenum (pars descendens, horizontalis, and ascendens) • Pancreas		• Colon ascendens and descendens • Rectum (upper 2/3)
Infraperitoneal/subperitoneal		• Vesica urinaria • Ureter distalis • Prostata	• Vesica seminalis • Cervix uteri	• Vagina • Rectum (lower 1/3)

Fig. 12.3 Peritoneal relationships

Midsagittal section through male pelvis, viewed from the left side.

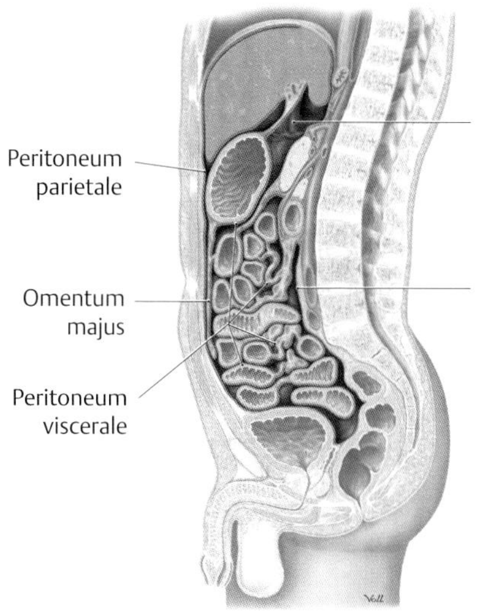
Omentum minus
(bursa omentalis)
Peritoneum
parietale
Peritoneum
parietale
Omentum
majus
Peritoneum
viscerale

A Peritoneal cavity. The peritoneum is shown in red.

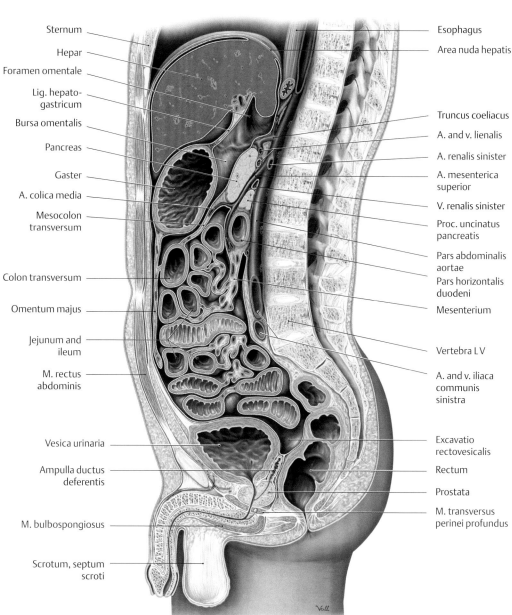

Sternum
Hepar
Foramen omentale
Lig. hepato-gastricum
Bursa omentalis
Pancreas
Gaster
A. colica media
Mesocolon transversum
Colon transversum
Omentum majus
Jejunum and ileum
M. rectus abdominis
Vesica urinaria
Ampulla ductus deferentis
M. bulbospongiosus
Scrotum, septum scroti
Esophagus
Area nuda hepatis
Truncus coeliacus
A. and v. lienalis
A. renalis sinister
A. mesenterica superior
V. renalis sinister
Proc. uncinatus pancreatis
Pars abdominalis aortae
Pars horizontalis duodeni
Mesenterium
Vertebra L V
A. and v. iliaca communis sinistra
Excavatio rectovesicalis
Rectum
Prostata
M. transversus perinei profundus

B Organs of the abdomen and pelvis.

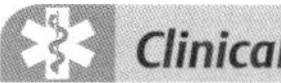

Clinical

Acute abdominal pain

Acute abdominal pain ("acute abdomen") may be so severe that the abdominal wall becomes extremely sensitive to touch ("guarding") and the intestines stop functioning. Causes include organ inflammation such as appendicitis, perforation due to a gastric ulcer (see p. 159), or organ blockage by a stone, tumor, etc. In women, gynecological processes or ectopic pregnancies may produce severe abdominal pain.

Cavitas Peritonealis & Greater Sac

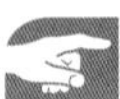

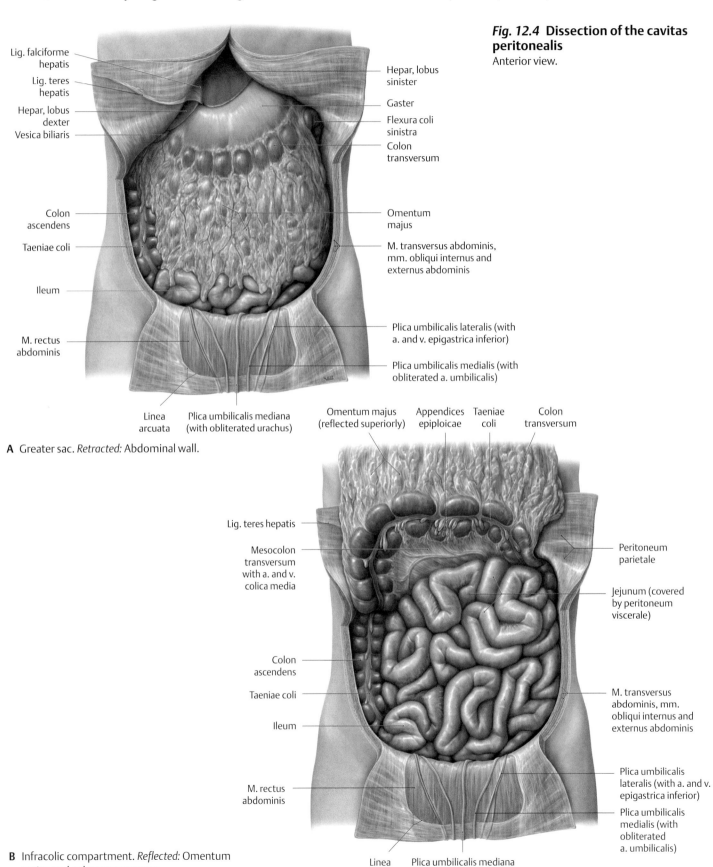

The largest part of the peritoneal cavity is the greater sac. The omentum majus is an apron-like fold of peritoneum suspended from curvatura major of gaster and covering the anterior surface of colon transversum. The colon transversum divides the peritoneal cavity into a supracolic compartment (hepar, vesica biliaris, and gaster) and an infracolic compartment (intestines).

Fig. 12.4 Dissection of the cavitas peritonealis
Anterior view.

Lig. falciforme hepatis
Lig. teres hepatis
Hepar, lobus dexter
Vesica biliaris
Colon ascendens
Taeniae coli
Ileum
M. rectus abdominis
Linea arcuata
Plica umbilicalis mediana (with obliterated urachus)
Hepar, lobus sinister
Gaster
Flexura coli sinistra
Colon transversum
Omentum majus
M. transversus abdominis, mm. obliqui internus and externus abdominis
Plica umbilicalis lateralis (with a. and v. epigastrica inferior)
Plica umbilicalis medialis (with obliterated a. umbilicalis)

A Greater sac. *Retracted:* Abdominal wall.

Omentum majus (reflected superiorly)
Appendices epiploicae
Taeniae coli
Colon transversum
Lig. teres hepatis
Mesocolon transversum with a. and v. colica media
Colon ascendens
Taeniae coli
Ileum
M. rectus abdominis
Linea arcuata
Plica umbilicalis mediana (with obliterated urachus)
Peritoneum parietale
Jejunum (covered by peritoneum viscerale)
M. transversus abdominis, mm. obliqui internus and externus abdominis
Plica umbilicalis lateralis (with a. and v. epigastrica inferior)
Plica umbilicalis medialis (with obliterated a. umbilicalis)

B Infracolic compartment. *Reflected:* Omentum majus and colon transversum.

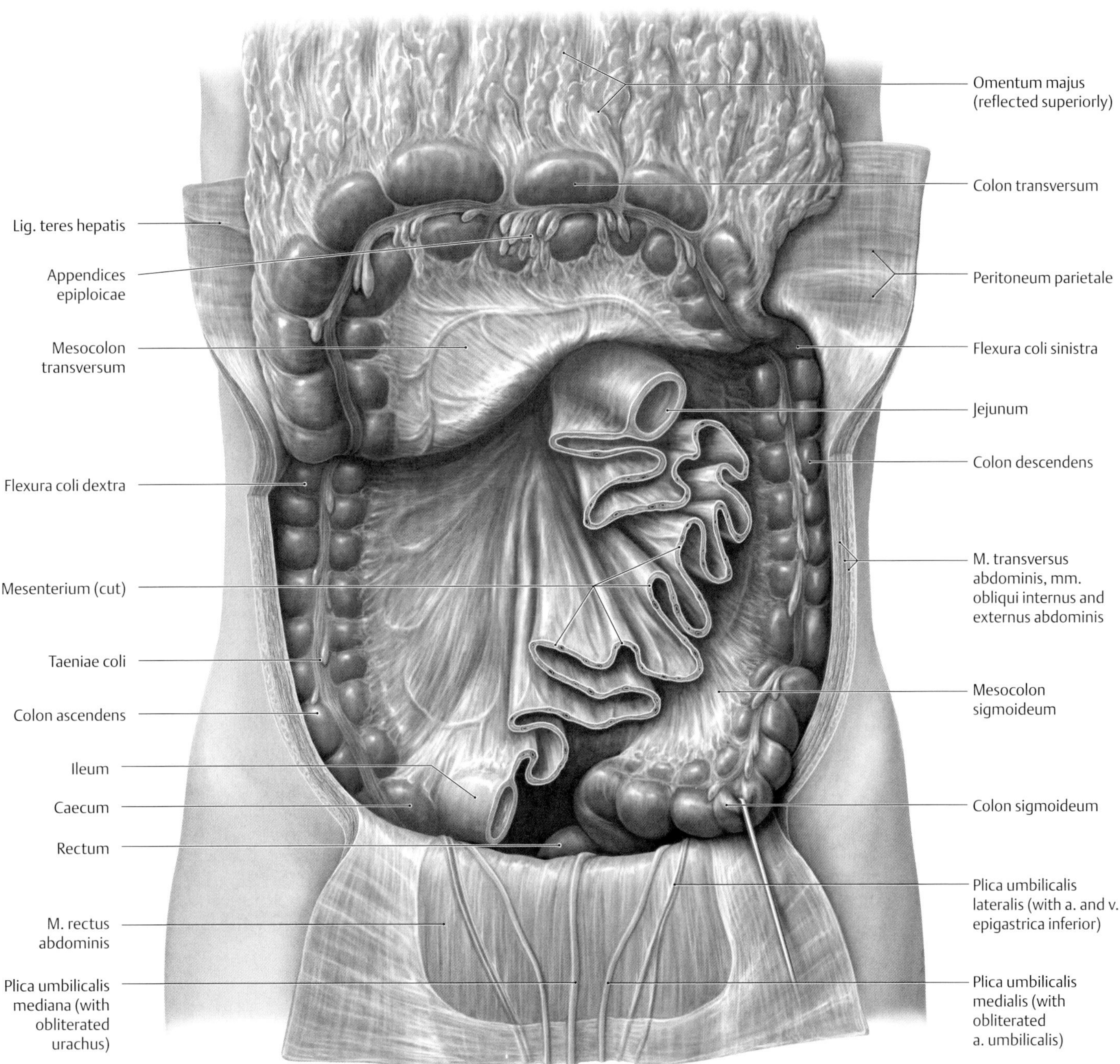

Omentum majus (reflected superiorly)
Colon transversum
Lig. teres hepatis
Appendices epiploicae
Peritoneum parietale
Mesocolon transversum
Flexura coli sinistra
Jejunum
Colon descendens
Flexura coli dextra
M. transversus abdominis, mm. obliqui internus and externus abdominis
Mesenterium (cut)
Taeniae coli
Mesocolon sigmoideum
Colon ascendens
Ileum
Caecum
Colon sigmoideum
Rectum
Plica umbilicalis lateralis (with a. and v. epigastrica inferior)
M. rectus abdominis
Plica umbilicalis mediana (with obliterated urachus)
Plica umbilicalis medialis (with obliterated a. umbilicalis)

C Mesenterium. *Reflected:* Omentum majus and colon transversum. *Removed:* Intraperitoneal intestinum tenue.

Bursa Omentalis

Fig. 12.5 Bursa omentalis (lesser sac)

Anterior view. Bursa omentalis is the portion of the peritoneal cavity located behind omentum minus and gaster.

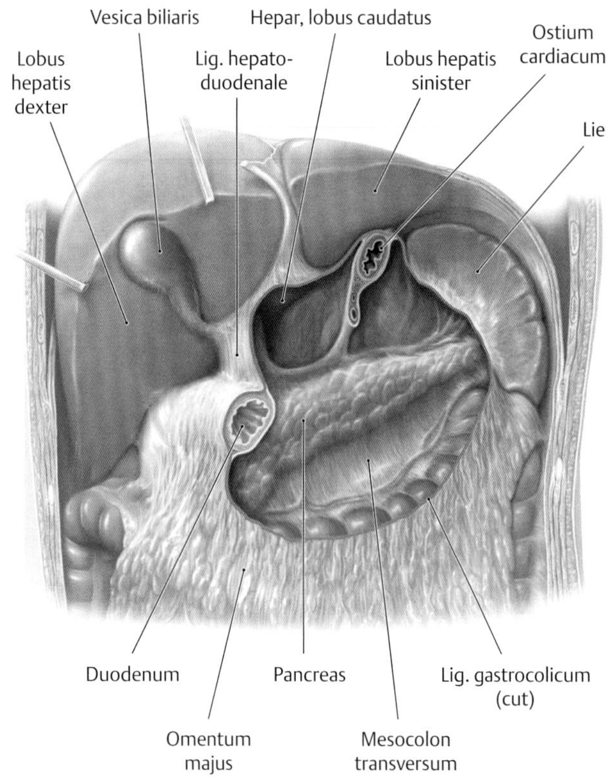

Vesica biliaris
Hepar, lobus caudatus
Ostium cardiacum
Lobus hepatis dexter
Lig. hepato-duodenale
Lobus hepatis sinister
Lien
Duodenum
Pancreas
Lig. gastrocolicum (cut)
Omentum majus
Mesocolon transversum

A Boundaries of bursa omentalis (omental bursa).

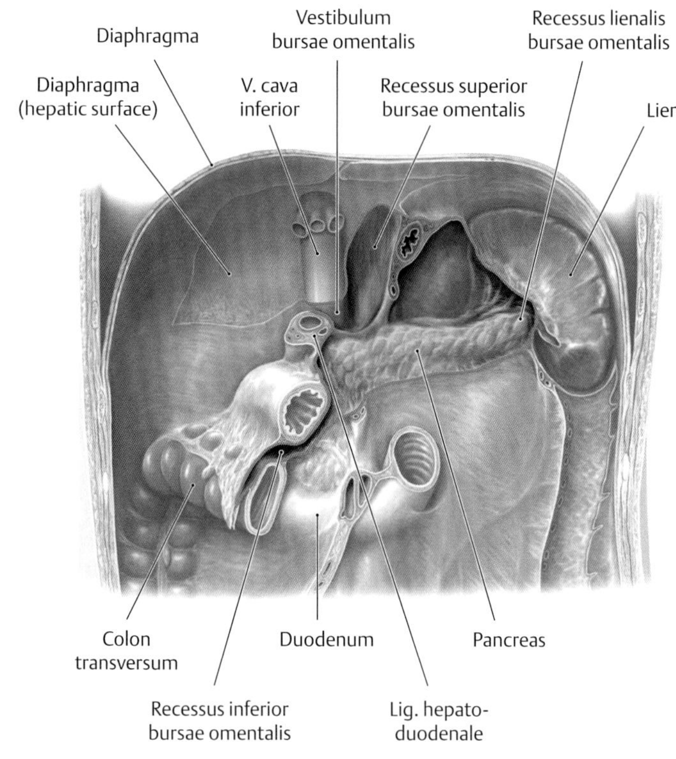

Diaphragma
Vestibulum bursae omentalis
Recessus lienalis bursae omentalis
Diaphragma (hepatic surface)
V. cava inferior
Recessus superior bursae omentalis
Lien
Colon transversum
Duodenum
Pancreas
Recessus inferior bursae omentalis
Lig. hepato-duodenale

B Posterior wall of bursa omentalis.

Fig. 12.6 Location of bursa omentalis

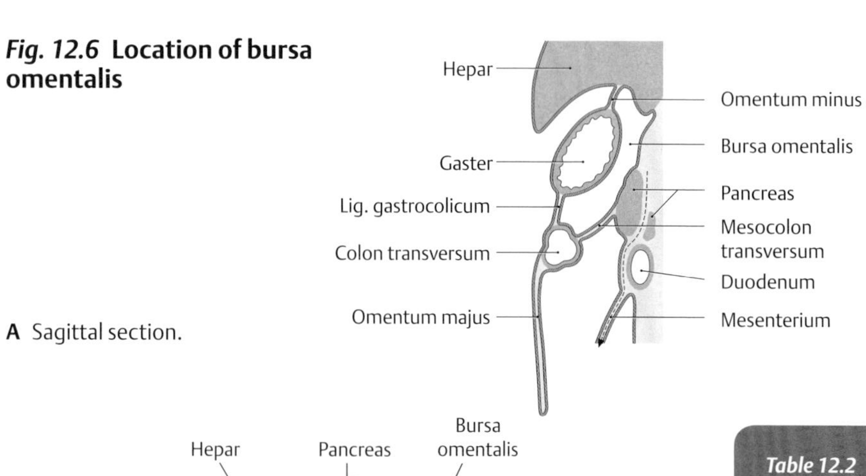

Hepar
Omentum minus
Bursa omentalis
Gaster
Pancreas
Lig. gastrocolicum
Mesocolon transversum
Colon transversum
Duodenum
Omentum majus
Mesenterium

A Sagittal section.

Hepar
Pancreas
Bursa omentalis
Gaster
Recessus lienalis bursae omentalis
Lien
V. cava inferior
Pars abdomi-nalis aortae
Ren sinister

B Transverse section, inferior view.

Table 12.2 Boundaries of the bursa omentalis (lesser sac)

Direction	Boundary	Recess
Anterior	Omentum minus, lig. gastrocolicum	–
Inferior	Mesocolon transversum	Recessus inferior
Superior	Hepar (with lobus caudatus)	Recessus superior
Posterior	Pancreas, aorta (pars abdominalis), truncus coeliacus, a./v. lienalis, lig. gastrosplenicum, glandula suprarenalis sinister, ren sinister (extremitas superior)	–
Right	Hepar, bulbus duodeni	–
Left	Lien, lig. gastrosplenicum	Recessus lienalis

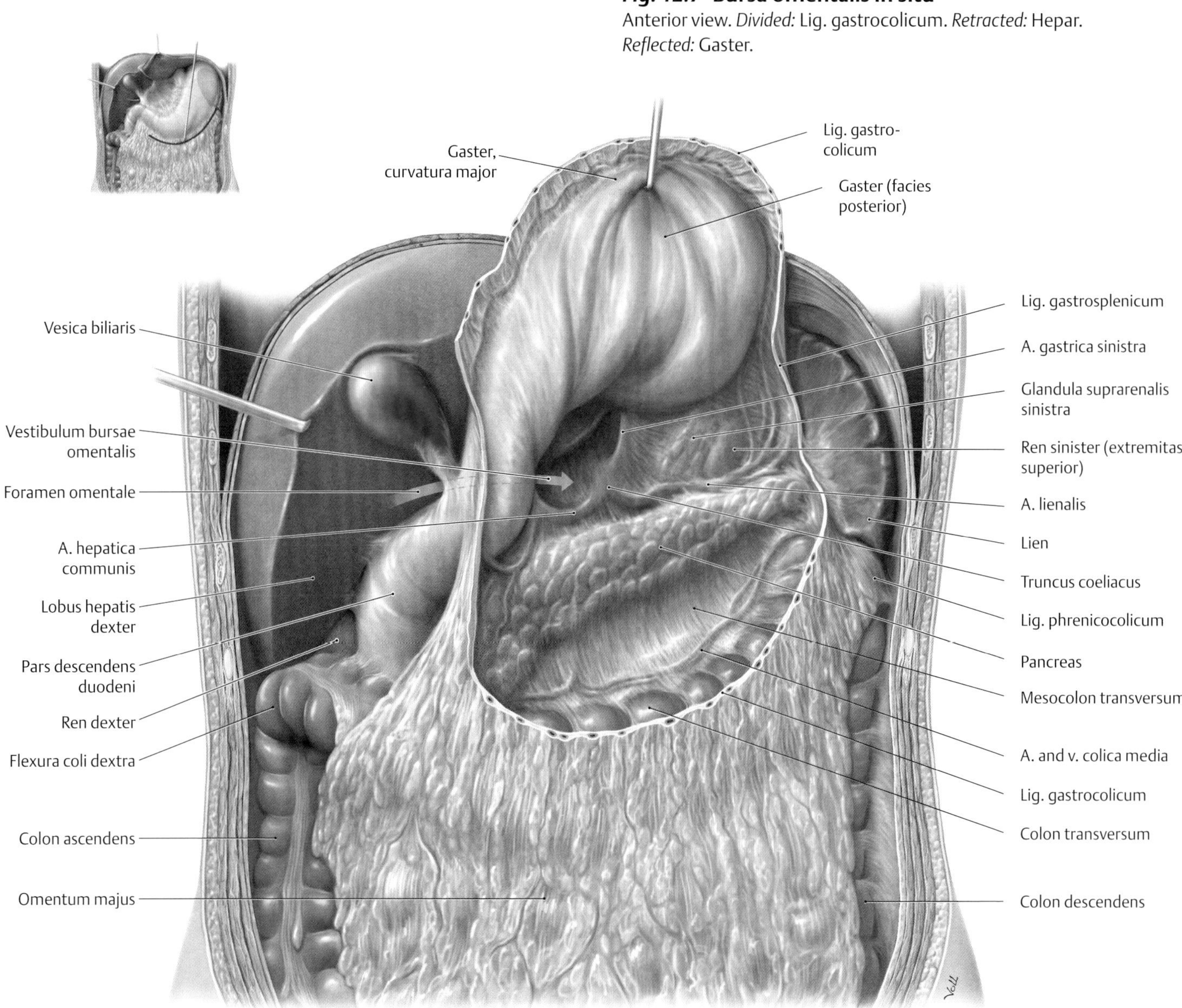

Gaster, curvatura major
Lig. gastro-colicum
Gaster (facies posterior)
Vesica biliaris
Vestibulum bursae omentalis
Foramen omentale
A. hepatica communis
Lobus hepatis dexter
Pars descendens duodeni
Ren dexter
Flexura coli dextra
Colon ascendens
Omentum majus
Lig. gastrosplenicum
A. gastrica sinistra
Glandula suprarenalis sinistra
Ren sinister (extremitas superior)
A. lienalis
Lien
Truncus coeliacus
Lig. phrenicocolicum
Pancreas
Mesocolon transversum
A. and v. colica media
Lig. gastrocolicum
Colon transversum
Colon descendens

Fig. 12.7 **Bursa omentalis in situ**
Anterior view. *Divided:* Lig. gastrocolicum. *Retracted:* Hepar. *Reflected:* Gaster.

Table 12.3 **Boundaries of the foramen omentale**

The communication between the cavitas peritonealis and bursa omentalis is the foramen omentale (epiploicum) (see arrow in Fig. 12.7).

Direction	Boundary
Anterior	Lig. hepatoduodenale with the v. portae, a. hepatica propria, and ductus choledochus
Inferior	Duodenum (pars superior)
Posterior	Vena cava inferior, diaphragma (crus dexter)
Superior	Hepar (lobus caudatus)

Mesenterium & Posterior Wall

Fig. 12.8 **Mesenterium and organs of the cavitas peritonealis**
Anterior view. *Removed:* Gaster, jejunum, and ileum. *Reflected:* Hepar.

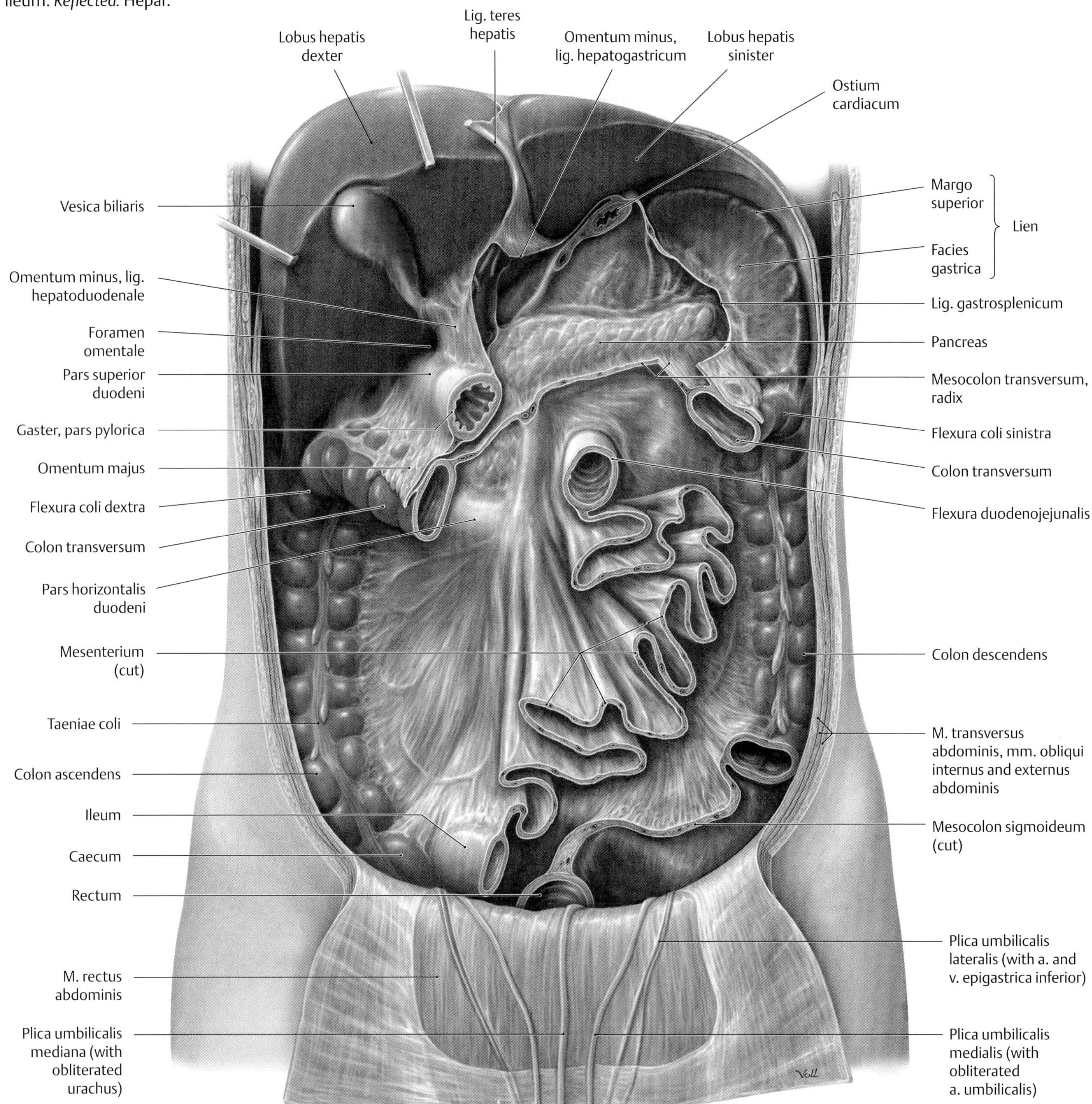
Lobus hepatis dexter
Lig. teres hepatis
Omentum minus, lig. hepatogastricum
Lobus hepatis sinister
Ostium cardiacum
Vesica biliaris
Omentum minus, lig. hepatoduodenale
Foramen omentale
Pars superior duodeni
Gaster, pars pylorica
Omentum majus
Flexura coli dextra
Colon transversum
Pars horizontalis duodeni
Mesenterium (cut)
Taeniae coli
Colon ascendens
Ileum
Caecum
Rectum
M. rectus abdominis
Plica umbilicalis mediana (with obliterated urachus)
Margo superior
Facies gastrica
Lien
Lig. gastrosplenicum
Pancreas
Mesocolon transversum, radix
Flexura coli sinistra
Colon transversum
Flexura duodenojejunalis
Colon descendens
M. transversus abdominis, mm. obliqui internus and externus abdominis
Mesocolon sigmoideum (cut)
Plica umbilicalis lateralis (with a. and v. epigastrica inferior)
Plica umbilicalis medialis (with obliterated a. umbilicalis)
Voll

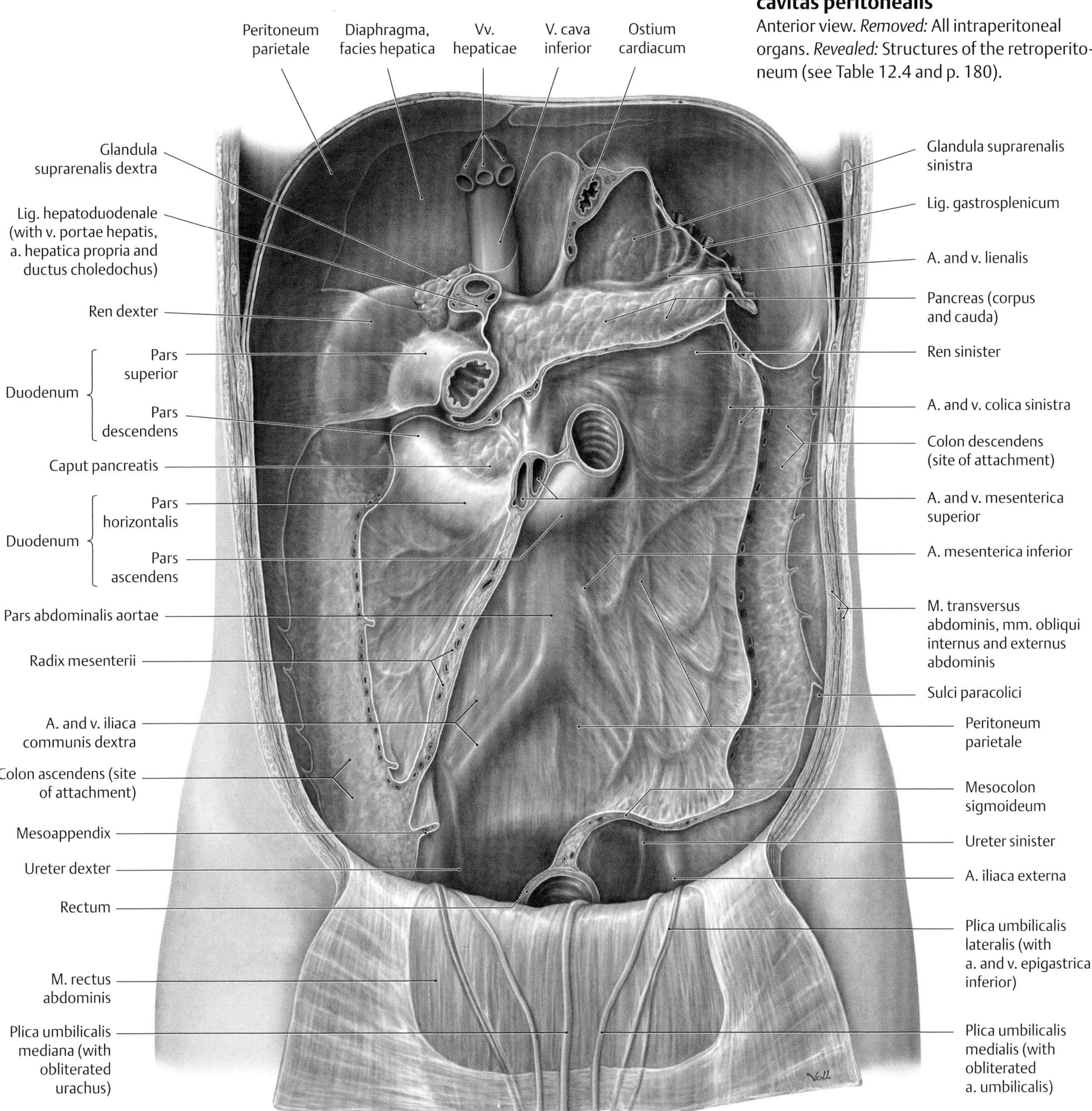

Peritoneum parietale
Diaphragma, facies hepatica
Vv. hepaticae
V. cava inferior
Ostium cardiacum
Glandula suprarenalis dextra
Lig. hepatoduodenale (with v. portae hepatis, a. hepatica propria and ductus choledochus)
Ren dexter
Duodenum
Pars superior
Pars descendens
Caput pancreatis
Duodenum
Pars horizontalis
Pars ascendens
Pars abdominalis aortae
Radix mesenterii
A. and v. iliaca communis dextra
Colon ascendens (site of attachment)
Mesoappendix
Ureter dexter
Rectum
M. rectus abdominis
Plica umbilicalis mediana (with obliterated urachus)
Glandula suprarenalis sinistra
Lig. gastrosplenicum
A. and v. lienalis
Pancreas (corpus and cauda)
Ren sinister
A. and v. colica sinistra
Colon descendens (site of attachment)
A. and v. mesenterica superior
A. mesenterica inferior
M. transversus abdominis, mm. obliqui internus and externus abdominis
Sulci paracolici
Peritoneum parietale
Mesocolon sigmoideum
Ureter sinister
A. iliaca externa
Plica umbilicalis lateralis (with a. and v. epigastrica inferior)
Plica umbilicalis medialis (with obliterated a. umbilicalis)

Fig. 12.9 **Posterior wall of the cavitas peritonealis**
Anterior view. *Removed:* All intraperitoneal organs. *Revealed:* Structures of the retroperitoneum (see Table 12.4 and p. 180).

Table 12.4 Structures of the retroperitoneum

See pp. 216, 228, 239 for neurovascular structures of the retroperitoneum.

Classification	Organs	Vessels	Nerves
Primarily retroperitoneal (Retroperitoneal when formed)	• Ren • Glandula suprarenalis • Ureter	• Aorta (pars abdominalis) • Vena cava inferior and tributaries • Vv. lumbalis ascendens • V. portae and tributaries • Nodi lymphatici lumbales, sacrales and iliaci • Trunci lumbales and cisterna chyli	• Plexus lumbalis branches ∘ N. iliohypogastricus ∘ N. ilioinguinalis ∘ N. genitofemoralis ∘ N. cutaneus femoris lateralis ∘ N. femoralis ∘ N. obturatorius • Truncus sympathicus • Autonomic ganglia and plexi
Secondarily retroperitoneal (Mesenterium lost during development)	• Pancreas • Duodenum (pars descendens and horizontalis; some of pars ascendens) • Colon ascendens and descendens • Caecum (portions; variable) • Rectum (upper 2/3)		

Contents of the Pelvis

Fig. 12.10 Male pelvis

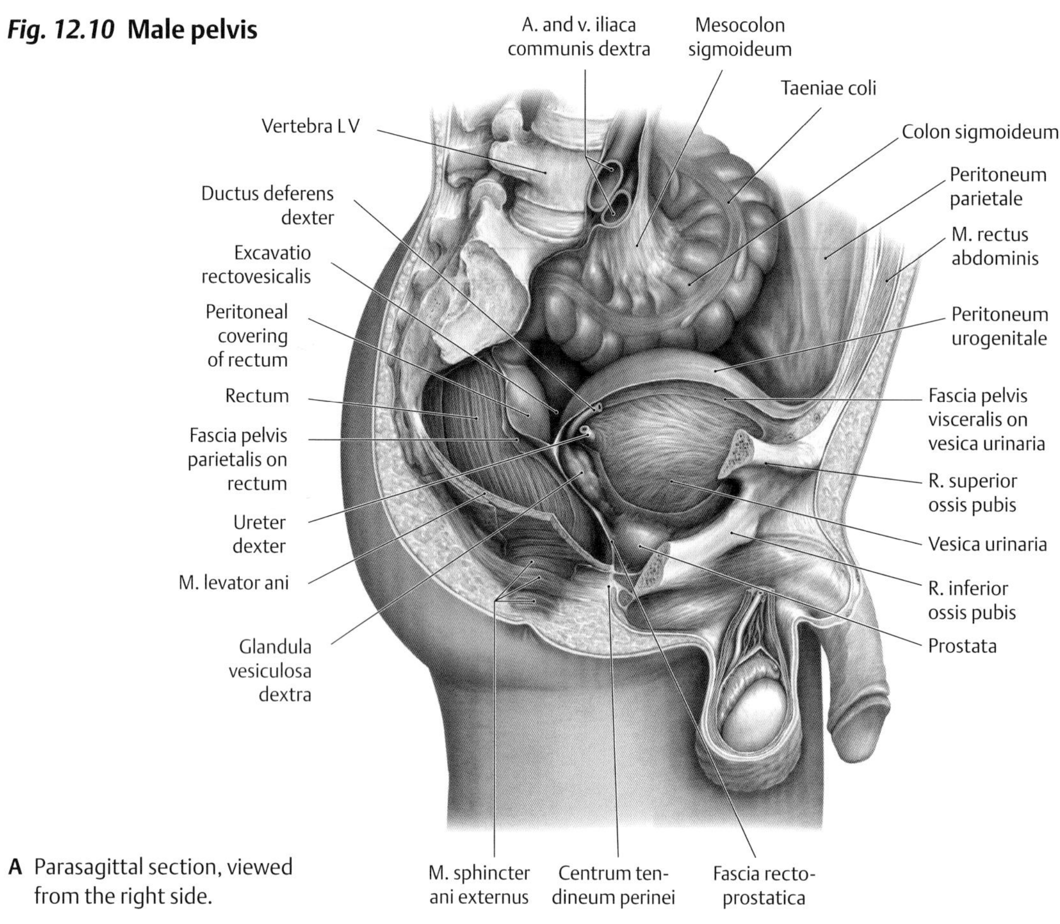
A. and v. iliaca communis dextra
Mesocolon sigmoideum
Taeniae coli
Colon sigmoideum
Peritoneum parietale
M. rectus abdominis
Peritoneum urogenitale
Fascia pelvis visceralis on vesica urinaria
R. superior ossis pubis
Vesica urinaria
R. inferior ossis pubis
Prostata
Vertebra LV
Ductus deferens dexter
Excavatio rectovesicalis
Peritoneal covering of rectum
Rectum
Fascia pelvis parietalis on rectum
Ureter dexter
M. levator ani
Glandula vesiculosa dextra
M. sphincter ani externus
Centrum tendineum perinei
Fascia rectoprostatica

A Parasagittal section, viewed from the right side.

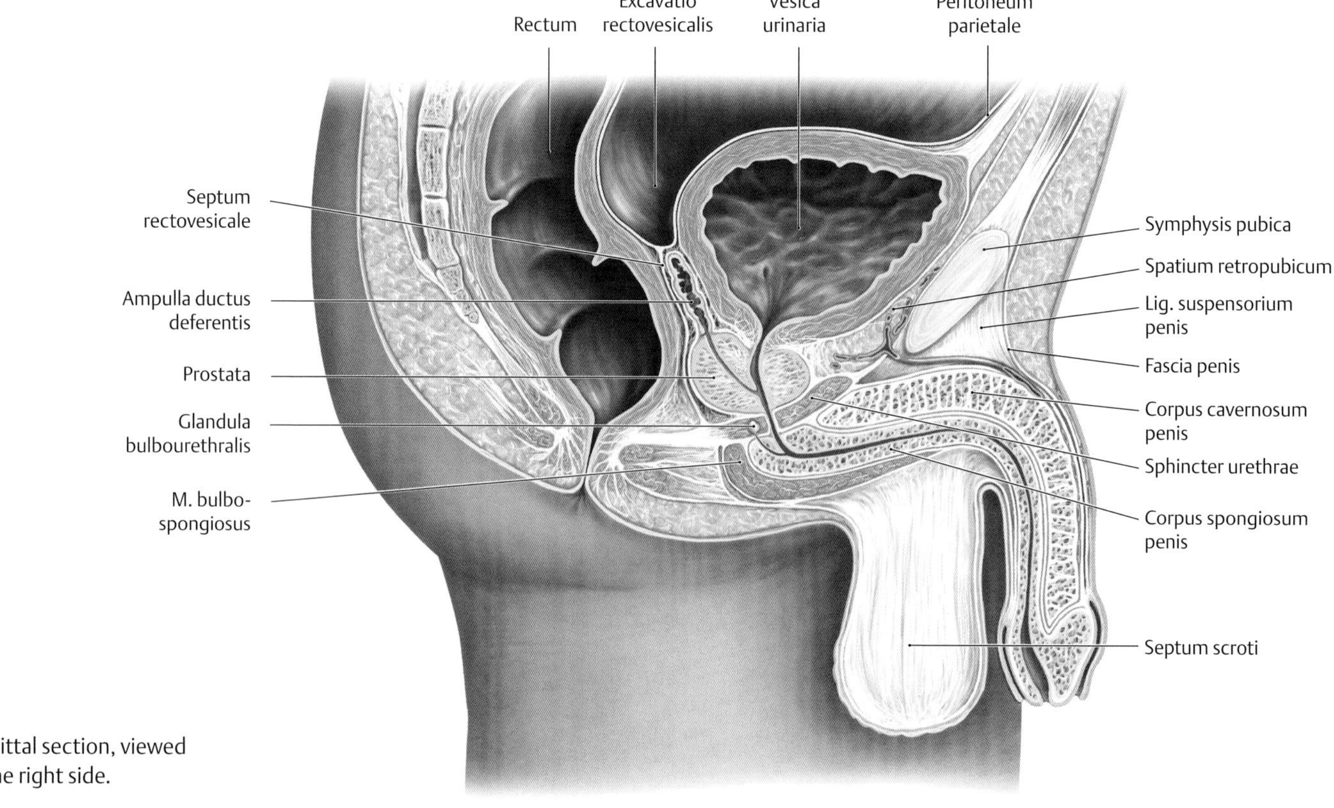
Rectum
Excavatio rectovesicalis
Vesica urinaria
Peritoneum parietale
Septum rectovesicale
Ampulla ductus deferentis
Prostata
Glandula bulbourethralis
M. bulbospongiosus
Symphysis pubica
Spatium retropubicum
Lig. suspensorium penis
Fascia penis
Corpus cavernosum penis
Sphincter urethrae
Corpus spongiosum penis
Septum scroti

B Midsagittal section, viewed from the right side.

Fig. 12.11 Female pelvis

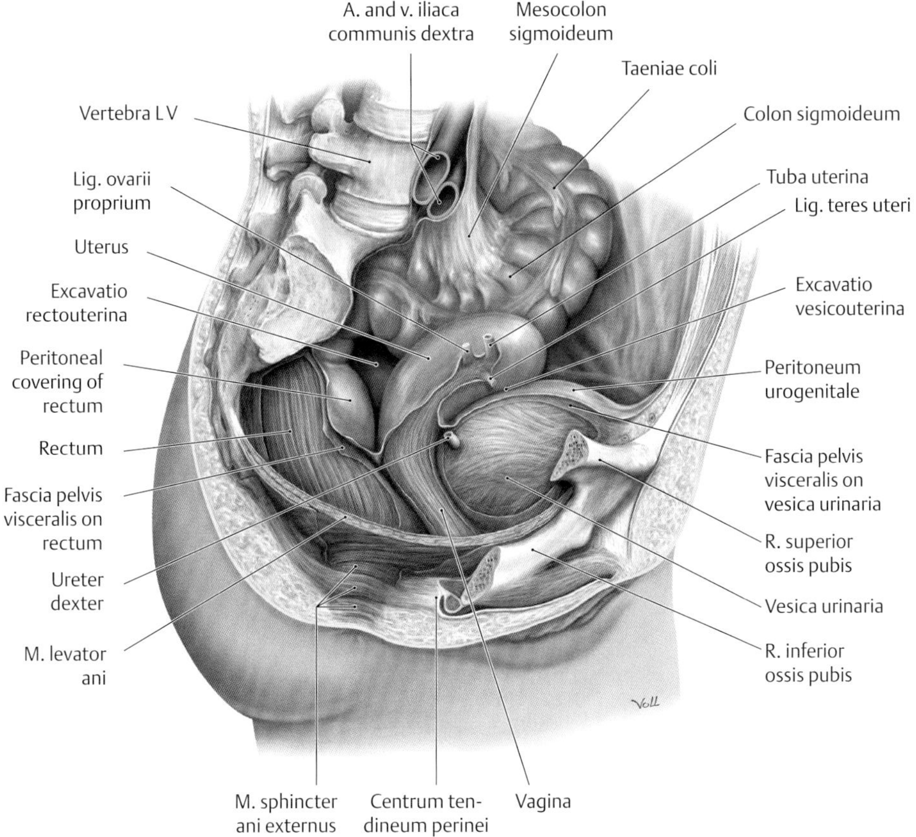
A. and v. iliaca communis dextra
Mesocolon sigmoideum
Taeniae coli
Vertebra LV
Colon sigmoideum
Tuba uterina
Lig. ovarii proprium
Lig. teres uteri
Uterus
Excavatio rectouterina
Excavatio vesicouterina
Peritoneal covering of rectum
Peritoneum urogenitale
Rectum
Fascia pelvis visceralis on vesica urinaria
Fascia pelvis visceralis on rectum
R. superior ossis pubis
Ureter dexter
Vesica urinaria
M. levator ani
R. inferior ossis pubis
M. sphincter ani externus
Centrum ten-dineum perinei
Vagina

A Parasagittal section, viewed from the right side.

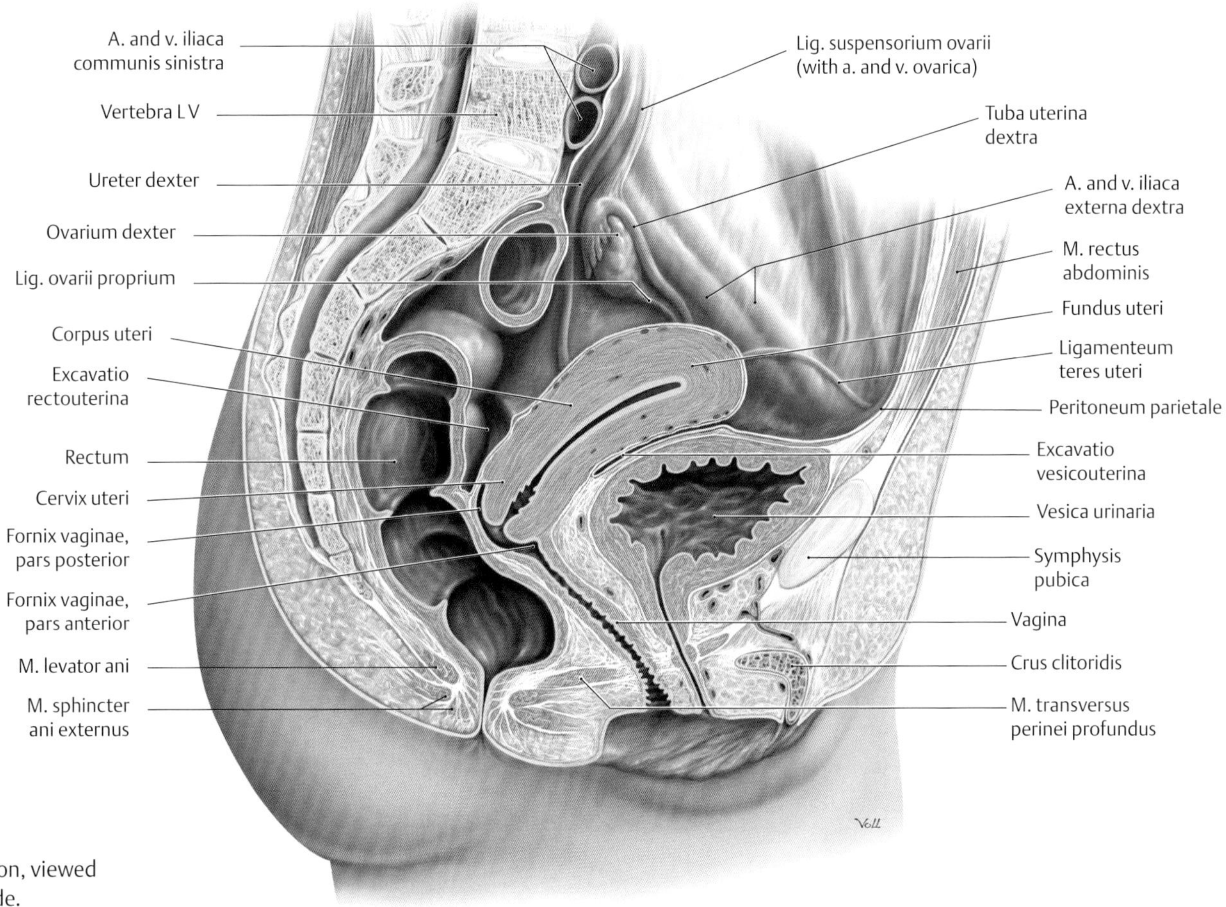
A. and v. iliaca communis sinistra
Lig. suspensorium ovarii (with a. and v. ovarica)
Vertebra LV
Tuba uterina dextra
Ureter dexter
A. and v. iliaca externa dextra
Ovarium dexter
M. rectus abdominis
Lig. ovarii proprium
Fundus uteri
Corpus uteri
Ligamenteum teres uteri
Excavatio rectouterina
Peritoneum parietale
Rectum
Excavatio vesicouterina
Cervix uteri
Vesica urinaria
Fornix vaginae, pars posterior
Symphysis pubica
Fornix vaginae, pars anterior
Vagina
M. levator ani
Crus clitoridis
M. sphincter ani externus
M. transversus perinei profundus

B Midsagittal section, viewed from the right side.

Peritoneal Relationships

Fig. 12.12 **Peritoneal relationships in the pelvis: Female**

Lig. latum uteri
Rectum
Excavatio rectouterina
Plica rectouterina
Lig. suspensorium ovarii
Tuba uterina
Ovarium sinister
Colon sigmoideum
Lig. ovarii proprium
Fossa paravesicalis
Anulus inguinalis profundus
Plica umbilicalis lateralis (with a. and v. epigastrica inferior)
M. rectus abdominis
Plica umbilicalis medialis (with obliterated a. umbilicalis)
Fossa supravesicalis
Plica umbilicalis mediana (with obliterated urachus)
Vesica urinaria
Plica vesicalis transversa
Excavatio vesicouterina
Lig. teres uteri
Peritoneum parietale
Fundus uteri
Caecum

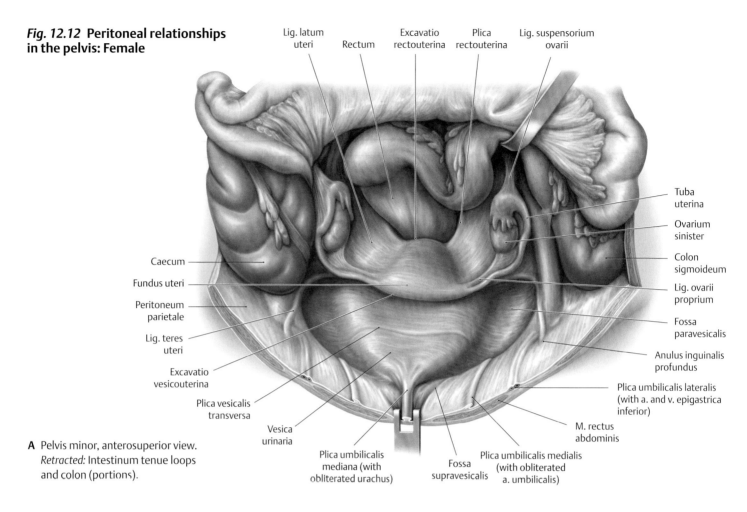

A Pelvis minor, anterosuperior view. *Retracted:* Intestinum tenue loops and colon (portions).

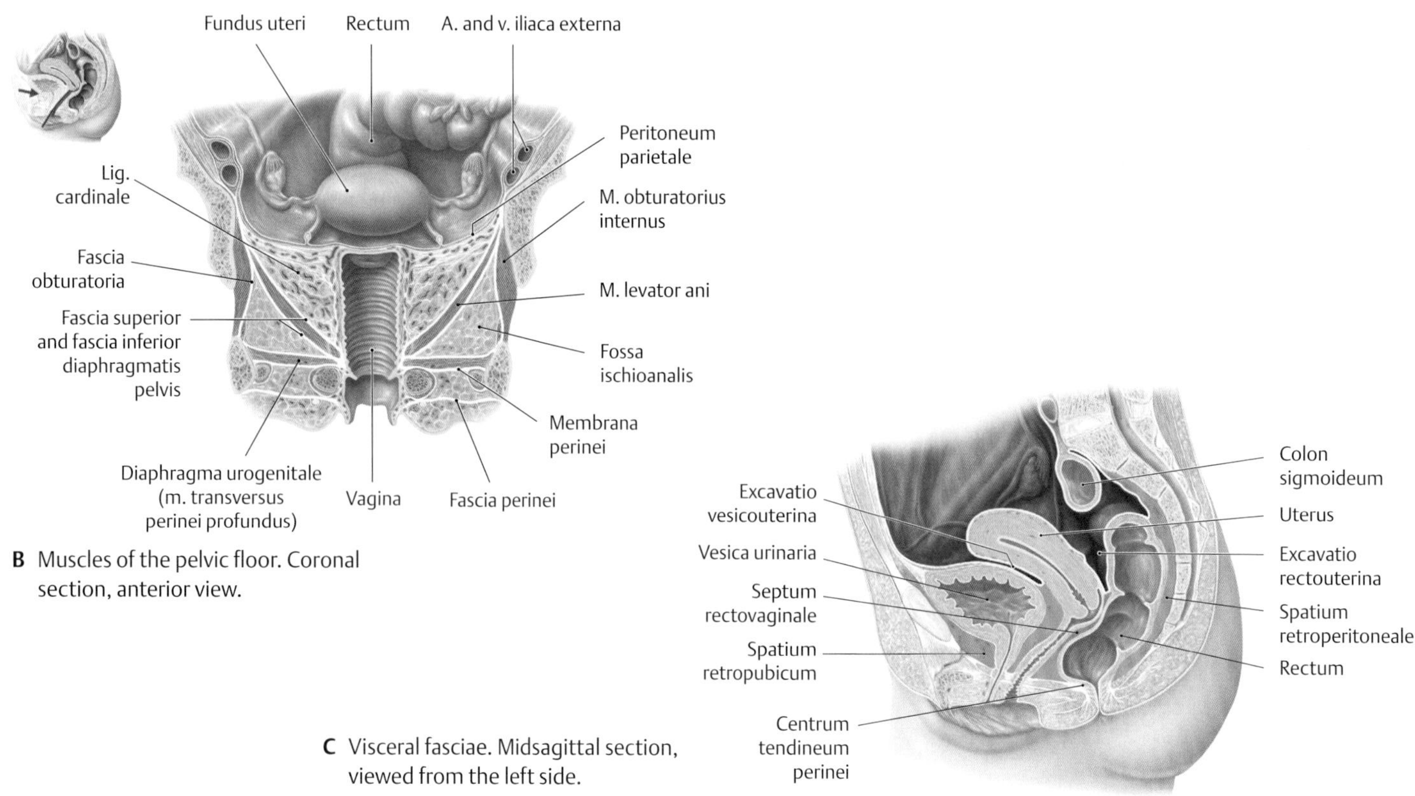
Fundus uteri
Rectum
A. and v. iliaca externa
Peritoneum parietale
M. obturatorius internus
M. levator ani
Fossa ischioanalis
Membrana perinei
Fascia perinei
Vagina
Diaphragma urogenitale (m. transversus perinei profundus)
Fascia superior and fascia inferior diaphragmatis pelvis
Fascia obturatoria
Lig. cardinale
Colon sigmoideum
Uterus
Excavatio rectouterina
Spatium retroperitoneale
Rectum
Excavatio vesicouterina
Vesica urinaria
Septum rectovaginale
Spatium retropubicum
Centrum tendineum perinei

B Muscles of the pelvic floor. Coronal section, anterior view.

C Visceral fasciae. Midsagittal section, viewed from the left side.

Fig. 12.13 Peritoneal relationships in the pelvis: Male

Ileum
Rectum
Excavatio rectovesicalis
Plica vesicalis transversa
Caecum
Peritoneum parietale
Ductus deferens
Appendix vermiformis
Fossa inguinalis lateralis
Vesica urinaria
Plica umbilicalis mediana (with underlying obliterated urachus)
M. rectus abdominis
Plica umbilicalis medialis (with underlying obliterated a. umbilicalis)
Plica umbilicalis lateralis (with a. and v. epigastrica inferior)
Colon sigmoideum

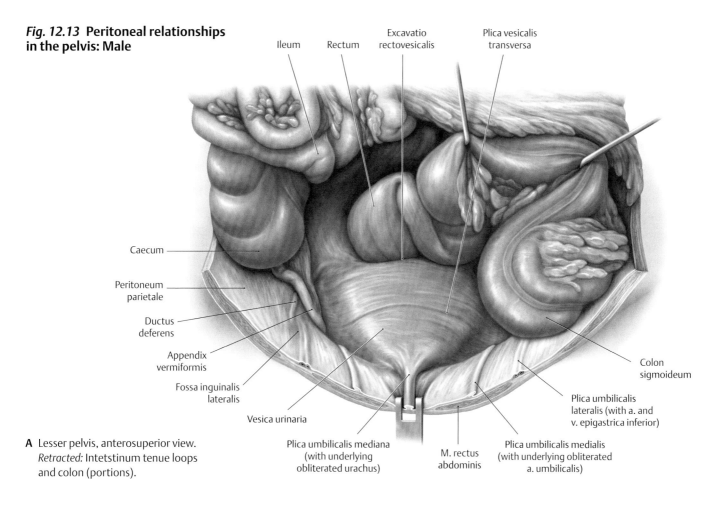

A Lesser pelvis, anterosuperior view. *Retracted:* Intetstinum tenue loops and colon (portions).

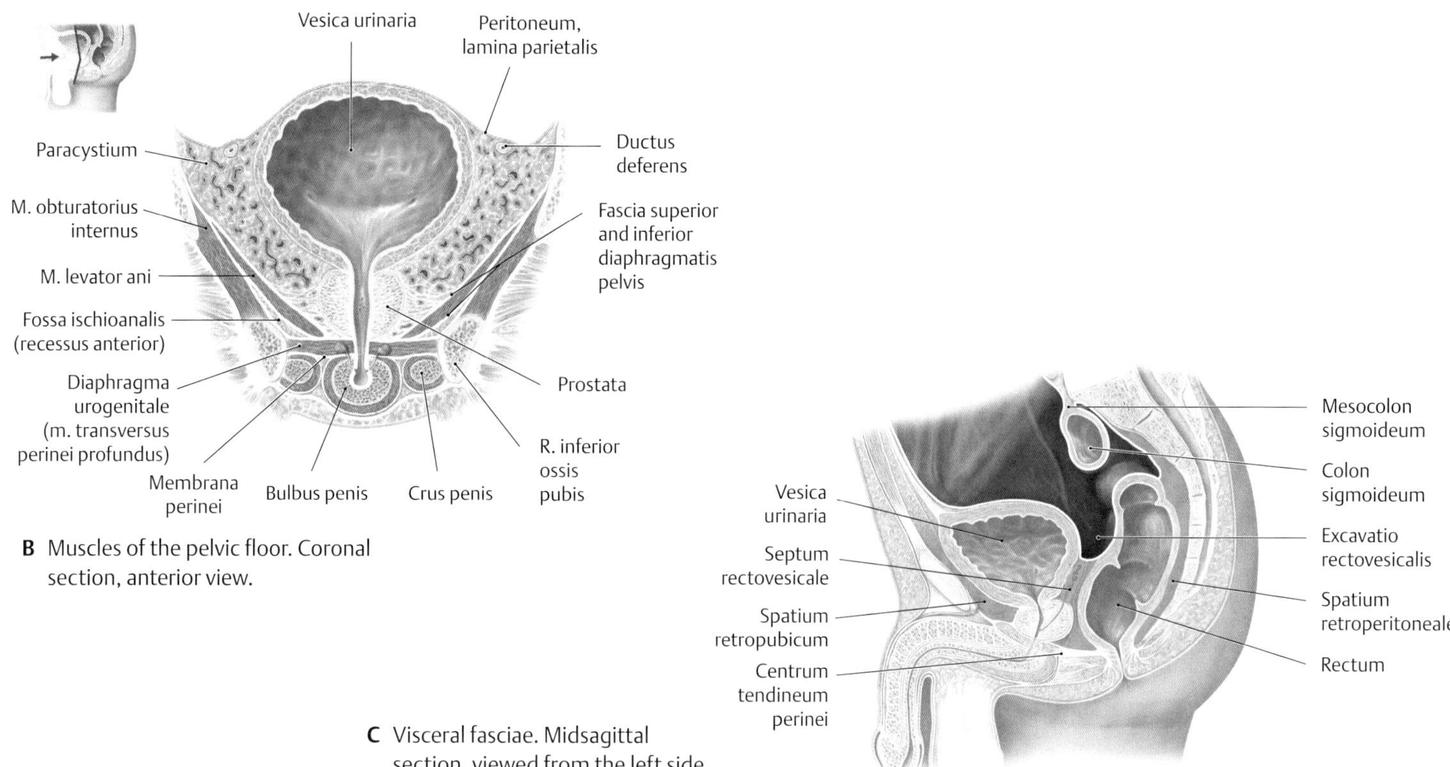
Vesica urinaria
Peritoneum, lamina parietalis
Paracystium
Ductus deferens
M. obturatorius internus
Fascia superior and inferior diaphragmatis pelvis
M. levator ani
Fossa ischioanalis (recessus anterior)
Prostata
Diaphragma urogenitale (m. transversus perinei profundus)
R. inferior ossis pubis
Membrana perinei
Bulbus penis
Crus penis
Mesocolon sigmoideum
Colon sigmoideum
Vesica urinaria
Excavatio rectovesicalis
Septum rectovesicale
Spatium retroperitoneale
Spatium retropubicum
Rectum
Centrum tendineum perinei

B Muscles of the pelvic floor. Coronal section, anterior view.

C Visceral fasciae. Midsagittal section, viewed from the left side.

Table 12.5 Divisions of the pelvis and perineum

The levels of the pelvis are determined by bony landmarks (crista iliaca and aperatura pelvis superior, see p. 126). The contents of the perineum are separated by the diaphragma pelvis and two fascial layers.

Crista iliaca		
Pelvis	**Pelvis major**	• Ileum (coils)
		• Caecum and appendix
		• Colon sigmoideum
		• A./v. iliaca communis and externa
		• Plexus lumbalis
	Aperatura pelvis superior	
	Pelvis minor	• Ureter distalis
		• Vesica urinaria
		• Rectum
		♀: Vagina, uterus, tuba uterina, and ovarium
		♂: Ductus deferens, glandula vesiculosa, and prostata
		• A./v. iliaca interna. and branches
		• Plexus sacralis
		• Plexus hypogastricus inferior
Diaphragma pelvis (m. levator ani with fascia diaphragmatica pelvis superior and inferior)		
Perineum	**Spatium perinei profundum**	• M. sphincter urethrae and m. transversus perinei profundus
		• Urethra (pars membranacea)
		• Vagina
		• Rectum
		• Glandula bulbourethralis
		• Fossa ischioanalis
		• A./v. pudenda interna, n. pudendus and branches
	Membrana perinei	
	Spatium perinei superficiale	• M. ischiocavernosus, m. bulbocavernosus, and m. transversus perinei superficialis
		• Urethra (pars spongiosa)
		• Clitoris and penis
		• A./v. pudenda interna, n. pudendus and branches
	Fascia perinealis (Colles') superficialis	
	Spatium (perineale) subcutaneum	• Fat
Cutis		

Fig. 12.14 **Pelvis and urogenital triangle**
Coronal section, anterior view.

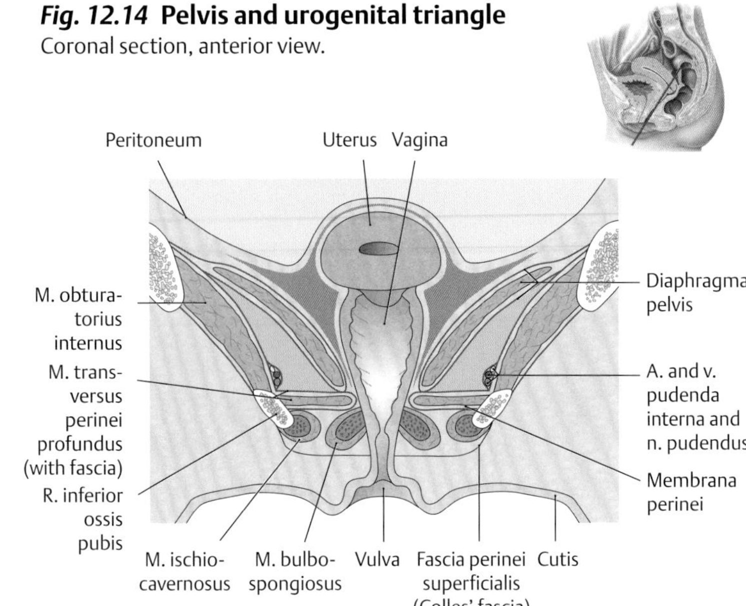

Peritoneum
Uterus
Vagina
M. obturatorius internus
M. transversus perinei profundus (with fascia)
R. inferior ossis pubis
M. ischiocavernosus
M. bulbospongiosus
Vulva
Fascia perinei superficialis (Colles' fascia)
Cutis
Diaphragma pelvis
A. and v. pudenda interna and n. pudendus
Membrana perinei

A Female.

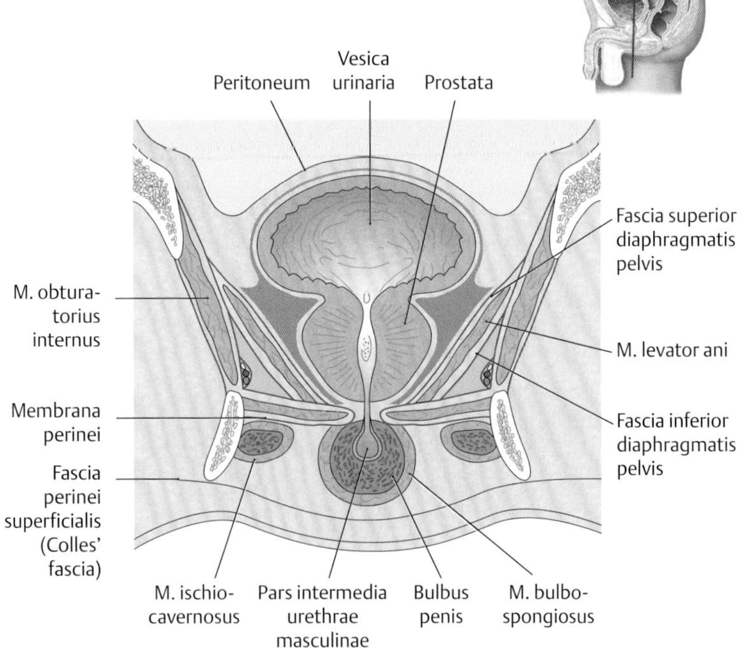

Peritoneum
Vesica urinaria
Prostata
M. obturatorius internus
Membrana perinei
Fascia perinei superficialis (Colles' fascia)
M. ischiocavernosus
Pars intermedia urethrae masculinae
Bulbus penis
M. bulbospongiosus
Fascia superior diaphragmatis pelvis
M. levator ani
Fascia inferior diaphragmatis pelvis

B Male.

- Cavitas peritonealis
- Subperitoneal space
- Fossa ischioanalis
- Fascia pelvis visceralis
- Fascia pelvis parietalis

Fig. 12.15 Pelvis: Coronal section
Anterior view.

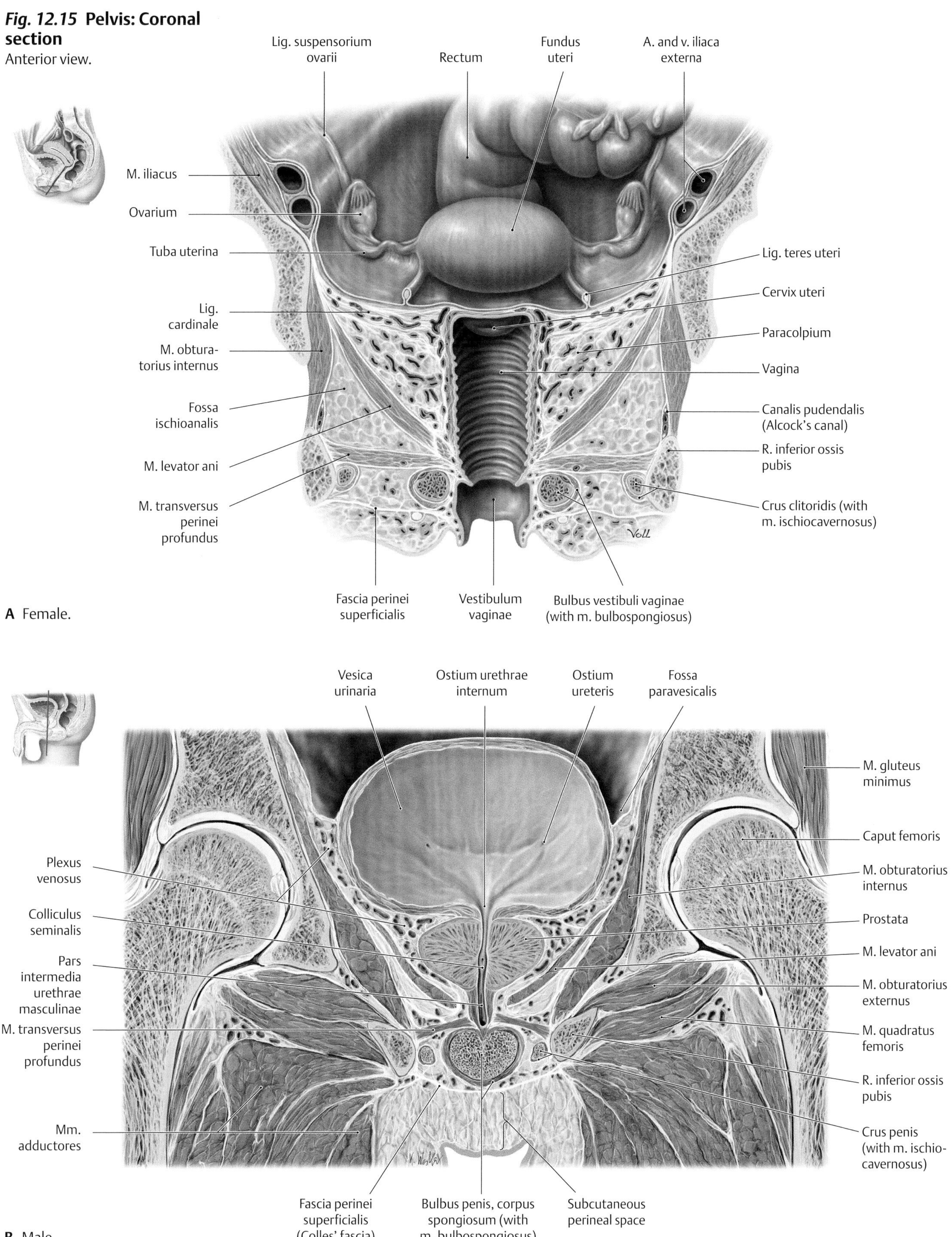
Lig. suspensorium ovarii
Rectum
Fundus uteri
A. and v. iliaca externa
M. iliacus
Ovarium
Tuba uterina
Lig. teres uteri
Cervix uteri
Lig. cardinale
Paracolpium
M. obturatorius internus
Vagina
Fossa ischioanalis
Canalis pudendalis (Alcock's canal)
R. inferior ossis pubis
M. levator ani
M. transversus perinei profundus
Crus clitoridis (with m. ischiocavernosus)
Fascia perinei superficialis
Vestibulum vaginae
Bulbus vestibuli vaginae (with m. bulbospongiosus)
Vesica urinaria
Ostium urethrae internum
Ostium ureteris
Fossa paravesicalis
M. gluteus minimus
Caput femoris
Plexus venosus
M. obturatorius internus
Colliculus seminalis
Prostata
Pars intermedia urethrae masculinae
M. levator ani
M. obturatorius externus
M. transversus perinei profundus
M. quadratus femoris
R. inferior ossis pubis
Mm. adductores
Crus penis (with m. ischio-cavernosus)
Fascia perinei superficialis (Colles' fascia)
Bulbus penis, corpus spongiosum (with m. bulbospongiosus)
Subcutaneous perineal space

A Female.

B Male.

Fig. 12.16 Abdomen: Transverse section
Inferior view.

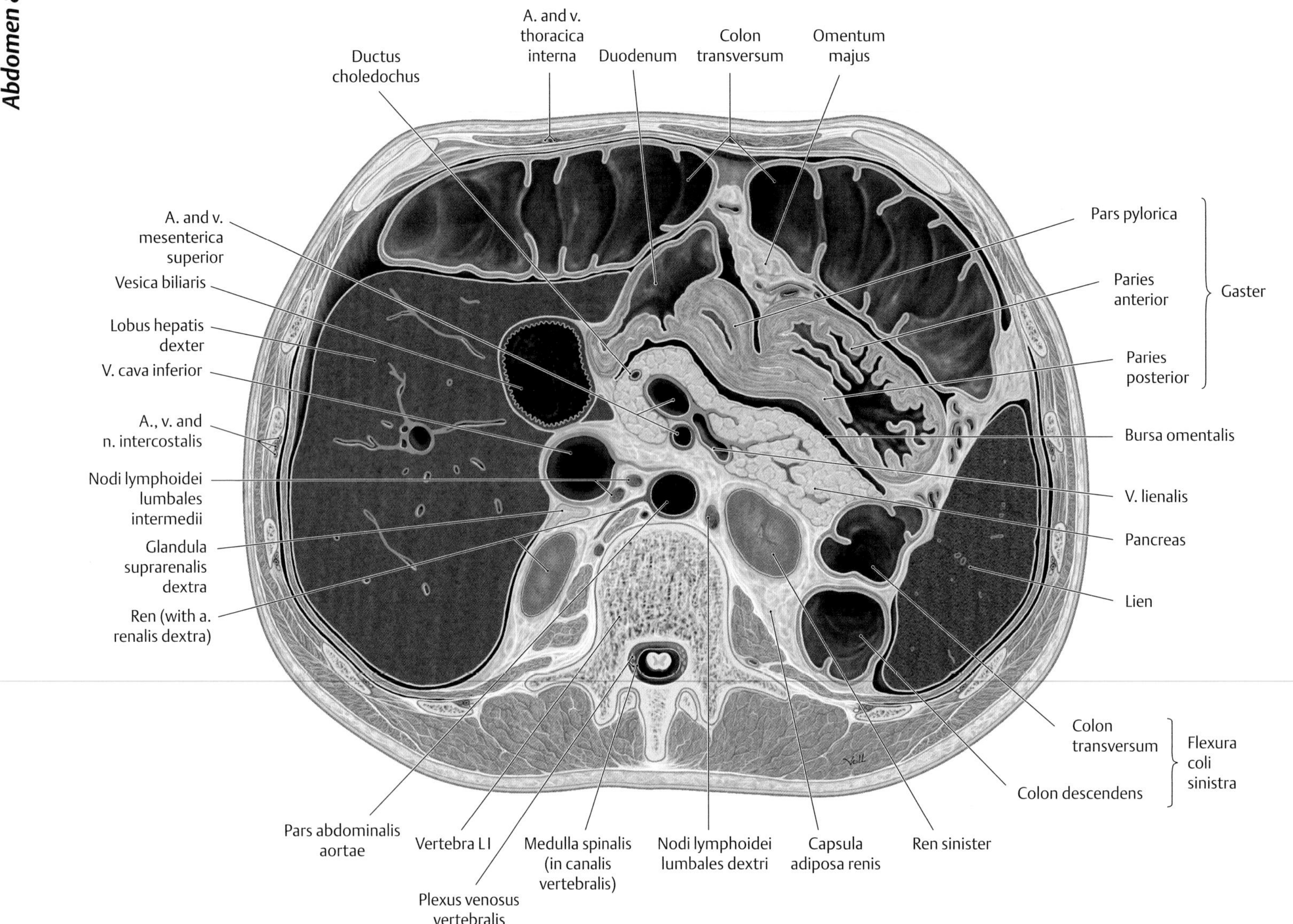
A. and v. thoracica interna
Ductus choledochus
Duodenum
Colon transversum
Omentum majus
A. and v. mesenterica superior
Vesica biliaris
Lobus hepatis dexter
V. cava inferior
A., v. and n. intercostalis
Nodi lymphoidei lumbales intermedii
Glandula suprarenalis dextra
Ren (with a. renalis dextra)
Pars pylorica
Paries anterior
Paries posterior
Gaster
Bursa omentalis
V. lienalis
Pancreas
Lien
Colon transversum
Colon descendens
Flexura coli sinistra
Pars abdominalis aortae
Vertebra L I
Plexus venosus vertebralis
Medulla spinalis (in canalis vertebralis)
Nodi lymphoidei lumbales dextri
Capsula adiposa renis
Ren sinister

Fig. 12.17 **Pelvis: Transverse section**
Inferior view.

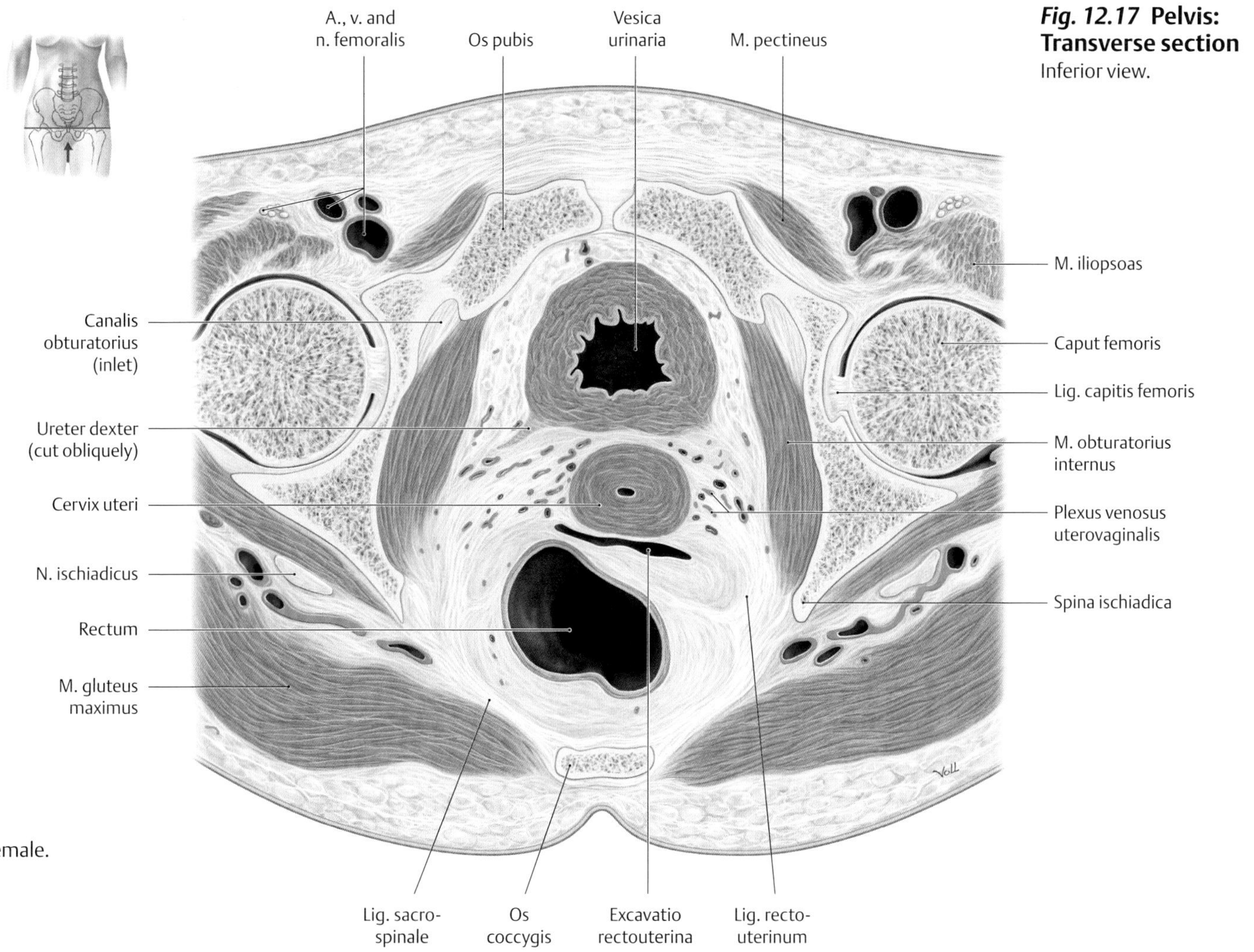

A., v. and n. femoralis
Os pubis
Vesica urinaria
M. pectineus
M. iliopsoas
Canalis obturatorius (inlet)
Caput femoris
Lig. capitis femoris
Ureter dexter (cut obliquely)
M. obturatorius internus
Cervix uteri
Plexus venosus uterovaginalis
N. ischiadicus
Spina ischiadica
Rectum
M. gluteus maximus
Lig. sacrospinale
Os coccygis
Excavatio rectouterina
Lig. rectouterinum

A Female.

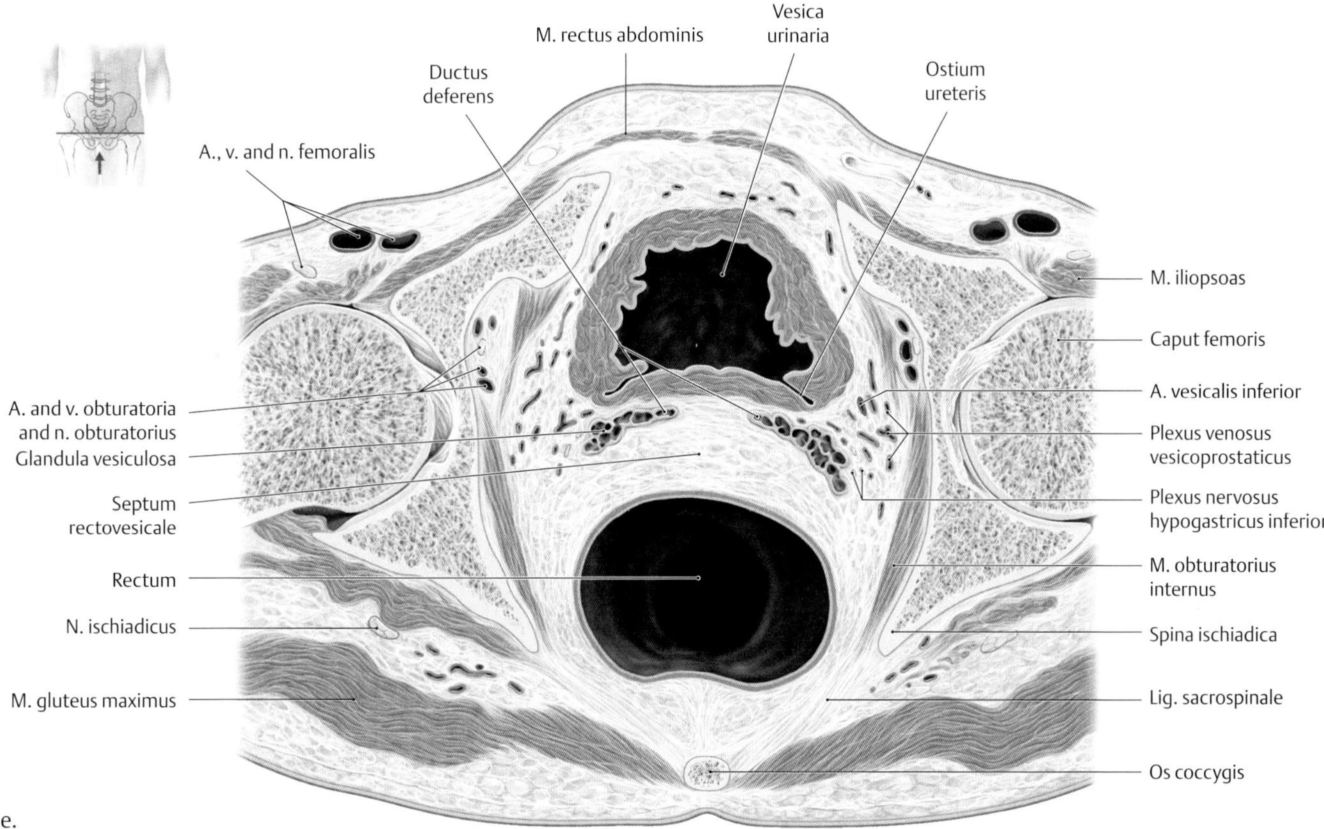
M. rectus abdominis
Vesica urinaria
Ductus deferens
Ostium ureteris
A., v. and n. femoralis
M. iliopsoas
Caput femoris
A. vesicalis inferior
A. and v. obturatoria and n. obturatorius
Glandula vesiculosa
Plexus venosus vesicoprostaticus
Septum rectovesicale
Plexus nervosus hypogastricus inferior
M. obturatorius internus
Rectum
N. ischiadicus
Spina ischiadica
M. gluteus maximus
Lig. sacrospinale
Os coccygis

B Male.

Gaster

Fig. 13.1 Gaster: Location

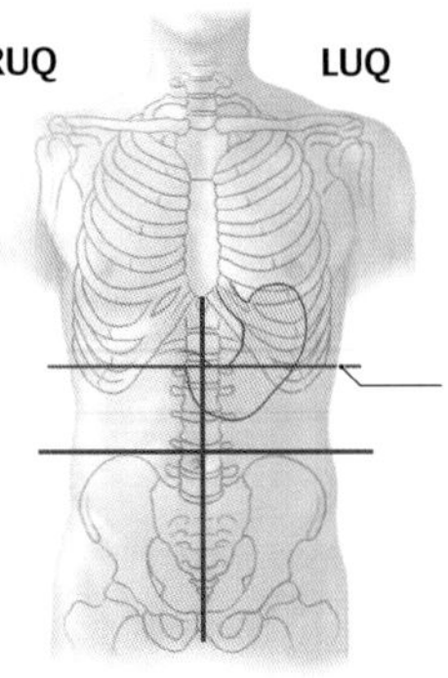

RUQ
LUQ
Planum trans-pyloricum

A Anterior view.

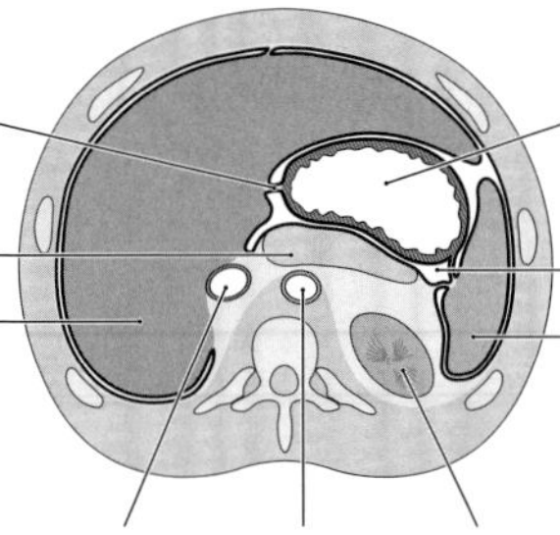

Omentum minus (lig. hepatogastricum)
Pancreas
Hepar
Gaster
Bursa omentalis
Lien
V. cava inferior
Pars abdominalis aortae
Ren sinister

B Transverse section, inferior view.

Fig. 13.2 Surfaces of gaster

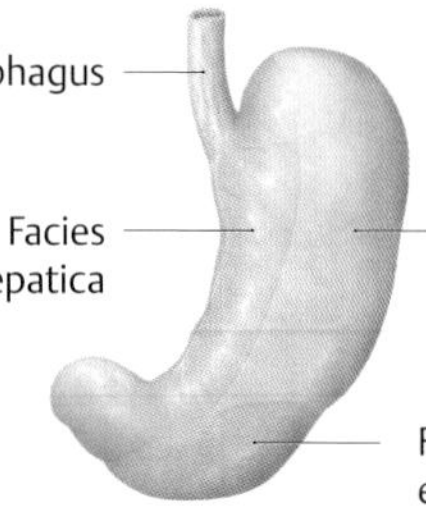

Esophagus
Facies hepatica
Facies phrenica
Facies epigastrica

A Anterior view.

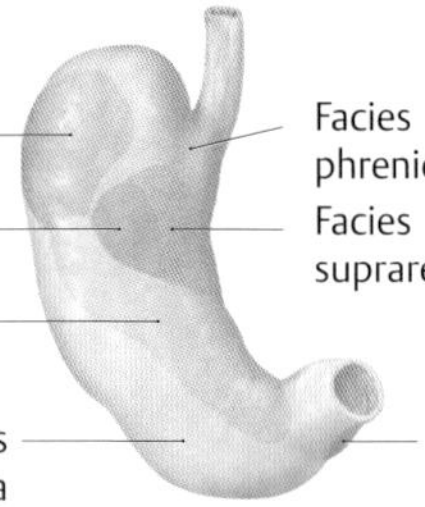

Facies splenica
Facies renalis
Facies pancreatica
Facies colomesocolica
Facies phrenica
Facies suprarenalis
Facies hepatica

B Posterior view.

Fig. 13.3 Gaster

Anterior view.

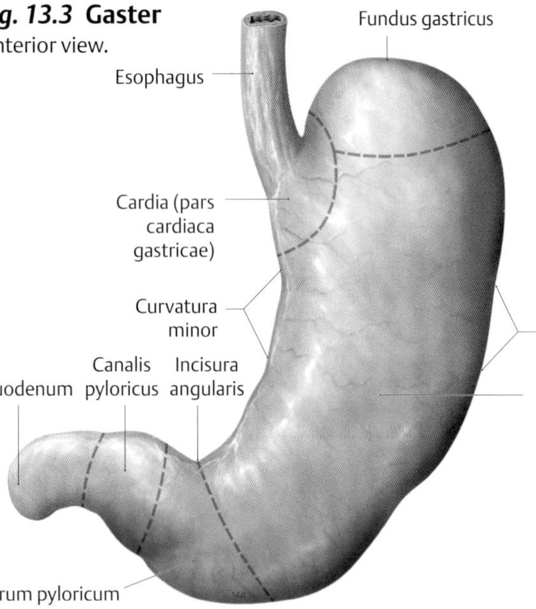

Fundus gastricus
Esophagus
Cardia (pars cardiaca gastricae)
Curvatura minor
Canalis pyloricus
Incisura angularis
Duodenum
Curvatura major
Corpus gastricum
Antrum pyloricum

A Anterior wall.

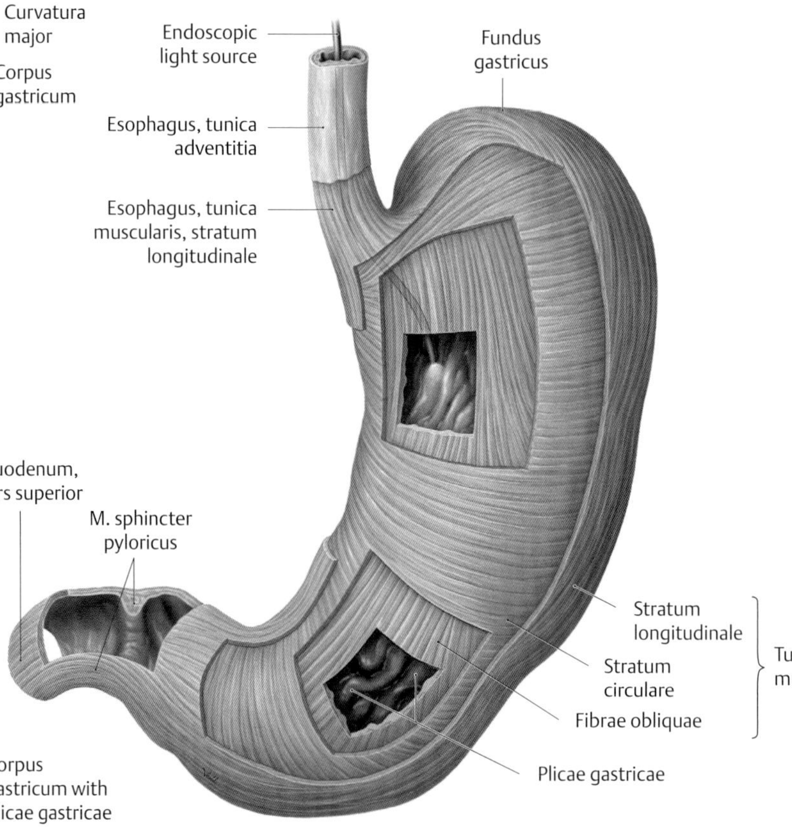

Endoscopic light source
Esophagus, tunica adventitia
Esophagus, tunica muscularis, stratum longitudinale
Fundus gastricus
Duodenum, pars superior
M. sphincter pyloricus
Stratum longitudinale
Stratum circulare
Fibrae obliquae
Tunica muscularis
Plicae gastricae

B Muscular layers. *Removed:* Serosa and subserosa. *Windowed:* Muscular coat.

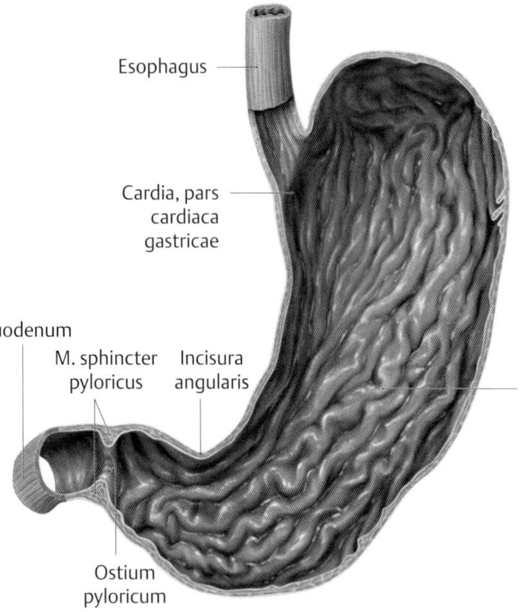

Esophagus
Cardia, pars cardiaca gastricae
Duodenum
M. sphincter pyloricus
Incisura angularis
Corpus gastricum with plicae gastricae
Ostium pyloricum

C Interior. *Removed:* Anterior wall.

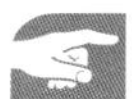

Gaster is found in the right and left upper quadrants. It is intraperitoneal, its mesenterium being omentum minus and omentum majus.

Fig. 13.4 Gaster in situ
Anterior view of the opened upper abdomen. Arrow indicates foramen omentale.

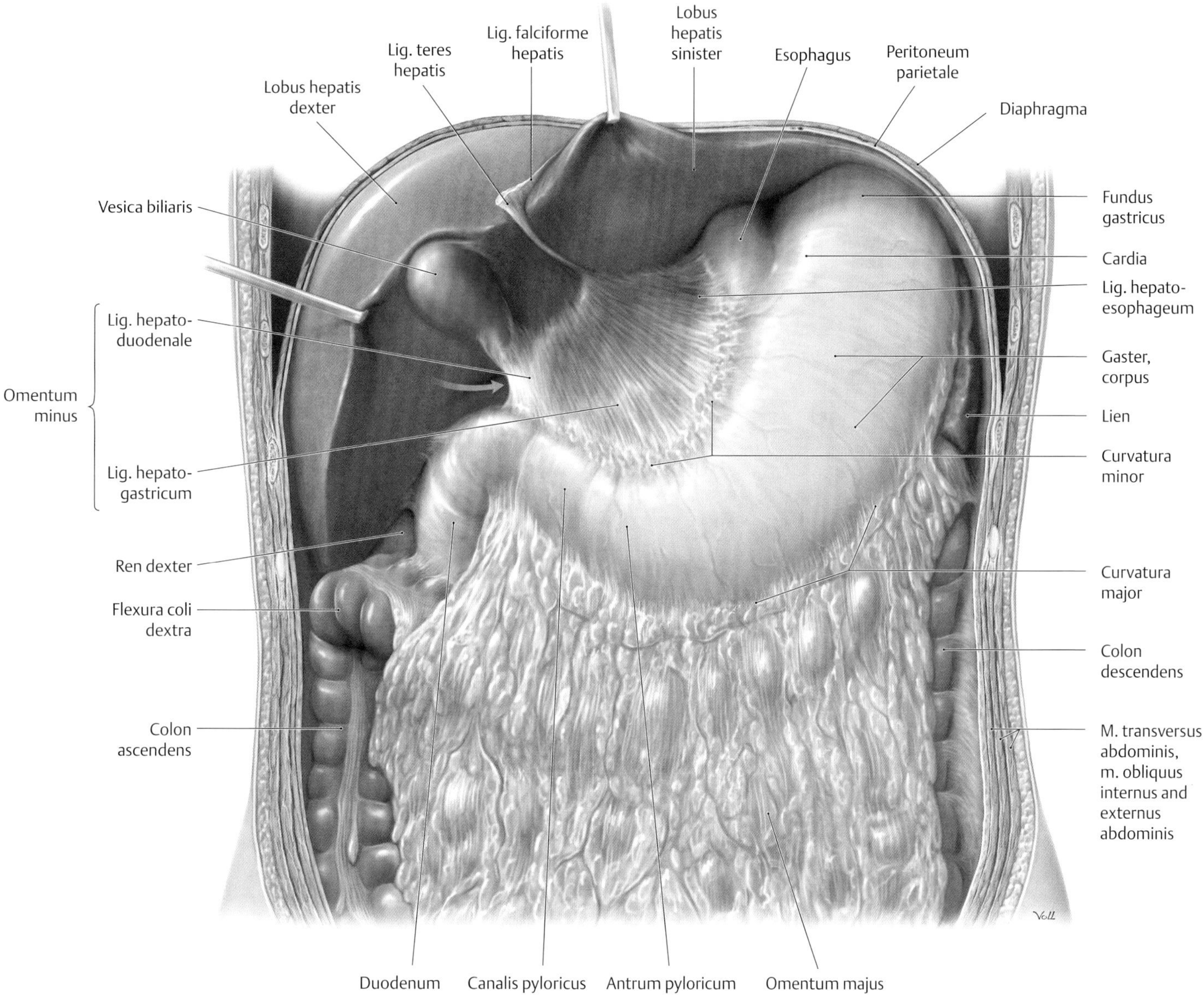

Lobus hepatis dexter
Lig. teres hepatis
Lig. falciforme hepatis
Lobus hepatis sinister
Esophagus
Peritoneum parietale
Diaphragma
Vesica biliaris
Omentum minus
Lig. hepato-duodenale
Lig. hepato-gastricum
Ren dexter
Flexura coli dextra
Colon ascendens
Fundus gastricus
Cardia
Lig. hepato-esophageum
Gaster, corpus
Lien
Curvatura minor
Curvatura major
Colon descendens
M. transversus abdominis, m. obliquus internus and externus abdominis
Duodenum
Canalis pyloricus
Antrum pyloricum
Omentum majus

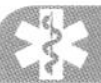

Clinical

Gastritis and ulcus ventriculi

Gastritis and ulcus ventriculi, the two most common diseases of the stomach, are associated with increased acid production and are caused by alcohol, drugs such as aspirin, and the bacterium *Helicobacter pylori*. Symptoms include lessened appetite, pain, and even bleeding, which manifests as black stool or dark brown material in vomit. Gastritis is limited to the inner surface of the stomach, while ulcus ventriculi extend into the stomach wall. The ulcus ventriculi in **C** is covered with fibrin and shows hematin spots.

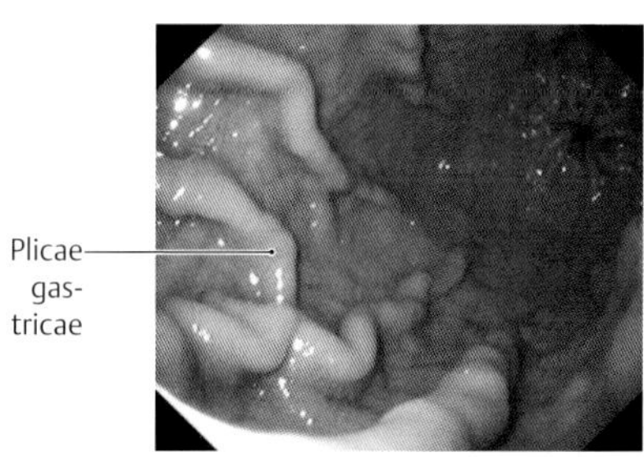
Plicae gastricae

A Body of normal gaster.

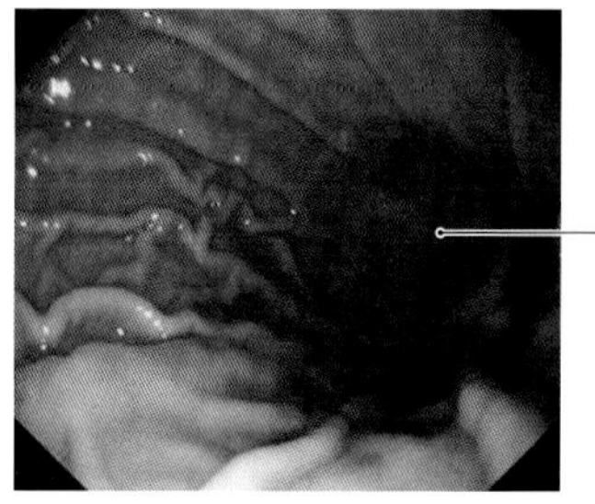
Antrum pyloricum

B Normal antrum pyloricum.

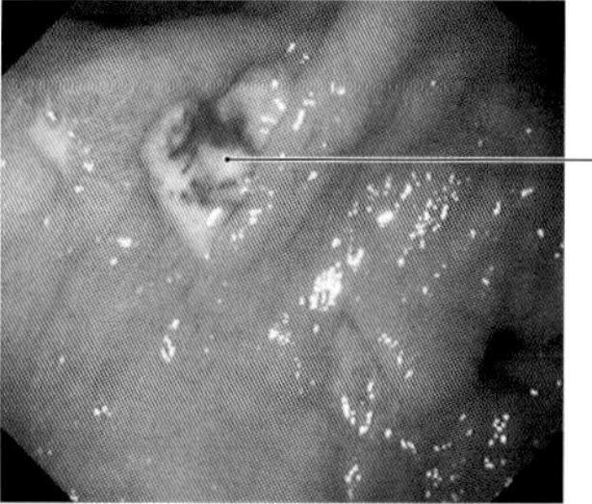
Ulcus ventriculi

C Ulcus ventriculi.

Duodenum

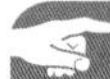

Intestinum tenue consists of the duodenum, jejunum, and ileum (see p. 162). The duodenum is primarily retroperitoneal and divided into four parts: superior, descending, horizontal, and ascending.

Fig. 13.5 Duodenum: Location
Anterior view.

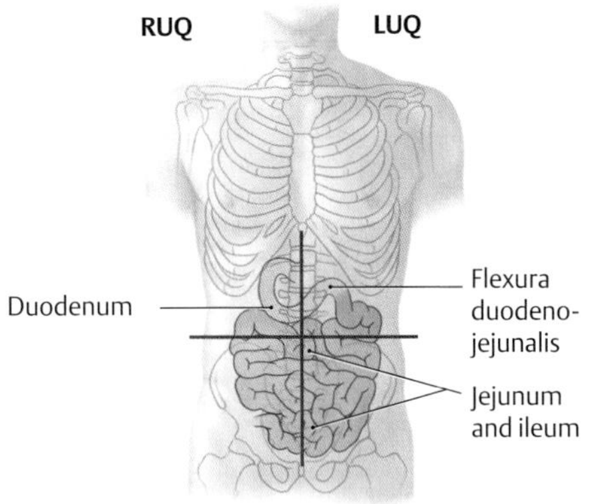
RUQ
LUQ
Duodenum
Flexura duodeno-jejunalis
Jejunum and ileum

Fig. 13.6 Parts of the duodenum
Anterior view.

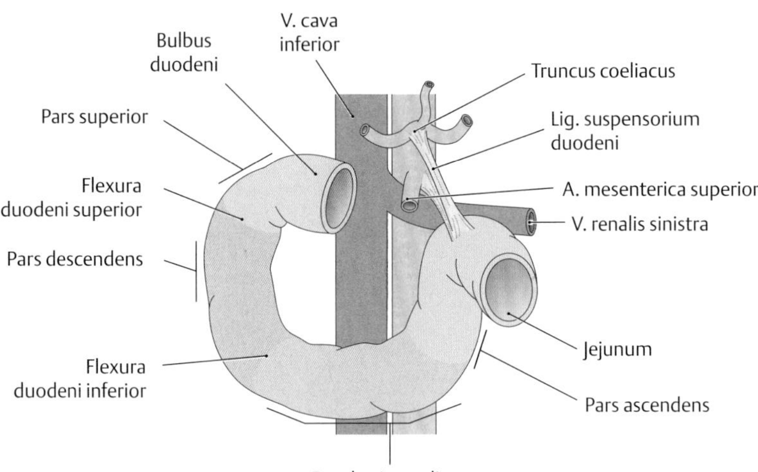
V. cava inferior
Bulbus duodeni
Truncus coeliacus
Pars superior
Lig. suspensorium duodeni
Flexura duodeni superior
A. mesenterica superior
V. renalis sinistra
Pars descendens
Jejunum
Flexura duodeni inferior
Pars ascendens
Pars horizontalis

Fig. 13.7 Duodenum
Anterior view with the anterior wall opened.

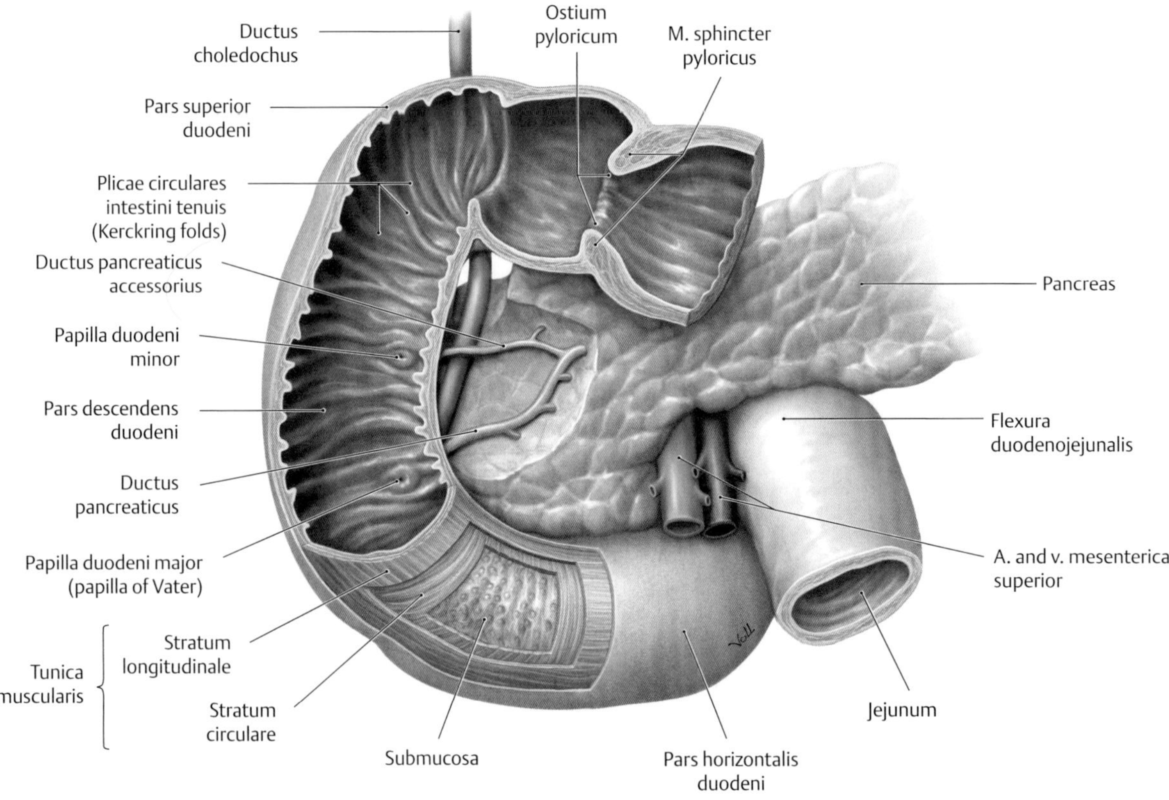
Ductus choledochus
Ostium pyloricum
M. sphincter pyloricus
Pars superior duodeni
Plicae circulares intestini tenuis (Kerckring folds)
Ductus pancreaticus accessorius
Pancreas
Papilla duodeni minor
Pars descendens duodeni
Flexura duodenojejunalis
Ductus pancreaticus
Papilla duodeni major (papilla of Vater)
A. and v. mesenterica superior
Tunica muscularis
Stratum longitudinale
Stratum circulare
Submucosa
Pars horizontalis duodeni
Jejunum

Fig. 13.8 Duodenum in situ

Anterior view. *Removed:* Gaster, hepar, intestinum tenue, and large portions of colon transversum. *Thinned:* Retroperitoneal fat and connective tissue.

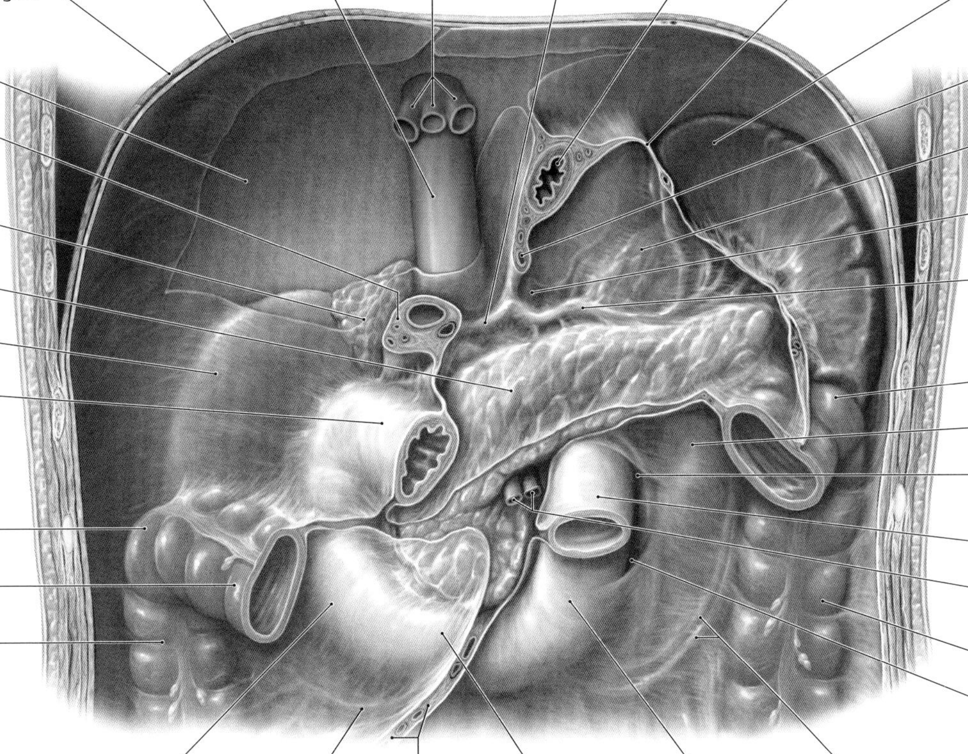

Peritoneum parietale
V. cava inferior
Vv. hepaticae
A. hepatica communis
Esophagus
Lig. phrenicosplenicum
Diaphragma
Lien
Hepatic surface of diaphragma
A. gastrica sinistra
Lig. hepato-duodenale (with v. portae hepatis)
Glandula suprarenalis sinistra
Glandula suprarenalis dextra
Pars abdominalis aortae
Pancreas
A. lienalis
Ren dexter
Flexura coli sinistra
Pars superior duodeni
Ren sinister
Recessus duodenalis superior
Flexura coli dextra
Jejunum
Colon transversum
A. and v. mesenterica superior
Colon ascendens
Colon descendens
Recessus duodenalis inferior
Pars descendens duodeni
A. colica dextra
Radix mesenterii
Pars horizontalis duodeni
Pars ascendens duodeni
A. and v. colica sinistra

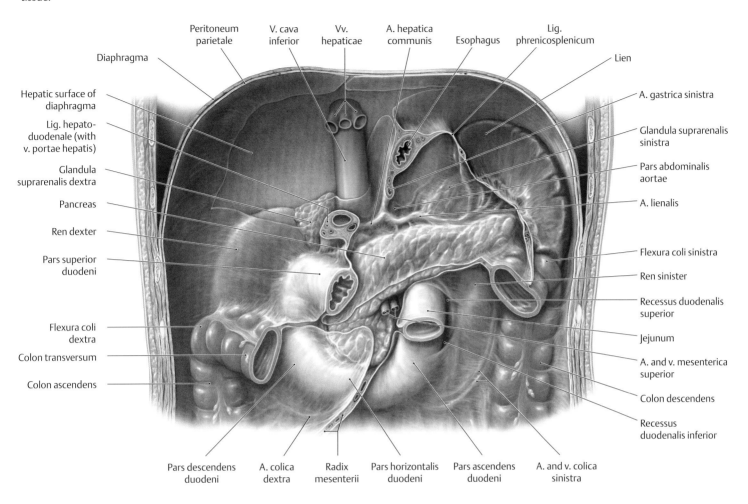

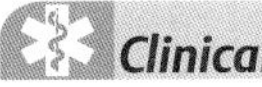

Clinical

Endoscopy of the papillary region

Two important ducts end in the papillary region of the duodenum: ductus choledocus and the ductus pancreaticus (see Fig. 13.7). These ducts may be examined by X-ray through endoscopic retrograde cholangiopancreatography (ERCP), in which dye is injected endoscopically into papilla duodeni major. Duodenal diverticula (generally harmless outpouchings) may complicate the procedure.

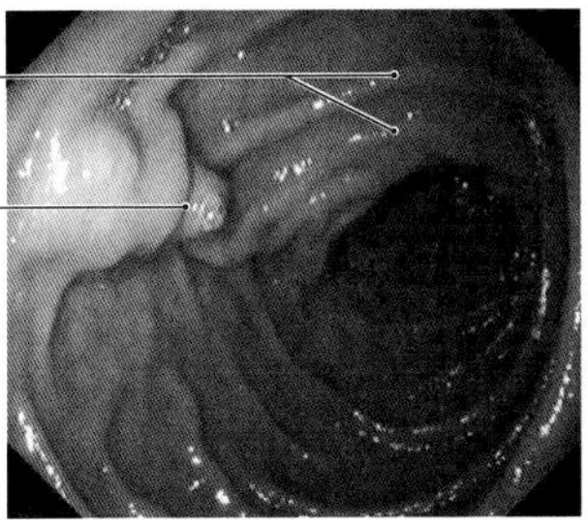

Plicae circulares intestini tenuis
Papillary region

A Endoscopic appearance.

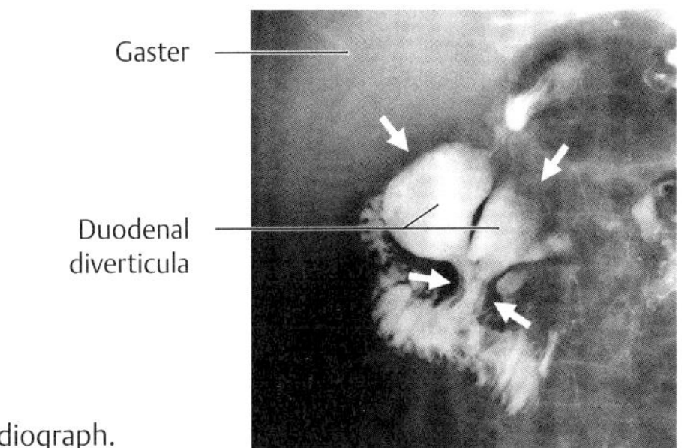

Gaster
Duodenal diverticula

B Radiograph.

Jejunum & Ileum

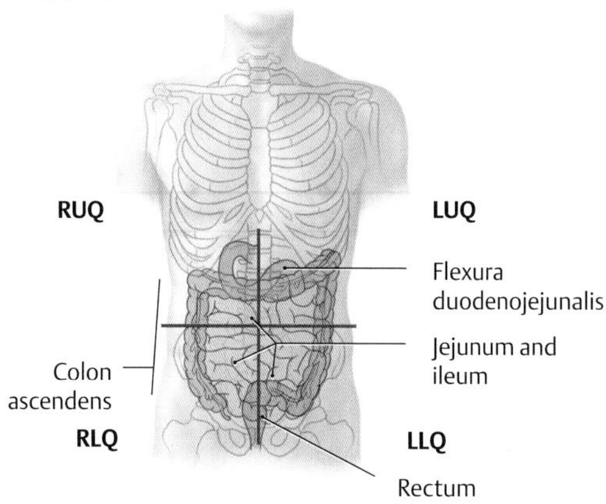
RUQ
LUQ
Flexura duodenojejunalis
Jejunum and ileum
Colon ascendens
RLQ
LLQ
Rectum

Fig. 13.9 **Jejunum and ileum: Location**
Anterior view. The intraperitoneal jejunum and ileum are enclosed by the mesentery proper.

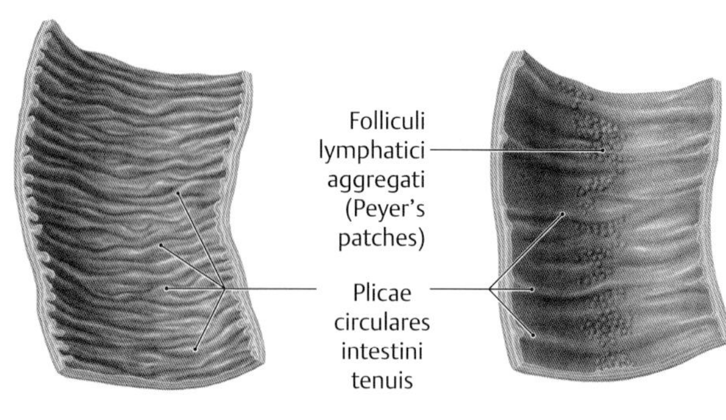
Folliculi lymphatici aggregati (Peyer's patches)
Plicae circulares intestini tenuis
A Jejunum.
B Ileum.

Fig. 13.10 **Wall structure of intestinum tenue**
Macroscopic views of the longitudinally opened small intestine.

Fig. 13.11 **Jejunum and ileum in situ**
Anterior view. *Reflected:* Colon transversum.

Omentum majus (reflected superiorly)
Appendices epiploicae
Taeniae coli
Colon transversum
Lig. teres hepatis
Mesocolon transversum (with a. and v. colica media)
Jejunum
Colon ascendens
Taeniae coli
Caecum
Ileum
M. transversus abdominis, m. obliquus internus and externus abdominis
Plica umbilicalis lateralis (with a. and v. epigastrica inferior)
M. rectus abdominis
Plica umbilicalis medialis (with obliterated a. umbilicalis)
Linea arcuata
Plica umbilicalis mediana (with obliterated urachus)

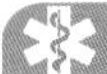

Clinical

Morbus Crohn

Mb. Crohn, a chronic inflammation of the digestive tract, occurs most often in the terminal ileum (30% of cases). Patients are generally young and suffer from abdominal pain, nausea, elevated body temperature, and diarrhea. Initially, these symptoms can be confused with appendicitis. Complications of Crohn's disease often include anal fistulae (**B**).

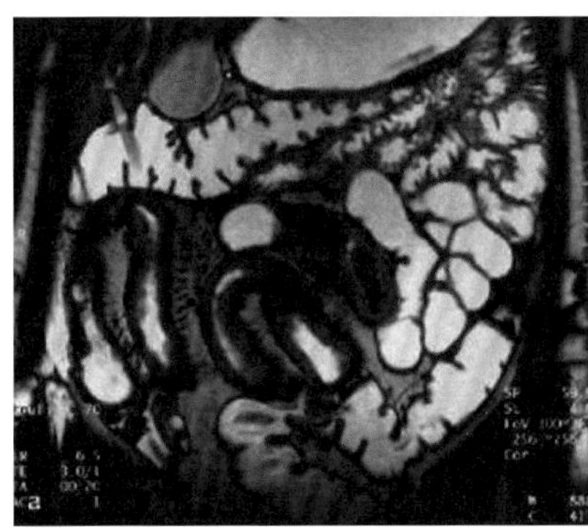

A MRI showing thickened wall of terminal ileum.

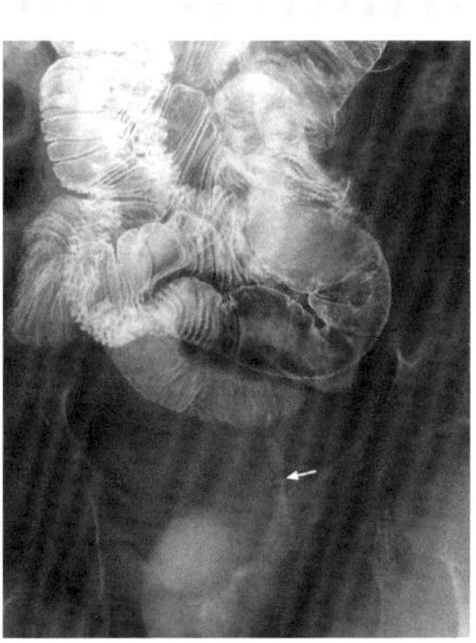

B Double-contrast radiograph. Arrow indicates fistula.

Fig. 13.12 Mesenterium of intestinum tenue

Anterior view. *Removed:* Gaster, jejunum, and ileum. *Reflected:* Hepar.

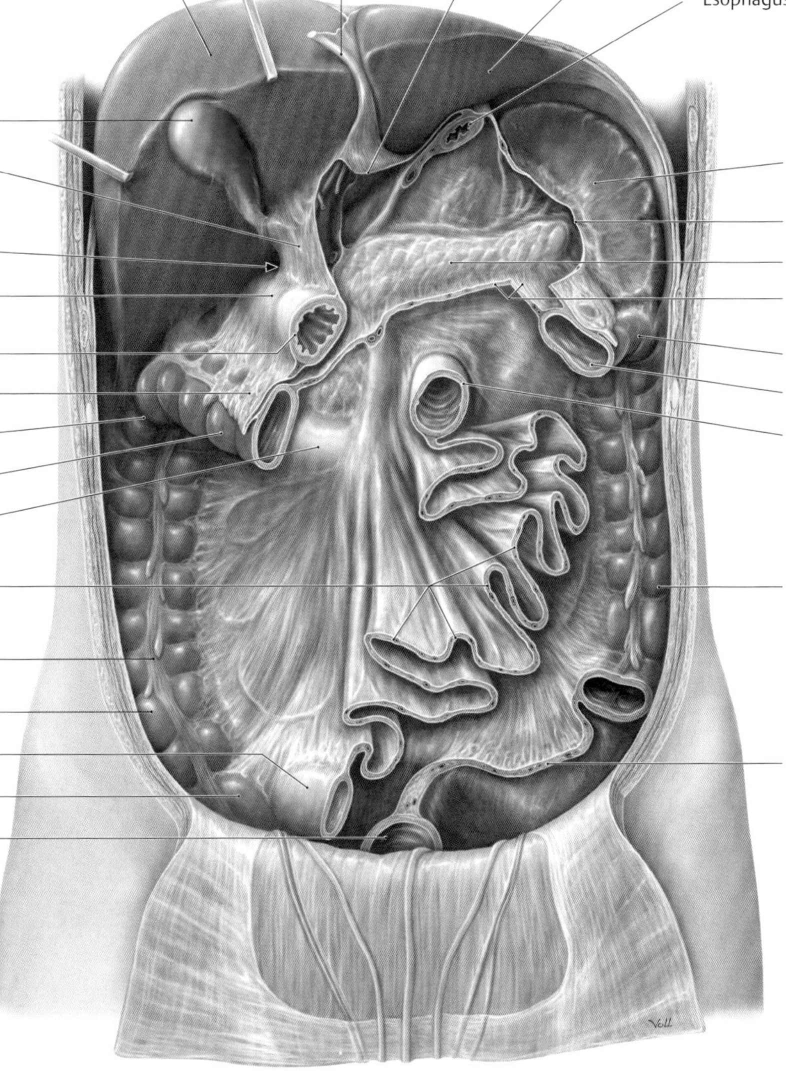

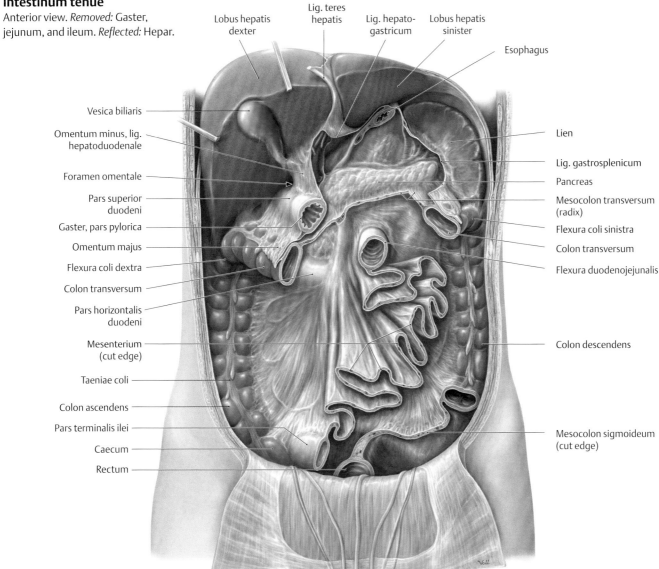

Lobus hepatis dexter
Lig. teres hepatis
Lig. hepato-gastricum
Lobus hepatis sinister
Esophagus
Vesica biliaris
Omentum minus, lig. hepatoduodenale
Foramen omentale
Pars superior duodeni
Gaster, pars pylorica
Omentum majus
Flexura coli dextra
Colon transversum
Pars horizontalis duodeni
Mesenterium (cut edge)
Taeniae coli
Colon ascendens
Pars terminalis ilei
Caecum
Rectum
Lien
Lig. gastrosplenicum
Pancreas
Mesocolon transversum (radix)
Flexura coli sinistra
Colon transversum
Flexura duodenojejunalis
Colon descendens
Mesocolon sigmoideum (cut edge)

Cecum, Appendix & Colon

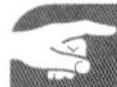

Intestinum crassum consists of the cecum, appendix, colon, and rectum (see p. 166). The colon is divided into four parts: ascendens, transversum, descendens, and sigmoideum. The appendix, colon transversum, and colon sigmoideum are intraperitoneal (suspended by the mesoappendix, mesocolon transversum, and mesocolon sigmoideum, respectively).

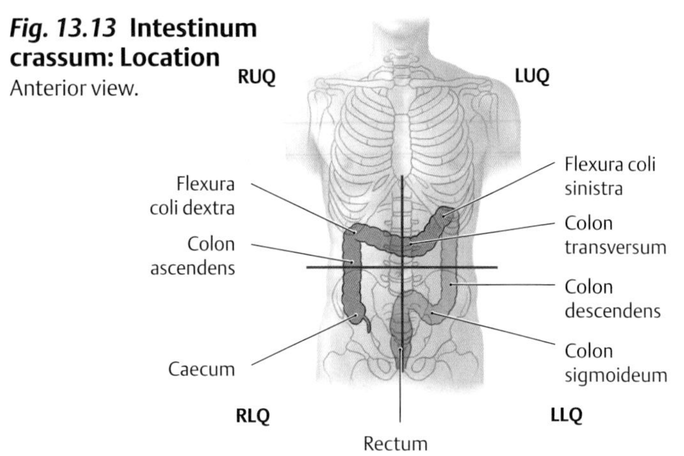
RUQ
LUQ
Flexura coli dextra
Colon ascendens
Caecum
Flexura coli sinistra
Colon transversum
Colon descendens
Colon sigmoideum
RLQ
LLQ
Rectum

Fig. 13.13 **Intestinum crassum: Location**
Anterior view.

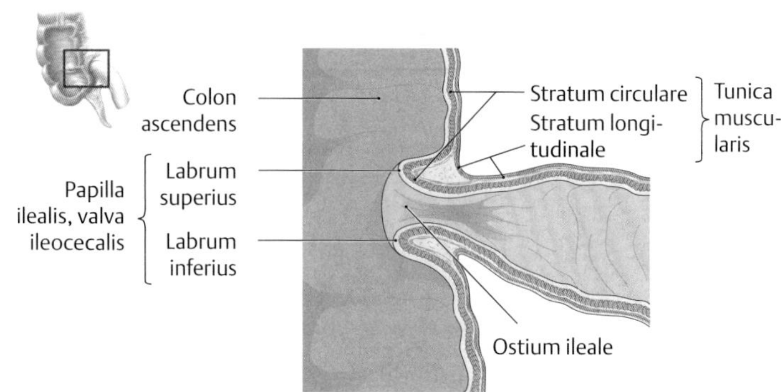
Colon ascendens
Papilla ilealis, valva ileocecalis
Labrum superius
Labrum inferius
Stratum circulare
Stratum longitudinale
Tunica muscularis
Ostium ileale

Fig. 13.14 **Ostium ileale**
Anterior view of longitudinal coronal section.

Fig. 13.15 **Intestinum crassum**
Anterior view.

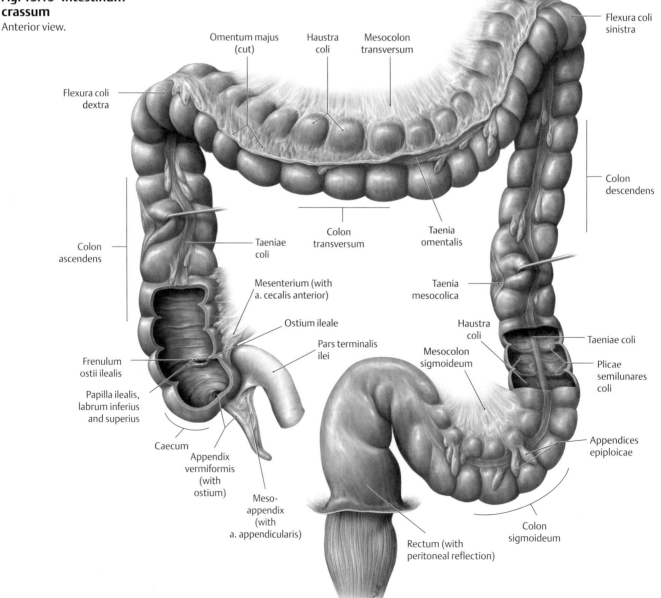

Omentum majus (cut)
Haustra coli
Mesocolon transversum
Flexura coli sinistra
Flexura coli dextra
Colon descendens
Colon ascendens
Taeniae coli
Colon transversum
Taenia omentalis
Mesenterium (with a. cecalis anterior)
Taenia mesocolica
Ostium ileale
Haustra coli
Pars terminalis ilei
Mesocolon sigmoideum
Taeniae coli
Frenulum ostii ilealis
Plicae semilunares coli
Papilla ilealis, labrum inferius and superius
Caecum
Appendices epiploicae
Appendix vermiformis (with ostium)
Meso-appendix (with a. appendicularis)
Colon sigmoideum
Rectum (with peritoneal reflection)

Fig. 13.16 Intestinum crassum in situ

Omentum majus
Colon transversum
Mesocolon transversum
Flexura coli sinistra (flexura coli splenica)
Jejunum
Flexura coli dextra (flexura coli hepatica)
Colon descendens
Mesenterium (cut)
Mesocolon sigmoideum
Colon ascendens
Colon sigmoideum
Ileum
Caecum
Rectum
M. rectus abdominis

A Anterior view. *Reflected:* Colon transversum and omentum majus. *Removed:* Intraperitoneal intestinum tenue.

R
Flexura coli sinistra
Flexura coli dextra
Colon transversum
Haustra coli
Os sacrum
Os ilium
Caecum
Colon sigmoideum

B Normal radiographic appearance. Double-contrast radiograph, anterior view.

Clinical

Colitis

Ulcerative colitis is a chronic inflammation of the large intestine, often starting in the rectum. Typical symptoms include diarrhea (sometimes with blood), pain, weight loss, and inflammation of other organs. Patients are also at higher risk for colorectal carcinomas.

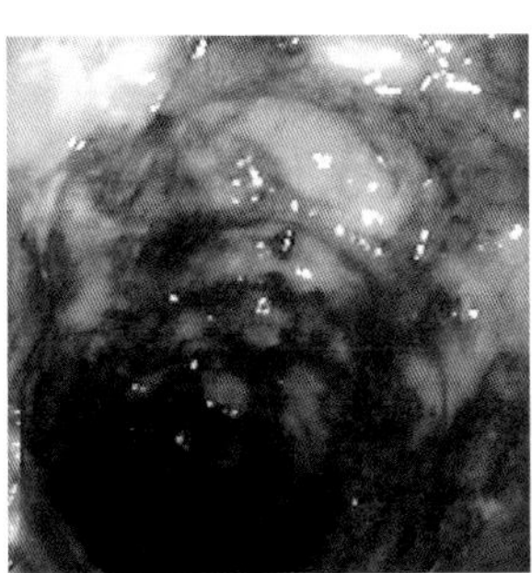

A Colonoscopy of ulcerative colitis.

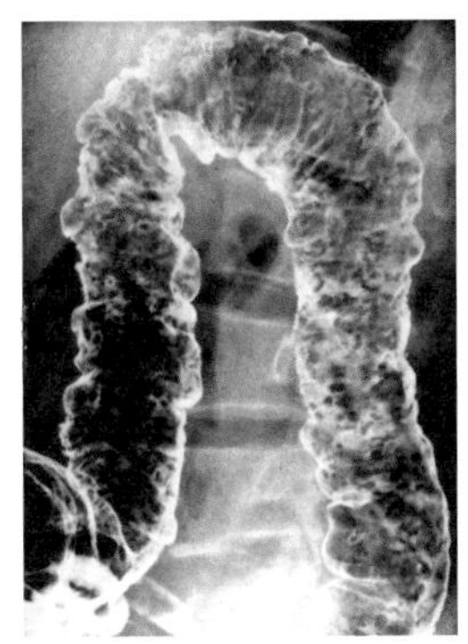

B Early-phase colitis. Residual normal mucosa appears as pseudopolyps.

Colon carcinoma

Malignant tumors of the colon and rectum are among the most frequent solid tumors. More than 90% occur in patients over the age of 50. In early stages, the tumor may be asymptomatic; later symptoms include loss of appetite, changes in bowel movements, and weight loss. Blood in the stools is particularly incriminating, necessitating a thorough examination. Hemorrhoids are not a sufficient explanation for blood in stools unless all other tests (including a colonoscopy) are negative.

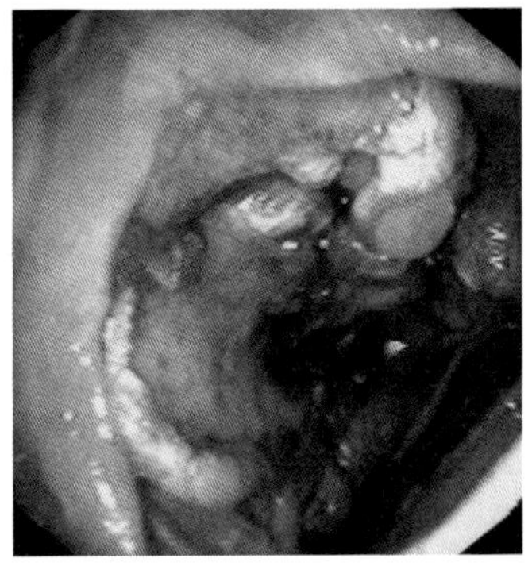

C Colonoscopy of colon carcinoma. The tumor partially blocks the lumen of the colon.

Rectum & Canalis Analis

Fig. 13.17 Rectum: Location

Fig. 13.18 Closure of the rectum

Left lateral view. M. puborectalis acts as a muscular sling that kinks the anorectal junction. It functions in the maintenance of fecal continence.

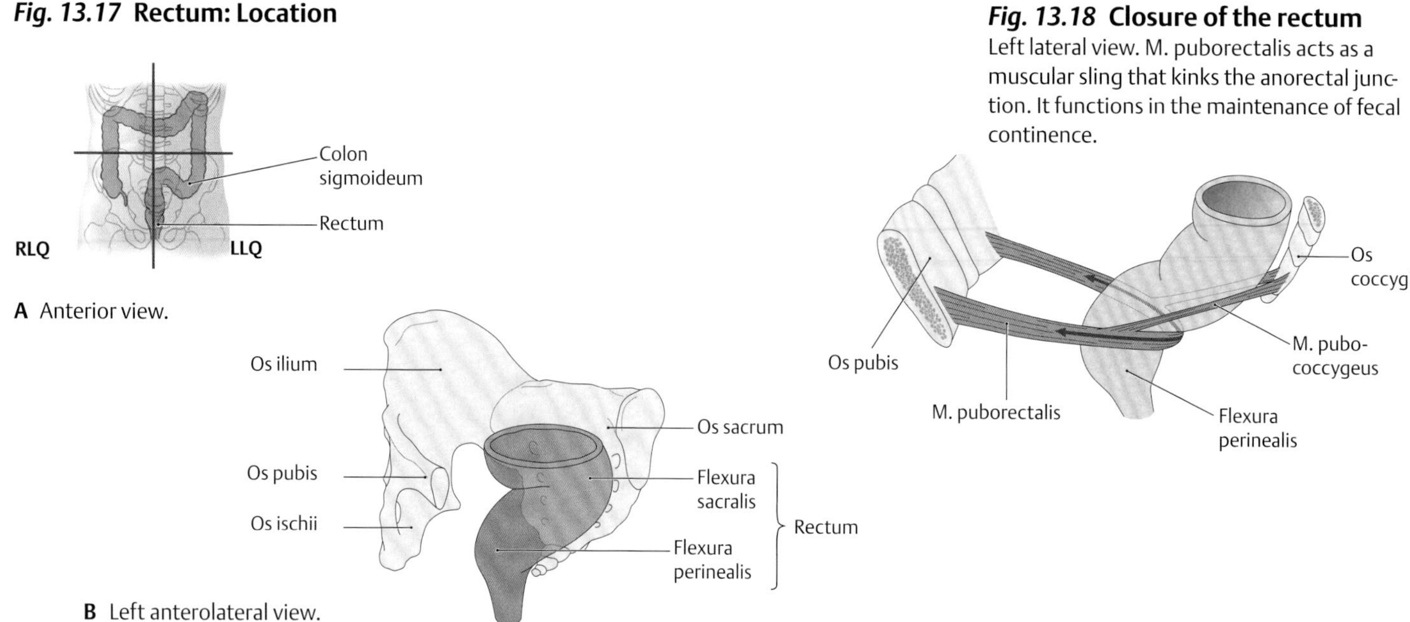

Colon sigmoideum
Rectum
RLQ
LLQ
Os ilium
Os pubis
Os ischii
Os sacrum
Flexura sacralis
Flexura perinealis
Rectum
Os coccygis
M. pubo-coccygeus
Os pubis
M. puborectalis
Flexura perinealis

A Anterior view.

B Left anterolateral view.

Fig. 13.19 Rectum in situ

Coronal section, anterior view of the female pelvis. The upper third of the rectum is covered with peritoneum viscerale on its anterior and lateral sides. The middle third is covered only anteriorly and the lower third is inferior to the peritoneum parietale.

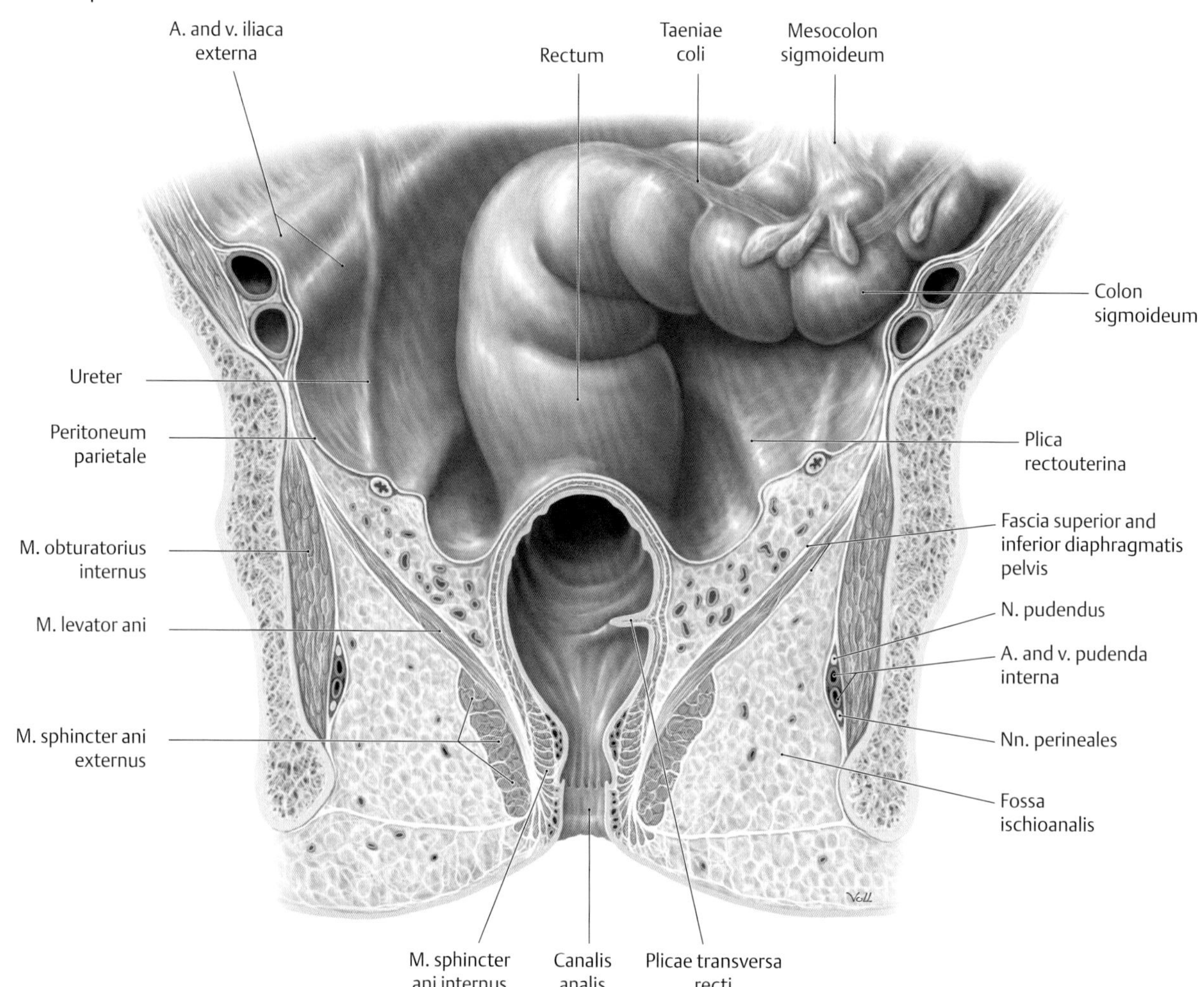

A. and v. iliaca externa
Rectum
Taeniae coli
Mesocolon sigmoideum
Colon sigmoideum
Ureter
Peritoneum parietale
Plica rectouterina
M. obturatorius internus
Fascia superior and inferior diaphragmatis pelvis
M. levator ani
N. pudendus
A. and v. pudenda interna
M. sphincter ani externus
Nn. perineales
Fossa ischioanalis
M. sphincter ani internus
Canalis analis
Plicae transversa recti

Fig. 13.20 **Rectum and canalis analis**
Coronal section, anterior view with the anterior wall removed.

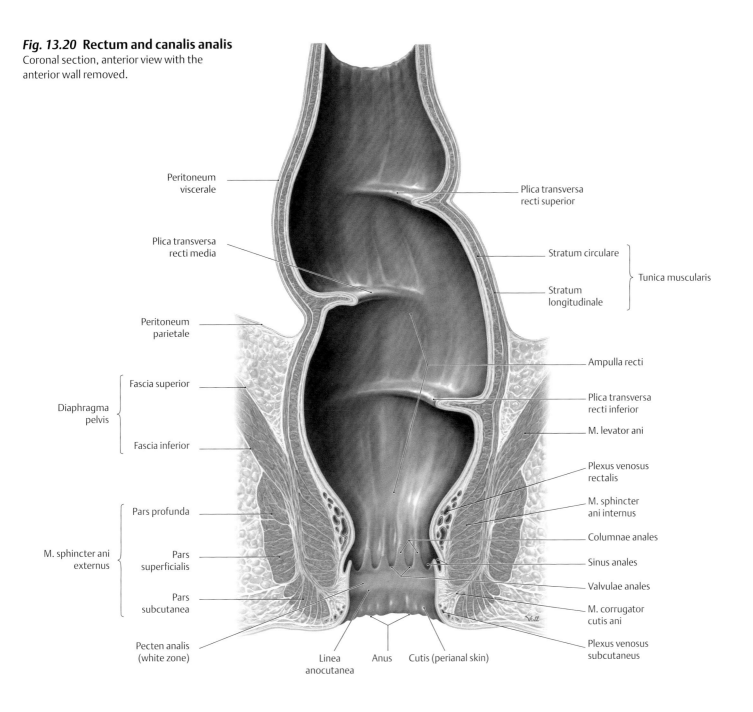

Peritoneum viscerale
Plica transversa recti superior
Plica transversa recti media
Stratum circulare
Stratum longitudinale
Tunica muscularis
Peritoneum parietale
Ampulla recti
Diaphragma pelvis
Fascia superior
Fascia inferior
Plica transversa recti inferior
M. levator ani
Plexus venosus rectalis
M. sphincter ani internus
M. sphincter ani externus
Pars profunda
Pars superficialis
Pars subcutanea
Columnae anales
Sinus anales
Valvulae anales
M. corrugator cutis ani
Pecten analis (white zone)
Linea anocutanea
Anus
Cutis (perianal skin)
Plexus venosus subcutaneus

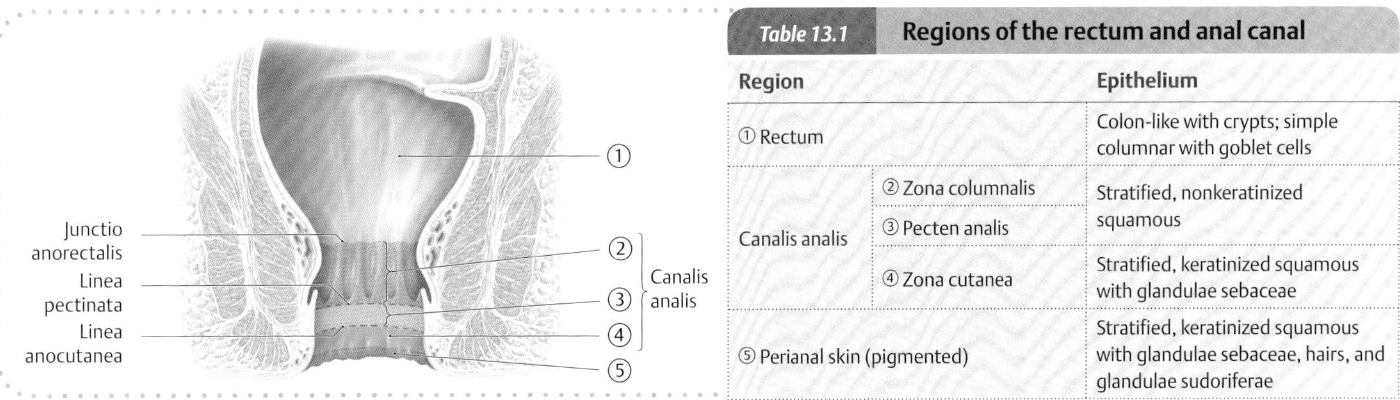

Junctio anorectalis
Linea pectinata
Linea anocutanea
①
②
③
④
⑤
Canalis analis

Table 13.1 Regions of the rectum and anal canal

Region		Epithelium
① Rectum		Colon-like with crypts; simple columnar with goblet cells
Canalis analis	② Zona columnalis	Stratified, nonkeratinized squamous
	③ Pecten analis	
	④ Zona cutanea	Stratified, keratinized squamous with glandulae sebaceae
⑤ Perianal skin (pigmented)		Stratified, keratinized squamous with glandulae sebaceae, hairs, and glandulae sudoriferae

Hepar: Overview

Fig. 13.21 Hepar: Location

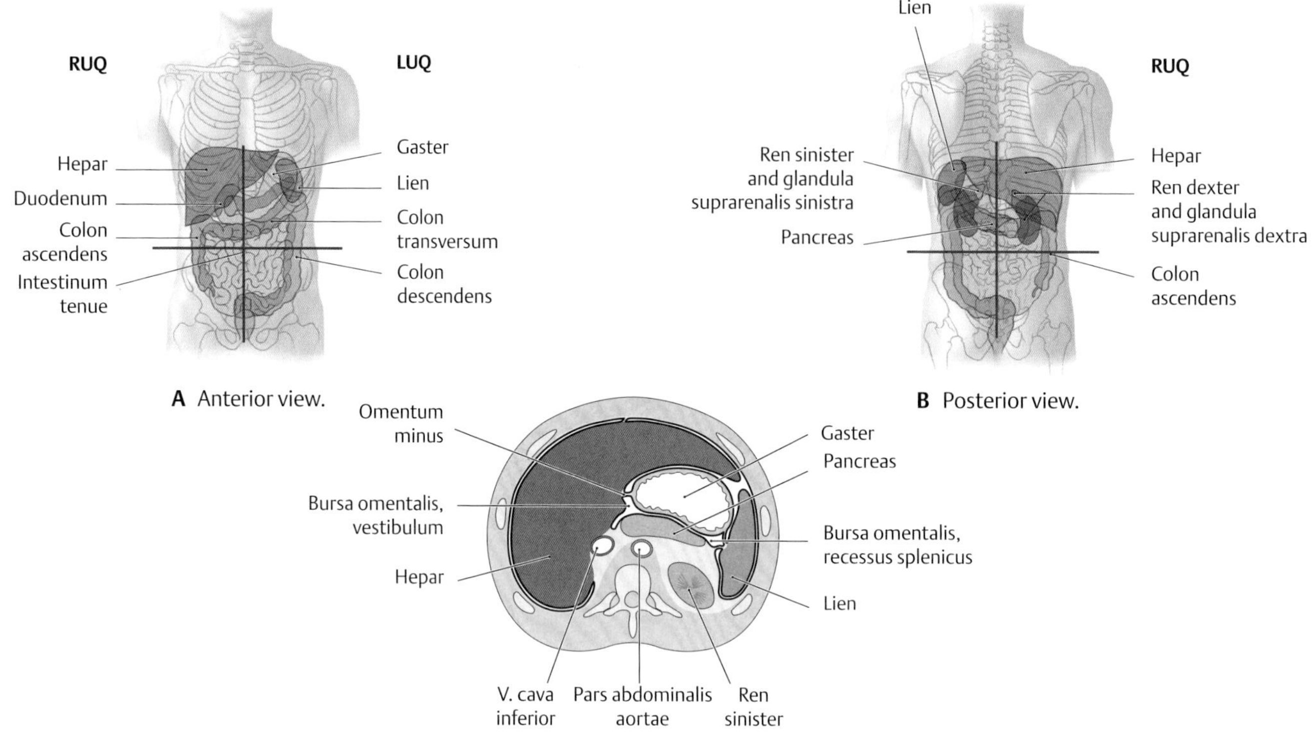
RUQ
LUQ
Hepar
Duodenum
Colon ascendens
Intestinum tenue
Gaster
Lien
Colon transversum
Colon descendens
Lien
RUQ
Ren sinister and glandula suprarenalis sinistra
Pancreas
Hepar
Ren dexter and glandula suprarenalis dextra
Colon ascendens
Omentum minus
Bursa omentalis, vestibulum
Hepar
Gaster
Pancreas
Bursa omentalis, recessus splenicus
Lien
V. cava inferior
Pars abdominalis aortae
Ren sinister

A Anterior view.

B Posterior view.

C Transverse section, inferior view.

Fig. 13.22 Hepar in situ

Anterior view with hepar retracted. *Removed:* Gaster, jejunum, and ileum. Hepar is intraperitoneal except for its "bare area" (see Fig. 13.26); its mestenterium include ligg. falciforme, coronarium, and triangulare (see Fig. 13.27).

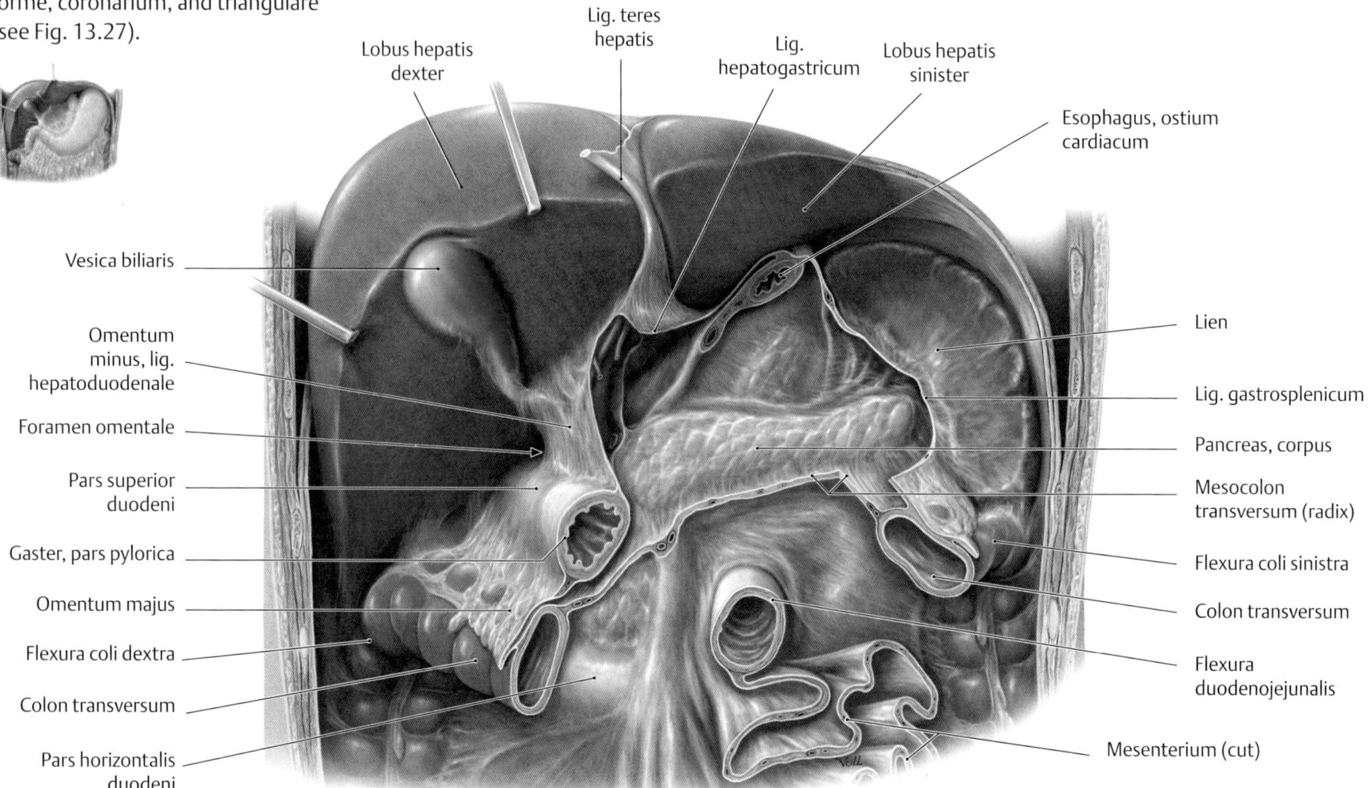
Lobus hepatis dexter
Lig. teres hepatis
Lig. hepatogastricum
Lobus hepatis sinister
Esophagus, ostium cardiacum
Vesica biliaris
Omentum minus, lig. hepatoduodenale
Foramen omentale
Pars superior duodeni
Gaster, pars pylorica
Omentum majus
Flexura coli dextra
Colon transversum
Pars horizontalis duodeni
Lien
Lig. gastrosplenicum
Pancreas, corpus
Mesocolon transversum (radix)
Flexura coli sinistra
Colon transversum
Flexura duodenojejunalis
Mesenterium (cut)

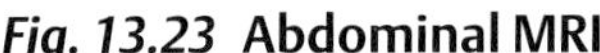

Fig. 13.23 **Abdominal MRI**
Inferior view.

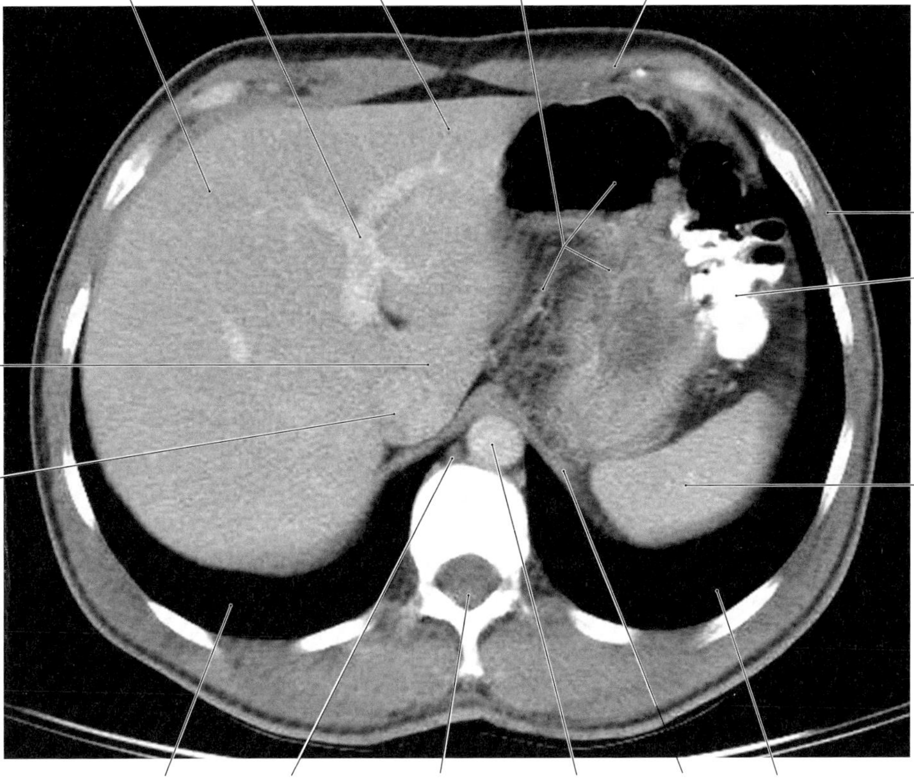

Lobus hepatis dexter
V. portae hepatis
Lobus hepatis sinister
Gaster (with a. gastrica sinistra)
M. rectus abdominis
M. obliquus externus abdominis
Flexura coli sinistra
Lobus caudatus hepatis
V. cava inferior
Lien
Pulmo dexter
V. azygos
Medulla spinalis (in canalis vertebralis)
Pars abdominalis aortae
Diaphragma
Pulmo sinister

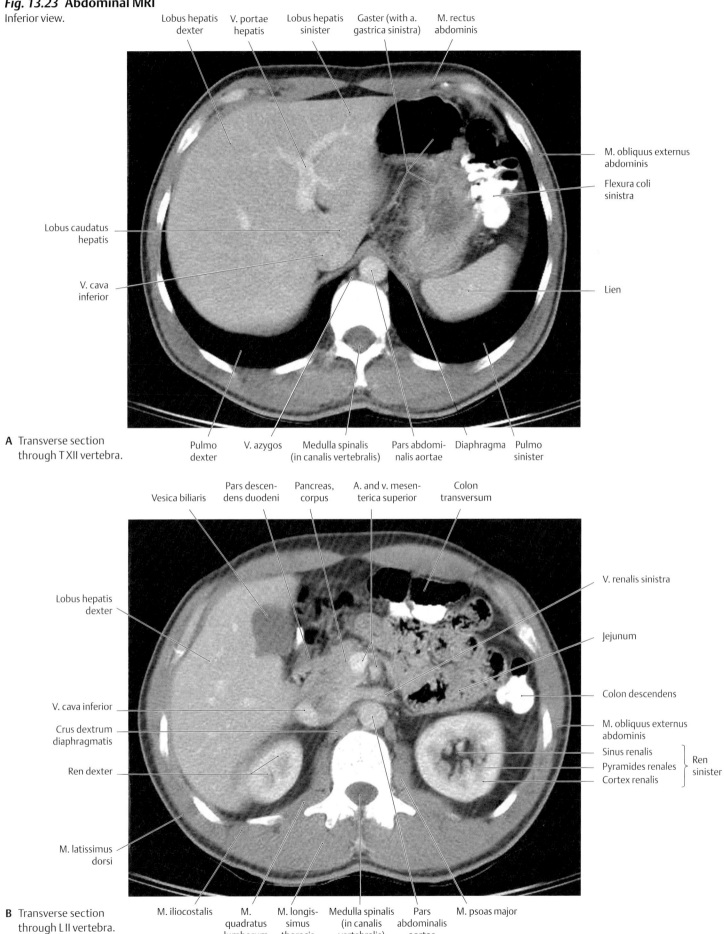

A Transverse section through T XII vertebra.

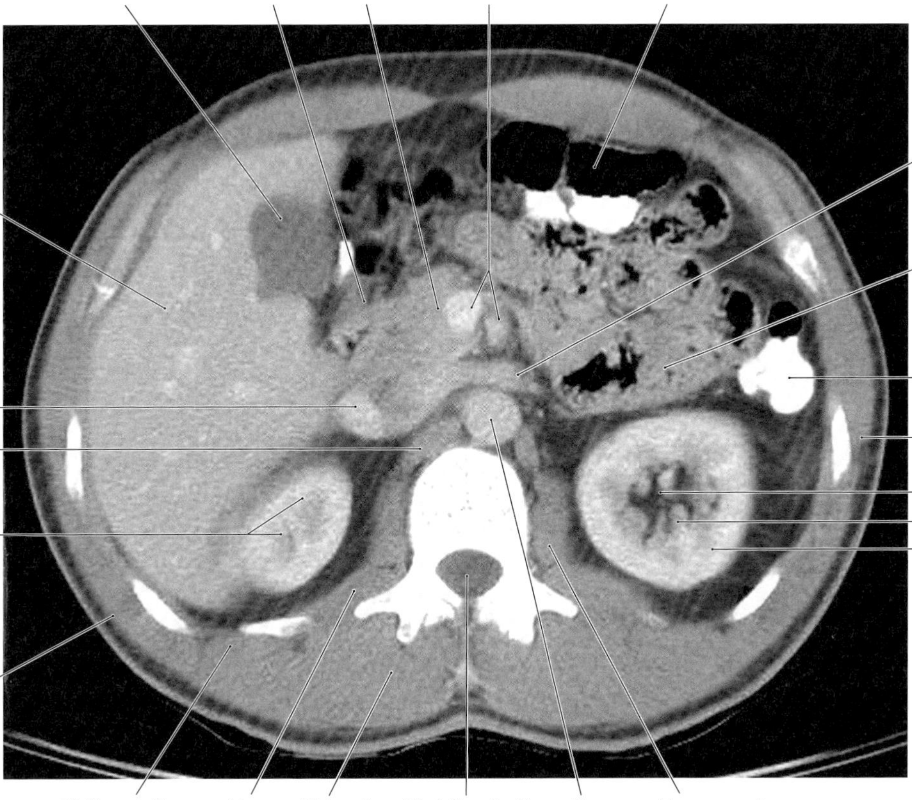

Vesica biliaris
Pars descendens duodeni
Pancreas, corpus
A. and v. mesenterica superior
Colon transversum
V. renalis sinistra
Lobus hepatis dexter
Jejunum
Colon descendens
V. cava inferior
Crus dextrum diaphragmatis
M. obliquus externus abdominis
Sinus renalis
Pyramides renales
Cortex renalis
Ren sinister
Ren dexter
M. latissimus dorsi
M. iliocostalis
M. quadratus lumborum
M. longissimus thoracis
Medulla spinalis (in canalis vertebralis)
Pars abdominalis aortae
M. psoas major

B Transverse section through L II vertebra.

Hepar: Segments & Lobes

Fig. 13.24 Segmentation of hepar

Anterior view. The components of the portal triad (a. hepatica propria, v. portae hepatis, and ductus hepaticus communis, see pp. 172, 219) divides the liver into hepatic segments (see Table 13.2).

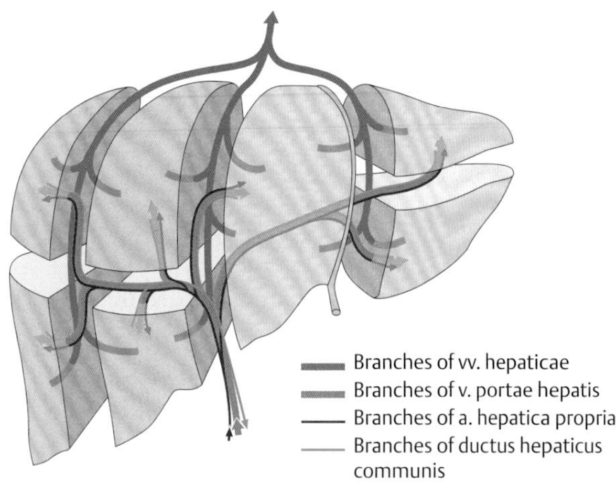
Branches of vv. hepaticae
Branches of v. portae hepatis
Branches of a. hepatica propria
Branches of ductus hepaticus communis

VIII
IV
II
VII
III
VI
Lig. teres hepatis
V

A Diaphragmatic surface, anterior view.

Appendix fibrosa hepatis
I
VII
II
V. cava inferior
VI
III
V
Lig. teres hepatis
IV
Vesica biliaris

B Visceral surface, inferior view.

Table 13.2 Hepatic segments

Part	Division	Segmentum	
Pars hepatis sinistra	Pars posterior	I	Lobus caudatus
	Divisio lateralis sinistra	II	Posterius laterale sinistrum
		III	Anterius laterale sinistrum
	Divisio medialis sinistra	IV	Mediale sinistrum
Pars hepatis dextra	Divisio medialis dextra	V	Anterius mediale dextrum
		VIII	Posterius mediale dextrum
	Divisio lateralis dextra	VII	Posterius laterale dextrum
		VI	Anterius laterale dextrum

Fig. 13.25 Hepar: Areas of organ contact

Visceral surface, inferior view.

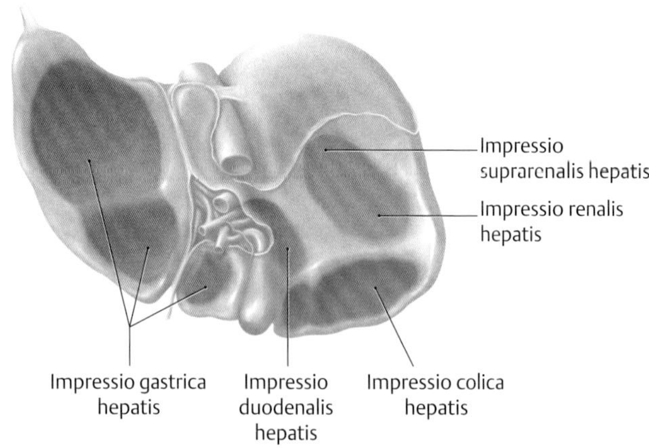
Impressio suprarenalis hepatis
Impressio renalis hepatis
Impressio gastrica hepatis
Impressio duodenalis hepatis
Impressio colica hepatis

Fig. 13.26 Attachment of hepar to diaphragma

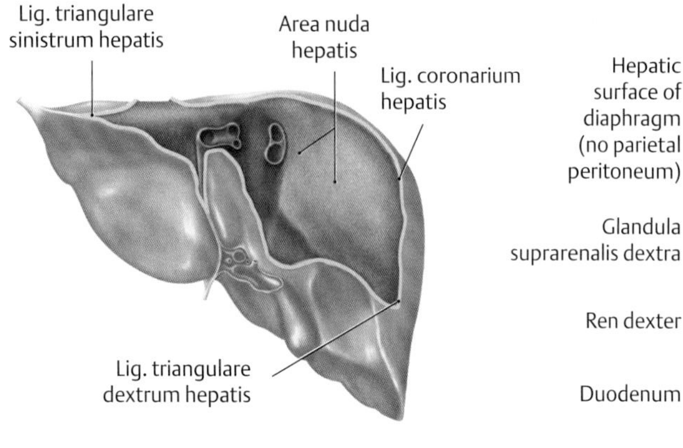
Lig. triangulare sinistrum hepatis
Area nuda hepatis
Lig. coronarium hepatis
Lig. triangulare dextrum hepatis

A Diaphragmatic surface of the liver, posterior view.

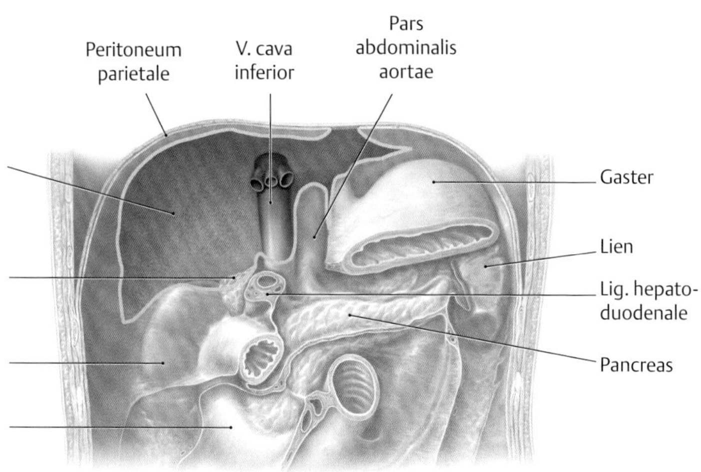
Peritoneum parietale
V. cava inferior
Pars abdominalis aortae
Hepatic surface of diaphragm (no parietal peritoneum)
Glandula suprarenalis dextra
Ren dexter
Duodenum
Gaster
Lien
Lig. hepato-duodenale
Pancreas

B Hepatic surface of the diaphragm, anterior view.

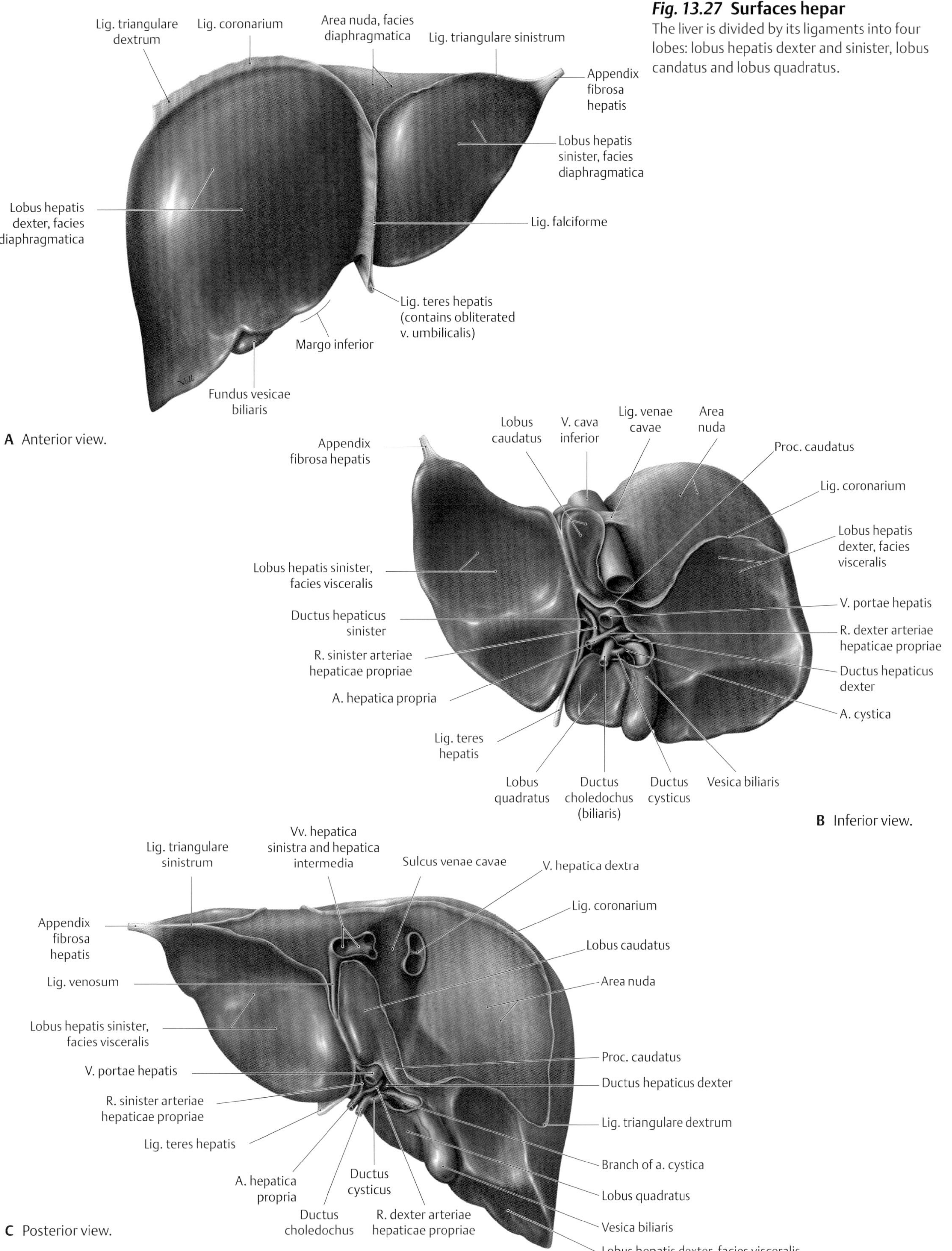
Lig. triangulare dextrum
Lig. coronarium
Area nuda, facies diaphragmatica
Lig. triangulare sinistrum
Appendix fibrosa hepatis
Lobus hepatis sinister, facies diaphragmatica
Lobus hepatis dexter, facies diaphragmatica
Lig. falciforme
Lig. teres hepatis (contains obliterated v. umbilicalis)
Margo inferior
Fundus vesicae biliaris
Appendix fibrosa hepatis
Lobus caudatus
V. cava inferior
Lig. venae cavae
Area nuda
Proc. caudatus
Lig. coronarium
Lobus hepatis dexter, facies visceralis
Lobus hepatis sinister, facies visceralis
V. portae hepatis
Ductus hepaticus sinister
R. dexter arteriae hepaticae propriae
R. sinister arteriae hepaticae propriae
Ductus hepaticus dexter
A. hepatica propria
A. cystica
Lig. teres hepatis
Lobus quadratus
Ductus choledochus (biliaris)
Ductus cysticus
Vesica biliaris
Lig. triangulare sinistrum
Vv. hepatica sinistra and hepatica intermedia
Sulcus venae cavae
V. hepatica dextra
Lig. coronarium
Appendix fibrosa hepatis
Lobus caudatus
Lig. venosum
Area nuda
Lobus hepatis sinister, facies visceralis
Proc. caudatus
V. portae hepatis
Ductus hepaticus dexter
R. sinister arteriae hepaticae propriae
Lig. triangulare dextrum
Lig. teres hepatis
Branch of a. cystica
A. hepatica propria
Ductus cysticus
Lobus quadratus
Vesica biliaris
Ductus choledochus
R. dexter arteriae hepaticae propriae
Lobus hepatis dexter, facies visceralis

A Anterior view.

B Inferior view.

C Posterior view.

Fig. 13.27 **Surfaces hepar**
The liver is divided by its ligaments into four lobes: lobus hepatis dexter and sinister, lobus candatus and lobus quadratus.

Vesica Biliaris & Bile Ducts

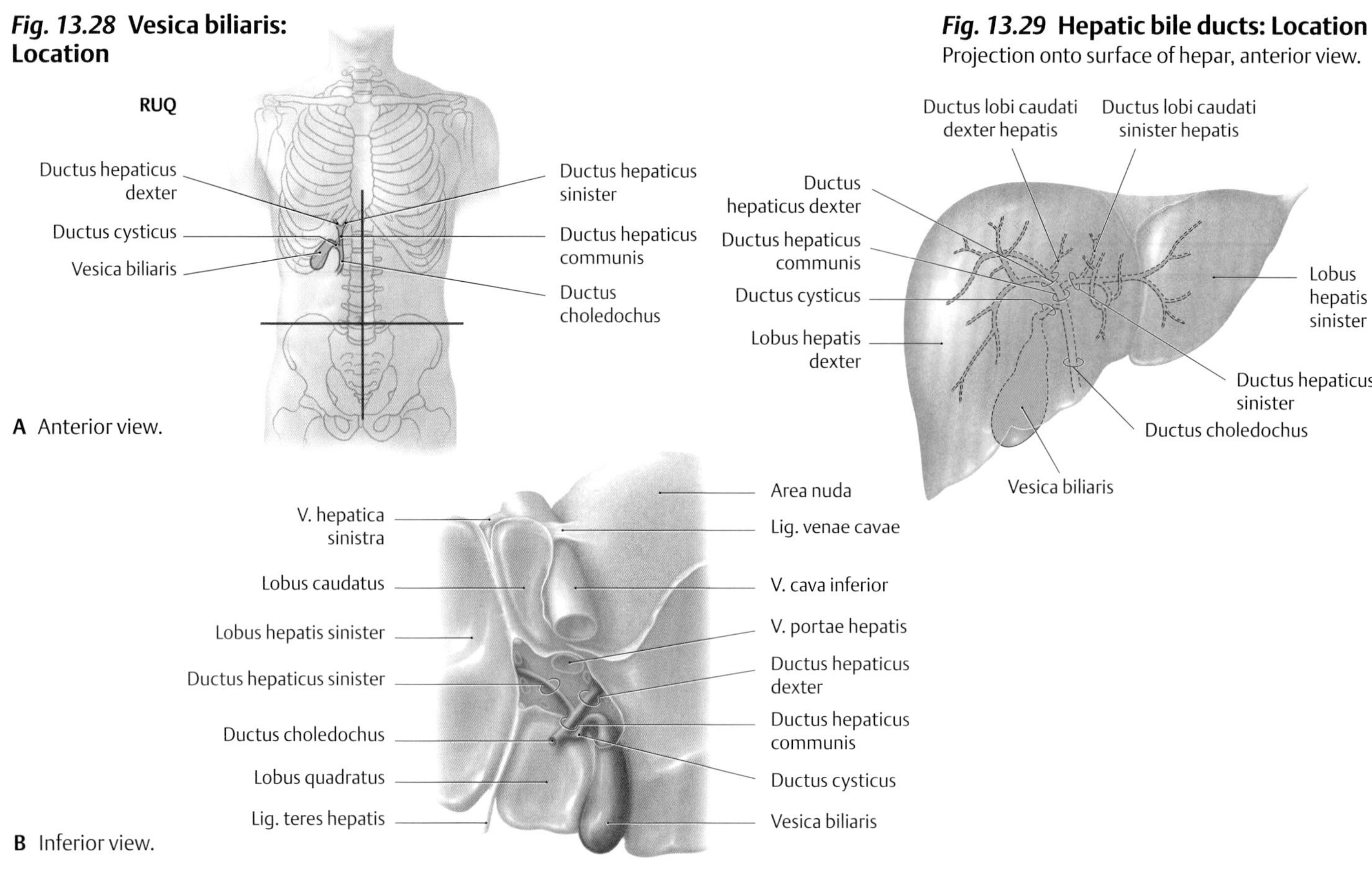
RUQ
Ductus hepaticus dexter
Ductus cysticus
Vesica biliaris
Ductus hepaticus sinister
Ductus hepaticus communis
Ductus choledochus
Ductus lobi caudati dexter hepatis
Ductus lobi caudati sinister hepatis
Ductus hepaticus dexter
Ductus hepaticus communis
Ductus cysticus
Lobus hepatis dexter
Lobus hepatis sinister
Ductus hepaticus sinister
Ductus choledochus
Vesica biliaris
V. hepatica sinistra
Lobus caudatus
Lobus hepatis sinister
Ductus hepaticus sinister
Ductus choledochus
Lobus quadratus
Lig. teres hepatis
Area nuda
Lig. venae cavae
V. cava inferior
V. portae hepatis
Ductus hepaticus dexter
Ductus hepaticus communis
Ductus cysticus
Vesica biliaris

Fig. 13.28 **Vesica biliaris: Location**

A Anterior view.

B Inferior view.

Fig. 13.29 **Hepatic bile ducts: Location**

Projection onto surface of hepar, anterior view.

Fig. 13.30 **Biliary sphincter system**

Duodenum (wall)
Ampulla hepato-pancreatica
M. sphincter ductus choledochi
M. sphincter ductus pancreatici
M. sphincter ampullae hepatopancreaticae

A Sphincters of the pancreatic and bile ducts.

Duodenum, tunica muscularis
Stratum longitudinale
Stratum circulare
Ductus choledochus
Longitudinal slips of duodenal muscle on ductus choledochus
M. sphincter ampullae hepato-pancreaticae
Ductus pancreaticus

B Sphincter system in the duodenal wall.

Fig. 13.31 **Extrahepatic bile ducts**

Anterior view. *Opened:* vesica biliaris and duodenum.

Ductus hepaticus dexter
Ductus cysticus
Vesica biliaris
Collum
Infundibulum
Corpus
Fundus
Papilla duodeni minor
Papilla duodeni major (papilla of Vater)
Pars descendens duodeni
Ductus hepaticus sinister
Ductus hepaticus communis
Pars superior duodeni
Ductus choledochus
Ductus pancreaticus accessorius
Ductus pancreaticus
Pars horizontalis duodeni

Fig. 13.32 **Biliary tract in situ**
Anterior view. *Removed:* Gaster, intestinum tenue, colon transversum, and large portions of hepar. The vesica biliaris is intraperitoneal, covered by peritoneum viscerale where it is not attached to hepar.

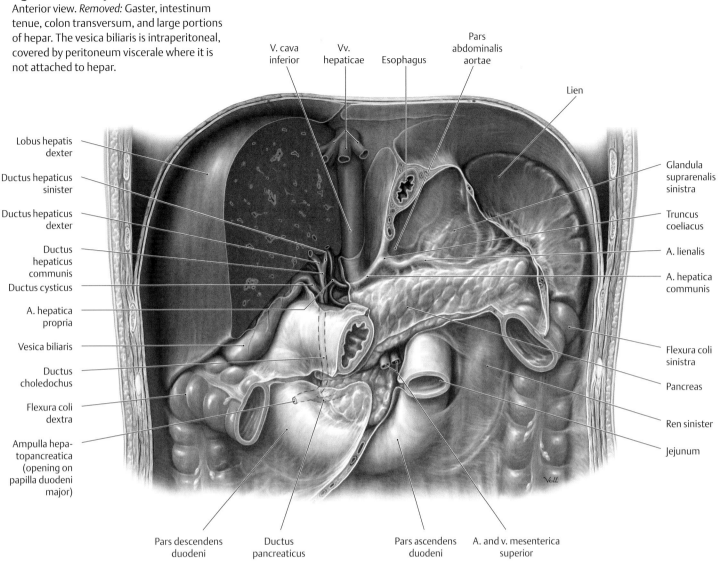

V. cava inferior
Vv. hepaticae
Esophagus
Pars abdominalis aortae
Lien
Lobus hepatis dexter
Ductus hepaticus sinister
Ductus hepaticus dexter
Ductus hepaticus communis
Ductus cysticus
A. hepatica propria
Vesica biliaris
Ductus choledochus
Flexura coli dextra
Ampulla hepatopancreatica (opening on papilla duodeni major)
Glandula suprarenalis sinistra
Truncus coeliacus
A. lienalis
A. hepatica communis
Flexura coli sinistra
Pancreas
Ren sinister
Jejunum
Pars descendens duodeni
Ductus pancreaticus
Pars ascendens duodeni
A. and v. mesenterica superior

Clinical

Obstruction of the ductus choledochus

As bile is stored and concentrated in vesica biliaris, certain substances, such as cholesterol, may crystallize, resulting in the formation of gallstones. Migration of gallstones into the ductus choledochus causes severe pain (colic). Gallstones may also block the ductus pancreaticus in the papillary regions, causing highly acute or even life-threatening pancreatitis.

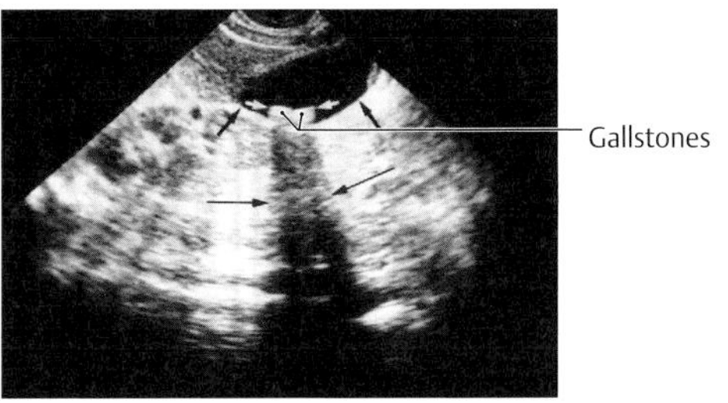
Gallstones

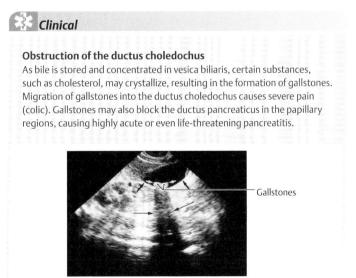

Ultrasound appearance of two gallstones. Black arrows mark the echo-free area behind the stones.

Pancreas & Lien

Fig. 13.33 **Pancreas and lien: Location**

RUQ
LUQ
Pancreas
Lien
Costa X

Gaster
Omentum minus (lig. hepato-gastricum)
Lig. gastro-splenicum
Bursa omentalis, recessus splenicus
Pancreas
Lig. splenorenale
Hepar
Lien
V. cava inferior
Pars abdominalis aortae
Ren sinister

A Anterior view. **B** Left lateral view. **C** Transverse section, inferior view.

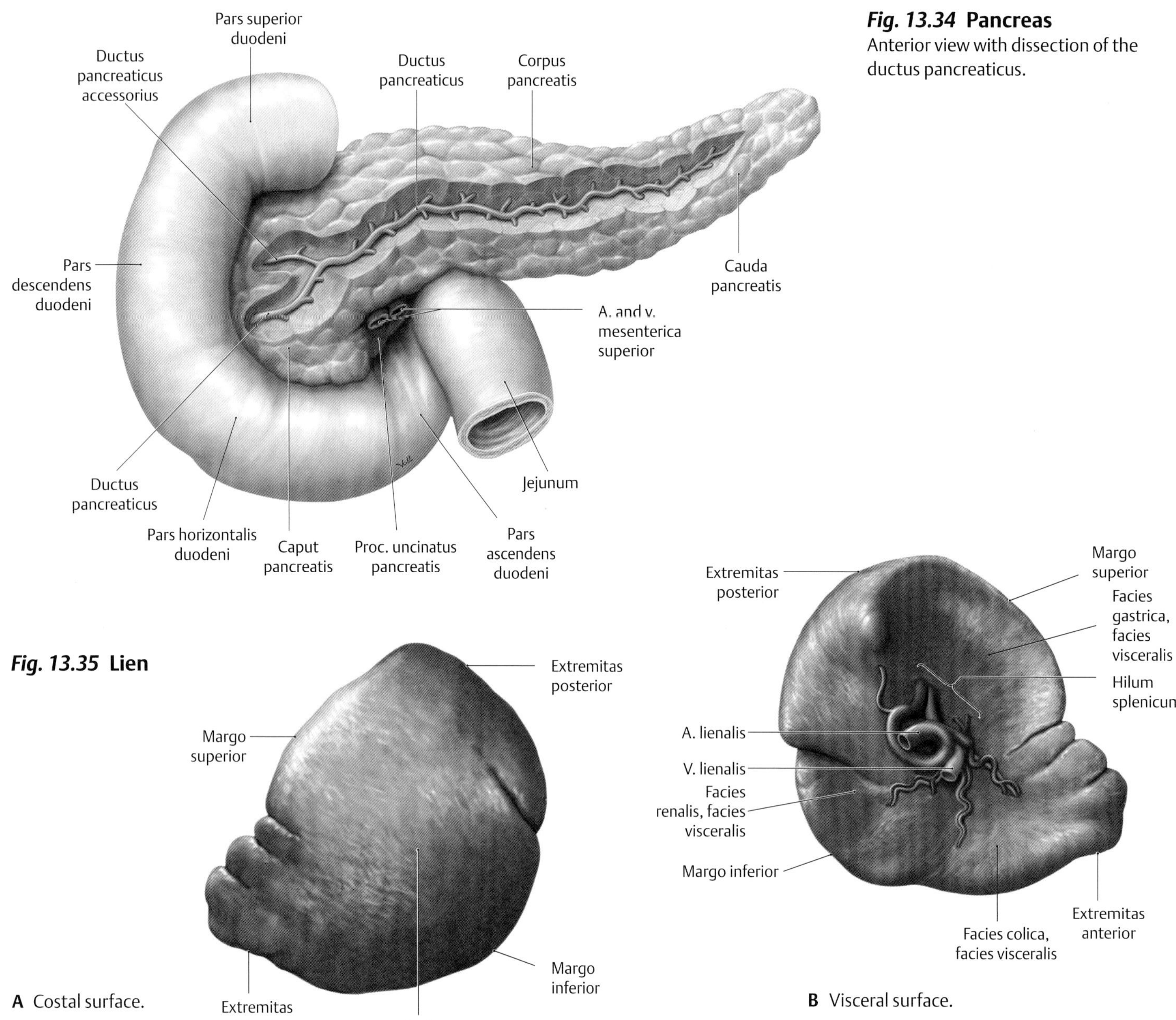
Pars superior duodeni
Ductus pancreaticus accessorius
Ductus pancreaticus
Corpus pancreatis
Pars descendens duodeni
Cauda pancreatis
A. and v. mesenterica superior
Ductus pancreaticus
Jejunum
Pars horizontalis duodeni
Caput pancreatis
Proc. uncinatus pancreatis
Pars ascendens duodeni
Extremitas posterior
Margo superior
Margo inferior
Extremitas anterior
Facies diaphragmatica
Extremitas posterior
Margo superior
Facies gastrica, facies visceralis
Hilum splenicum
A. lienalis
V. lienalis
Facies renalis, facies visceralis
Margo inferior
Extremitas anterior
Facies colica, facies visceralis

Fig. 13.34 **Pancreas**
Anterior view with dissection of the ductus pancreaticus.

Fig. 13.35 **Lien**

A Costal surface.

B Visceral surface.

Fig. 13.36 **Pancreas and lien in situ**

Anterior view. *Removed:* Hepar, gaster, intestinum tenue, and intestinum crassum. The pancreas is retroperitoneal, while lien is intraperitoneal.

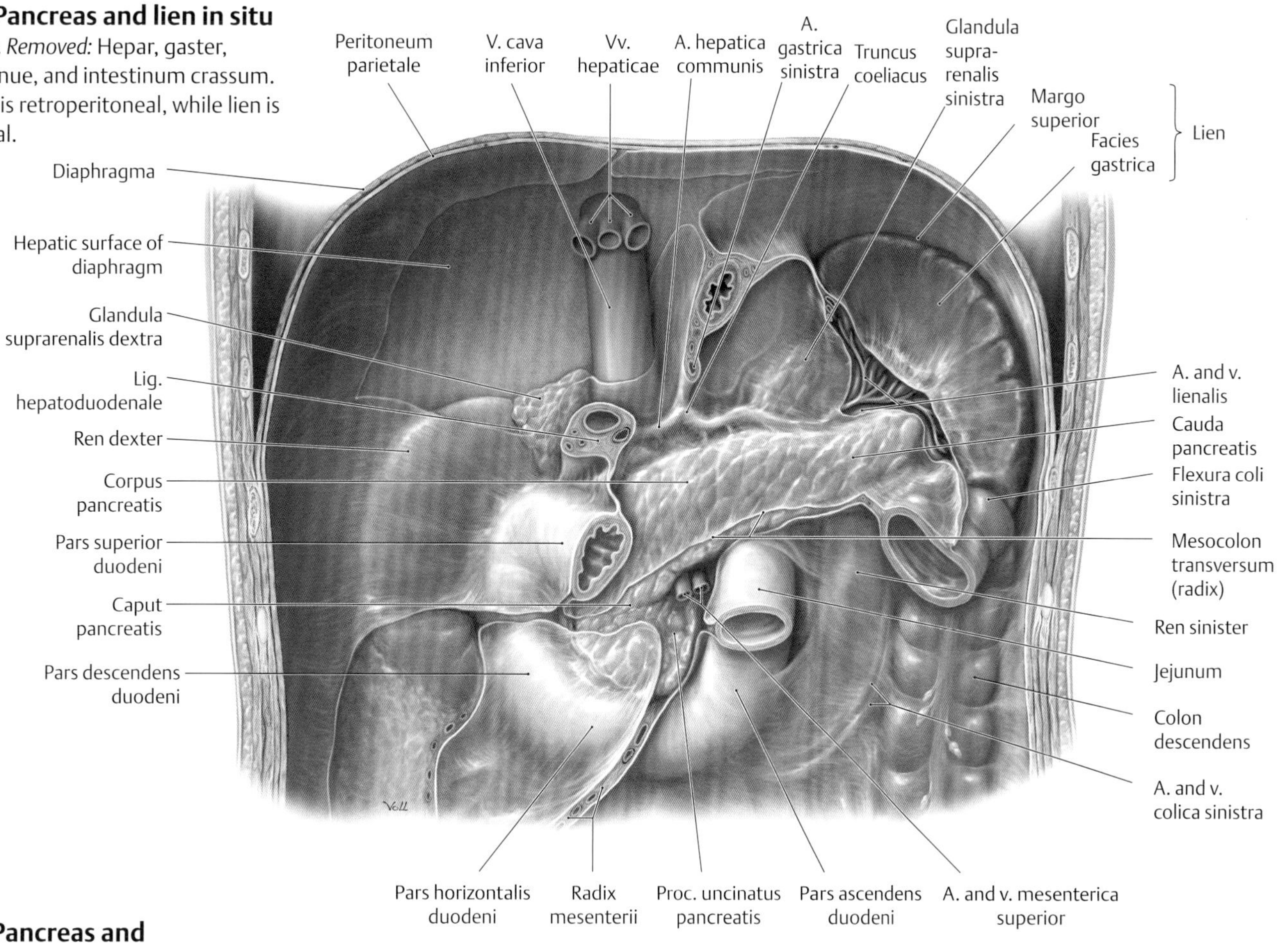

Peritoneum parietale
V. cava inferior
Vv. hepaticae
A. hepatica communis
A. gastrica sinistra
Truncus coeliacus
Glandula suprarenalis sinistra
Margo superior
Facies gastrica
Lien
Diaphragma
Hepatic surface of diaphragm
Glandula suprarenalis dextra
Lig. hepatoduodenale
Ren dexter
Corpus pancreatis
Pars superior duodeni
Caput pancreatis
Pars descendens duodeni
A. and v. lienalis
Cauda pancreatis
Flexura coli sinistra
Mesocolon transversum (radix)
Ren sinister
Jejunum
Colon descendens
A. and v. colica sinistra
Pars horizontalis duodeni
Radix mesenterii
Proc. uncinatus pancreatis
Pars ascendens duodeni
A. and v. mesenterica superior

Fig. 13.37 **Pancreas and lien: Transverse section**

Inferior view. Section through L I vertebra.

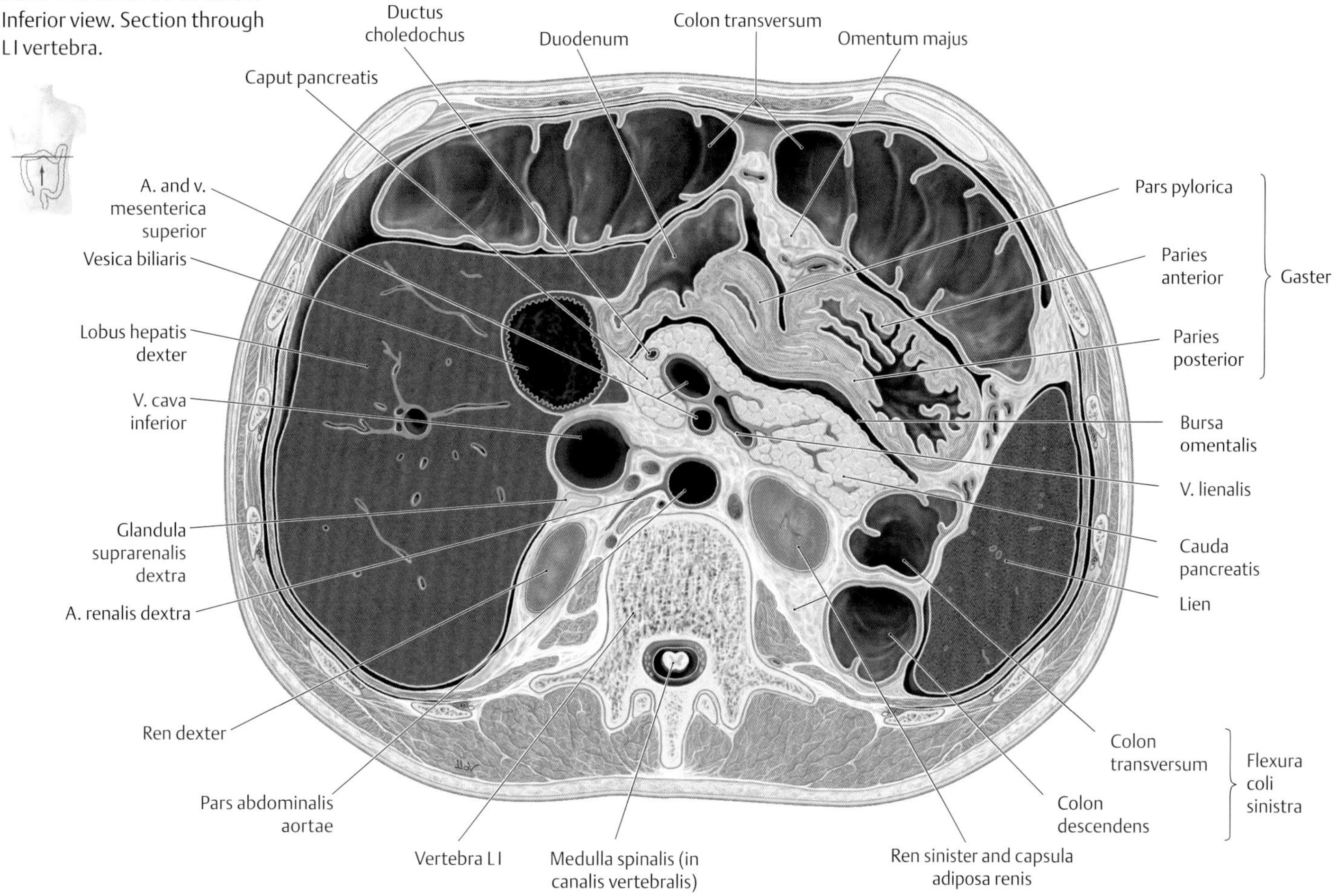

Ductus choledochus
Duodenum
Colon transversum
Omentum majus
Caput pancreatis
A. and v. mesenterica superior
Vesica biliaris
Lobus hepatis dexter
V. cava inferior
Glandula suprarenalis dextra
A. renalis dextra
Ren dexter
Pars abdominalis aortae
Vertebra L I
Medulla spinalis (in canalis vertebralis)
Ren sinister and capsula adiposa renis
Pars pylorica
Paries anterior
Paries posterior
Gaster
Bursa omentalis
V. lienalis
Cauda pancreatis
Lien
Colon transversum
Colon descendens
Flexura coli sinistra

Renes & Glandulae Suprarenales: Overview

Fig. 13.38 Renes gll. suprarenales: Location

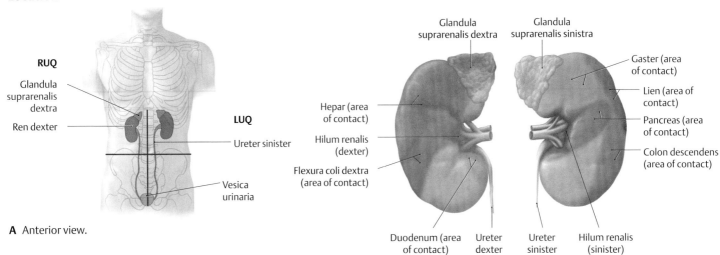

RUQ

Glandula suprarenalis dextra

Ren dexter

LUQ

Ureter sinister

Vesica urinaria

A Anterior view.

Costa XII

N. subcostalis

Ren dexter

N. iliohypogastricus

N. ilioinguinalis

B Posterior view with the trunk wall opened.

Fig. 13.39 Renes: Areas of organ contact

Anterior view.

Glandula suprarenalis dextra

Glandula suprarenalis sinistra

Hepar (area of contact)

Hilum renalis (dexter)

Flexura coli dextra (area of contact)

Gaster (area of contact)

Lien (area of contact)

Pancreas (area of contact)

Colon descendens (area of contact)

Duodenum (area of contact)

Ureter dexter

Ureter sinister

Hilum renalis (sinister)

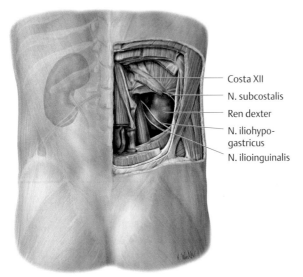

Fig. 13.40 Ren dexter in the renal bed

Sagittal section through the right renal bed.

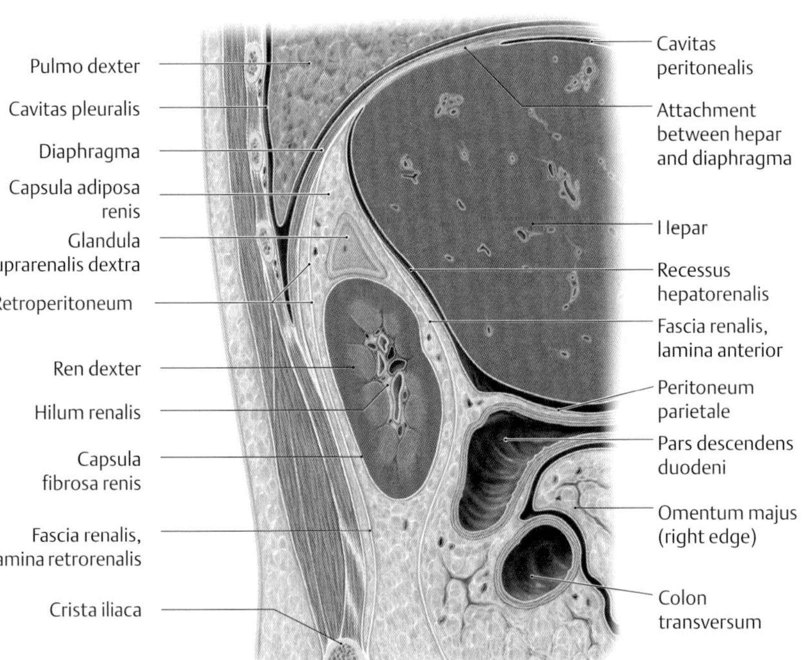

Pulmo dexter
Cavitas pleuralis
Diaphragma
Capsula adiposa renis
Glandula suprarenalis dextra
Retroperitoneum
Ren dexter
Hilum renalis
Capsula fibrosa renis
Fascia renalis, lamina retrorenalis
Crista iliaca
Cavitas peritonealis
Attachment between hepar and diaphragma
Hepar
Recessus hepatorenalis
Fascia renalis, lamina anterior
Peritoneum parietale
Pars descendens duodeni
Omentum majus (right edge)
Colon transversum

Fig. 13.41 Glandula suprarenalis

Anterior view.

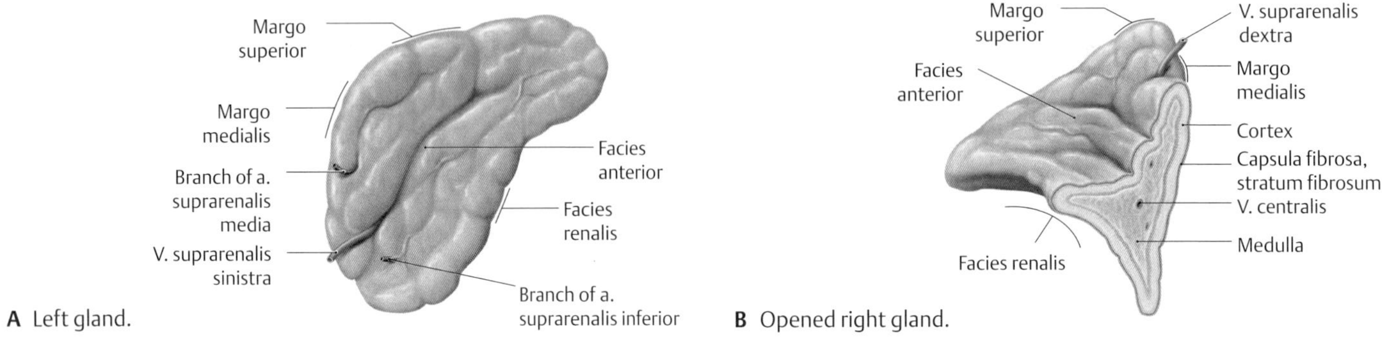

Margo superior
Margo medialis
Branch of a. suprarenalis media
V. suprarenalis sinistra
Facies anterior
Facies renalis
Branch of a. suprarenalis inferior
Margo superior
Facies anterior
Facies renalis
V. suprarenalis dextra
Margo medialis
Cortex
Capsula fibrosa, stratum fibrosum
V. centralis
Medulla

A Left gland.

B Opened right gland.

Fig. 13.42 Renes and gll. suprarenales in the retroperitoneum

Anterior view. Both renes and gll. suprarenales are retroperitoneal.

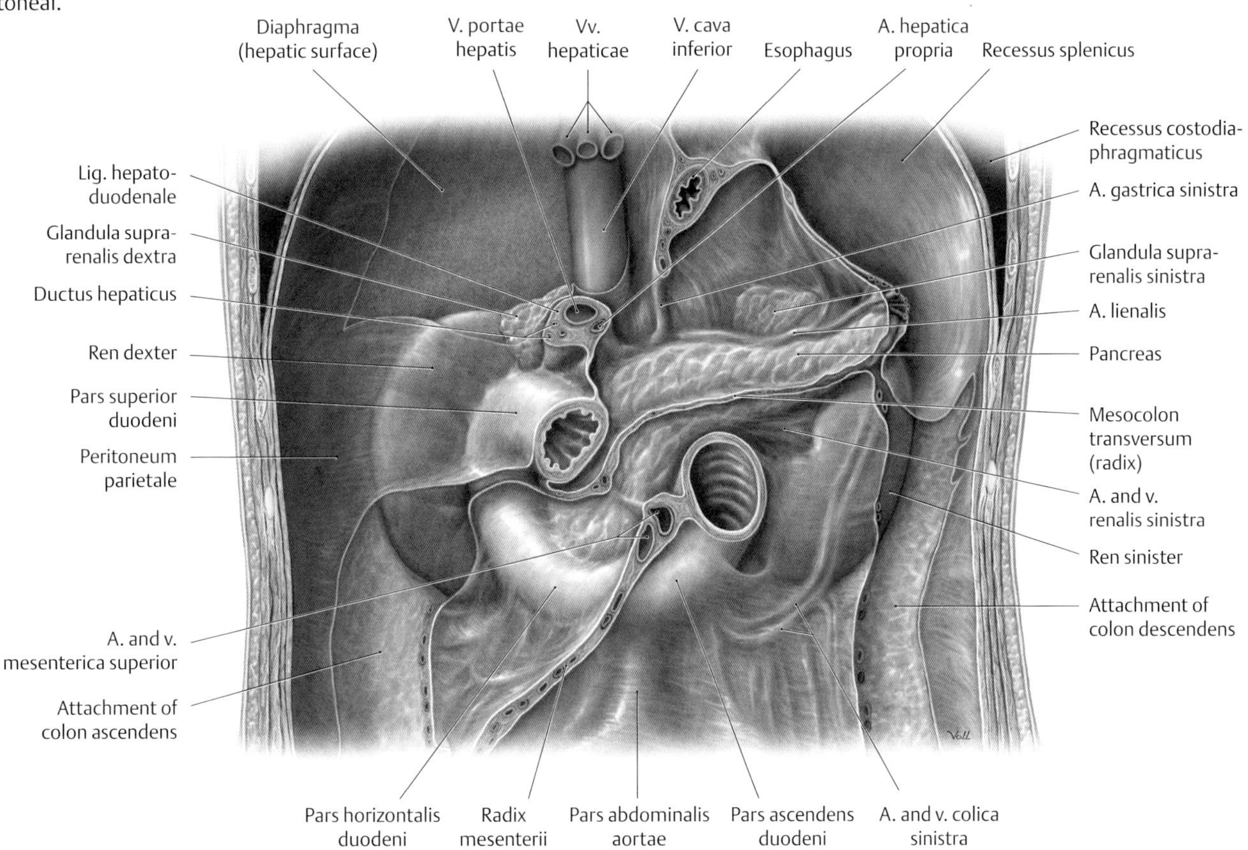
Diaphragma (hepatic surface)
V. portae hepatis
Vv. hepaticae
V. cava inferior
Esophagus
A. hepatica propria
Recessus splenicus
Recessus costodia-phragmaticus
A. gastrica sinistra
Glandula supra-renalis sinistra
A. lienalis
Pancreas
Mesocolon transversum (radix)
A. and v. renalis sinistra
Ren sinister
Attachment of colon descendens
Lig. hepato-duodenale
Glandula supra-renalis dextra
Ductus hepaticus
Ren dexter
Pars superior duodeni
Peritoneum parietale
A. and v. mesenterica superior
Attachment of colon ascendens
Pars horizontalis duodeni
Radix mesenterii
Pars abdominalis aortae
Pars ascendens duodeni
A. and v. colica sinistra

A _Removed:_ Intraperitoneal organs, along with portions of the colon ascendens and descendens.

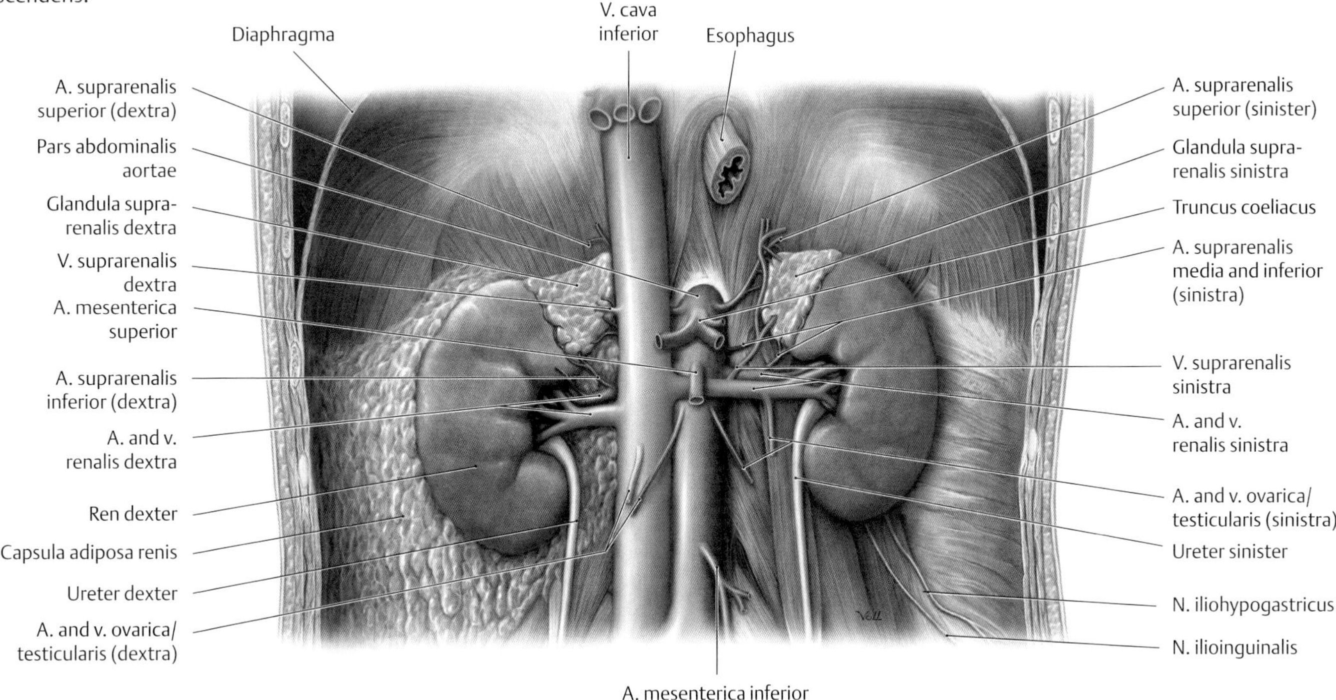
Diaphragma
V. cava inferior
Esophagus
A. suprarenalis superior (dextra)
Pars abdominalis aortae
Glandula supra-renalis dextra
V. suprarenalis dextra
A. mesenterica superior
A. suprarenalis inferior (dextra)
A. and v. renalis dextra
Ren dexter
Capsula adiposa renis
Ureter dexter
A. and v. ovarica/ testicularis (dextra)
A. suprarenalis superior (sinister)
Glandula supra-renalis sinistra
Truncus coeliacus
A. suprarenalis media and inferior (sinistra)
V. suprarenalis sinistra
A. and v. renalis sinistra
A. and v. ovarica/ testicularis (sinistra)
Ureter sinister
N. iliohypogastricus
N. ilioinguinalis
A. mesenterica inferior

B _Removed:_ Peritoneum, lien, and gastrointestinal organs, along with fat capsule (left side). _Retracted:_ Esophagus.

Renes & Glandulae Suprarenales: Features

Fig. 13.43 Ren dexter and gl. suprarenalis
Anterior view. *Removed:* Capsula adiposa renis.
Retracted: V. cava inferior.

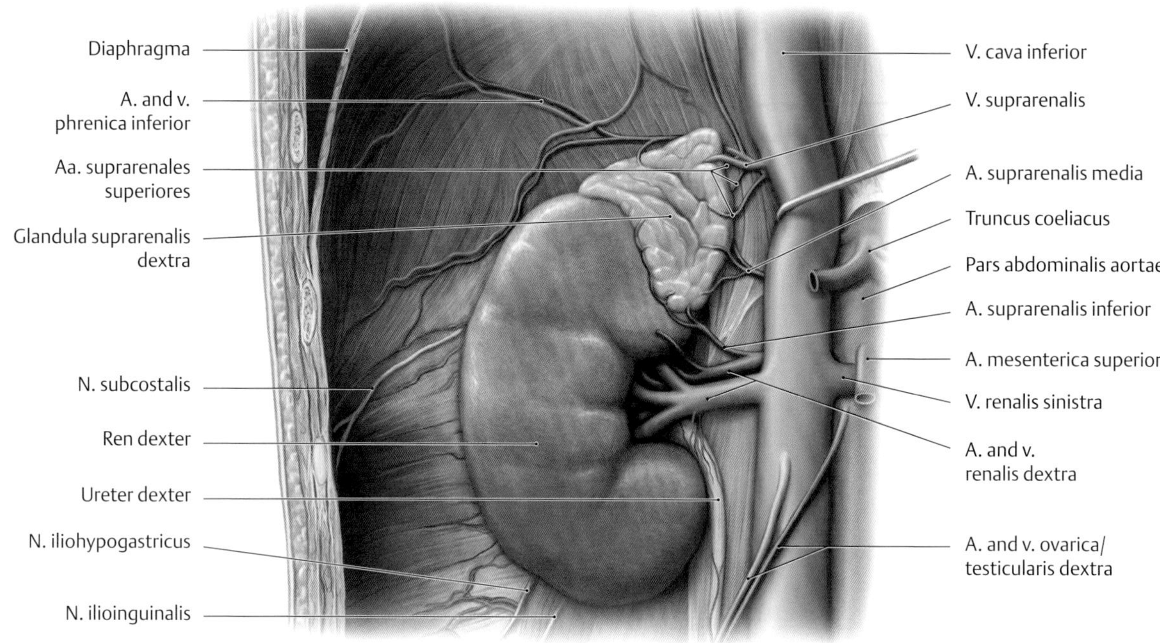
Diaphragma
A. and v. phrenica inferior
Aa. suprarenales superiores
Glandula suprarenalis dextra
N. subcostalis
Ren dexter
Ureter dexter
N. iliohypogastricus
N. ilioinguinalis
V. cava inferior
V. suprarenalis
A. suprarenalis media
Truncus coeliacus
Pars abdominalis aortae
A. suprarenalis inferior
A. mesenterica superior
V. renalis sinistra
A. and v. renalis dextra
A. and v. ovarica/ testicularis dextra

Fig. 13.45 Ren: Structure
Ren dexter with gl. suprarenalis.

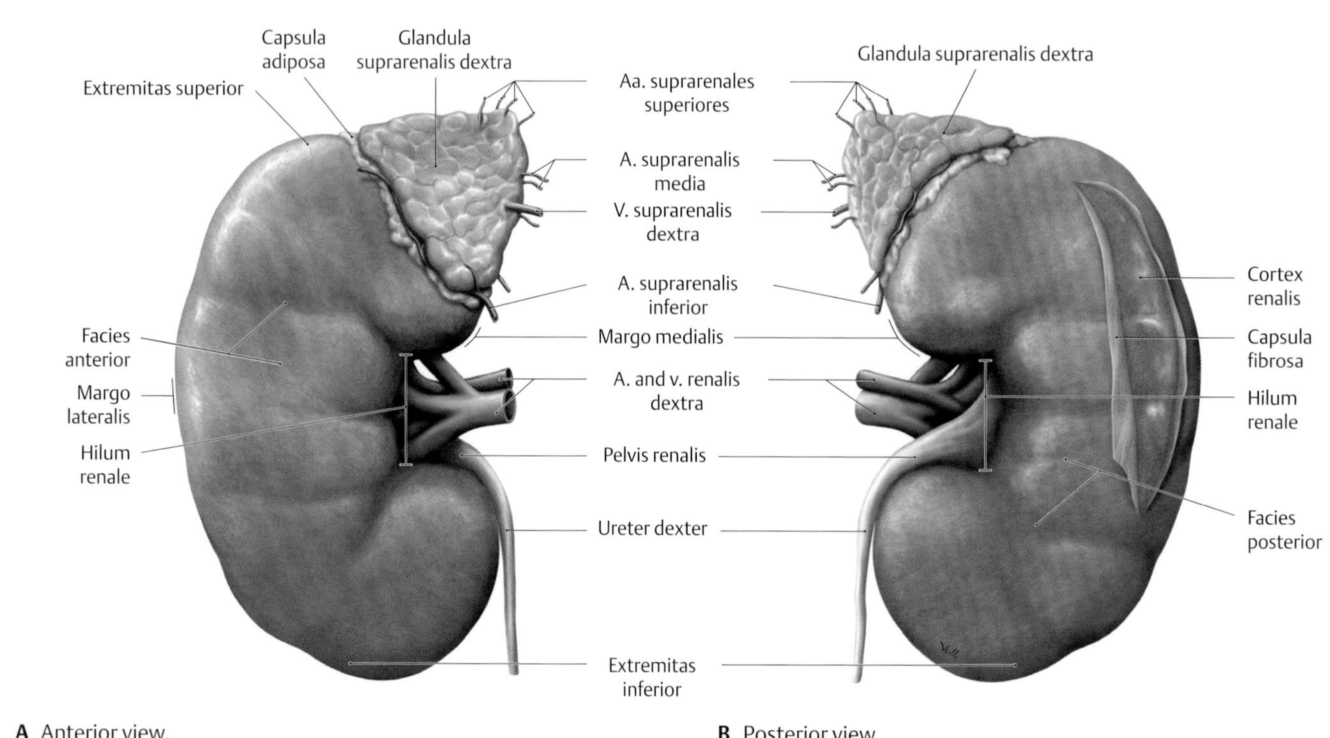
Capsula adiposa
Glandula suprarenalis dextra
Extremitas superior
Facies anterior
Margo lateralis
Hilum renale
Aa. suprarenales superiores
A. suprarenalis media
V. suprarenalis dextra
A. suprarenalis inferior
Margo medialis
A. and v. renalis dextra
Pelvis renalis
Ureter dexter
Extremitas inferior
Glandula suprarenalis dextra
Cortex renalis
Capsula fibrosa
Hilum renale
Facies posterior

A Anterior view.

B Posterior view.

Fig. 13.44 **Ren sinister and gl. suprarenalis**
Anterior view. *Removed:* Capsula adiposa renis.
Retracted: Pancreas.

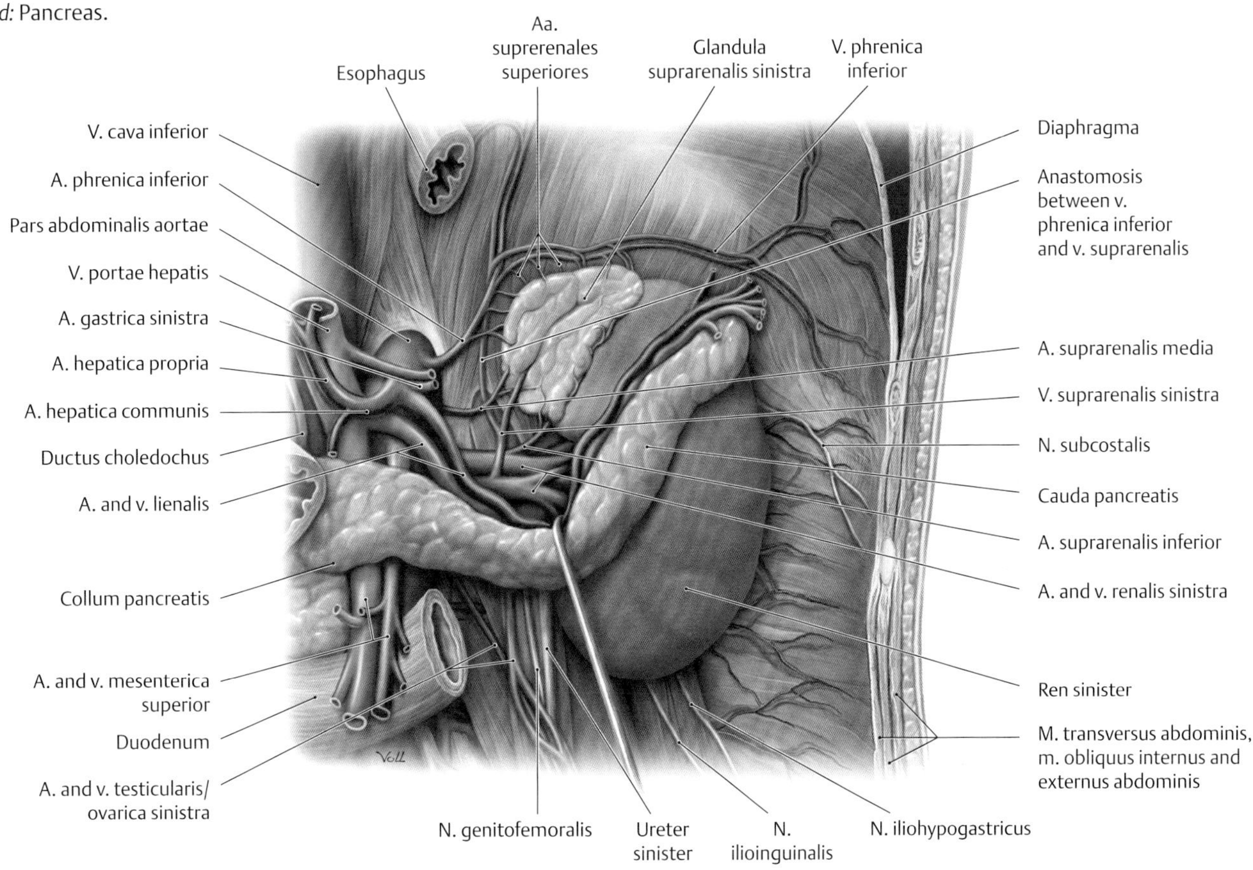
Esophagus
Aa. suprerenales superiores
Glandula suprarenalis sinistra
V. phrenica inferior
V. cava inferior
A. phrenica inferior
Pars abdominalis aortae
V. portae hepatis
A. gastrica sinistra
A. hepatica propria
A. hepatica communis
Ductus choledochus
A. and v. lienalis
Collum pancreatis
A. and v. mesenterica superior
Duodenum
A. and v. testicularis/ ovarica sinistra
Diaphragma
Anastomosis between v. phrenica inferior and v. suprarenalis
A. suprarenalis media
V. suprarenalis sinistra
N. subcostalis
Cauda pancreatis
A. suprarenalis inferior
A. and v. renalis sinistra
Ren sinister
M. transversus abdominis, m. obliquus internus and externus abdominis
N. genitofemoralis
Ureter sinister
N. ilioinguinalis
N. iliohypogastricus

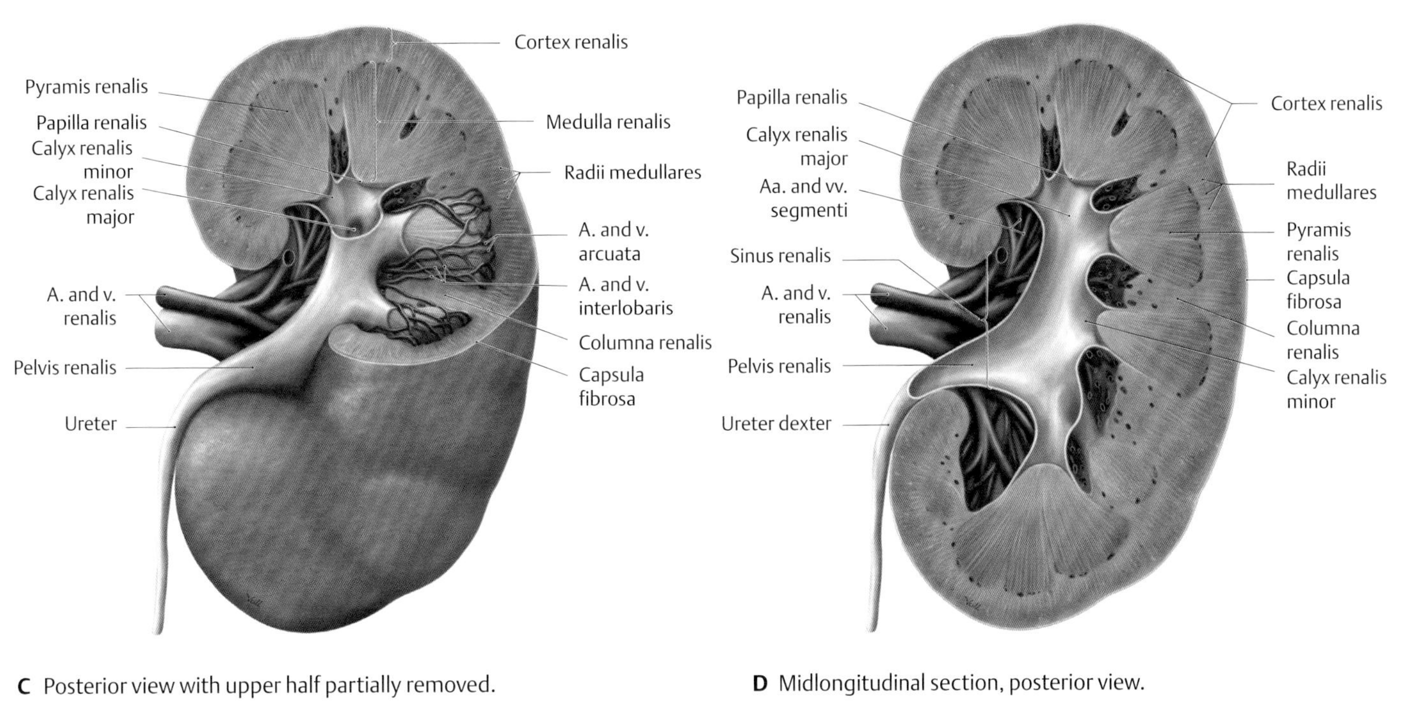
Cortex renalis
Pyramis renalis
Papilla renalis
Calyx renalis minor
Calyx renalis major
Medulla renalis
Radii medullares
A. and v. arcuata
A. and v. interlobaris
Columna renalis
Capsula fibrosa
A. and v. renalis
Pelvis renalis
Ureter
Papilla renalis
Calyx renalis major
Aa. and vv. segmenti
Sinus renalis
A. and v. renalis
Pelvis renalis
Ureter dexter
Cortex renalis
Radii medullares
Pyramis renalis
Capsula fibrosa
Columna renalis
Calyx renalis minor

C Posterior view with upper half partially removed.

D Midlongitudinal section, posterior view.

Ureter

The ureters cross a. iliaca communis at its bifurcation into aa. iliaca externa and interna.

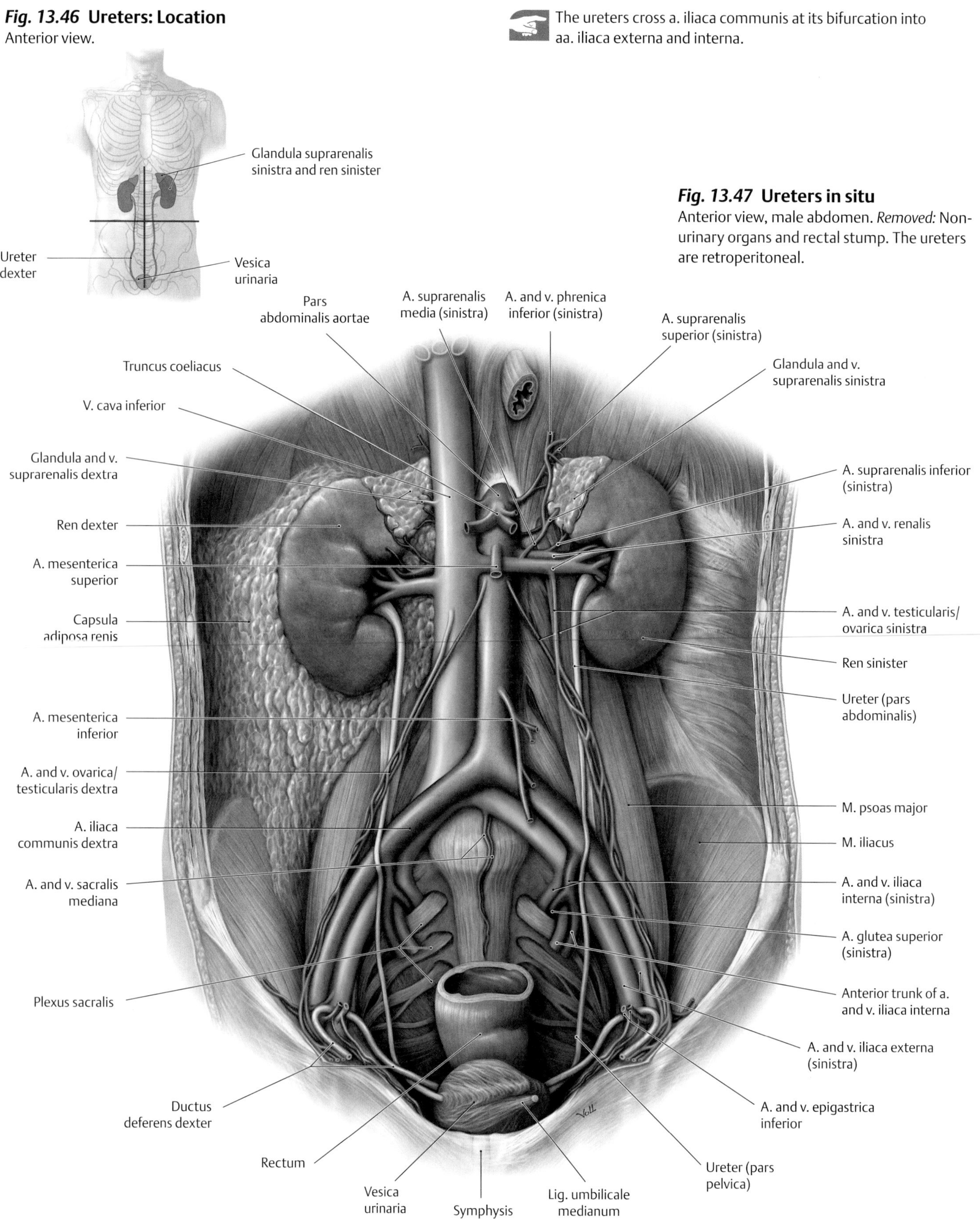

Glandula suprarenalis sinistra and ren sinister
Ureter dexter
Vesica urinaria
Pars abdominalis aortae
A. suprarenalis media (sinistra)
A. and v. phrenica inferior (sinistra)
A. suprarenalis superior (sinistra)
Glandula and v. suprarenalis sinistra
Truncus coeliacus
V. cava inferior
Glandula and v. suprarenalis dextra
Ren dexter
A. mesenterica superior
Capsula adiposa renis
A. mesenterica inferior
A. and v. ovarica/ testicularis dextra
A. iliaca communis dextra
A. and v. sacralis mediana
Plexus sacralis
Ductus deferens dexter
Rectum
Vesica urinaria
Symphysis pubica
Lig. umbilicale medianum
Ureter (pars pelvica)
A. and v. epigastrica inferior
A. and v. iliaca externa (sinistra)
Anterior trunk of a. and v. iliaca interna
A. glutea superior (sinistra)
A. and v. iliaca interna (sinistra)
M. iliacus
M. psoas major
Ureter (pars abdominalis)
Ren sinister
A. and v. testicularis/ ovarica sinistra
A. and v. renalis sinistra
A. suprarenalis inferior (sinistra)

Fig. 13.46 **Ureters: Location**
Anterior view.

Fig. 13.47 **Ureters in situ**
Anterior view, male abdomen. *Removed:* Non-urinary organs and rectal stump. The ureters are retroperitoneal.

Fig. 13.48 Ureter in the male pelvis
Superior view.

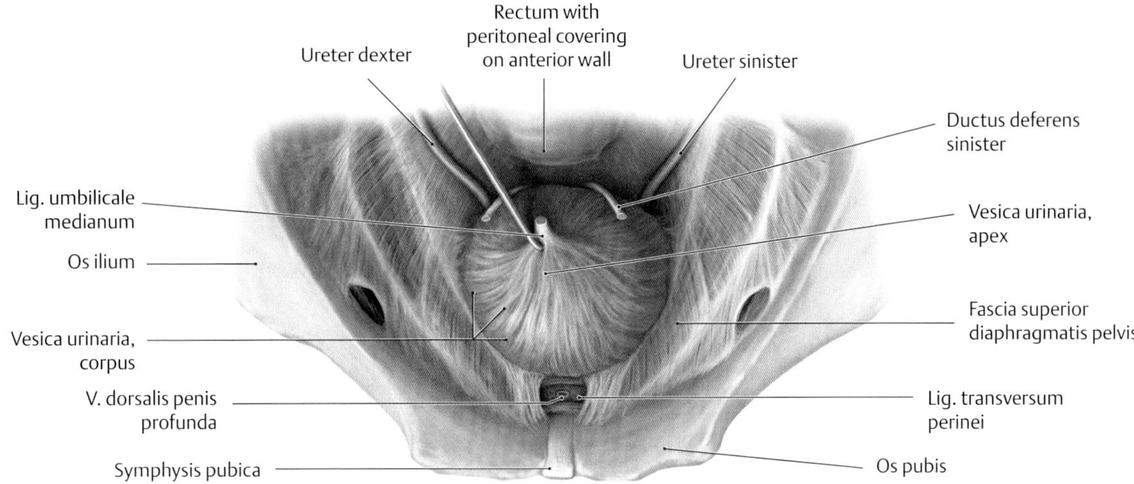
Rectum with peritoneal covering on anterior wall
Ureter dexter
Ureter sinister
Ductus deferens sinister
Lig. umbilicale medianum
Vesica urinaria, apex
Os ilium
Fascia superior diaphragmatis pelvis
Vesica urinaria, corpus
V. dorsalis penis profunda
Lig. transversum perinei
Symphysis pubica
Os pubis

Fig. 13.49 Ureter in the female pelvis
Superior view.

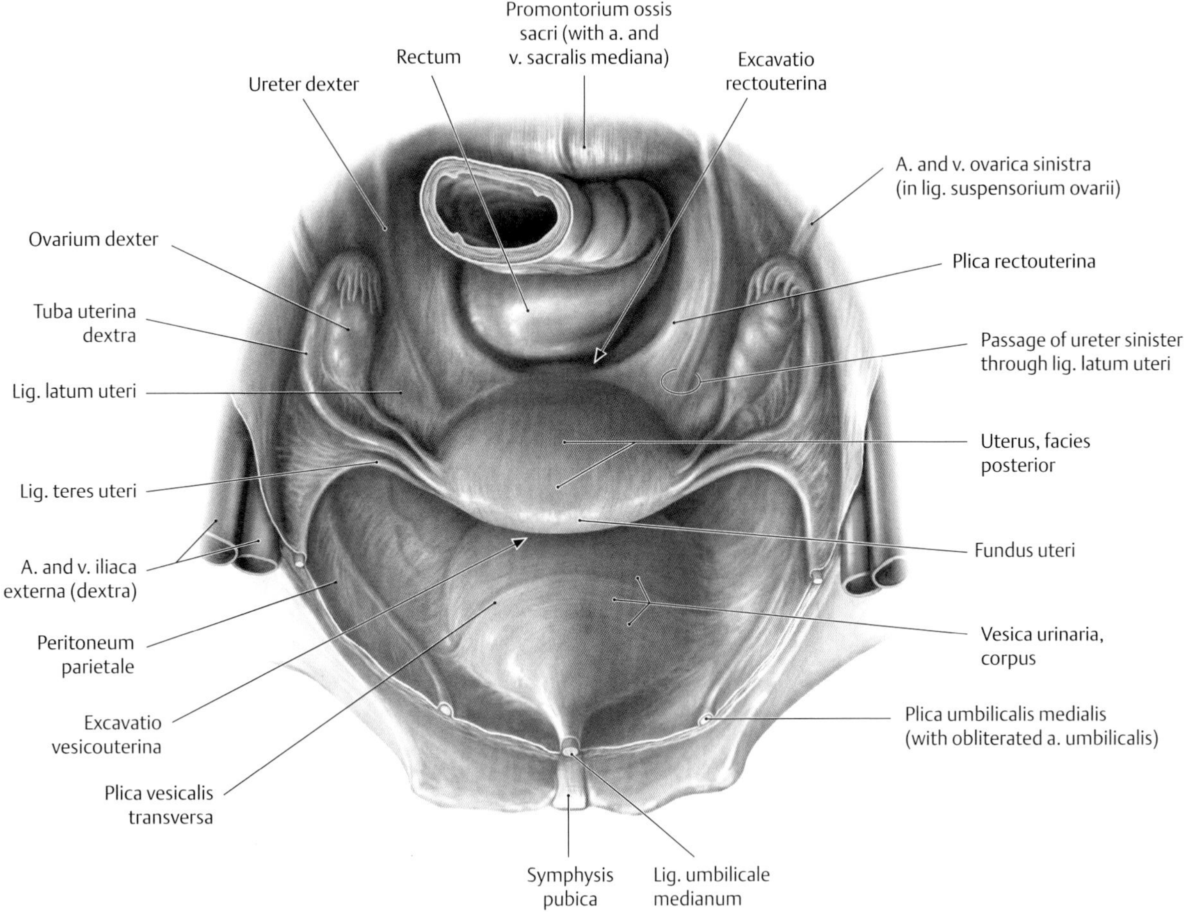
Promontorium ossis sacri (with a. and v. sacralis mediana)
Rectum
Ureter dexter
Excavatio rectouterina
A. and v. ovarica sinistra (in lig. suspensorium ovarii)
Ovarium dexter
Plica rectouterina
Tuba uterina dextra
Passage of ureter sinister through lig. latum uteri
Lig. latum uteri
Uterus, facies posterior
Lig. teres uteri
Fundus uteri
A. and v. iliaca externa (dextra)
Vesica urinaria, corpus
Peritoneum parietale
Excavatio vesicouterina
Plica umbilicalis medialis (with obliterated a. umbilicalis)
Plica vesicalis transversa
Symphysis pubica
Lig. umbilicale medianum

Vesica Urinaria

Fig. 13.50 **Male vesica urinaria**

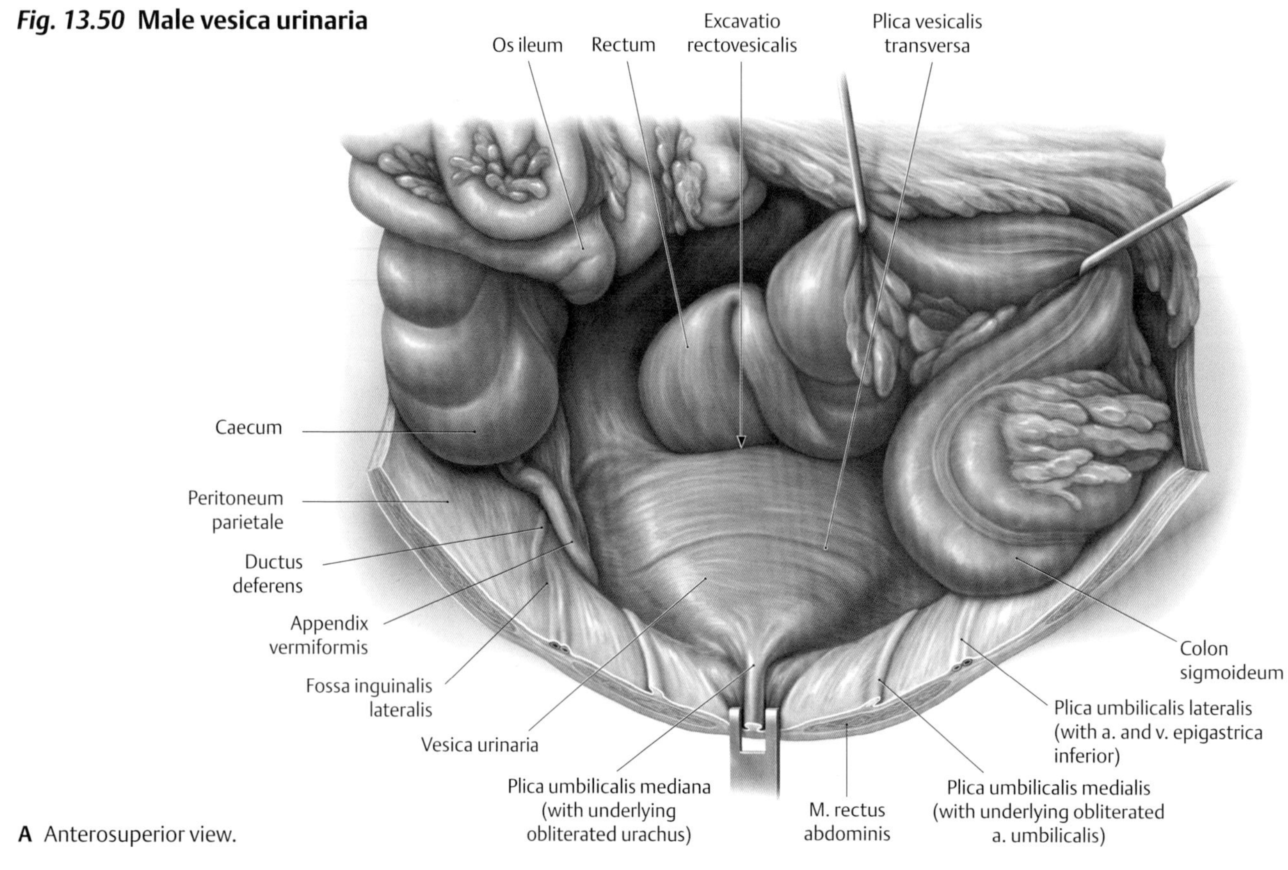
Os ileum
Rectum
Excavatio rectovesicalis
Plica vesicalis transversa
Caecum
Peritoneum parietale
Ductus deferens
Appendix vermiformis
Fossa inguinalis lateralis
Vesica urinaria
Plica umbilicalis mediana (with underlying obliterated urachus)
M. rectus abdominis
Plica umbilicalis medialis (with underlying obliterated a. umbilicalis)
Plica umbilicalis lateralis (with a. and v. epigastrica inferior)
Colon sigmoideum

A Anterosuperior view.

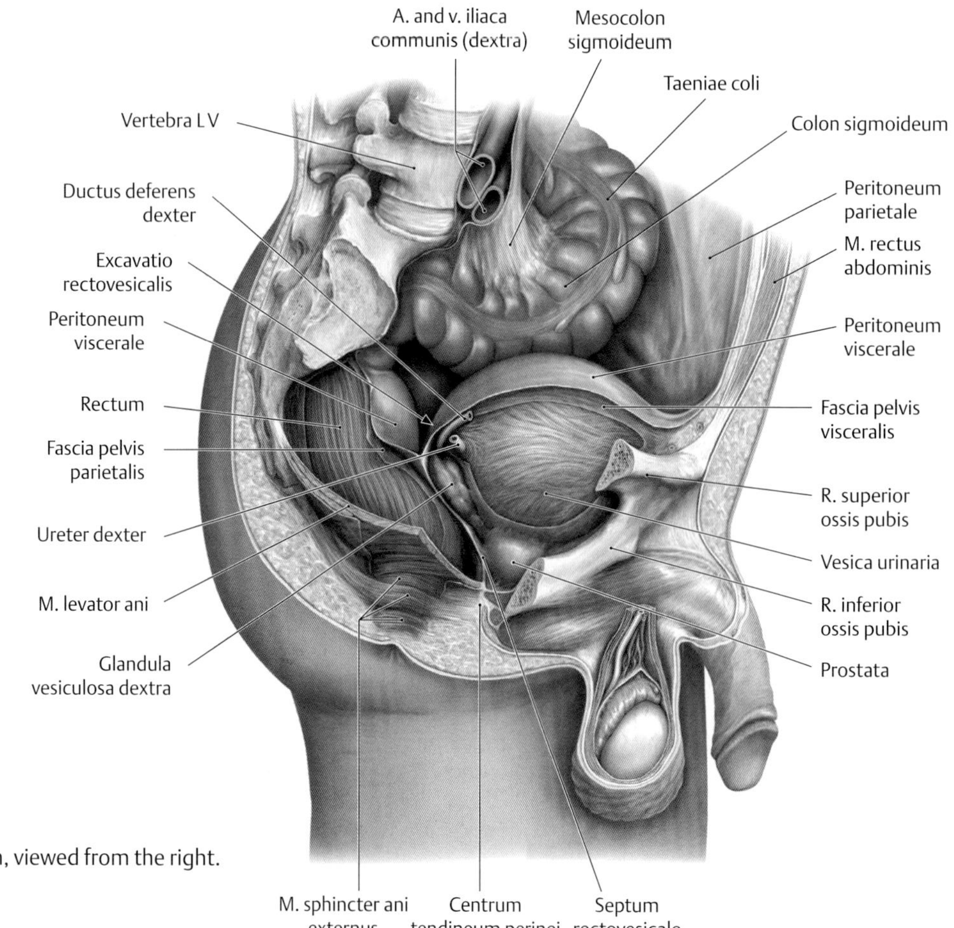
A. and v. iliaca communis (dextra)
Mesocolon sigmoideum
Taeniae coli
Colon sigmoideum
Vertebra LV
Ductus deferens dexter
Excavatio rectovesicalis
Peritoneum viscerale
Rectum
Fascia pelvis parietalis
Ureter dexter
M. levator ani
Glandula vesiculosa dextra
Peritoneum parietale
M. rectus abdominis
Peritoneum viscerale
Fascia pelvis visceralis
R. superior ossis pubis
Vesica urinaria
R. inferior ossis pubis
Prostata
M. sphincter ani externus
Centrum tendineum perinei
Septum rectovesicale

B Parasagittal section, viewed from the right.

Vesica urinaria is retropubic and retroperitoneal in location.

Fig. 13.51 Female vesica urinaria

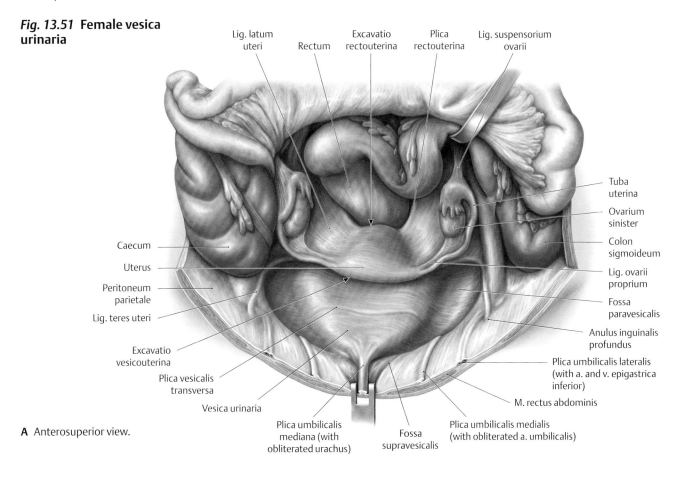

Lig. latum uteri
Rectum
Excavatio rectouterina
Plica rectouterina
Lig. suspensorium ovarii
Tuba uterina
Ovarium sinister
Colon sigmoideum
Lig. ovarii proprium
Fossa paravesicalis
Anulus inguinalis profundus
Plica umbilicalis lateralis (with a. and v. epigastrica inferior)
M. rectus abdominis
Plica umbilicalis medialis (with obliterated a. umbilicalis)
Fossa supravesicalis
Plica umbilicalis mediana (with obliterated urachus)
Vesica urinaria
Plica vesicalis transversa
Excavatio vesicouterina
Lig. teres uteri
Peritoneum parietale
Uterus
Caecum

A Anterosuperior view.

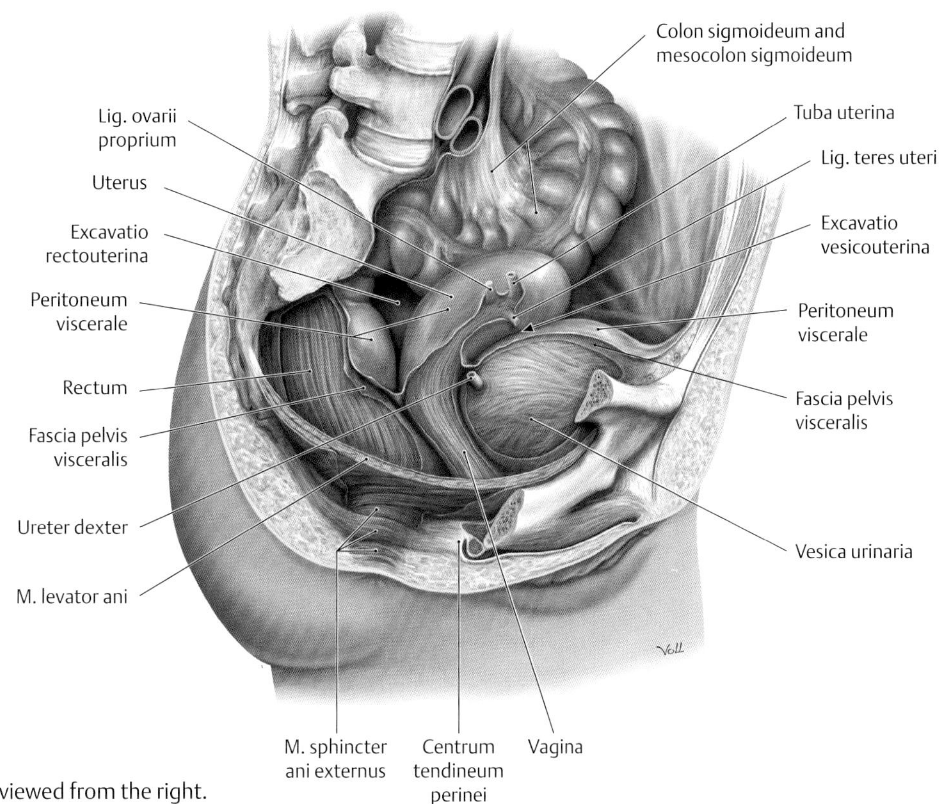
Colon sigmoideum and mesocolon sigmoideum
Tuba uterina
Lig. teres uteri
Excavatio vesicouterina
Peritoneum viscerale
Fascia pelvis visceralis
Vesica urinaria
Lig. ovarii proprium
Uterus
Excavatio rectouterina
Peritoneum viscerale
Rectum
Fascia pelvis visceralis
Ureter dexter
M. levator ani
M. sphincter ani externus
Centrum tendineum perinei
Vagina

B Parasagittal section, viewed from the right.

Vesica Urinaria & Urethra

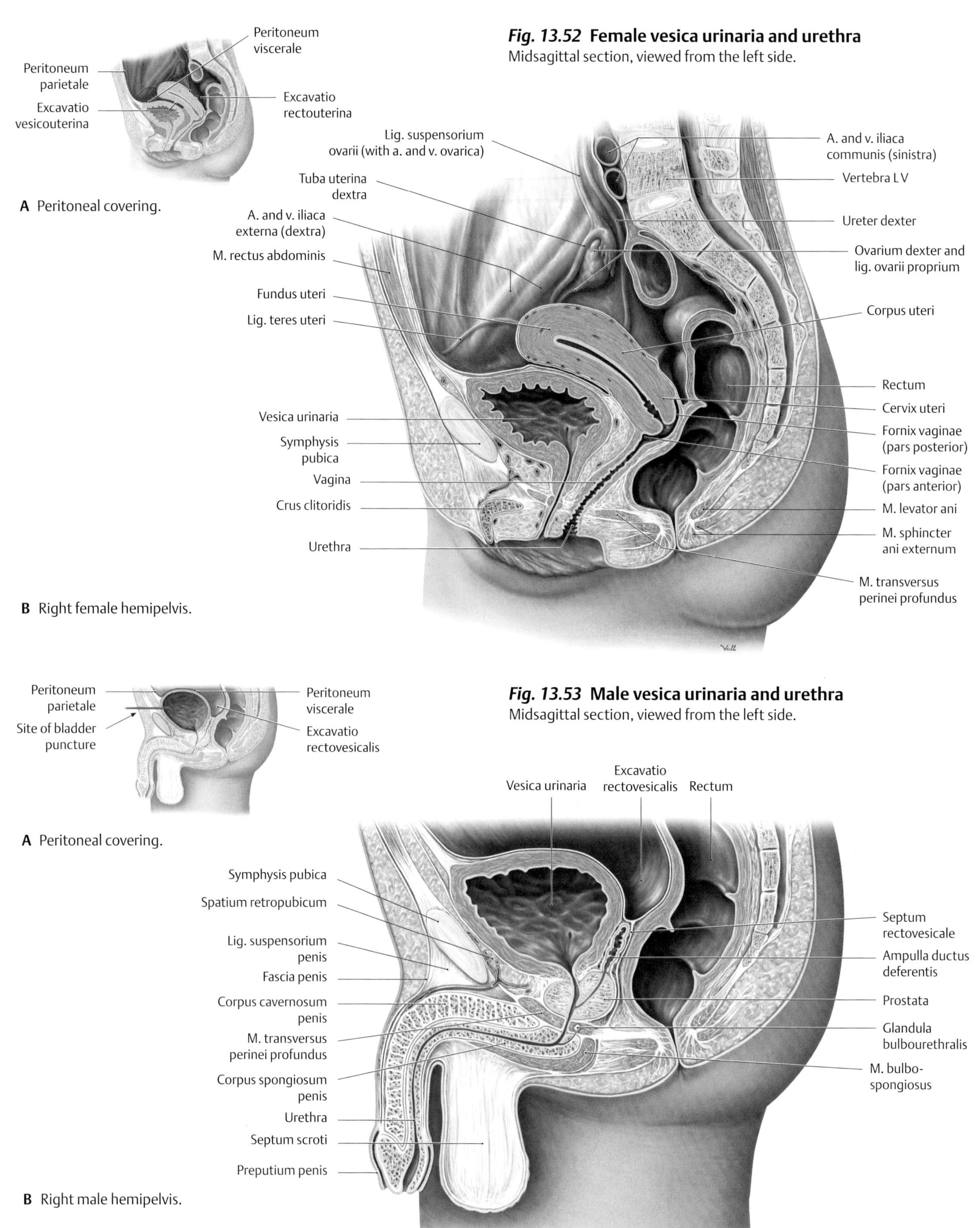
Peritoneum parietale
Peritoneum viscerale
Excavatio vesicouterina
Excavatio rectouterina
Lig. suspensorium ovarii (with a. and v. ovarica)
Tuba uterina dextra
A. and v. iliaca externa (dextra)
M. rectus abdominis
Fundus uteri
Lig. teres uteri
Vesica urinaria
Symphysis pubica
Vagina
Crus clitoridis
Urethra
A. and v. iliaca communis (sinistra)
Vertebra L V
Ureter dexter
Ovarium dexter and lig. ovarii proprium
Corpus uteri
Rectum
Cervix uteri
Fornix vaginae (pars posterior)
Fornix vaginae (pars anterior)
M. levator ani
M. sphincter ani externum
M. transversus perinei profundus
Peritoneum parietale
Site of bladder puncture
Peritoneum viscerale
Excavatio rectovesicalis
Vesica urinaria
Excavatio rectovesicalis
Rectum
Symphysis pubica
Spatium retropubicum
Lig. suspensorium penis
Fascia penis
Corpus cavernosum penis
M. transversus perinei profundus
Corpus spongiosum penis
Urethra
Septum scroti
Preputium penis
Septum rectovesicale
Ampulla ductus deferentis
Prostata
Glandula bulbourethralis
M. bulbo-spongiosus

Fig. 13.52 Female vesica urinaria and urethra
Midsagittal section, viewed from the left side.

A Peritoneal covering.

B Right female hemipelvis.

Fig. 13.53 Male vesica urinaria and urethra
Midsagittal section, viewed from the left side.

A Peritoneal covering.

B Right male hemipelvis.

Fig. 13.54 Wall structure

Anterior view of coronal section.

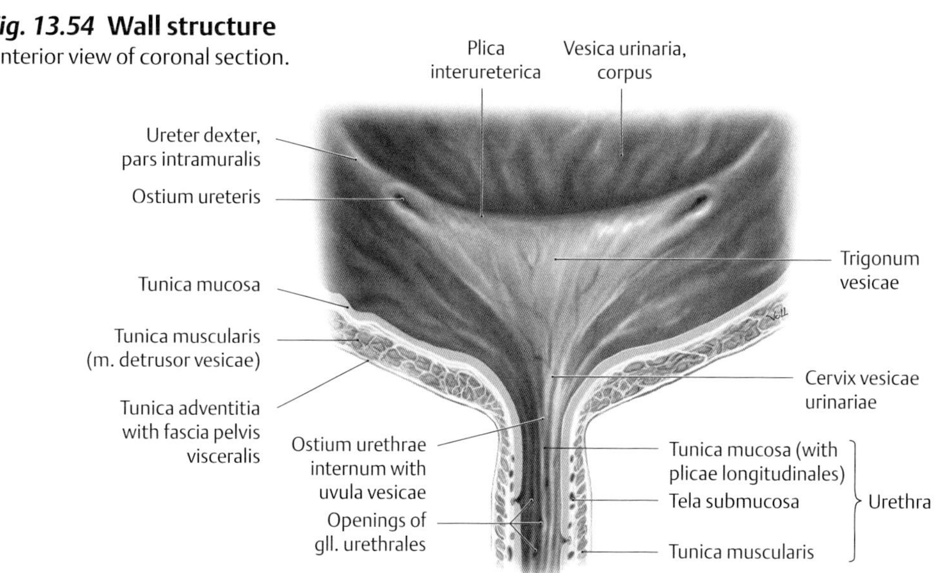
Plica interureterica
Vesica urinaria, corpus
Ureter dexter, pars intramuralis
Ostium ureteris
Trigonum vesicae
Tunica mucosa
Tunica muscularis (m. detrusor vesicae)
Cervix vesicae urinariae
Tunica adventitia with fascia pelvis visceralis
Ostium urethrae internum with uvula vesicae
Tunica mucosa (with plicae longitudinales)
Tela submucosa
Urethra
Openings of gll. urethrales
Tunica muscularis

Fig. 13.55 Vesica urinaria and urethra

Anterior view.

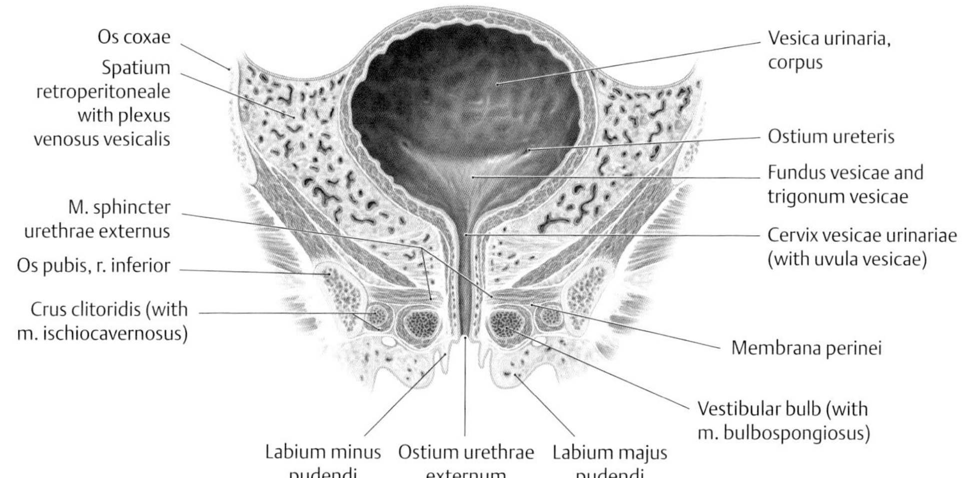
Os coxae
Spatium retroperitoneale with plexus venosus vesicalis
Vesica urinaria, corpus
Ostium ureteris
Fundus vesicae and trigonum vesicae
M. sphincter urethrae externus
Cervix vesicae urinariae (with uvula vesicae)
Os pubis, r. inferior
Crus clitoridis (with m. ischiocavernosus)
Membrana perinei
Vestibular bulb (with m. bulbospongiosus)
Labium minus pudendi
Ostium urethrae externum
Labium majus pudendi

A Female pelvis in coronal section.

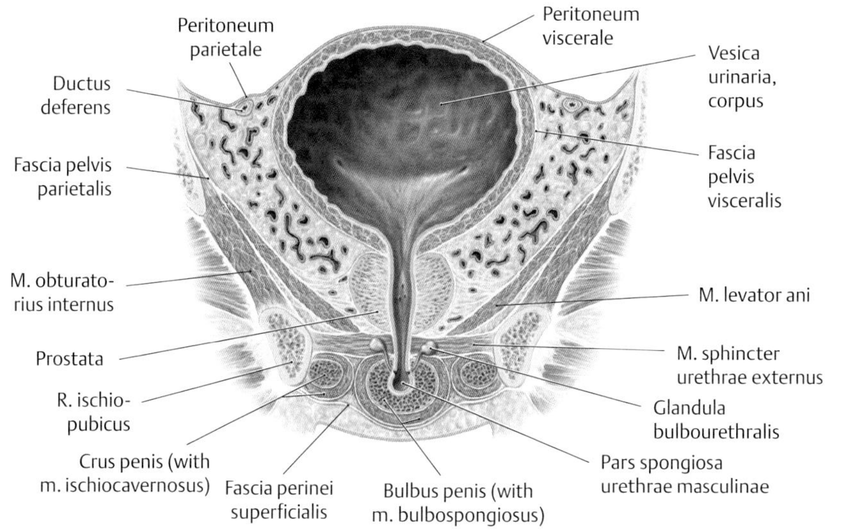
Peritoneum parietale
Peritoneum viscerale
Ductus deferens
Vesica urinaria, corpus
Fascia pelvis parietalis
Fascia pelvis visceralis
M. obturatorius internus
M. levator ani
Prostata
M. sphincter urethrae externus
R. ischiopubicus
Glandula bulbourethralis
Crus penis (with m. ischiocavernosus)
Fascia perinei superficialis
Bulbus penis (with m. bulbospongiosus)
Pars spongiosa urethrae masculinae

B Male pelvis in coronal section.

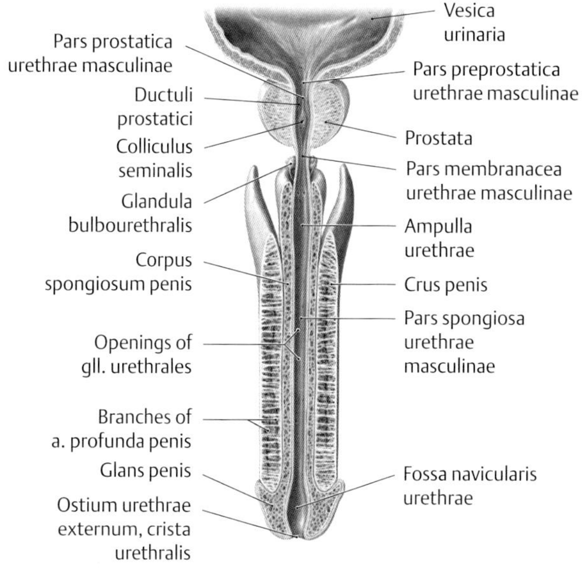
Vesica urinaria
Pars prostatica urethrae masculinae
Pars preprostatica urethrae masculinae
Ductuli prostatici
Prostata
Colliculus seminalis
Pars membranacea urethrae masculinae
Glandula bulbourethralis
Ampulla urethrae
Corpus spongiosum penis
Crus penis
Pars spongiosa urethrae masculinae
Openings of gll. urethrales
Branches of a. profunda penis
Glans penis
Fossa navicularis urethrae
Ostium urethrae externum, crista urethralis

C Male urethra in longitudinal section.

Overview of the Genital Organs

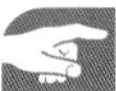

The genital organs can be classified topographically (external versus internal), functionally (Tables 14.1 and 14.2), or ontogenetically (see p. 204).

Table 14.1 Female genital organs

	Organ		Function
Internal genitalia	Ovarium		Germ cell and hormone production
	Tuba (fallopii) uterina		Site of conception and transport organ for zygote
	Uterus		Organ of incubation and parturition
	Vagina (pars superior)		Organ of copulation and parturition
External genitalia	Vulva	Vagina (vestibulum)	
		Labia majora and minora	Copulatory organ
		Clitoris	
		Glandula vestibularis minor and major	Production of secretions
		Mons pubis	Protection of the os pubis

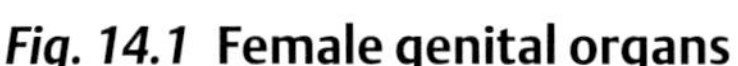

Fig. 14.1 **Female genital organs**

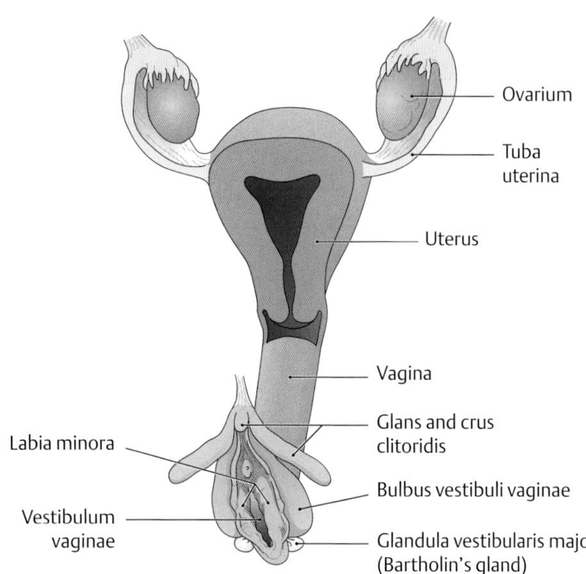
Ovarium
Tuba uterina
Uterus
Vagina
Glans and crus clitoridis
Labia minora
Bulbus vestibuli vaginae
Vestibulum vaginae
Glandula vestibularis major (Bartholin's gland)

A Internal and external genitalia.

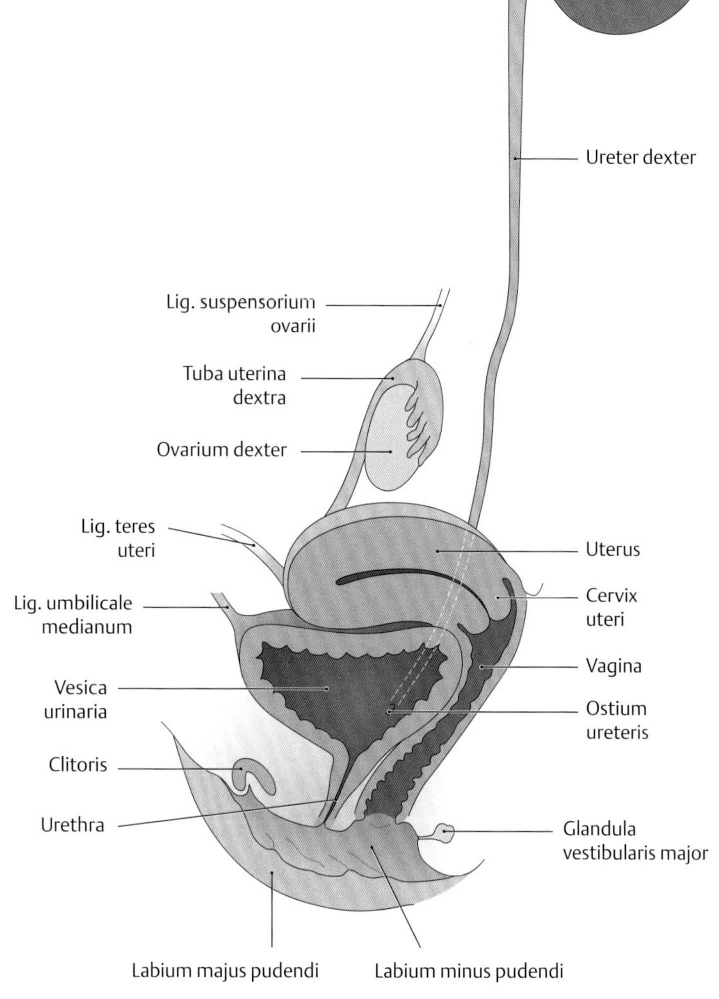
Ren dexter
Ureter dexter
Lig. suspensorium ovarii
Tuba uterina dextra
Ovarium dexter
Lig. teres uteri
Uterus
Lig. umbilicale medianum
Cervix uteri
Vagina
Vesica urinaria
Ostium ureteris
Clitoris
Urethra
Glandula vestibularis major
Labium majus pudendi
Labium minus pudendi

B Urogenital system. *Note:* The female urinary and genital tracts are functionally separate, though topographically close.

Table 14.2 Male genital organs

	Organ		Function
Internal genitalia	Testis		Germ cell and hormone production
	Epididymis		Reservoir for sperm
	Ductus deferens		Transport organ for sperm
	Accessory sex glands	Prostata	Production of secretions (semen)
		Glandula vesiculosa	
		Glandula bulbourethralis	
External genitalia	Penis		Copulatory and urinary organ
	Urethra		Urinary organ and transport organ for sperm
	Skrotum		Protection of testis
	Coverings of the testis		

Fig. 14.2 Male genital organs

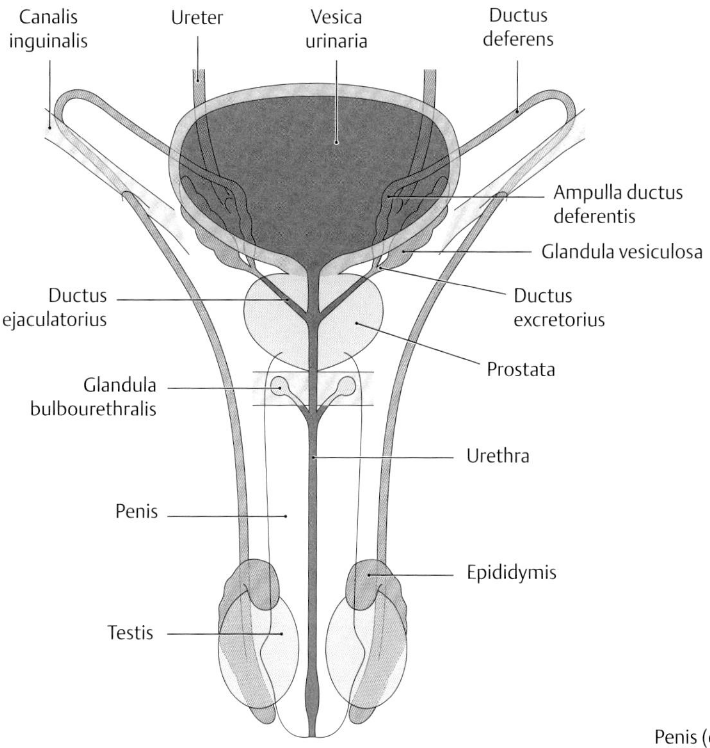

A Seminiferous structures.

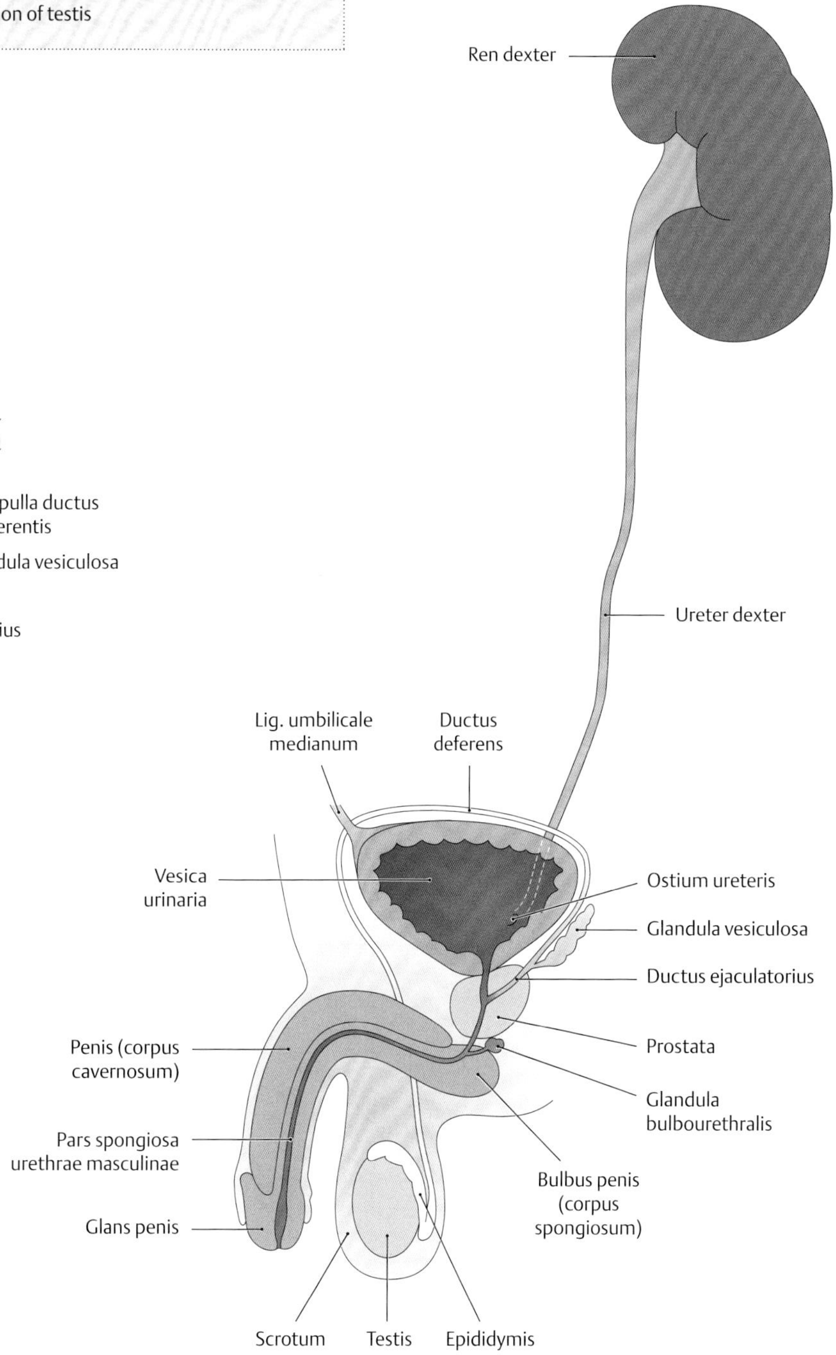

B Urogenital system. *Note:* The male urethra serves as a common urinary and genital passage.

Uterus & Ovaries

Fig. 14.3 Female internal genitalia

The uterus and ovaria are suspended by the mesovarium and mesometrium (portions of lig. latum uteri).

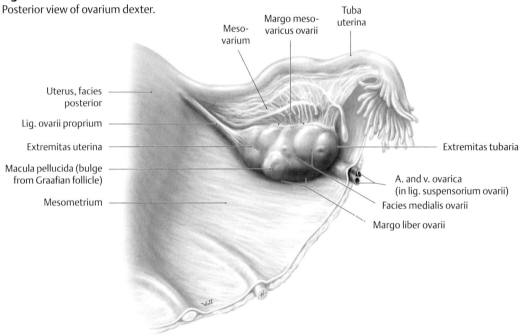

Bifurcatio aortae
A. iliaca communis
A. iliaca externa
A. iliaca interna

A Location. Anterior view.

Peritoneal covering
Tuba uterina
Mesosalpinx
Mesovarium
Ovarium
Mesometrium
Germinal epithelial covering

B Mesenterium. Sagittal section. Lig. latum uteri is a combination of the mesosalpinx, mesovarium, amd mesometrium.

Fig. 14.4 Ovarium

Posterior view of ovarium dexter.

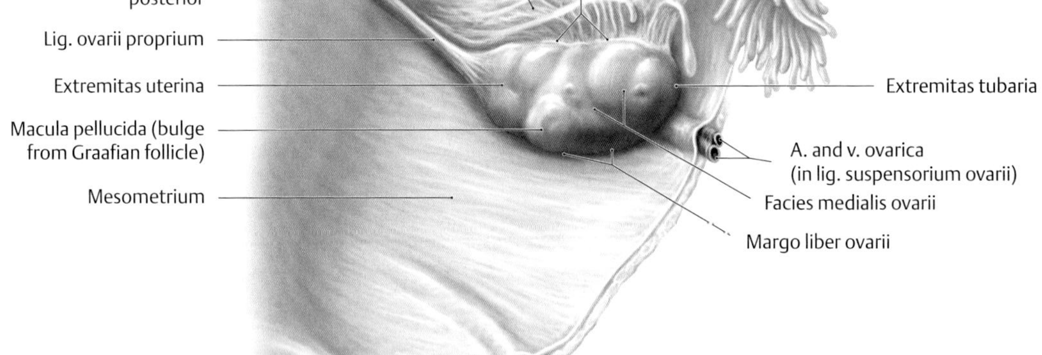

Meso-varium
Margo meso-varicus ovarii
Tuba uterina
Uterus, facies posterior
Lig. ovarii proprium
Extremitas uterina
Macula pellucida (bulge from Graafian follicle)
Mesometrium
Extremitas tubaria
A. and v. ovarica (in lig. suspensorium ovarii)
Facies medialis ovarii
Margo liber ovarii

Fig. 14.5 Curvature of the uterus

Midsagittal section, left lateral view. The position of the uterus can be described in terms of flexion (①) and version (②).

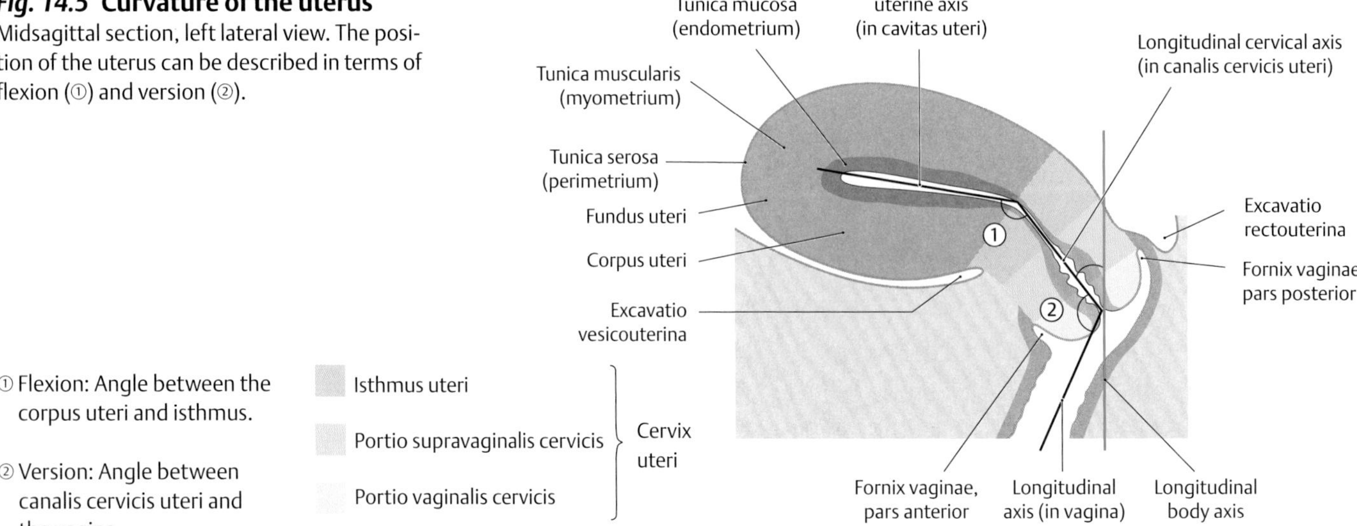

Tunica mucosa (endometrium)
Longitudinal uterine axis (in cavitas uteri)
Longitudinal cervical axis (in canalis cervicis uteri)
Tunica muscularis (myometrium)
Tunica serosa (perimetrium)
Fundus uteri
Corpus uteri
Excavatio vesicouterina
Excavatio rectouterina
Fornix vaginae, pars posterior
①
②
Fornix vaginae, pars anterior
Longitudinal axis (in vagina)
Longitudinal body axis
Isthmus uteri
Portio supravaginalis cervicis
Portio vaginalis cervicis
Cervix uteri

① Flexion: Angle between the corpus uteri and isthmus.

② Version: Angle between canalis cervicis uteri and the vagina.

Fig. 14.6 Uterus and tuba uterina

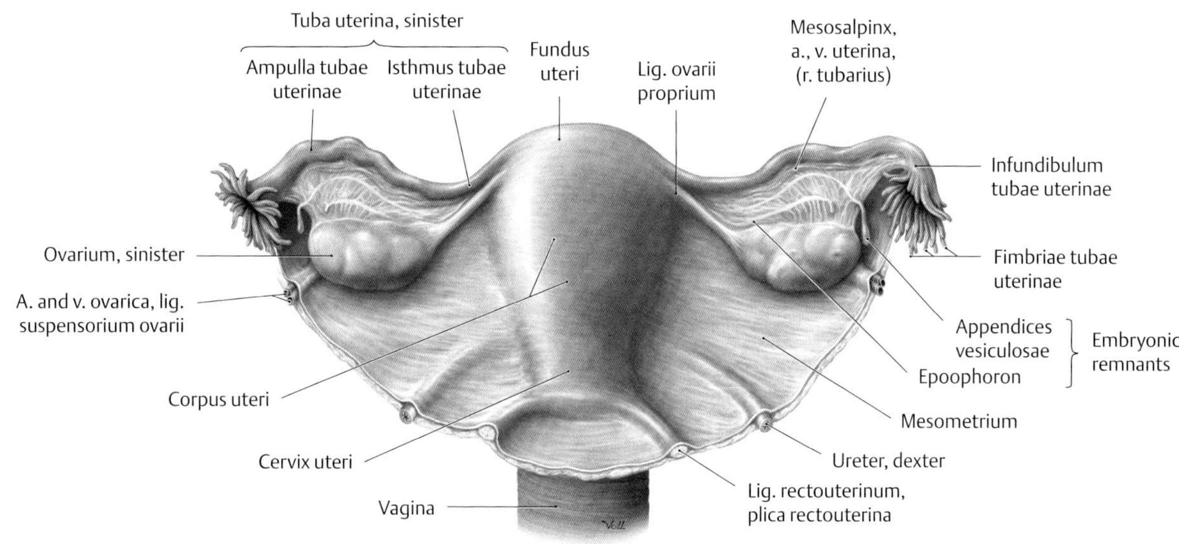
Tuba uterina, sinister
Ampulla tubae uterinae
Isthmus tubae uterinae
Fundus uteri
Lig. ovarii proprium
Mesosalpinx, a., v. uterina, (r. tubarius)
Infundibulum tubae uterinae
Fimbriae tubae uterinae
Ovarium, sinister
A. and v. ovarica, lig. suspensorium ovarii
Appendices vesiculosae
Epoophoron
Embryonic remnants
Corpus uteri
Mesometrium
Cervix uteri
Ureter, dexter
Vagina
Lig. rectouterinum, plica rectouterina

A Posterosuperior view.

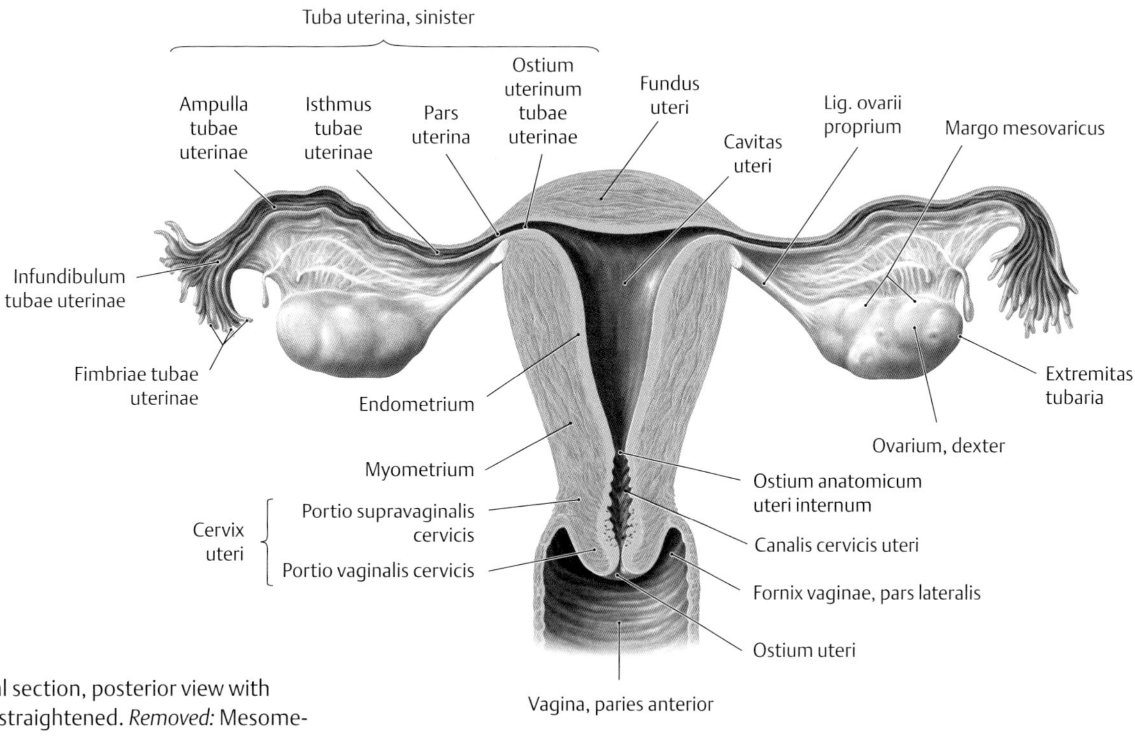
Tuba uterina, sinister
Ampulla tubae uterinae
Isthmus tubae uterinae
Pars uterina
Ostium uterinum tubae uterinae
Fundus uteri
Cavitas uteri
Lig. ovarii proprium
Margo mesovaricus
Infundibulum tubae uterinae
Fimbriae tubae uterinae
Endometrium
Extremitas tubaria
Ovarium, dexter
Myometrium
Ostium anatomicum uteri internum
Cervix uteri
Portio supravaginalis cervicis
Portio vaginalis cervicis
Canalis cervicis uteri
Fornix vaginae, pars lateralis
Ostium uteri
Vagina, paries anterior

B Coronal section, posterior view with uterus straightened. *Removed:* Mesometrium.

Clinical

Ectopic pregnancy

After fertilization, the ovum usually implants in the wall of the uterine cavity. However, it may become implanted at other sites (e.g., tuba uterina or even the cavitas peritoneale). Tubal pregnancies, the most common type of ectopic pregnancy, pose the risk of tubal wall rupture and potentially life-threatening bleeding into the peritoneal cavity. Tubal pregnancies are promoted by adhesion of the tubal mucosa, mostly due to inflammation.

Vagina

Fig. 14.7 Location

Midsagittal section, left lateral view.

Excavatio vesicouterina
Tunica serosa
Corpus uteri
Cervix uteri, portio vaginalis cervicis
Vesica urinaria
Vagina, pars anterior
Urethra
Septum vesicovaginale
Ostium vaginae
Vestibulum vaginae, labium minus pudendi
Excavatio rectouterina
Cervix uteri, portio supravaginalis cervicis
Pars posterior
Pars anterior
Fornix vaginae
Vagina, paries posterior
Rectum
Fascia rectovaginalis (septum rectovaginale)
M. transversus perinei profundus

Fig. 14.8 Structure

Posteriorly angled coronal section, posterior view.

Ostium uteri, labium posterius
Ostium uteri, labium anterius
Columna rugarum anterior
Vagina, paries anterior
Ostium urethrae externum
Clitoris
Cervix uteri, portio supravaginalis cervicis
Ostium uteri
Rugae vaginales
Carina urethralis vaginae
Vestibulum vaginae

Fig. 14.9 Cervix uteri: Transverse section

Inferior view.

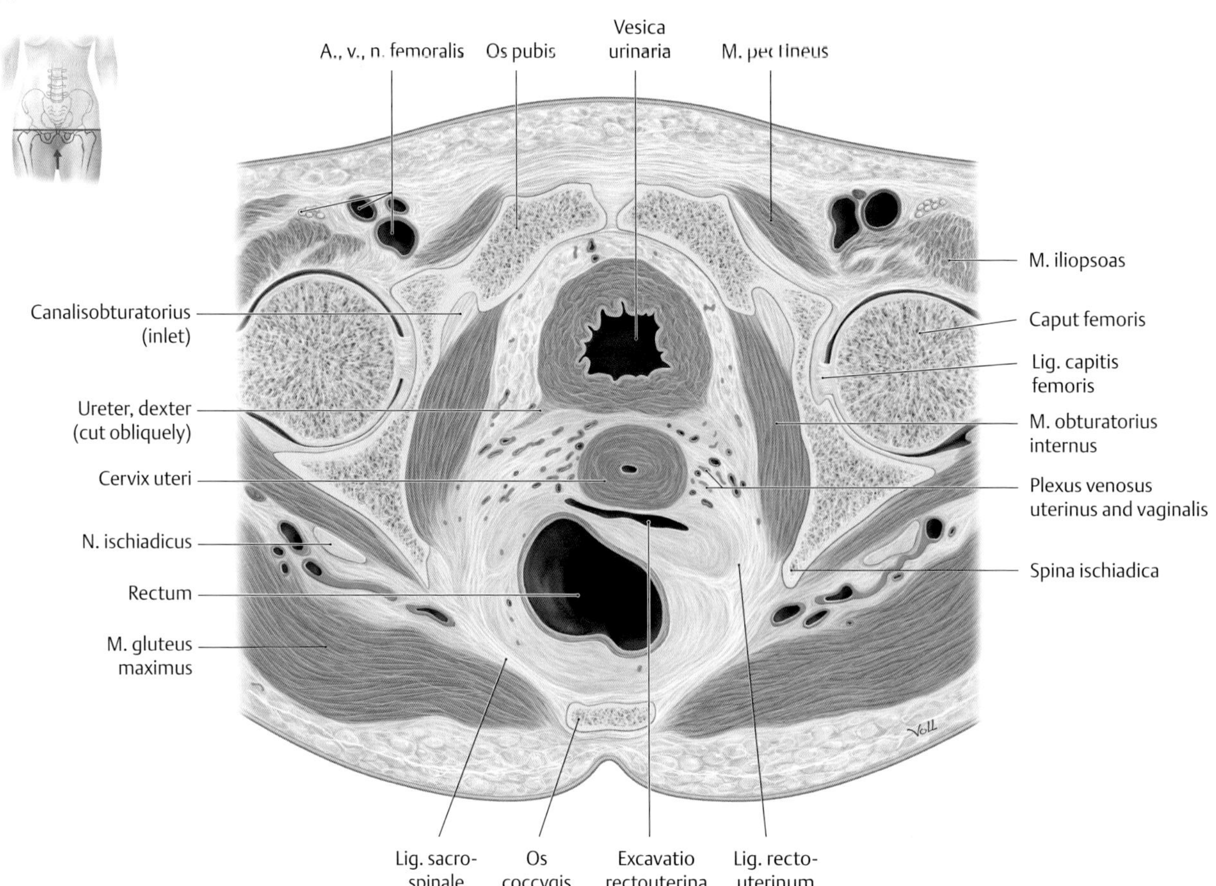
A., v., n. femoralis
Os pubis
Vesica urinaria
M. pectineus
M. iliopsoas
Caput femoris
Lig. capitis femoris
M. obturatorius internus
Plexus venosus uterinus and vaginalis
Spina ischiadica
Canalisobturatorius (inlet)
Ureter, dexter (cut obliquely)
Cervix uteri
N. ischiadicus
Rectum
M. gluteus maximus
Lig. sacrospinale
Os coccygis
Excavatio rectouterina
Lig. rectouterinum

Fig. 14.10 Female genital organs: Coronal section

Anterior view. The vagina is both pelvic and perineal in location. It is also retroperitoneal.

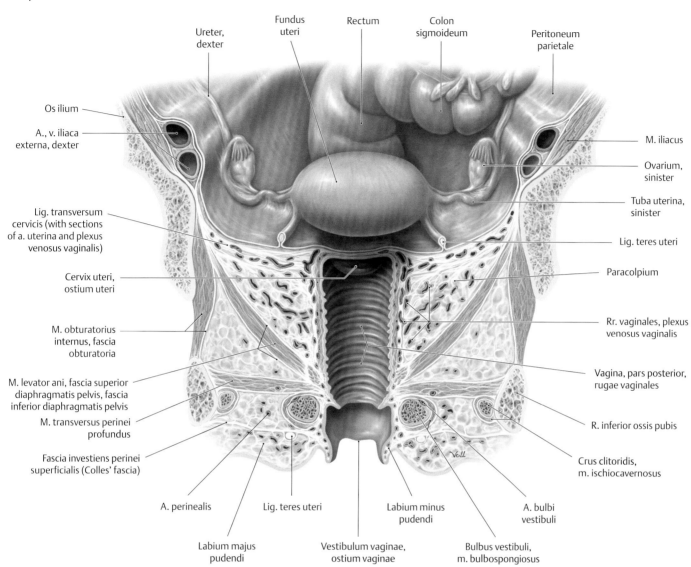

Ureter, dexter
Fundus uteri
Rectum
Colon sigmoideum
Peritoneum parietale
Os ilium
A., v. iliaca externa, dexter
M. iliacus
Ovarium, sinister
Tuba uterina, sinister
Lig. transversum cervicis (with sections of a. uterina and plexus venosus vaginalis)
Lig. teres uteri
Cervix uteri, ostium uteri
Paracolpium
M. obturatorius internus, fascia obturatoria
Rr. vaginales, plexus venosus vaginalis
M. levator ani, fascia superior diaphragmatis pelvis, fascia inferior diaphragmatis pelvis
Vagina, pars posterior, rugae vaginales
M. transversus perinei profundus
R. inferior ossis pubis
Fascia investiens perinei superficialis (Colles' fascia)
Crus clitoridis, m. ischiocavernosus
A. perinealis
Lig. teres uteri
Labium minus pudendi
A. bulbi vestibuli
Labium majus pudendi
Vestibulum vaginae, ostium vaginae
Bulbus vestibuli, m. bulbospongiosus

Fig. 14.11 Vagina: Location in the pelvic floor

Inferior view.

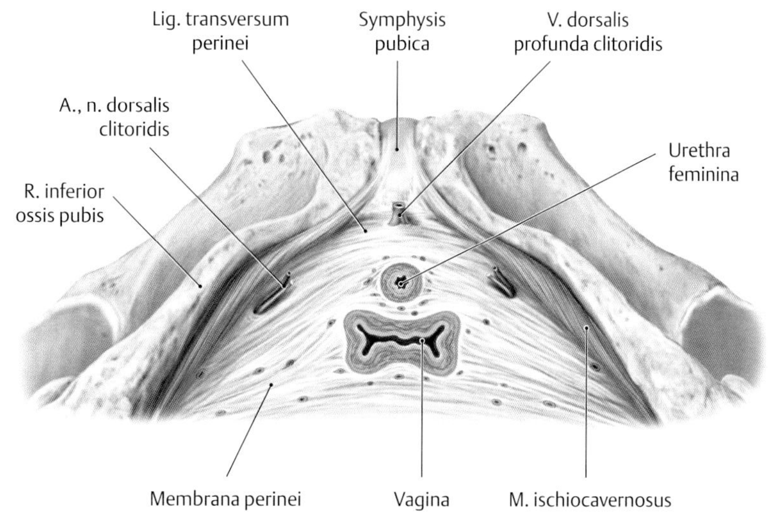
Lig. transversum perinei
Symphysis pubica
V. dorsalis profunda clitoridis
A., n. dorsalis clitoridis
Urethra feminina
R. inferior ossis pubis
Membrana perinei
Vagina
M. ischiocavernosus

Female External Genitalia

Fig. 14.12 **Female external genitalia**
Lithotomy position with labia minora separated.

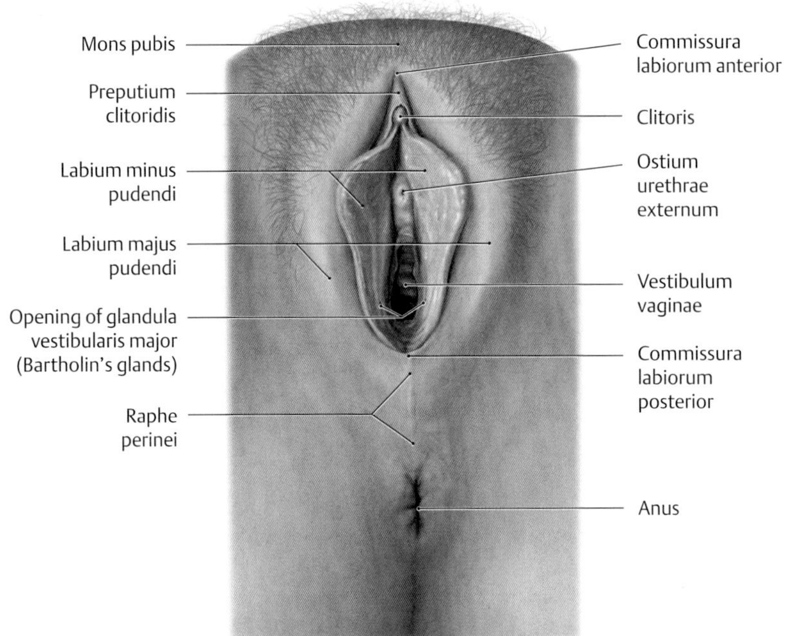
Mons pubis
Preputium clitoridis
Labium minus pudendi
Labium majus pudendi
Opening of glandula vestibularis major (Bartholin's glands)
Raphe perinei
Commissura labiorum anterior
Clitoris
Ostium urethrae externum
Vestibulum vaginae
Commissura labiorum posterior
Anus

Fig. 14.13 **Vestibulum vaginae and vestibular glands**
Lithotomy position with labia separated.

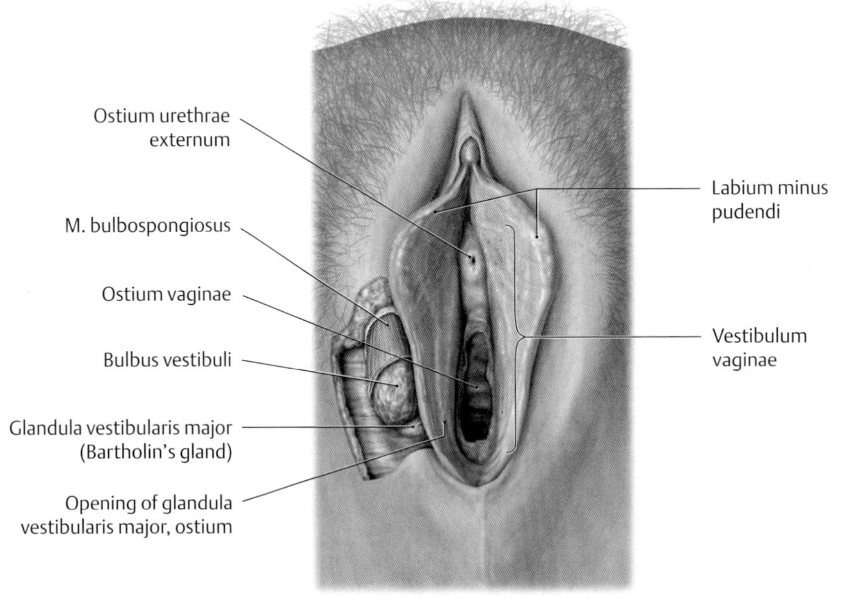
Ostium urethrae externum
M. bulbospongiosus
Ostium vaginae
Bulbus vestibuli
Glandula vestibularis major (Bartholin's gland)
Opening of glandula vestibularis major, ostium
Labium minus pudendi
Vestibulum vaginae

Fig. 14.14 Erectile muscles and tissue: Female
Lithotomy position. *Removed:* Labia, skin, and membrana perinei; erectile muscles (left side).

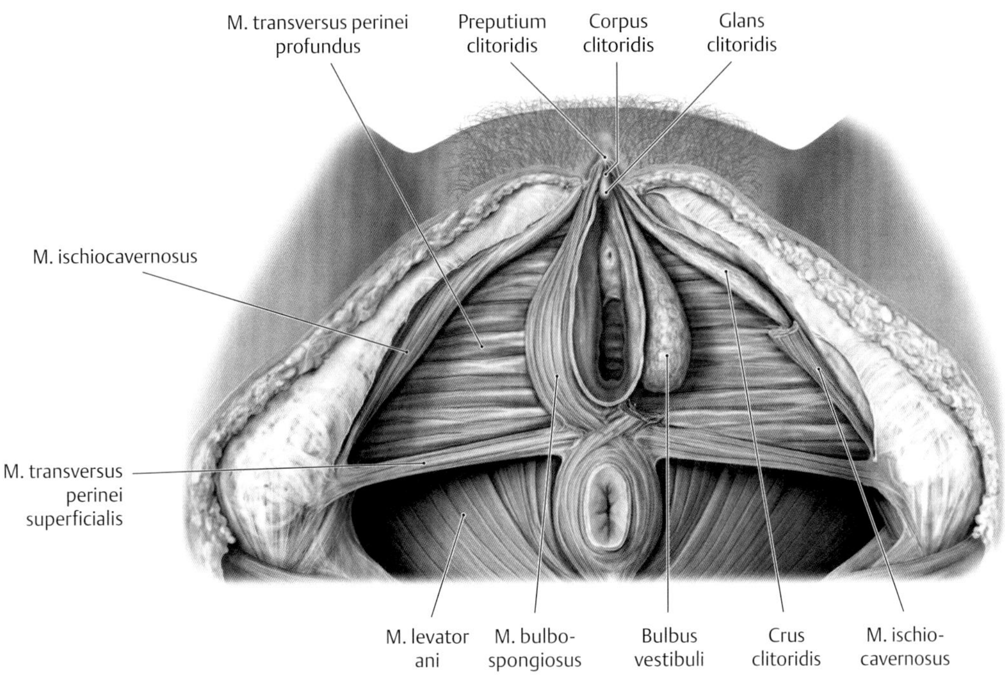
M. transversus perinei profundus
Preputium clitoridis
Corpus clitoridis
Glans clitoridis
M. ischiocavernosus
M. transversus perinei superficialis
M. levator ani
M. bulbo-spongiosus
Bulbus vestibuli
Crus clitoridis
M. ischio-cavernosus

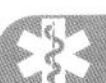

Clinical

Episiotomy

Episiotomy is a common obstetric procedure used to enlarge the birth canal during the expulsive stage of labor. The procedure is generally used to expedite the delivery of a baby at risk for hypoxia during the expulsive stage. Alternately, if the perineal skin turns white (indicating diminished blood flow), there is imminent danger of perineal laceration, and an episiotomy is often performed. More lateral incisions gain more room, but they are more difficult to repair.

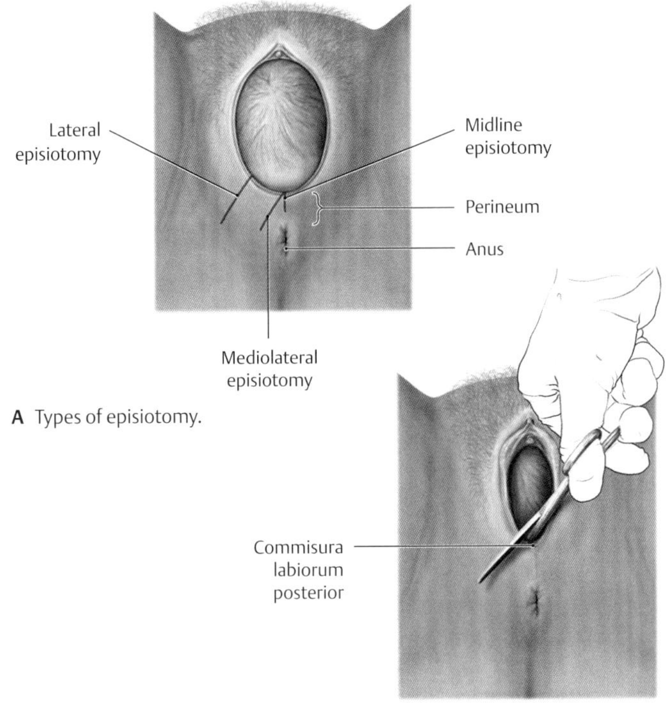
Lateral episiotomy
Midline episiotomy
Perineum
Anus
Mediolateral episiotomy
Commisura labiorum posterior

A Types of episiotomy.

B Mediolateral episiotomy at height of contraction.

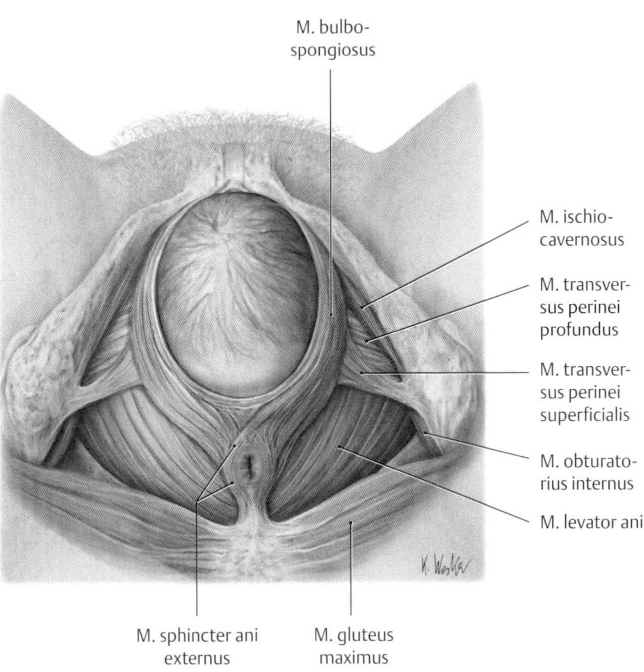
M. bulbo-spongiosus
M. ischio-cavernosus
M. transver-sus perinei profundus
M. transver-sus perinei superficialis
M. obturato-rius internus
M. levator ani
M. sphincter ani externus
M. gluteus maximus

C Pelvic floor with crowning of fetal head.

Neurovasculature of the Female Genitalia

Fig. 14.15 Nerves of the female perineum and genitalia

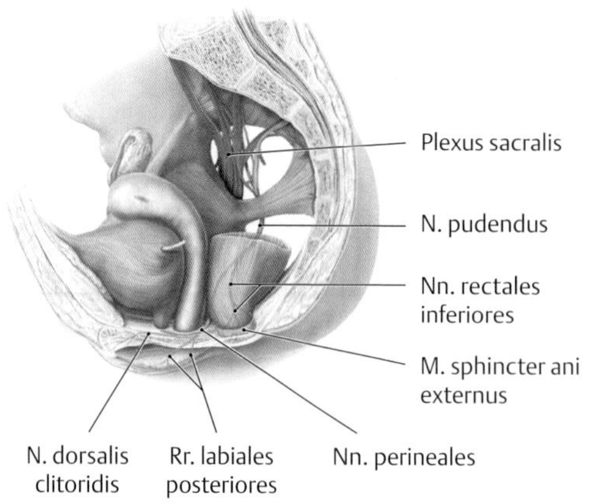

Plexus sacralis
N. pudendus
Nn. rectales inferiores
M. sphincter ani externus
N. dorsalis clitoridis
Rr. labiales posteriores
Nn. perineales

A Nerve supply to the female external genitalia. Lesser pelvis, left lateral view.

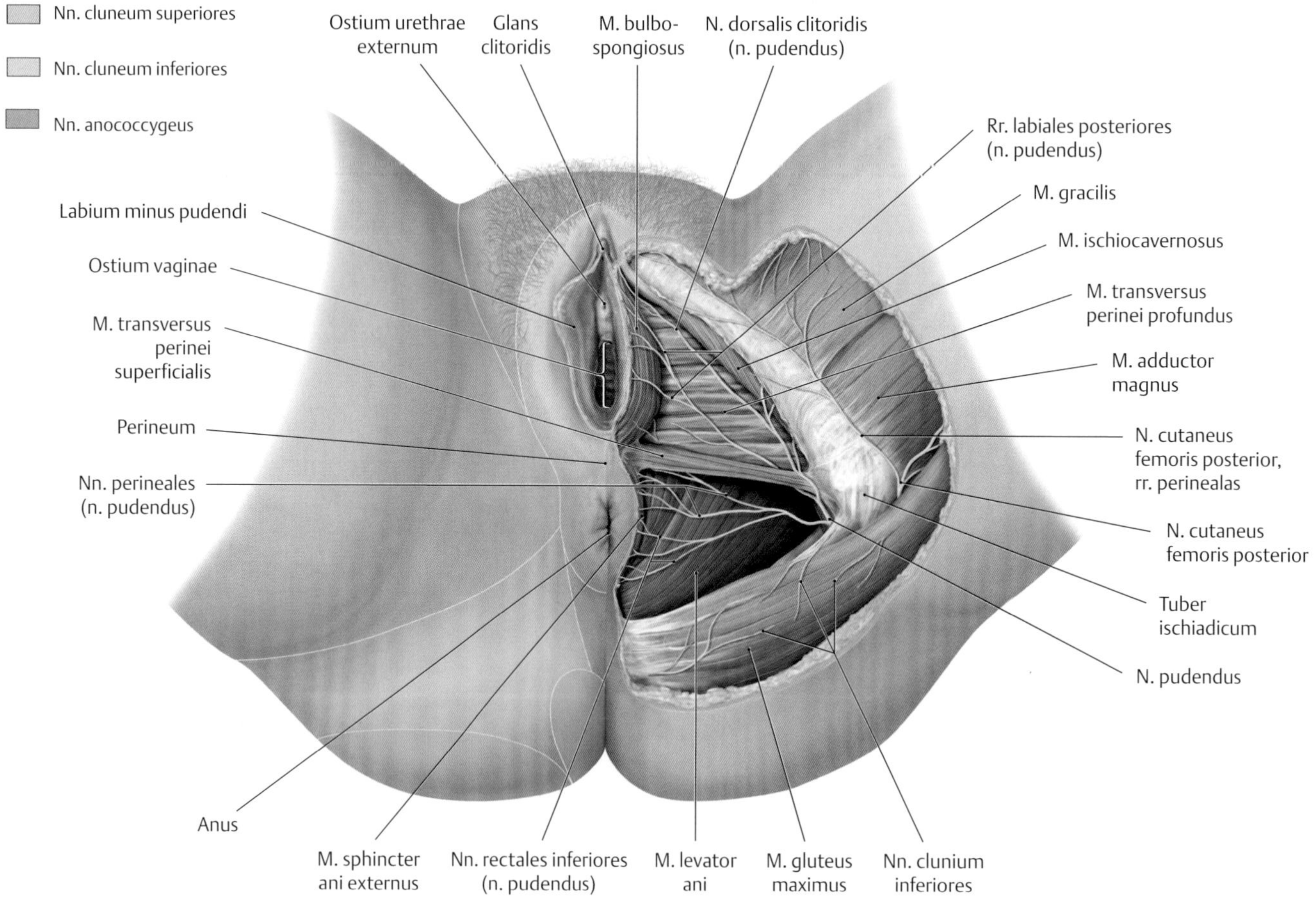

N. ilioinguinalis and n. genitofemoralis, r. genitalis
N. pudendus
N. cutaneus femoris posterior
Nn. cluneum medii
Nn. cluneum superiores
Nn. cluneum inferiores
Nn. anococcygeus
Ostium urethrae externum
Glans clitoridis
M. bulbo-spongiosus
N. dorsalis clitoridis (n. pudendus)
Rr. labiales posteriores (n. pudendus)
M. gracilis
M. ischiocavernosus
M. transversus perinei profundus
M. adductor magnus
N. cutaneus femoris posterior, rr. perinealas
N. cutaneus femoris posterior
Tuber ischiadicum
N. pudendus
Labium minus pudendi
Ostium vaginae
M. transversus perinei superficialis
Perineum
Nn. perineales (n. pudendus)
Anus
M. sphincter ani externus
Nn. rectales inferiores (n. pudendus)
M. levator ani
M. gluteus maximus
Nn. clunium inferiores

B Sensory innervation of the female perineum. Lithotomy position.

Fig. 14.16 **Blood vessels of the female external genitalia**
Inferior view.

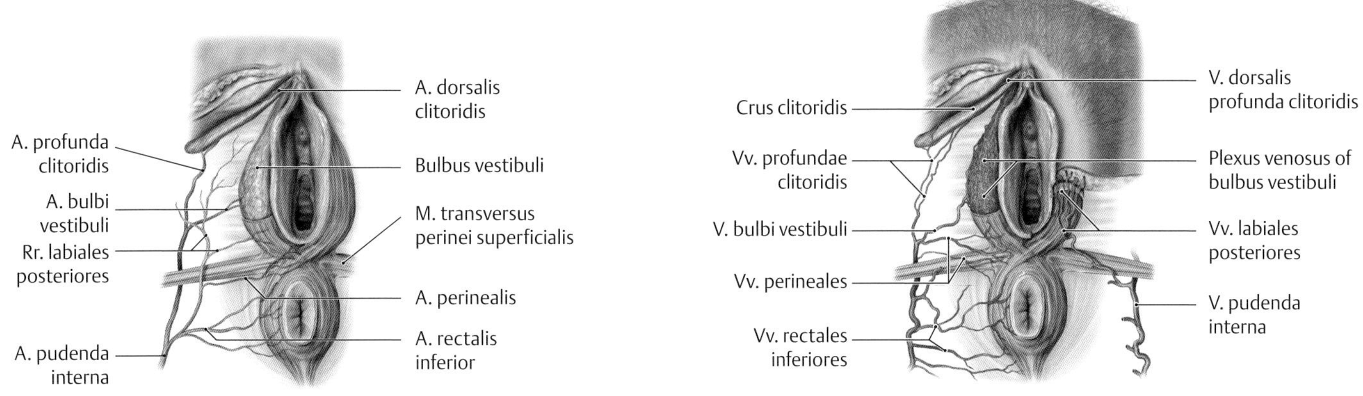
A. dorsalis clitoridis
A. profunda clitoridis
Bulbus vestibuli
A. bulbi vestibuli
M. transversus perinei superficialis
Rr. labiales posteriores
A. perinealis
A. rectalis inferior
A. pudenda interna
Crus clitoridis
V. dorsalis profunda clitoridis
Vv. profundae clitoridis
Plexus venosus of bulbus vestibuli
V. bulbi vestibuli
Vv. labiales posteriores
Vv. perineales
V. pudenda interna
Vv. rectales inferiores

A Arterial supply.

B Venous drainage.

Fig. 14.17 **Neurovasculature of the female perineum**
Lithotomy position.

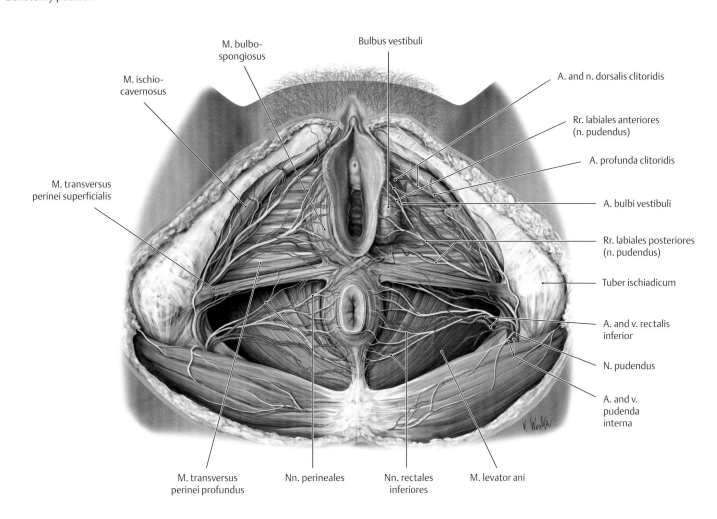

M. bulbo-spongiosus
Bulbus vestibuli
M. ischio-cavernosus
A. and n. dorsalis clitoridis
Rr. labiales anteriores (n. pudendus)
A. profunda clitoridis
M. transversus perinei superficialis
A. bulbi vestibuli
Rr. labiales posteriores (n. pudendus)
Tuber ischiadicum
A. and v. rectalis inferior
N. pudendus
A. and v. pudenda interna
M. transversus perinei profundus
Nn. perineales
Nn. rectales inferiores
M. levator ani

Penis, Scrotum & Funiculus Spermaticus

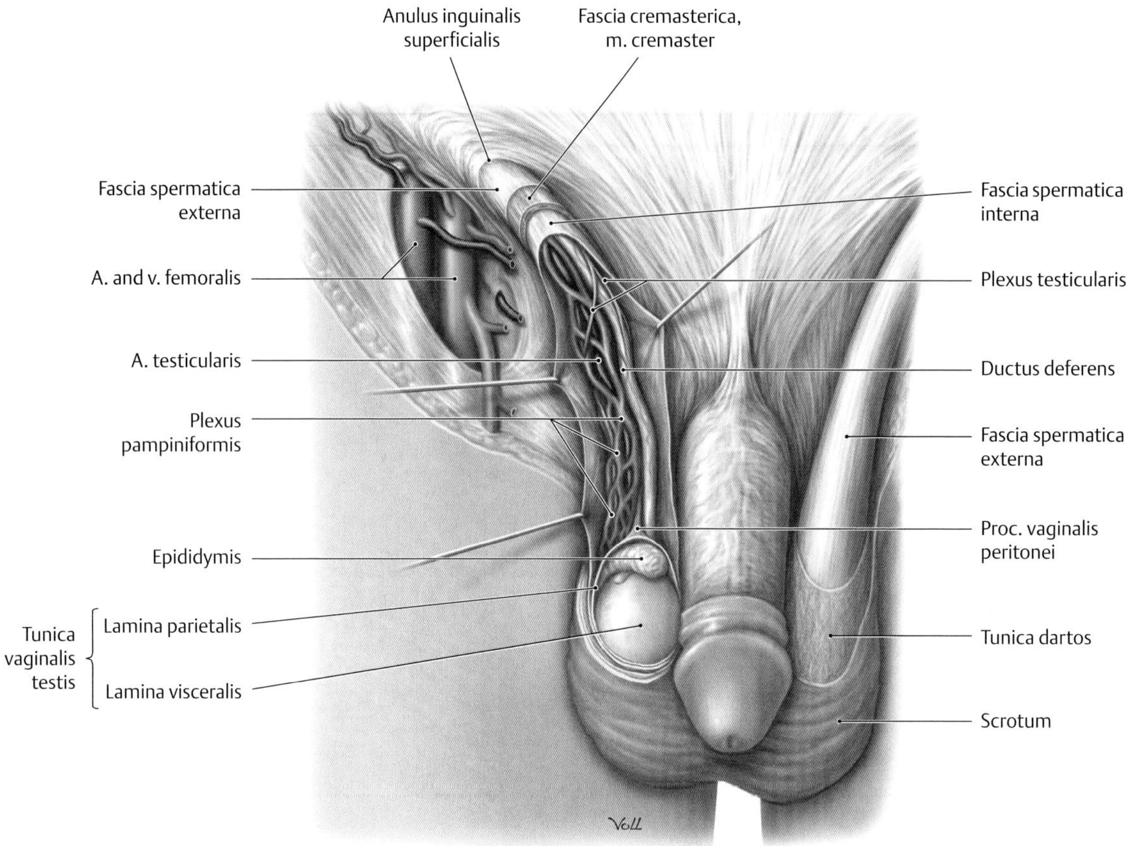
Anulus inguinalis superficialis
Fascia cremasterica, m. cremaster
Fascia spermatica externa
A. and v. femoralis
A. testicularis
Plexus pampiniformis
Epididymis
Tunica vaginalis testis
Lamina parietalis
Lamina visceralis
Fascia spermatica interna
Plexus testicularis
Ductus deferens
Fascia spermatica externa
Proc. vaginalis peritonei
Tunica dartos
Scrotum

Fig. 14.18 **Penis, scrotum, and funiculus spermaticus**
Anterior view. *Removed:* Skin over the scrotum and funiculus spermaticus.

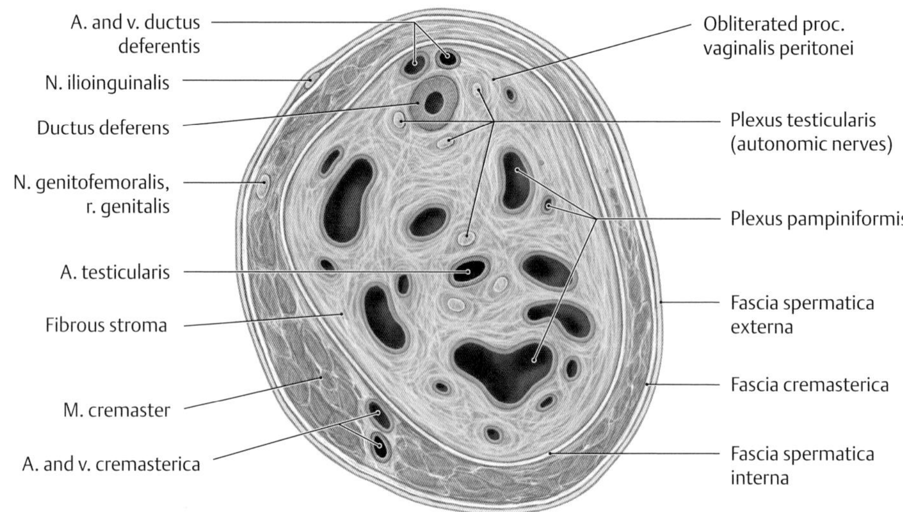
A. and v. ductus deferentis
N. ilioinguinalis
Ductus deferens
N. genitofemoralis, r. genitalis
A. testicularis
Fibrous stroma
M. cremaster
A. and v. cremasterica
Obliterated proc. vaginalis peritonei
Plexus testicularis (autonomic nerves)
Plexus pampiniformis
Fascia spermatica externa
Fascia cremasterica
Fascia spermatica interna

Fig. 14.19 **Funiculus spermaticus: Contents**
Cross section.

Fig. 14.20 Penis

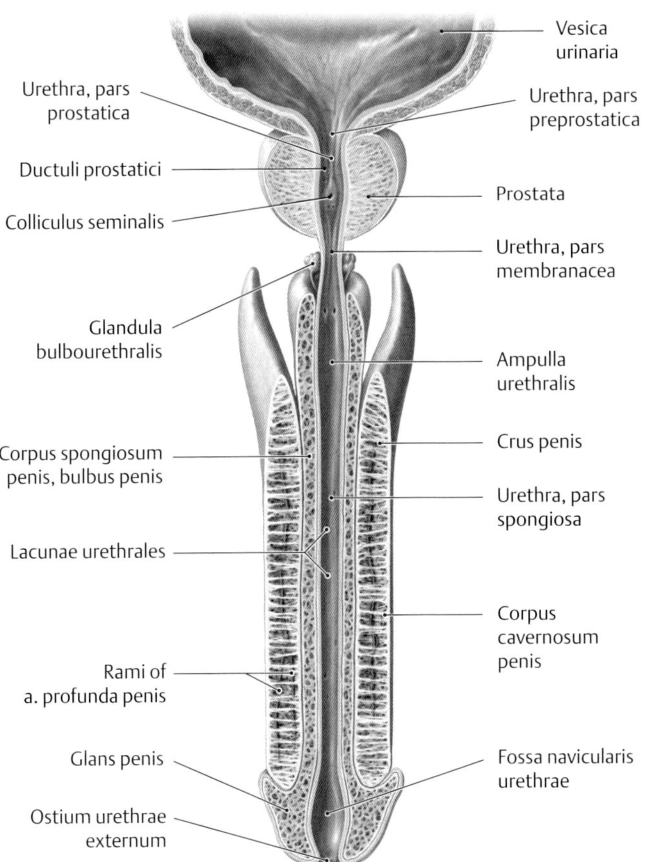
Vesica urinaria
Urethra, pars prostatica
Urethra, pars preprostatica
Ductuli prostatici
Prostata
Colliculus seminalis
Urethra, pars membranacea
Glandula bulbourethralis
Ampulla urethralis
Crus penis
Corpus spongiosum penis, bulbus penis
Urethra, pars spongiosa
Lacunae urethrales
Corpus cavernosum penis
Rami of a. profunda penis
Glans penis
Fossa navicularis urethrae
Ostium urethrae externum

A Longitudinal section.

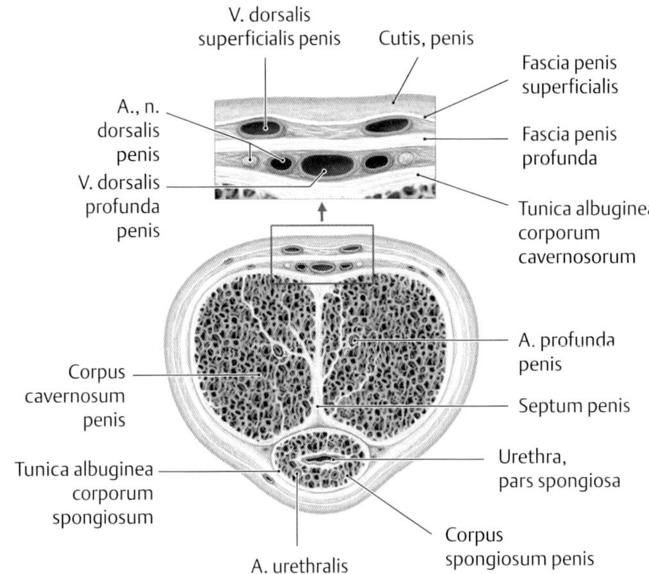
V. dorsalis superficialis penis
Cutis, penis
Fascia penis superficialis
A., n. dorsalis penis
Fascia penis profunda
V. dorsalis profunda penis
Tunica albuginea corporum cavernosorum
A. profunda penis
Corpus cavernosum penis
Septum penis
Tunica albuginea corporum spongiosum
Urethra, pars spongiosa
Corpus spongiosum penis
A. urethralis

B Cross section through corpus penis.

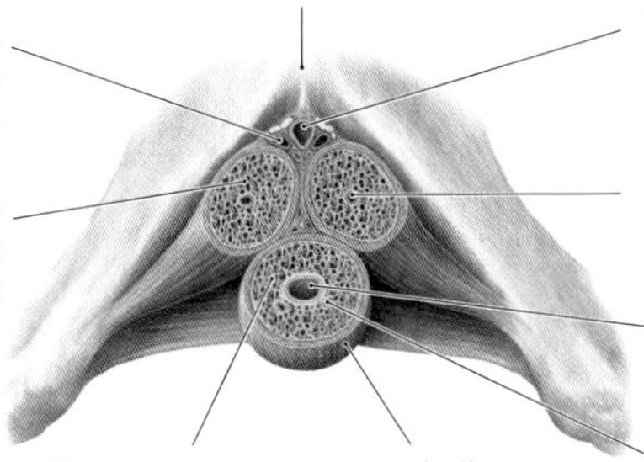

Symphysis pubica
A. and n. dorsalis penis
V. dorsalis profunda penis
Corpus cavernosum penis
A. profunda penis
Urethra, pars spongiosa
Bulbus penis, corpus spongiosum penis
M. bulbo-spongiosus
A. urethralis

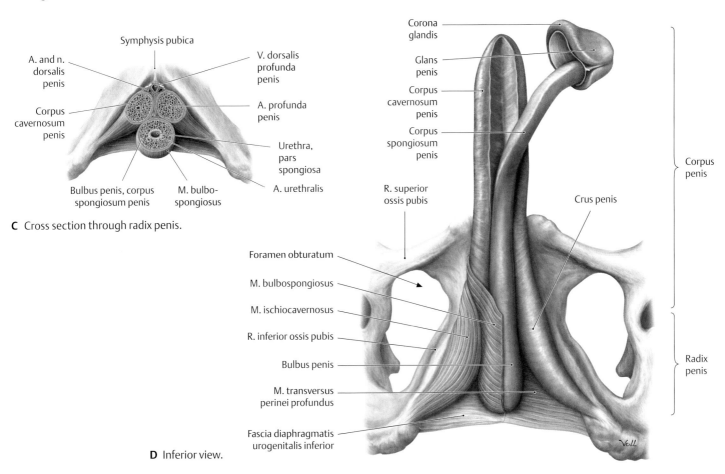

C Cross section through radix penis.

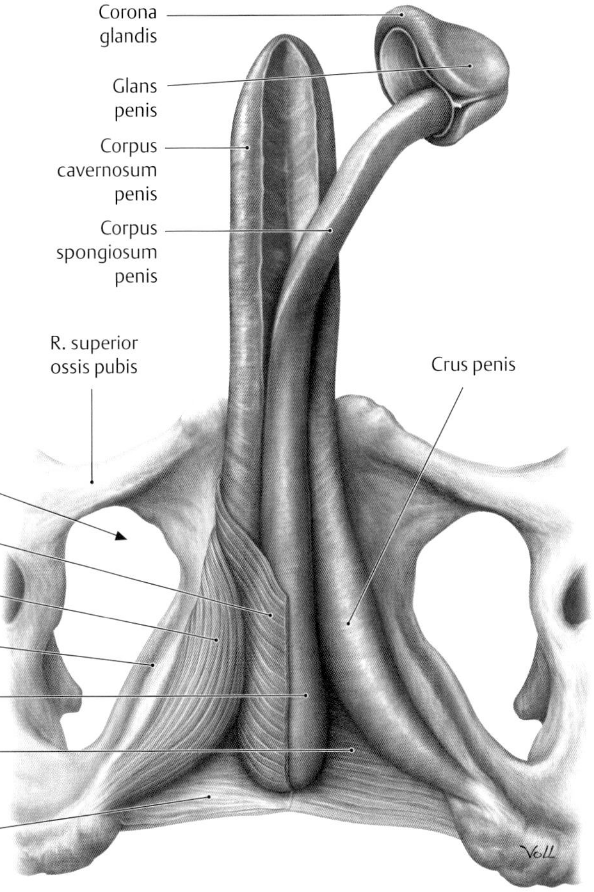

Corona glandis
Glans penis
Corpus cavernosum penis
Corpus spongiosum penis
Corpus penis
R. superior ossis pubis
Crus penis
Foramen obturatum
M. bulbospongiosus
M. ischiocavernosus
R. inferior ossis pubis
Radix penis
Bulbus penis
M. transversus perinei profundus
Fascia diaphragmatis urogenitalis inferior

D Inferior view.

Testis & Epididymis

Fig. 14.21 **Testis and epididymis**
Left lateral view.

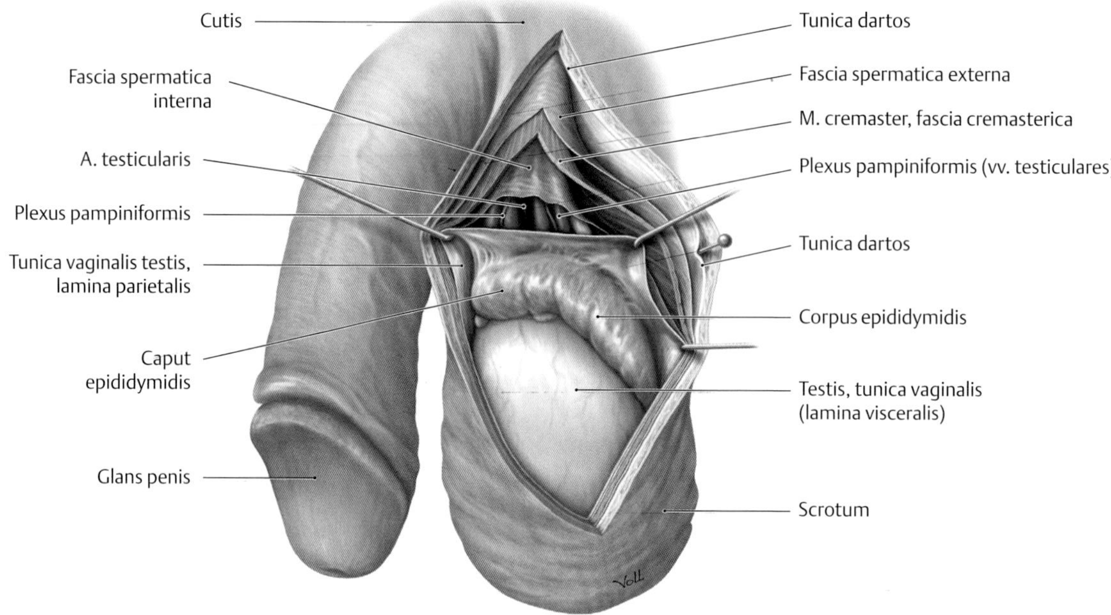
Cutis
Fascia spermatica interna
A. testicularis
Plexus pampiniformis
Tunica vaginalis testis, lamina parietalis
Caput epididymidis
Glans penis
Tunica dartos
Fascia spermatica externa
M. cremaster, fascia cremasterica
Plexus pampiniformis (vv. testiculares)
Tunica dartos
Corpus epididymidis
Testis, tunica vaginalis (lamina visceralis)
Scrotum

A Testis and epididymis in situ.

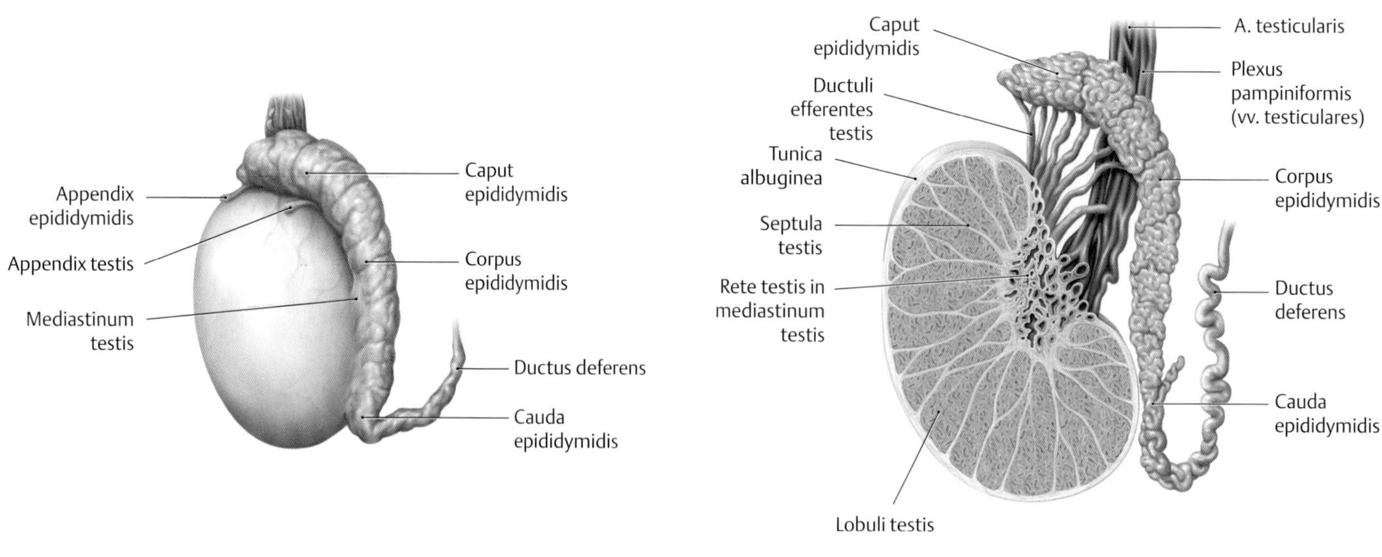
Appendix epididymidis
Appendix testis
Mediastinum testis
Caput epididymidis
Corpus epididymidis
Ductus deferens
Cauda epididymidis
Caput epididymidis
Ductuli efferentes testis
Tunica albuginea
Septula testis
Rete testis in mediastinum testis
Lobuli testis
A. testicularis
Plexus pampiniformis (vv. testiculares)
Corpus epididymidis
Ductus deferens
Cauda epididymidis

B Surface anatomy of the testis and epididymis.

C Sagittal section.

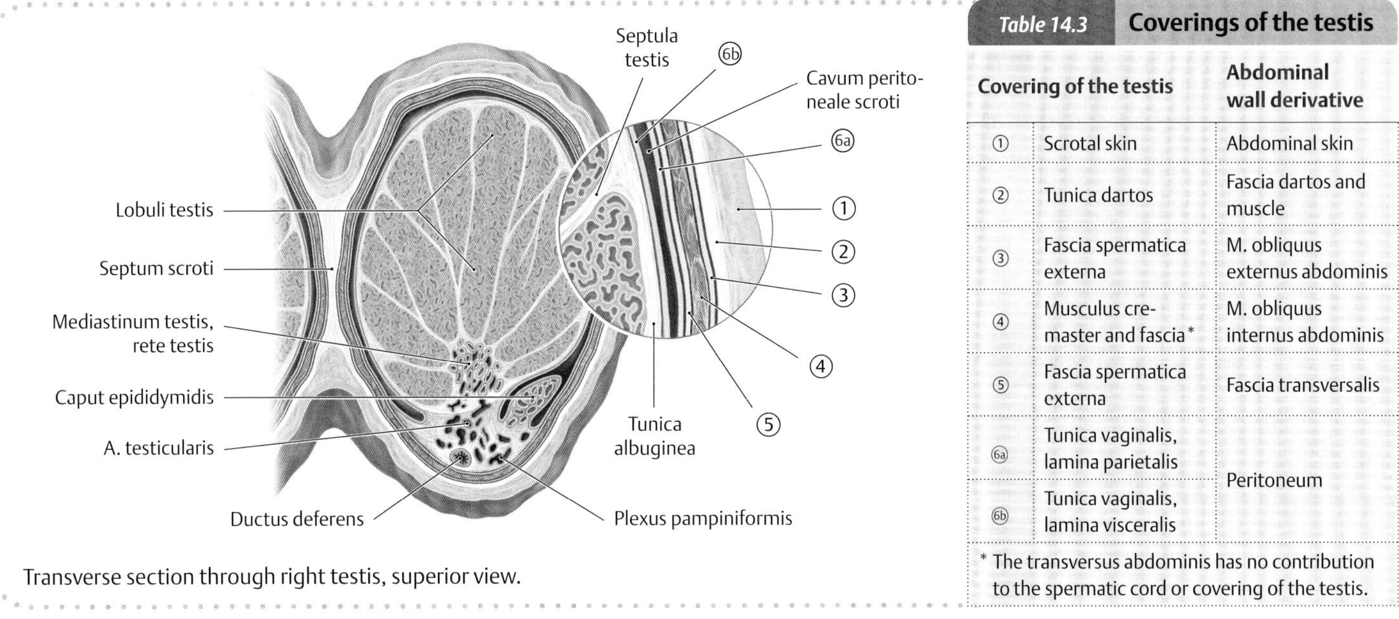
Septula testis
6b
Cavum perito-neale scroti
6a
1
2
3
4
5
Lobuli testis
Septum scroti
Mediastinum testis, rete testis
Caput epididymidis
A. testicularis
Ductus deferens
Tunica albuginea
Plexus pampiniformis

Transverse section through right testis, superior view.

Table 14.3 Coverings of the testis

	Covering of the testis	Abdominal wall derivative
①	Scrotal skin	Abdominal skin
②	Tunica dartos	Fascia dartos and muscle
③	Fascia spermatica externa	M. obliquus externus abdominis
④	Musculus cremaster and fascia*	M. obliquus internus abdominis
⑤	Fascia spermatica externa	Fascia transversalis
⑥a	Tunica vaginalis, lamina parietalis	Peritoneum
⑥b	Tunica vaginalis, lamina visceralis	

* The transversus abdominis has no contribution to the spermatic cord or covering of the testis.

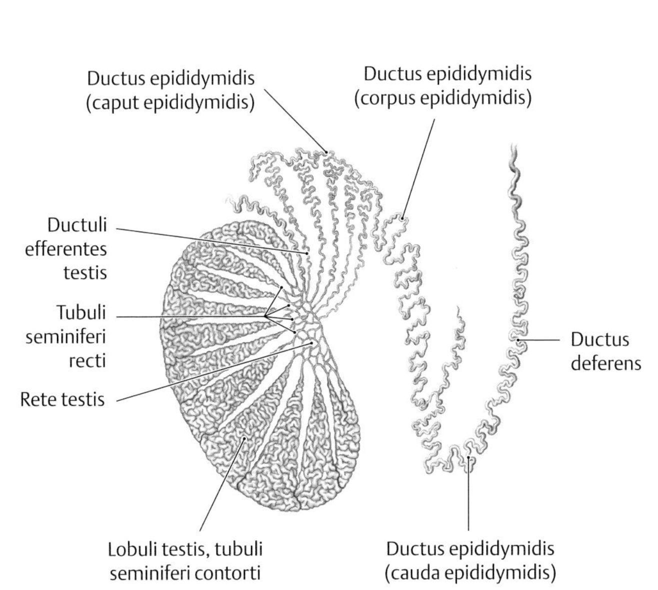
Ductus epididymidis (caput epididymidis)
Ductus epididymidis (corpus epididymidis)
Ductuli efferentes testis
Tubuli seminiferi recti
Rete testis
Ductus deferens
Lobuli testis, tubuli seminiferi contorti
Ductus epididymidis (cauda epididymidis)

D Tubuli seminiferi.

Fig. 14.22 **Blood vessels of the testis**
Left lateral view.

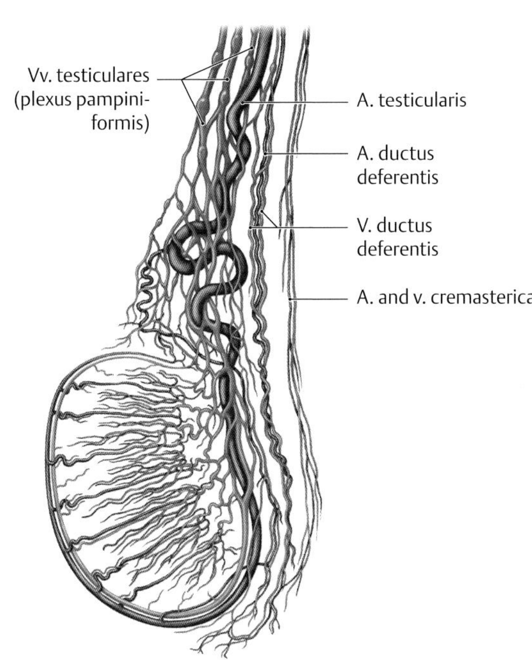
Vv. testiculares (plexus pampini-formis)
A. testicularis
A. ductus deferentis
V. ductus deferentis
A. and v. cremasterica

Male Accessory Sex Glands

Fig. 14.23 Accessory sex glands

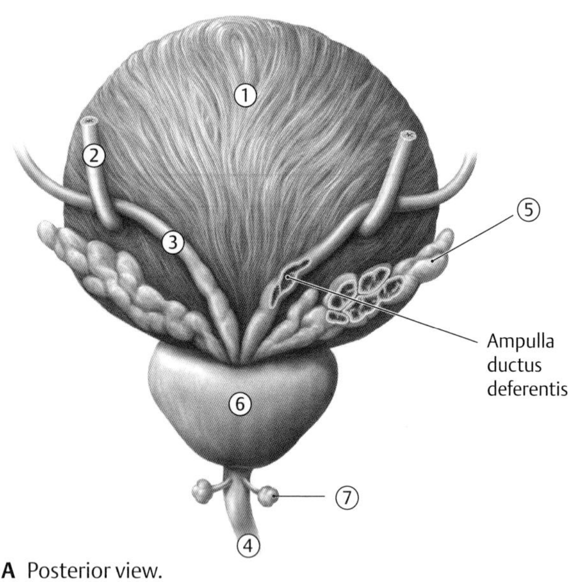

①
②
③
⑤
Ampulla ductus deferentis
⑥
⑦
④

A Posterior view.

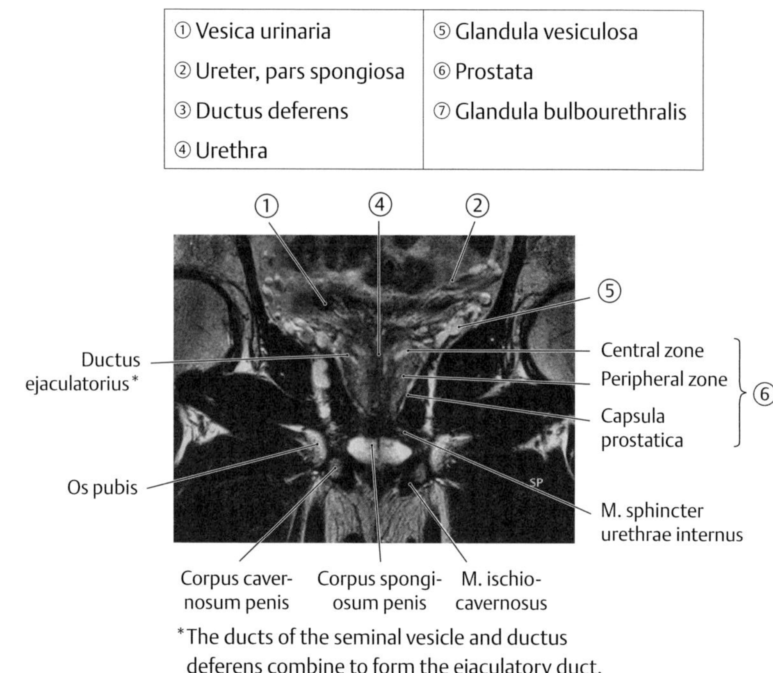

① Vesica urinaria
② Ureter, pars spongiosa
③ Ductus deferens
④ Urethra
⑤ Glandula vesiculosa
⑥ Prostata
⑦ Glandula bulbourethralis
①
④
②
⑤
Ductus ejaculatorius*
Central zone
Peripheral zone
Capsula prostatica
⑥
Os pubis
M. sphincter urethrae internus
Corpus cavernosum penis
Corpus spongiosum penis
M. ischiocavernosus

*The ducts of the seminal vesicle and ductus deferens combine to form the ejaculatory duct.

B MRI. Coronal section, anterior view.

Fig. 14.24 Prostata

The prostata may be divided anatomically (top row) or clinically (bottom row).

Cervix vesicae

Prostata

Colliculus seminalis

Capsula prostatica

Glandula bulbourethralis

M. transversus perinei profundus

Pars prostatica

Pars membranacea

Urethra

Pars spongiosa

Basis prostatae

Apex prostatae

Capsula prostatica

Urethra

Isthmus prostatae

Lobus prostatae sinister

Lobus prostatae dexter

Ductus ejaculatorius, ostia

Ductus ejaculatorius, dexter

Ductus ejaculatorius, ostia

Colliculus seminalis

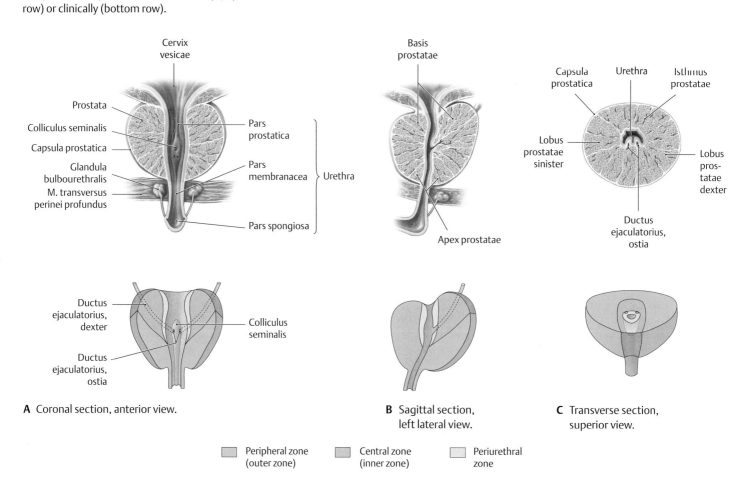

A Coronal section, anterior view.

B Sagittal section, left lateral view.

C Transverse section, superior view.

Peripheral zone (outer zone)

Central zone (inner zone)

Periurethral zone

Fig. 14.25 **Prostata in situ**
Sagittal section through the male pelvis, left lateral view.

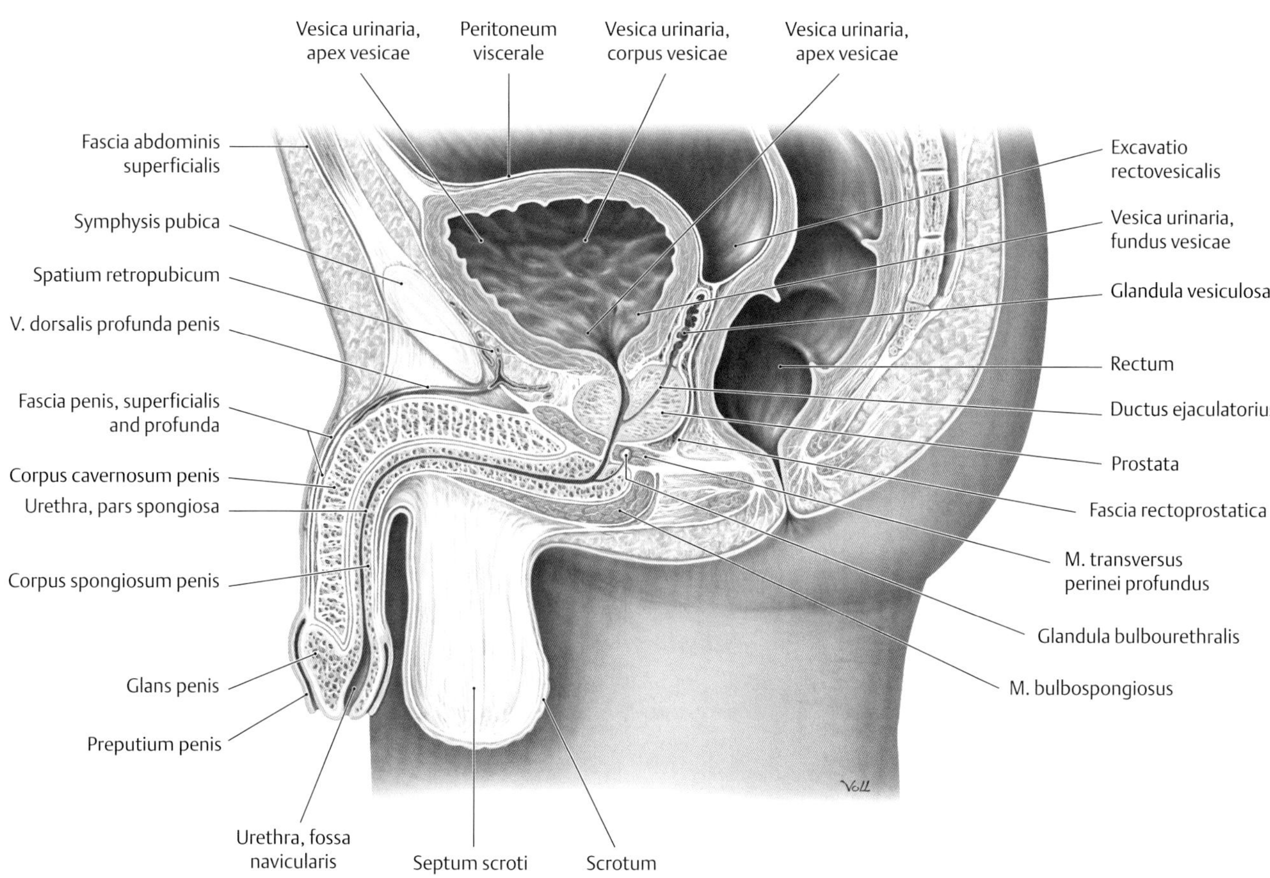
Vesica urinaria, apex vesicae
Peritoneum viscerale
Vesica urinaria, corpus vesicae
Vesica urinaria, apex vesicae
Fascia abdominis superficialis
Symphysis pubica
Spatium retropubicum
V. dorsalis profunda penis
Fascia penis, superficialis and profunda
Corpus cavernosum penis
Urethra, pars spongiosa
Corpus spongiosum penis
Glans penis
Preputium penis
Urethra, fossa navicularis
Septum scroti
Scrotum
Excavatio rectovesicalis
Vesica urinaria, fundus vesicae
Glandula vesiculosa
Rectum
Ductus ejaculatorius
Prostata
Fascia rectoprostatica
M. transversus perinei profundus
Glandula bulbourethralis
M. bulbospongiosus
Voll

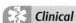

Clinical

Prostatic carcinoma and hypertrophy

Prostatic carcinoma is one of the most common malignant tumors in older men, often growing at a subcapsular location in the peripheral zone of the prostate. Unlike benign prostatic hyperplasia, which begins in the central part of the gland, prostatic carcinoma does not cause urinary outflow obstruction in its early stages. Being in the peripheral zone, the tumor is palpable as a firm mass through the anterior wall of the rectum during rectal examination.

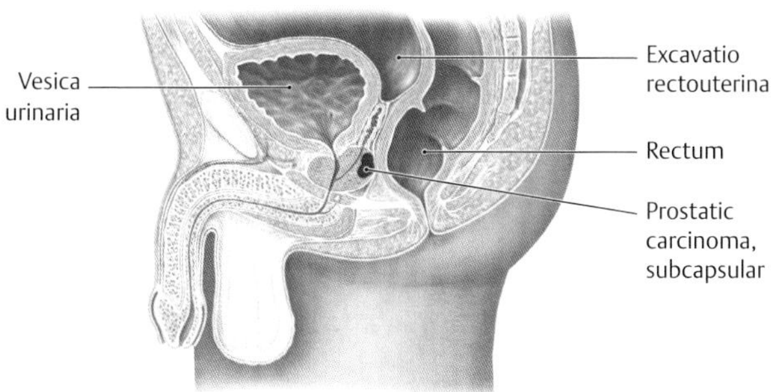
Vesica urinaria
Excavatio rectouterina
Rectum
Prostatic carcinoma, subcapsular

A Common site of prostatic carcinoma.

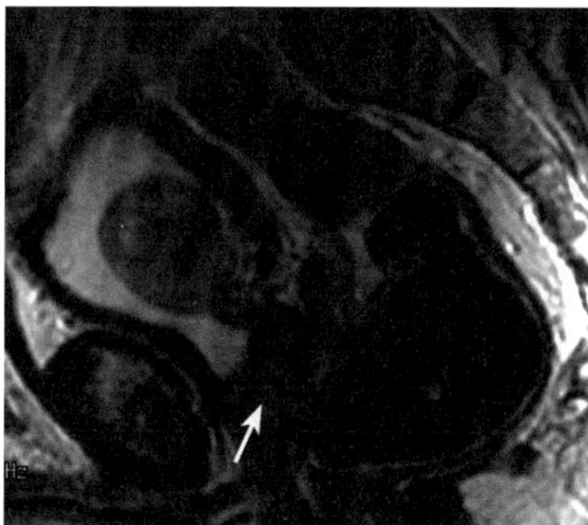

B Prostatic carcinoma (arrow) with bladder infiltration.

In certain prostate diseases, especially cancer, increased amounts of a protein, prostate-specific antigen or PSA, appear in the blood. This protein can be measured by a simple blood test.

Neurovasculature of the Male Genitalia

Fig. 14.26 **Neurovasculature of the male genitalia**
Left lateral view.

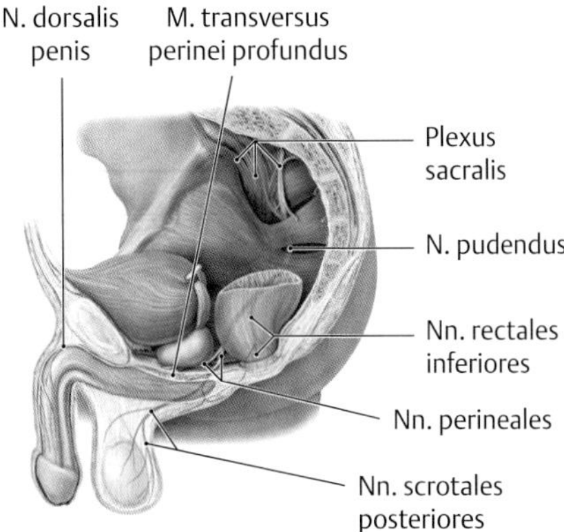

N. dorsalis penis
M. transversus perinei profundus
Plexus sacralis
N. pudendus
Nn. rectales inferiores
Nn. perineales
Nn. scrotales posteriores

A Nerve supply.

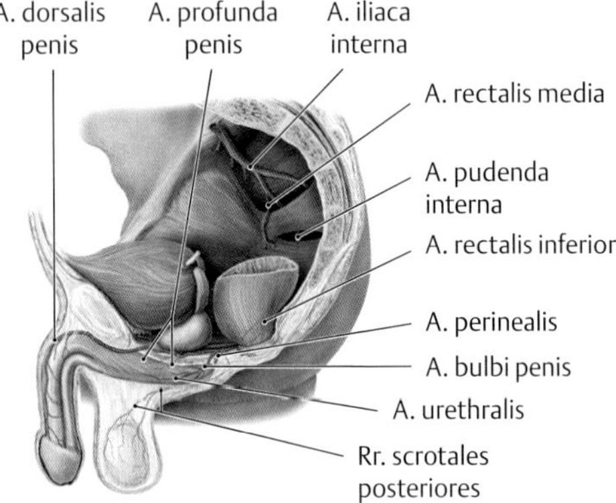

A. dorsalis penis
A. profunda penis
A. iliaca interna
A. rectalis media
A. pudenda interna
A. rectalis inferior
A. perinealis
A. bulbi penis
A. urethralis
Rr. scrotales posteriores

B Arterial supply.

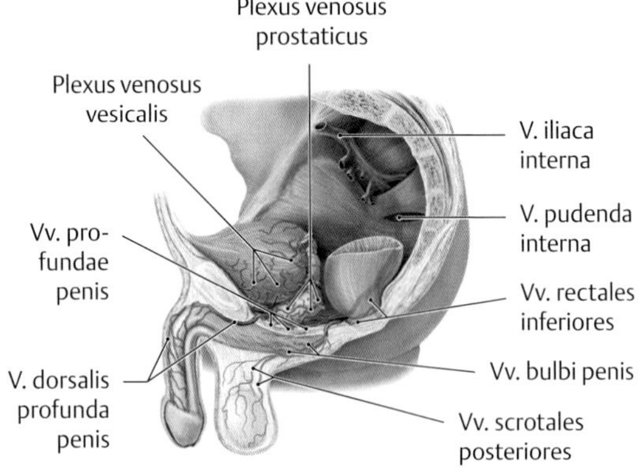

Plexus venosus prostaticus
Plexus venosus vesicalis
Vv. profundae penis
V. dorsalis profunda penis
V. iliaca interna
V. pudenda interna
Vv. rectales inferiores
Vv. bulbi penis
Vv. scrotales posteriores

C Venous drainage.

Fig. 14.27 **Neurovasculature of the penis and scrotum**

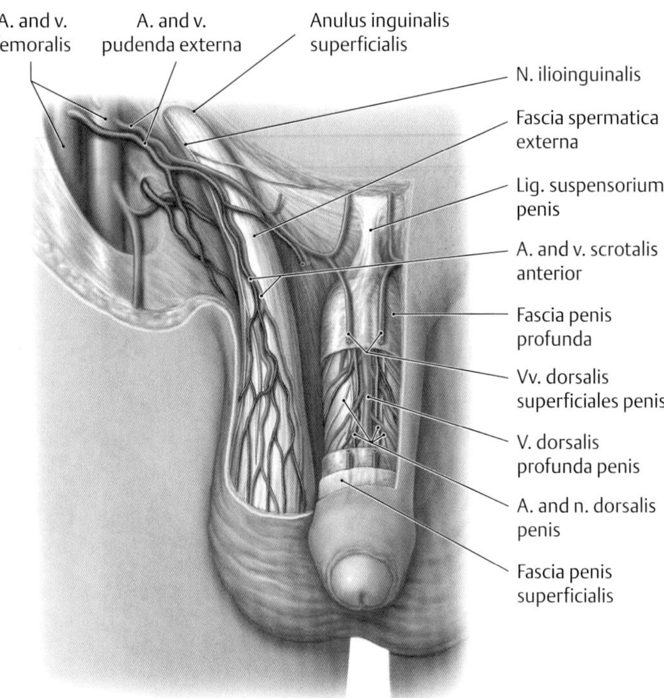

A. and v. femoralis
A. and v. pudenda externa
Anulus inguinalis superficialis
N. ilioinguinalis
Fascia spermatica externa
Lig. suspensorium penis
A. and v. scrotalis anterior
Fascia penis profunda
Vv. dorsalis superficiales penis
V. dorsalis profunda penis
A. and n. dorsalis penis
Fascia penis superficialis

A Anterior view. *Partially removed:* Skin and fascia.

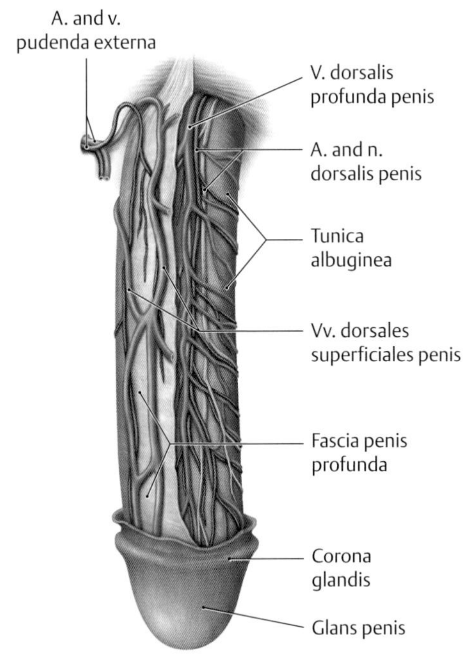

A. and v. pudenda externa
V. dorsalis profunda penis
A. and n. dorsalis penis
Tunica albuginea
Vv. dorsales superficiales penis
Fascia penis profunda
Corona glandis
Glans penis

B Dorsal vasculature of the penis.

Fig. 14.28 Nerves of the male perineum and genitalia

Lithotomy position.

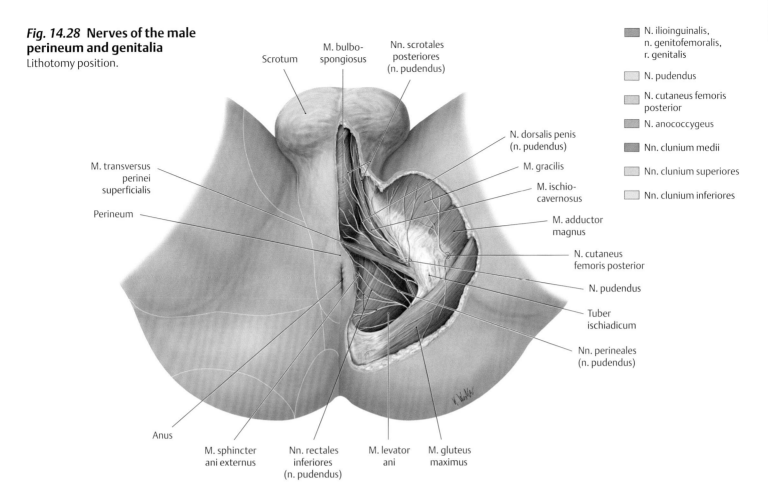

Scrotum
M. bulbo-spongiosus
Nn. scrotales posteriores (n. pudendus)
M. transversus perinei superficialis
Perineum
N. dorsalis penis (n. pudendus)
M. gracilis
M. ischio-cavernosus
M. adductor magnus
N. cutaneus femoris posterior
N. pudendus
Tuber ischiadicum
Nn. perineales (n. pudendus)
Anus
M. sphincter ani externus
Nn. rectales inferiores (n. pudendus)
M. levator ani
M. gluteus maximus

N. ilioinguinalis, n. genitofemoralis, r. genitalis
N. pudendus
N. cutaneus femoris posterior
N. anococcygeus
Nn. clunium medii
Nn. clunium superiores
Nn. clunium inferiores

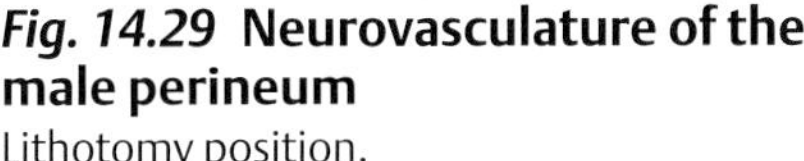

Fig. 14.29 Neurovasculature of the male perineum

Lithotomy position.

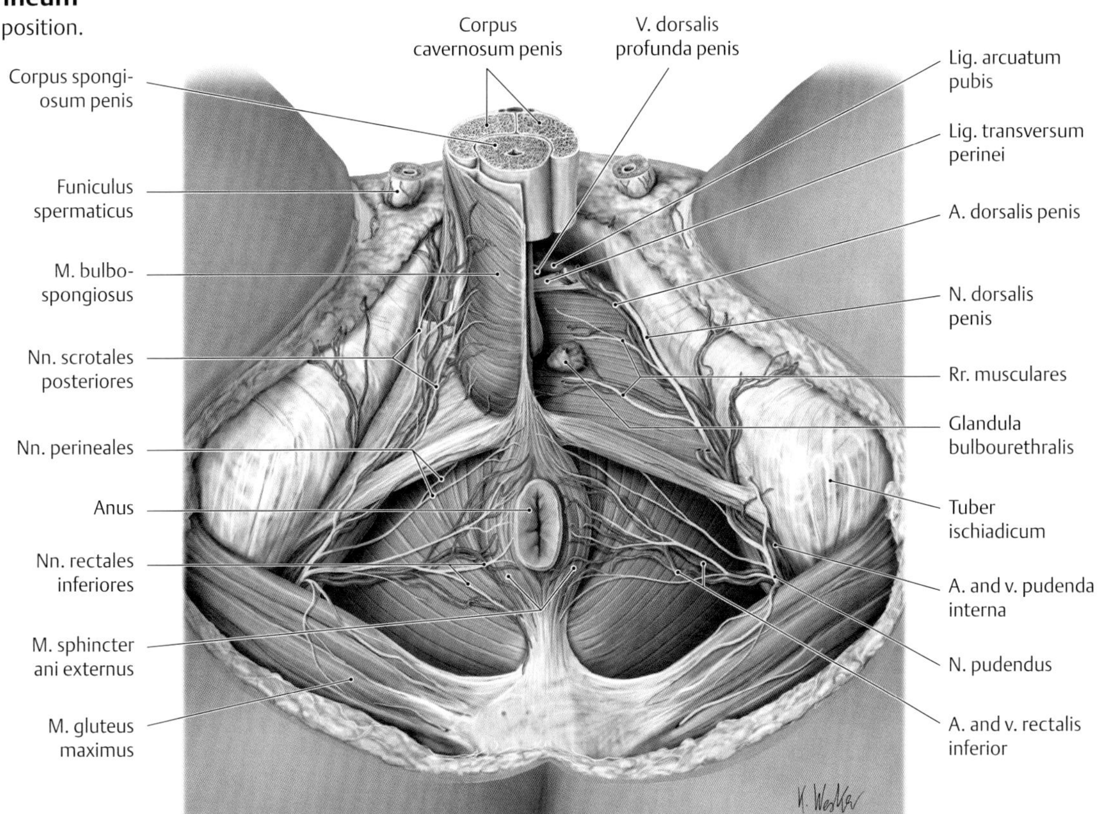
Corpus cavernosum penis
V. dorsalis profunda penis
Corpus spongiosum penis
Funiculus spermaticus
M. bulbo-spongiosus
Nn. scrotales posteriores
Nn. perineales
Anus
Nn. rectales inferiores
M. sphincter ani externus
M. gluteus maximus
Lig. arcuatum pubis
Lig. transversum perinei
A. dorsalis penis
N. dorsalis penis
Rr. musculares
Glandula bulbourethralis
Tuber ischiadicum
A. and v. pudenda interna
N. pudendus
A. and v. rectalis inferior

Development of the Genitalia

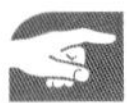

The male and female genitalia are derived from a common gonadal primordium.

Fig. 14.30 **Development of the external genitalia**

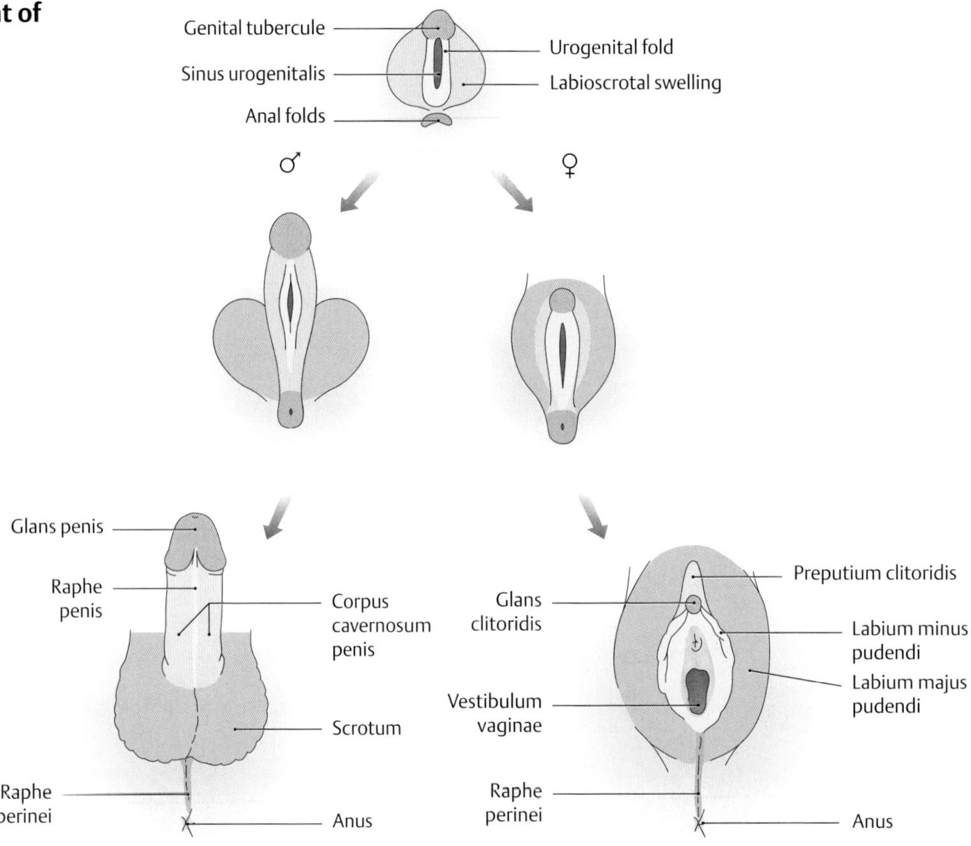
Genital tubercule
Sinus urogenitalis
Anal folds
Urogenital fold
Labioscrotal swelling
♂
♀
Glans penis
Raphe penis
Corpus cavernosum penis
Scrotum
Raphe perinei
Anus
Glans clitoridis
Vestibulum vaginae
Raphe perinei
Preputium clitoridis
Labium minus pudendi
Labium majus pudendi
Anus

Fig. 14.31 **Descent of the testis**
Left lateral view.

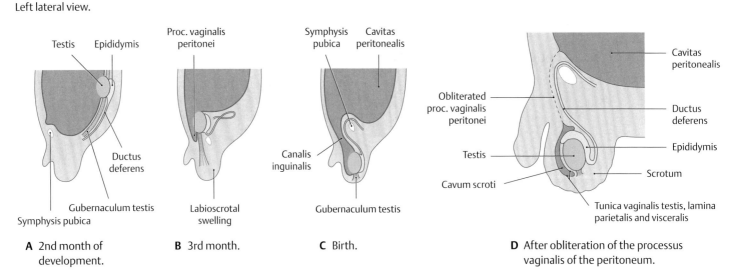

Testis
Epididymis
Ductus deferens
Gubernaculum testis
Symphysis pubica

A 2nd month of development.

Proc. vaginalis peritonei
Labioscrotal swelling

B 3rd month.

Symphysis pubica
Cavitas peritonealis
Canalis inguinalis
Gubernaculum testis

C Birth.

Obliterated proc. vaginalis peritonei
Testis
Cavum scroti
Cavitas peritonealis
Ductus deferens
Epididymis
Scrotum
Tunica vaginalis testis, lamina parietalis and visceralis

D After obliteration of the processus vaginalis of the peritoneum.

Fig. 14.32 Development of the internal genitalia
Anterior view.

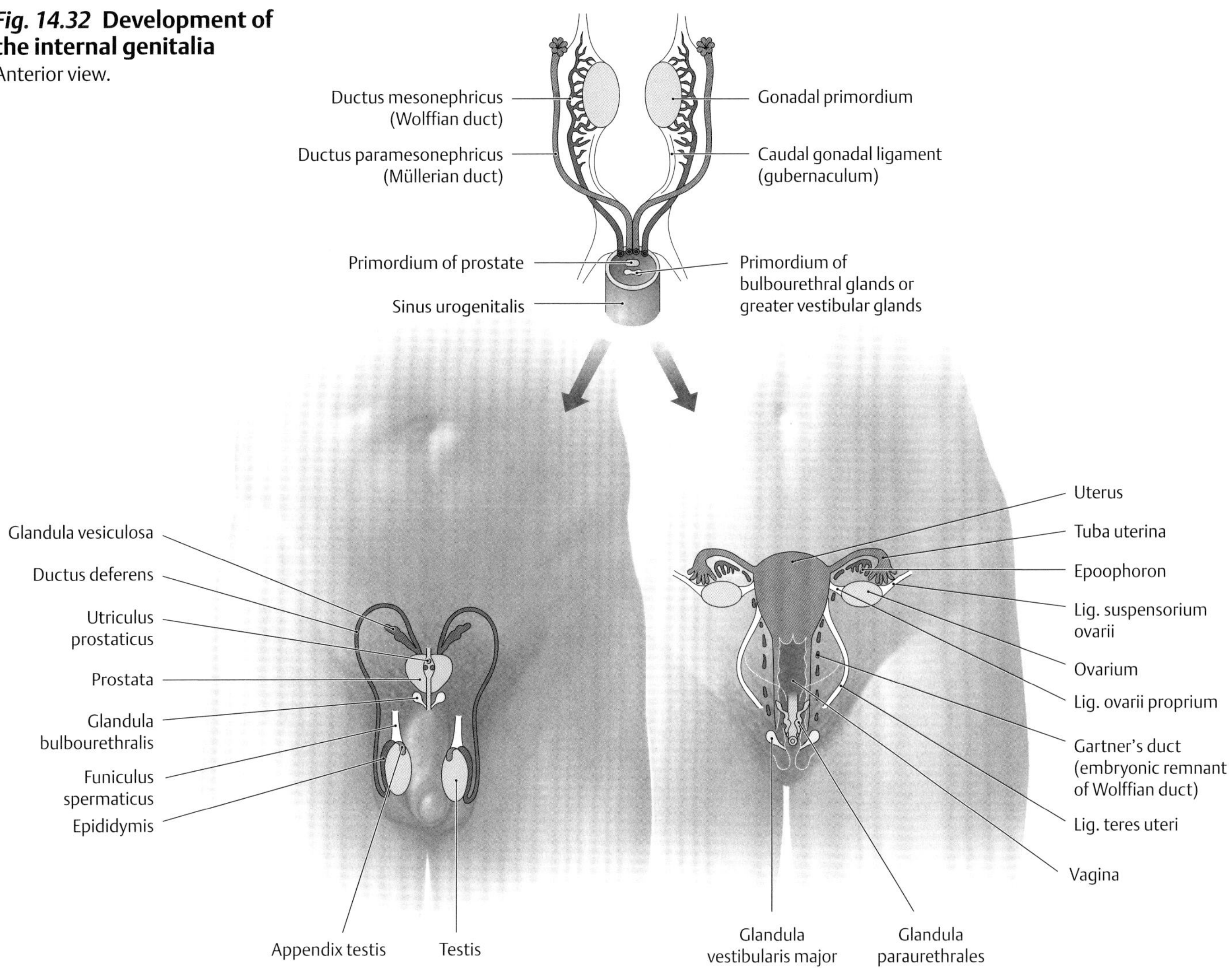

Ductus mesonephricus (Wolffian duct)
Gonadal primordium
Ductus paramesonephricus (Müllerian duct)
Caudal gonadal ligament (gubernaculum)
Primordium of prostate
Primordium of bulbourethral glands or greater vestibular glands
Sinus urogenitalis
Glandula vesiculosa
Ductus deferens
Utriculus prostaticus
Prostata
Glandula bulbourethralis
Funiculus spermaticus
Epididymis
Appendix testis
Testis
Uterus
Tuba uterina
Epoophoron
Lig. suspensorium ovarii
Ovarium
Lig. ovarii proprium
Gartner's duct (embryonic remnant of Wolffian duct)
Lig. teres uteri
Vagina
Glandula vestibularis major
Glandula paraurethrales

A Genetically male embryo (testicular primordium).

B Genetically female embryo (ovarian primordium).

Table 14.4 Derivatives of embryonic urogenital structures

Nonfunctioning remnants in italics. Structures common to both sexes in bold.

Rudiment	Male structure	Female structure
Undifferentiated gonad	Testis	Ovarium
Cortex	Tubuli seminiferi	Folliculi
Medulla	Rete testis	Stroma ovarii
Mesonephric ductule	Ductuli efferentis testis, *paradidymis*	*Epo- and paroöphoron*
Mesonephric (Wolffian) duct	**Ureter, pelvis renalis and calices, collecting ducts**	
	Ductus epididymidis, ductus deferens, ductus ejaculatorius, glandula vesiculosa	–
Paramesonephric (Müllerian) duct	*Appendix testis*	Tuba uterina, uterus, vagina (superior portion), *Morgagni's hydatids*
Sinus urogenitalis	**Vesica urinaria, urethra**	
	Prostata, glandula bulbourethralis, *utriculus prostaticus*	Vagina (inferior portion), glandula vestibularis minor and major
Phallus (tuberculum genitalis)	Corpus cavernosum penis	Clitoris, glans clitoridis
Genital folds	Glans of penis, *raphe penis*	Labia minora, *bulbus vestibularis*
Labioscrotal swellings	Skrotum	Labia majora
Gubernaculum	*Gubernaculum testis*	Lig. ovarium proprium, lig. teres uteri
Tuberculum genitalis (of Müller)	*Colliculus seminalis*	*Hymen*

Arteries of the Abdomen

Fig. 15.1 Aorta abdominalis and major branches

Anterior view. The aorta abdominalis enters the abdomen at the T XII level through hiatus aortae of the diaphragm (see p. 54). Before bifurcating at L IV into its terminal branches, a. iliaca communis, the aorta abdominalis gives off a. renalis (see p. 209) and three major trunks that supply the organs of the alimentary canal:

Truncus coeliacus: Supplies the structures of the foregut, the anterior portion of the alimentary canal. The foregut consists of the esophagus (distal half), gaster, duodenum (proximal half), hepar, vesica biliaris, and pancreas (superior portion).

A. mesenterica superior: Supplies the structures of the midgut: the duodenum (distal half), jejunum and ileum, cecum and appendix, colon ascendens and transversum, and right colic (hepatic) flexure.

A. mesenterica inferior: Supplies the structures of the hindgut: the colon transversum (distal third), left colic (splenic) flexure, colon descendens and sigmoiden, rectum, and canalis analis (upper part).

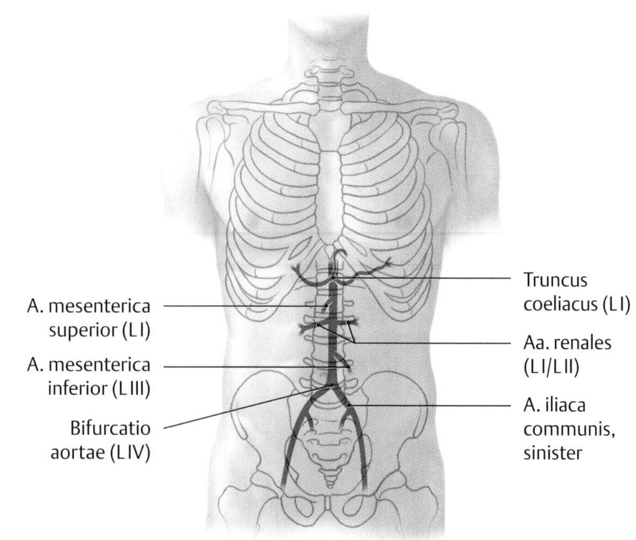
A. mesenterica superior (L I)
A. mesenterica inferior (L III)
Bifurcatio aortae (L IV)
Truncus coeliacus (L I)
Aa. renales (L I/L II)
A. iliaca communis, sinister

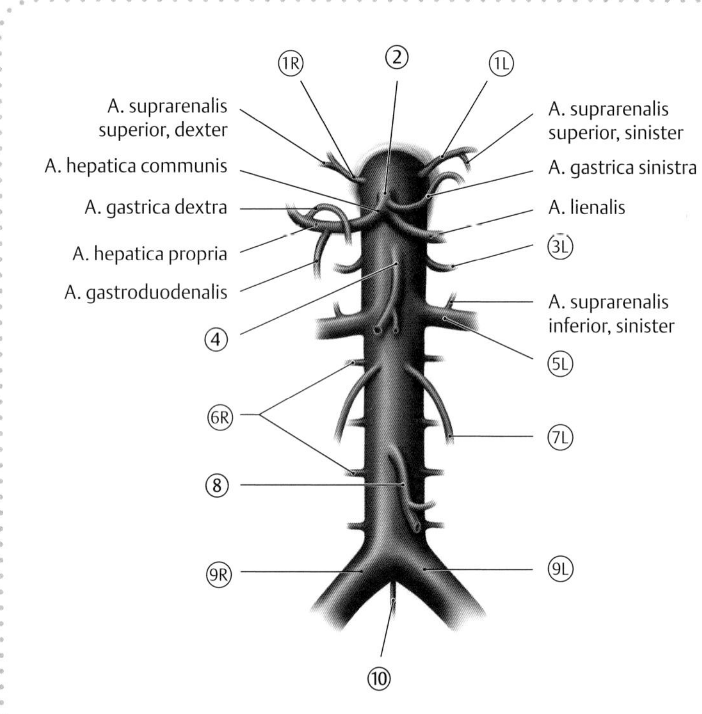
1R
2
1L
A. suprarenalis superior, dexter
A. hepatica communis
A. gastrica dextra
A. hepatica propria
A. gastroduodenalis
4
6R
8
9R
10
A. suprarenalis superior, sinister
A. gastrica sinistra
A. lienalis
3L
A. suprarenalis inferior, sinister
5L
7L
9L

Table 15.1 Branches of the aorta abdominalis

The aorta abdominalis gives rise to three major unpaired trunks (bold) and the unpaired a. sacralis mediana, as well as six paired branches.

Branch from aorta abdominalis			Branches	
1R	1L	A. phrenica inferior (paired)	A. suprarenalis superior	
2		**Truncus coeliacus**	A. gastrica sinister	
			A. lienalis	
			A. hepatica communis	A. hepatica propria
				A. gastrica dextra
				A. gastroduodenalis
3R	3L	A. suprarenalis media (paired)		
4		**A. mesenterica superior**		
5R	5L	A. renalis (paired)	A. suprarenalis inferior	
6R	6L	Aa. lumbales (1st through 4th, paired)		
7R	7L	A. testicularis/ovarica (paired)		
8		**A. mesenterica inferior**		
9R	9L	A. iliaca communis (paired)	A. iliaca externa	
			A. iliaca interna	
10		A. sacralis mediana		

Fig. 15.2 Truncus coeliacus

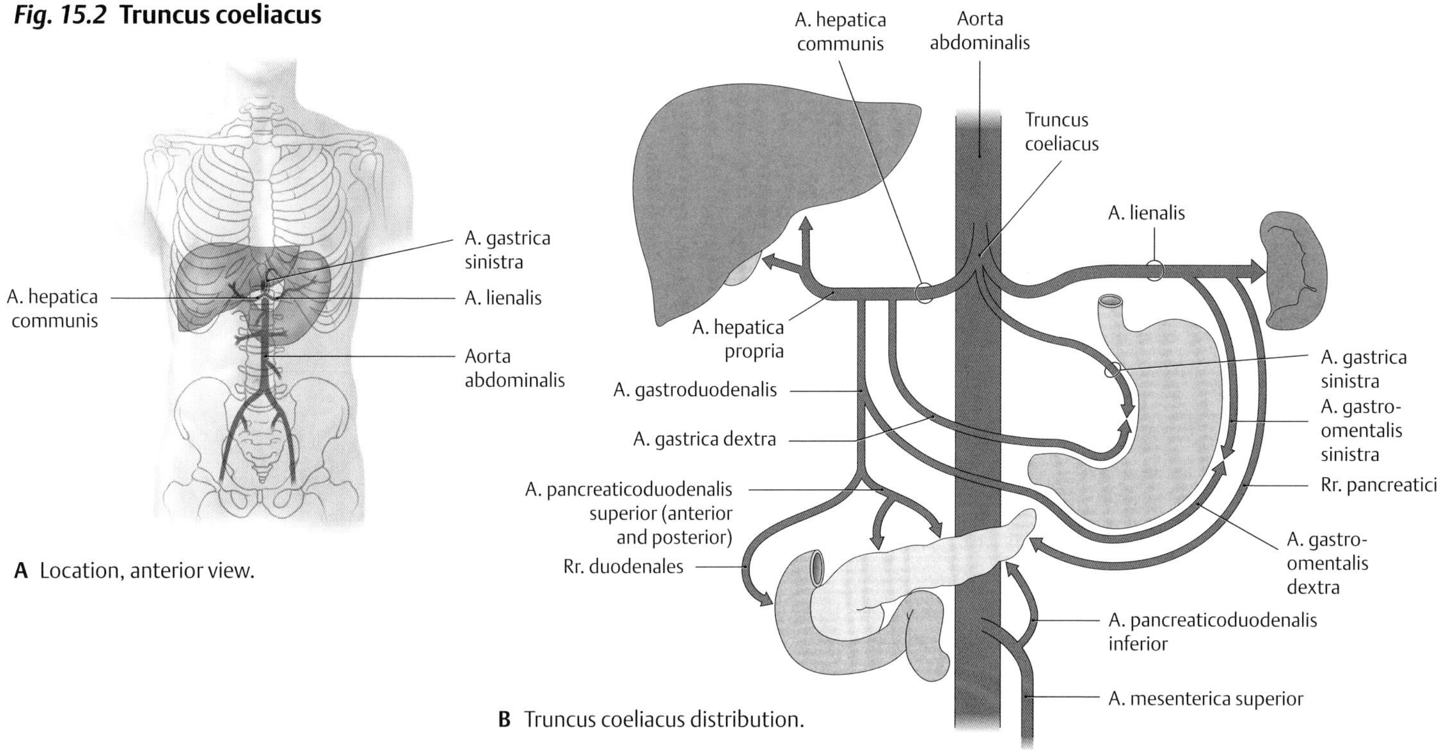
A. gastrica sinistra
A. hepatica communis
A. lienalis
Aorta abdominalis
A. hepatica communis
Aorta abdominalis
Truncus coeliacus
A. lienalis
A. hepatica propria
A. gastroduodenalis
A. gastrica dextra
A. pancreaticoduodenalis superior (anterior and posterior)
Rr. duodenales
A. gastrica sinistra
A. gastro-omentalis sinistra
Rr. pancreatici
A. gastro-omentalis dextra
A. pancreaticoduodenalis inferior
A. mesenterica superior

A Location, anterior view.

B Truncus coeliacus distribution.

Fig. 15.3 A. mesenterica superior

Anterior view.

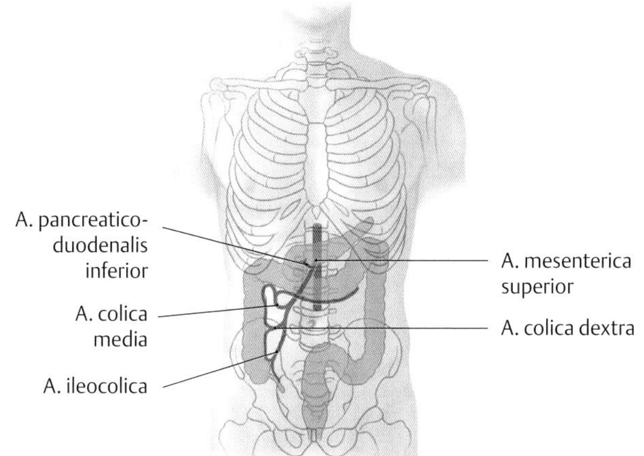
A. pancreatico-duodenalis inferior
A. colica media
A. ileocolica
A. mesenterica superior
A. colica dextra

Fig. 15.4 A. mesenterica inferior

Anterior view.

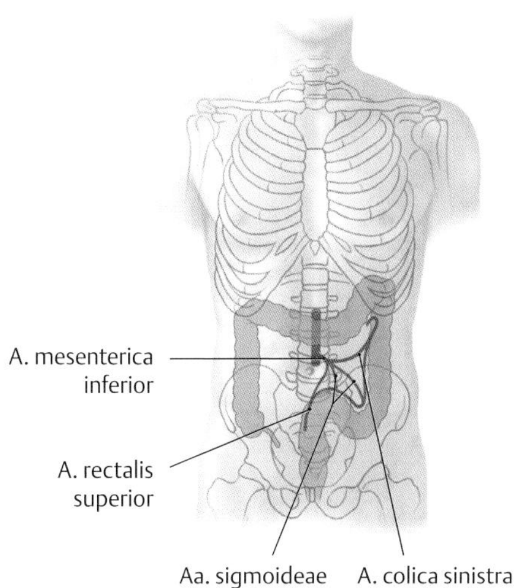
A. mesenterica inferior
A. rectalis superior
Aa. sigmoideae
A. colica sinistra

Fig. 15.5 Aorta abdominalis anastomoses

The three major arterial anastomoses of the abdomen deliver blood to intestinal areas deprived of their normal blood supply.

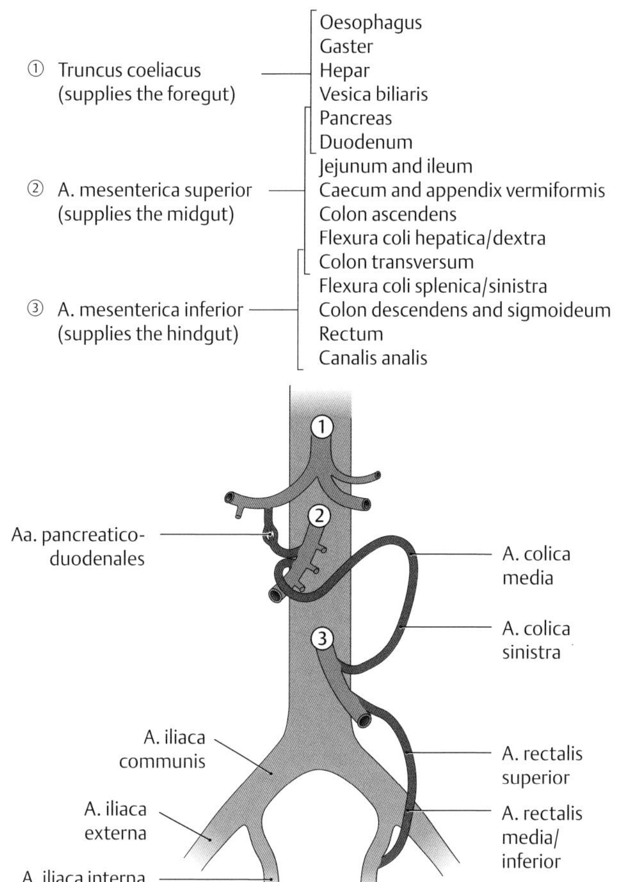
① Truncus coeliacus (supplies the foregut)
② A. mesenterica superior (supplies the midgut)
③ A. mesenterica inferior (supplies the hindgut)
Oesophagus
Gaster
Hepar
Vesica biliaris
Pancreas
Duodenum
Jejunum and ileum
Caecum and appendix vermiformis
Colon ascendens
Flexura coli hepatica/dextra
Colon transversum
Flexura coli splenica/sinistra
Colon descendens and sigmoideum
Rectum
Canalis analis
1
2
3
Aa. pancreatico-duodenales
A. colica media
A. colica sinistra
A. iliaca communis
A. iliaca externa
A. iliaca interna
A. rectalis superior
A. rectalis media/inferior

Aorta Abdominalis & Arteriae Renales

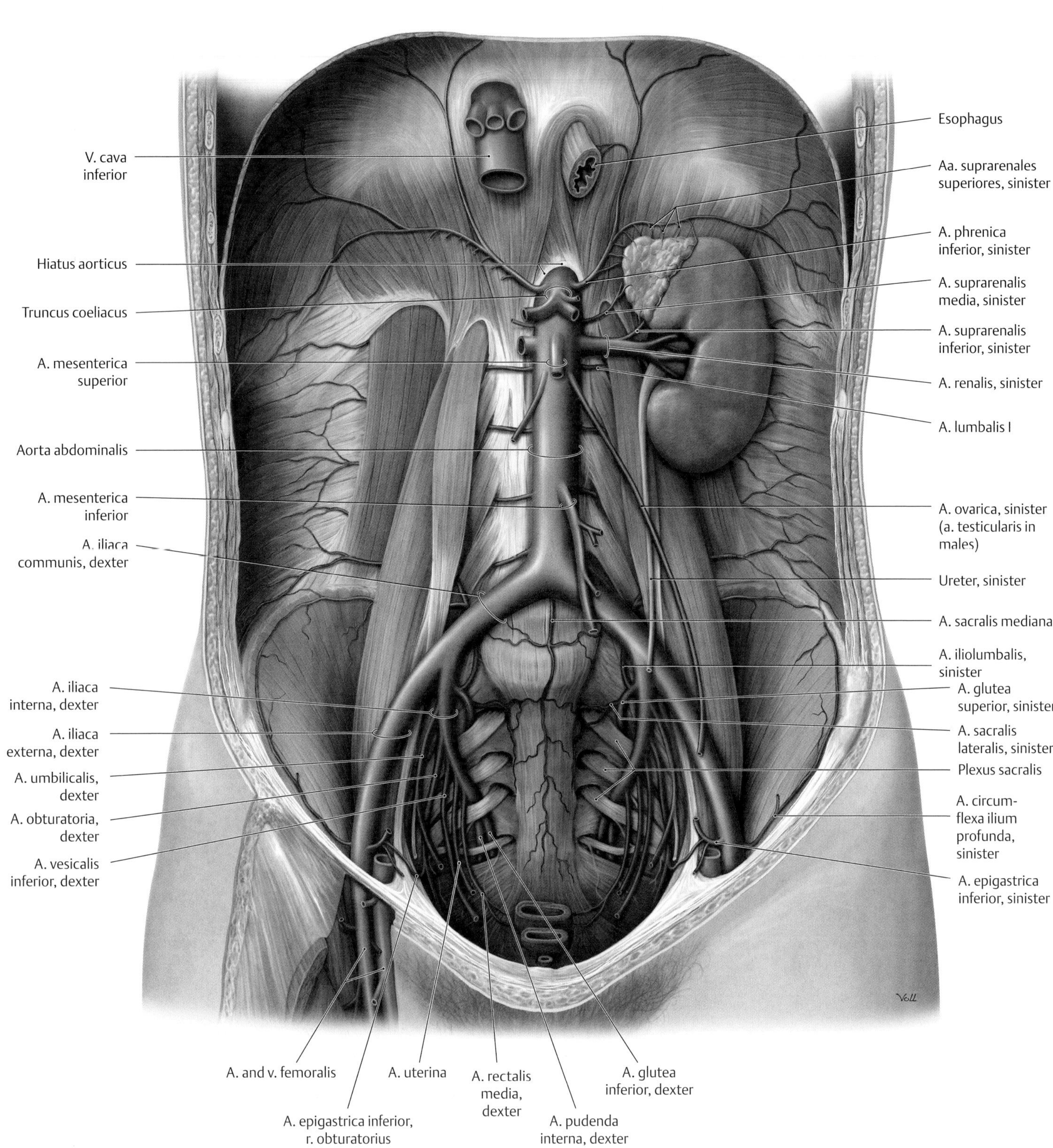
Esophagus
V. cava inferior
Aa. suprarenales superiores, sinister
A. phrenica inferior, sinister
Hiatus aorticus
A. suprarenalis media, sinister
Truncus coeliacus
A. suprarenalis inferior, sinister
A. mesenterica superior
A. renalis, sinister
A. lumbalis I
Aorta abdominalis
A. mesenterica inferior
A. ovarica, sinister (a. testicularis in males)
A. iliaca communis, dexter
Ureter, sinister
A. sacralis mediana
A. iliolumbalis, sinister
A. iliaca interna, dexter
A. glutea superior, sinister
A. iliaca externa, dexter
A. sacralis lateralis, sinister
A. umbilicalis, dexter
Plexus sacralis
A. obturatoria, dexter
A. circumflexa ilium profunda, sinister
A. vesicalis inferior, dexter
A. epigastrica inferior, sinister
A. and v. femoralis
A. uterina
A. rectalis media, dexter
A. glutea inferior, dexter
A. epigastrica inferior, r. obturatorius
A. pudenda interna, dexter
Voll

***Fig. 15.6* Aorta abdominalis**
Anterior view of the female abdomen. *Removed:* Abdominal organs and peritoneum. The aorta abdominalis is the distal continuation of the aorta thoracica (see p. 68). It enters the abdomen at the T XII level and bifurcates into a. iliaca communis at L IV.

Fig. 15.7 Arterine renales

Ren sinister, anterior view. Aa. renales arise at approximately the level of L II. Each renal artery divides into an anterior and a posterior rami. The anterior rami further divides into four segmental arteries (circled).

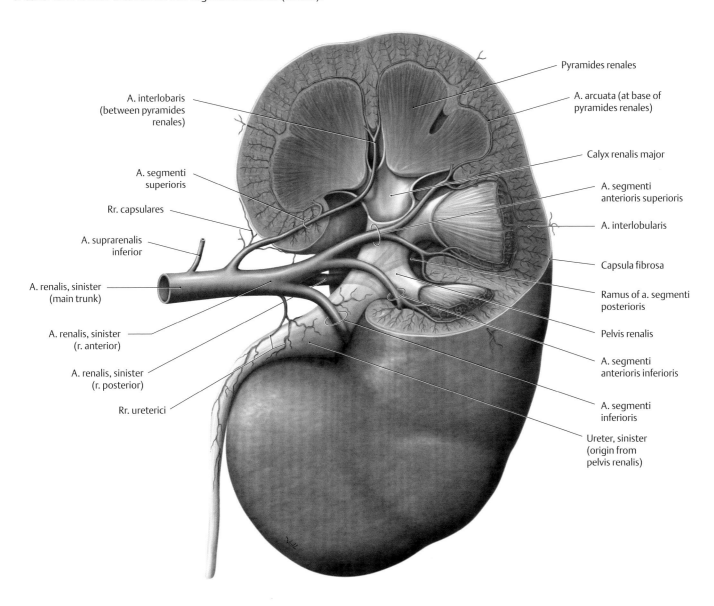

A. interlobaris (between pyramides renales)
A. segmenti superioris
Rr. capsulares
A. suprarenalis inferior
A. renalis, sinister (main trunk)
A. renalis, sinister (r. anterior)
A. renalis, sinister (r. posterior)
Rr. ureterici
Pyramides renales
A. arcuata (at base of pyramides renales)
Calyx renalis major
A. segmenti anterioris superioris
A. interlobularis
Capsula fibrosa
Ramus of a. segmenti posterioris
Pelvis renalis
A. segmenti anterioris inferioris
A. segmenti inferioris
Ureter, sinister (origin from pelvis renalis)

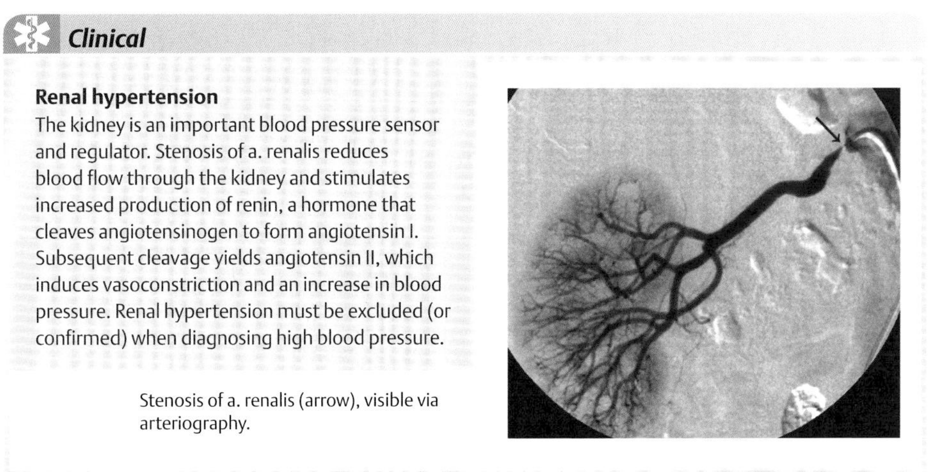

Clinical

Renal hypertension

The kidney is an important blood pressure sensor and regulator. Stenosis of a. renalis reduces blood flow through the kidney and stimulates increased production of renin, a hormone that cleaves angiotensinogen to form angiotensin I. Subsequent cleavage yields angiotensin II, which induces vasoconstriction and an increase in blood pressure. Renal hypertension must be excluded (or confirmed) when diagnosing high blood pressure.

Stenosis of a. renalis (arrow), visible via arteriography.

Truncus Coeliacus

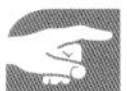
The distribution of truncus coeliacus is shown on p. 207.

Fig. 15.8 Truncus coeliacus: Gaster, hepar, and vesica biliaris
Anterior view. *Opened:* Omentum minus. *Incised:* Omentum majus. Truncus coeliacus arises from the aorta abdominalis at about the level of L I.

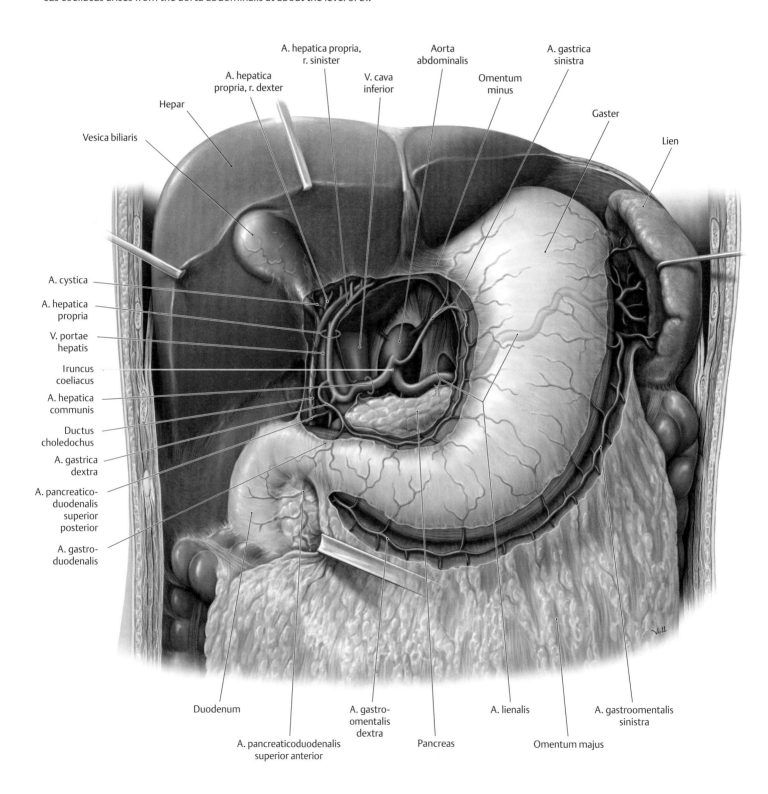

A. hepatica propria, r. sinister
Aorta abdominalis
A. gastrica sinistra
A. hepatica propria, r. dexter
V. cava inferior
Omentum minus
Hepar
Gaster
Vesica biliaris
Lien
A. cystica
A. hepatica propria
V. portae hepatis
Truncus coeliacus
A. hepatica communis
Ductus choledochus
A. gastrica dextra
A. pancreatico-duodenalis superior posterior
A. gastro-duodenalis
Duodenum
A. gastro-omentalis dextra
A. lienalis
A. gastroomentalis sinistra
A. pancreaticoduodenalis superior anterior
Pancreas
Omentum majus

Fig. 15.9 **Truncus coeliacus: Pancreas, duodenum, and lien**
Anterior view. *Removed:* Gaster (body) and omentum minus.

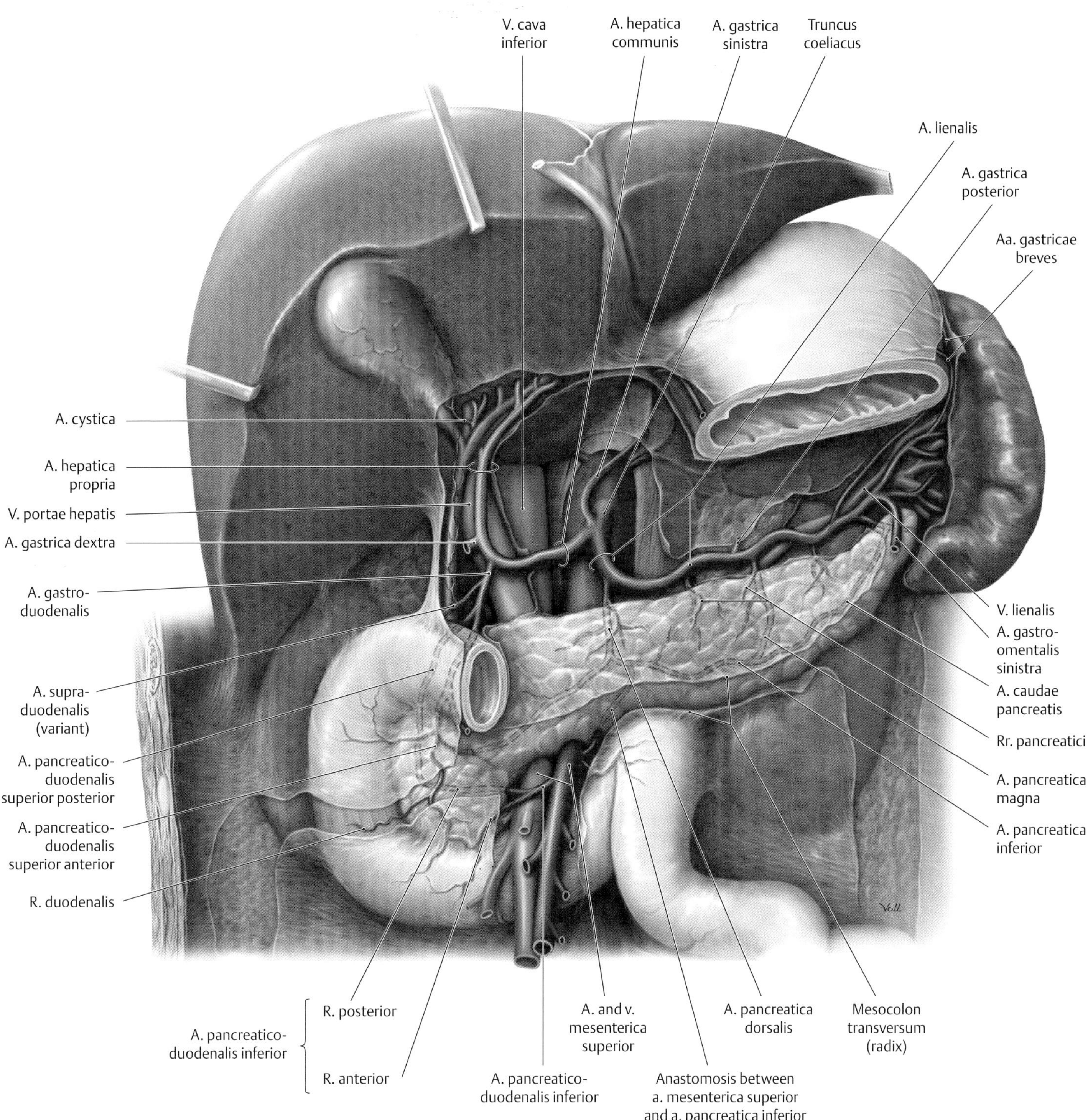
V. cava inferior
A. hepatica communis
A. gastrica sinistra
Truncus coeliacus
A. lienalis
A. gastrica posterior
Aa. gastricae breves
A. cystica
A. hepatica propria
V. portae hepatis
A. gastrica dextra
A. gastro-duodenalis
A. supra-duodenalis (variant)
A. pancreatico-duodenalis superior posterior
A. pancreatico-duodenalis superior anterior
R. duodenalis
V. lienalis
A. gastro-omentalis sinistra
A. caudae pancreatis
Rr. pancreatici
A. pancreatica magna
A. pancreatica inferior
A. pancreatico-duodenalis inferior
R. posterior
R. anterior
A. and v. mesenterica superior
A. pancreatico-duodenalis inferior
A. pancreatica dorsalis
Anastomosis between a. mesenterica superior and a. pancreatica inferior
Mesocolon transversum (radix)
Voll

Arteriae Mesenterica Superior & Inferior

Fig. 15.10 **A. mesenterica superior**
Anterior view. *Partially removed:* Gaster and peritoneum.
Note: A. colica media has been truncated (see Fig. 15.11). Aa. mesenterica superior and inferior arise from the aorta opposite L II and L III, respectively.

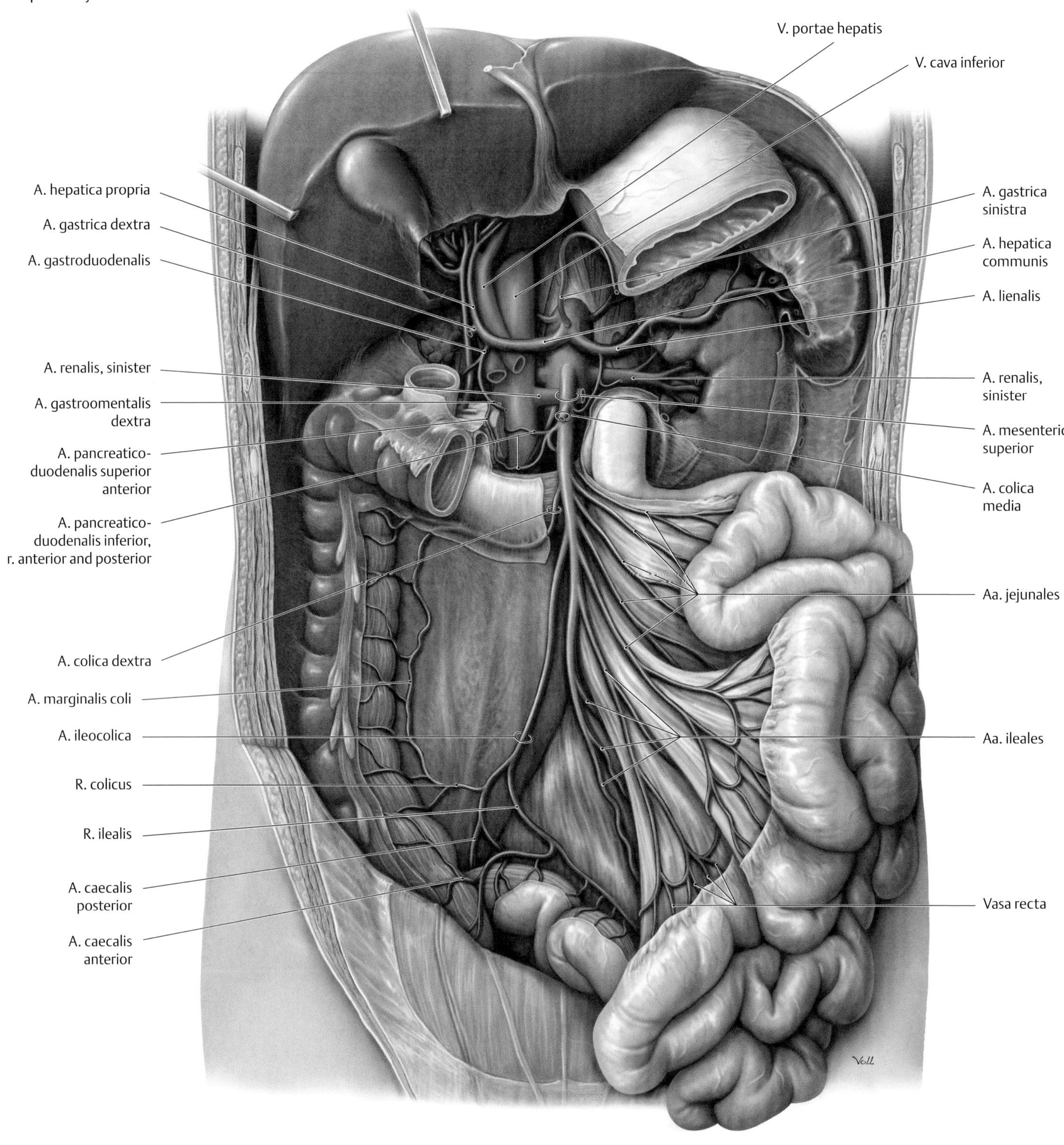
V. portae hepatis
V. cava inferior
A. hepatica propria
A. gastrica dextra
A. gastroduodenalis
A. renalis, sinister
A. gastroomentalis dextra
A. pancreatico-duodenalis superior anterior
A. pancreatico-duodenalis inferior, r. anterior and posterior
A. colica dextra
A. marginalis coli
A. ileocolica
R. colicus
R. ilealis
A. caecalis posterior
A. caecalis anterior
A. gastrica sinistra
A. hepatica communis
A. lienalis
A. renalis, sinister
A. mesenterica superior
A. colica media
Aa. jejunales
Aa. ileales
Vasa recta
Voll

Fig. 15.11 **A. mesenterica inferior**
Anterior view. *Removed:* Jejunum and ileum. *Reflected:* Colon transversum.

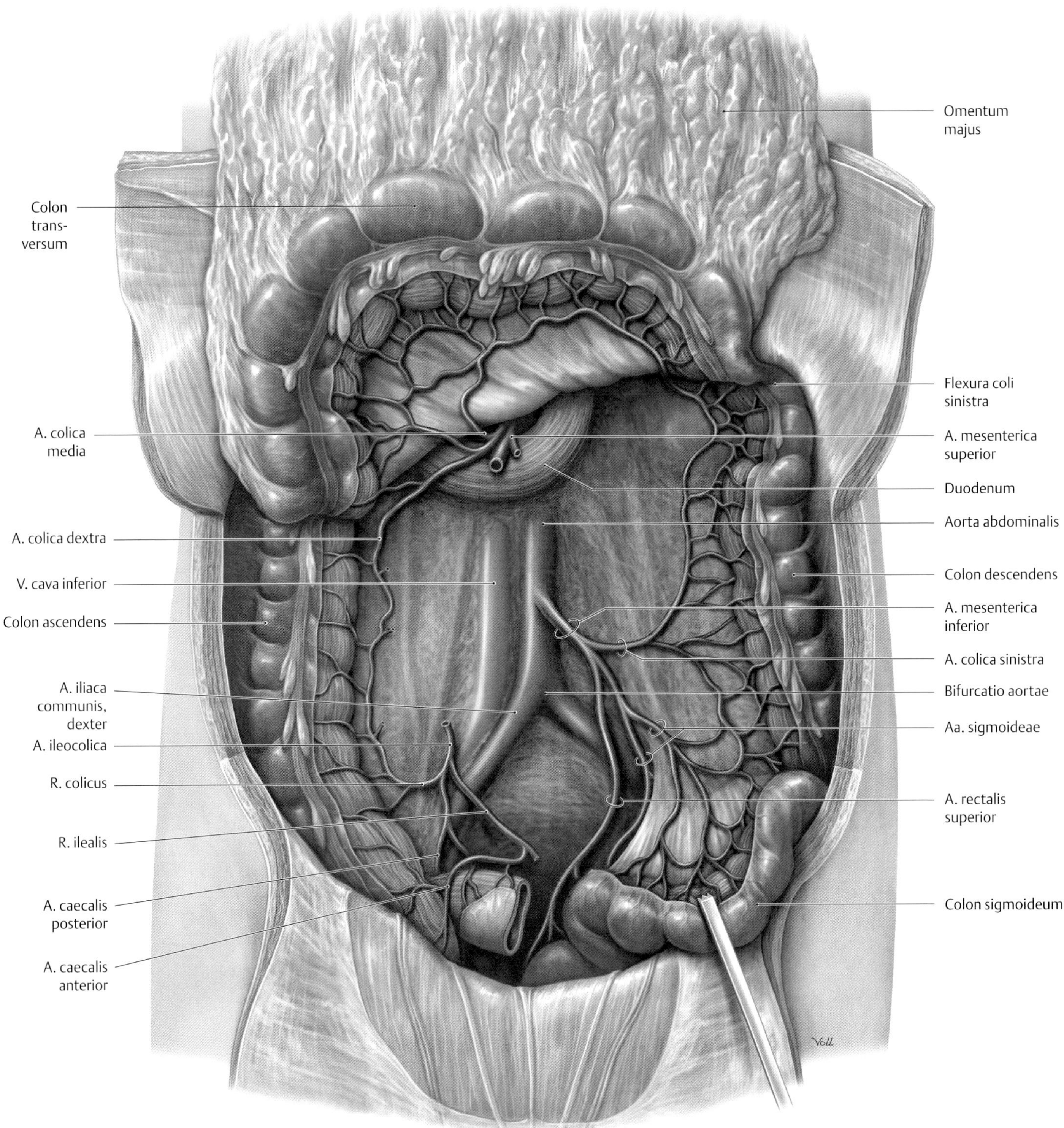
Omentum majus
Colon transversum
Flexura coli sinistra
A. colica media
A. mesenterica superior
Duodenum
Aorta abdominalis
A. colica dextra
Colon descendens
V. cava inferior
Colon ascendens
A. mesenterica inferior
A. colica sinistra
Bifurcatio aortae
A. iliaca communis, dexter
Aa. sigmoideae
A. ileocolica
R. colicus
A. rectalis superior
R. ilealis
A. caecalis posterior
Colon sigmoideum
A. caecalis anterior
Voll

Veins of the Abdomen

Fig. 15.12 **V. cava inferior: Location**
Anterior view.

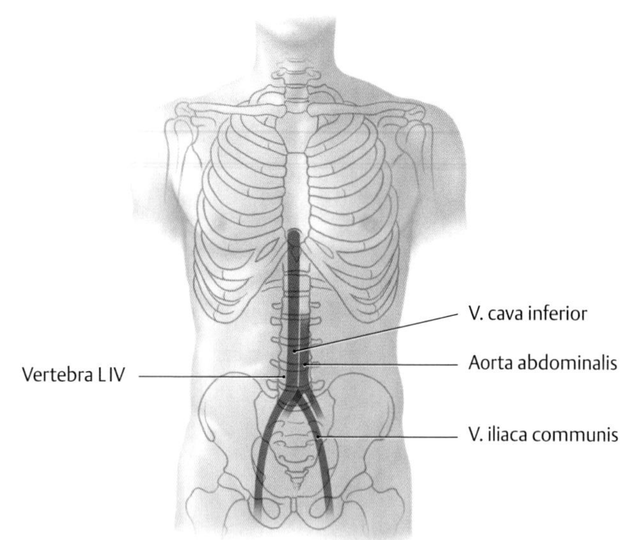
V. cava inferior
Aorta abdominalis
Vertebra LIV
V. iliaca communis

Fig. 15.13 **Tributaries of the vv. renales**
Anterior view.

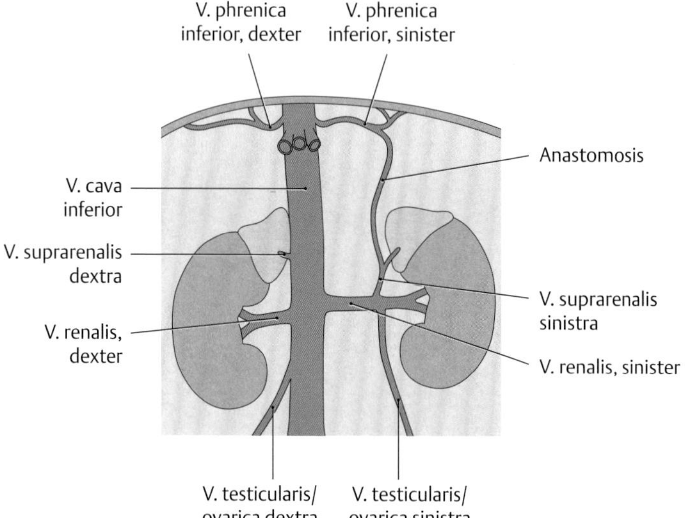
V. phrenica inferior, dexter
V. phrenica inferior, sinister
Anastomosis
V. cava inferior
V. suprarenalis dextra
V. suprarenalis sinistra
V. renalis, dexter
V. renalis, sinister
V. testicularis/ ovarica dextra
V. testicularis/ ovarica sinistra

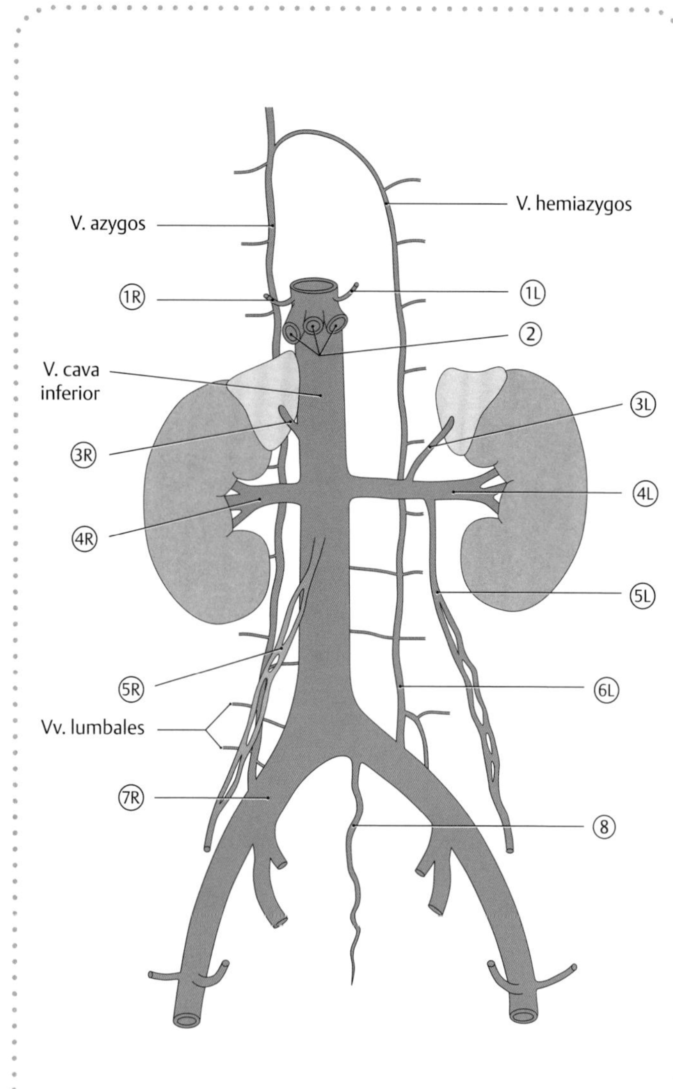
V. azygos
V. hemiazygos
1R
1L
2
V. cava inferior
3L
3R
4L
4R
5L
5R
6L
Vv. lumbales
7R
8

Table 15.2		Tributaries of the inferior vena cava
1R	1L	Vv. phrenicae inferiores (paired)
2		Vv. hepaticae (3)
3R	3L	Vv. suprarenales (the right vena is a direct tributary)
4R	4L	Vv. renales (paired)
5R	5L	Vv. testicularis/ovarica (the right vena is a direct tributary)
6R	6L	Vv. lumbales ascendens (paired)
7R	7L	Vv. iliacae communes (paired)
8		V. sacralis mediana

Fig. 15.14 **V. portae hepatis**

V. portae hepatis (see p. 218) drains venous blood from the abdominopelvic organs supplied by truncus coeliacus and aa. mesenterica superior and inferior.

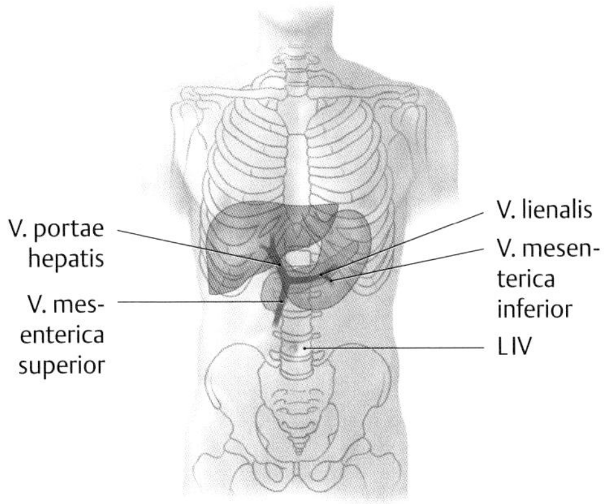
V. portae hepatis
V. mes-enterica superior
V. lienalis
V. mesen-terica inferior
LIV

A Location, anterior view.

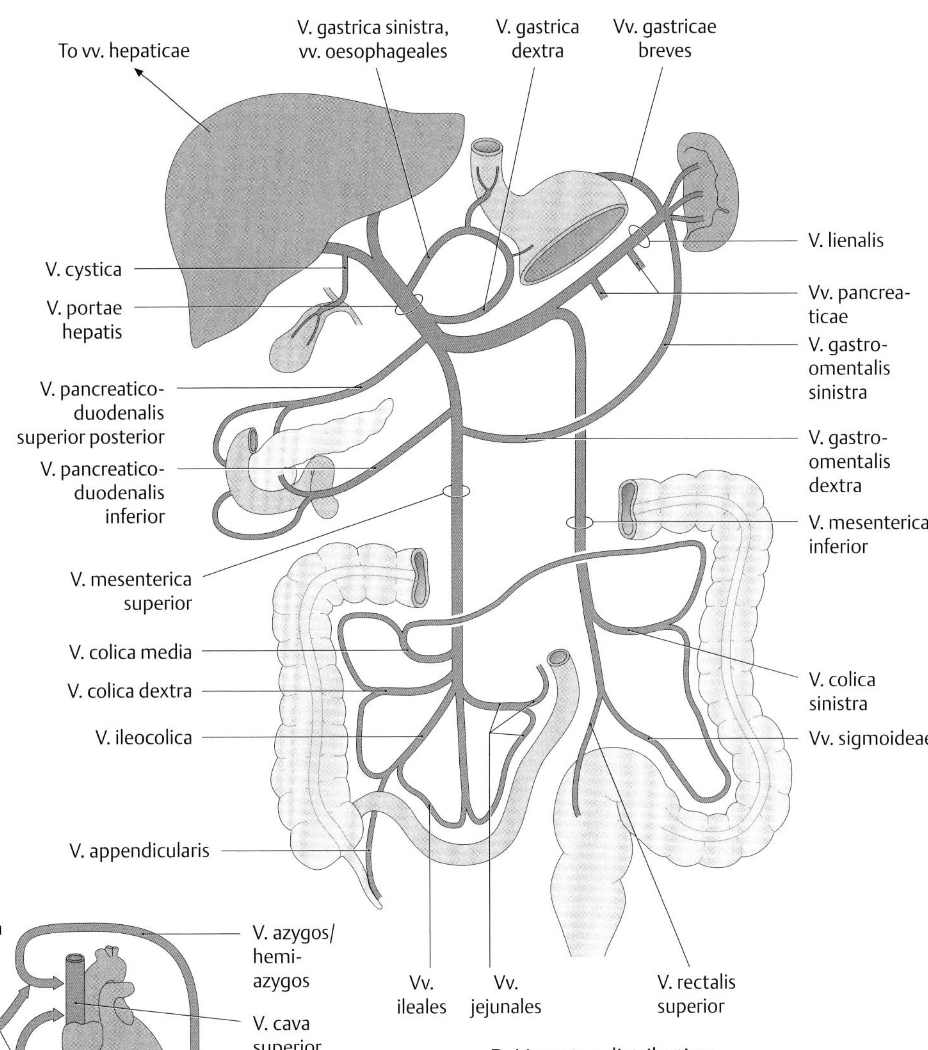
To vv. hepaticae
V. gastrica sinistra, vv. oesophageales
V. gastrica dextra
Vv. gastricae breves
V. lienalis
V. cystica
V. portae hepatis
Vv. pancreaticae
V. gastro-omentalis sinistra
V. pancreatico-duodenalis superior posterior
V. gastro-omentalis dextra
V. pancreatico-duodenalis inferior
V. mesenterica inferior
V. mesenterica superior
V. colica media
V. colica sinistra
V. colica dextra
V. ileocolica
Vv. sigmoideae
V. appendicularis
Vv. ileales
Vv. jejunales
V. rectalis superior

B V. portae distribution.

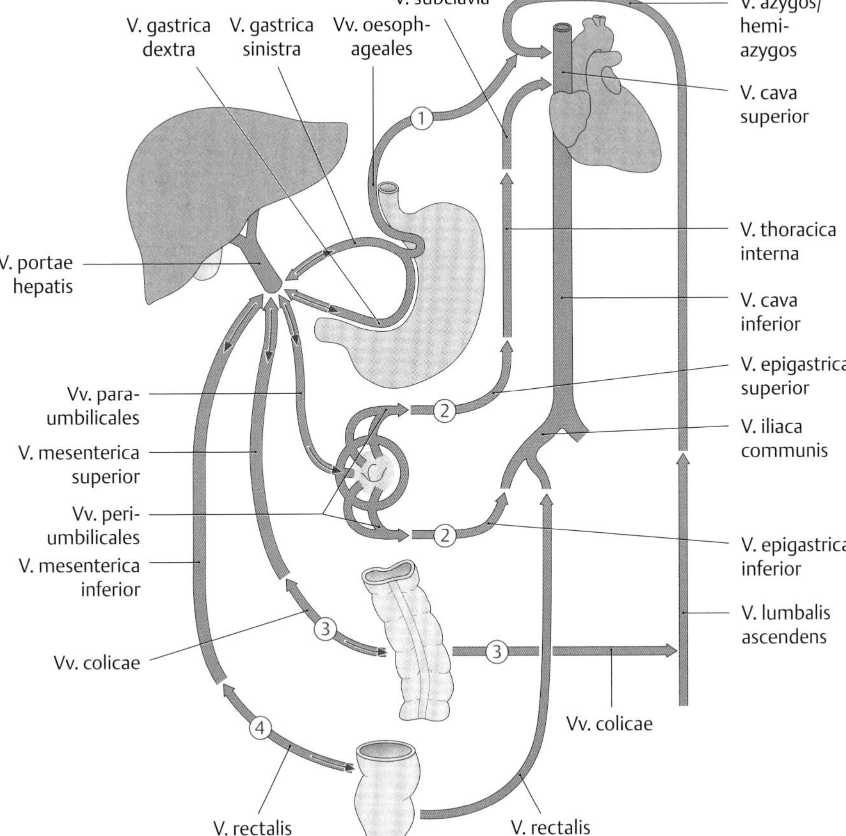
V. gastrica dextra
V. gastrica sinistra
Vv. oesoph-ageales
V. subclavia
V. azygos/hemi-azygos
V. cava superior
V. portae hepatis
V. thoracica interna
V. cava inferior
Vv. para-umbilicales
V. epigastrica superior
V. mesenterica superior
V. iliaca communis
Vv. peri-umbilicales
V. epigastrica inferior
V. mesenterica inferior
V. lumbalis ascendens
Vv. colicae
Vv. colicae
V. rectalis superior
V. rectalis inferor/media
1
2
2
3
3
4

C Collateral pathways (portosystemic collaterals). When the portal system is compromised, nutrient-laden blood may be transported to the heart via the venae cavae without passing through hepar. Red arrows indicate flow reversal.

Clinical

Cancer metastases

Tumors in the region drained by v. rectalis superior may spread through the portal venous system to the capillary bed of hepar (hepatic metastasis). Tumors drained by vv. rectalis media and inferior may metastasize to the capillary bed of the lung (pulmonary metastasis) via the v. cava inferior and right heart.

Vena Cava Inferior & Venae Renales

Fig. 15.15 Vena cava inferior
Anterior view of the female abdomen. *Removed:* All organs (except ren and gl. suprarenalis sinister).

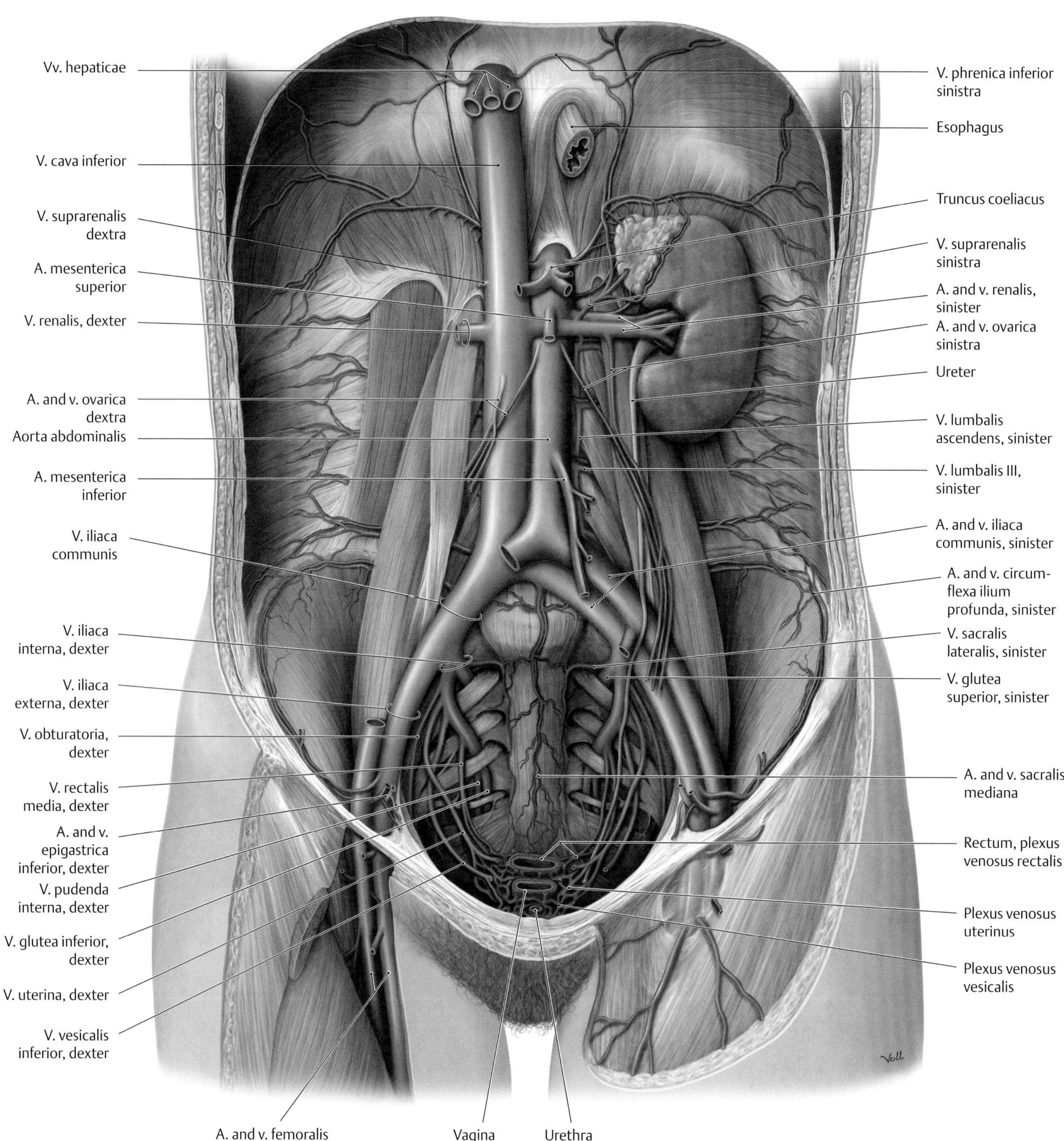
Vv. hepaticae
V. cava inferior
V. suprarenalis dextra
A. mesenterica superior
V. renalis, dexter
A. and v. ovarica dextra
Aorta abdominalis
A. mesenterica inferior
V. iliaca communis
V. iliaca interna, dexter
V. iliaca externa, dexter
V. obturatoria, dexter
V. rectalis media, dexter
A. and v. epigastrica inferior, dexter
V. pudenda interna, dexter
V. glutea inferior, dexter
V. uterina, dexter
V. vesicalis inferior, dexter
A. and v. femoralis
Vagina
Urethra
V. phrenica inferior sinistra
Esophagus
Truncus coeliacus
V. suprarenalis sinistra
A. and v. renalis, sinister
A. and v. ovarica sinistra
Ureter
V. lumbalis ascendens, sinister
V. lumbalis III, sinister
A. and v. iliaca communis, sinister
A. and v. circum-flexa ilium profunda, sinister
V. sacralis lateralis, sinister
V. glutea superior, sinister
A. and v. sacralis mediana
Rectum, plexus venosus rectalis
Plexus venosus uterinus
Plexus venosus vesicalis

Fig. 15.16 **Vv. renales**

Anterior view. See p. 209 for aa. renales in isolation.

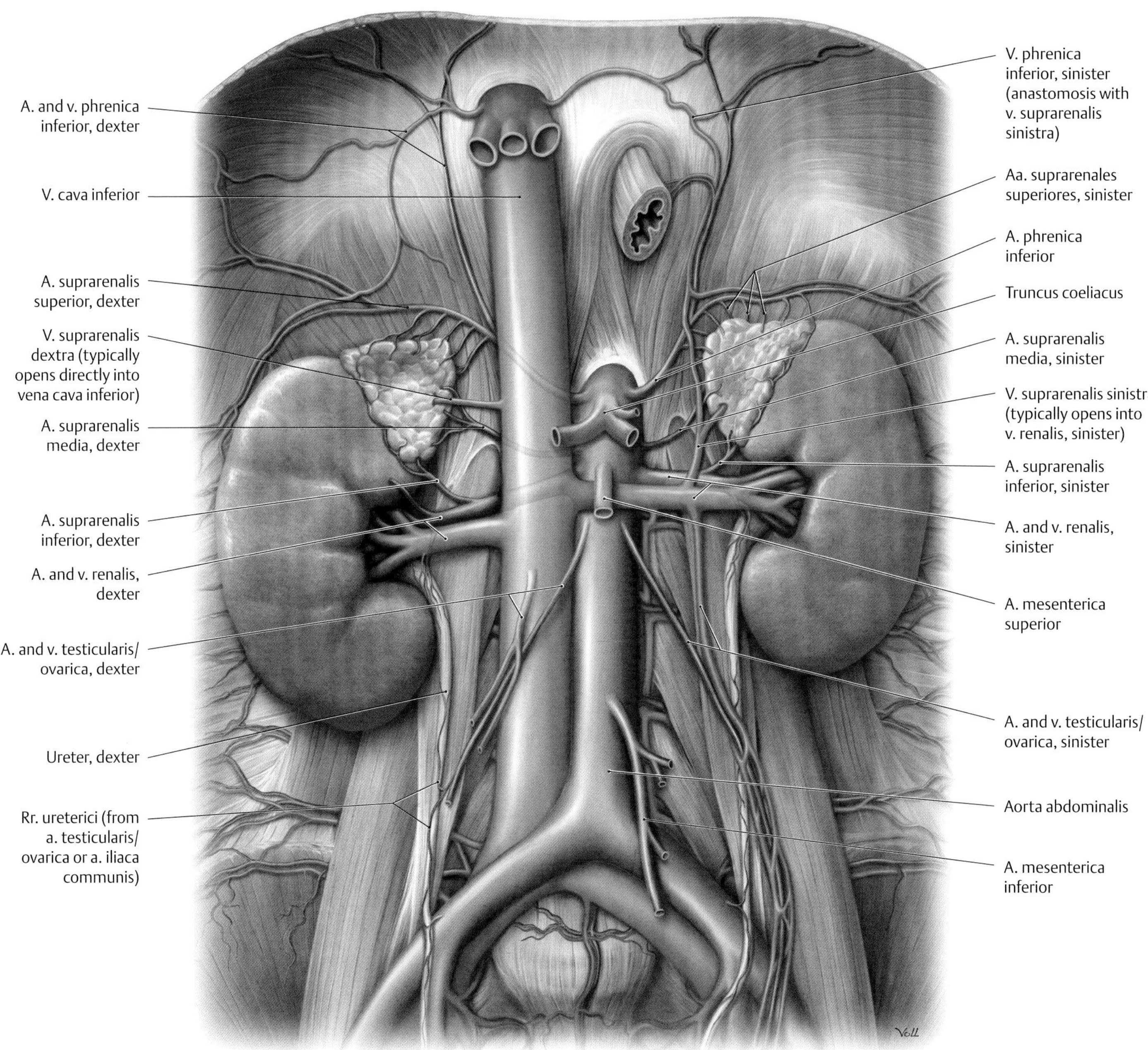
A. and v. phrenica inferior, dexter
V. cava inferior
A. suprarenalis superior, dexter
V. suprarenalis dextra (typically opens directly into vena cava inferior)
A. suprarenalis media, dexter
A. suprarenalis inferior, dexter
A. and v. renalis, dexter
A. and v. testicularis/ ovarica, dexter
Ureter, dexter
Rr. ureterici (from a. testicularis/ ovarica or a. iliaca communis)
V. phrenica inferior, sinister (anastomosis with v. suprarenalis sinistra)
Aa. suprarenales superiores, sinister
A. phrenica inferior
Truncus coeliacus
A. suprarenalis media, sinister
V. suprarenalis sinistra (typically opens into v. renalis, sinister)
A. suprarenalis inferior, sinister
A. and v. renalis, sinister
A. mesenterica superior
A. and v. testicularis/ ovarica, sinister
Aorta abdominalis
A. mesenterica inferior
Voll

Vena Portae Hepatis

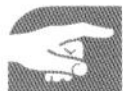

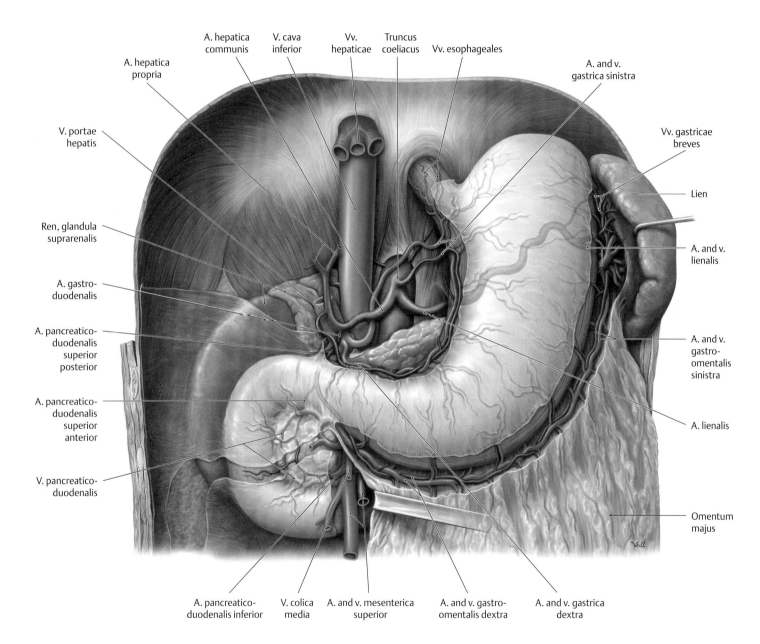

V. portae hepatis is typically formed by the union of v. mesenterica superior and v. lienalis posterior to the neck of the pancreas. The distribution of v. portae hepatis is shown on p. 215.

Fig. 15.17 V. portae hepatis: Gaster and duodenum
Anterior view. *Removed:* Hepar, omentum minus, and peritoneum. *Opened:* Omentum majus.

A. hepatica propria
V. portae hepatis
Ren, glandula suprarenalis
A. gastroduodenalis
A. pancreaticoduodenalis superior posterior
A. pancreaticoduodenalis superior anterior
V. pancreaticoduodenalis
A. hepatica communis
V. cava inferior
Vv. hepaticae
Truncus coeliacus
Vv. esophageales
A. and v. gastrica sinistra
Vv. gastricae breves
Lien
A. and v. lienalis
A. and v. gastroomentalis sinistra
A. lienalis
Omentum majus
A. pancreaticoduodenalis inferior
V. colica media
A. and v. mesenterica superior
A. and v. gastroomentalis dextra
A. and v. gastrica dextra

Fig. 15.18 **V. portae hepatis: Pancreas and lien**
Anterior view. *Partially removed:* Gaster, pancreas, and peritoneum.

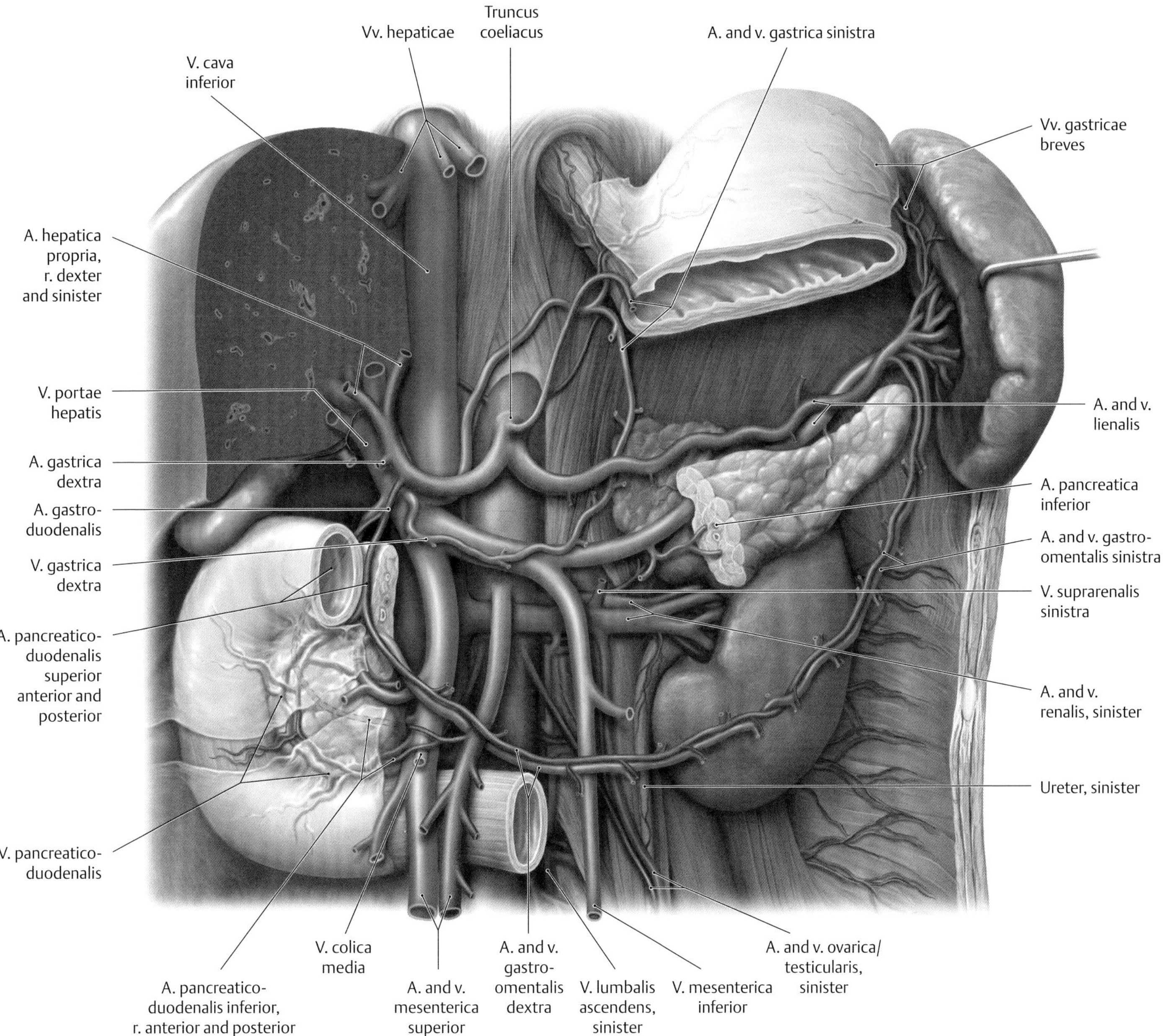
Truncus coeliacus
Vv. hepaticae
A. and v. gastrica sinistra
V. cava inferior
Vv. gastricae breves
A. hepatica propria, r. dexter and sinister
V. portae hepatis
A. and v. lienalis
A. gastrica dextra
A. pancreatica inferior
A. gastro-duodenalis
A. and v. gastro-omentalis sinistra
V. gastrica dextra
V. suprarenalis sinistra
A. pancreatico-duodenalis superior anterior and posterior
A. and v. renalis, sinister
Ureter, sinister
V. pancreatico-duodenalis
V. colica media
A. and v. gastro-omentalis dextra
A. and v. ovarica/ testicularis, sinister
A. pancreatico-duodenalis inferior, r. anterior and posterior
A. and v. mesenterica superior
V. lumbalis ascendens, sinister
V. mesenterica inferior

Venae Mesenterica Superior & Inferior

Fig. 15.19 **V. mesenterica superior**
Anterior view. *Partially removed:* Gaster, pancreas, peritoneum, mesenterium, and colon transversum. *Displaced:* Intestinum tenue.

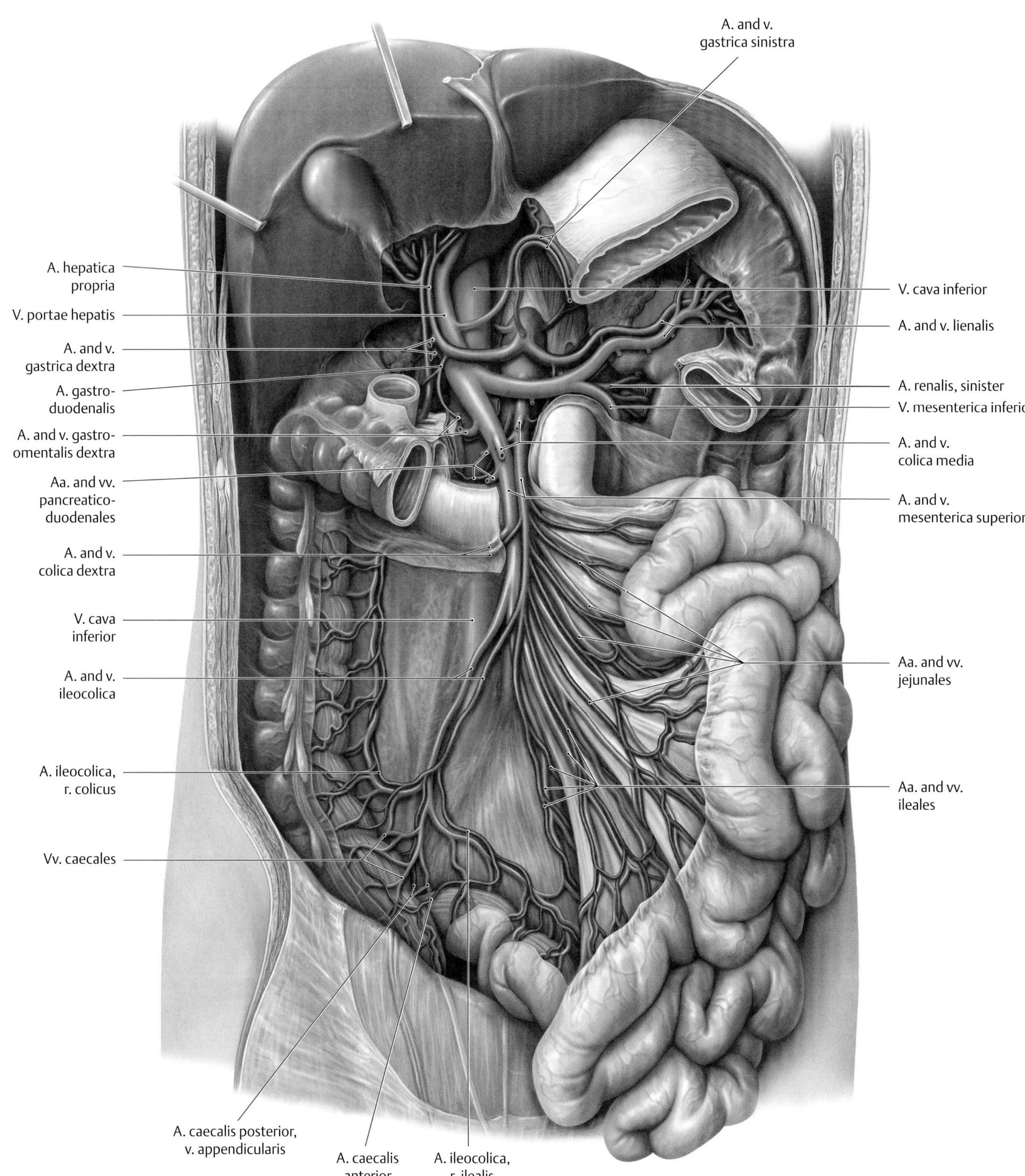
A. and v. gastrica sinistra
A. hepatica propria
V. portae hepatis
A. and v. gastrica dextra
A. gastroduodenalis
A. and v. gastroomentalis dextra
Aa. and vv. pancreaticoduodenales
A. and v. colica dextra
V. cava inferior
A. and v. ileocolica
A. ileocolica, r. colicus
Vv. caecales
A. caecalis posterior, v. appendicularis
A. caecalis anterior
A. ileocolica, r. ilealis
V. cava inferior
A. and v. lienalis
A. renalis, sinister
V. mesenterica inferior
A. and v. colica media
A. and v. mesenterica superior
Aa. and vv. jejunales
Aa. and vv. ileales

Fig. 15.20 **V. mesenterica inferior**
Anterior view. *Removed:* Gaster, pancreas, intestinum tenue, and peritoneum.

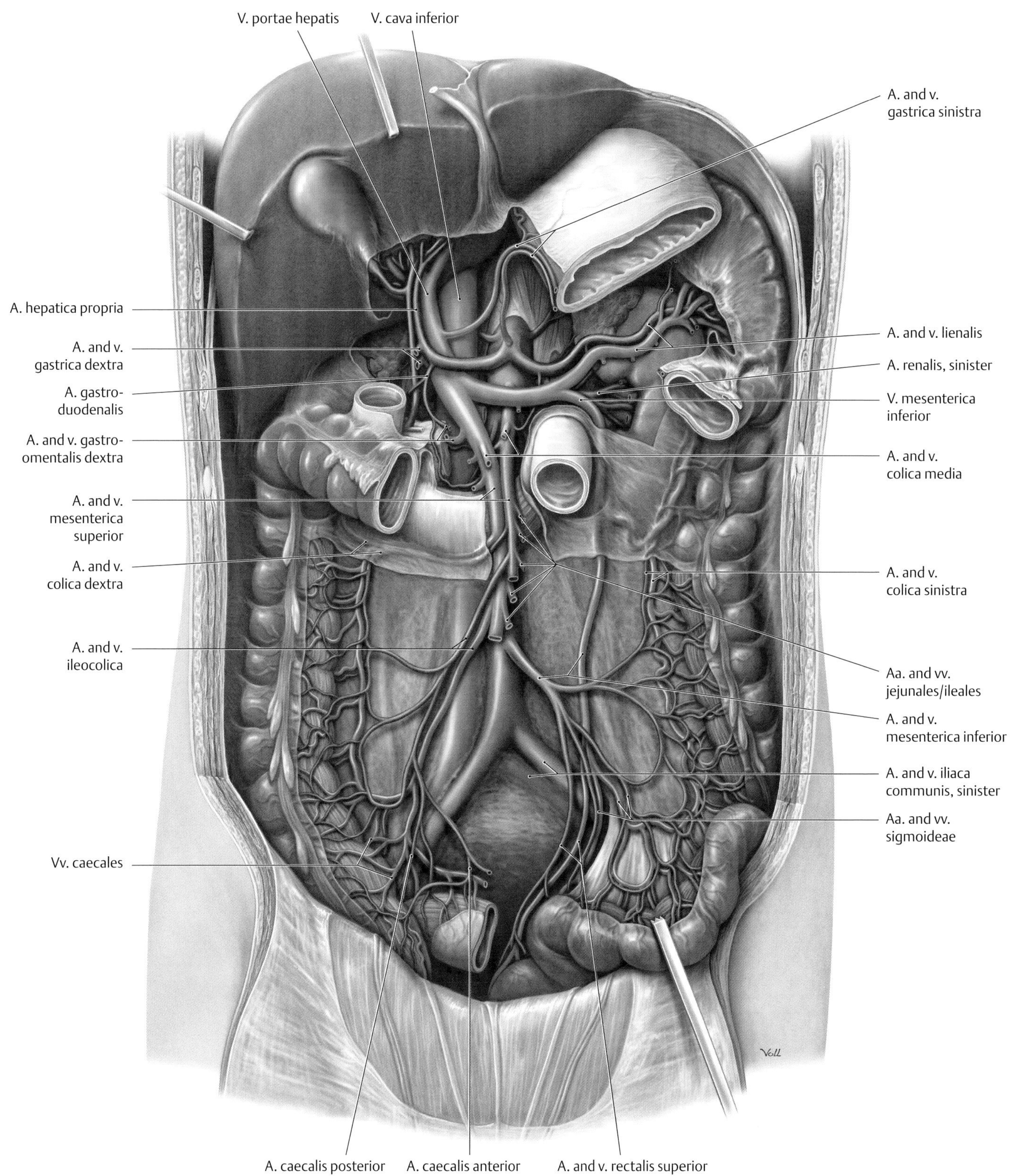
V. portae hepatis
V. cava inferior
A. and v. gastrica sinistra
A. hepatica propria
A. and v. gastrica dextra
A. gastro-duodenalis
A. and v. gastro-omentalis dextra
A. and v. mesenterica superior
A. and v. colica dextra
A. and v. ileocolica
Vv. caecales
A. and v. lienalis
A. renalis, sinister
V. mesenterica inferior
A. and v. colica media
A. and v. colica sinistra
Aa. and vv. jejunales/ileales
A. and v. mesenterica inferior
A. and v. iliaca communis, sinister
Aa. and vv. sigmoideae
A. caecalis posterior
A. caecalis anterior
A. and v. rectalis superior

Arteries & Veins of the Pelvis

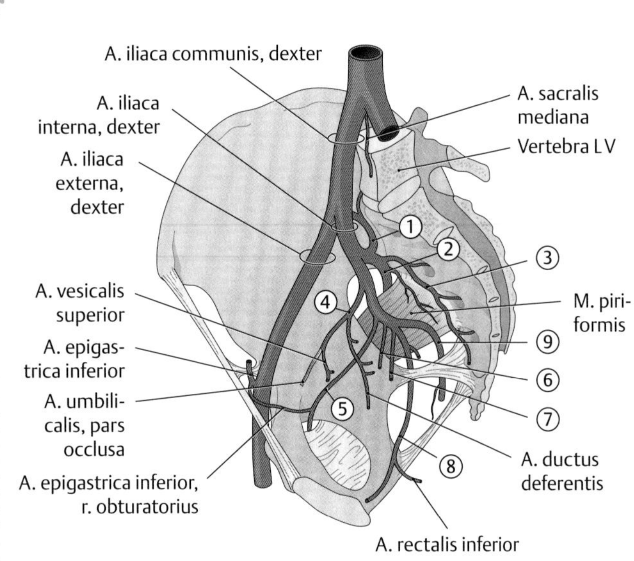
A. iliaca communis, dexter
A. iliaca interna, dexter
A. iliaca externa, dexter
A. vesicalis superior
A. epigas-trica inferior
A. umbili-calis, pars occlusa
A. epigastrica inferior, r. obturatorius
A. sacralis mediana
Vertebra LV
M. piri-formis
A. ductus deferentis
A. rectalis inferior
1
2
3
4
5
6
7
8
9

A Male pelvis.

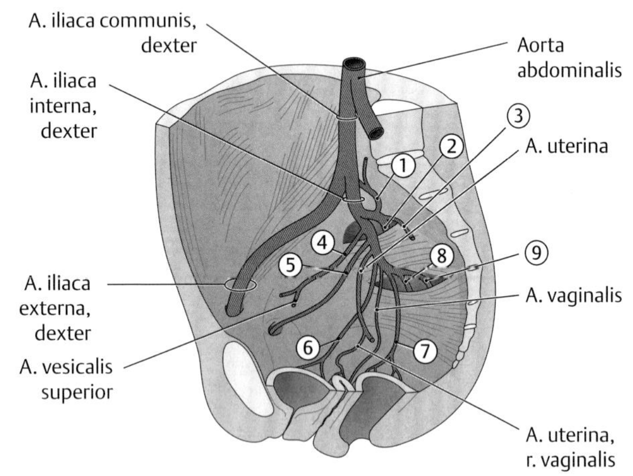
A. iliaca communis, dexter
A. iliaca interna, dexter
A. iliaca externa, dexter
A. vesicalis superior
Aorta abdominalis
A. uterina
A. vaginalis
A. uterina, r. vaginalis
1
2
3
4
5
6
7
8
9

B Female pelvis.

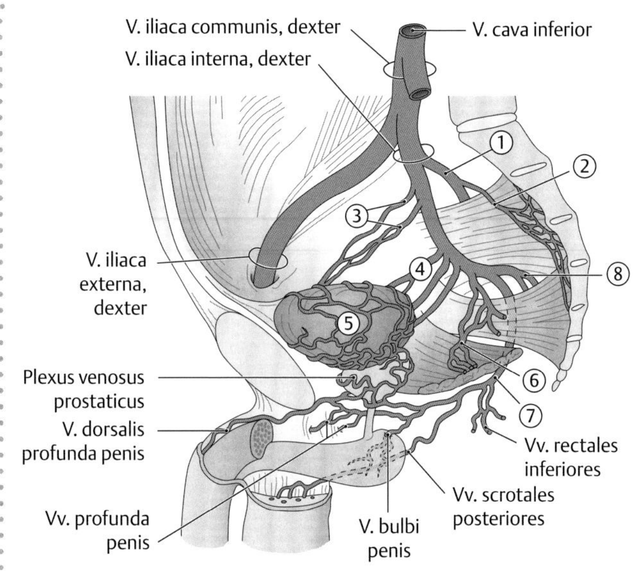
V. iliaca communis, dexter
V. iliaca interna, dexter
V. cava inferior
V. iliaca externa, dexter
Plexus venosus prostaticus
V. dorsalis profunda penis
Vv. profunda penis
V. bulbi penis
Vv. scrotales posteriores
Vv. rectales inferiores
1
2
3
4
5
6
7
8

A Male pelvis.

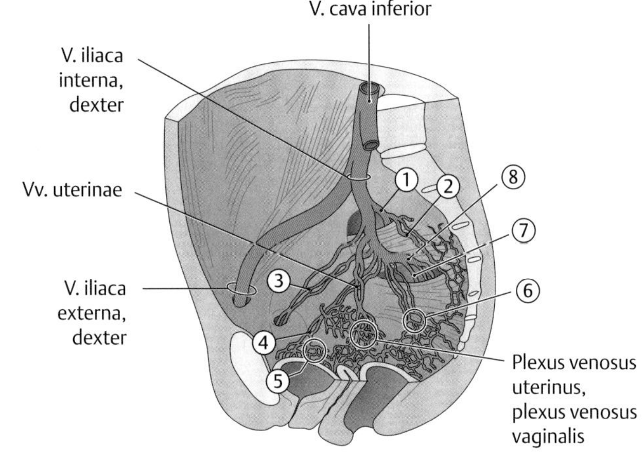
V. cava inferior
V. iliaca interna, dexter
Vv. uterinae
V. iliaca externa, dexter
Plexus venosus uterinus, plexus venosus vaginalis
1
2
3
4
5
6
7
8

B Female pelvis.

Table 15.3 Branches of the A. iliaca interna

The A. iliaca interna gives off five parietal (pelvic wall) and four visceral (pelvic organs) branches.* Parietal branches are shown in italics.

Branches		
①	*A. iliolumbalis*	
②	*A. glutea superior*	
③	*A. sacralis lateralis*	
④	A. umbilicalis	A. ductus deferentis
		A. vesicalis superior
⑤	*A. obturatoria*	
⑥	A. vesicalis inferior	
⑦	A. rectalis media	
⑧	A. pudenda interna	A. rectalis inferior
⑨	*A. glutaea inferior*	

* In the female pelvis, a. uterina and a. vaginalis may arise directly from a. iliaca interna.

Table 15.4 Venous drainage of the pelvis

Tributaries	
①	V. glutaea superior
②	V. sacralis lateralis
③	Vv. obturatoriae
④	Vv. vesicales
⑤	Plexus venosus vesicalis
⑥	Vv. rectales mediae (plexus venosus rectalis) (also vv. rectales inferior/superior, not shown)
⑦	V. pudenda interna
⑧	Vv. glutaea inferiores

The male pelvis also contains a plexus venosus prostaticus and venae draining the penis and scrotum. The female pelvis contains vv. uterinae and plexus venosus vaginalis.

Fig. 15.21 Blood vessels of the pelvis

Idealized right hemipelvis, left lateral view.

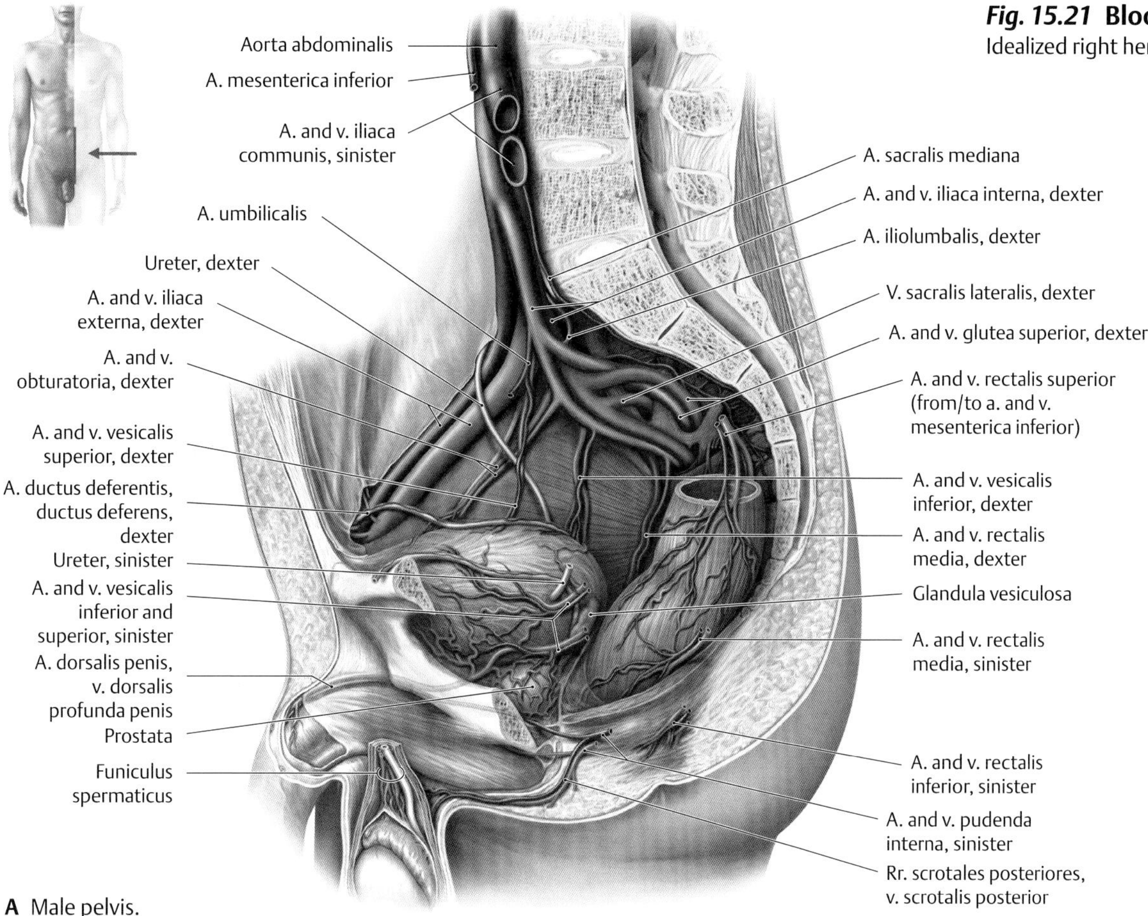
Aorta abdominalis
A. mesenterica inferior
A. and v. iliaca communis, sinister
A. umbilicalis
Ureter, dexter
A. and v. iliaca externa, dexter
A. and v. obturatoria, dexter
A. and v. vesicalis superior, dexter
A. ductus deferentis, ductus deferens, dexter
Ureter, sinister
A. and v. vesicalis inferior and superior, sinister
A. dorsalis penis, v. dorsalis profunda penis
Prostata
Funiculus spermaticus
A. sacralis mediana
A. and v. iliaca interna, dexter
A. iliolumbalis, dexter
V. sacralis lateralis, dexter
A. and v. glutea superior, dexter
A. and v. rectalis superior (from/to a. and v. mesenterica inferior)
A. and v. vesicalis inferior, dexter
A. and v. rectalis media, dexter
Glandula vesiculosa
A. and v. rectalis media, sinister
A. and v. rectalis inferior, sinister
A. and v. pudenda interna, sinister
Rr. scrotales posteriores, v. scrotalis posterior

A Male pelvis.

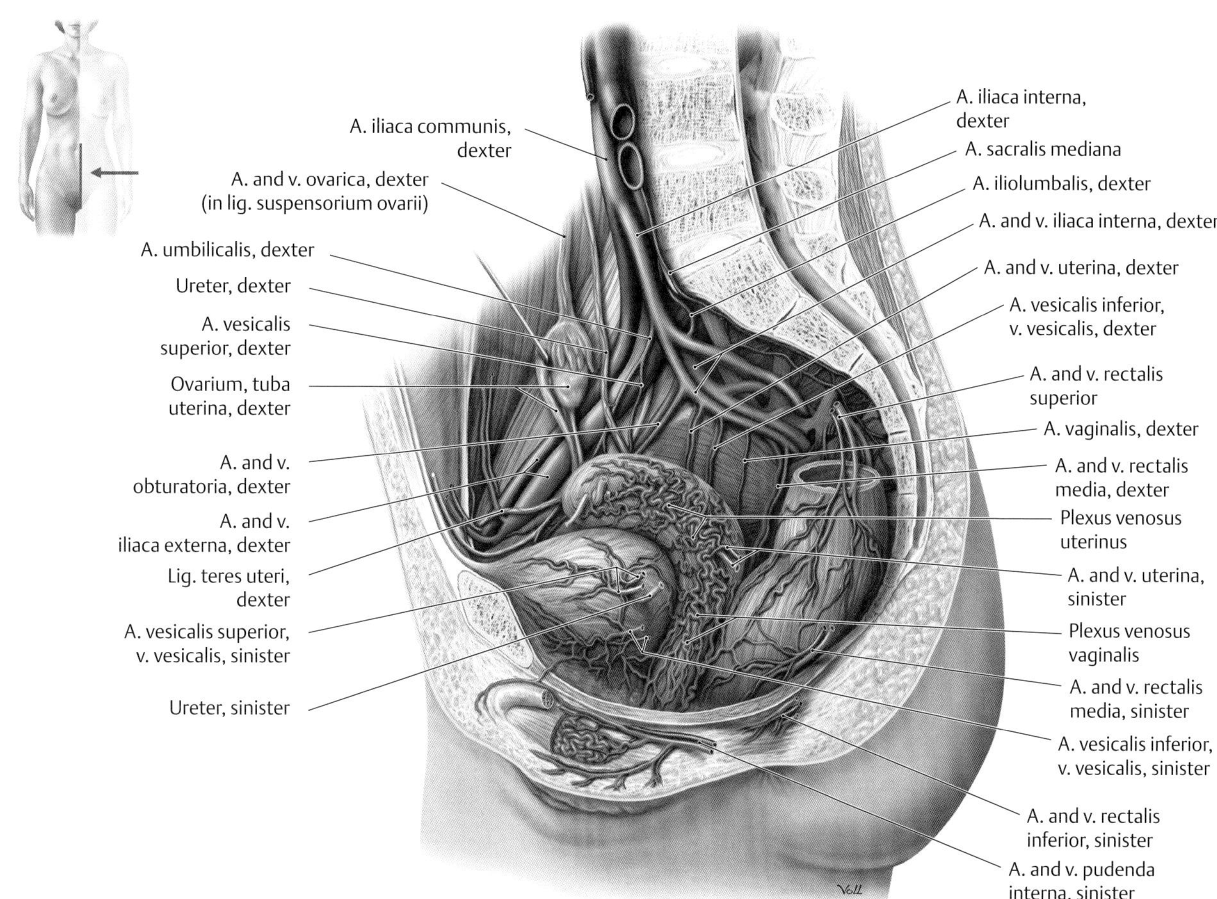
A. iliaca communis, dexter
A. and v. ovarica, dexter (in lig. suspensorium ovarii)
A. umbilicalis, dexter
Ureter, dexter
A. vesicalis superior, dexter
Ovarium, tuba uterina, dexter
A. and v. obturatoria, dexter
A. and v. iliaca externa, dexter
Lig. teres uteri, dexter
A. vesicalis superior, v. vesicalis, sinister
Ureter, sinister
A. iliaca interna, dexter
A. sacralis mediana
A. iliolumbalis, dexter
A. and v. iliaca interna, dexter
A. and v. uterina, dexter
A. vesicalis inferior, v. vesicalis, dexter
A. and v. rectalis superior
A. vaginalis, dexter
A. and v. rectalis media, dexter
Plexus venosus uterinus
A. and v. uterina, sinister
Plexus venosus vaginalis
A. and v. rectalis media, sinister
A. vesicalis inferior, v. vesicalis, sinister
A. and v. rectalis inferior, sinister
A. and v. pudenda interna, sinister

B Female pelvis.

Arteries & Veins of the Rectum & Genitalia

Fig. 15.22 Blood vessels of the rectum

Posterior view. The main blood supply to the rectum is from aa. rectales superiores; the aa. rectales mediae serve as an anastomosis between aa. rectales superior and inferior.

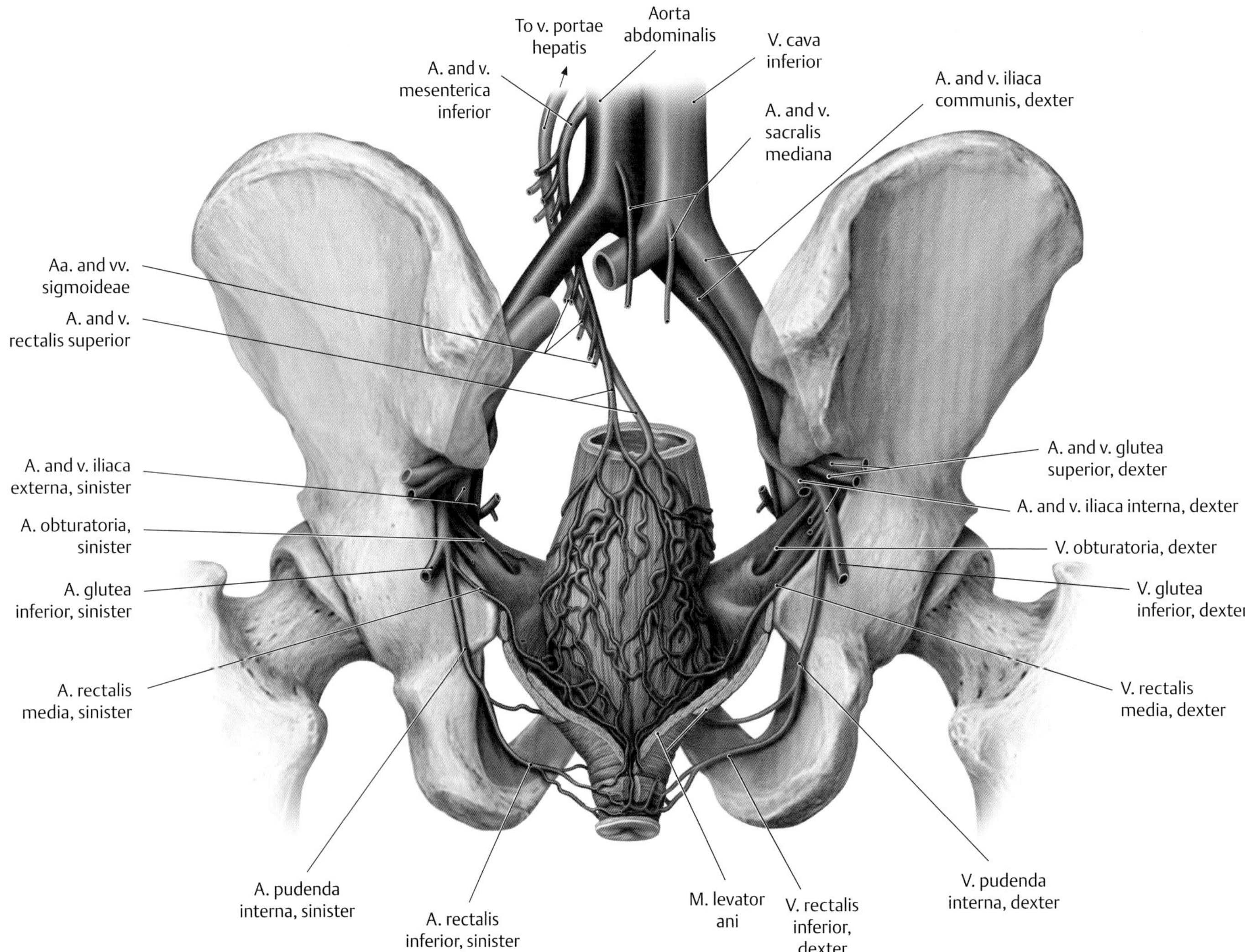
To v. portae hepatis
Aorta abdominalis
V. cava inferior
A. and v. mesenterica inferior
A. and v. iliaca communis, dexter
A. and v. sacralis mediana
Aa. and vv. sigmoideae
A. and v. rectalis superior
A. and v. iliaca externa, sinister
A. obturatoria, sinister
A. glutea inferior, sinister
A. rectalis media, sinister
A. and v. glutea superior, dexter
A. and v. iliaca interna, dexter
V. obturatoria, dexter
V. glutea inferior, dexter
V. rectalis media, dexter
A. pudenda interna, sinister
A. rectalis inferior, sinister
M. levator ani
V. rectalis inferior, dexter
V. pudenda interna, dexter

Fig. 15.23 Blood vessels of the genitalia

Anterior view.

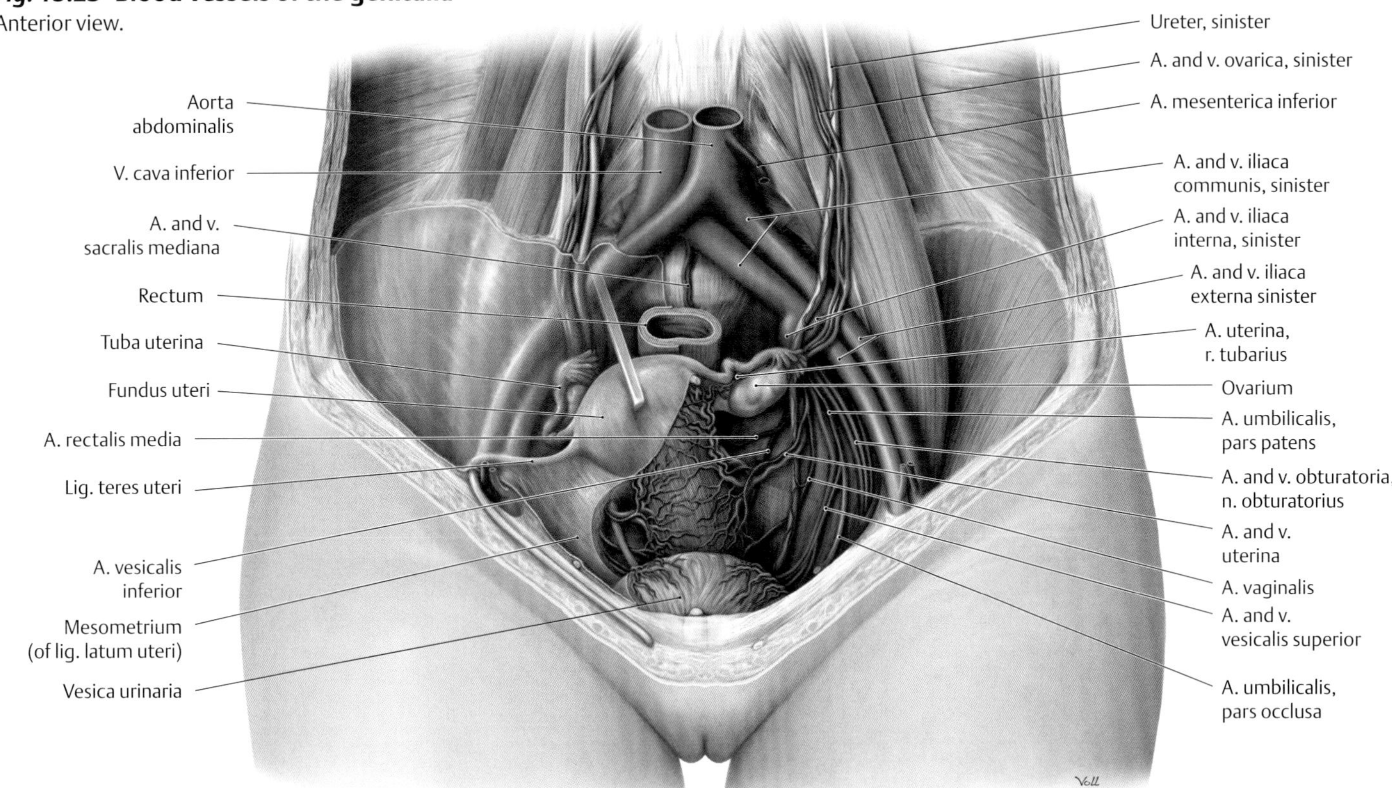
Aorta abdominalis
V. cava inferior
A. and v. sacralis mediana
Rectum
Tuba uterina
Fundus uteri
A. rectalis media
Lig. teres uteri
A. vesicalis inferior
Mesometrium (of lig. latum uteri)
Vesica urinaria
Ureter, sinister
A. and v. ovarica, sinister
A. mesenterica inferior
A. and v. iliaca communis, sinister
A. and v. iliaca interna, sinister
A. and v. iliaca externa sinister
A. uterina, r. tubarius
Ovarium
A. umbilicalis, pars patens
A. and v. obturatoria, n. obturatorius
A. and v. uterina
A. vaginalis
A. and v. vesicalis superior
A. umbilicalis, pars occlusa

A Female pelvis. *Removed:* Peritoneum (left side). *Displaced:* Uterus.

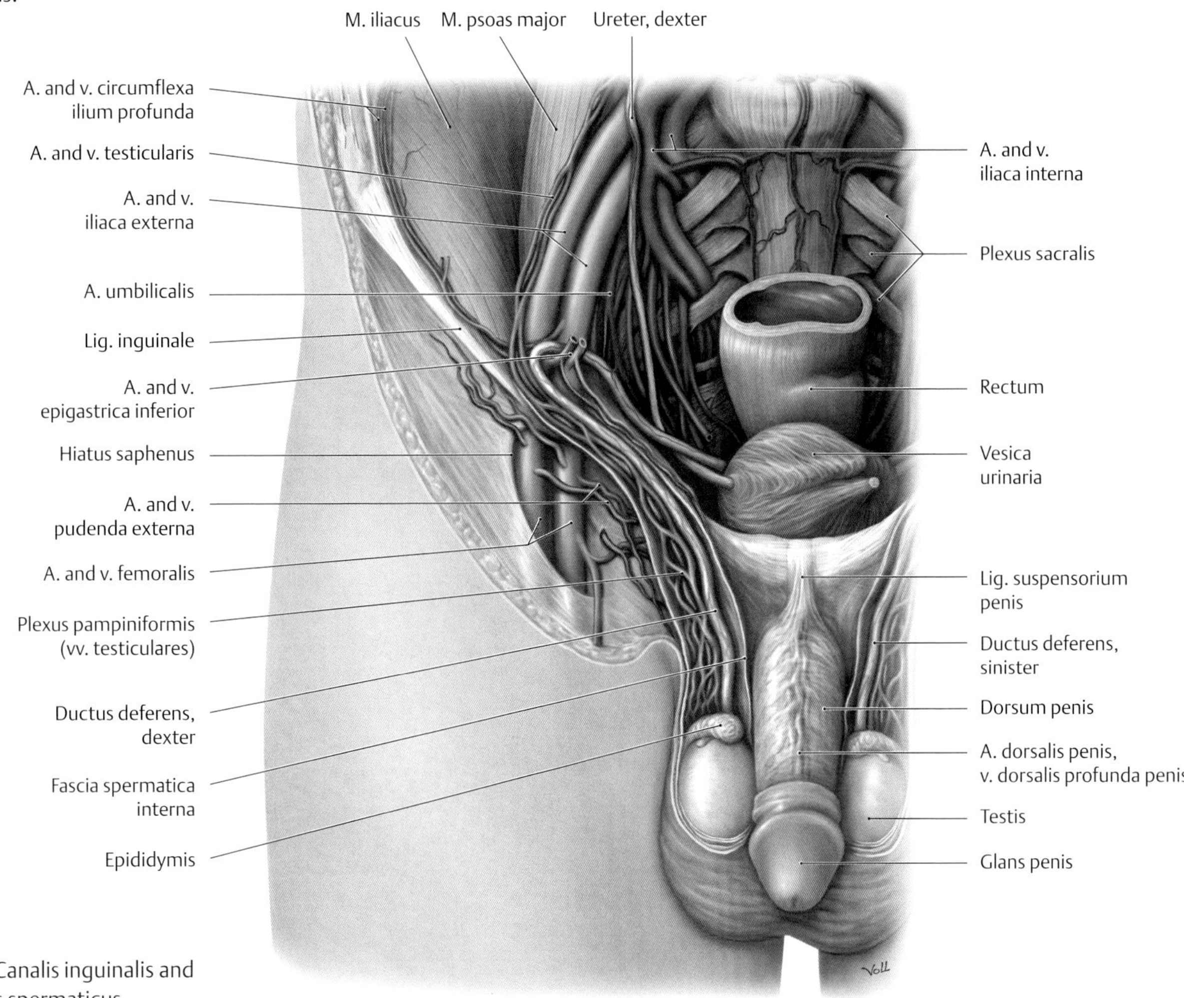
M. iliacus
M. psoas major
Ureter, dexter
A. and v. circumflexa ilium profunda
A. and v. testicularis
A. and v. iliaca externa
A. umbilicalis
Lig. inguinale
A. and v. epigastrica inferior
Hiatus saphenus
A. and v. pudenda externa
A. and v. femoralis
Plexus pampiniformis (vv. testiculares)
Ductus deferens, dexter
Fascia spermatica interna
Epididymis
A. and v. iliaca interna
Plexus sacralis
Rectum
Vesica urinaria
Lig. suspensorium penis
Ductus deferens, sinister
Dorsum penis
A. dorsalis penis, v. dorsalis profunda penis
Testis
Glans penis

B Male pelvis. *Opened:* Canalis inguinalis and coverings of funiculus spermaticus.

Lymph Nodes of the Abdomen & Pelvis

Fig. 16.1 **Lymphatic drainage of the internal organs**

See Table 16.1 for numbering. Lymph drainage from the abdomen, pelvis, and lower limb ultimately passes through the lumbar lymph nodes (clinically: aortic nodes). The lumbar lymph nodes consist of the right (caval) and left lateral aortic nodes, the preaortic nodes, and the retroaortic nodes. Efferent lymph vessels from the lumbar and preaortic nodes form trunci lumbales and intestinalis, respectively. Trunci lumbales and intestinalis terminate into the cisterna chyli.

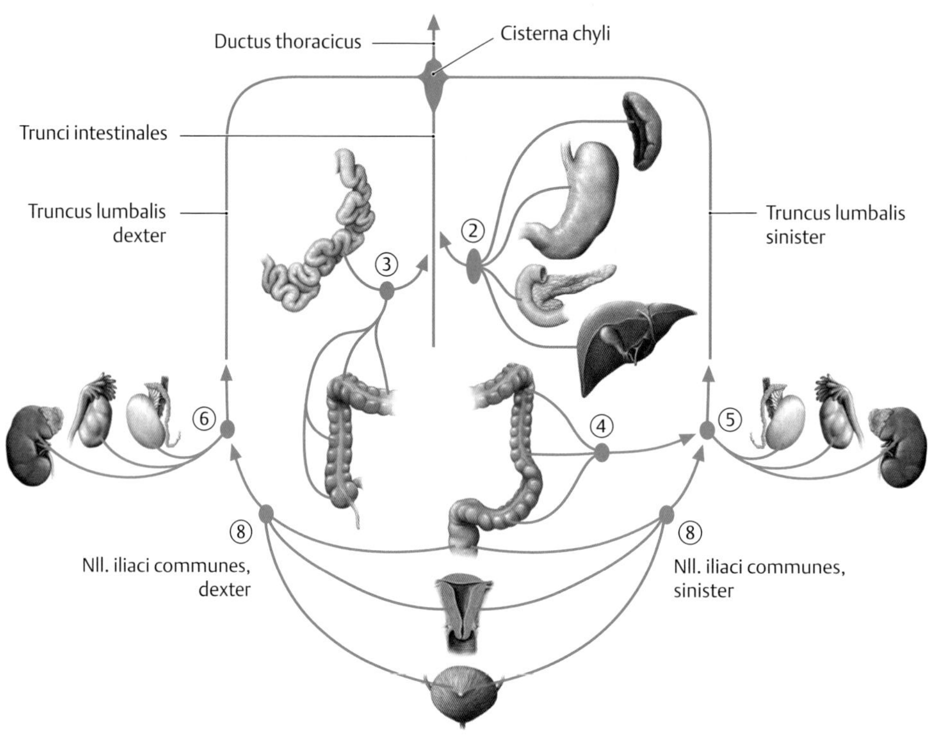
Ductus thoracicus
Cisterna chyli
Trunci intestinales
Truncus lumbalis dexter
Truncus lumbalis sinister
②
③
④
⑤
⑥
⑧
Nll. iliaci communes, dexter
⑧
Nll. iliaci communes, sinister

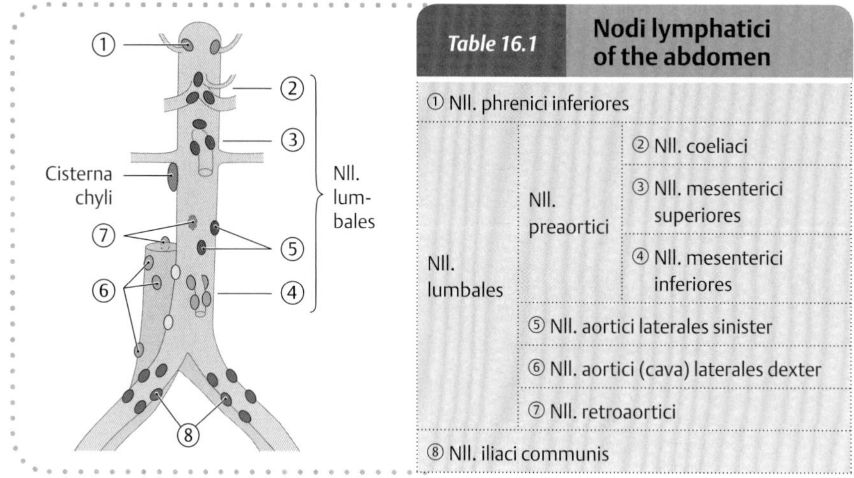
①
②
③
Cisterna chyli
⑦
⑥
⑤
④
Nll. lum-bales
⑧

Table 16.1	Nodi lymphatici of the abdomen	
① Nll. phrenici inferiores		
Nll. lumbales	Nll. preaortici	② Nll. coeliaci
		③ Nll. mesenterici superiores
		④ Nll. mesenterici inferiores
	⑤ Nll. aortici laterales sinister	
	⑥ Nll. aortici (cava) laterales dexter	
	⑦ Nll. retroaortici	
⑧ Nll. iliaci communis		

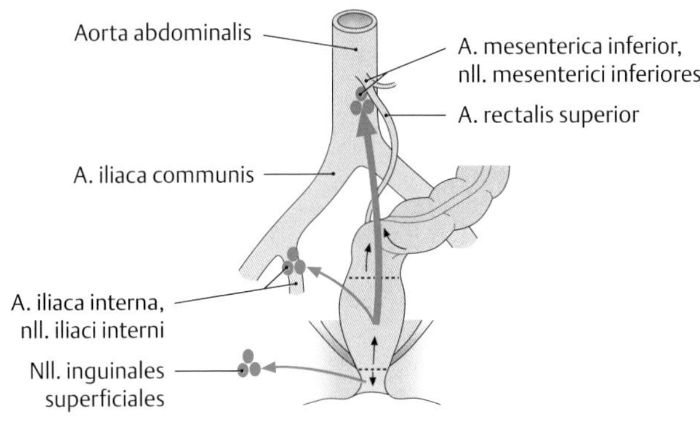

Aorta abdominalis
A. mesenterica inferior, nll. mesenterici inferiores
A. rectalis superior
A. iliaca communis
A. iliaca interna, nll. iliaci interni
Nll. inguinales superficiales

Fig. 16.2 **Lymphatic drainage of the rectum**
Anterior view.

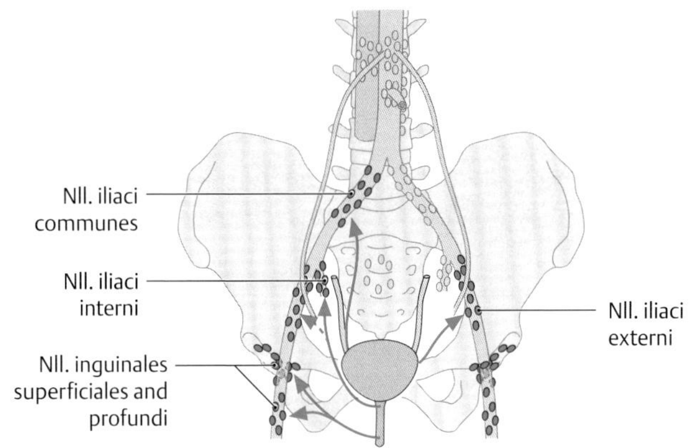

Nll. iliaci communes
Nll. iliaci interni
Nll. inguinales superficiales and profundi
Nll. iliaci externi

Fig. 16.3 **Lymphatic drainage of vesica urinaria and urethra**
Anterior view.

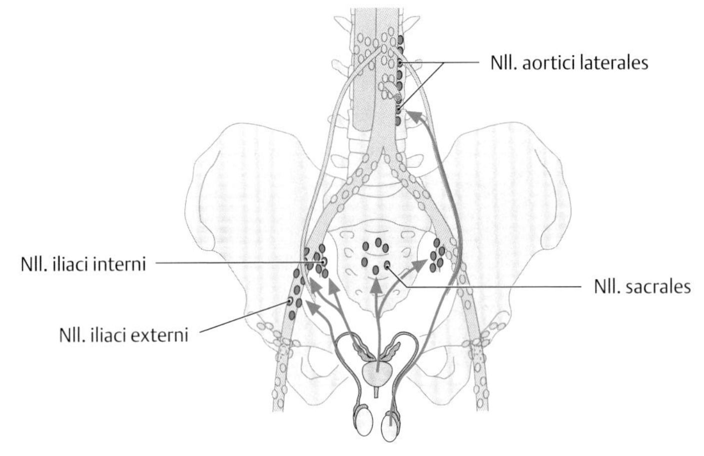

Nll. aortici laterales
Nll. iliaci interni
Nll. sacrales
Nll. iliaci externi

Fig. 16.4 **Lymphatic drainage of the male genitalia**
Anterior view.

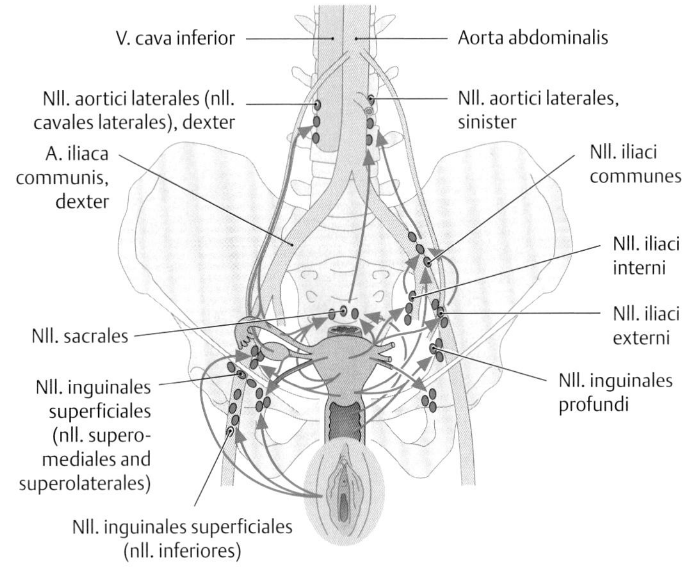

V. cava inferior
Aorta abdominalis
Nll. aortici laterales (nll. cavales laterales), dexter
Nll. aortici laterales, sinister
A. iliaca communis, dexter
Nll. iliaci communes
Nll. iliaci interni
Nll. iliaci externi
Nll. sacrales
Nll. inguinales superficiales (nll. superomediales and superolaterales)
Nll. inguinales profundi
Nll. inguinales superficiales (nll. inferiores)

Fig. 16.5 **Lymphatic drainage of the female genitalia**
Anterior view.

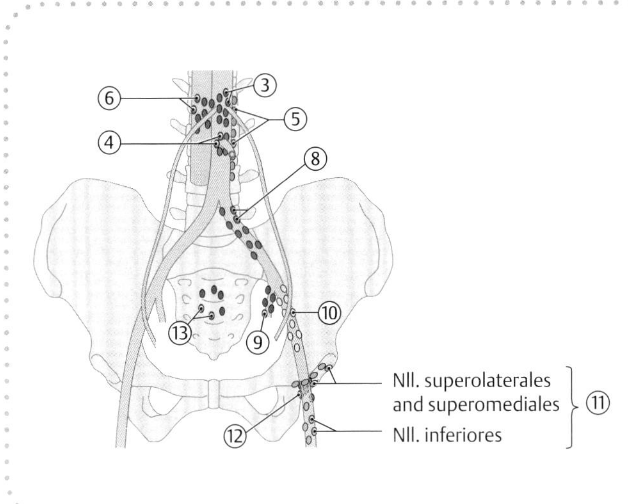

6
3
5
4
8
10
13
9
Nll. superolaterales and superomediales
11
Nll. inferiores
12

Table 16.2	**Nodi lymphatici of the pelvis**
Numbers continued from Table 16.1.	
Nll. preaortici	③ Nll. mesenterici superiores
	④ Nll. mesenterici inferiores
⑤ Nll. aortici laterales sinister	
⑥ Nll. aortici (cava) laterales dexter	
⑧ Nll. iliaci communis	
⑨ Nll. iliaci interni	
⑩ Nll. iliaci externi	
⑪ Nll. inguinales superficiales	Horizontal group
	Vertical group
⑫ Nll. inguinales profundi	
⑬ Nll. sacrales	

Lymph Nodes of the Posterior Abdominal Wall

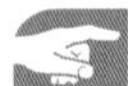

Lymph nodes in the abdomen and pelvis may be classified as either parietal or visceral. The majority of the parietal lymph nodes are located on the posterior abdominal wall.

Fig. 16.6 Parietal lymph nodes in the abdomen and pelvis
Anterior view. *Removed:* All visceral structures (except vessels).

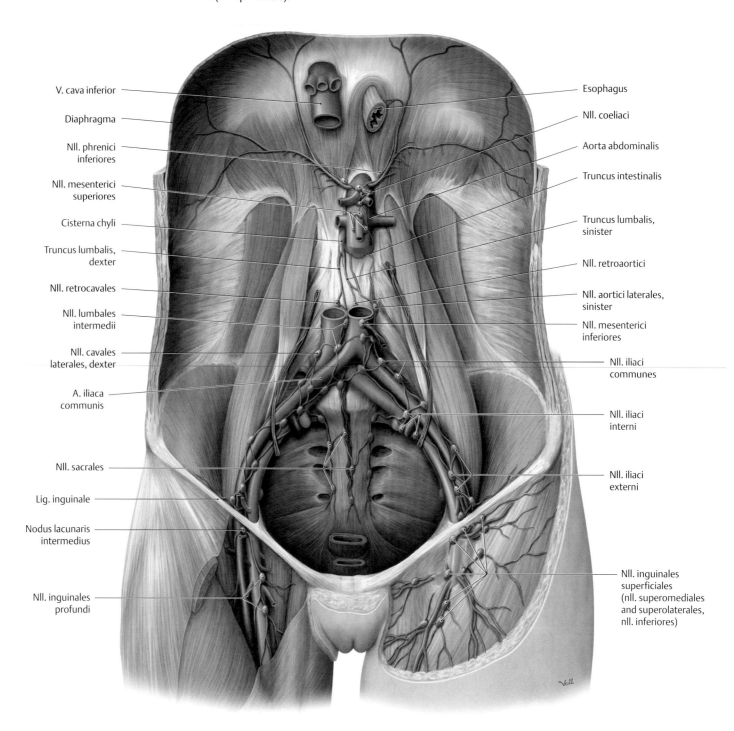

V. cava inferior
Diaphragma
Nll. phrenici inferiores
Nll. mesenterici superiores
Cisterna chyli
Truncus lumbalis, dexter
Nll. retrocavales
Nll. lumbales intermedii
Nll. cavales laterales, dexter
A. iliaca communis
Nll. sacrales
Lig. inguinale
Nodus lacunaris intermedius
Nll. inguinales profundi
Esophagus
Nll. coeliaci
Aorta abdominalis
Truncus intestinalis
Truncus lumbalis, sinister
Nll. retroaortici
Nll. aortici laterales, sinister
Nll. mesenterici inferiores
Nll. iliaci communes
Nll. iliaci interni
Nll. iliaci externi
Nll. inguinales superficiales (nll. superomediales and superolaterales, nll. inferiores)
Voll

Fig. 16.7 **Lymphatic nodes of the urinary organs**
Anterior view.

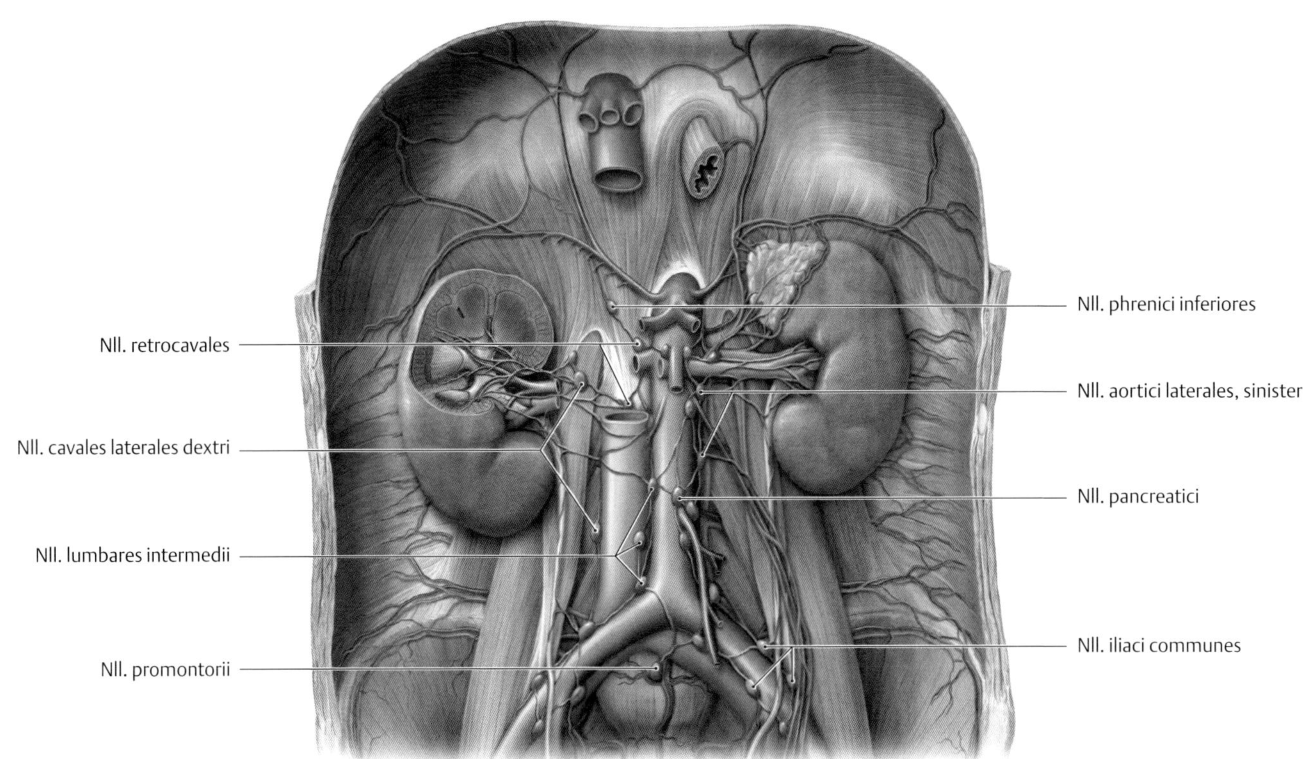
Nll. retrocavales
Nll. cavales laterales dextri
Nll. lumbares intermedii
Nll. promontorii
Nll. phrenici inferiores
Nll. aortici laterales, sinister
Nll. pancreatici
Nll. iliaci communes

Fig. 16.8 **Drainage of renes (with pelvic organs)**

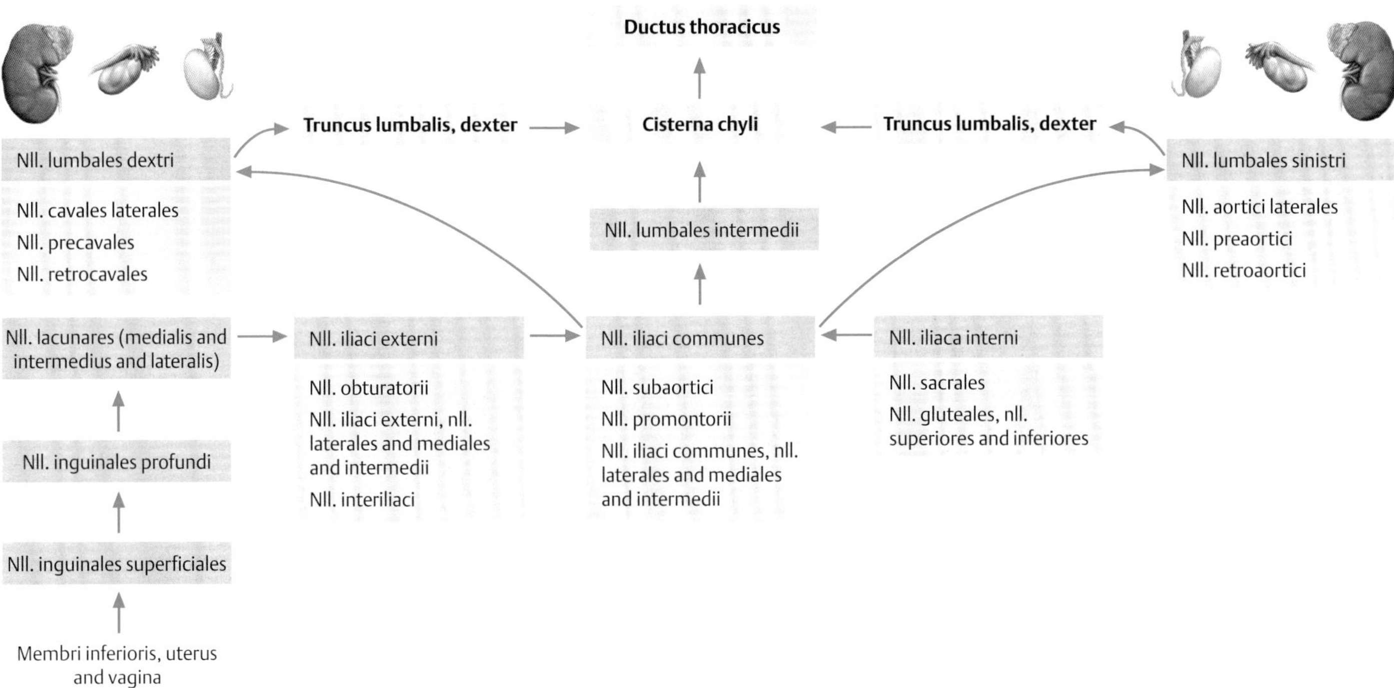
Ductus thoracicus
Truncus lumbalis, dexter
Cisterna chyli
Truncus lumbalis, dexter
Nll. lumbales dextri
Nll. cavales laterales
Nll. precavales
Nll. retrocavales
Nll. lumbales intermedii
Nll. lumbales sinistri
Nll. aortici laterales
Nll. preaortici
Nll. retroaortici
Nll. lacunares (medialis and intermedius and lateralis)
Nll. iliaci externi
Nll. iliaci communes
Nll. iliaca interni
Nll. obturatorii
Nll. iliaci externi, nll. laterales and mediales and intermedii
Nll. interiliaci
Nll. subaortici
Nll. promontorii
Nll. iliaci communes, nll. laterales and mediales and intermedii
Nll. sacrales
Nll. gluteales, nll. superiores and inferiores
Nll. inguinales profundi
Nll. inguinales superficiales
Membri inferioris, uterus and vagina

Lymph Nodes of the Anterior Abdominal Organs

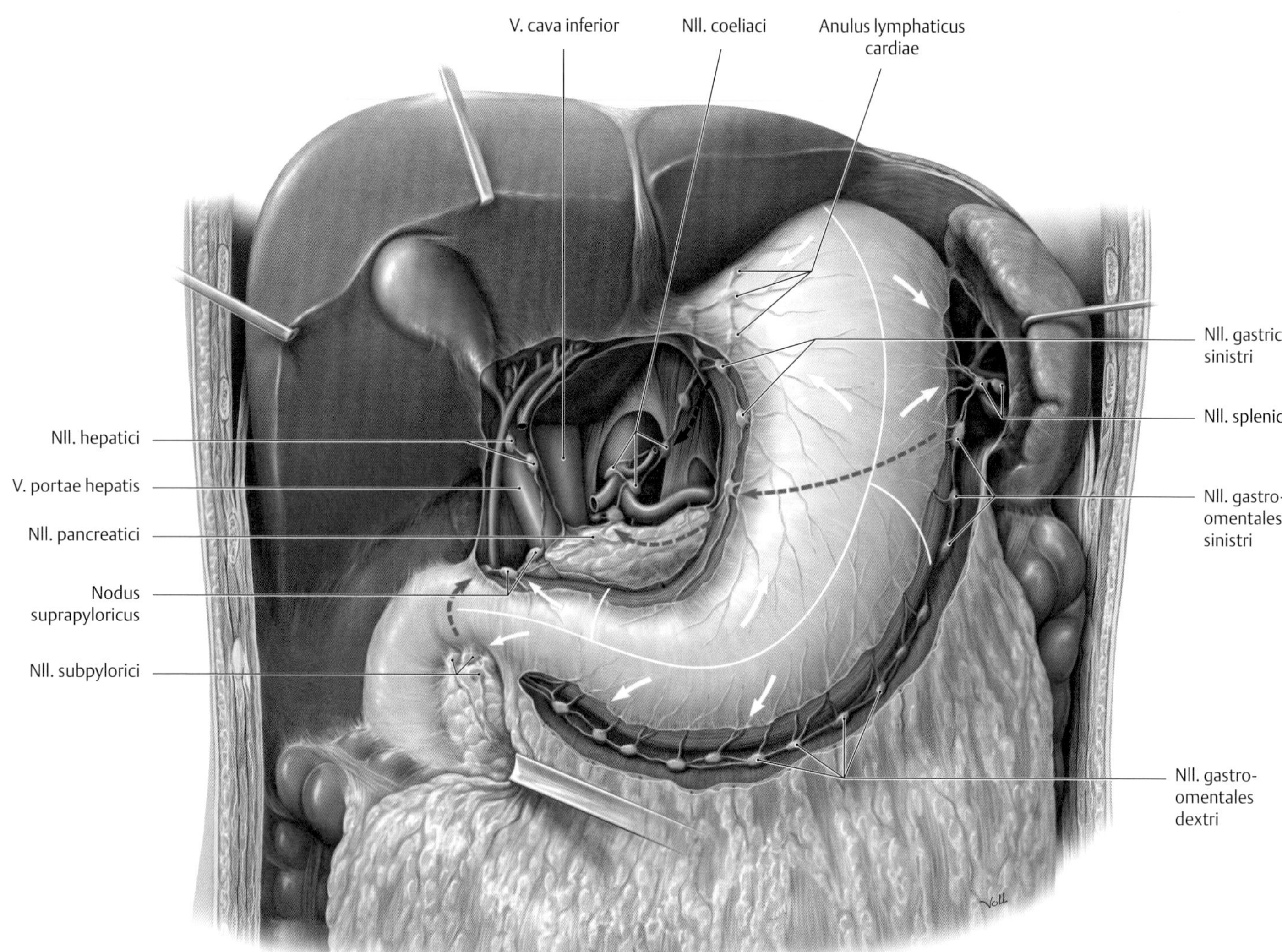
V. cava inferior
Nll. coeliaci
Anulus lymphaticus cardiae
Nll. gastrici sinistri
Nll. splenici
Nll. gastro-omentales sinistri
Nll. hepatici
V. portae hepatis
Nll. pancreatici
Nodus suprapyloricus
Nll. subpylorici
Nll. gastro-omentales dextri

Fig. 16.9 **Lymph nodes of gaster and hepar**
Anterior view. *Removed:* Omentum minus. *Opened:* Omentum majus. Arrows show direction of lymphatic drainage.

Fig. 16.10 **Lymph nodes of lien, pancreas, and duodenum**

Anterior view. *Removed:* Gaster and colon.

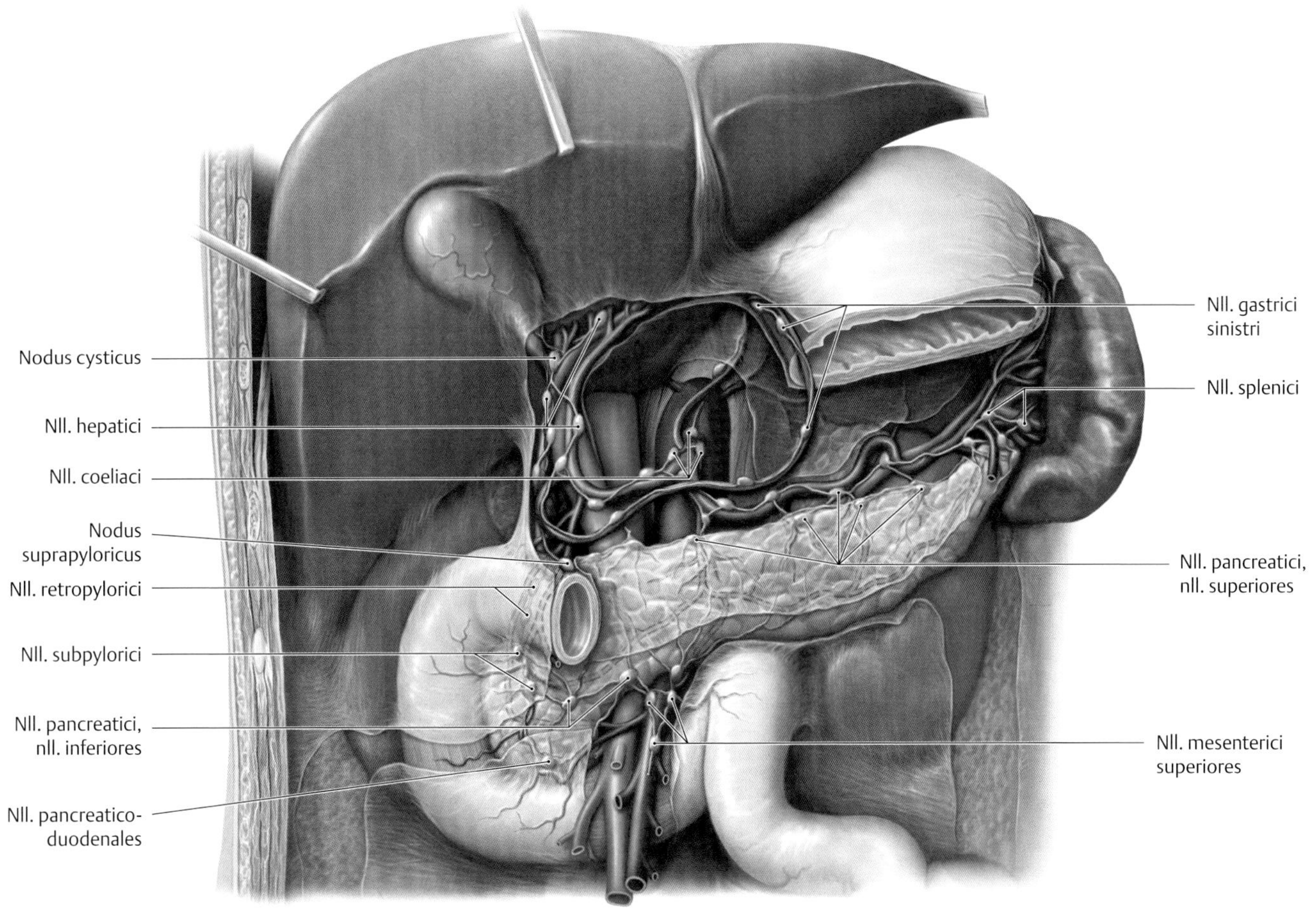

Nodus cysticus
Nll. hepatici
Nll. coeliaci
Nodus suprapyloricus
Nll. retropylorici
Nll. subpylorici
Nll. pancreatici, nll. inferiores
Nll. pancreaticoduodenales
Nll. gastrici sinistri
Nll. splenici
Nll. pancreatici, nll. superiores
Nll. mesenterici superiores

Fig. 16.11 **Lymphatic drainage of gaster, hepar, lien, pancreas, and duodenum**

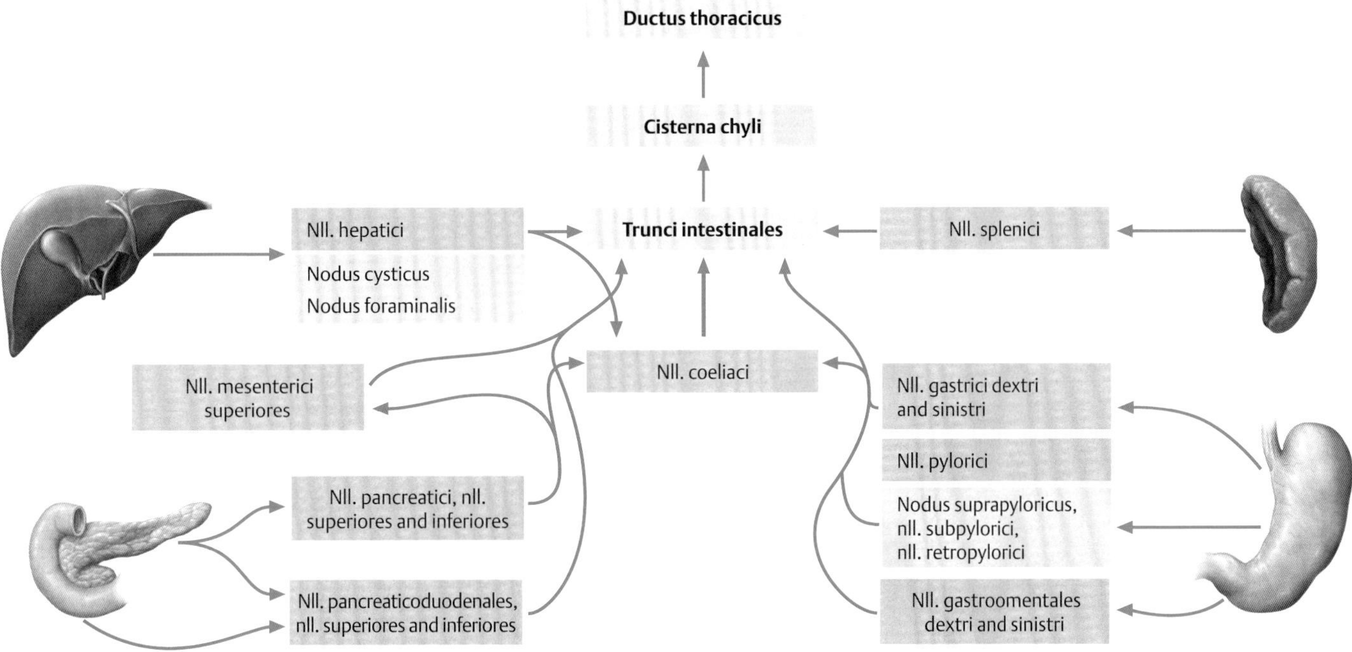

Ductus thoracicus
Cisterna chyli
Nll. hepatici
Nodus cysticus
Nodus foraminalis
Trunci intestinales
Nll. splenici
Nll. mesenterici superiores
Nll. coeliaci
Nll. gastrici dextri and sinistri
Nll. pylorici
Nodus suprapyloricus, nll. subpylorici, nll. retropylorici
Nll. pancreatici, nll. superiores and inferiores
Nll. pancreaticoduodenales, nll. superiores and inferiores
Nll. gastroomentales dextri and sinistri

Lymph Nodes of the Intestines

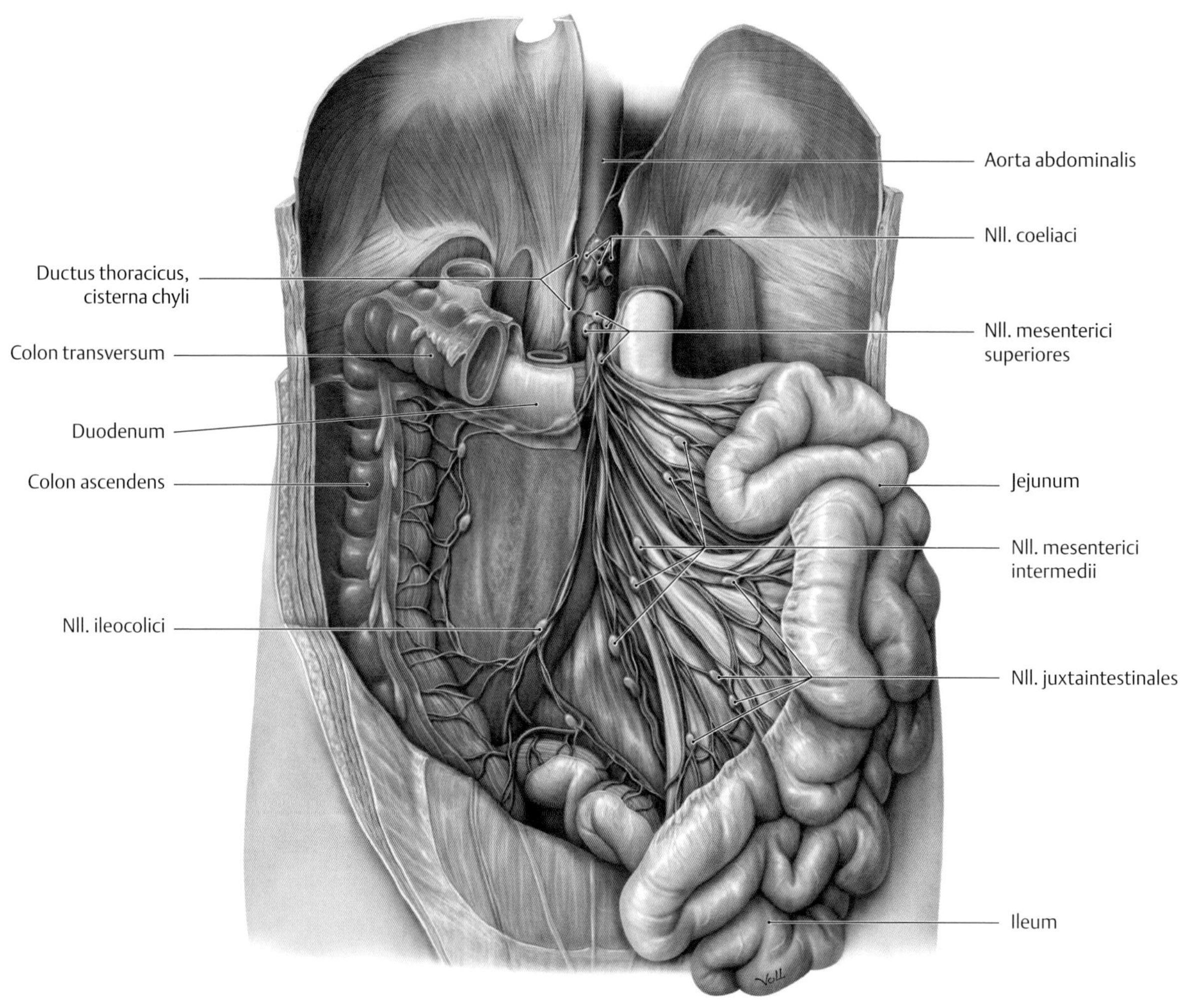
Aorta abdominalis
Nll. coeliaci
Ductus thoracicus, cisterna chyli
Nll. mesenterici superiores
Colon transversum
Duodenum
Colon ascendens
Jejunum
Nll. mesenterici intermedii
Nll. ileocolici
Nll. juxtaintestinales
Ileum

Fig. 16.12 **Lymph nodes of the jejunum and ileum**
Anterior view. *Removed:* Gaster, hepar, pancreas, and colon.

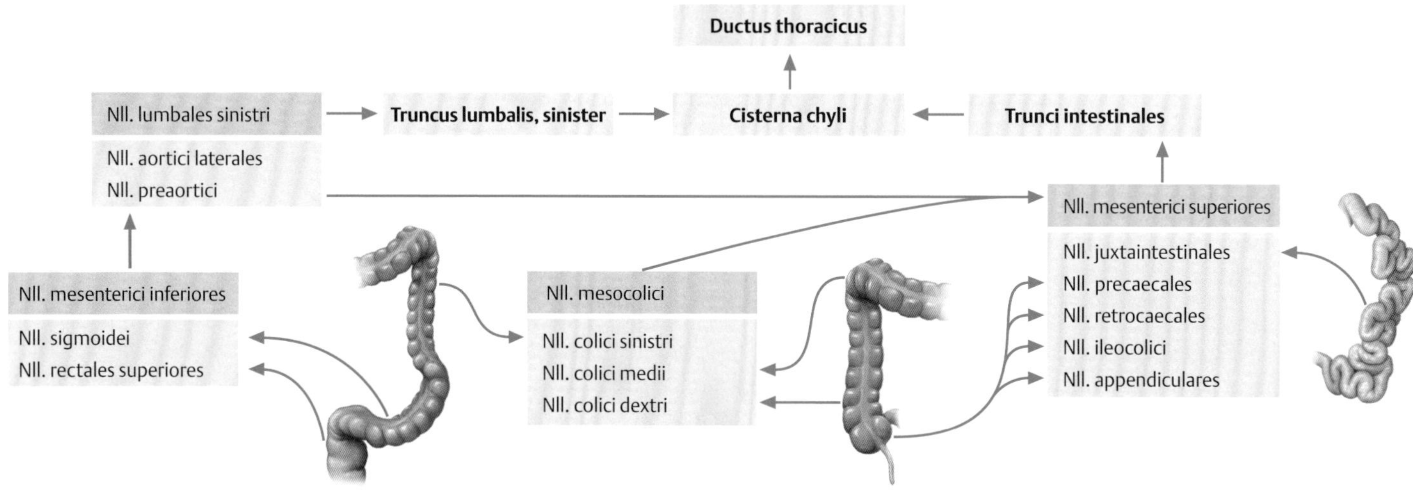
Ductus thoracicus
Nll. lumbales sinistri
Truncus lumbalis, sinister
Cisterna chyli
Trunci intestinales
Nll. aortici laterales
Nll. preaortici
Nll. mesenterici superiores
Nll. juxtaintestinales
Nll. precaecales
Nll. retrocaecales
Nll. ileocolici
Nll. appendiculares
Nll. mesenterici inferiores
Nll. sigmoidei
Nll. rectales superiores
Nll. mesocolici
Nll. colici sinistri
Nll. colici medii
Nll. colici dextri

Fig. 16.13 **Lymphatic drainage of the intestines**

Fig. 16.14 **Lymph nodes of intestinum crassum**
Anterior view. *Reflected:* Colon transversum and omentum majus.

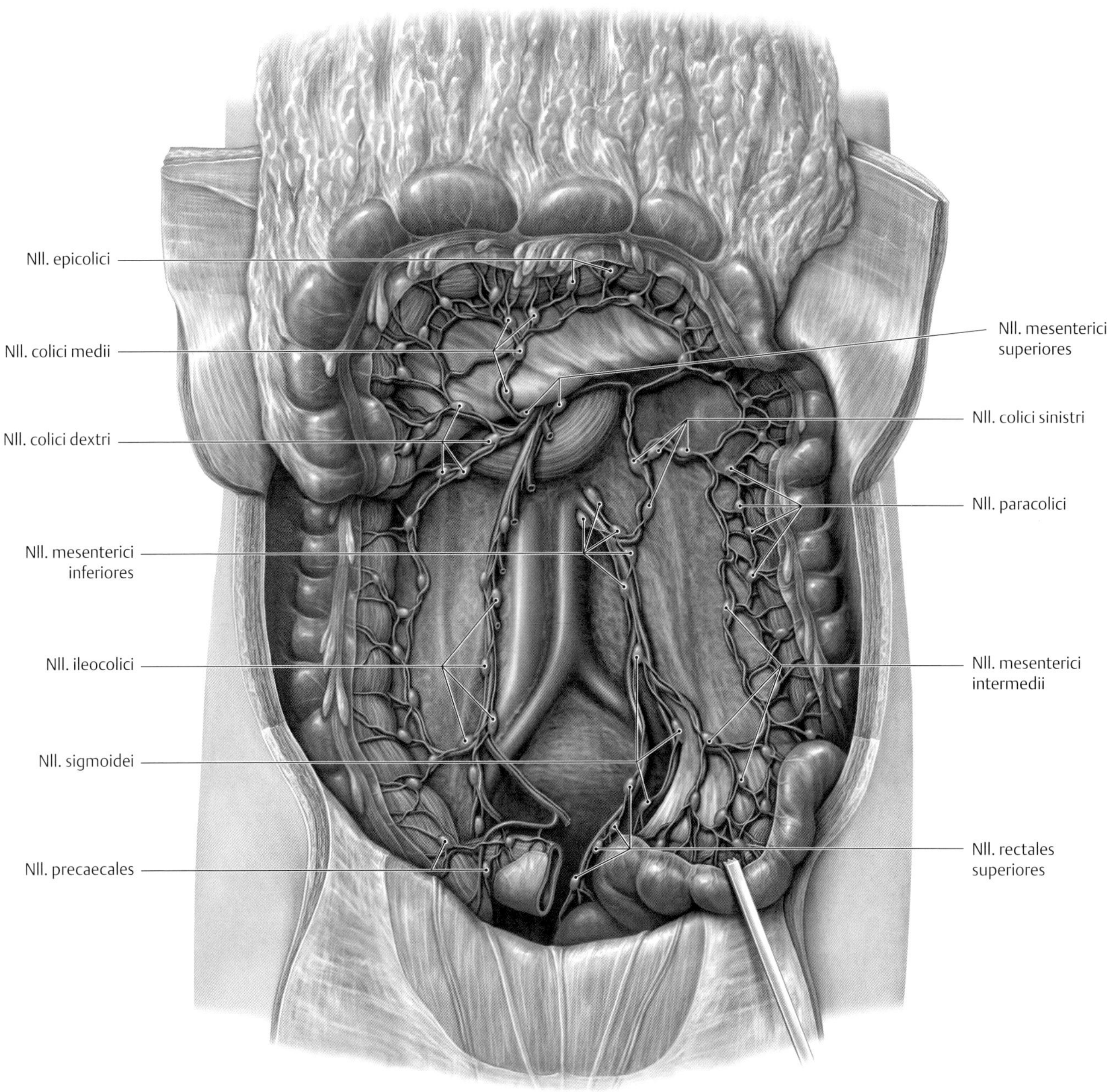
Nll. epicolici
Nll. colici medii
Nll. colici dextri
Nll. mesenterici inferiores
Nll. ileocolici
Nll. sigmoidei
Nll. precaecales
Nll. mesenterici superiores
Nll. colici sinistri
Nll. paracolici
Nll. mesenterici intermedii
Nll. rectales superiores

Lymph Nodes of the Genitalia

Fig. 16.15 Lymph nodes of the male genitalia
Anterior view. *Removed:* Gastrointestinal tract (except rectal stump) and peritoneum.

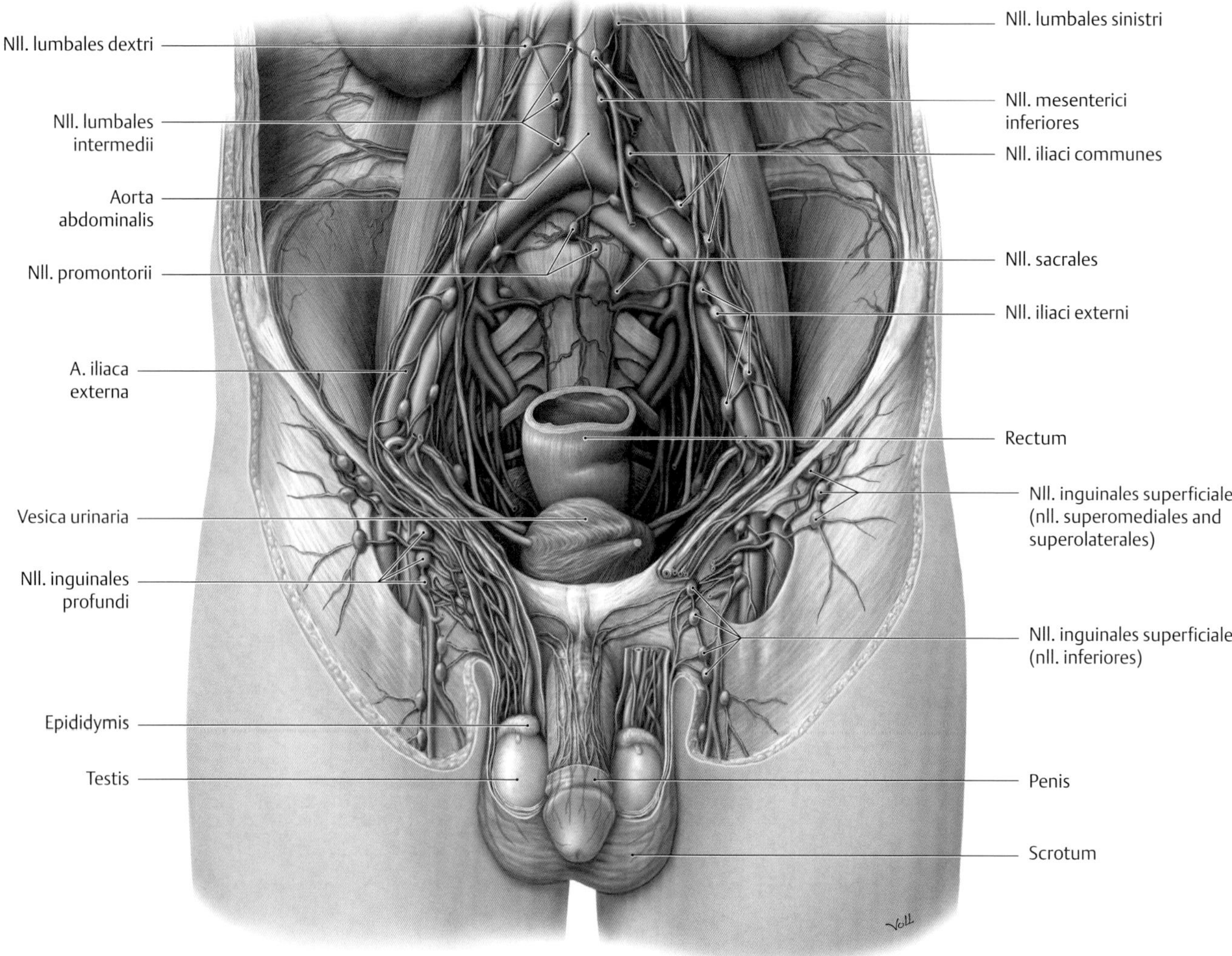

Nll. lumbales dextri
Nll. lumbales intermedii
Aorta abdominalis
Nll. promontorii
A. iliaca externa
Vesica urinaria
Nll. inguinales profundi
Epididymis
Testis
Nll. lumbales sinistri
Nll. mesenterici inferiores
Nll. iliaci communes
Nll. sacrales
Nll. iliaci externi
Rectum
Nll. inguinales superficiales (nll. superomediales and superolaterales)
Nll. inguinales superficiales (nll. inferiores)
Penis
Scrotum

Fig. 16.16 Lymph nodes of the female genitalia

Anterior view. *Removed:* Gastrointestinal tract (except rectal stump) and peritoneum. *Retracted:* Uterus.

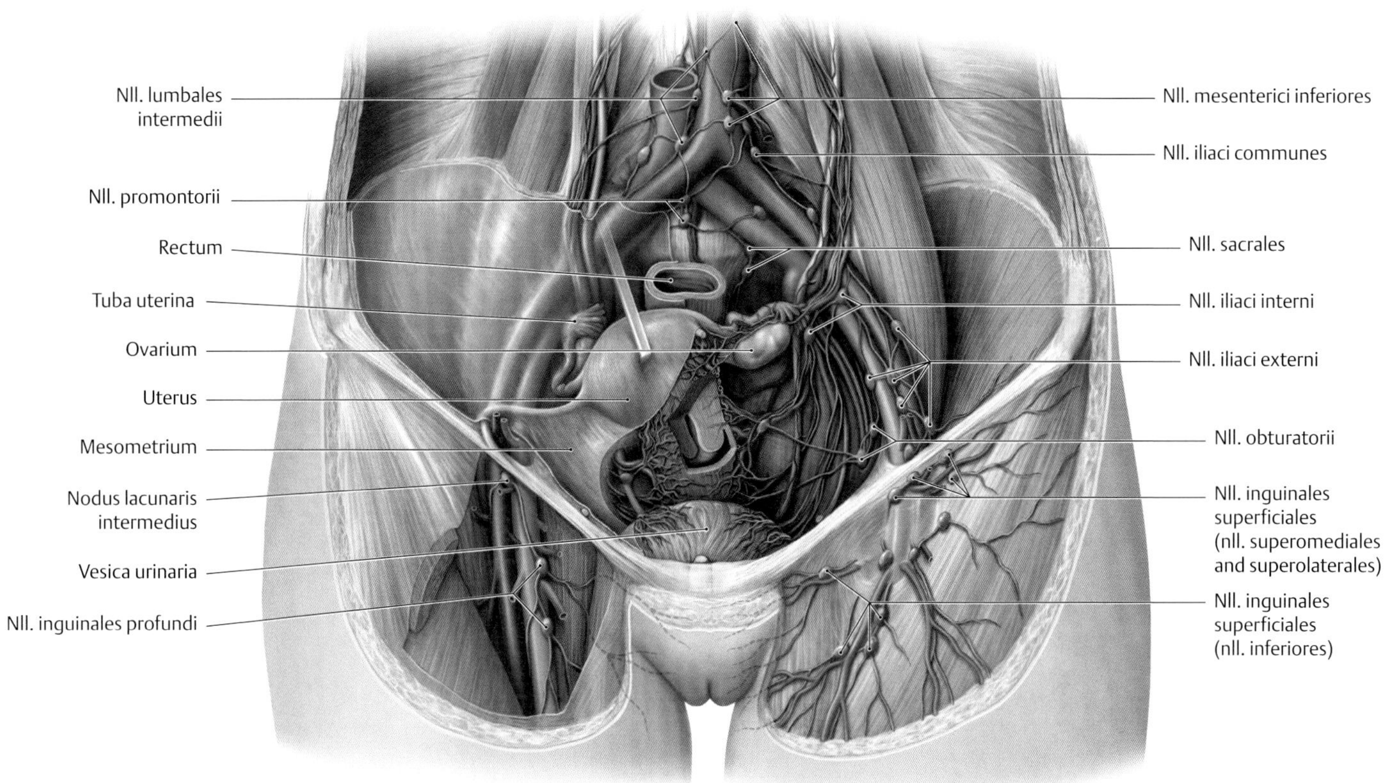
Nll. lumbales intermedii
Nll. promontorii
Rectum
Tuba uterina
Ovarium
Uterus
Mesometrium
Nodus lacunaris intermedius
Vesica urinaria
Nll. inguinales profundi
Nll. mesenterici inferiores
Nll. iliaci communes
Nll. sacrales
Nll. iliaci interni
Nll. iliaci externi
Nll. obturatorii
Nll. inguinales superficiales (nll. superomediales and superolaterales)
Nll. inguinales superficiales (nll. inferiores)

Fig. 16.17 Lymphatic drainage of the pelvic organs

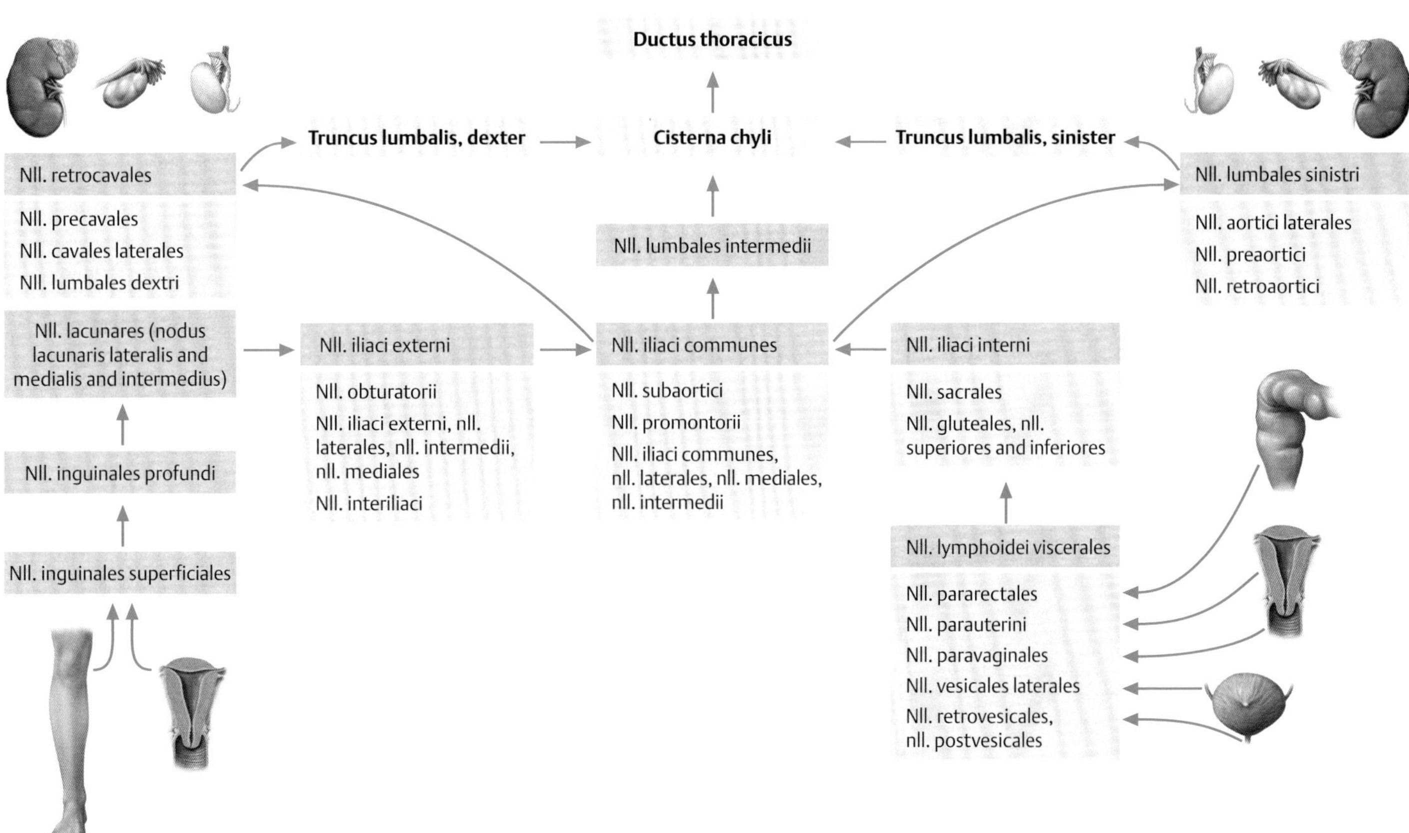
Ductus thoracicus
Truncus lumbalis, dexter
Cisterna chyli
Truncus lumbalis, sinister
Nll. retrocavales
Nll. precavales
Nll. cavales laterales
Nll. lumbales dextri
Nll. lumbales intermedii
Nll. lumbales sinistri
Nll. aortici laterales
Nll. preaortici
Nll. retroaortici
Nll. lacunares (nodus lacunaris lateralis and medialis and intermedius)
Nll. iliaci externi
Nll. obturatorii
Nll. iliaci externi, nll. laterales, nll. intermedii, nll. mediales
Nll. interiliaci
Nll. iliaci communes
Nll. subaortici
Nll. promontorii
Nll. iliaci communes, nll. laterales, nll. mediales, nll. intermedii
Nll. iliaci interni
Nll. sacrales
Nll. gluteales, nll. superiores and inferiores
Nll. inguinales profundi
Nll. inguinales superficiales
Nll. lymphoidei viscerales
Nll. pararectales
Nll. parauterini
Nll. paravaginales
Nll. vesicales laterales
Nll. retrovesicales, nll. postvesicales

Plexus Autonomicus

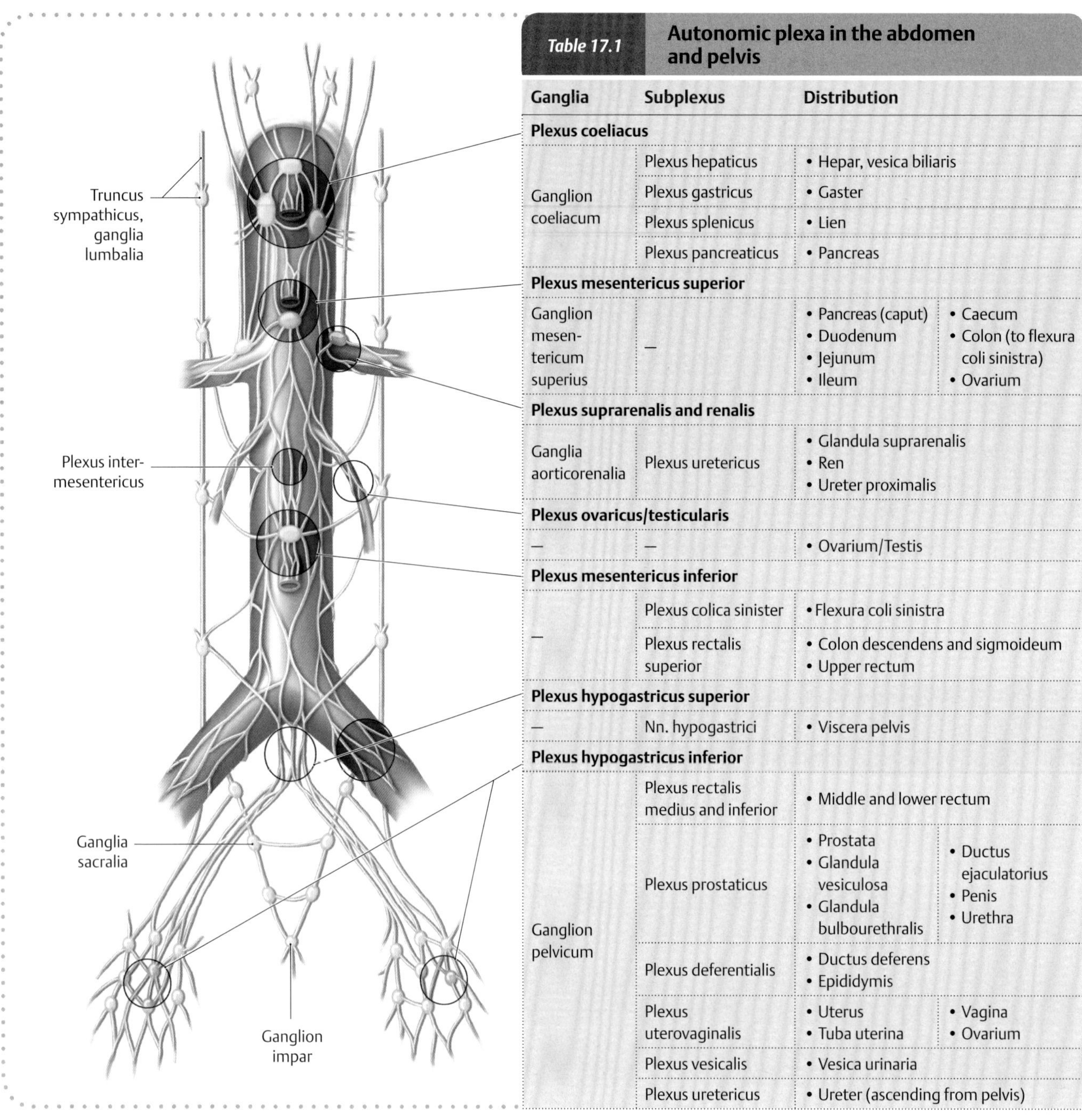
Truncus sympathicus, ganglia lumbalia
Plexus inter-mesentericus
Ganglia sacralia
Ganglion impar

Table 17.1 Autonomic plexa in the abdomen and pelvis

Ganglia	Subplexus	Distribution
Plexus coeliacus		
Ganglion coeliacum	Plexus hepaticus	• Hepar, vesica biliaris
	Plexus gastricus	• Gaster
	Plexus splenicus	• Lien
	Plexus pancreaticus	• Pancreas
Plexus mesentericus superior		
Ganglion mesen-tericum superius	–	• Pancreas (caput) • Duodenum • Jejunum • Ileum • Caecum • Colon (to flexura coli sinistra) • Ovarium
Plexus suprarenalis and renalis		
Ganglia aorticorenalia	Plexus uretericus	• Glandula suprarenalis • Ren • Ureter proximalis
Plexus ovaricus/testicularis		
–	–	• Ovarium/Testis
Plexus mesentericus inferior		
–	Plexus colica sinister	• Flexura coli sinistra
	Plexus rectalis superior	• Colon descendens and sigmoideum • Upper rectum
Plexus hypogastricus superior		
–	Nn. hypogastrici	• Viscera pelvis
Plexus hypogastricus inferior		
Ganglion pelvicum	Plexus rectalis medius and inferior	• Middle and lower rectum
	Plexus prostaticus	• Prostata • Glandula vesiculosa • Glandula bulbourethralis • Ductus ejaculatorius • Penis • Urethra
	Plexus deferentialis	• Ductus deferens • Epididymis
	Plexus uterovaginalis	• Uterus • Tuba uterina • Vagina • Ovarium
	Plexus vesicalis	• Vesica urinaria
	Plexus uretericus	• Ureter (ascending from pelvis)

***Fig. 17.1* Plexus autonomicus in the abdomen and pelvis**
Anterior view of the male abdomen. *Removed:* Peritoneum and majority of gaster.

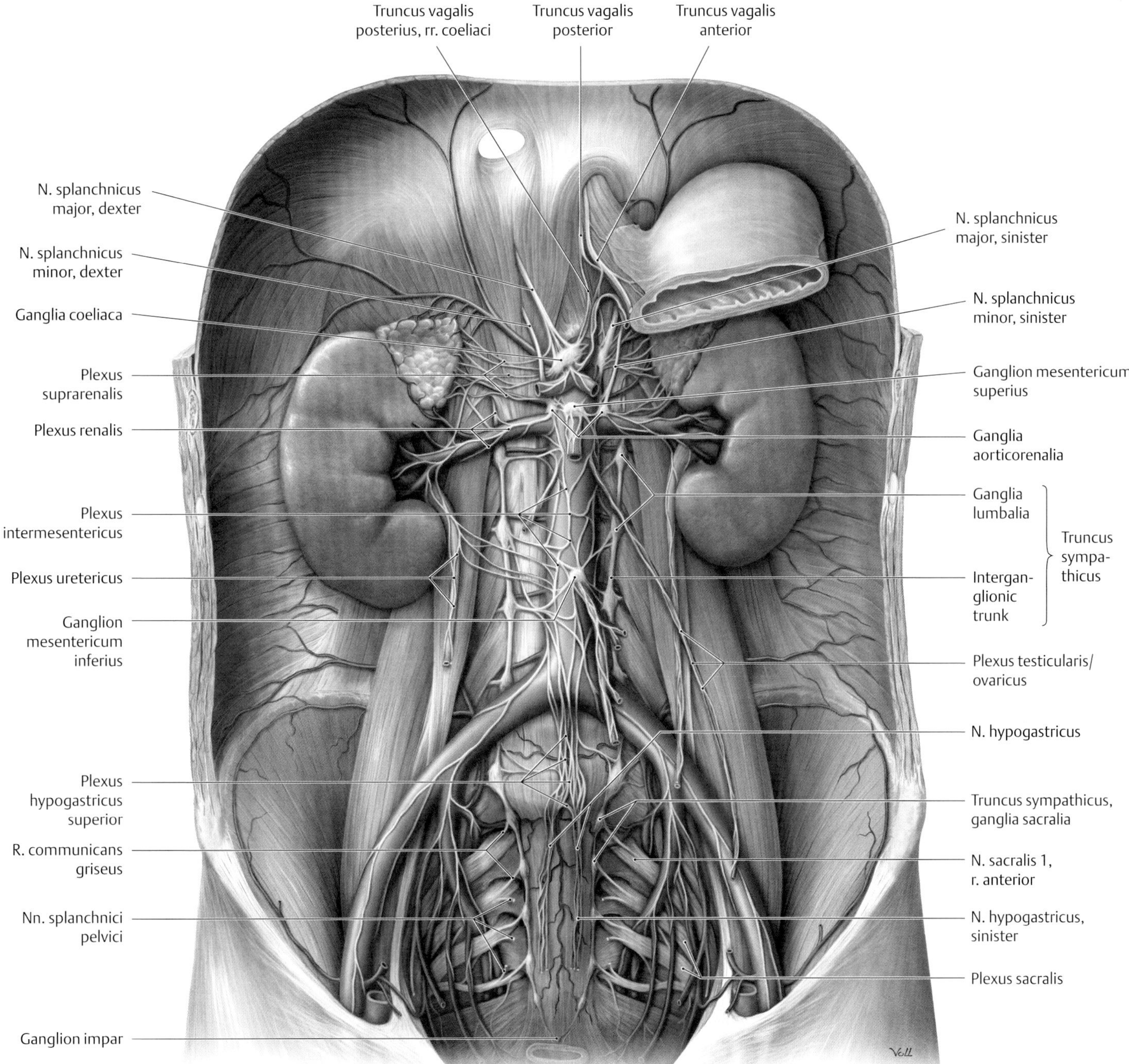
Truncus vagalis posterius, rr. coeliaci
Truncus vagalis posterior
Truncus vagalis anterior
N. splanchnicus major, dexter
N. splanchnicus minor, dexter
Ganglia coeliaca
Plexus suprarenalis
Plexus renalis
Plexus intermesentericus
Plexus uretericus
Ganglion mesentericum inferius
Plexus hypogastricus superior
R. communicans griseus
Nn. splanchnici pelvici
Ganglion impar
N. splanchnicus major, sinister
N. splanchnicus minor, sinister
Ganglion mesentericum superius
Ganglia aorticorenalia
Ganglia lumbalia
Intergan-glionic trunk
Truncus sympa-thicus
Plexus testicularis/ ovaricus
N. hypogastricus
Truncus sympathicus, ganglia sacralia
N. sacralis 1, r. anterior
N. hypogastricus, sinister
Plexus sacralis

Innervation of the Abdominal Organs

Fig. 17.2 Innervation of the anterior abdominal organs
Anterior view. *Removed:* Omentum minus, colon ascendens, and parts of colon transversum. *Opened:* Bursa omentalis. Trunci vagalis anterior and posterior each produce a r. coeliacus, r. hepaticus and r. pyloricus, and a plexus gastricus. See p. 245 for schematic.

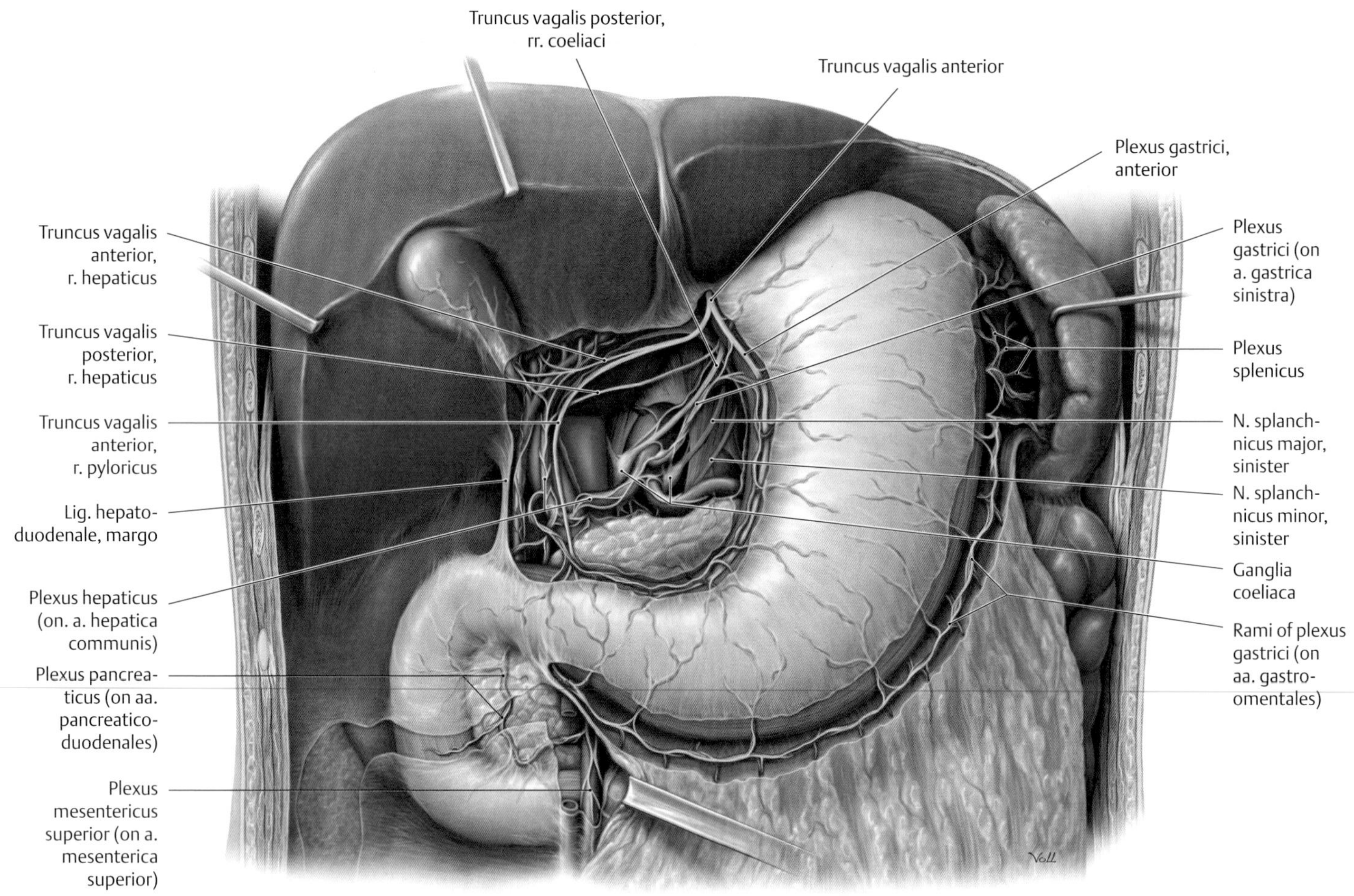
Truncus vagalis posterior, rr. coeliaci
Truncus vagalis anterior
Plexus gastrici, anterior
Truncus vagalis anterior, r. hepaticus
Plexus gastrici (on a. gastrica sinistra)
Truncus vagalis posterior, r. hepaticus
Plexus splenicus
Truncus vagalis anterior, r. pyloricus
N. splanchnicus major, sinister
Lig. hepatoduodenale, margo
N. splanchnicus minor, sinister
Ganglia coeliaca
Plexus hepaticus (on. a. hepatica communis)
Rami of plexus gastrici (on aa. gastroomentales)
Plexus pancreaticus (on aa. pancreaticoduodenales)
Plexus mesentericus superior (on a. mesenterica superior)
Voll

Fig. 17.3 Innervation of the urinary organs
Anterior view of the male abdomen and pelvis. *Removed:* Abdominal organs and peritoneum. See p. 246 for schematic.

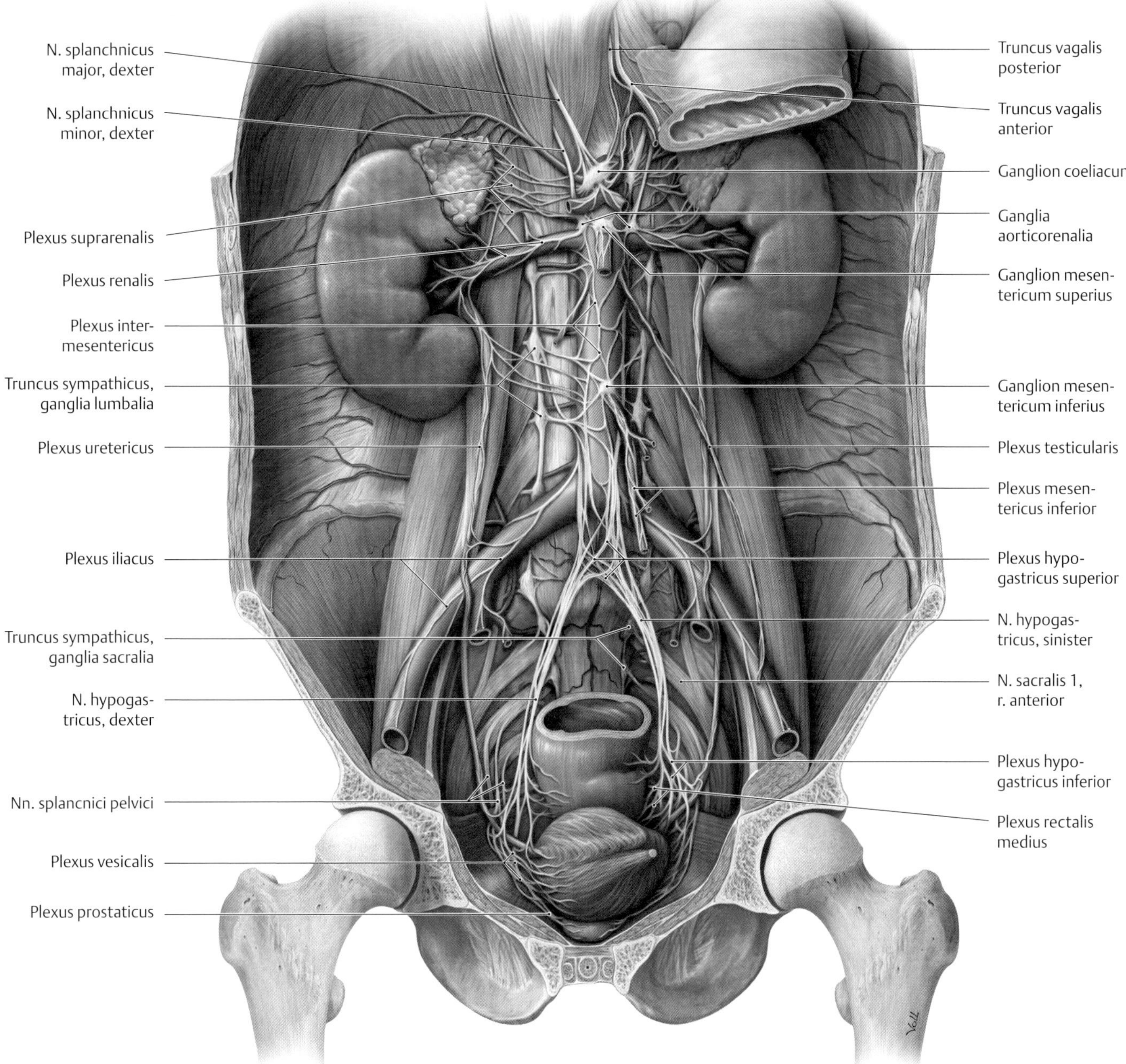
N. splanchnicus major, dexter
N. splanchnicus minor, dexter
Plexus suprarenalis
Plexus renalis
Plexus inter-mesentericus
Truncus sympathicus, ganglia lumbalia
Plexus uretericus
Plexus iliacus
Truncus sympathicus, ganglia sacralia
N. hypogas-tricus, dexter
Nn. splancnici pelvici
Plexus vesicalis
Plexus prostaticus
Truncus vagalis posterior
Truncus vagalis anterior
Ganglion coeliacum
Ganglia aorticorenalia
Ganglion mesen-tericum superius
Ganglion mesen-tericum inferius
Plexus testicularis
Plexus mesen-tericus inferior
Plexus hypo-gastricus superior
N. hypogas-tricus, sinister
N. sacralis 1, r. anterior
Plexus hypo-gastricus inferior
Plexus rectalis medius

Innervation of the Intestines

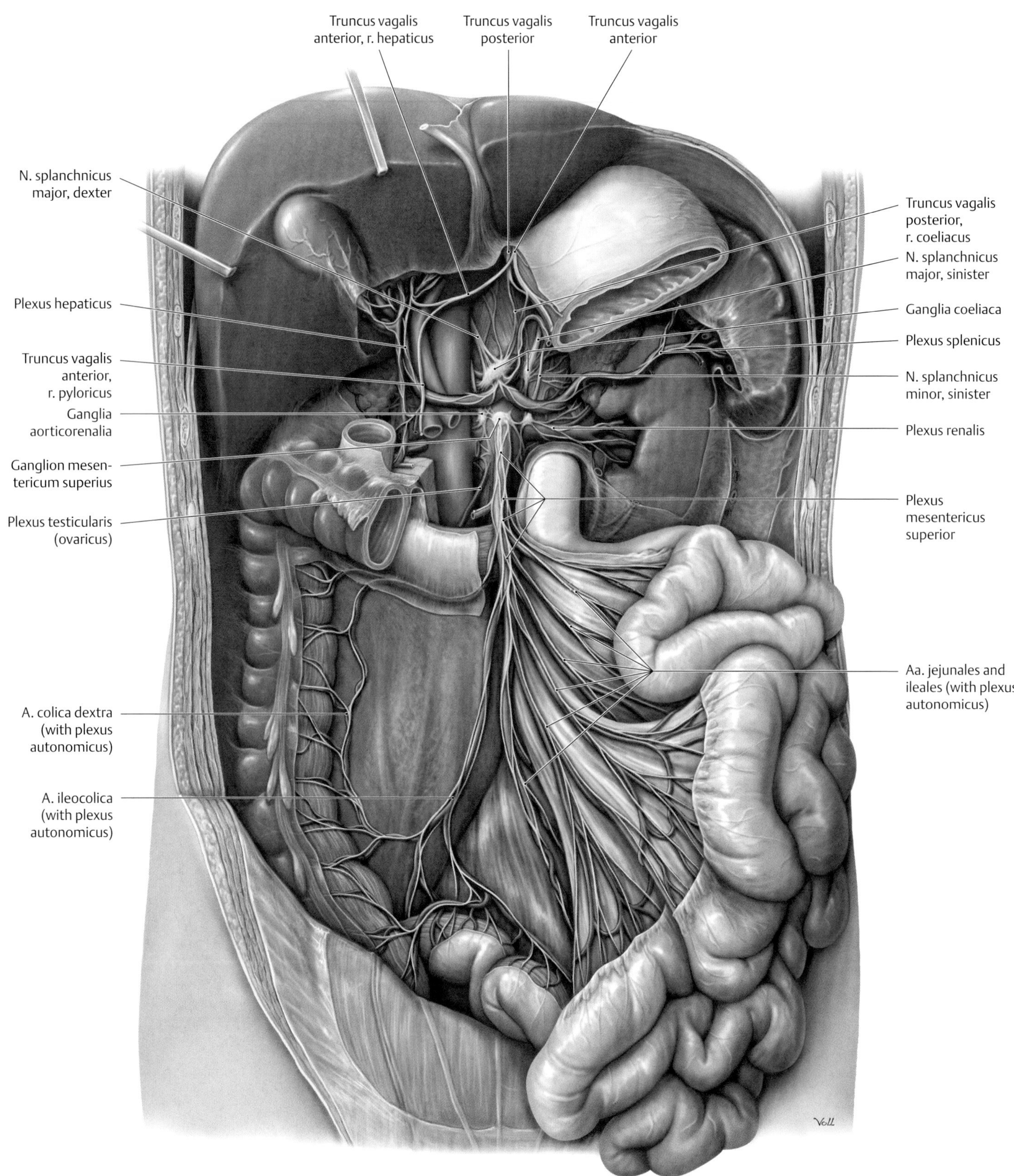

Truncus vagalis anterior, r. hepaticus
Truncus vagalis posterior
Truncus vagalis anterior
N. splanchnicus major, dexter
Plexus hepaticus
Truncus vagalis anterior, r. pyloricus
Ganglia aorticorenalia
Ganglion mesentericum superius
Plexus testicularis (ovaricus)
A. colica dextra (with plexus autonomicus)
A. ileocolica (with plexus autonomicus)
Truncus vagalis posterior, r. coeliacus
N. splanchnicus major, sinister
Ganglia coeliaca
Plexus splenicus
N. splanchnicus minor, sinister
Plexus renalis
Plexus mesentericus superior
Aa. jejunales and ileales (with plexus autonomicus)
Voll

Fig. 17.4 **Innervation of the intestinum tenue**
Anterior view. *Partially removed:* Gaster, pancreas, and colon transversum (distal part). See p. 245 for schematic.

Fig. 17.5 Innervation of the intestinum crassum
Anterior view. *Removed:* Jejunum and ileum. *Reflected:* Colon transversum and sigmoideum. See p. 245 for schematic.

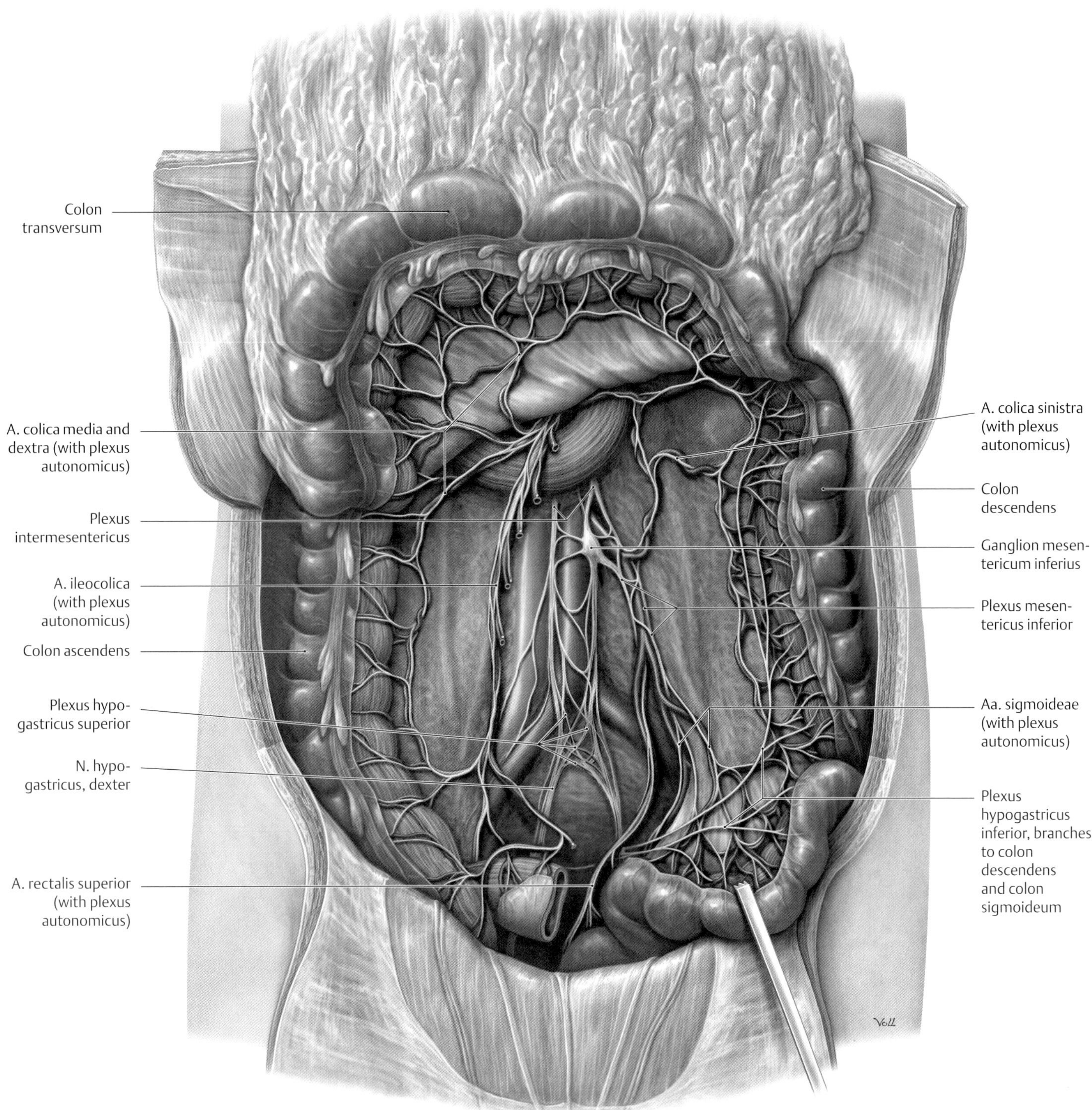

Colon transversum
A. colica media and dextra (with plexus autonomicus)
Plexus intermesentericus
A. ileocolica (with plexus autonomicus)
Colon ascendens
Plexus hypogastricus superior
N. hypogastricus, dexter
A. rectalis superior (with plexus autonomicus)
A. colica sinistra (with plexus autonomicus)
Colon descendens
Ganglion mesentericum inferius
Plexus mesentericus inferior
Aa. sigmoideae (with plexus autonomicus)
Plexus hypogastricus inferior, branches to colon descendens and colon sigmoideum

Innervation of the Pelvis

Fig. 17.6 **Innervation of the female pelvis**
Right pelvis, left lateral view. *Reflected:* Uterus and rectum.
See p. 247 for schematic.

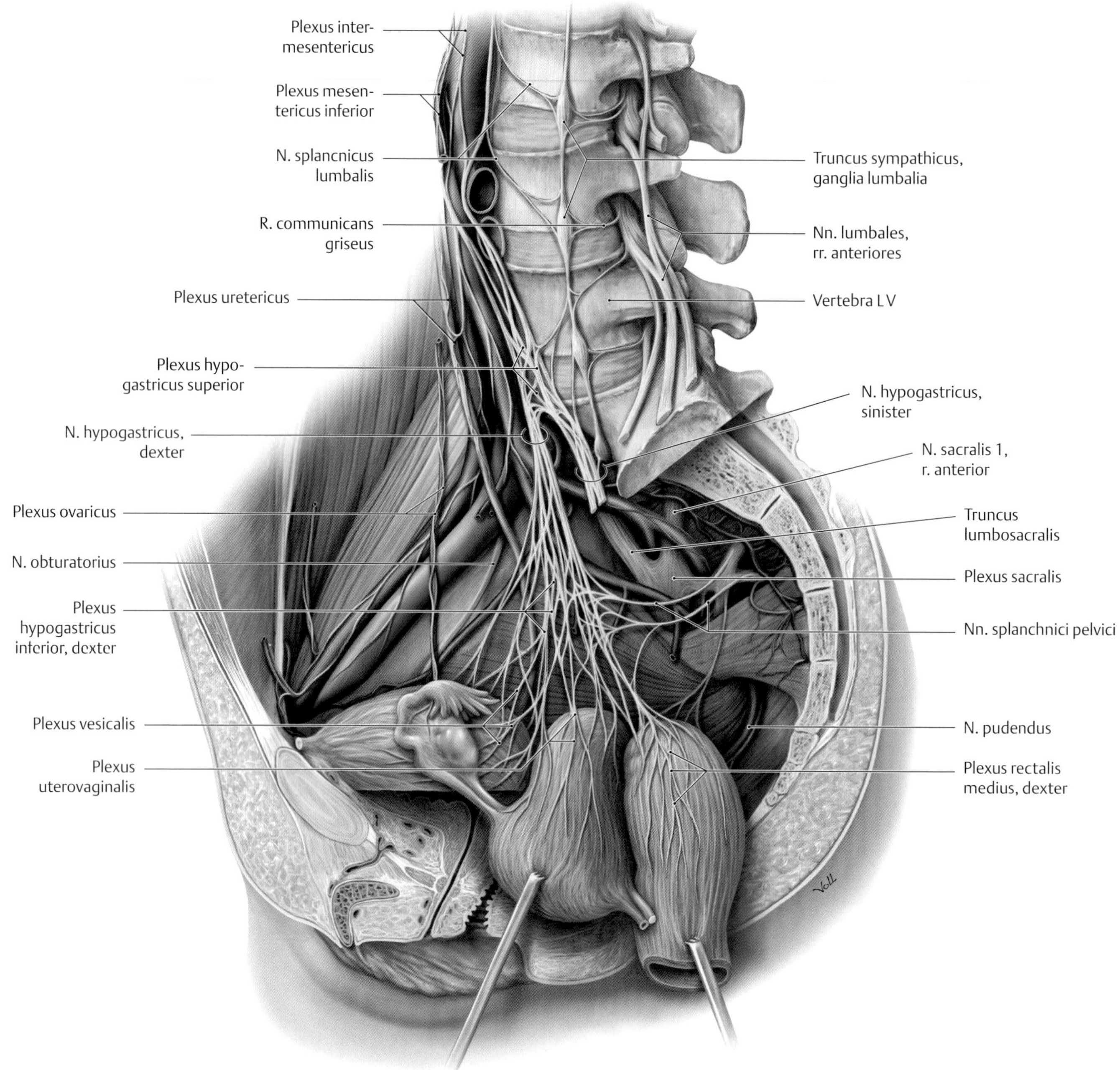
Plexus inter-
mesentericus
Plexus mesen-
tericus inferior
N. splancnicus
lumbalis
R. communicans
griseus
Plexus uretericus
Plexus hypo-
gastricus superior
N. hypogastricus,
dexter
Plexus ovaricus
N. obturatorius
Plexus
hypogastricus
inferior, dexter
Plexus vesicalis
Plexus
uterovaginalis
Truncus sympathicus,
ganglia lumbalia
Nn. lumbales,
rr. anteriores
Vertebra LV
N. hypogastricus,
sinister
N. sacralis 1,
r. anterior
Truncus
lumbosacralis
Plexus sacralis
Nn. splanchnici pelvici
N. pudendus
Plexus rectalis
medius, dexter

Fig. 17.7 **Innervation of the male pelvis**
Right pelvis, left lateral view. See p. 247 for schematic.

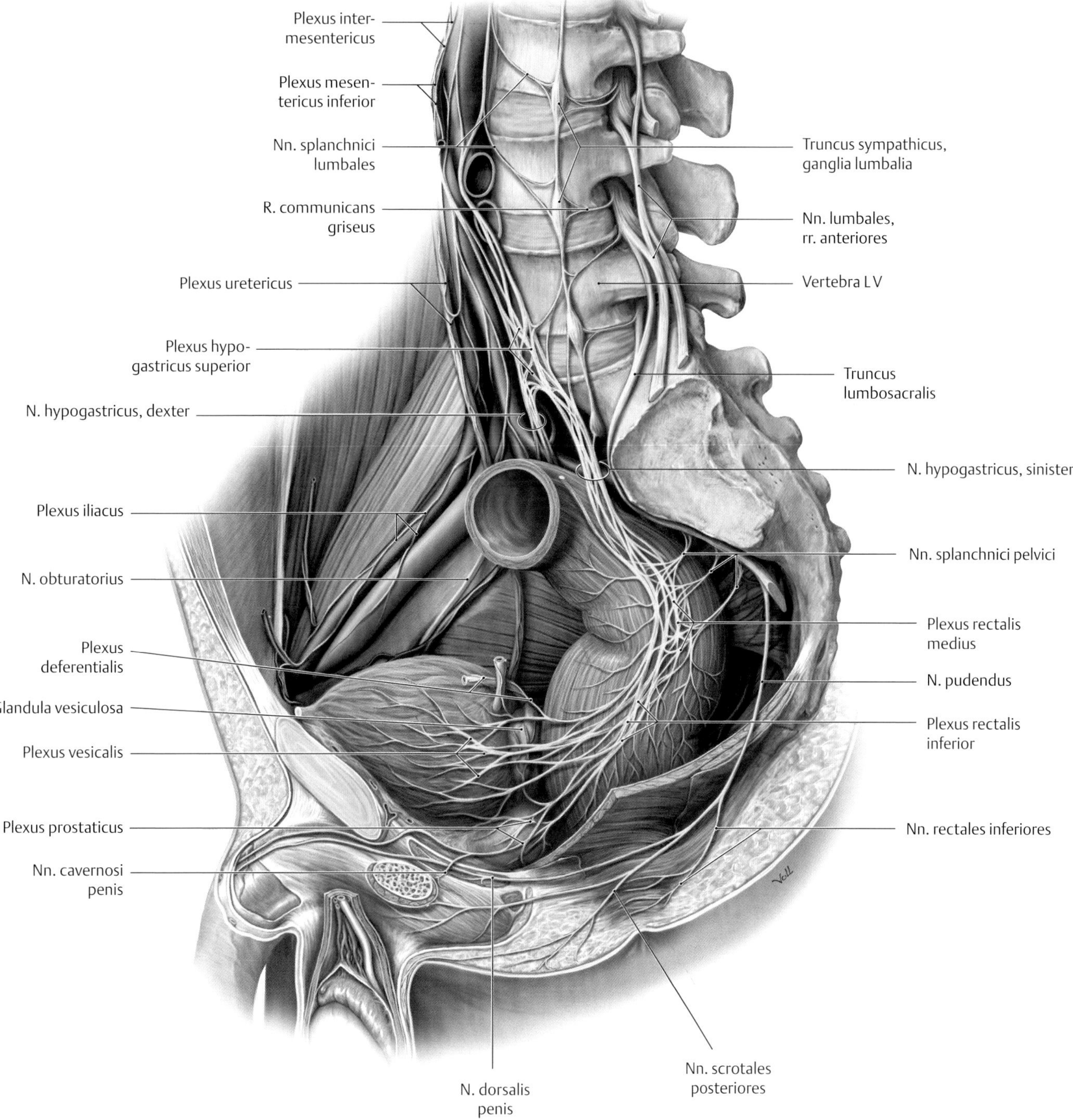
Plexus inter-mesentericus
Plexus mesen-tericus inferior
Nn. splanchnici lumbales
R. communicans griseus
Plexus uretericus
Plexus hypo-gastricus superior
N. hypogastricus, dexter
Plexus iliacus
N. obturatorius
Plexus deferentialis
Glandula vesiculosa
Plexus vesicalis
Plexus prostaticus
Nn. cavernosi penis
Truncus sympathicus, ganglia lumbalia
Nn. lumbales, rr. anteriores
Vertebra LV
Truncus lumbosacralis
N. hypogastricus, sinister
Nn. splanchnici pelvici
Plexus rectalis medius
N. pudendus
Plexus rectalis inferior
Nn. rectales inferiores
N. dorsalis penis
Nn. scrotales posteriores

Autonomic Innervation: Overview

Fig. 17.8 Sympathetic and parasympathetic nervous systems in the abdomen and pelvis

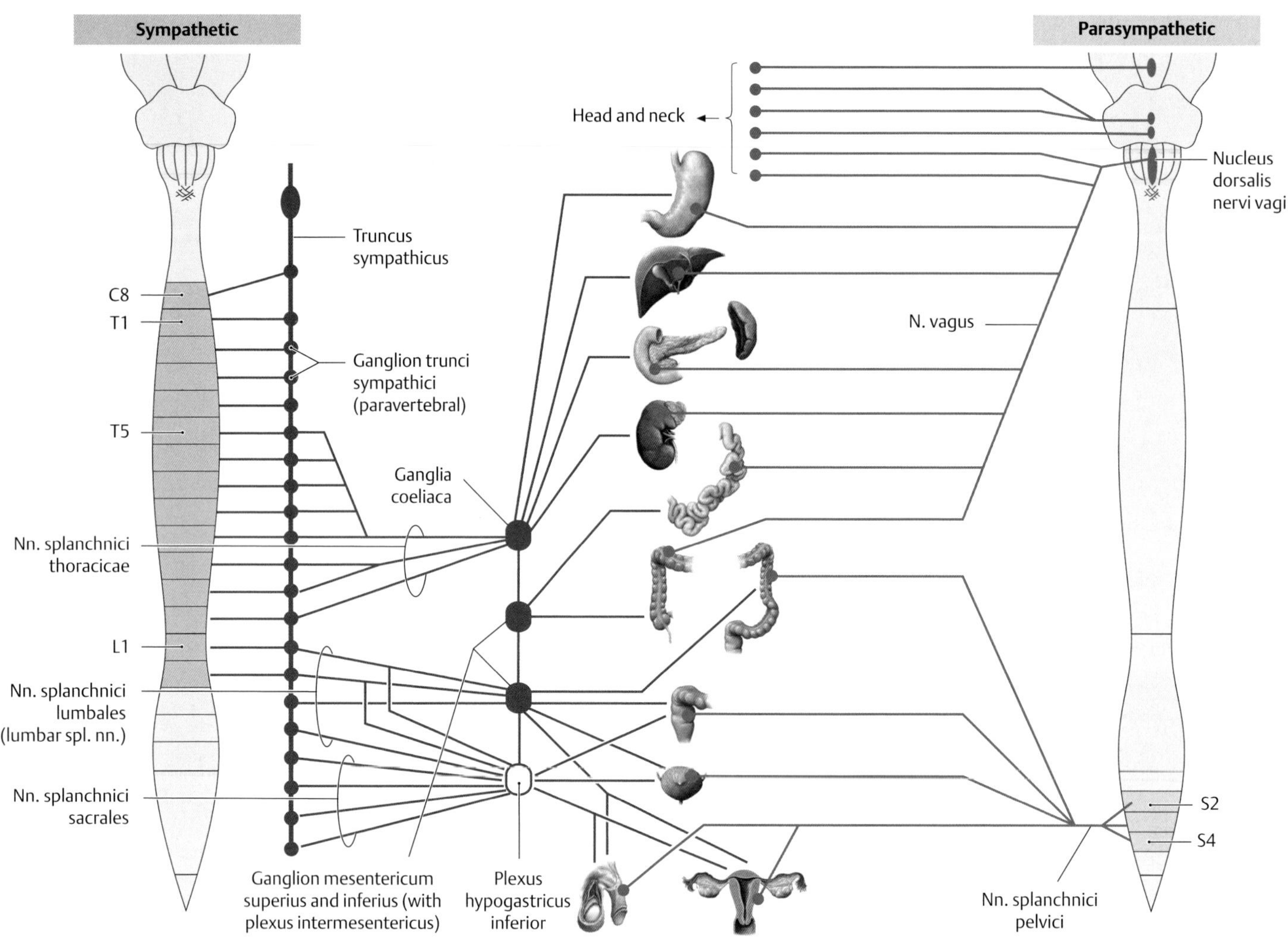
Sympathetic
Parasympathetic
Head and neck
Nucleus dorsalis nervi vagi
Truncus sympathicus
C8
T1
Ganglion trunci sympathici (paravertebral)
N. vagus
T5
Ganglia coeliaca
Nn. splanchnici thoracicae
L1
Nn. splanchnici lumbales (lumbar spl. nn.)
Nn. splanchnici sacrales
S2
S4
Ganglion mesentericum superius and inferius (with plexus intermesentericus)
Plexus hypogastricus inferior
Nn. splanchnici pelvici

A Sympathetic nervous system.

B Parasympathetic nervous system.

Table 17.2 Effects of the autonomic nervous system in the abdomen and pelvis

Organ (organ system)		Sympathetic effect	Parasympathetic effect
Gastrointestinal tract	Longitudinal and circular muscle fibers	Decreases motility	Increases motility
	Musculi sphincteri	Contraction	Relaxation
	Glandulae	Decreases secretions	Increases secretions
Capsula splenica		Contraction	No effect
Hepar		Increases glycogenolysis/gluconeogenesis	
Pancreas	Endocrine pancreas	Decreases insulin secretion	
	Exocrine pancreas	Decreases secretion	Increases secretion
Vesica urinaria	M. detrusor vesicae	Relaxation	Contraction
	Functional bladder sphincter	Contraction	Inhibits contraction
Glandula vesiculosa and ductus deferens		Contraction (ejakulation)	No effect
Uterus		Contraction or relaxation, depending on hormonal status	
Arteriae		Vasoconstriction	Vasodilation of the arteriae of the penis and clitoris (erection)
Glandula suprarenalis (medulla)		Release of adrenalin	No effect
Urinary tract	Ren	Vasokonstriction (decreases urine formation)	Vasodilation

Fig. 17.9 **Autonomic innervation of the intraperitoneal organs**

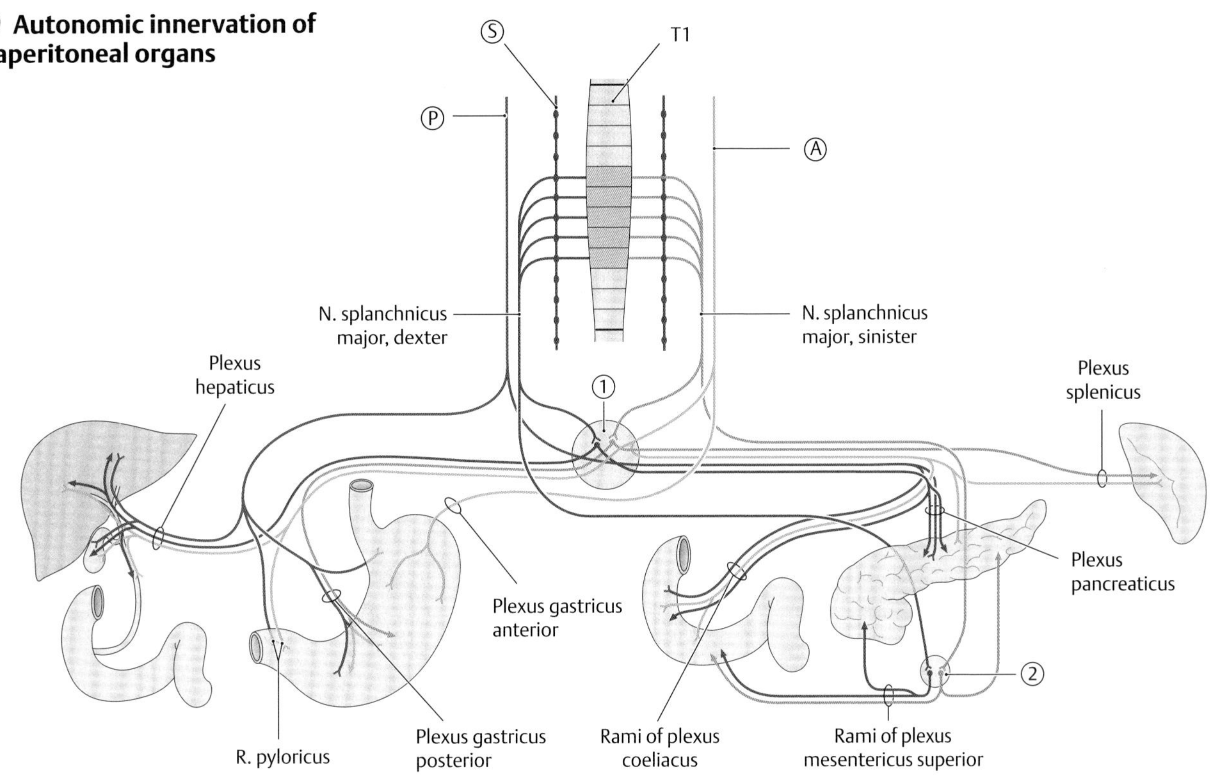
Ⓢ
T1
Ⓟ
Ⓐ
N. splanchnicus major, dexter
N. splanchnicus major, sinister
Plexus hepaticus
①
Plexus splenicus
Plexus pancreaticus
Plexus gastricus anterior
②
R. pyloricus
Plexus gastricus posterior
Rami of plexus coeliacus
Rami of plexus mesentericus superior

A Innervation of the foregut. As the left and right nn. vagus descend along the esophagus, they become truncus vagalis anterior and posterior, respectively. Each trunk produces a r. coeliacus, r. pyloricus and r. hepaticus, and a plexus gastricus.

Ⓢ	Truncus sympathicus
Ⓟ	Truncus vagalis posterior (n. vagus, dexter)
Ⓐ	Truncus vagalis anterior (n. vagus, sinister)
①	Ganglia coeliaca
②	Ganglion mesentericum superius
③	Ganglion mesentericum inferius
④	N. splanchnicus major (T5–T9)
⑤	N. splanchnicus minor (T10–T11)
⑥	N. splanchnicus imus (T12)
⑦	Nn. splanchnici lumbales (L1–L2)
⑧	Nn. splanchnici lumbales (from ganglia lumbalia 3–4)
⑨	Nn. splanchnici sacrales (from ganglia sacralia 1–3)
⑩	Nn. splanchnici pelvici (S2–S4)

Ⓢ
Ⓟ
T5
Nn. splanchnici thoracica
T10
T12
L1
Nn. splanchnici lumbales
S2
④ ⑤ ⑥ ⑦ ⑧* ⑨* ⑩
① ② ③
Plexus mesentericus superior
Plexus mesentericus inferior
Plexus rectalis superior
Plexus rectalis medius
Plexus hypogastricus inferior, ganglia pelvica
Plexus rectalis inferior

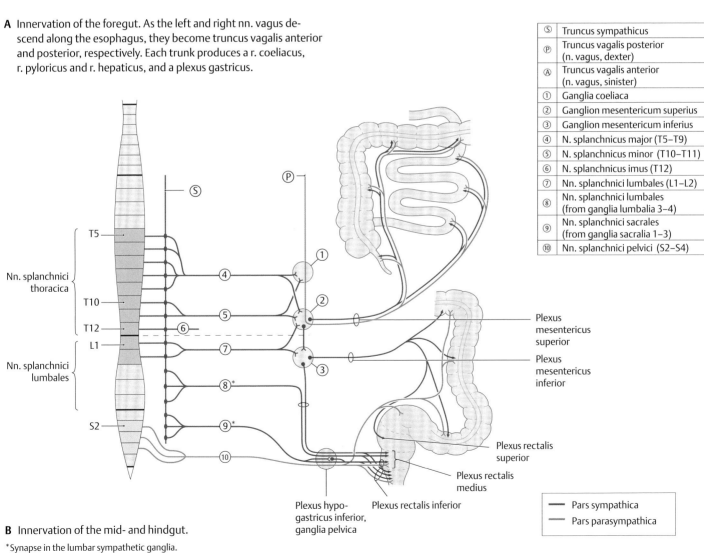

Pars sympathica
Pars parasympathica

B Innervation of the mid- and hindgut.

*Synapse in the lumbar sympathetic ganglia.

Autonomic Innervation: Urinary & Genital Organs

Fig. 17.10 Autonomic innervation of the urinary organs

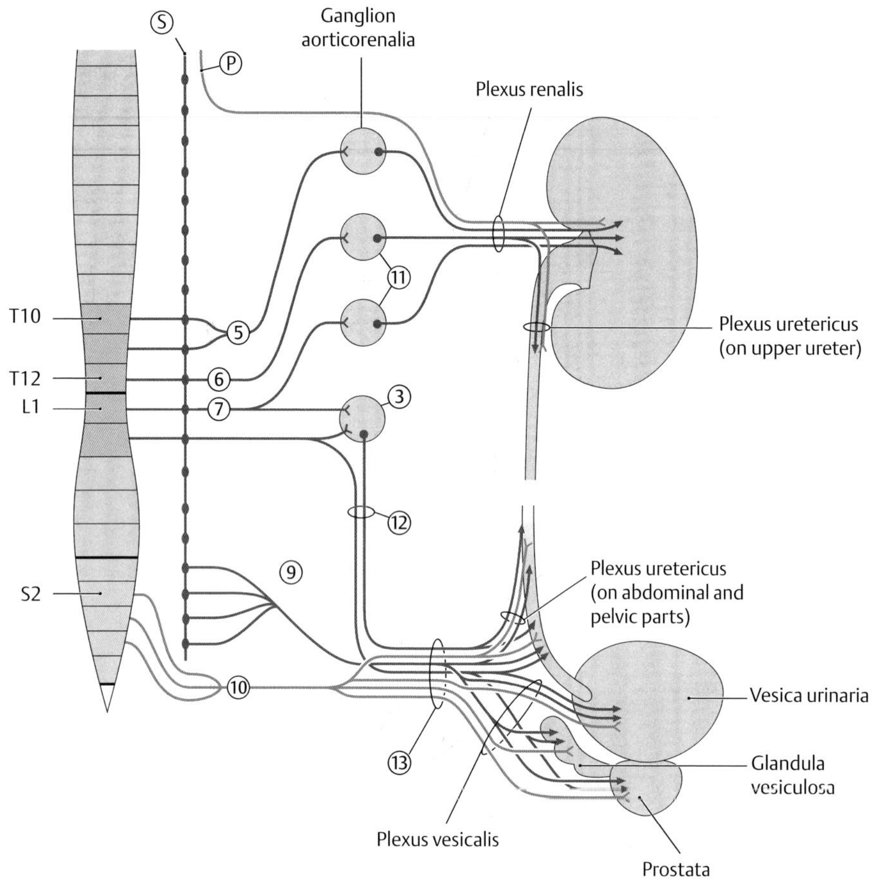

Ⓢ
Ⓟ
Ganglion aorticorenalia
Plexus renalis
T10
T12
L1
S2
⑤
⑥
⑦
③
⑪
⑫
⑨
⑩
⑬
Plexus uretericus (on upper ureter)
Plexus uretericus (on abdominal and pelvic parts)
Vesica urinaria
Glandula vesiculosa
Plexus vesicalis
Prostata

—	Pars sympathica
—	Pars parasympathica

Numbering continued from p. 245.	
Ⓢ	Truncus sympathicus
Ⓟ	Truncus vagalis posterior (n. vagus, dexter)
③	Ganglion mesentericum inferius
⑤	N. splanchnicus minor (T10–T11)
⑥	N. splanchnicus imus (T12)
⑦	Nn. splanchnici lumbales (L1–L2)
⑨	Nn. splanchnici sacrales (from ganglia sacralia 1–3)
⑩	Nn. splanchnici pelvici (S2–S4)
⑪	Ganglia renalia
⑫	Plexus hypogastricus superior
⑬	Plexus hypogastricus inferior

Clinical

Referred pain from the internal organs

The convergence of somatic and visceral afferent fibers to a common level of the spinal cord confuses the relationship between the perceived and actual sites of pain, a phenomenon known as referred pain. Pain impulses from a particular organ are consistently projected to the same well-defined skin area.

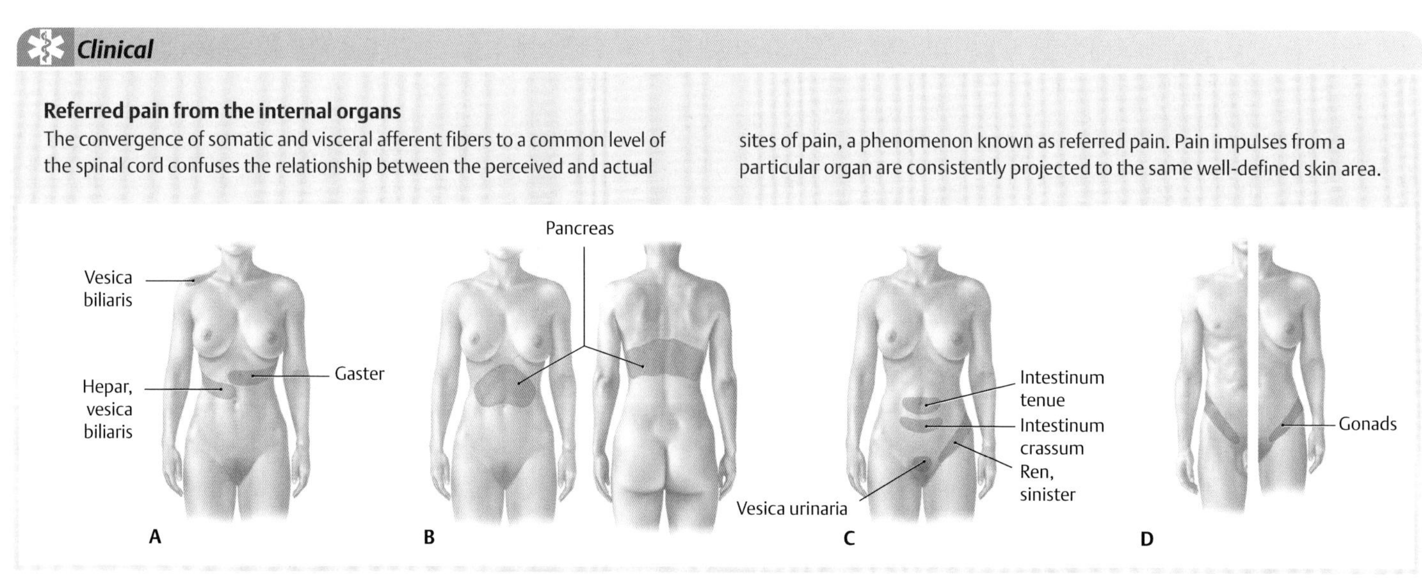

Vesica biliaris
Hepar, vesica biliaris
Gaster
Pancreas
Intestinum tenue
Intestinum crassum
Ren, sinister
Vesica urinaria
Gonads
A
B
C
D

Fig. 17.11 Autonomic innervation of the genitalia

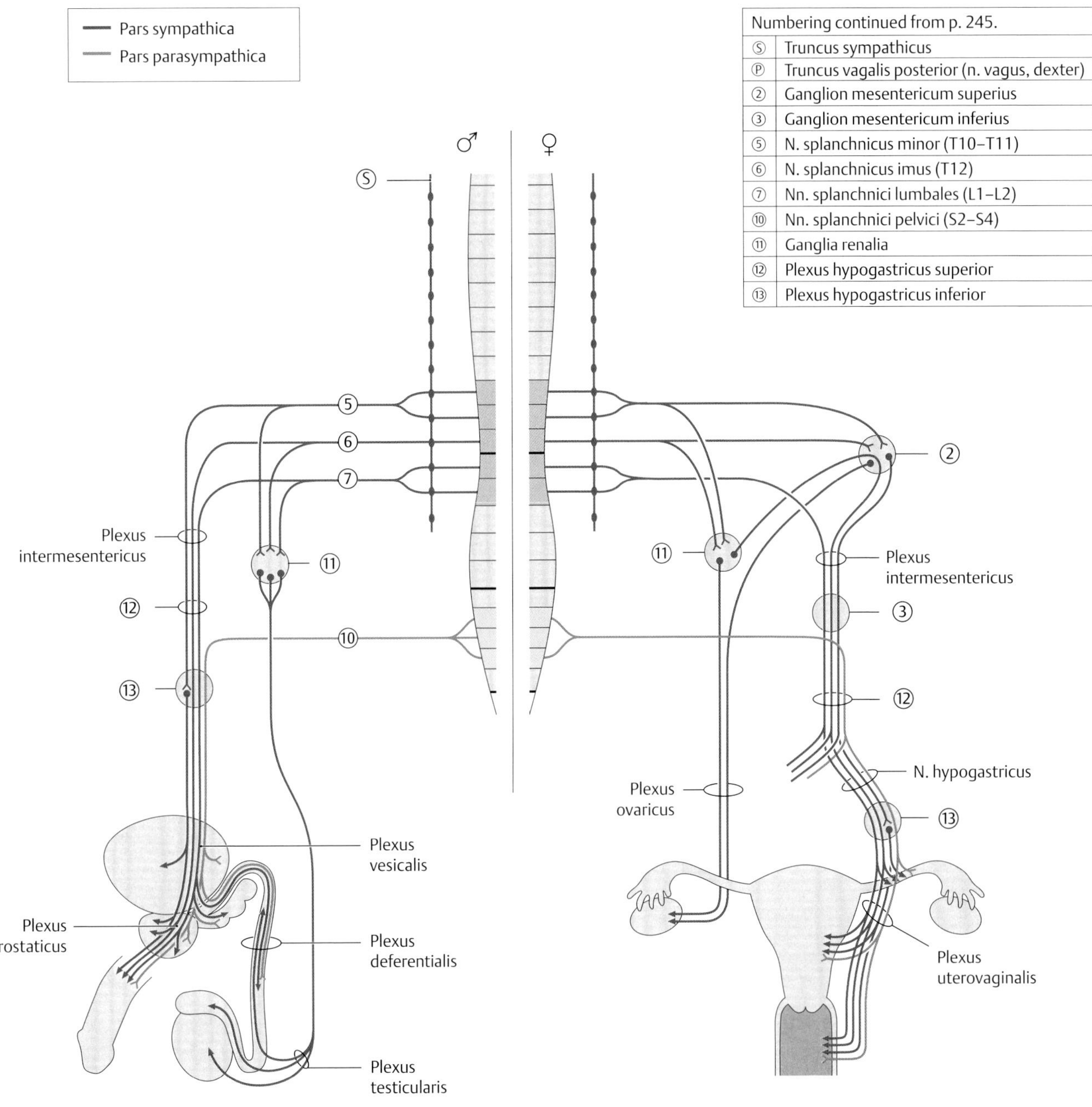

Pars sympathica
Pars parasympathica
Numbering continued from p. 245.
Ⓢ Truncus sympathicus
Ⓟ Truncus vagalis posterior (n. vagus, dexter)
② Ganglion mesentericum superius
③ Ganglion mesentericum inferius
⑤ N. splanchnicus minor (T10–T11)
⑥ N. splanchnicus imus (T12)
⑦ Nn. splanchnici lumbales (L1–L2)
⑩ Nn. splanchnici pelvici (S2–S4)
⑪ Ganglia renalia
⑫ Plexus hypogastricus superior
⑬ Plexus hypogastricus inferior
♂
♀
Ⓢ
⑤
⑥
⑦
Plexus intermesentericus
⑪
⑫
⑩
⑬
②
③
N. hypogastricus
Plexus ovaricus
Plexus vesicalis
Plexus prostaticus
Plexus deferentialis
Plexus testicularis
Plexus uterovaginalis

A Male genitalia.

B Female genitalia.

Surface Anatomy

Fig. 18.1 **Palpable structures in the abdomen and pelvis**
Anterior view. See pp. 40–41 for structures of the back.

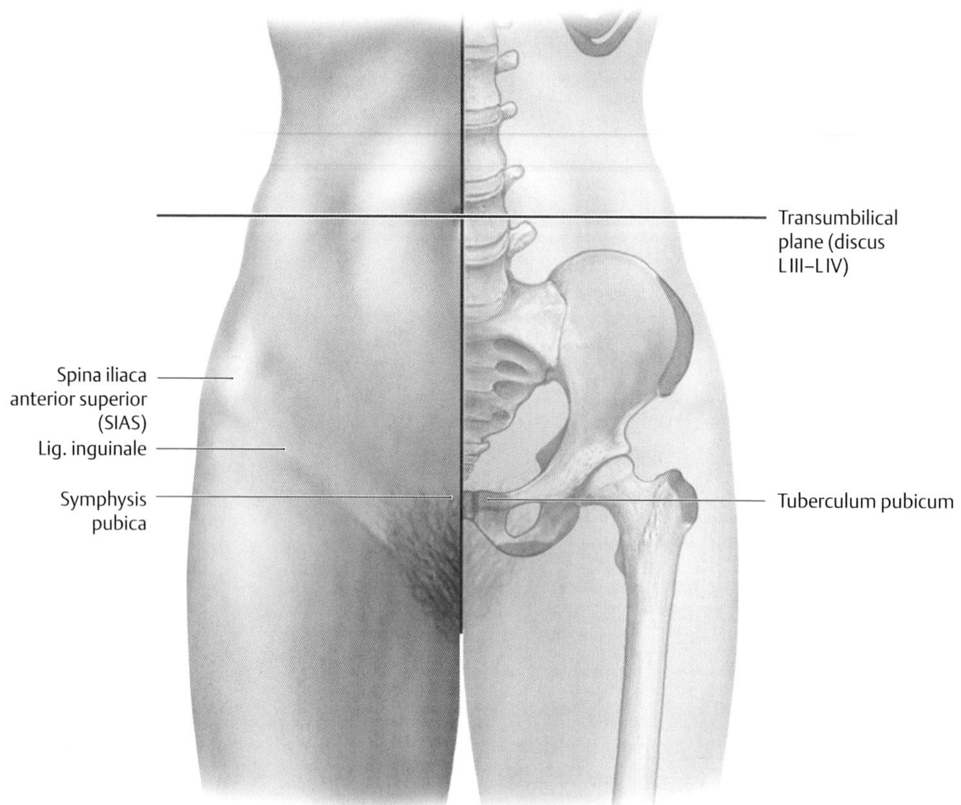
Transumbilical plane (discus LIII–LIV)
Spina iliaca anterior superior (SIAS)
Lig. inguinale
Symphysis pubica
Tuberculum pubicum

A Bony prominences.

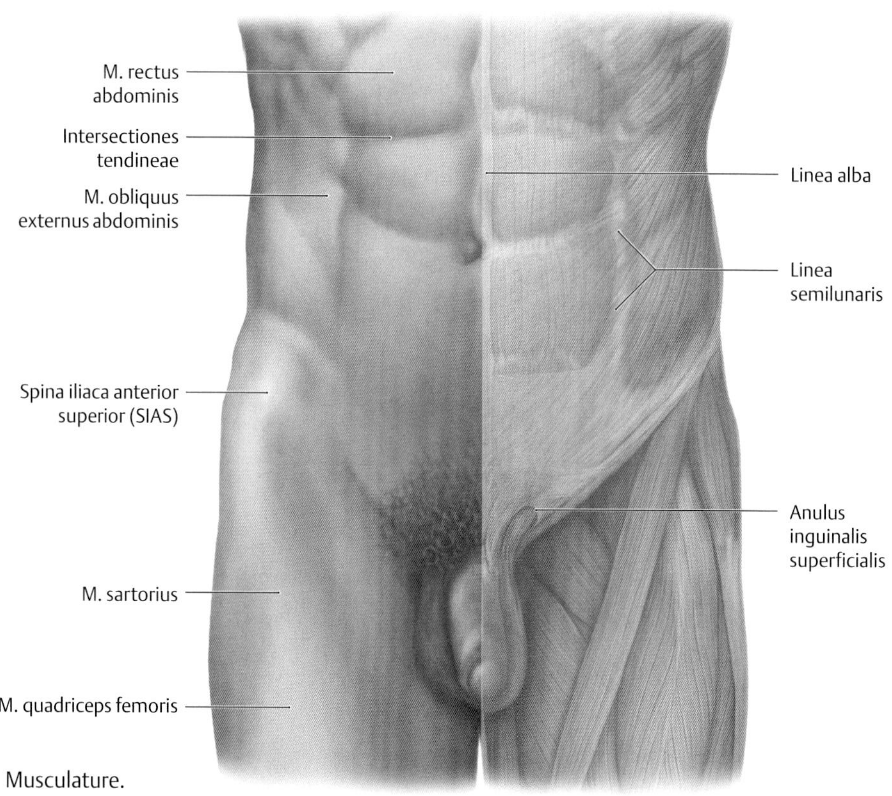
M. rectus abdominis
Intersectiones tendineae
M. obliquus externus abdominis
Linea alba
Linea semilunaris
Spina iliaca anterior superior (SIAS)
Anulus inguinalis superficialis
M. sartorius
M. quadriceps femoris

B Musculature.

Fig. 18.2 **Surface anatomy of the abdomen and pelvis**
Anterior view. See pp. 40–41 for structures of the back.

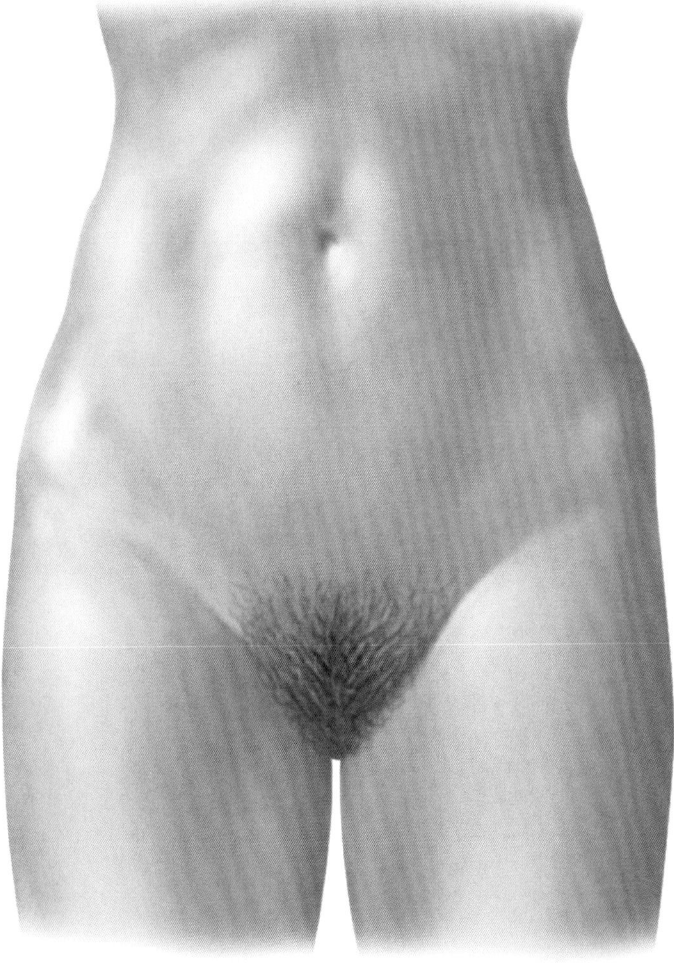

A Female abdomen and pelvis.

Q1: How would this patient's abdomen be subdivided for descriptive purposes into four quadrants? Name five organs in each quadrant.

Q2: A patient's inguinal region shows a slight swelling just superior to the middle of the inguinal region. What factors (age, anatomical) might assist you in determining if this is a direct or indirect inguinal hernia?

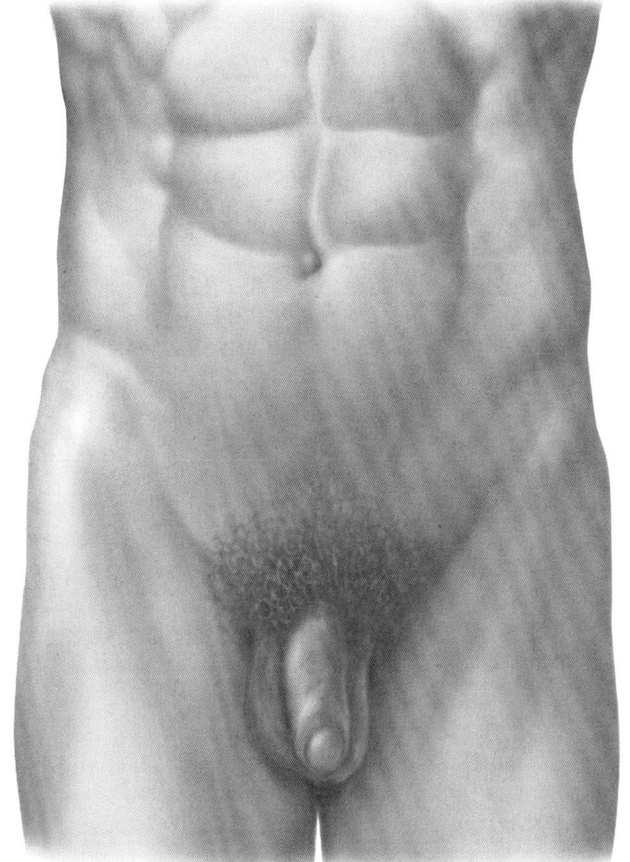

B Male abdomen and pelvis.

See answers beginning on p. 626.

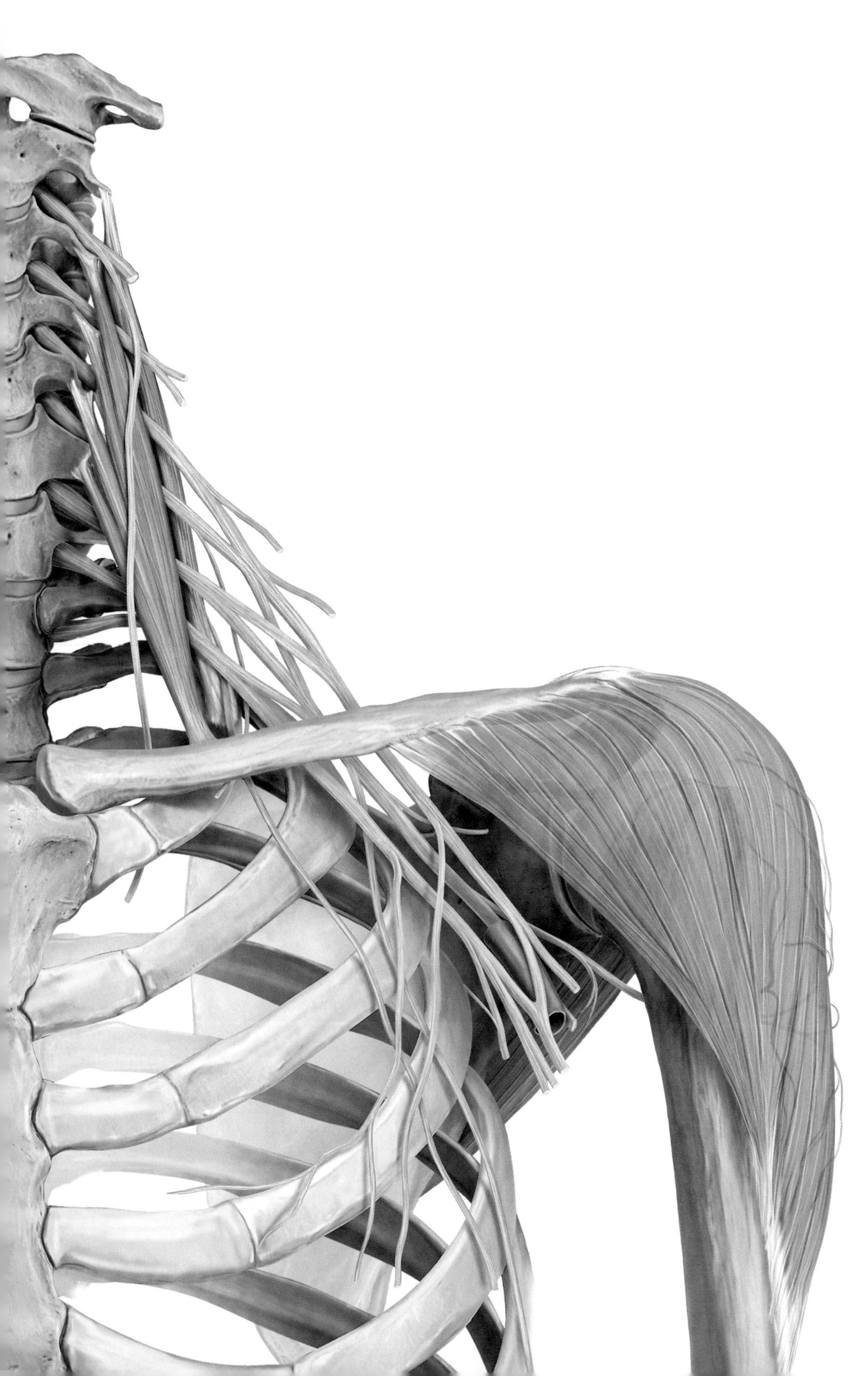

Upper Limb

19 Shoulder & Arm

Bones of the Upper Limb 252
Clavicula & Scapula 254
Humerus 256
Joints of the Shoulder 258
Joints of the Shoulder: Articulatio Humeri 260
Subacromial Space & Bursae 262
Anterior Muscles of the Shoulder & Arm (I) 264
Anterior Muscles of the Shoulder & Arm (II) 266
Posterior Muscles of the Shoulder & Arm (I) 268
Posterior Muscles of the Shoulder & Arm (II) 270
Muscle Facts (I) 272
Muscle Facts (II) 274
Muscle Facts (III) 276
Muscle Facts (IV) 278

20 Elbow & Forearm

Radius & Ulna 280
Articulatio Cubiti 282
Ligaments of Articulatio Cubiti 284
Radioulnar Joints 286
Muscles of the Forearm (I) 288
Muscles of the Forearm (II) 290
Muscle Facts (I) 292
Muscle Facts (II) 294
Muscle Facts (III) 296

21 Wrist & Hand

Bones of the Wrist & Hand 298
Joints of the Wrist & Hand 300
Ligaments of the Wrist & Hand 302
Ligaments of the Fingers 304
Muscles of the Hand: Superficial & Middle Layers 306
Muscles of the Hand: Middle & Deep Layers 308
Dorsum of the Hand 310
Muscle Facts (I) 312
Muscle Facts (II) 314

22 Neurovasculature

Arteries of the Upper Limb 316
Veins & Lymphatics of the Upper Limb 318
Nerves of Plexus Brachialis 320
Supraclavicular Branches & Fasciculus Posterior 322
Fasciculus Posterior: N. Axillaris & N. Radialis 324
Fasciculus Medialis & Fasciculus Lateralis 326
N. Medianus & N. Ulnaris 328
Superficial Veins & Nerves of the Upper Limb 330
Posterior Shoulder & Axilla 332
Anterior Shoulder 334
Topography of the Axilla 336
Topography of the Brachial & Cubital Regions 338
Topography of the Forearm 340
Topography of the Carpal Region 342
Topography of the Palm of the Hand 344
Topography of the Dorsum of the Hand 346
Transverse Sections 348

23 Surface Anatomy

Surface Anatomy (I) 350
Surface Anatomy (II) 352

Bones of the Upper Limb

Fig. 19.1 Skeleton of the upper limb

Right limb. The upper limb is subdivided into three regions: arm, forearm, and hand. The shoulder girdle (clavicula and scapula) joins the upper limb to the thorax at articulatio sternoclavicularis.

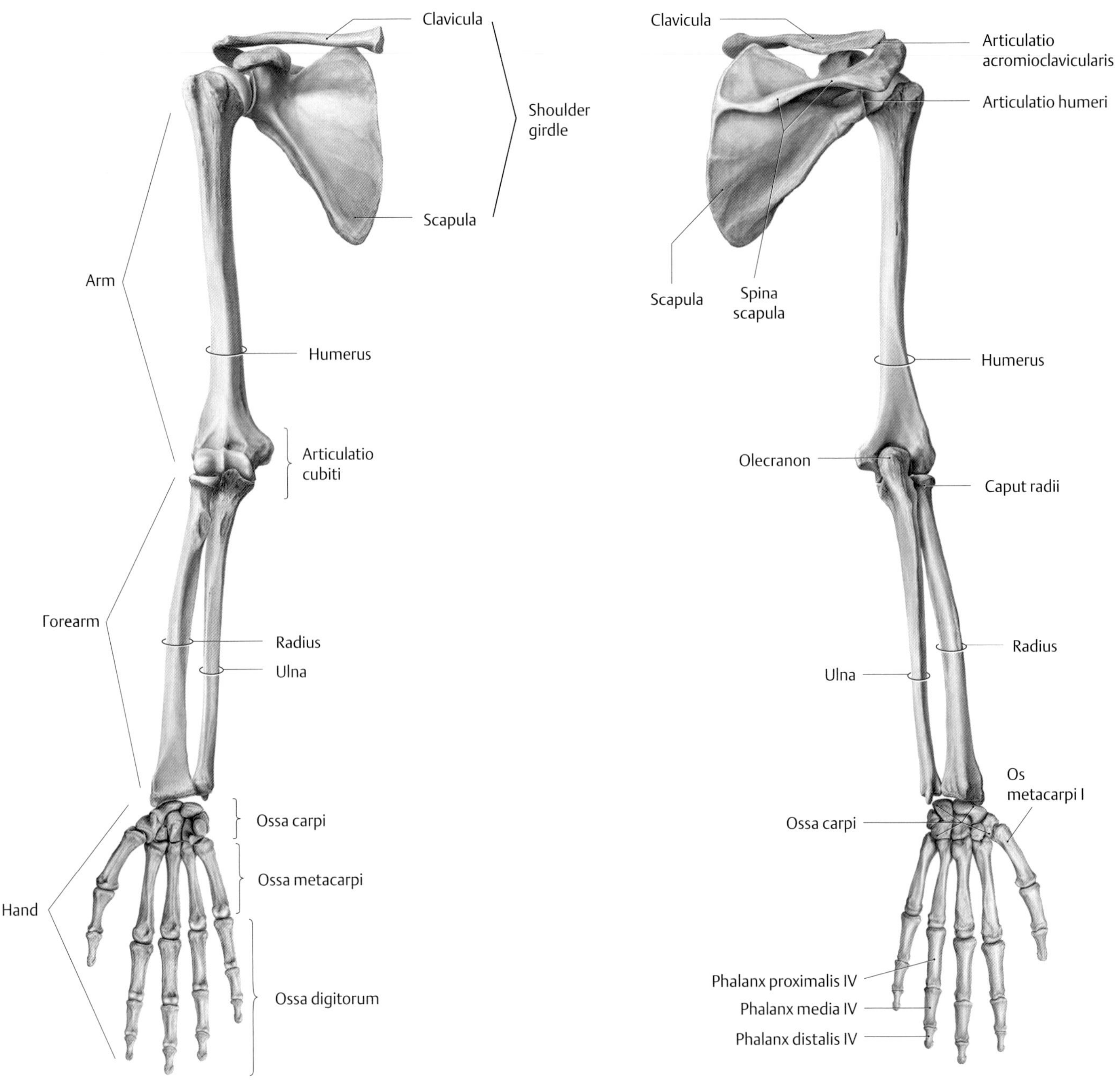
Clavicula
Shoulder girdle
Scapula
Arm
Humerus
Articulatio cubiti
Forearm
Radius
Ulna
Ossa carpi
Ossa metacarpi
Hand
Ossa digitorum
Clavicula
Articulatio acromioclavicularis
Articulatio humeri
Scapula
Spina scapula
Humerus
Olecranon
Caput radii
Radius
Ulna
Os metacarpi I
Ossa carpi
Phalanx proximalis IV
Phalanx media IV
Phalanx distalis IV

A Anterior view.

B Posterior view.

Fig. 19.2 **Palpable bony prominences**

Except for the os lunatum and os trapezoideum, all of the bones in the upper limb are palpable to some degree through the skin and soft tissues.

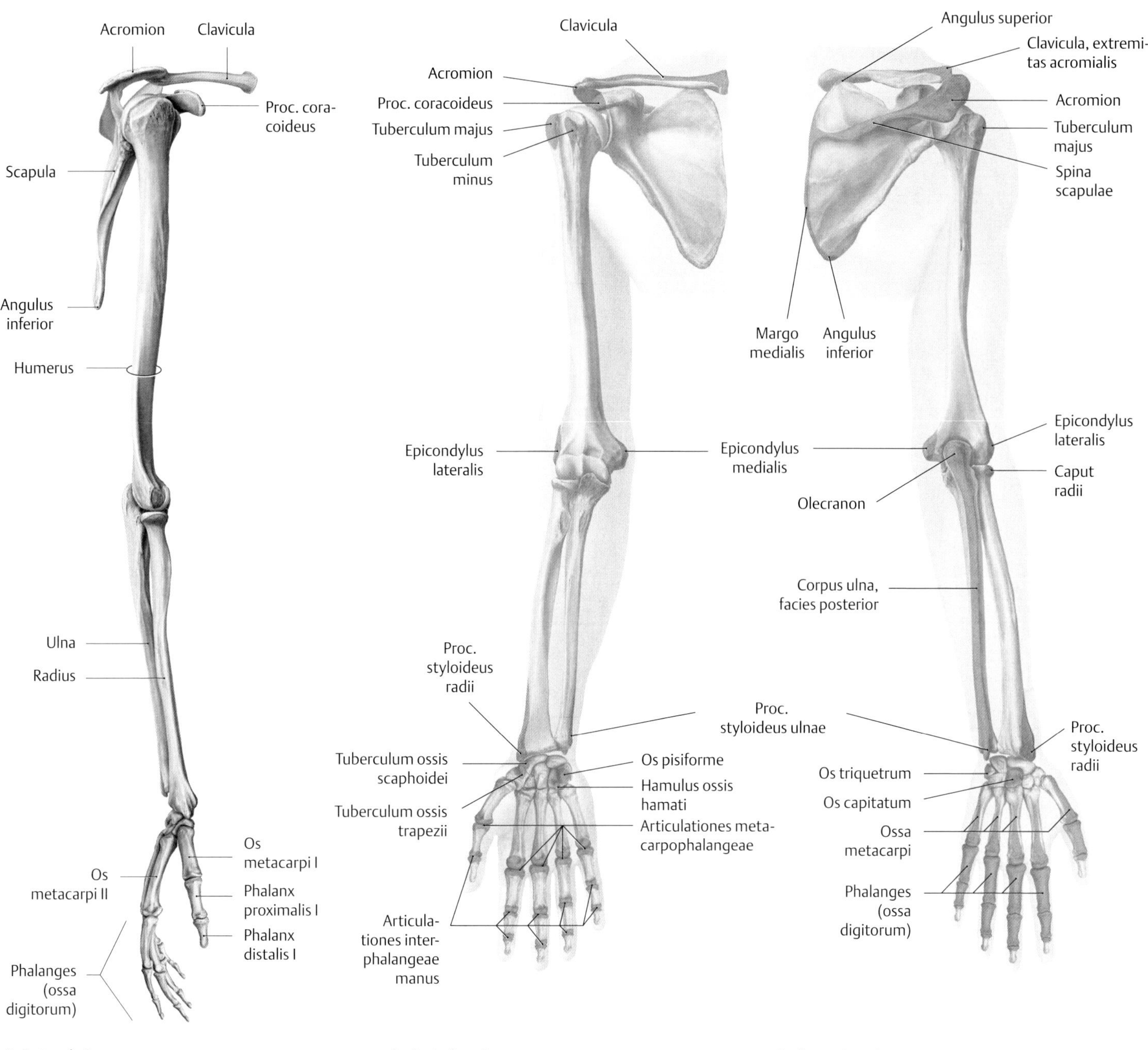

Acromion
Clavicula
Proc. coracoideus
Scapula
Angulus inferior
Humerus
Ulna
Radius
Os metacarpi I
Os metacarpi II
Phalanx proximalis I
Phalanx distalis I
Phalanges (ossa digitorum)
Clavicula
Acromion
Proc. coracoideus
Tuberculum majus
Tuberculum minus
Epicondylus lateralis
Epicondylus medialis
Proc. styloideus radii
Proc. styloideus ulnae
Tuberculum ossis scaphoidei
Tuberculum ossis trapezii
Os pisiforme
Hamulus ossis hamati
Articulationes metacarpophalangeae
Articulationes interphalangeae manus
Angulus superior
Clavicula, extremitas acromialis
Acromion
Tuberculum majus
Spina scapulae
Margo medialis
Angulus inferior
Epicondylus lateralis
Caput radii
Olecranon
Corpus ulna, facies posterior
Proc. styloideus radii
Os triquetrum
Os capitatum
Ossa metacarpi
Phalanges (ossa digitorum)

C Lateral view.

A Anterior view.

B Posterior view.

Clavicula & Scapula

The shoulder girdle (clavicula and scapula) connects the bones of the upper limb to the thoracic cage. Whereas the pelvic girdle (paired hip bones) is firmly integrated into the axial skeleton (see p. 358), the shoulder girdle is extremely mobile.

Fig. 19.3 Clavicula

Right clavicula. The S-shaped clavicle is visible and palpable along its entire length (generally 12 to 15 cm). Its medial end articulates with sternum at articulatio sternoclavicularis (see p. 258). Its lateral end articulates with scapula at articulatio acromioclavicularis (see p. 259).

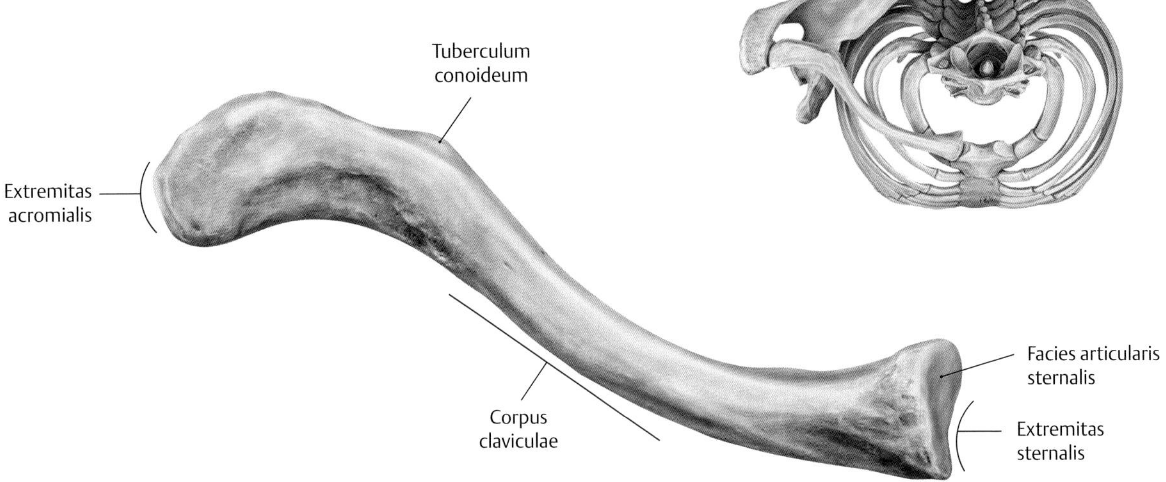
Tuberculum conoideum
Extremitas acromialis
Facies articularis sternalis
Corpus claviculae
Extremitas sternalis

A Superior view.

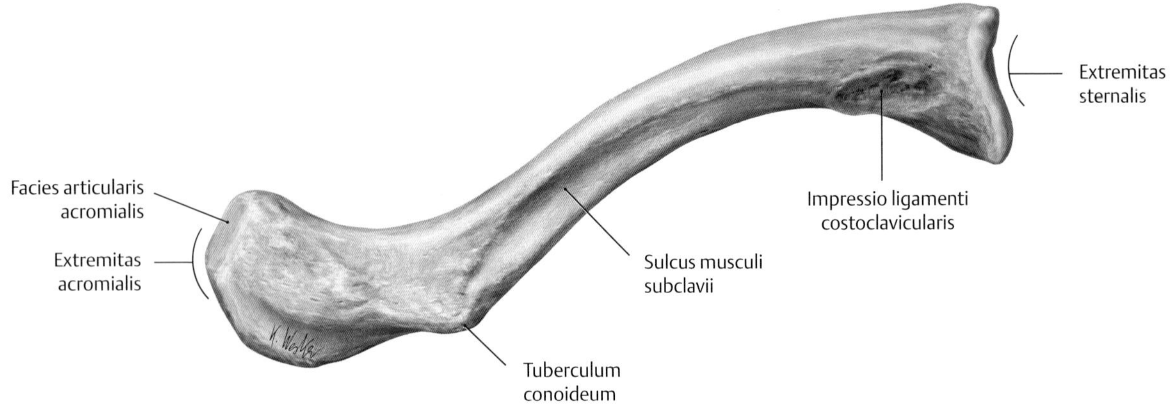
Extremitas sternalis
Facies articularis acromialis
Extremitas acromialis
Impressio ligamenti costoclavicularis
Sulcus musculi subclavii
Tuberculum conoideum

B Inferior view.

Clinical

Foramen scapulae

Lig. transversum scapulae superius (see p. 259) may become ossified, transforming incisura scapulae into an anomalous bony canal, foramen scapulae. This can lead to compression of n. suprascapularis as it passes through the canal (see p. 333).

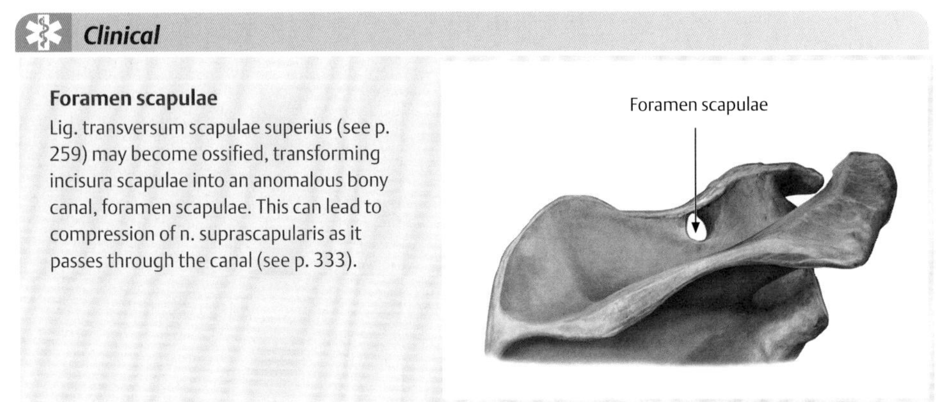
Foramen scapulae

Fig. 19.4 Scapula

Right scapula. In its normal anatomical position, the scapula extends from costa II to costa VII.

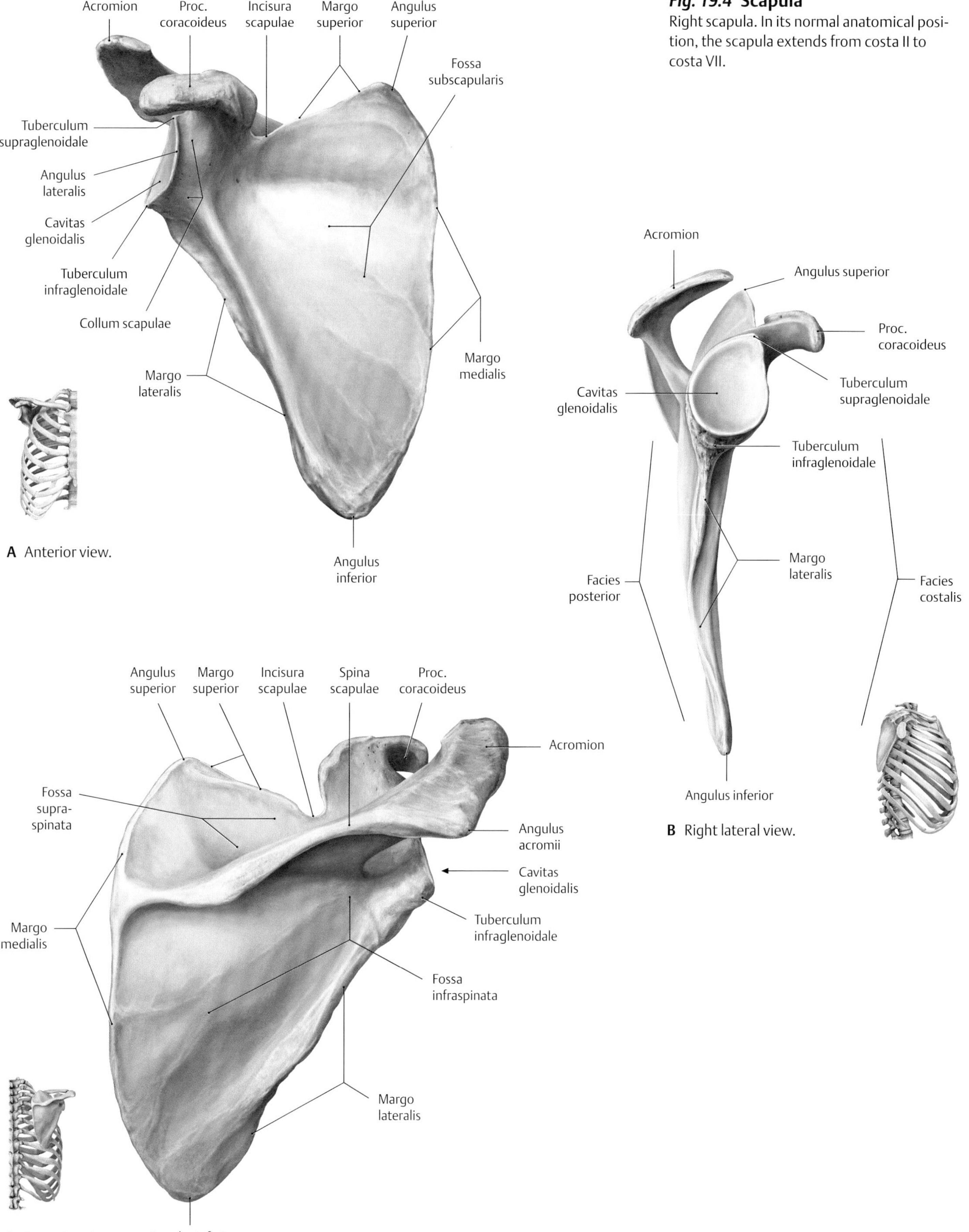

Acromion
Proc. coracoideus
Incisura scapulae
Margo superior
Angulus superior
Fossa subscapularis
Tuberculum supraglenoidale
Angulus lateralis
Cavitas glenoidalis
Tuberculum infraglenoidale
Collum scapulae
Margo lateralis
Margo medialis
Angulus inferior
Acromion
Angulus superior
Proc. coracoideus
Cavitas glenoidalis
Tuberculum supraglenoidale
Tuberculum infraglenoidale
Margo lateralis
Facies posterior
Facies costalis
Angulus inferior
Angulus superior
Margo superior
Incisura scapulae
Spina scapulae
Proc. coracoideus
Acromion
Fossa supra-spinata
Angulus acromii
Cavitas glenoidalis
Tuberculum infraglenoidale
Margo medialis
Fossa infraspinata
Margo lateralis
Angulus inferior

A Anterior view.

B Right lateral view.

C Posterior view.

Humerus

Fig. 19.5 Humerus
Right humerus. The caput humeri articulates with scapula at articulatio humeri (see p. 258). The capitulum and trochlea humeri articulate with radius and ulna, respectively, at articulatio cubiti (see p. 282).

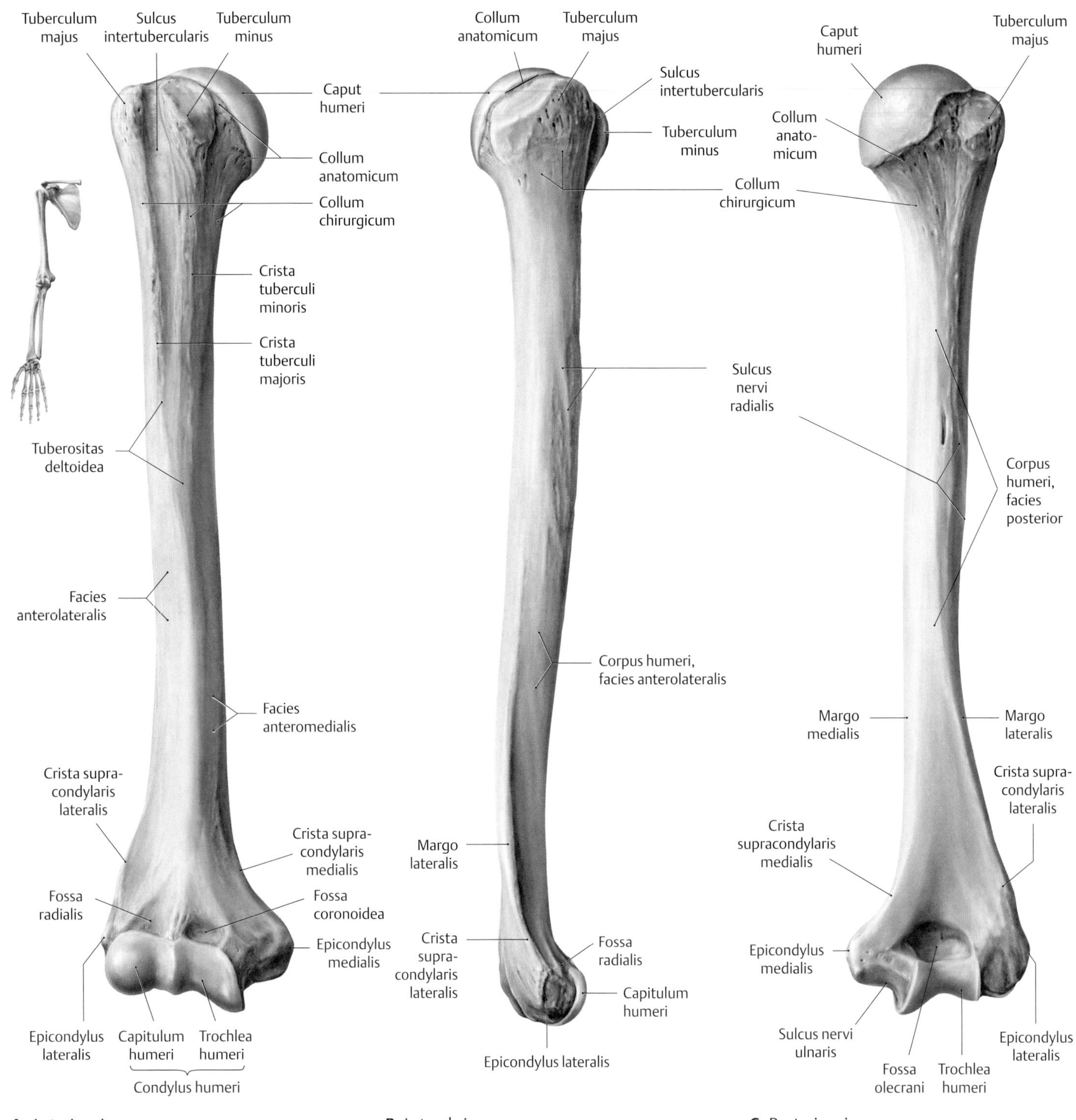
Tuberculum majus
Sulcus intertubercularis
Tuberculum minus
Caput humeri
Collum anatomicum
Collum chirurgicum
Crista tuberculi minoris
Crista tuberculi majoris
Tuberositas deltoidea
Facies anterolateralis
Facies anteromedialis
Crista supra-condylaris lateralis
Crista supra-condylaris medialis
Fossa radialis
Fossa coronoidea
Epicondylus medialis
Epicondylus lateralis
Capitulum humeri
Trochlea humeri
Condylus humeri
Collum anatomicum
Tuberculum majus
Sulcus intertubercularis
Tuberculum minus
Collum chirurgicum
Sulcus nervi radialis
Corpus humeri, facies anterolateralis
Margo lateralis
Crista supra-condylaris lateralis
Fossa radialis
Capitulum humeri
Epicondylus lateralis
Caput humeri
Tuberculum majus
Collum anato-micum
Corpus humeri, facies posterior
Margo medialis
Margo lateralis
Crista supra-condylaris lateralis
Crista supracondylaris medialis
Epicondylus medialis
Sulcus nervi ulnaris
Fossa olecrani
Trochlea humeri
Epicondylus lateralis

A Anterior view.

B Lateral view.

C Posterior view.

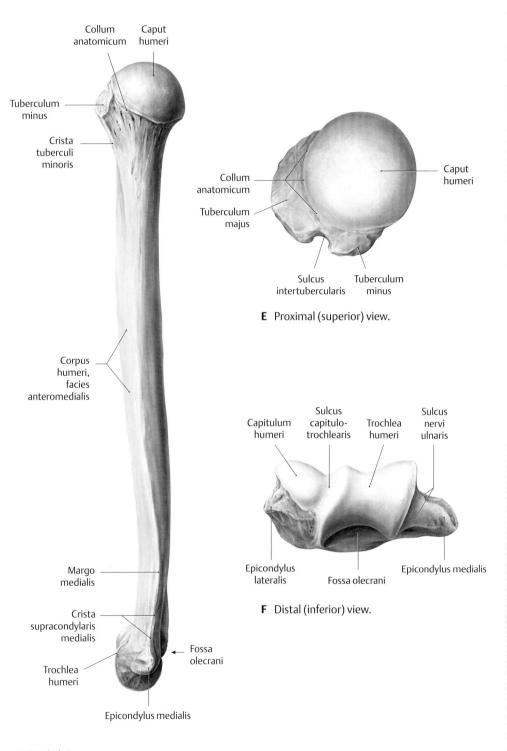

Collum anatomicum
Caput humeri
Tuberculum minus
Crista tuberculi minoris
Corpus humeri, facies anteromedialis
Margo medialis
Crista supracondylaris medialis
Fossa olecrani
Trochlea humeri
Epicondylus medialis

D Medial view.

Collum anatomicum
Tuberculum majus
Caput humeri
Sulcus intertubercularis
Tuberculum minus

E Proximal (superior) view.

Capitulum humeri
Sulcus capitulo-trochlearis
Trochlea humeri
Sulcus nervi ulnaris
Epicondylus lateralis
Fossa olecrani
Epicondylus medialis

F Distal (inferior) view.

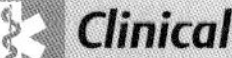

Clinical

Fractures of the humerus

Anterior view. Fractures of the proximal humerus are very common and occur predominantly in older patients who sustain a fall onto the outstretched arm or directly onto the shoulder. Three main types are distinguished.

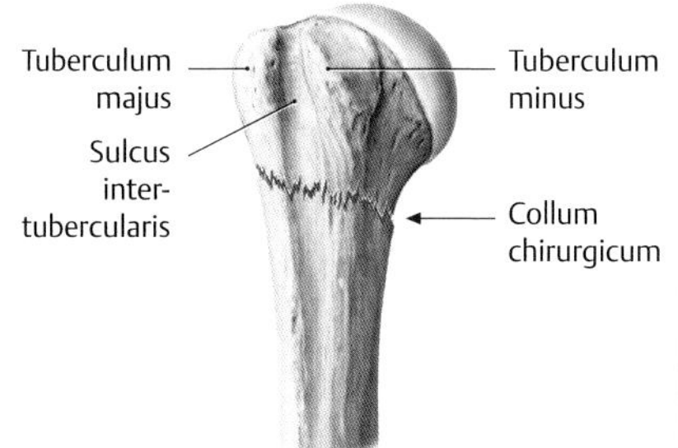
Tuberculum majus
Sulcus inter-tubercularis
Tuberculum minus
Collum chirurgicum

A Extra-articular fracture.

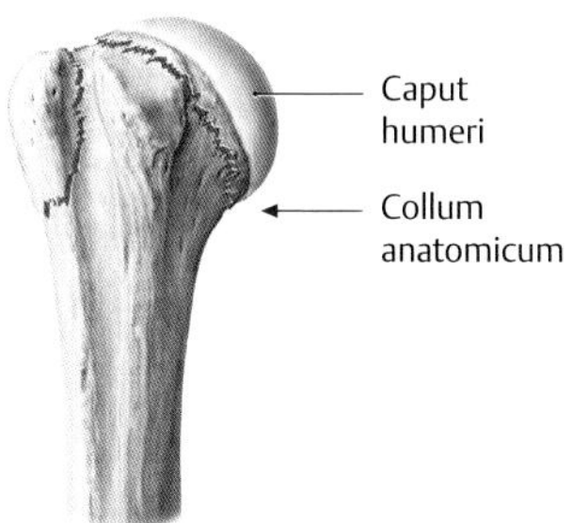
Caput humeri
Collum anatomicum

B Intra-articular fracture.

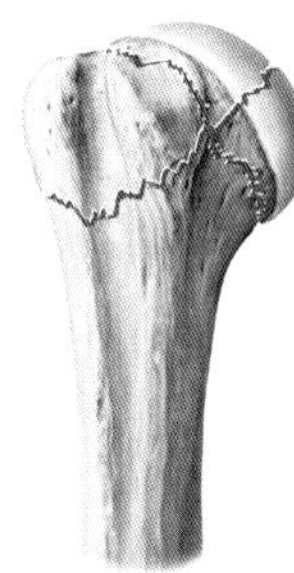

C Comminuted fracture.

Extra-articular fractures and intra-articular fractures are often accompanied by injuries of the blood vessels that supply the humeral head (aa. circumflexa humeri anterior and posterior), with an associated risk of post-traumatic avascular necrosis.

Fractures of the humeral shaft and distal humerus are frequently associated with damage to the radial nerve.

Joints of the Shoulder

Fig. 19.6 **Joints of the shoulder: Overview**
Right shoulder, anterior view.

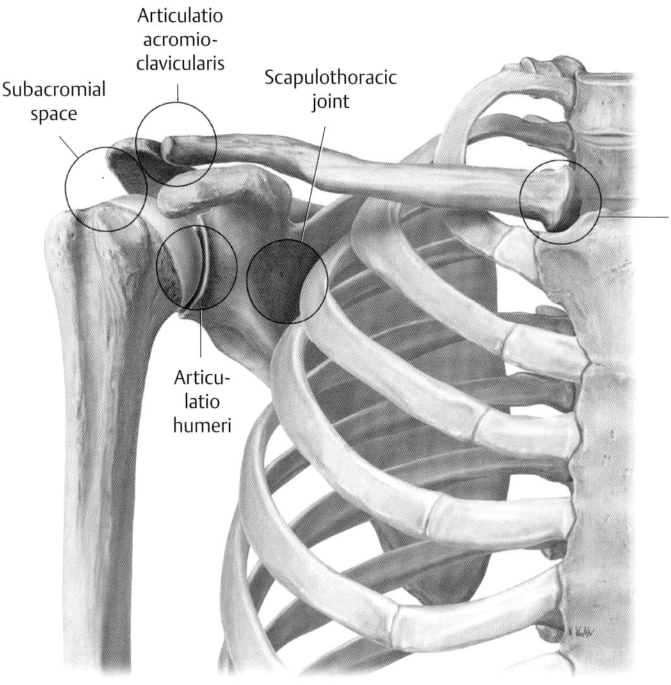
Articulatio
acromio-
clavicularis
Subacromial
space
Scapulothoracic
joint
Articulatio
sternocla-
vicularis
Articu-
latio
humeri

Fig. 19.7 **Joints of the shoulder girdle**
Right side, superior view.

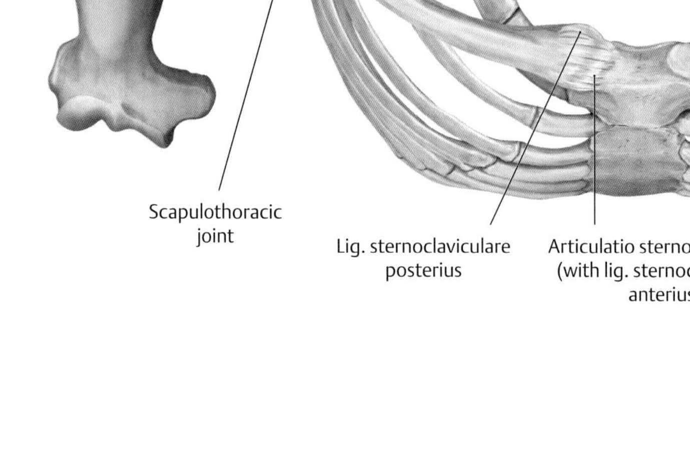
Articulatio
acromioclavicularis (with
lig. acromioclaviculare)
Lig. coraco-
acromiale
Articulatio
humeri
Scapulothoracic
joint
Lig. sternoclaviculare
posterius
Articulatio sternoclavicularis
(with lig. sternoclaviculare
anterius)

Fig. 19.8 **Scapulothoracic joint**
Right side, superior view. In all movements of the shoulder girdle, scapula glides on a curved surface of loose connective tissue between m. serratus anterior and m. subscapularis. This surface can be considered a scapulothoracic joint.

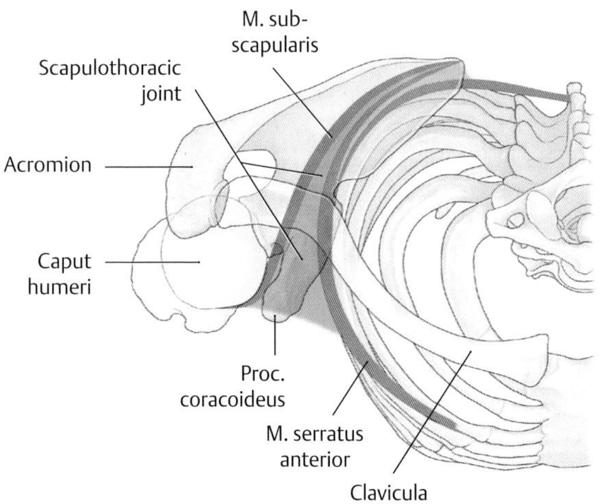
M. sub-
scapularis
Scapulothoracic
joint
Acromion
Caput
humeri
Proc.
coracoideus
M. serratus
anterior
Clavicula

Fig. 19.9 Articulatio sterno-clavicularis
Anterior view with sternum coronally sectioned (left). *Note:* A fibrocartilaginous discus articularis compensates for the mismatch of surfaces between the two saddle-shaped articular facets of clavicula and manubrium sterni.

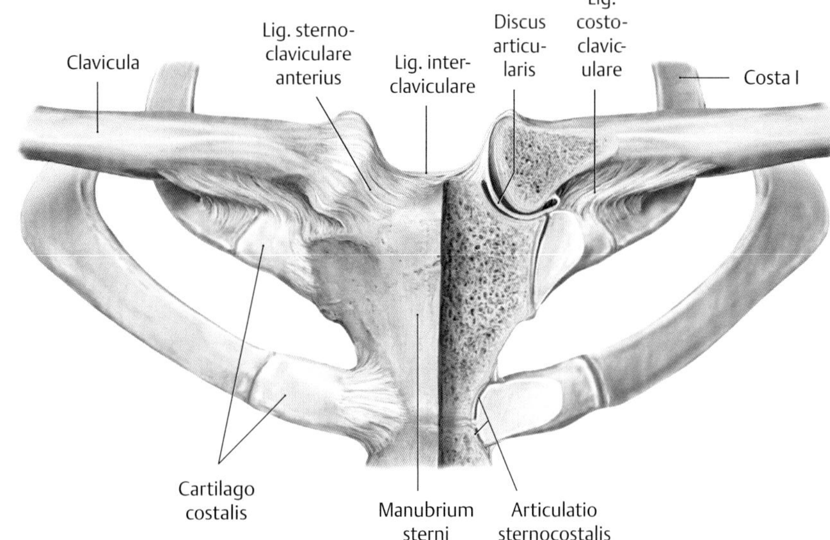
Clavicula
Lig. sterno-claviculare anterius
Lig. inter-claviculare
Discus articu-laris
Lig. costo-clavic-ulare
Costa I
Cartilago costalis
Manubrium sterni
Articulatio sternocostalis

Fig. 19.10 Articulatio acromio-clavicularis
Anterior view. Articulatio acromioclavicularis is a plane joint. Because the articulating surfaces are flat, they must be held in place by strong ligaments, greatly limiting the mobility of the joint.

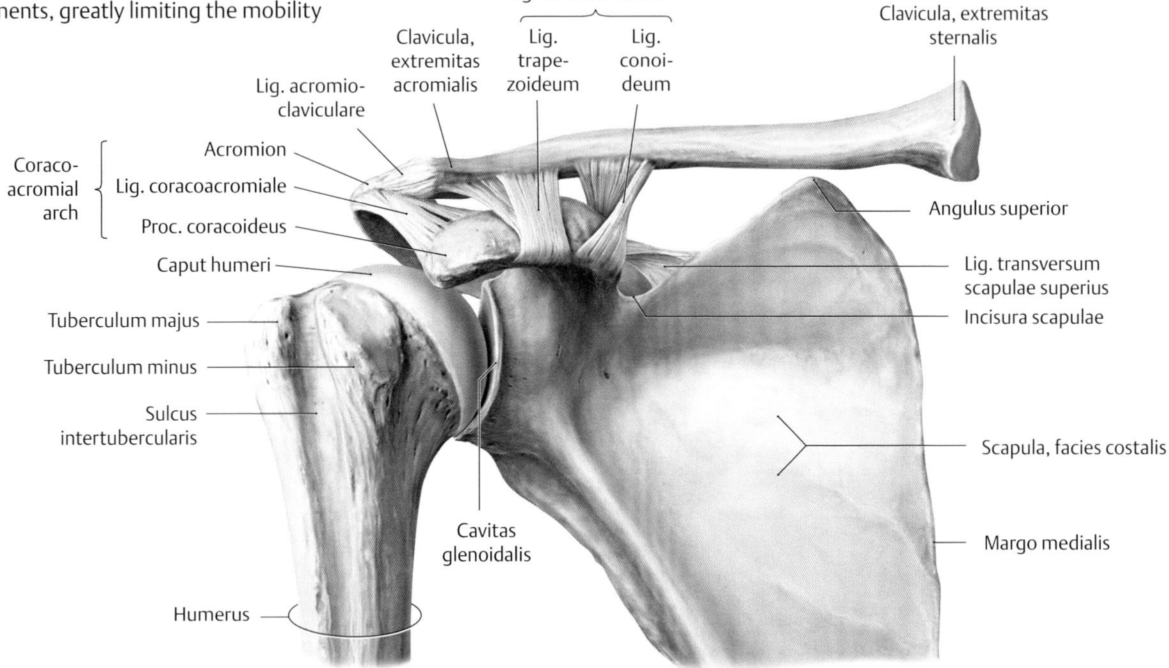
Lig. coracoclaviculare
Clavicula, extremitas sternalis
Clavicula, extremitas acromialis
Lig. trape-zoideum
Lig. conoi-deum
Lig. acromio-claviculare
Coraco-acromial arch
Acromion
Lig. coracoacromiale
Proc. coracoideus
Caput humeri
Angulus superior
Lig. transversum scapulae superius
Incisura scapulae
Tuberculum majus
Tuberculum minus
Sulcus intertubercularis
Scapula, facies costalis
Cavitas glenoidalis
Margo medialis
Humerus

Clinical

Injuries of articulatio acromioclavicularis

A fall onto the outstretched arm or shoulder frequently causes dislocation of articulatio acromioclavicularis and damage to Ligg. coracoclaviculare and acromioclaviculare.

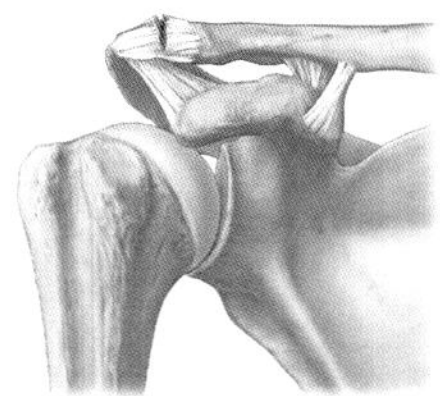

A Stretching of ligaments.

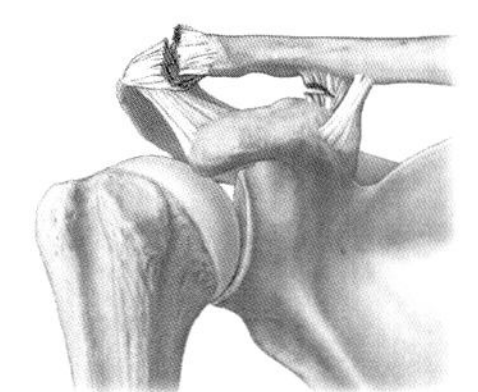

B Rupture of Lig. acromioclaviculare.

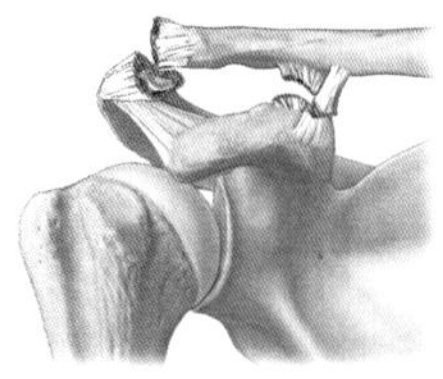

C Complete dislocation of articulatio acromioclavicularis.

Joints of the Shoulder: Articulatio Humeri

Fig. 19.11 **Articulatio humeri: Bony elements**
Right shoulder.

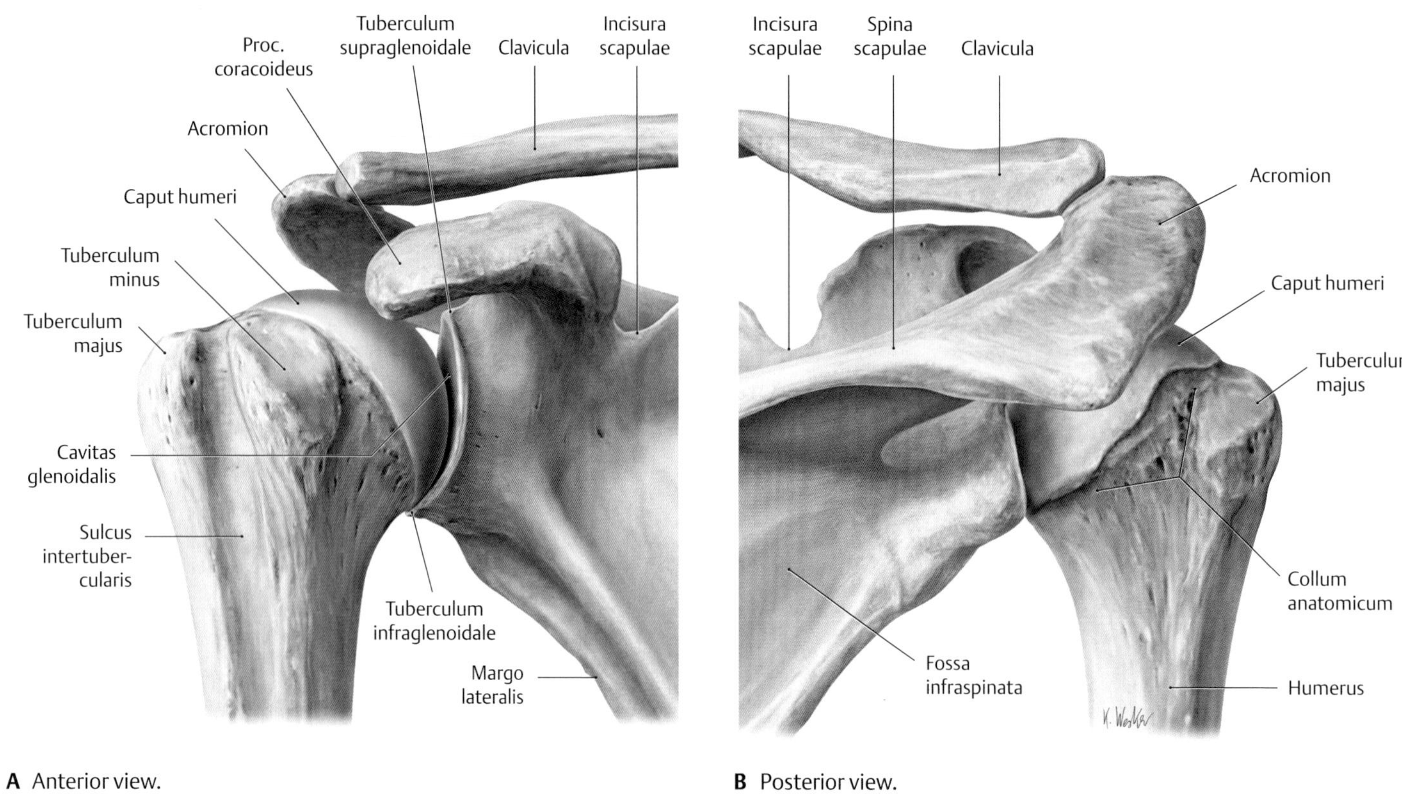
Tuberculum supraglenoidale
Proc. coracoideus
Clavicula
Incisura scapulae
Acromion
Caput humeri
Tuberculum minus
Tuberculum majus
Cavitas glenoidalis
Sulcus intertuber-cularis
Tuberculum infraglenoidale
Margo lateralis
Incisura scapulae
Spina scapulae
Clavicula
Acromion
Caput humeri
Tuberculum majus
Collum anatomicum
Fossa infraspinata
Humerus

A Anterior view.

B Posterior view.

Fig. 19.12 **Radiograph of the shoulder**
Anteroposterior view.

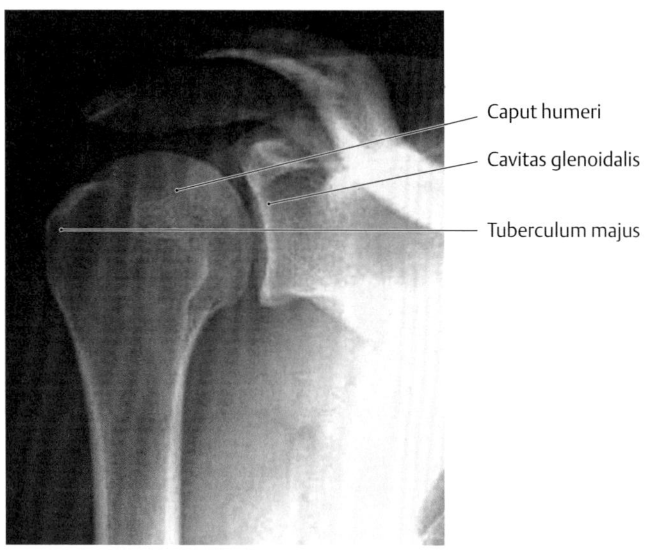
Caput humeri
Cavitas glenoidalis
Tuberculum majus

Fig. 19.13 Articulatio humeri: Capsule and ligaments

Right shoulder.

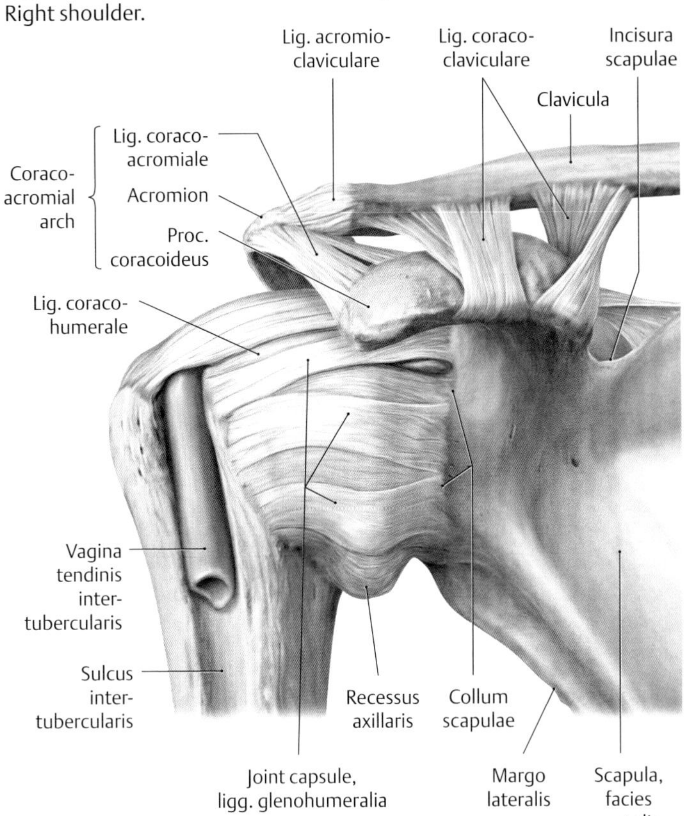
Lig. acromio-
claviculare
Lig. coraco-
claviculare
Incisura
scapulae
Clavicula
Coraco-
acromial
arch
Lig. coraco-
acromiale
Acromion
Proc.
coracoideus
Lig. coraco-
humerale
Vagina
tendinis
inter-
tubercularis
Sulcus
inter-
tubercularis
Recessus
axillaris
Collum
scapulae
Joint capsule,
ligg. glenohumeralia
Margo
lateralis
Scapula,
facies
costalis

A Anterior view.

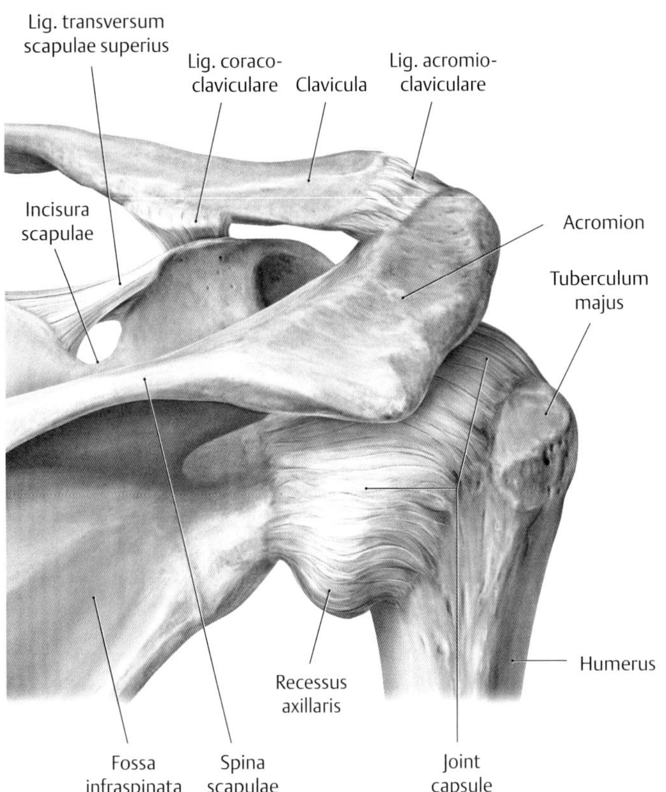
Lig. transversum
scapulae superius
Lig. coraco-
claviculare
Clavicula
Lig. acromio-
claviculare
Incisura
scapulae
Acromion
Tuberculum
majus
Humerus
Recessus
axillaris
Fossa
infraspinata
Spina
scapulae
Joint
capsule

B Posterior view.

Fig. 19.14 Articulatio humeri: Joint cavity

Anterior view.

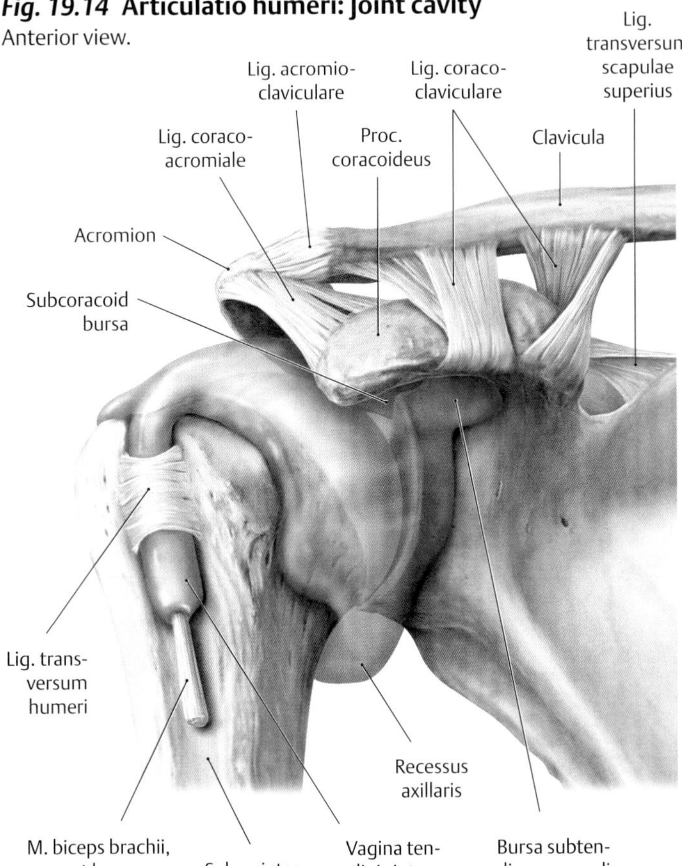
Lig.
transversum
scapulae
superius
Lig. acromio-
claviculare
Lig. coraco-
claviculare
Lig. coraco-
acromiale
Proc.
coracoideus
Clavicula
Acromion
Subcoracoid
bursa
Lig. trans-
versum
humeri
Recessus
axillaris
M. biceps brachii,
caput longum
tendon
Sulcus inter-
tubercularis
Vagina ten-
dinis inter-
tubercularis
Bursa subten-
dinea musculi
subscapularis

Fig. 19.15 MRI of the shoulder

Coronal section, anterior view.

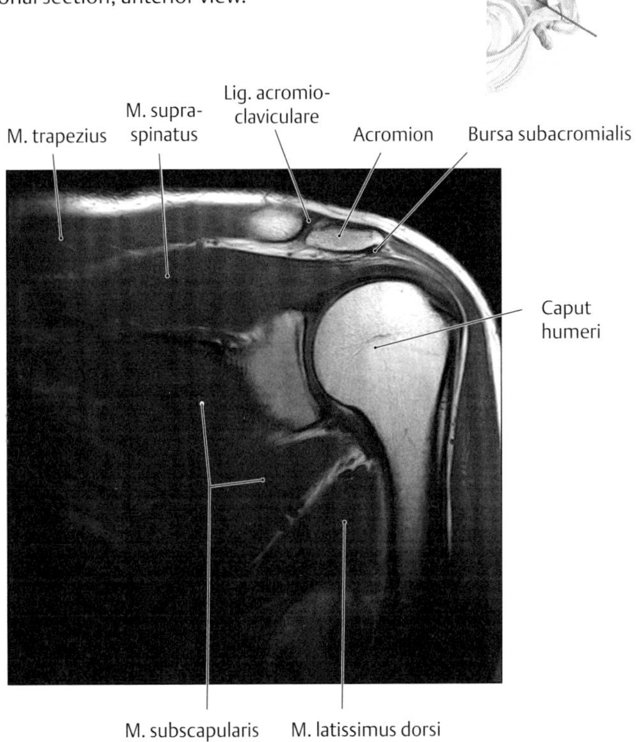
M. trapezius
M. supra-
spinatus
Lig. acromio-
claviculare
Acromion
Bursa subacromialis
Caput
humeri
M. subscapularis
M. latissimus dorsi

Subacromial Space & Bursae

Fig. 19.16 Subacromial space

Right shoulder.

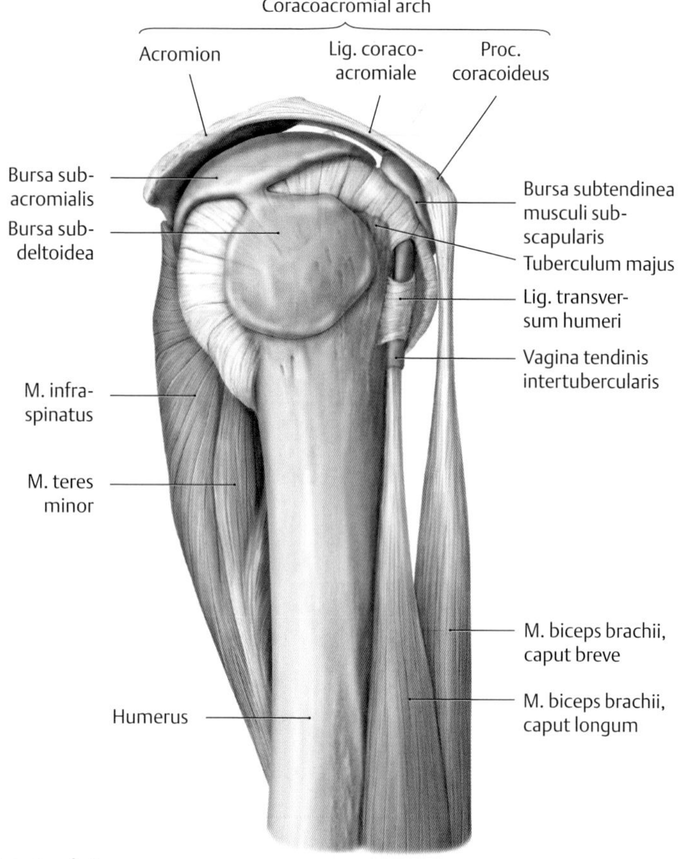

Coracoacromial arch
Acromion
Lig. coraco-acromiale
Proc. coracoideus
Bursa sub-acromialis
Bursa sub-deltoidea
Bursa subtendinea musculi sub-scapularis
Tuberculum majus
Lig. transver-sum humeri
Vagina tendinis intertubercularis
M. infra-spinatus
M. teres minor
M. biceps brachii, caput breve
M. biceps brachii, caput longum
Humerus

A Lateral view.

Fig. 19.17 Bursa subacromialis and cavitas glenoidalis

Right shoulder, lateral view of sagittal section with humerus removed.

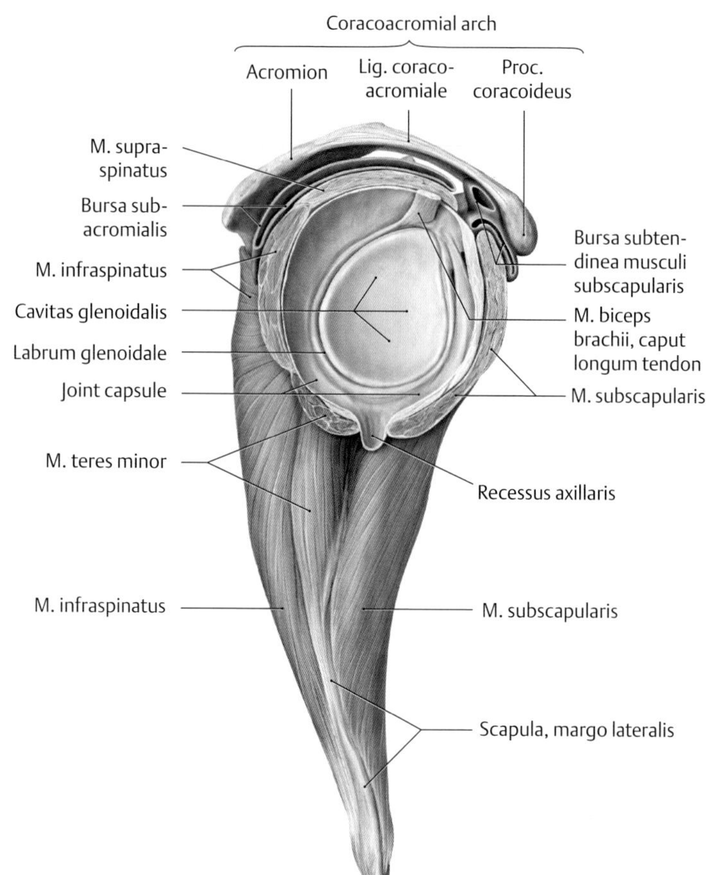

Coracoacromial arch
Acromion
Lig. coraco-acromiale
Proc. coracoideus
M. supra-spinatus
Bursa sub-acromialis
M. infraspinatus
Cavitas glenoidalis
Labrum glenoidale
Joint capsule
M. teres minor
Bursa subten-dinea musculi subscapularis
M. biceps brachii, caput longum tendon
M. subscapularis
Recessus axillaris
M. infraspinatus
M. subscapularis
Scapula, margo lateralis

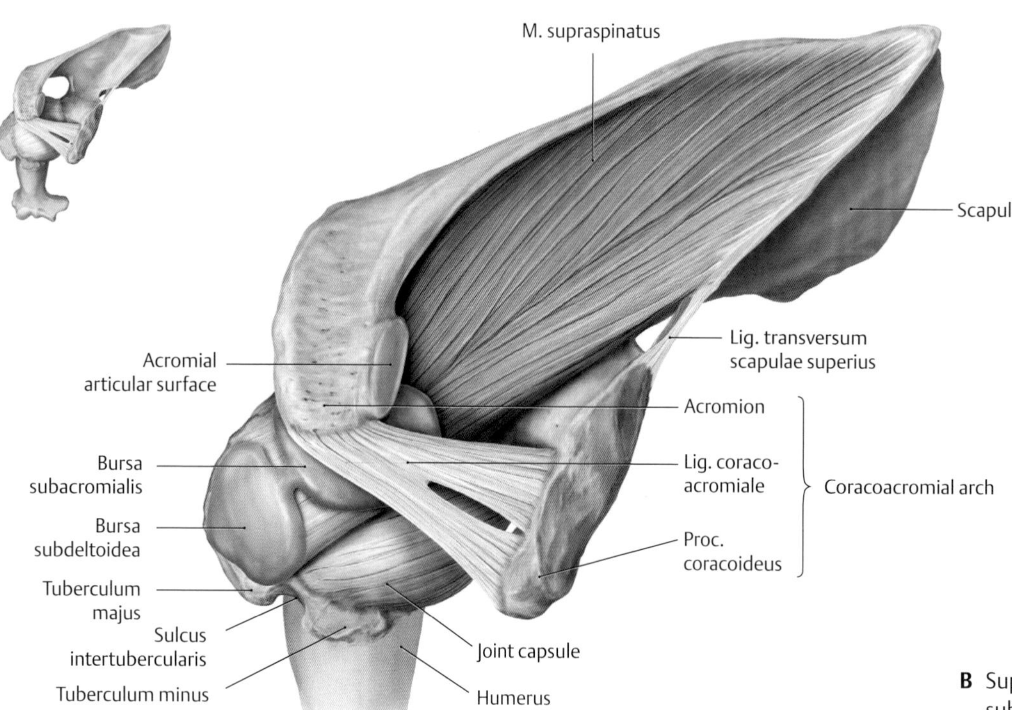

M. supraspinatus
Scapula
Lig. transversum scapulae superius
Acromial articular surface
Acromion
Lig. coraco-acromiale
Coracoacromial arch
Proc. coracoideus
Bursa subacromialis
Bursa subdeltoidea
Tuberculum majus
Sulcus intertubercularis
Tuberculum minus
Joint capsule
Humerus

B Superior view. Note the position of bursa subacromialis between m. supraspinatus and the coracoacromial arch.

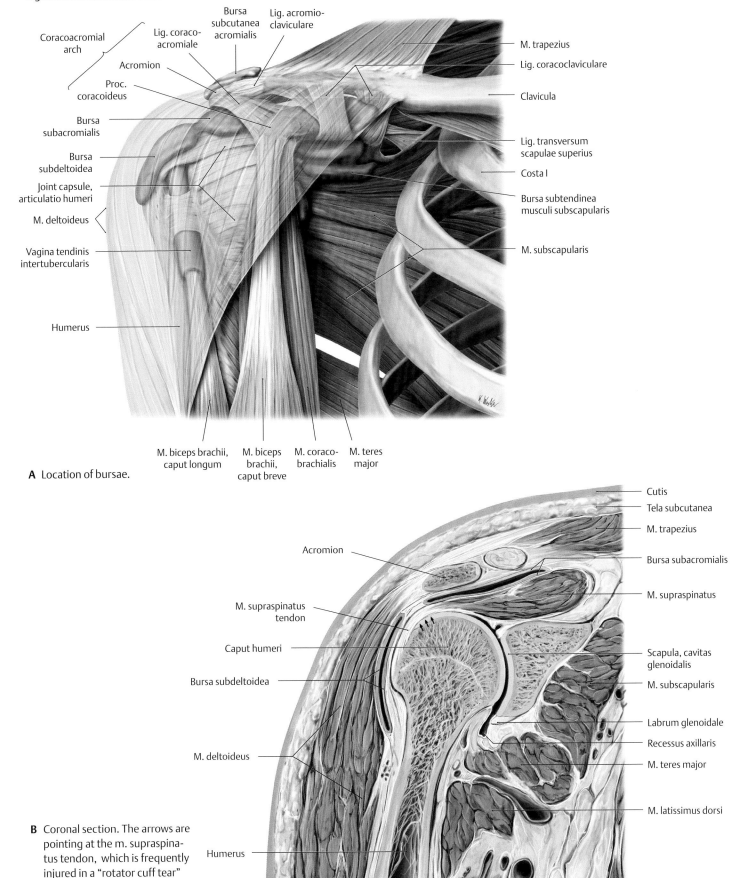

Fig. 19.18 **Bursae subacromialis and subdeltoidea**

Right shoulder, anterior view.

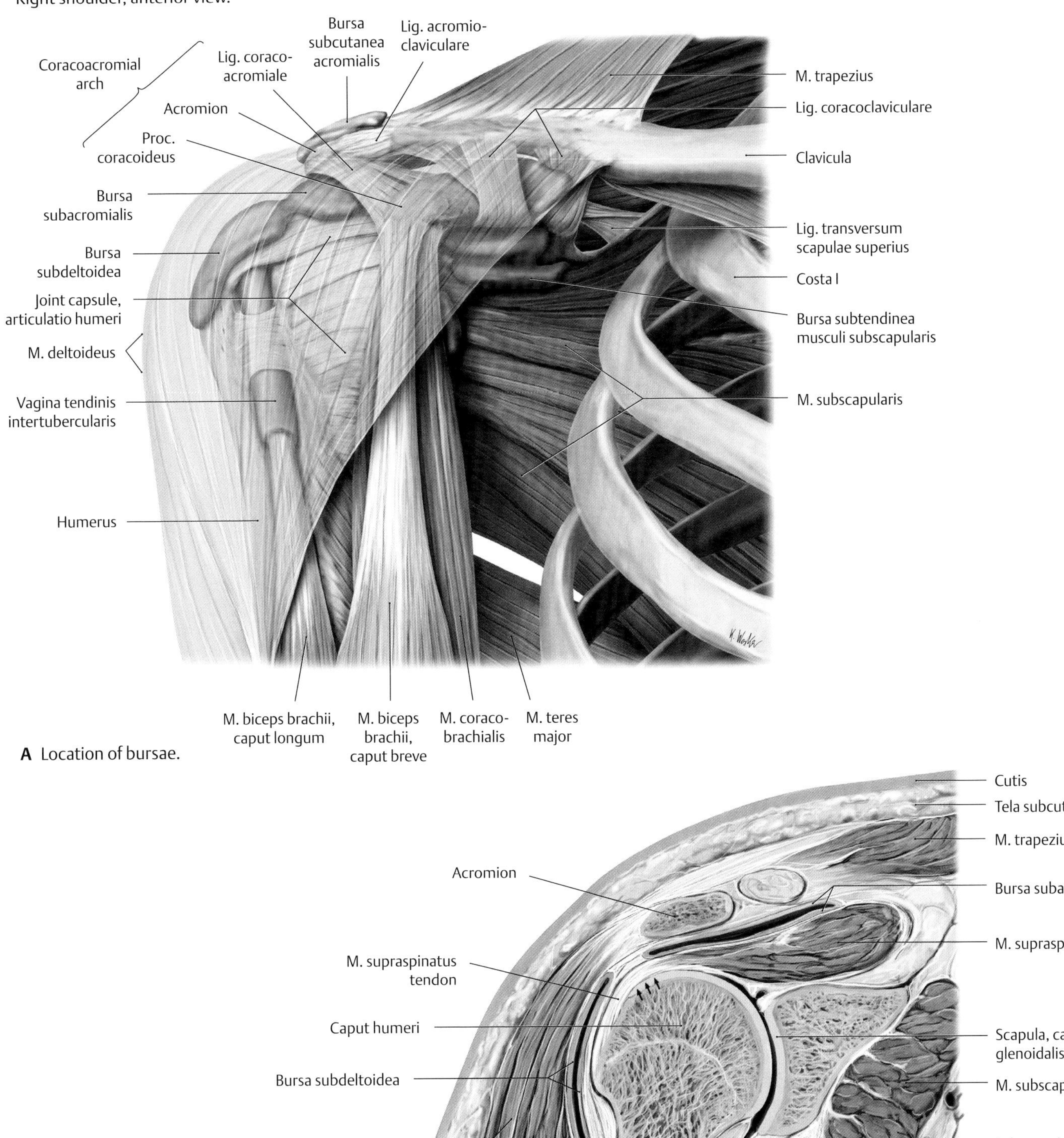
Coracoacromial arch
Lig. coraco-acromiale
Bursa subcutanea acromialis
Lig. acromio-claviculare
Acromion
Proc. coracoideus
Bursa subacromialis
Bursa subdeltoidea
Joint capsule, articulatio humeri
M. deltoideus
Vagina tendinis intertubercularis
Humerus
M. trapezius
Lig. coracoclaviculare
Clavicula
Lig. transversum scapulae superius
Costa I
Bursa subtendinea musculi subscapularis
M. subscapularis
M. biceps brachii, caput longum
M. biceps brachii, caput breve
M. coraco-brachialis
M. teres major

A Location of bursae.

Cutis
Tela subcutanea
M. trapezius
Acromion
Bursa subacromialis
M. supraspinatus
M. supraspinatus tendon
Caput humeri
Scapula, cavitas glenoidalis
Bursa subdeltoidea
M. subscapularis
Labrum glenoidale
Recessus axillaris
M. deltoideus
M. teres major
M. latissimus dorsi
Humerus

B Coronal section. The arrows are pointing at the m. supraspinatus tendon, which is frequently injured in a “rotator cuff tear” (for rotator cuff, see p. 273).

Anterior Muscles of the Shoulder & Arm (I)

Fig. 19.19 **Anterior muscles**
Right side, anterior view. Muscle origins (O) are shown in red, insertions (I) in blue.

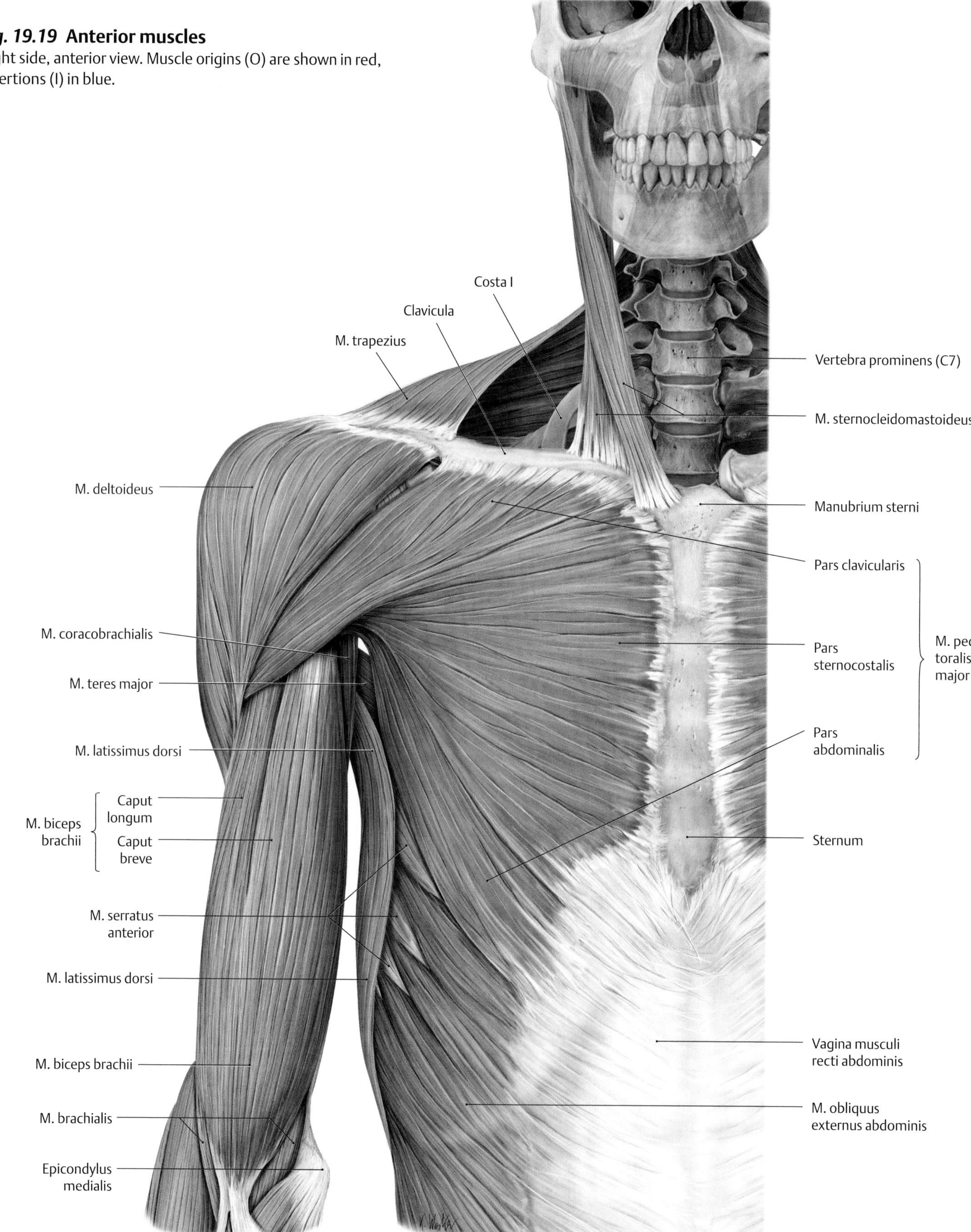
Costa I
Clavicula
M. trapezius
Vertebra prominens (C7)
M. sternocleidomastoideus
M. deltoideus
Manubrium sterni
Pars clavicularis
M. coracobrachialis
Pars sternocostalis
M. pectoralis major
M. teres major
Pars abdominalis
M. latissimus dorsi
M. biceps brachii
Caput longum
Caput breve
Sternum
M. serratus anterior
M. latissimus dorsi
Vagina musculi recti abdominis
M. biceps brachii
M. brachialis
M. obliquus externus abdominis
Epicondylus medialis

A Superficial dissection.

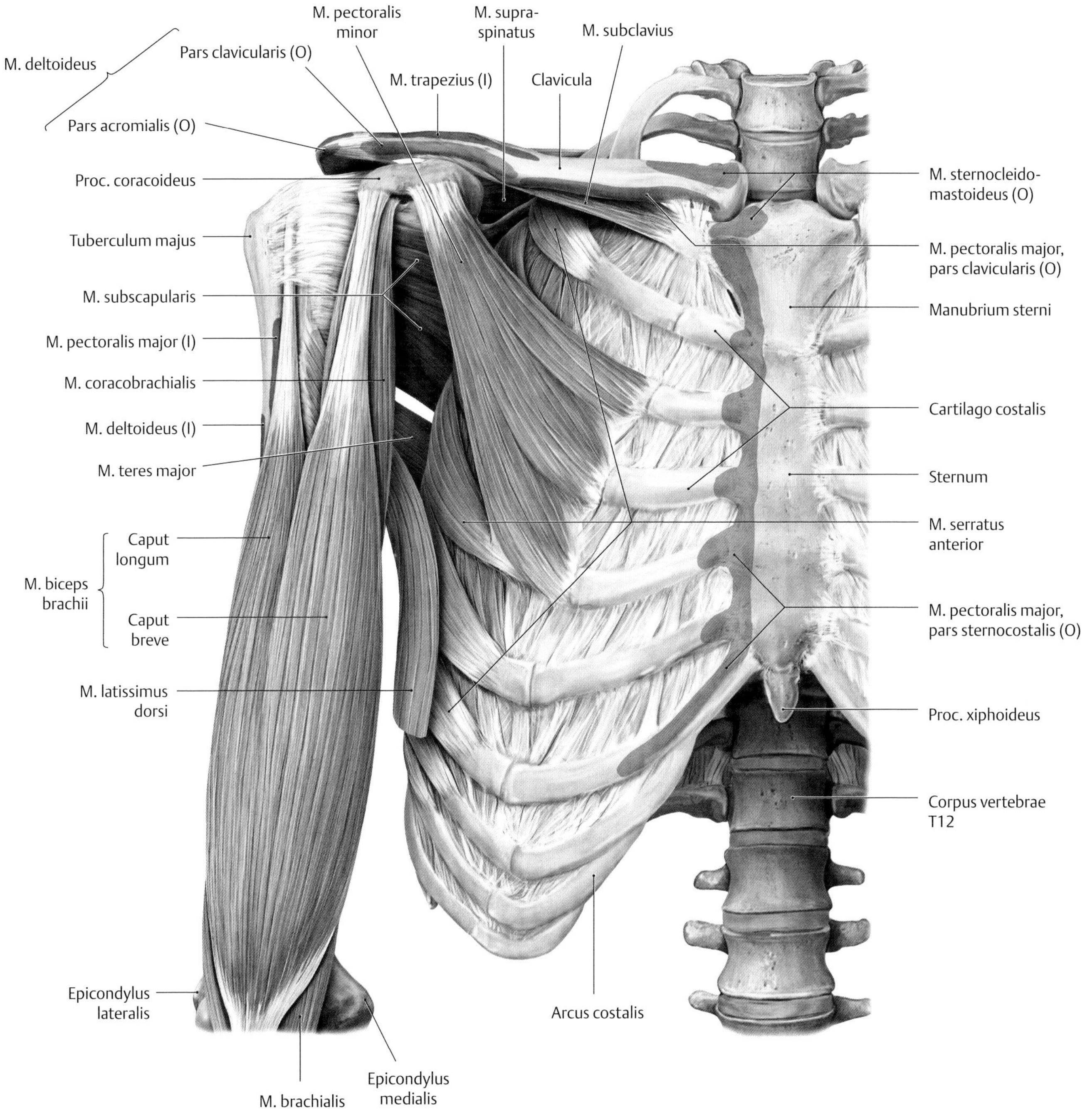
M. deltoideus
Pars clavicularis (O)
Pars acromialis (O)
M. pectoralis minor
M. supra-spinatus
M. subclavius
M. trapezius (I)
Clavicula
Proc. coracoideus
Tuberculum majus
M. subscapularis
M. pectoralis major (I)
M. coracobrachialis
M. deltoideus (I)
M. teres major
M. biceps brachii
Caput longum
Caput breve
M. latissimus dorsi
Epicondylus lateralis
M. brachialis
Epicondylus medialis
Arcus costalis
M. sternocleido-mastoideus (O)
M. pectoralis major, pars clavicularis (O)
Manubrium sterni
Cartilago costalis
Sternum
M. serratus anterior
M. pectoralis major, pars sternocostalis (O)
Proc. xiphoideus
Corpus vertebrae T12

B Deep dissection. *Removed:* M. sternocleidomastoideus, m. trapezius, m. pectoralis major, m. deltoideus, and m. obliquus externus abdominis.

Anterior Muscles of the Shoulder & Arm (II)

***Fig. 19.20* Anterior dissection**
Right arm, anterior view. Muscle origins (O) are shown in red, insertions (I) in blue.

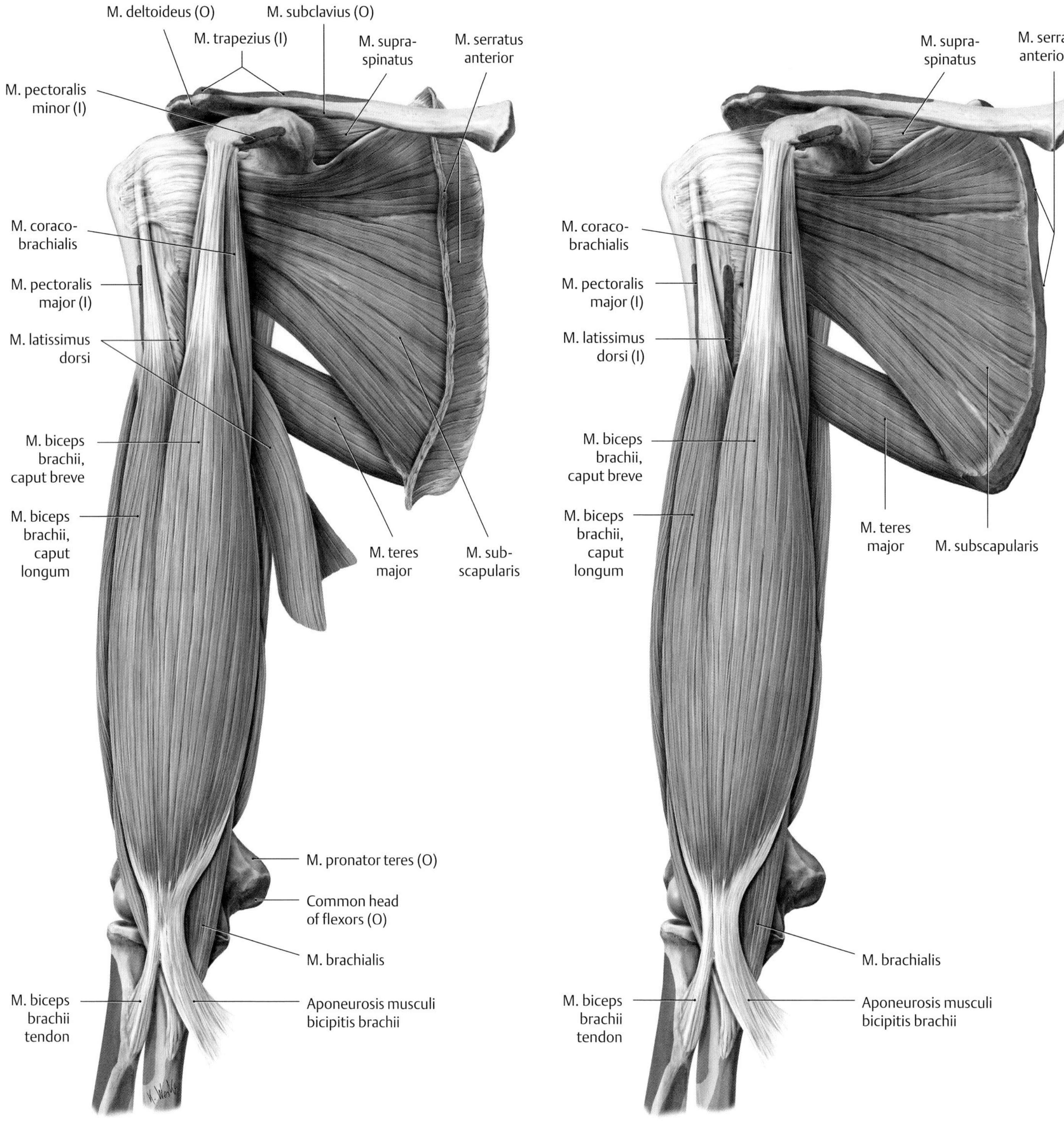
M. deltoideus (O)
M. subclavius (O)
M. trapezius (I)
M. supra-spinatus
M. serratus anterior
M. pectoralis minor (I)
M. coraco-brachialis
M. pectoralis major (I)
M. latissimus dorsi
M. biceps brachii, caput breve
M. biceps brachii, caput longum
M. teres major
M. sub-scapularis
M. pronator teres (O)
Common head of flexors (O)
M. brachialis
M. biceps brachii tendon
Aponeurosis musculi bicipitis brachii
M. supra-spinatus
M. serratus anterior (I)
M. coraco-brachialis
M. pectoralis major (I)
M. latissimus dorsi (I)
M. biceps brachii, caput breve
M. biceps brachii, caput longum
M. teres major
M. subscapularis
M. brachialis
M. biceps brachii tendon
Aponeurosis musculi bicipitis brachii

A *Removed:* Thoracic skeleton. *Partially removed:* M. latissimus dorsi and m. serratus anterior.

B *Removed:* M. latissimus dorsi and m. serratus anterior.

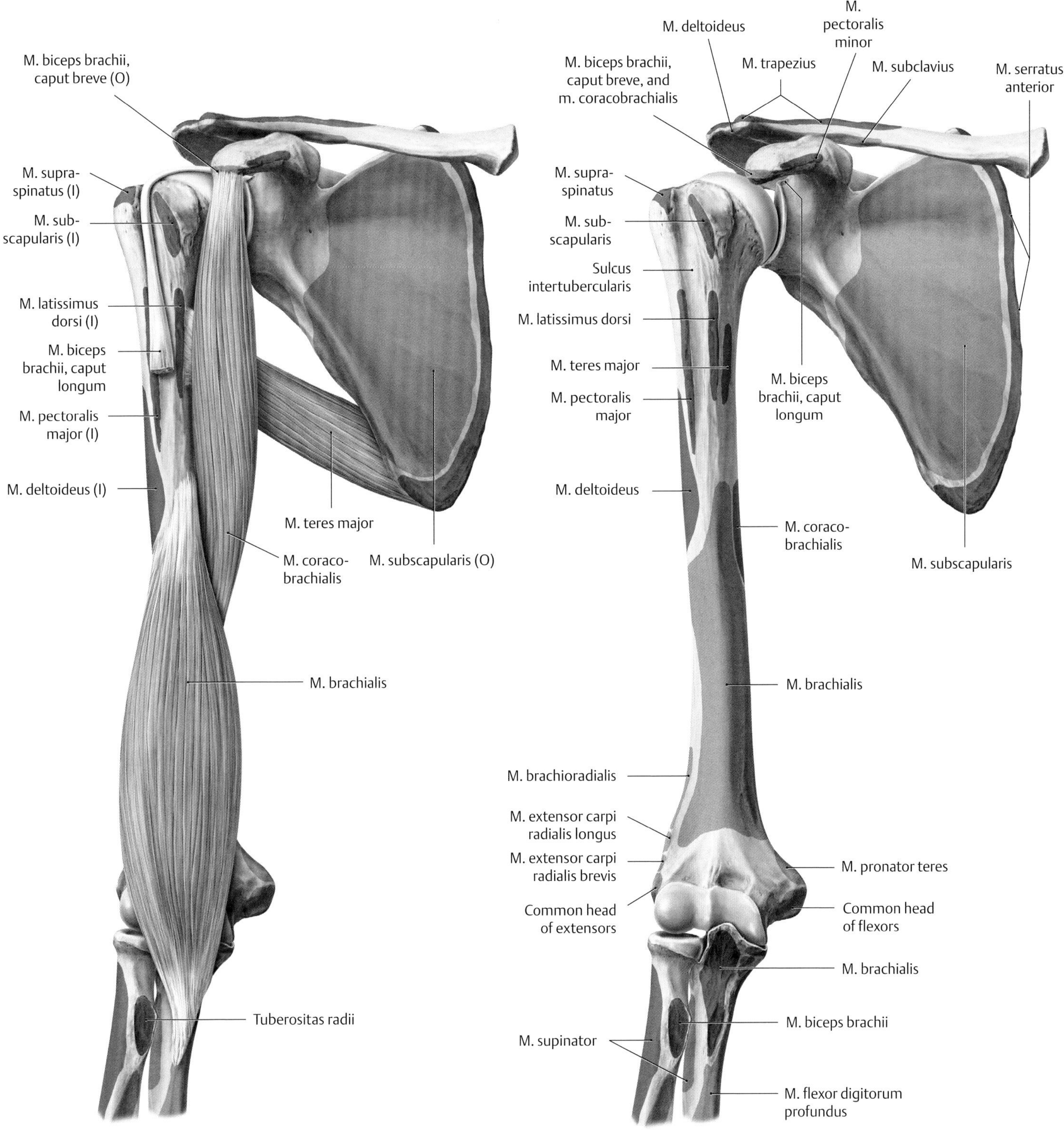
M. biceps brachii, caput breve (O)
M. supra-spinatus (I)
M. sub-scapularis (I)
M. latissimus dorsi (I)
M. biceps brachii, caput longum
M. pectoralis major (I)
M. deltoideus (I)
M. teres major
M. coraco-brachialis
M. subscapularis (O)
M. brachialis
Tuberositas radii
M. deltoideus
M. pectoralis minor
M. biceps brachii, caput breve, and m. coracobrachialis
M. trapezius
M. subclavius
M. serratus anterior
M. supra-spinatus
M. sub-scapularis
Sulcus intertubercularis
M. latissimus dorsi
M. teres major
M. pectoralis major
M. biceps brachii, caput longum
M. deltoideus
M. coraco-brachialis
M. subscapularis
M. brachialis
M. brachioradialis
M. extensor carpi radialis longus
M. extensor carpi radialis brevis
M. pronator teres
Common head of extensors
Common head of flexors
M. brachialis
M. biceps brachii
M. supinator
M. flexor digitorum profundus

C *Removed:* M. subscapularis and m. supraspinatus. *Partially removed:* M. biceps brachii.

D *Removed:* M. biceps brachii, m. coracobrachialis, and m. teres major.

Posterior Muscles of the Shoulder & Arm (I)

Fig. 19.21 **Posterior muscles**
Right side, posterior view.

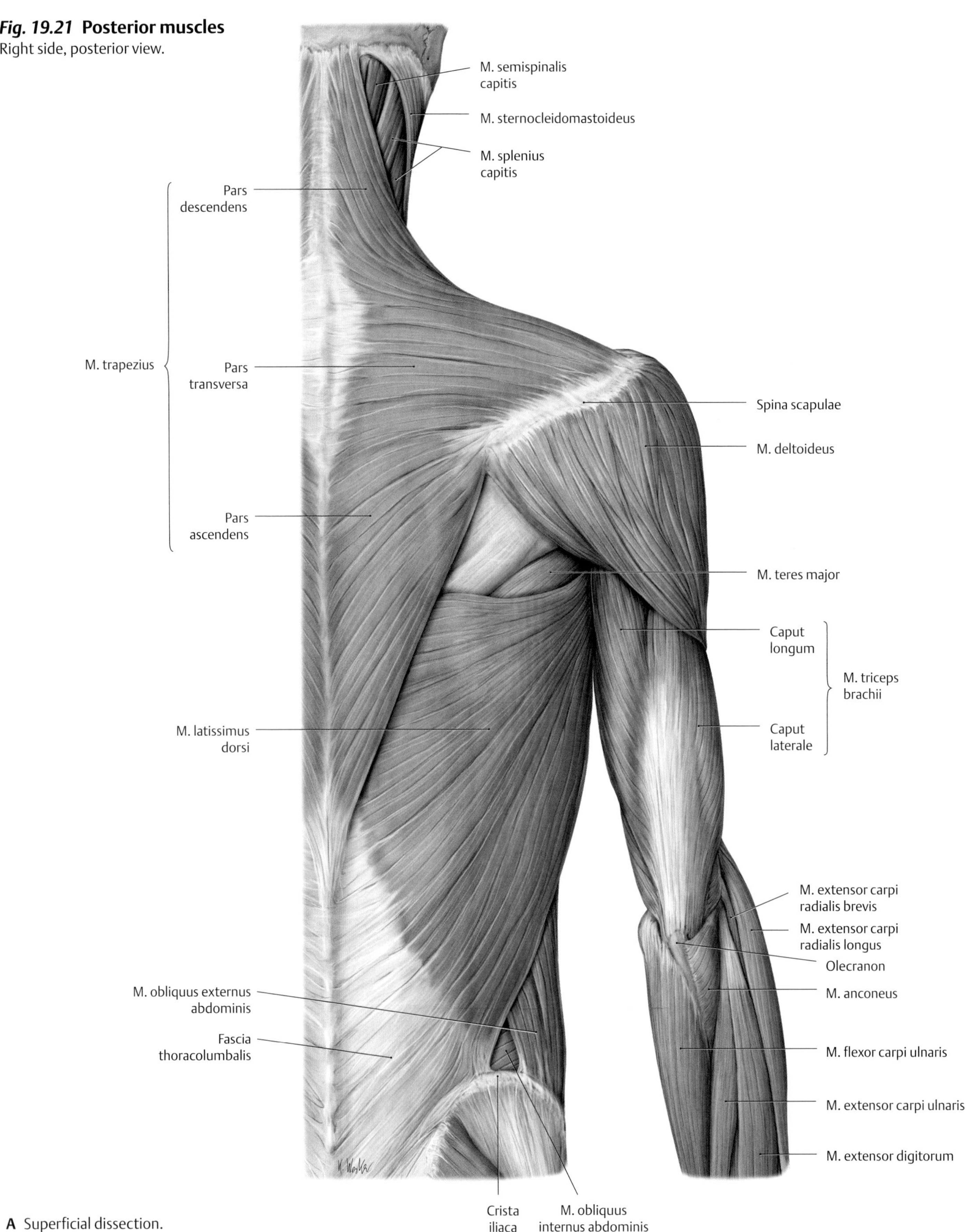
M. semispinalis capitis
M. sternocleidomastoideus
M. splenius capitis
M. trapezius
Pars descendens
Pars transversa
Pars ascendens
Spina scapulae
M. deltoideus
M. teres major
Caput longum
Caput laterale
M. triceps brachii
M. latissimus dorsi
M. extensor carpi radialis brevis
M. extensor carpi radialis longus
Olecranon
M. anconeus
M. obliquus externus abdominis
Fascia thoracolumbalis
M. flexor carpi ulnaris
M. extensor carpi ulnaris
M. extensor digitorum
Crista iliaca
M. obliquus internus abdominis

A Superficial dissection.

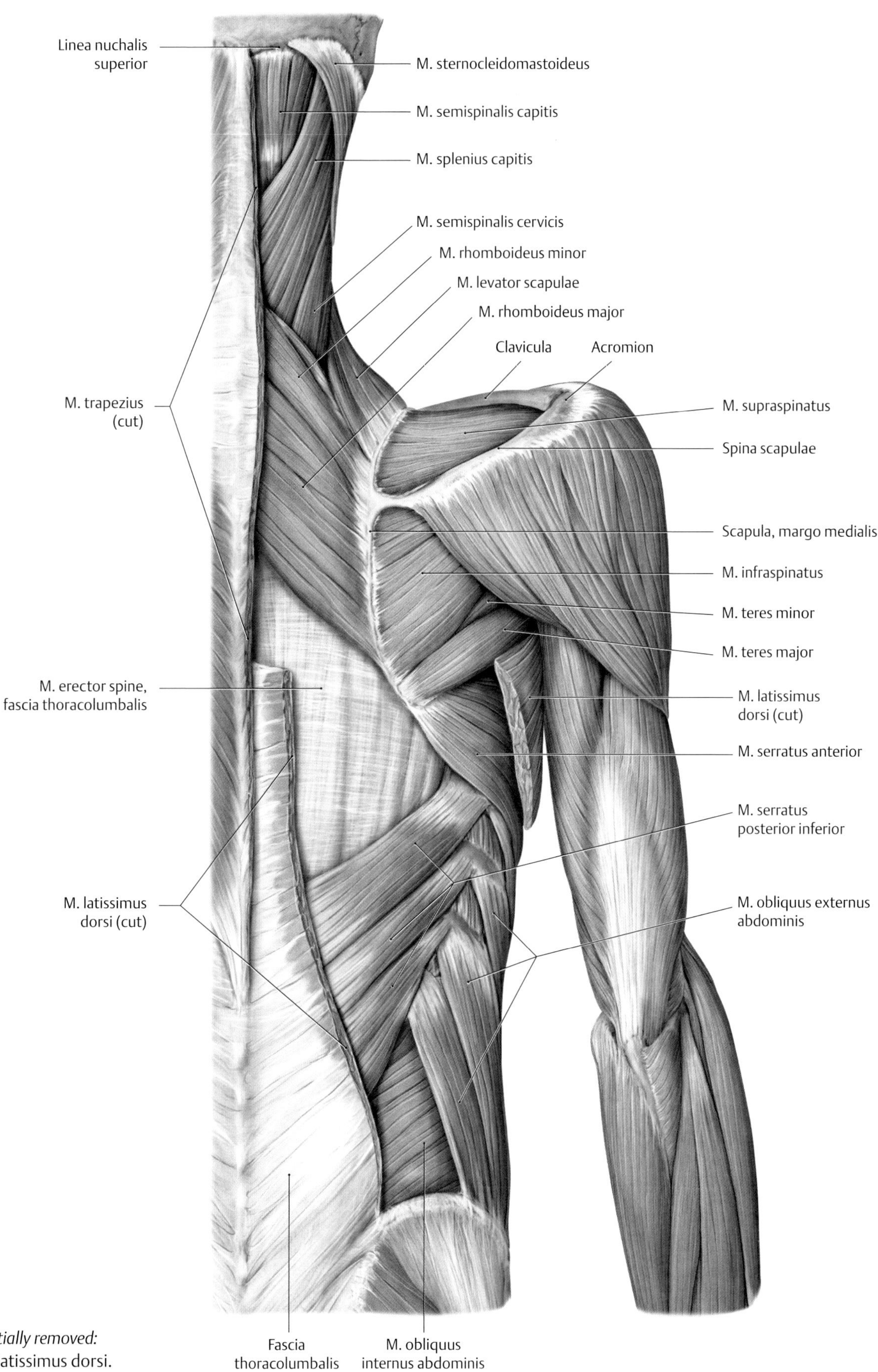
Linea nuchalis superior
M. sternocleidomastoideus
M. semispinalis capitis
M. splenius capitis
M. semispinalis cervicis
M. rhomboideus minor
M. levator scapulae
M. rhomboideus major
Clavicula
Acromion
M. trapezius (cut)
M. supraspinatus
Spina scapulae
Scapula, margo medialis
M. infraspinatus
M. teres minor
M. teres major
M. erector spine, fascia thoracolumbalis
M. latissimus dorsi (cut)
M. serratus anterior
M. serratus posterior inferior
M. latissimus dorsi (cut)
M. obliquus externus abdominis
Fascia thoracolumbalis
M. obliquus internus abdominis

B Deep dissection. *Partially removed:* M. trapezius and m. latissimus dorsi.

Posterior Muscles of the Shoulder & Arm (II)

Fig. 19.22 **Posterior dissection**
Right arm, posterior view. Muscle origins (O) are shown in red, insertions (I) in blue.

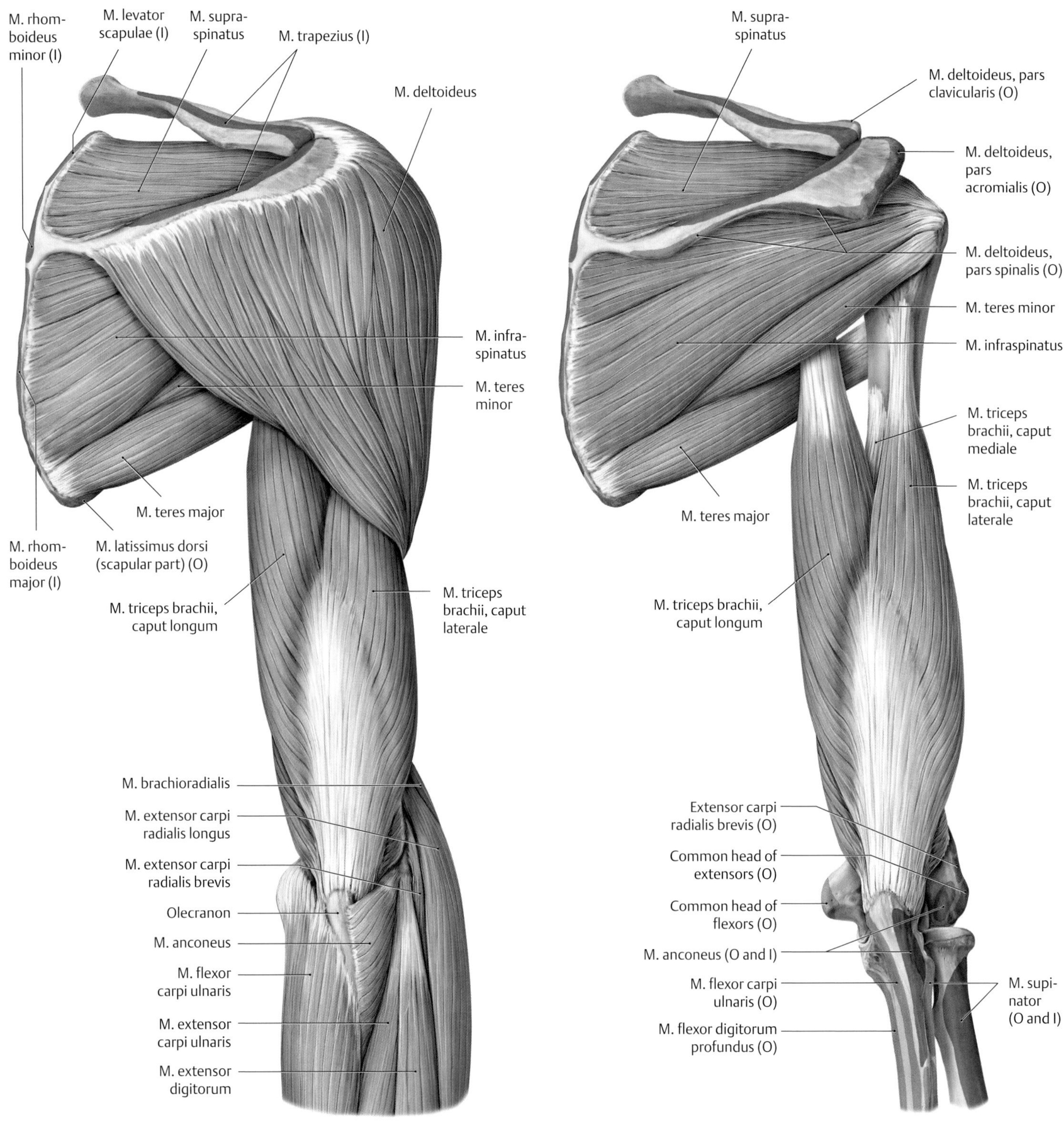

M. rhomboideus minor (I)
M. levator scapulae (I)
M. supraspinatus
M. trapezius (I)
M. deltoideus
M. infraspinatus
M. teres minor
M. teres major
M. rhomboideus major (I)
M. latissimus dorsi (scapular part) (O)
M. triceps brachii, caput longum
M. triceps brachii, caput laterale
M. brachioradialis
M. extensor carpi radialis longus
M. extensor carpi radialis brevis
Olecranon
M. anconeus
M. flexor carpi ulnaris
M. extensor carpi ulnaris
M. extensor digitorum
M. supraspinatus
M. deltoideus, pars clavicularis (O)
M. deltoideus, pars acromialis (O)
M. deltoideus, pars spinalis (O)
M. teres minor
M. infraspinatus
M. triceps brachii, caput mediale
M. triceps brachii, caput laterale
M. teres major
M. triceps brachii, caput longum
Extensor carpi radialis brevis (O)
Common head of extensors (O)
Common head of flexors (O)
M. anconeus (O and I)
M. flexor carpi ulnaris (O)
M. flexor digitorum profundus (O)
M. supinator (O and I)

A *Removed:* Mm. rhomboideus major and minor, m. serratus anterior, and m. levator scapulae.

B *Removed:* M. deltoideus and forearm muscles.

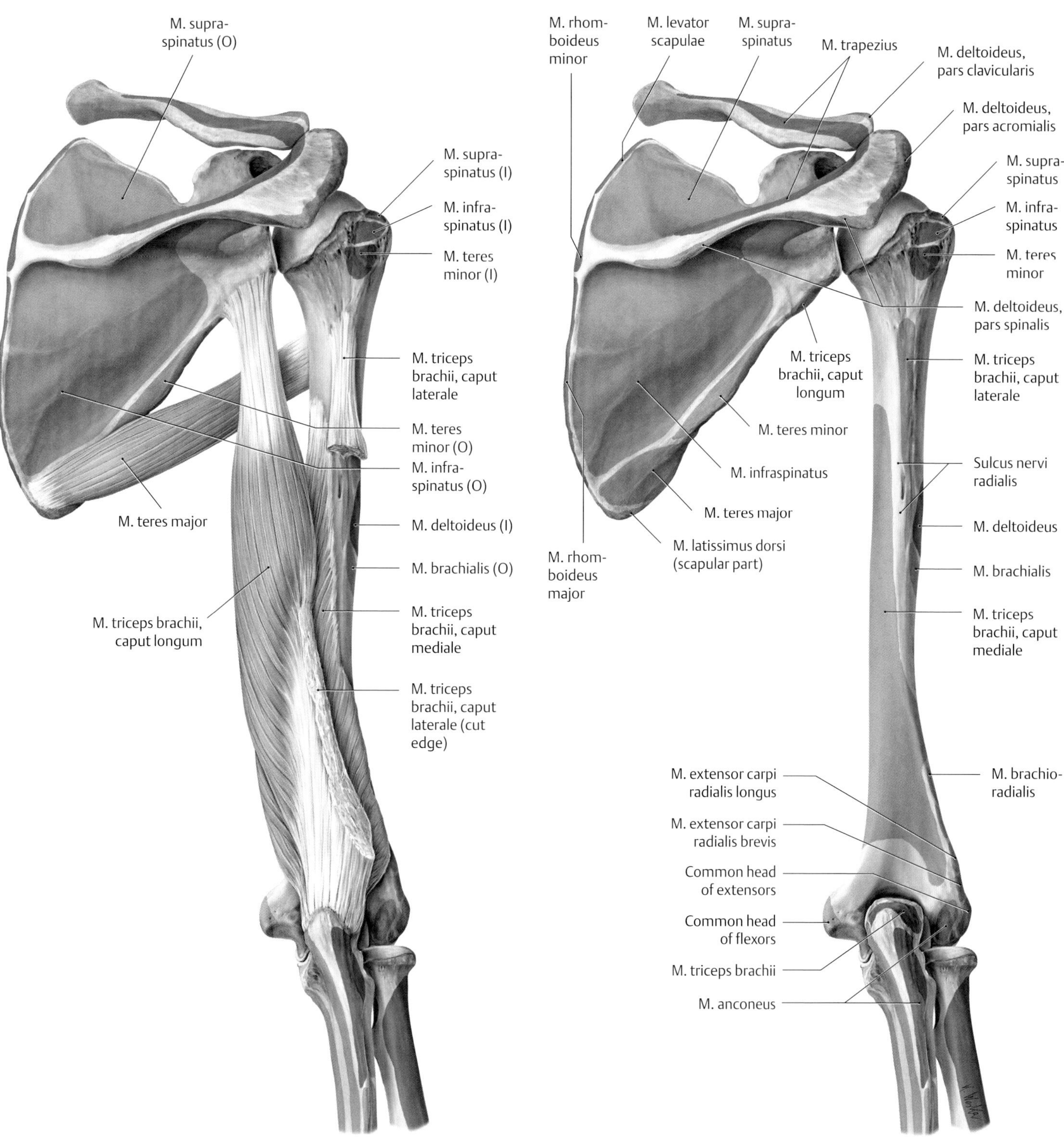

M. supra-
spinatus (O)
M. supra-
spinatus (I)
M. infra-
spinatus (I)
M. teres
minor (I)
M. triceps
brachii, caput
laterale
M. teres
minor (O)
M. infra-
spinatus (O)
M. teres major
M. deltoideus (I)
M. brachialis (O)
M. triceps brachii,
caput longum
M. triceps
brachii, caput
mediale
M. triceps
brachii, caput
laterale (cut
edge)
M. rhom-
boideus
minor
M. levator
scapulae
M. supra-
spinatus
M. trapezius
M. deltoideus,
pars clavicularis
M. deltoideus,
pars acromialis
M. supra-
spinatus
M. infra-
spinatus
M. teres
minor
M. deltoideus,
pars spinalis
M. triceps
brachii, caput
longum
M. triceps
brachii, caput
laterale
M. teres minor
Sulcus nervi
radialis
M. infraspinatus
M. teres major
M. deltoideus
M. latissimus dorsi
(scapular part)
M. rhom-
boideus
major
M. brachialis
M. triceps
brachii, caput
mediale
M. extensor carpi
radialis longus
M. brachio-
radialis
M. extensor carpi
radialis brevis
Common head
of extensors
Common head
of flexors
M. triceps brachii
M. anconeus

C *Removed:* M. supraspinatus, m. infraspinatus, and m. teres minor. *Partially removed:* M. triceps brachii.

D *Removed:* M. triceps brachii and m. teres major.

Muscle Facts (I)

The actions of the three parts of m. deltoideus depend on their relationship to the position of the humerus and its axis of motion. At less than 60 degrees, the muscles act as adductors, but at greater than 60 degrees, they act as abductors. As a result, the parts of m. deltoideus can act antagonistically as well as synergistically.

Fig. 19.23 **M. deltoideus**
Right shoulder.

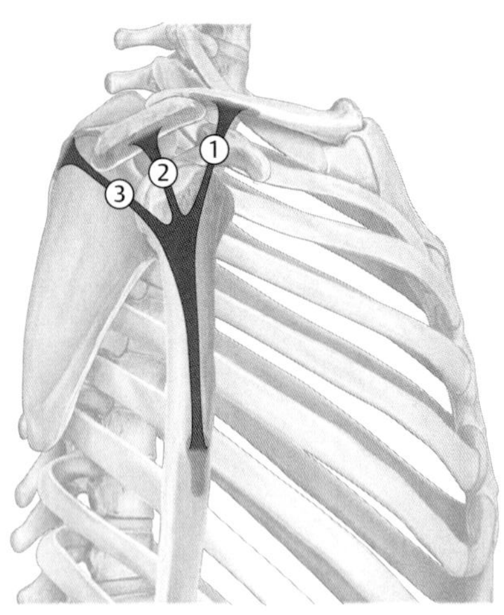
1
2
3

A Parts of the m. deltoideus, right lateral view.

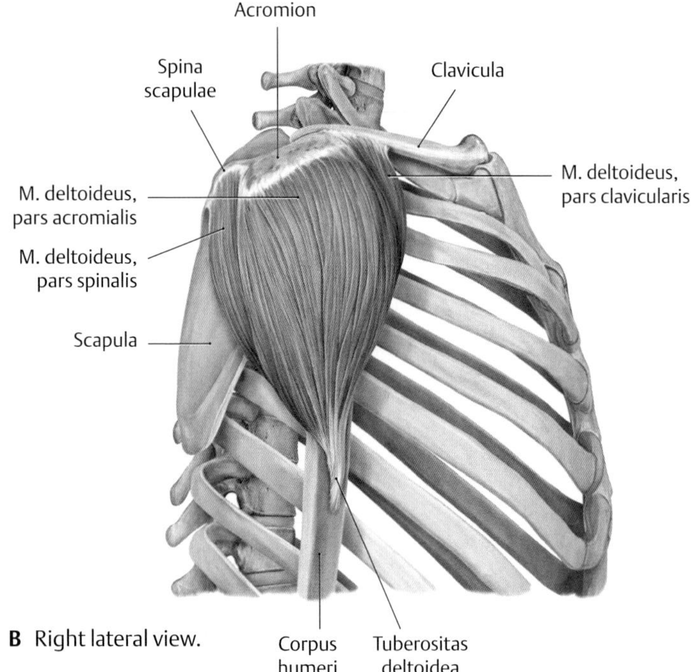
Acromion
Spina scapulae
Clavicula
M. deltoideus, pars acromialis
M. deltoideus, pars clavicularis
M. deltoideus, pars spinalis
Scapula
Corpus humeri
Tuberositas deltoidea

B Right lateral view.

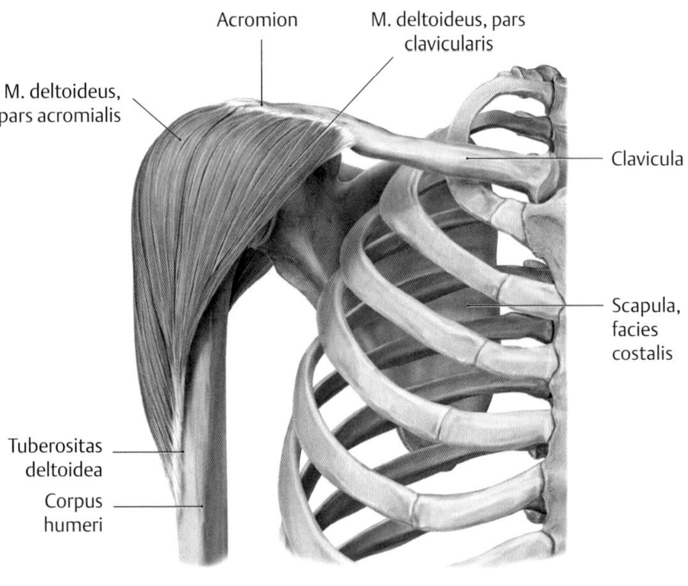
Acromion
M. deltoideus, pars clavicularis
M. deltoideus, pars acromialis
Clavicula
Scapula, facies costalis
Tuberositas deltoidea
Corpus humeri

C Anterior view.

Clavicula
Proc. coracoideus
M. deltoideus, pars clavicularis
Acromion
M. deltoideus, pars acromialis
Spina scapulae
M. deltoideus, pars spinalis
Scapula, facies posterior
Tuberositas deltoidea
Corpus humeri

D Posterior view.

Table 19.1 **Parts of the M. deltoideus**

Muscle		Origin	Insertion	Innervation	Action*
M. deltoideus	① Pars clavicularis	Lateral one third of clavicula	Humerus (Tuberositas deltoidea)	N. axillaris (C5, C6)	Flexion, internal rotation, adduction
	② Pars acromialis	Acromion			Abduction
	③ Pars spinalis	Spina scapulae			Extension, external rotation, adduction

* Between 60 and 90 degrees of abduction, Pars clavicularis and Pars spinalis assist the Pars acromialis with abduction.

Fig. 19.24 Rotator cuff

Right shoulder. The rotator cuff consists of four muscles: M. supraspinatus, m. infraspinatus, m. teres minor, and m. subscapularis.

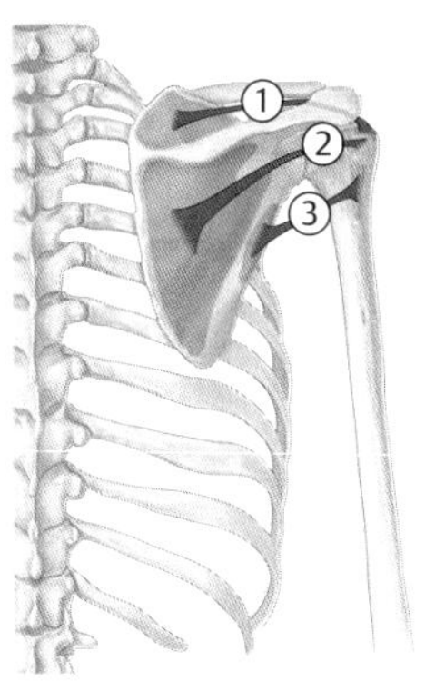

①
②
③

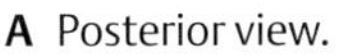

A Posterior view.

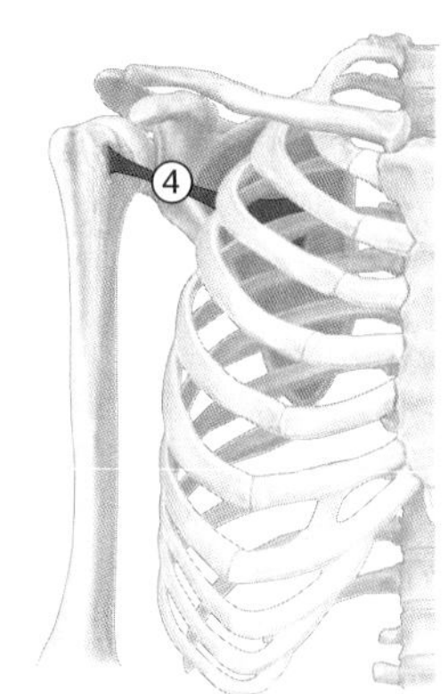

④

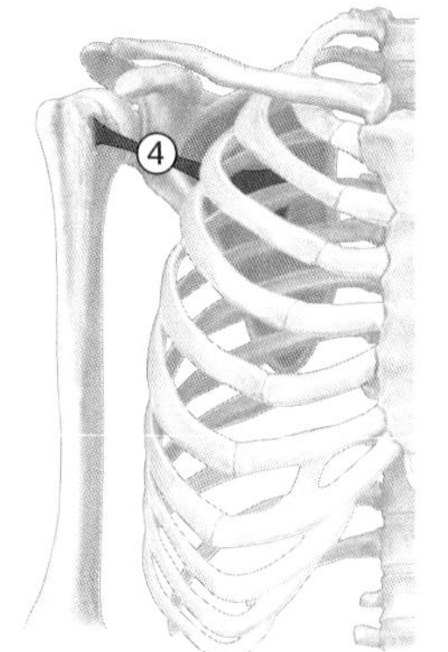

B Anterior view.

Acromion
Proc. coracoideus
Incisura scapulae
M. supraspinatus
Margo superior
Angulus superior
Tuberculum majus
Tuberculum minus
Sulcus intertubercularis
Crista tuberculi majoris
Crista tuberculi minoris
Corpus humeri
Margo medialis
M. subscapularis
Angulus inferior

C Anterior view.

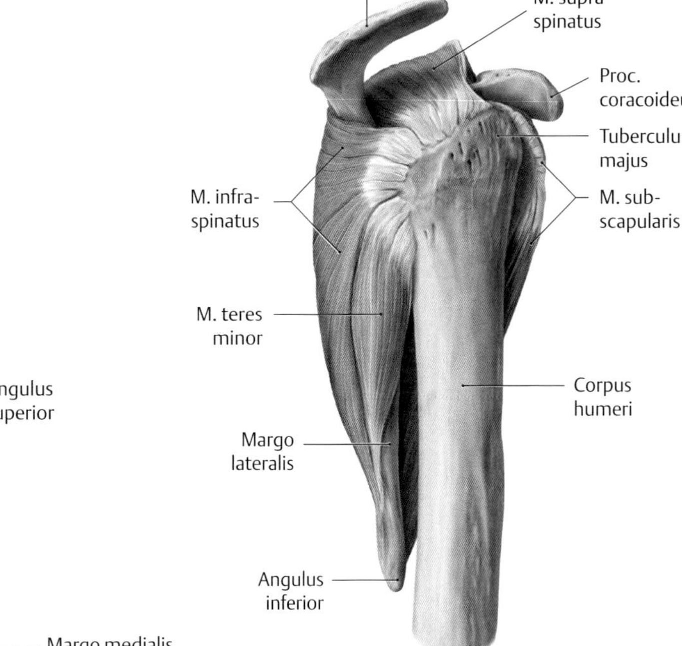

Acromion
M. supraspinatus
Proc. coracoideus
Tuberculum majus
M. infraspinatus
M. subscapularis
M. teres minor
Corpus humeri
Margo lateralis
Angulus inferior

D Lateral view.

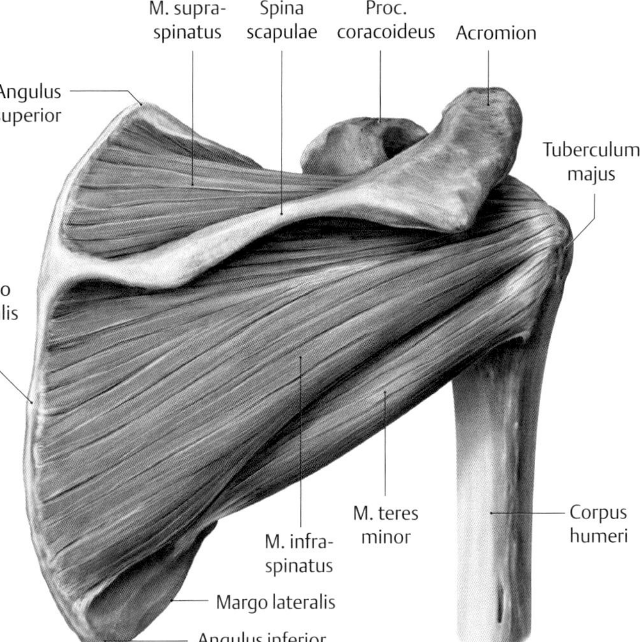

M. supraspinatus
Spina scapulae
Proc. coracoideus
Acromion
Angulus superior
Tuberculum majus
Margo medialis
M. teres minor
M. infraspinatus
Corpus humeri
Margo lateralis
Angulus inferior

E Posterior view.

Table 19.2 Muscles of the rotator cuff

Muscle	Origin		Insertion		Innervation	Action
① M. supraspinatus	Scapula	Fossa supraspinata scapulae	Humerus	Tuberculum majus humeri	N. suprascapularis (C4–C6)	Abduction
② M. infraspinatus		Fossa infraspinata scapulae				External rotation
③ M. teres minor		Margo lateralis scapulae			N. axillaris (C5, C6)	External rotation, weak adduction
④ M. subscapularis		Fossa subscapularis scapulae		Tuberculum minus humeri	N. subscapularis (C5, C6)	Internal rotation

Muscle Facts (II)

Fig. 19.25 **M. pectoralis major and m. coracobrachialis**
Anterior view.

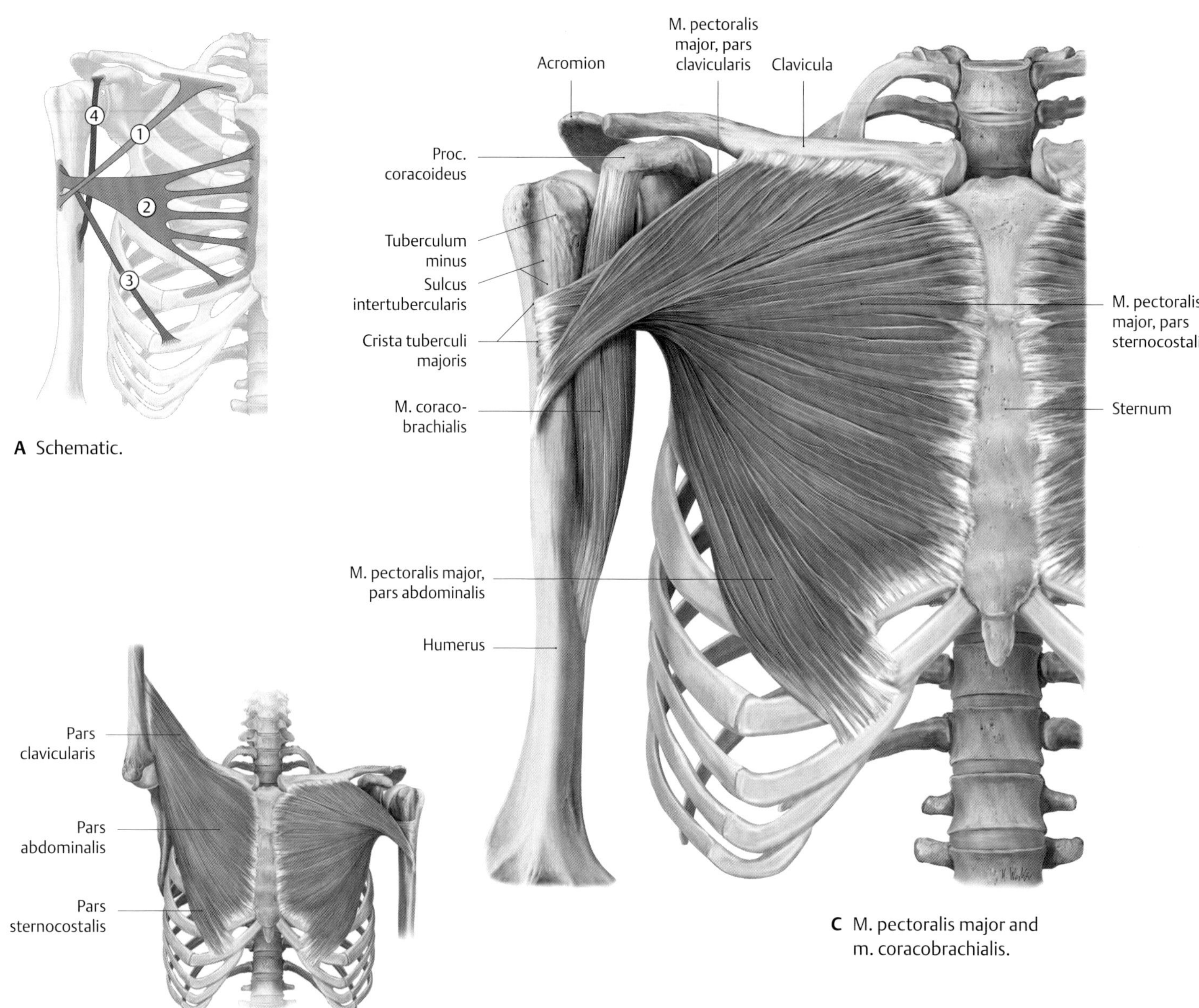

④
①
②
③
Acromion
M. pectoralis major, pars clavicularis
Clavicula
Proc. coracoideus
Tuberculum minus
Sulcus intertubercularis
Crista tuberculi majoris
M. coraco-brachialis
M. pectoralis major, pars abdominalis
Humerus
M. pectoralis major, pars sternocostalis
Sternum
Pars clavicularis
Pars abdominalis
Pars sternocostalis

A Schematic.

B M. pectoralis major in neutral position (left) and elevation (right).

C M. pectoralis major and m. coracobrachialis.

Table 19.3 **M. pectoralis major and M. coracobrachialis**

Muscle		Origin	Insertion	Innervation	Action
M. pectoralis major	① Pars clavicularis	Clavicula (medial half)	Humerus (crista tuberculi majoris humeri)	Nn. pectorales mediales et laterales (C5–T1)	Entire muscle: adduction, internal rotation Pars clavicularis and pars sternocostalis: flexion; assist in respiration when shoulder is fixed
	② Pars sternocostalis	Sternum and cartilagines costales 1–6			
	③ Pars abdominalis	Rectus sheath (anterior layer)			
④ M. coracobrachialis		Scapula (proc. coracoideus scapulae)	Humerus (crista tuberculis minoris)	N. musculo-cutaneous (C6, C7)	Flexion, adduction, internal rotation

Fig. 19.26 **M. subclavius and m. pectoralis minor**

Right side, anterior view.

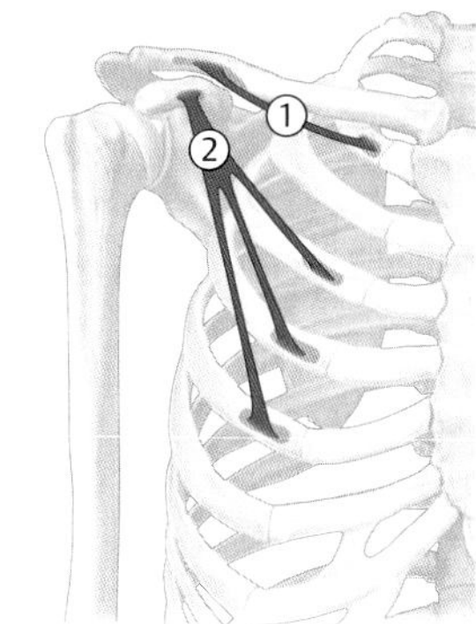

①
②

A Schematic.

Clavicula
Costa I
Acromion
Proc. coracoideus
M. subclavius
M. pectoralis minor
Costa III–V

B M. subclavius and m. pectoralis minor.

Fig. 19.27 **M. serratus anterior**

Right lateral view.

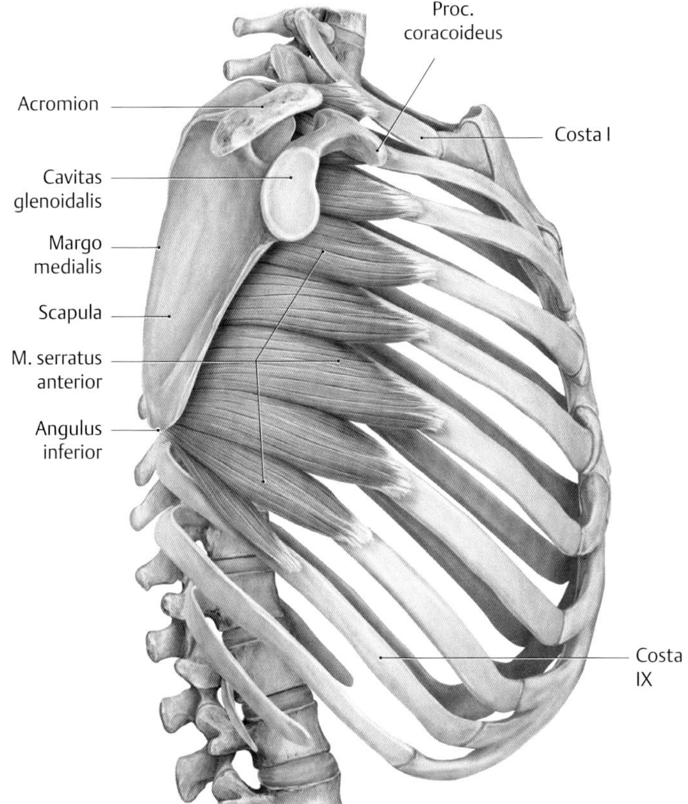

Proc. coracoideus
Acromion
Costa I
Cavitas glenoidalis
Margo medialis
Scapula
M. serratus anterior
Angulus inferior
Costa IX

A M. serratus anterior.

③
④
⑤

B Schematic.

Table 19.4	M. subclavius, m. pectoralis minor, and m. serratus anterior				
Muscle		**Origin**	**Insertion**	**Innervation**	**Action**
① M. subclavius		Costa I	Clavicula (inferior surface)	N. subclavius (C5, C6)	Steadies the clavicula in the articulatio sternoclavicularis
② M. pectoralis minor		Costa III–V	Proc. coracoideus scapulae	Nn. pectorales mediales et laterales	Draws scapula downward, causing inferior angle to move posteromedially; rotates glenoid inferiorly; assists in respiration
M. serratus anterior	③ Pars superior	Costa I–IX	Scapula (margo medialis)	N. thoracicus longus (C5–C7)	Pars superior: lowers the raised arm
	④ Pars intermedia				Entire muscle: draws scapula laterally forward; elevates ribs when shoulder is fixed
	⑤ Pars inferior				Pars inferior: rotates scapula laterally

Muscle Facts (III)

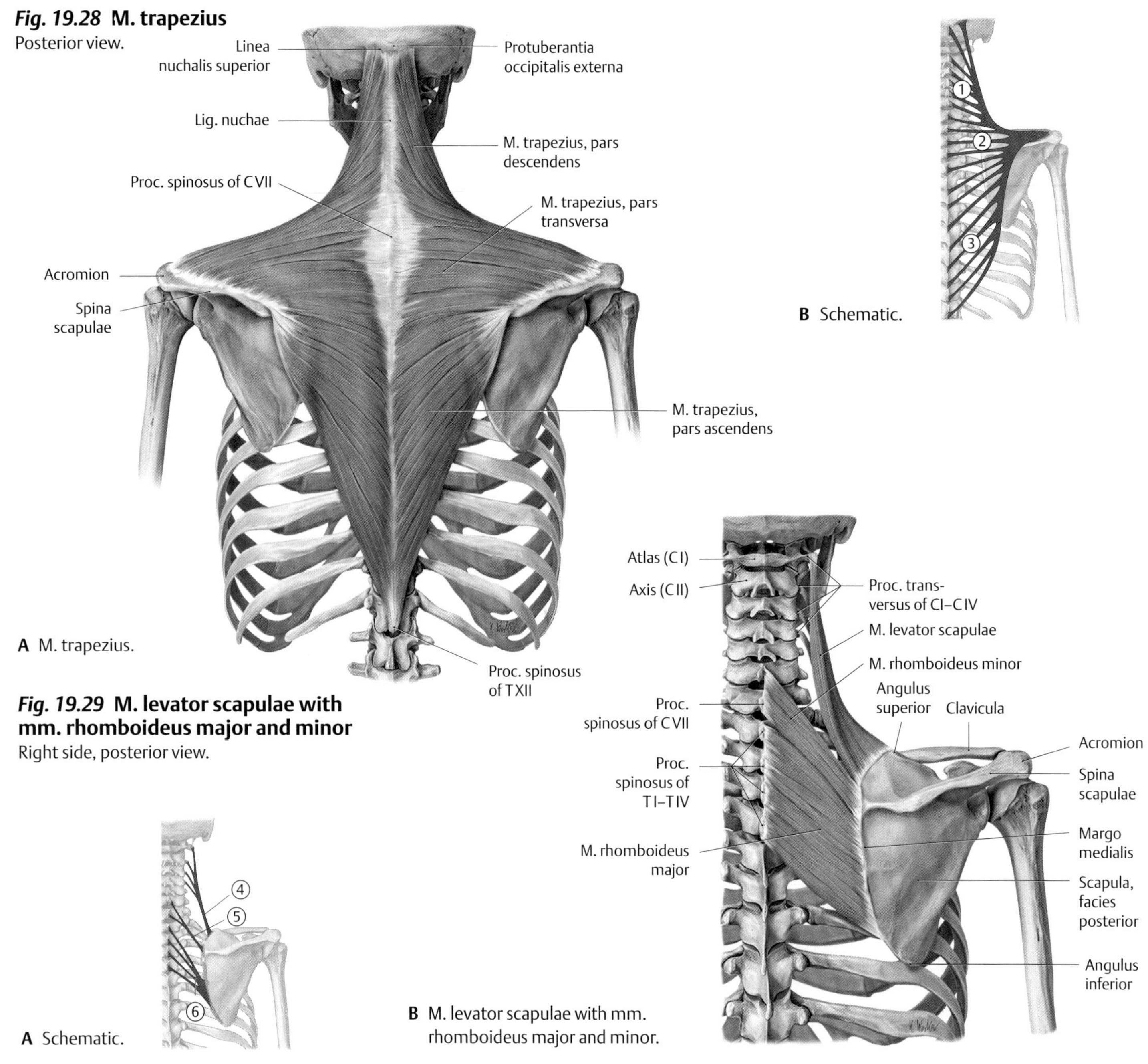

Linea nuchalis superior
Protuberantia occipitalis externa
Lig. nuchae
M. trapezius, pars descendens
Proc. spinosus of C VII
M. trapezius, pars transversa
Acromion
Spina scapulae
M. trapezius, pars ascendens
Proc. spinosus of T XII
Atlas (C I)
Axis (C II)
Proc. transversus of CI–C IV
M. levator scapulae
M. rhomboideus minor
Angulus superior
Clavicula
Proc. spinosus of C VII
Acromion
Proc. spinosus of T I–T IV
Spina scapulae
Margo medialis
M. rhomboideus major
Scapula, facies posterior
Angulus inferior

Fig. 19.28 M. trapezius
Posterior view.

A M. trapezius.

B Schematic.

Fig. 19.29 M. levator scapulae with mm. rhomboideus major and minor
Right side, posterior view.

A Schematic.

B M. levator scapulae with mm. rhomboideus major and minor.

Table 19.5 M. trapezius, m. levator scapulae, and m. rhomboideus major and minor

Muscle		Origin	Insertion	Innervation	Action
M. trapezius	① Pars descendens	Protuberantia occipitalis ext.; procc. spinosi of C I–C VII	Clavicula (lateral one third)	N. accessorius (CN XI); Plexus cervicalis (C3–C4)	Draws scapula obliquely upward; rotates cavitas glenoidalis superiorly; tilts head to same side and rotates it to opposite
	② Pars transversa	Aponeurosis at T I–T IV Proc. spinosus	Acromion		Draws scapula medially
	③ Pars ascendens	Procc. spinosi of T V–T XII	Spina scapulae		Draws scapula medially downward
					Entire muscle: steadies scapula on thorax
④ M. levator scapulae		Procc. transversi of C I–C IV	Angulus superior scapulae	N. dorsalis scapulae (C4–C5)	Draws scapula medially upward while moving angulus inferior medially; inclines neck to same side
⑤ M. rhomboideus minor		Procc. spinosi of C VI, C VII	Medial border of scapula above (minor) and below (major) spina scapulae		Steadies scapula; draws scapula medially upward
⑥ M. rhomboideus major		Procc. spinosi of T I–T IV vertebrae			

CN = cranial nerve.

Fig. 19.30 M. latissimus dorsi and m. teres major
Posterior view.

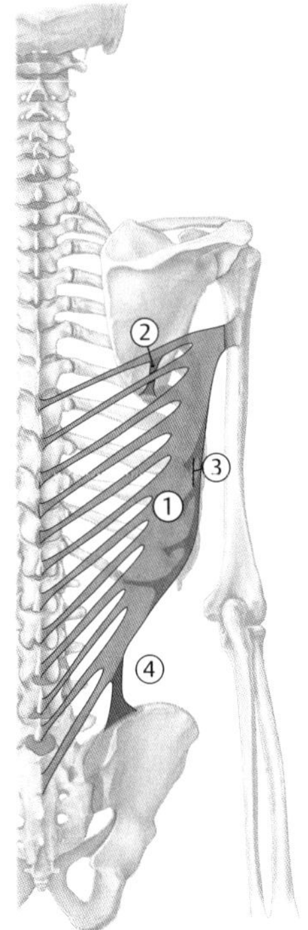
②
③
①
④

A M. latissimus dorsi.

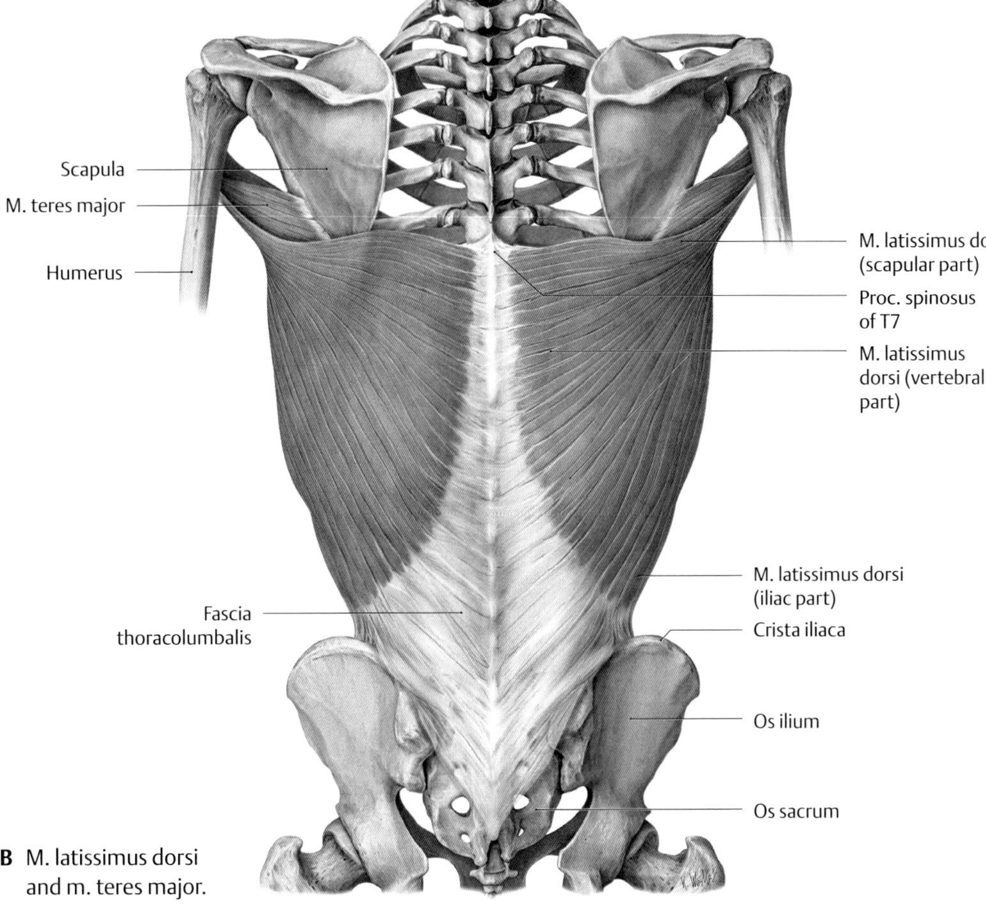
Scapula
M. teres major
Humerus
M. latissimus dorsi (scapular part)
Proc. spinosus of T7
M. latissimus dorsi (vertebral part)
M. latissimus dorsi (iliac part)
Crista iliaca
Fascia thoracolumbalis
Os ilium
Os sacrum

B M. latissimus dorsi and m. teres major.

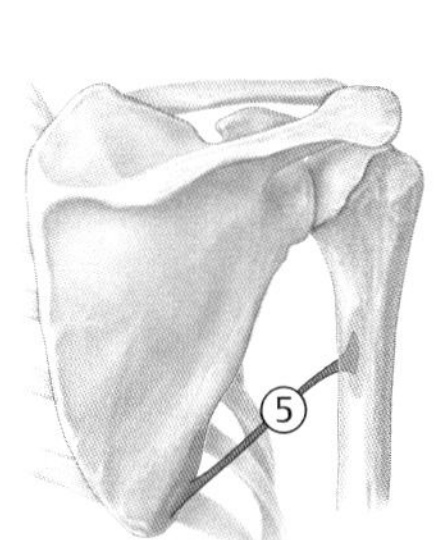
⑤

C M. teres major.

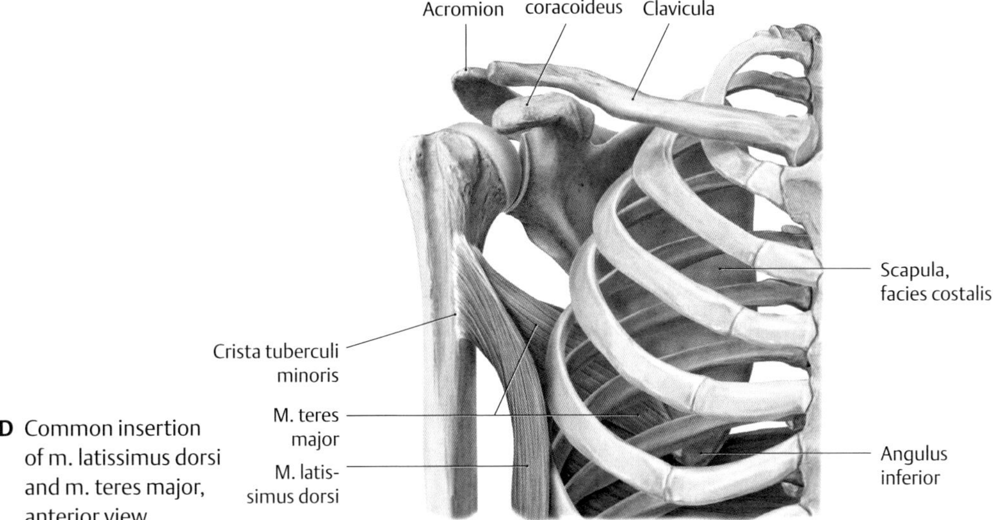
Acromion
Proc. coracoideus
Clavicula
Scapula, facies costalis
Crista tuberculi minoris
M. teres major
M. latissimus dorsi
Angulus inferior

D Common insertion of m. latissimus dorsi and m. teres major, anterior view.

Table 19.6 M. latissimus dorsi and M. teres major

Muscle		Origin	Insertion	Innervation	Action
M. latissimus dorsi	① Pars vertebralis	Procc. spinosi of T VII–T XII vertebrae thoracicae; fascia thoracolumbalis	Humerus (crista tuberculis minoris)	N. thoracodorsalis (C6–C8)	Internal rotation, adduction, extension, respiration (“cough muscle”)
	② Pars scapularis	Angulus inferior scapulae			
	③ Pars costalis	Costa IX–XII			
	④ Pars iliaca	Crista iliaca (posterior one third)			
⑤ M. teres major		Angulus inferior scapulae		N. subscapularis (C5–C7)	Internal rotation, adduction, extension

Muscle Facts (IV)

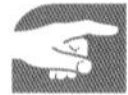

The anterior and posterior muscles of the arm may be classified respectively as flexors and extensors relative to the movement of the elbow joint. Although m. coracobrachialis is topographically part of the anterior compartment, it is functionally grouped with the muscles of the shoulder (see p. 274).

Fig. 19.31 M. biceps brachii and m. brachialis
Right arm, anterior view.

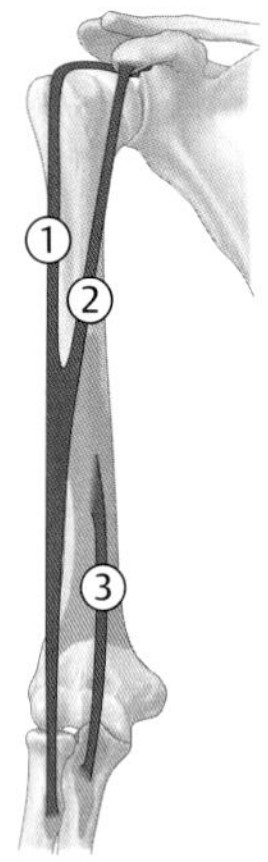

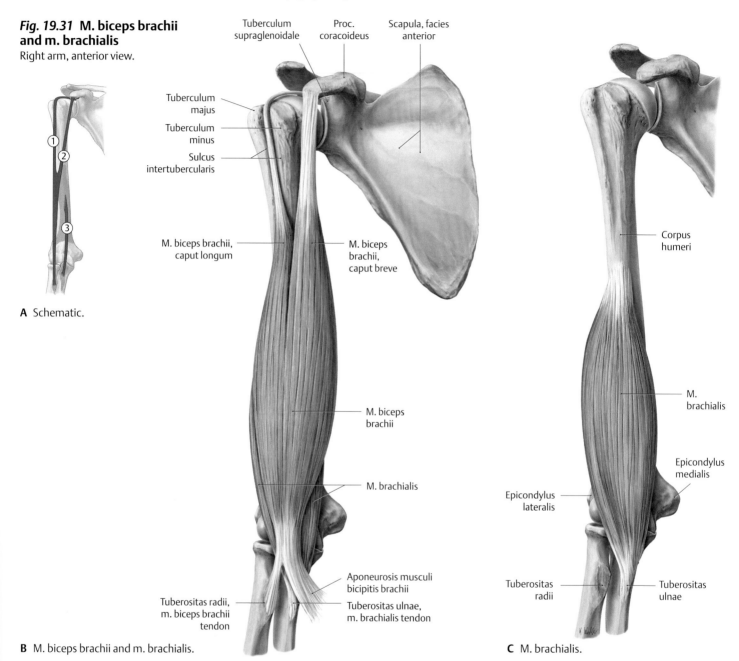

①
②
③

A Schematic.

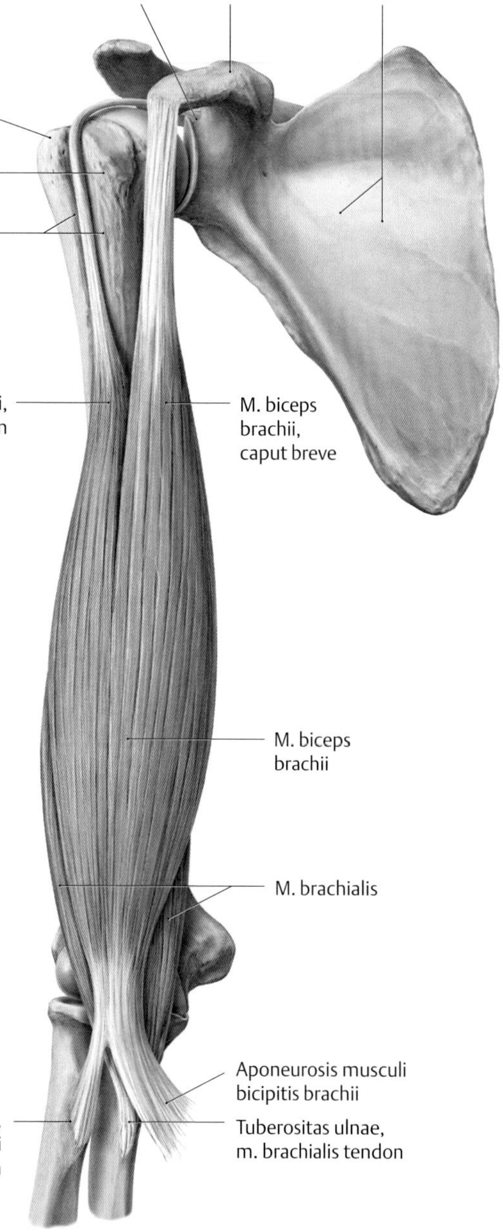

Tuberculum supraglenoidale
Proc. coracoideus
Scapula, facies anterior
Tuberculum majus
Tuberculum minus
Sulcus intertubercularis
M. biceps brachii, caput longum
M. biceps brachii, caput breve
M. biceps brachii
M. brachialis
Aponeurosis musculi bicipitis brachii
Tuberositas radii, m. biceps brachii tendon
Tuberositas ulnae, m. brachialis tendon

B M. biceps brachii and m. brachialis.

Corpus humeri
M. brachialis
Epicondylus medialis
Epicondylus lateralis
Tuberositas radii
Tuberositas ulnae

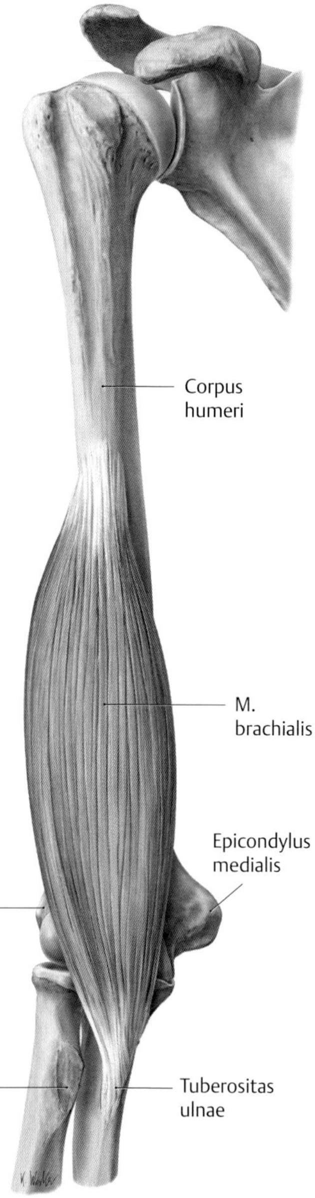

C M. brachialis.

Table 19.7 Anterior group: M. biceps brachii and M. brachialis

Muscle		Origin	Insertion	Innervation	Action
M. biceps brachii	① Caput longum	Tuberculum supraglenoidale scapulae	Tuberositas radii	N. musculocutaneous (C5–C6)	Articulatio cubiti: flexion; supination* Shoulder joint: flexion; stabilization of humeral head during m. deltoideus contraction; abduction and internal rotation of the humerus
	② Caput breve	Proc. scapulae			
③ M. brachialis		Humerus (distal half of anterior surface)	Tuberositas ulnae	N. musculocutaneous (C5–C6) and N. radialis (C7, minor)	Flexion at the Articulatio cubiti

* *Note:* When the elbow is flexed, the M. biceps brachii acts as a powerful supinator because the lever arm is almost perpendicular to the axis of pronation/supination.

Fig. 19.32 **M. triceps brachii and m. anconeus**
Right arm, posterior view.

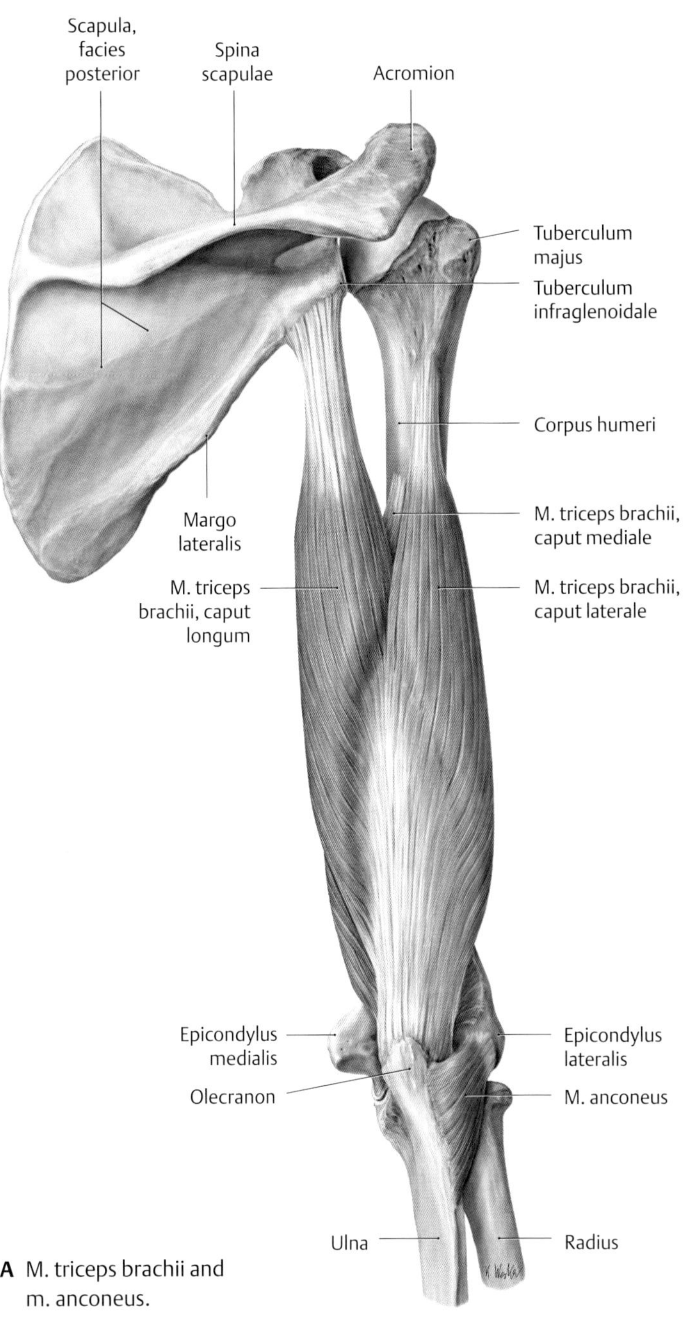
Scapula, facies posterior
Spina scapulae
Acromion
Tuberculum majus
Tuberculum infraglenoidale
Corpus humeri
Margo lateralis
M. triceps brachii, caput mediale
M. triceps brachii, caput longum
M. triceps brachii, caput laterale
Epicondylus medialis
Epicondylus lateralis
Olecranon
M. anconeus
Ulna
Radius

A M. triceps brachii and m. anconeus.

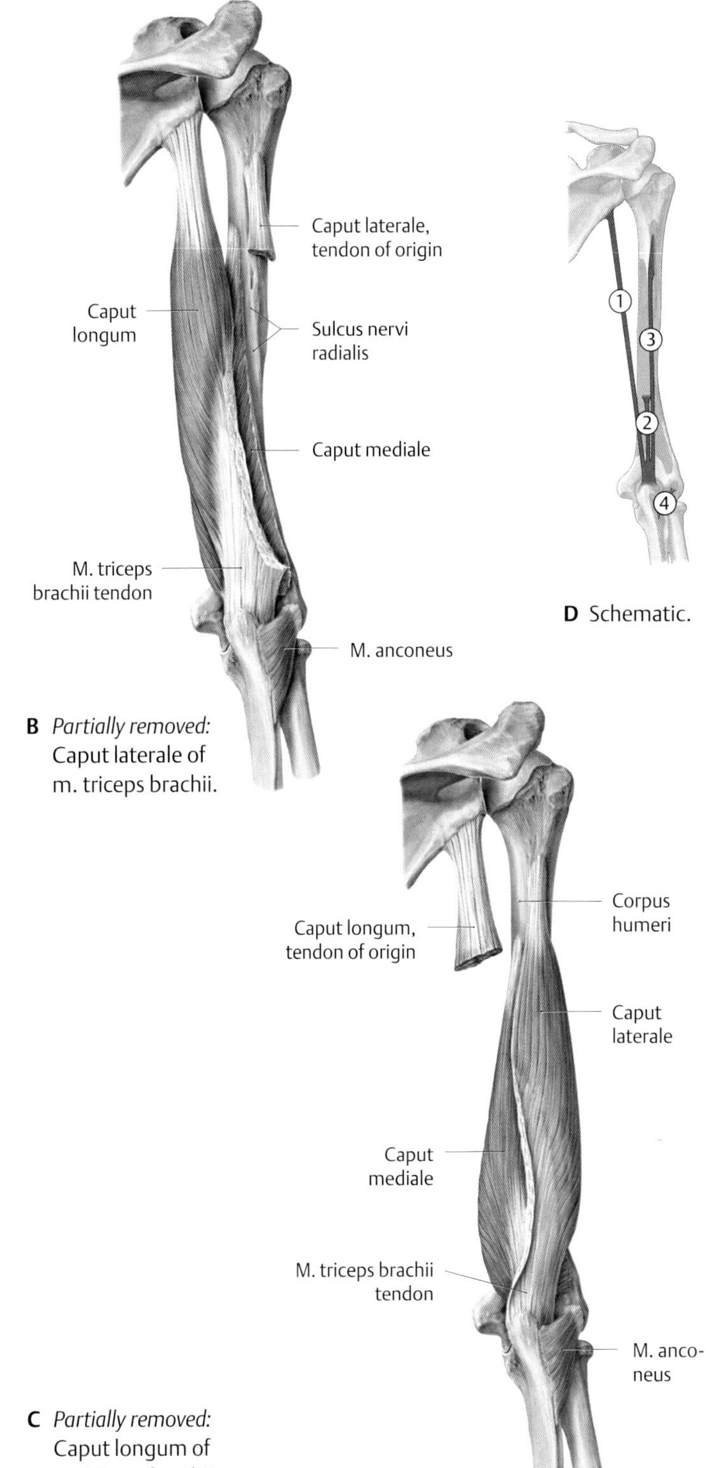
Caput laterale, tendon of origin
Caput longum
Sulcus nervi radialis
Caput mediale
M. triceps brachii tendon
M. anconeus
1
2
3
4
Corpus humeri
Caput longum, tendon of origin
Caput laterale
Caput mediale
M. triceps brachii tendon
M. anco-neus

B *Partially removed:* Caput laterale of m. triceps brachii.

C *Partially removed:* Caput longum of m. triceps brachii.

D Schematic.

Table 19.8 **Posterior group: M. triceps brachii and M. anconeus**

Muscle		Origin	Insertion	Innervation	Action
M. triceps brachii	① Caput longum	Tuberculum infraglenoidale scapulae	Olecranon ulnae	N. radialis (C6–C8)	Articulatio cubiti: extension Articulatio humeri, Caput longum: extension and adduction
	② Caput mediale	Posterior humerus, distal to sulcus radialis; septum intermuscularis medialis			
	③ Caput laterale	Posterior humerus, proximal to sulcus radialis; lateral to septum intermuscularis			
④ M. anconeus		Epicondylus lateralis humeri (variance: posterior joint capsule)	Olecranon ulnae (radial surface)		Extends the elbow and tightens its joint

Radius & Ulna

Fig. 20.1 **Radius and ulna**
Right forearm.

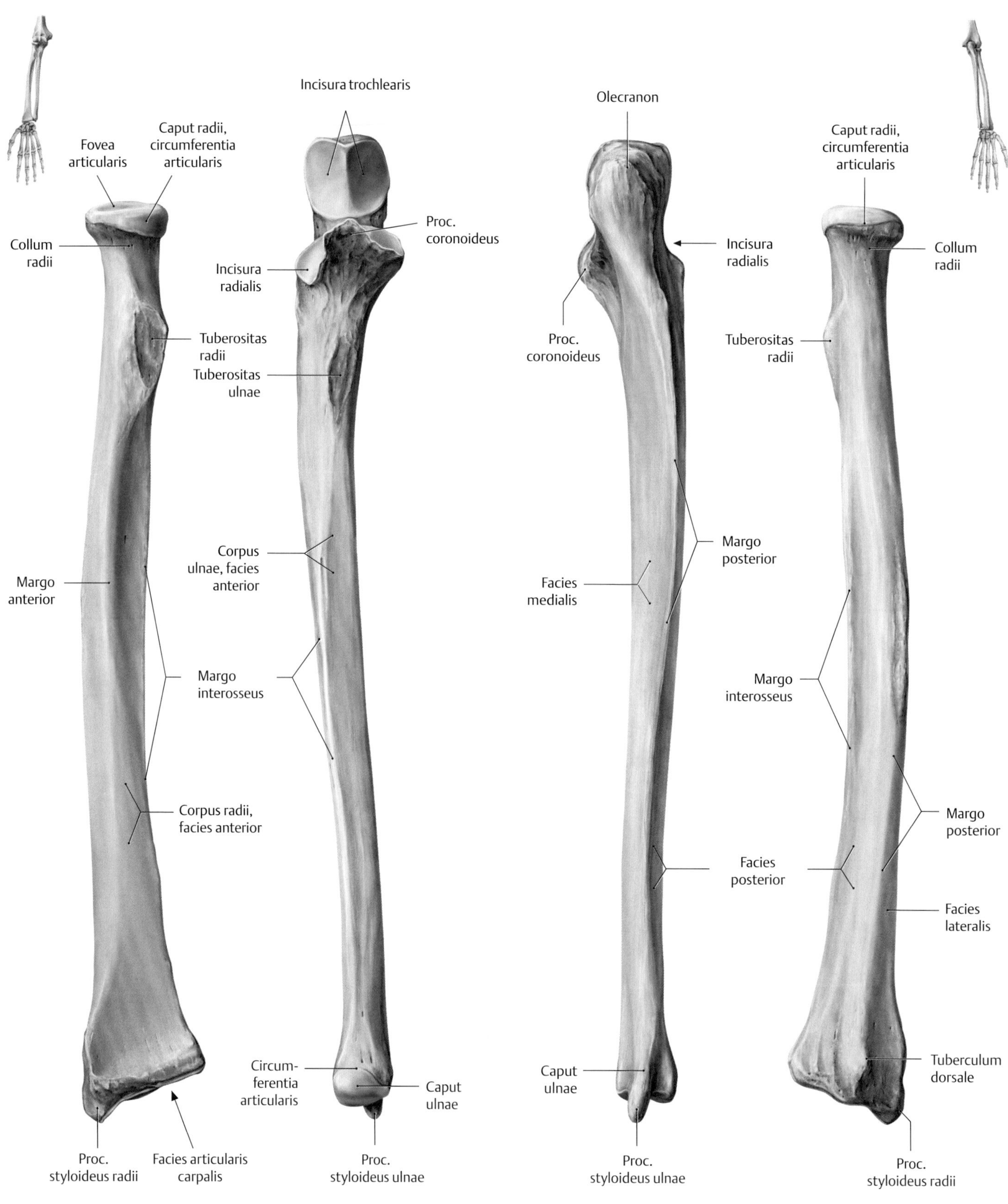
Fovea articularis
Caput radii, circumferentia articularis
Collum radii
Tuberositas radii
Margo anterior
Corpus radii, facies anterior
Proc. styloideus radii
Facies articularis carpalis
Incisura trochlearis
Proc. coronoideus
Incisura radialis
Tuberositas ulnae
Corpus ulnae, facies anterior
Margo interosseus
Circum-ferentia articularis
Caput ulnae
Proc. styloideus ulnae
Olecranon
Incisura radialis
Proc. coronoideus
Margo posterior
Facies medialis
Facies posterior
Caput ulnae
Proc. styloideus ulnae
Caput radii, circumferentia articularis
Collum radii
Tuberositas radii
Margo interosseus
Margo posterior
Facies posterior
Facies lateralis
Tuberculum dorsale
Proc. styloideus radii

A Anterior view.

B Posterior view.

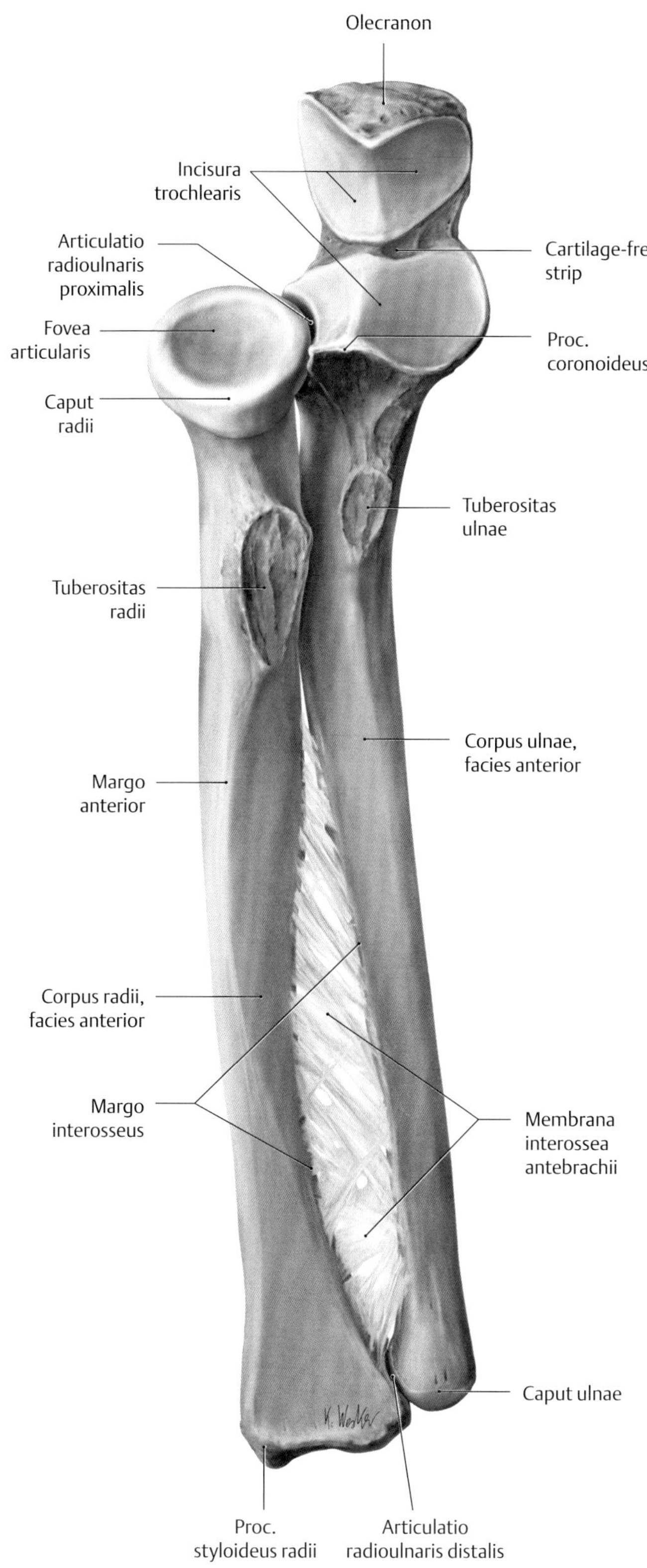

Olecranon
Incisura trochlearis
Articulatio radioulnaris proximalis
Fovea articularis
Caput radii
Cartilage-free strip
Proc. coronoideus
Tuberositas ulnae
Tuberositas radii
Corpus ulnae, facies anterior
Margo anterior
Corpus radii, facies anterior
Margo interosseus
Membrana interossea antebrachii
Caput ulnae
Proc. styloideus radii
Articulatio radioulnaris distalis

C Anterosuperior view.

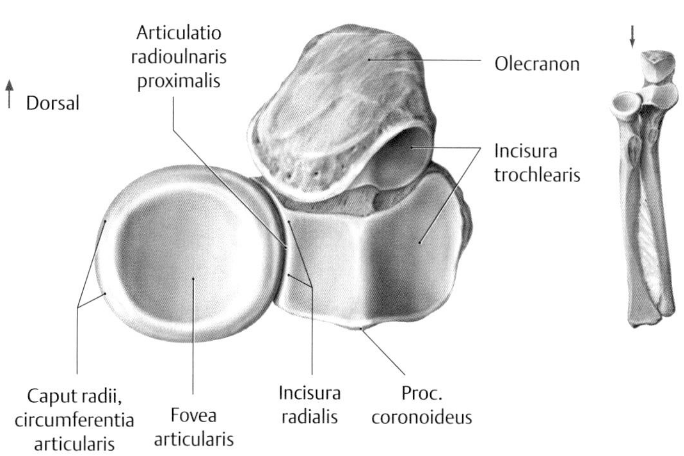

Dorsal
Articulatio radioulnaris proximalis
Olecranon
Incisura trochlearis
Caput radii, circumferentia articularis
Fovea articularis
Incisura radialis
Proc. coronoideus

D Proximal view.

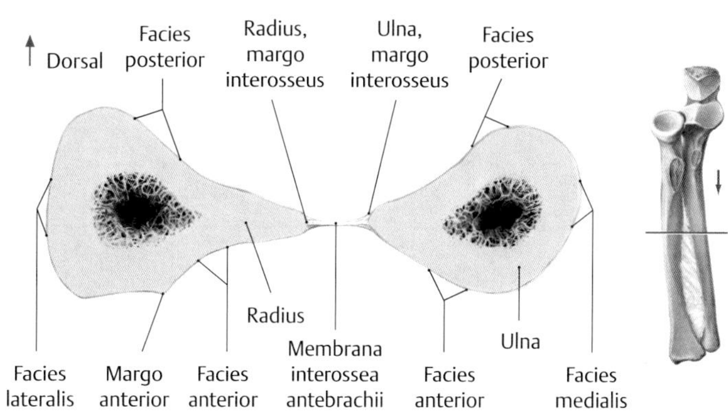

Dorsal
Facies posterior
Radius, margo interosseus
Ulna, margo interosseus
Facies posterior
Radius
Ulna
Facies lateralis
Margo anterior
Facies anterior
Membrana interossea antebrachii
Facies anterior
Facies medialis

E Transverse section, proximal view.

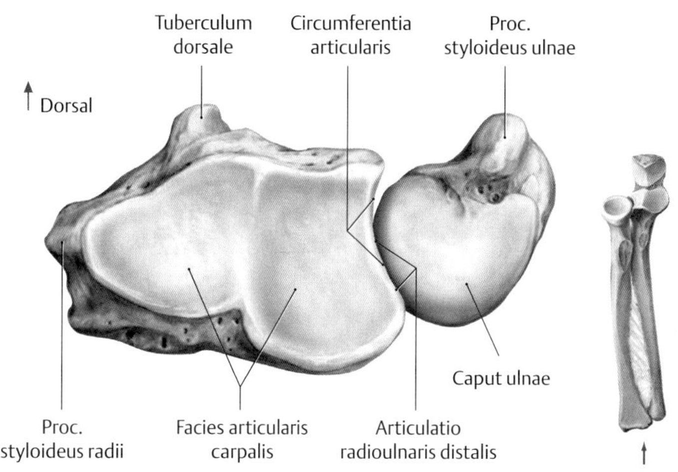

Dorsal
Tuberculum dorsale
Circumferentia articularis
Proc. styloideus ulnae
Caput ulnae
Proc. styloideus radii
Facies articularis carpalis
Articulatio radioulnaris distalis

F Distal view.

Articulatio Cubiti

***Fig. 20.2* Articulatio cubiti**
Right limb. The elbow consists of three articulations between the humerus, ulna, and radius: articulatio humeroulnaris, articulatio humeroradialis, and articulatio radioulnaris proximalis.

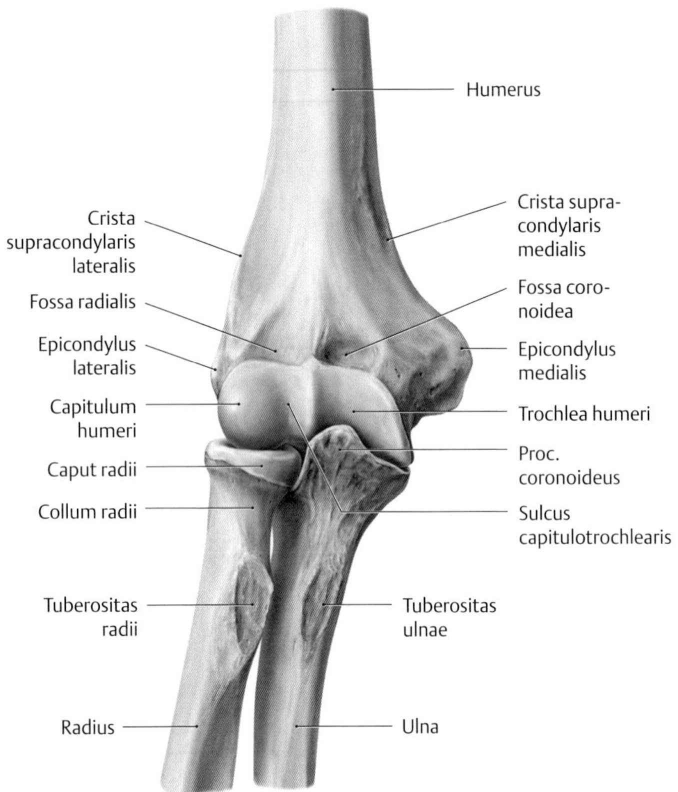
Humerus
Crista supracondylaris lateralis
Crista supra-condylaris medialis
Fossa radialis
Fossa coro-noidea
Epicondylus lateralis
Epicondylus medialis
Capitulum humeri
Trochlea humeri
Caput radii
Proc. coronoideus
Collum radii
Sulcus capitulotrochlearis
Tuberositas radii
Tuberositas ulnae
Radius
Ulna

A Anterior view.

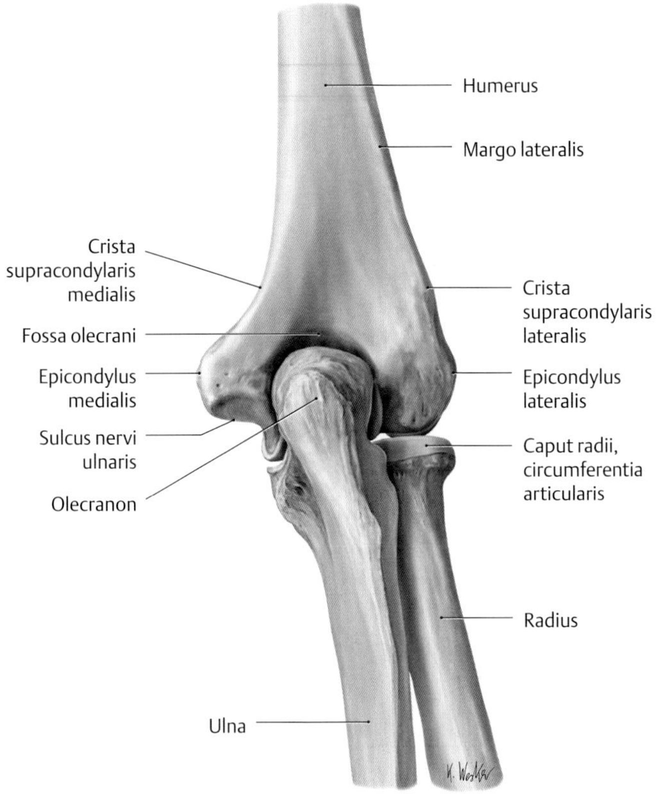

Humerus
Margo lateralis
Crista supracondylaris medialis
Crista supracondylaris lateralis
Fossa olecrani
Epicondylus medialis
Epicondylus lateralis
Sulcus nervi ulnaris
Caput radii, circumferentia articularis
Olecranon
Radius
Ulna

B Posterior view.

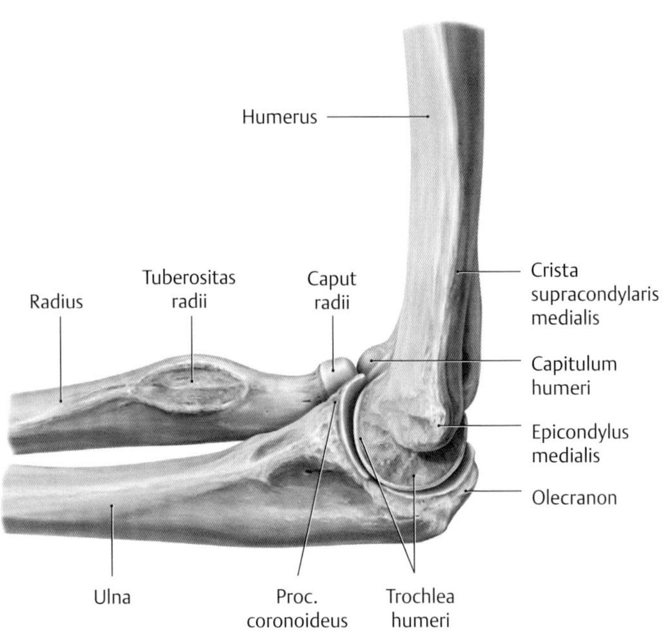
Humerus
Radius
Tuberositas radii
Caput radii
Crista supracondylaris medialis
Capitulum humeri
Epicondylus medialis
Olecranon
Ulna
Proc. coronoideus
Trochlea humeri

C Medial view.

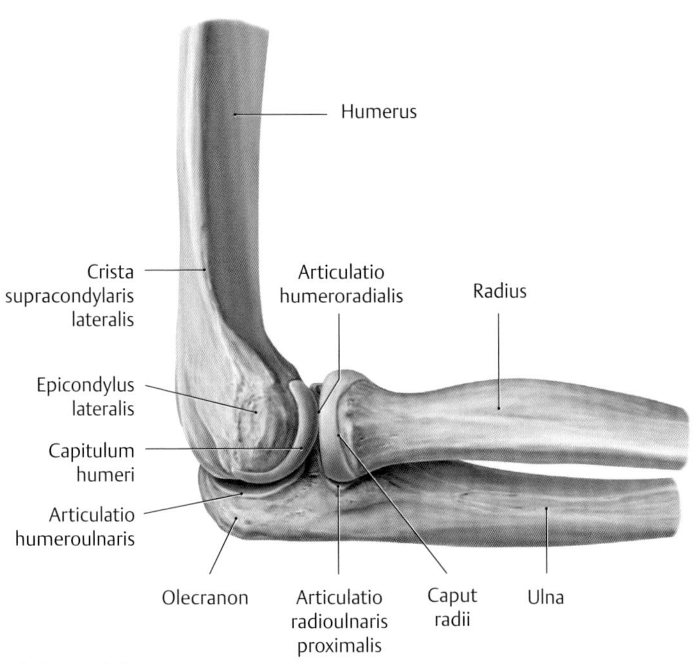
Humerus
Crista supracondylaris lateralis
Articulatio humeroradialis
Radius
Epicondylus lateralis
Capitulum humeri
Articulatio humeroulnaris
Olecranon
Articulatio radioulnaris proximalis
Caput radii
Ulna

D Lateral view.

Fig. 20.3 MRI of articulatio cubiti

Sagittal section.

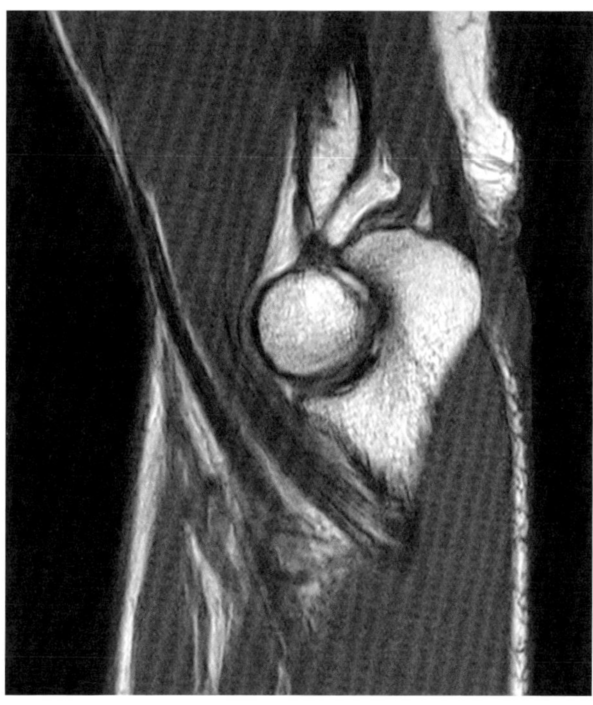

Fig. 20.4 Articulatio humeroulnaris

Sagittal section through articulatio humeroulnaris, medial view.

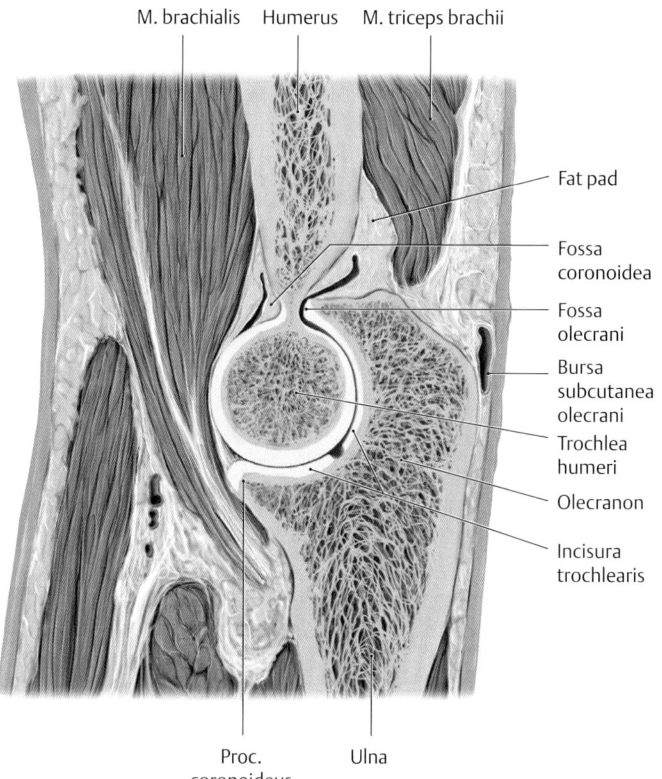
M. brachialis
Humerus
M. triceps brachii
Fat pad
Fossa coronoidea
Fossa olecrani
Bursa subcutanea olecrani
Trochlea humeri
Olecranon
Incisura trochlearis
Proc. coronoideus
Ulna

Clinical

Assessing elbow injuries

The fat pads between the fibrous capsule and synovial membrane are part of the normal anatomy of the elbow joint. The anterior pad is most readily seen on a sagittal MRI while the posterior pad is often hidden within the bony fossa (Fig. 20.3). With an effusion of the joint space, the inferior edge of the anterior pad appears concave as it gets pushed superiorly by the intra-articular fluid. This causes the pad to resemble the shape of a ship's sail, thus creating a characteristic "sail sign." The alignment of the prominences in the elbow also aids in the identification of fractures and dislocations.

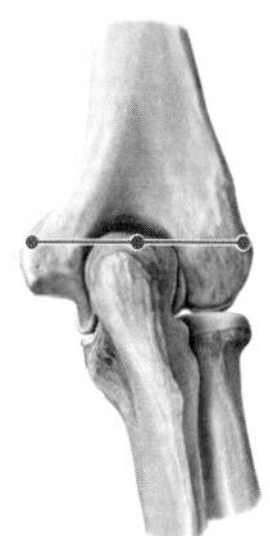

A Posterior view of extended elbow: The epicondyles and olecranon lie in a straight line.

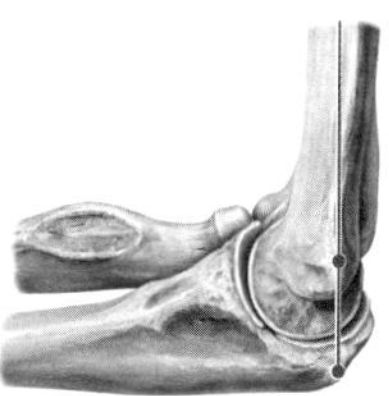

B Lateral view of flexed elbow: The epicondyles and olecranon lie in a straight line.

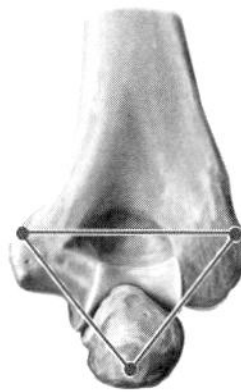

C Posterior view of flexed elbow: The two epicondyles and the tip of the olecranon form an equilateral triangle. Fractures and dislocations alter the shape of the triangle.

Ligaments of Articulatio Cubiti

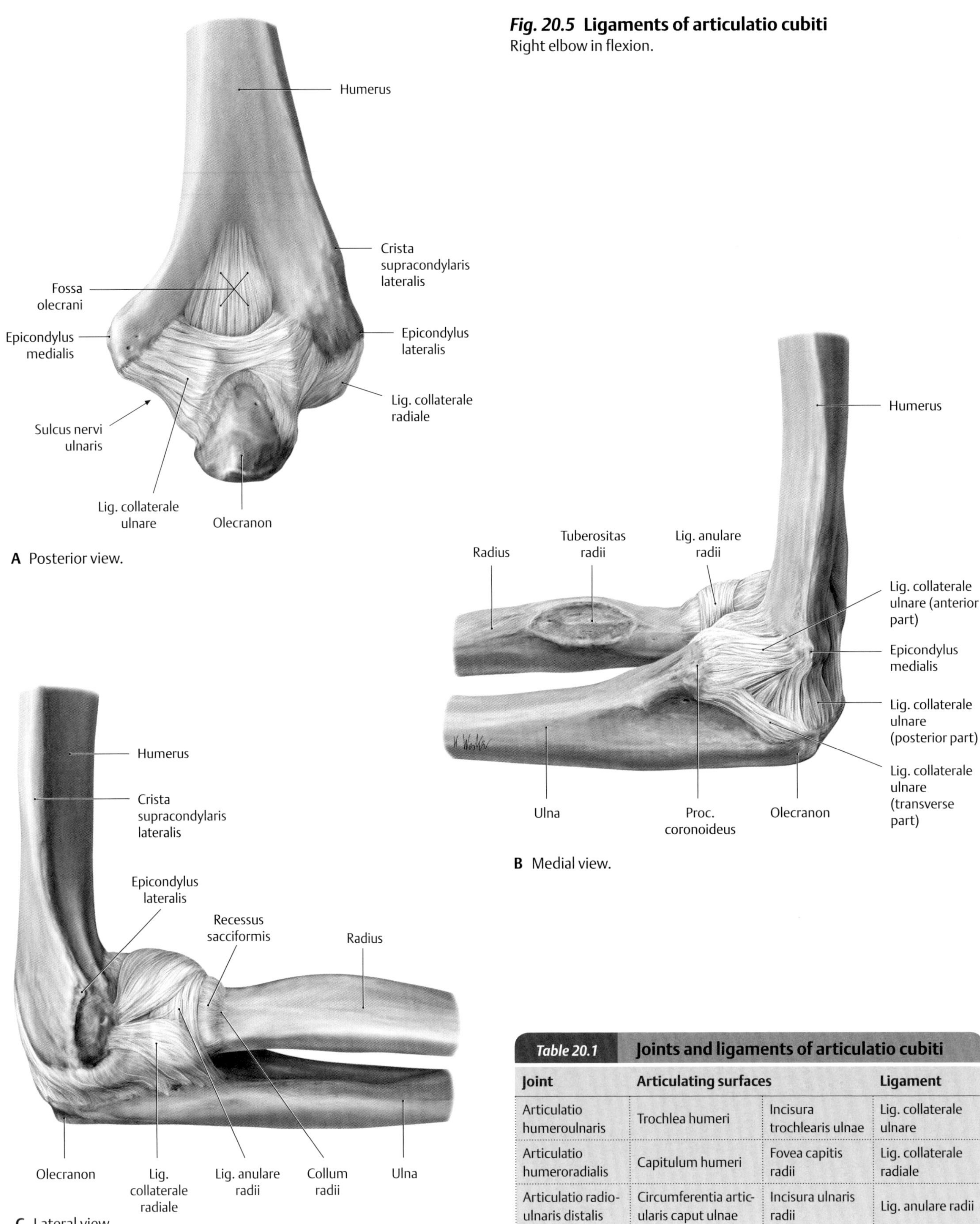
Humerus
Crista supracondylaris lateralis
Fossa olecrani
Epicondylus medialis
Epicondylus lateralis
Lig. collaterale radiale
Sulcus nervi ulnaris
Lig. collaterale ulnare
Olecranon
Radius
Tuberositas radii
Lig. anulare radii
Humerus
Lig. collaterale ulnare (anterior part)
Epicondylus medialis
Lig. collaterale ulnare (posterior part)
Lig. collaterale ulnare (transverse part)
Ulna
Proc. coronoideus
Olecranon
Humerus
Crista supracondylaris lateralis
Epicondylus lateralis
Recessus sacciformis
Radius
Olecranon
Lig. collaterale radiale
Lig. anulare radii
Collum radii
Ulna

Fig. 20.5 **Ligaments of articulatio cubiti**
Right elbow in flexion.

A Posterior view.

B Medial view.

C Lateral view.

Table 20.1 Joints and ligaments of articulatio cubiti

Joint	Articulating surfaces		Ligament
Articulatio humeroulnaris	Trochlea humeri	Incisura trochlearis ulnae	Lig. collaterale ulnare
Articulatio humeroradialis	Capitulum humeri	Fovea capitis radii	Lig. collaterale radiale
Articulatio radio-ulnaris distalis	Circumferentia articularis caput ulnae	Incisura ulnaris radii	Lig. anulare radii

Fig. 20.6 Joint capsule of articulatio cubiti

Right elbow in extension, anterior view.

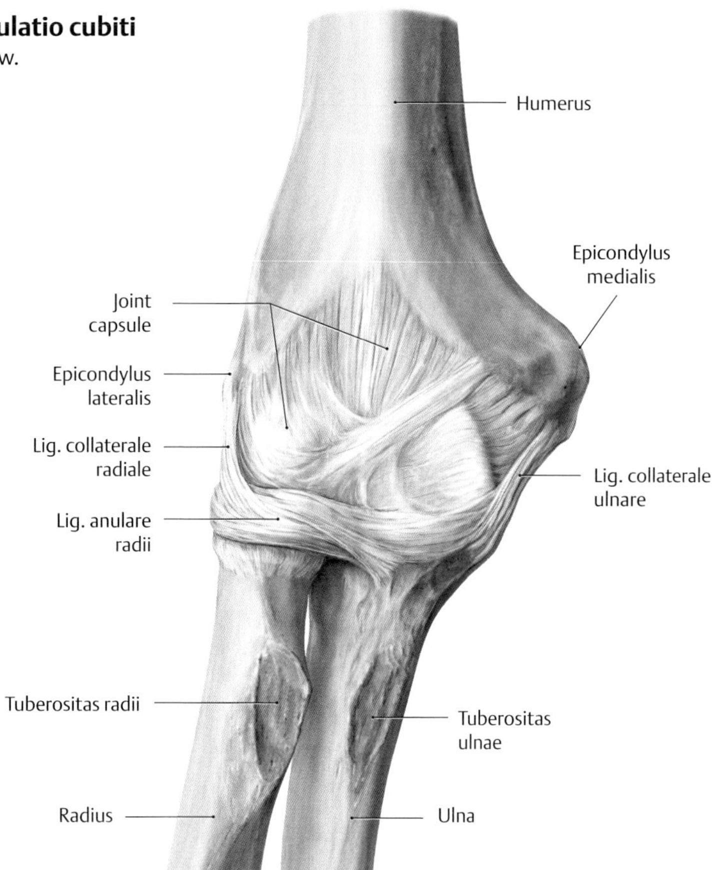
Humerus
Epicondylus medialis
Joint capsule
Epicondylus lateralis
Lig. collaterale radiale
Lig. collaterale ulnare
Lig. anulare radii
Tuberositas radii
Tuberositas ulnae
Radius
Ulna

A Intact joint capsule.

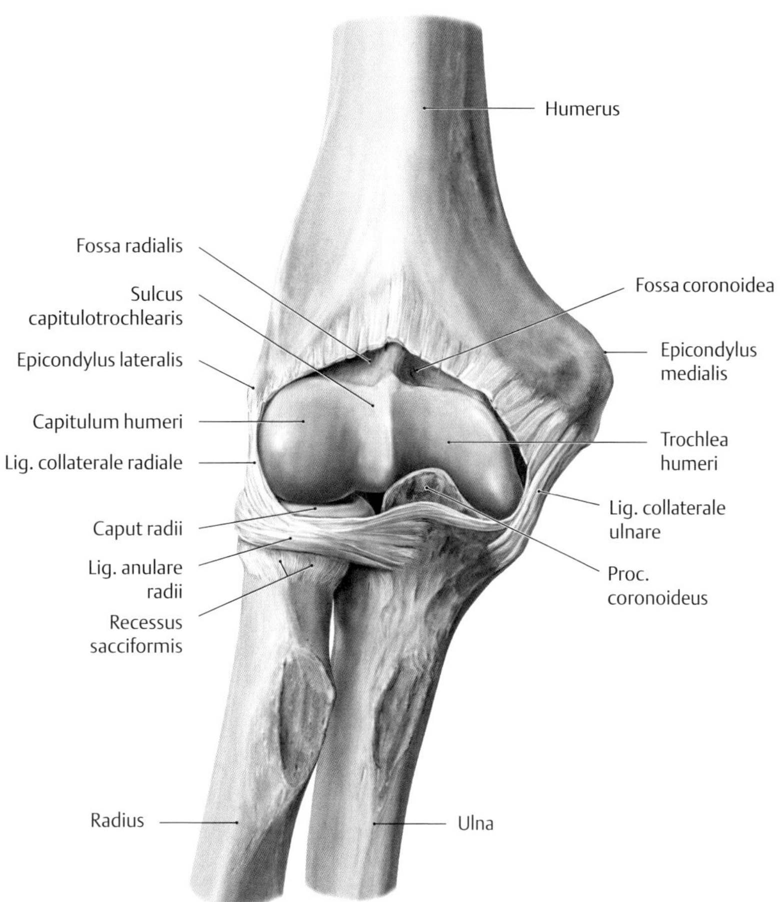
Humerus
Fossa radialis
Fossa coronoidea
Sulcus capitulotrochlearis
Epicondylus lateralis
Epicondylus medialis
Capitulum humeri
Trochlea humeri
Lig. collaterale radiale
Caput radii
Lig. collaterale ulnare
Lig. anulare radii
Proc. coronoideus
Recessus sacciformis
Radius
Ulna

B Windowed joint capsule.

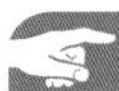

Radioulnar Joints

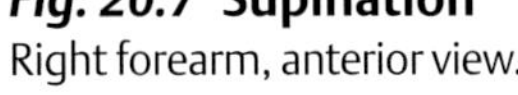

Articulatio radioulnaris proximalis and articulatio radioulnaris distalis function together to enable pronation and supination movements of the hand. The joints are functionally linked by membrana interossea antebrachii. The axis for pronation and supination runs obliquely from the center of capitulum humeri through the center of fovea articularis radii down to processus styloideus ulnae.

Fig. 20.7 **Supination**
Right forearm, anterior view.

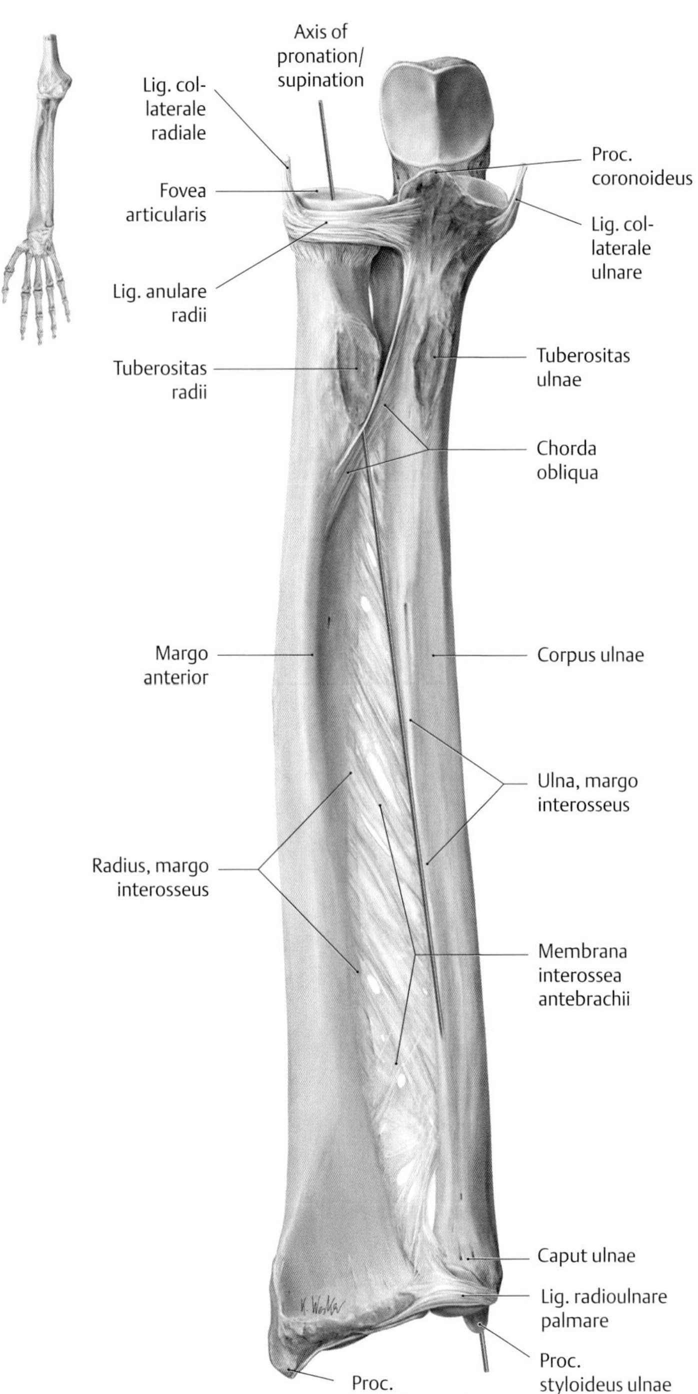

Axis of pronation/ supination
Lig. collaterale radiale
Fovea articularis
Lig. anulare radii
Tuberositas radii
Proc. coronoideus
Lig. collaterale ulnare
Tuberositas ulnae
Chorda obliqua
Margo anterior
Corpus ulnae
Ulna, margo interosseus
Radius, margo interosseus
Membrana interossea antebrachii
Caput ulnae
Lig. radioulnare palmare
Proc. styloideus ulnae
Proc. styloideus radii

Fig. 20.8 **Pronation**
Right forearm, anterior view.

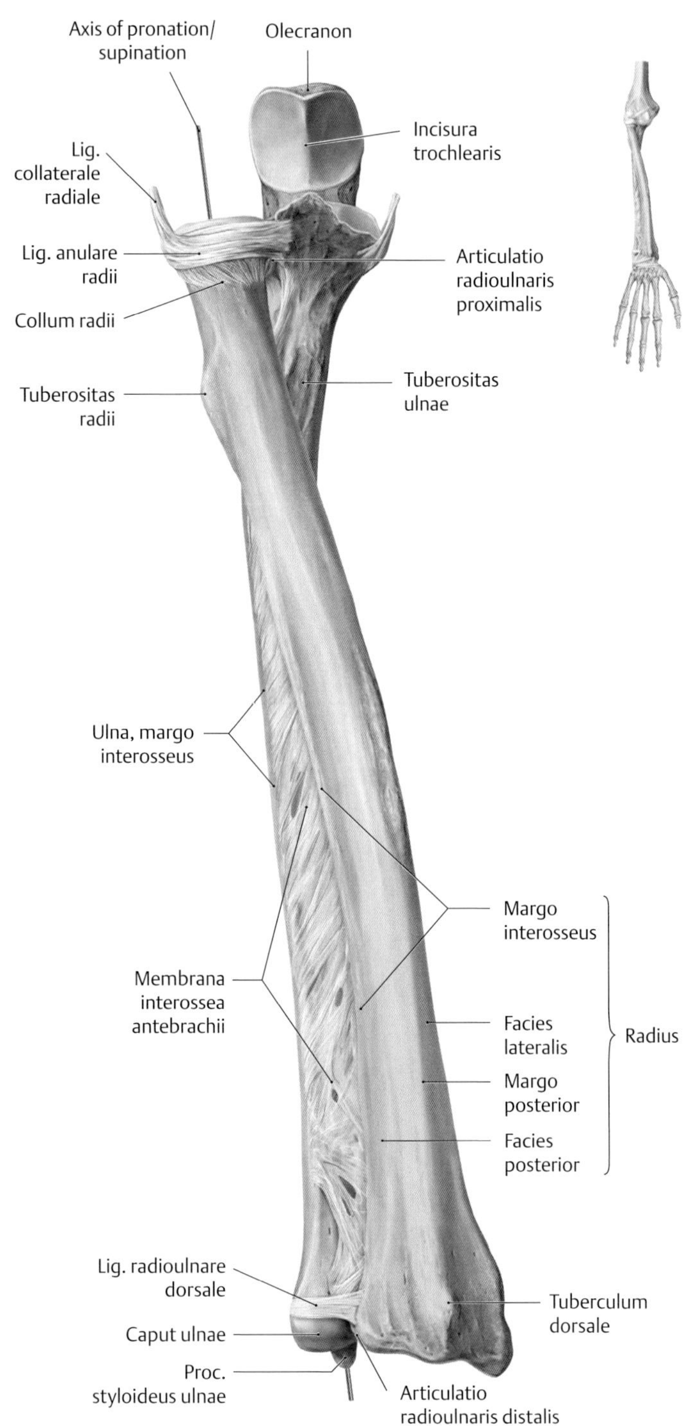

Axis of pronation/ supination
Olecranon
Incisura trochlearis
Lig. collaterale radiale
Lig. anulare radii
Collum radii
Articulatio radioulnaris proximalis
Tuberositas radii
Tuberositas ulnae
Ulna, margo interosseus
Margo interosseus
Facies lateralis
Margo posterior
Facies posterior
Radius
Membrana interossea antebrachii
Lig. radioulnare dorsale
Caput ulnae
Proc. styloideus ulnae
Tuberculum dorsale
Articulatio radioulnaris distalis

Clinical

Subluxation of caput radii ("nursemaid's elbow")

When small children are abruptly pulled up by their arm, the immature caput radii can dislocate from the lig. anulare radii, resulting in painful pronation.

Fig. 20.9 Articulatio radioulnaris proximalis

Right elbow, proximal (superior) view.

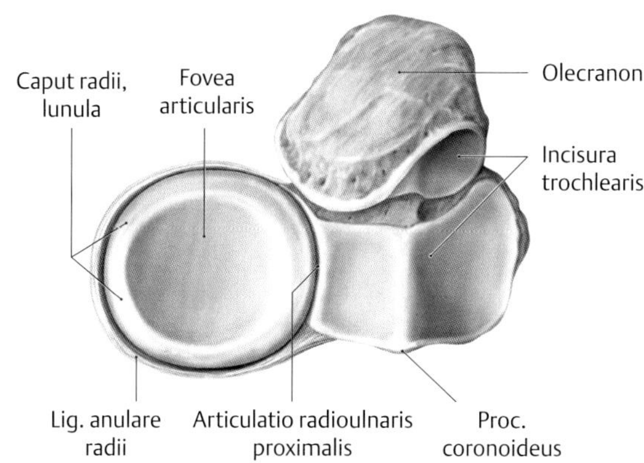
Caput radii, lunula
Fovea articularis
Olecranon
Incisura trochlearis
Lig. anulare radii
Articulatio radioulnaris proximalis
Proc. coronoideus

A Proximal articular surfaces of radius and ulna.

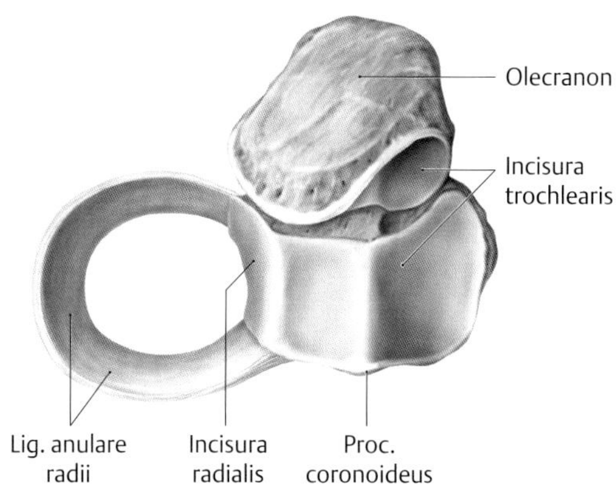
Olecranon
Incisura trochlearis
Lig. anulare radii
Incisura radialis
Proc. coronoideus

B Radius removed.

Clinical

Radius fracture

Falls onto the outstretched arm often result in fractures of the distal radius. In a "Colles' fracture," the distal fragment is tilted dorsally.

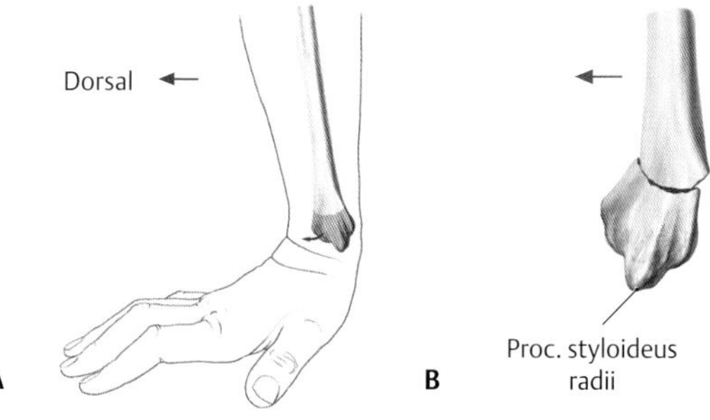
Dorsal
A
B
Proc. styloideus radii

Fig. 20.10 Rotation of articulatio radioulnaris distalis

Right forearm, distal view of articular surfaces of radius and ulna. The ligg. radioulnare dorsale and palmare stabilize articulatio radioulnaris distalis.

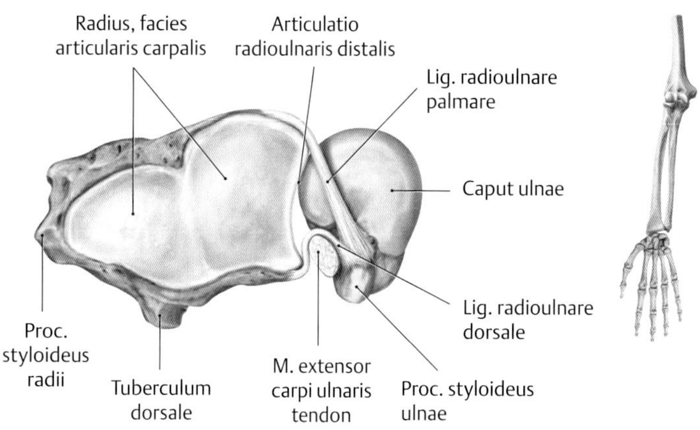
Radius, facies articularis carpalis
Articulatio radioulnaris distalis
Lig. radioulnare palmare
Caput ulnae
Lig. radioulnare dorsale
Proc. styloideus radii
Tuberculum dorsale
M. extensor carpi ulnaris tendon
Proc. styloideus ulnae

A Supination.

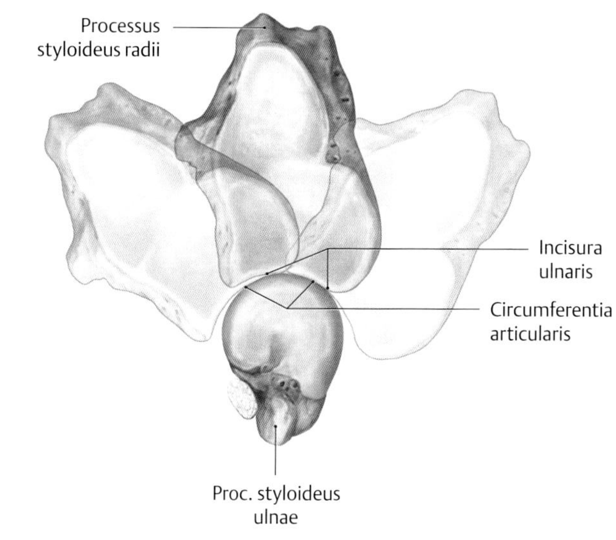
Processus styloideus radii
Incisura ulnaris
Circumferentia articularis
Proc. styloideus ulnae

B Semipronation.

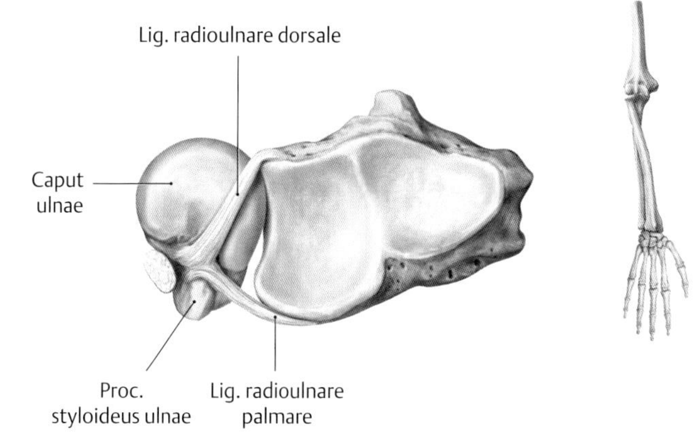
Lig. radioulnare dorsale
Caput ulnae
Proc. styloideus ulnae
Lig. radioulnare palmare

C Pronation.

Muscles of the Forearm (I)

Fig. 20.11 **Anterior muscles**
Right forearm, anterior view. Muscle origins (O) are shown in red, insertions (I) in blue.

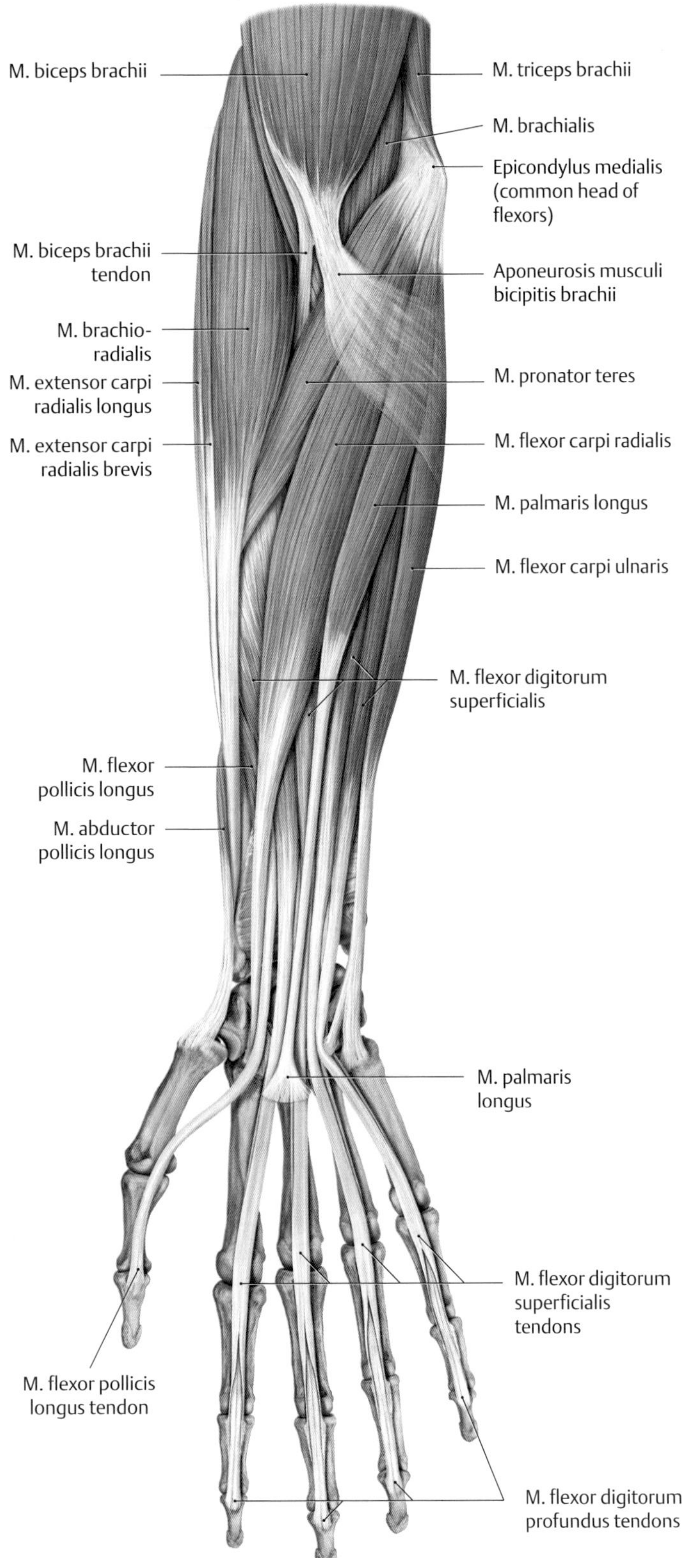
M. biceps brachii
M. triceps brachii
M. brachialis
Epicondylus medialis (common head of flexors)
M. biceps brachii tendon
Aponeurosis musculi bicipitis brachii
M. brachio-radialis
M. extensor carpi radialis longus
M. pronator teres
M. extensor carpi radialis brevis
M. flexor carpi radialis
M. palmaris longus
M. flexor carpi ulnaris
M. flexor digitorum superficialis
M. flexor pollicis longus
M. abductor pollicis longus
M. palmaris longus
M. flexor digitorum superficialis tendons
M. flexor pollicis longus tendon
M. flexor digitorum profundus tendons

A Superficial flexors and radialis group.

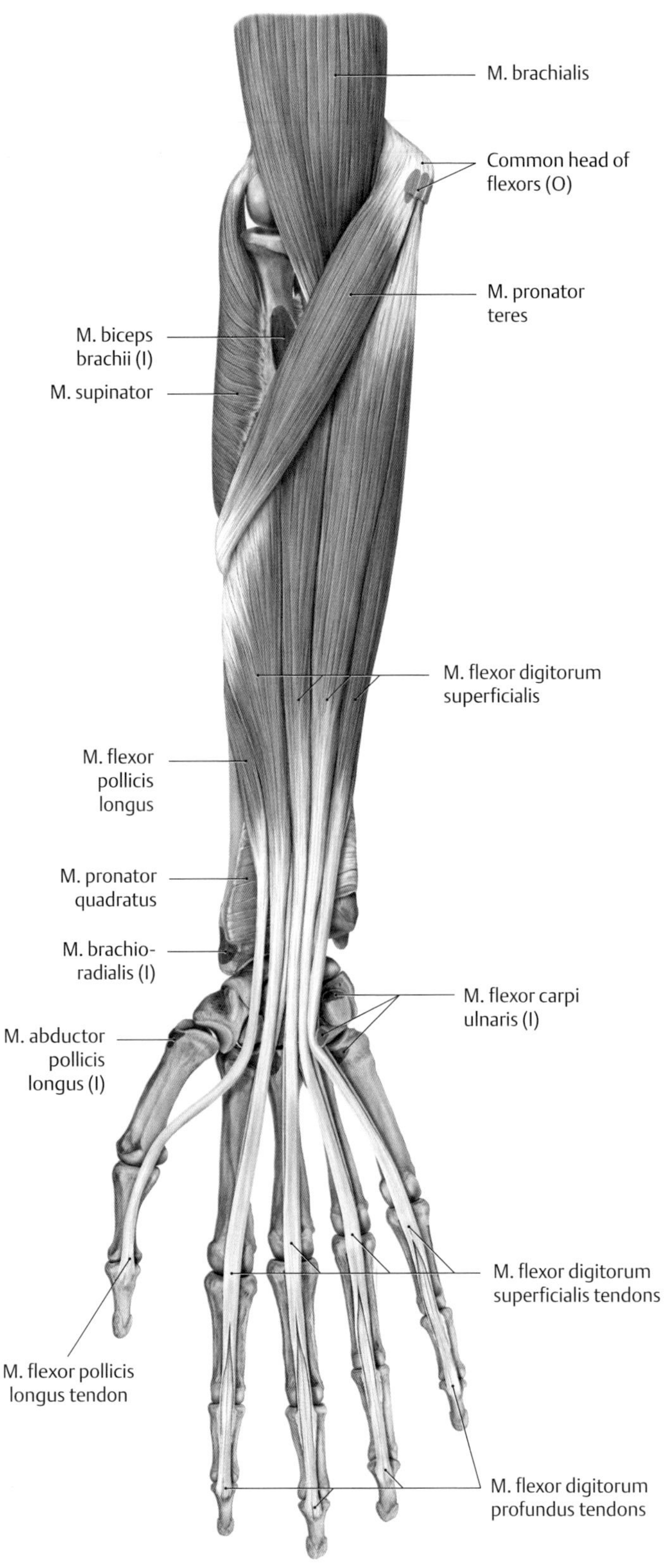
M. brachialis
Common head of flexors (O)
M. pronator teres
M. biceps brachii (I)
M. supinator
M. flexor digitorum superficialis
M. flexor pollicis longus
M. pronator quadratus
M. brachio-radialis (I)
M. flexor carpi ulnaris (I)
M. abductor pollicis longus (I)
M. flexor digitorum superficialis tendons
M. flexor pollicis longus tendon
M. flexor digitorum profundus tendons

B *Removed:* Radialis group (m. brachioradialis, m. extensor carpi radialis longus, and m. extensor carpi radialis brevis), m. flexor carpi radialis, m. flexor carpi ulnaris, m. abductor pollicis longus, m. palmaris longus, and m. biceps brachii.

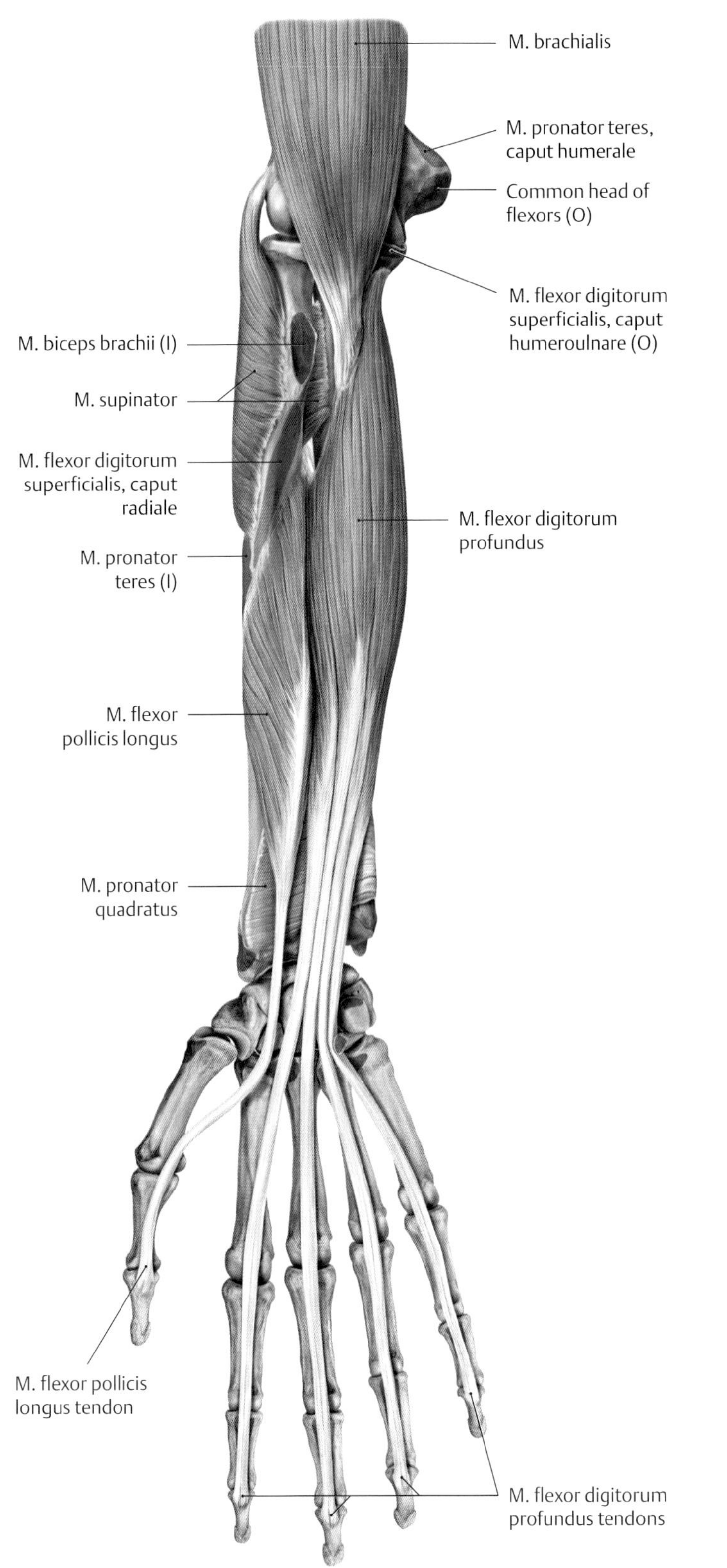
M. brachialis
M. pronator teres, caput humerale
Common head of flexors (O)
M. flexor digitorum superficialis, caput humeroulnare (O)
M. biceps brachii (I)
M. supinator
M. flexor digitorum superficialis, caput radiale
M. flexor digitorum profundus
M. pronator teres (I)
M. flexor pollicis longus
M. pronator quadratus
M. flexor pollicis longus tendon
M. flexor digitorum profundus tendons

C *Removed:* M. pronator teres and m. flexor digitorum superficialis.

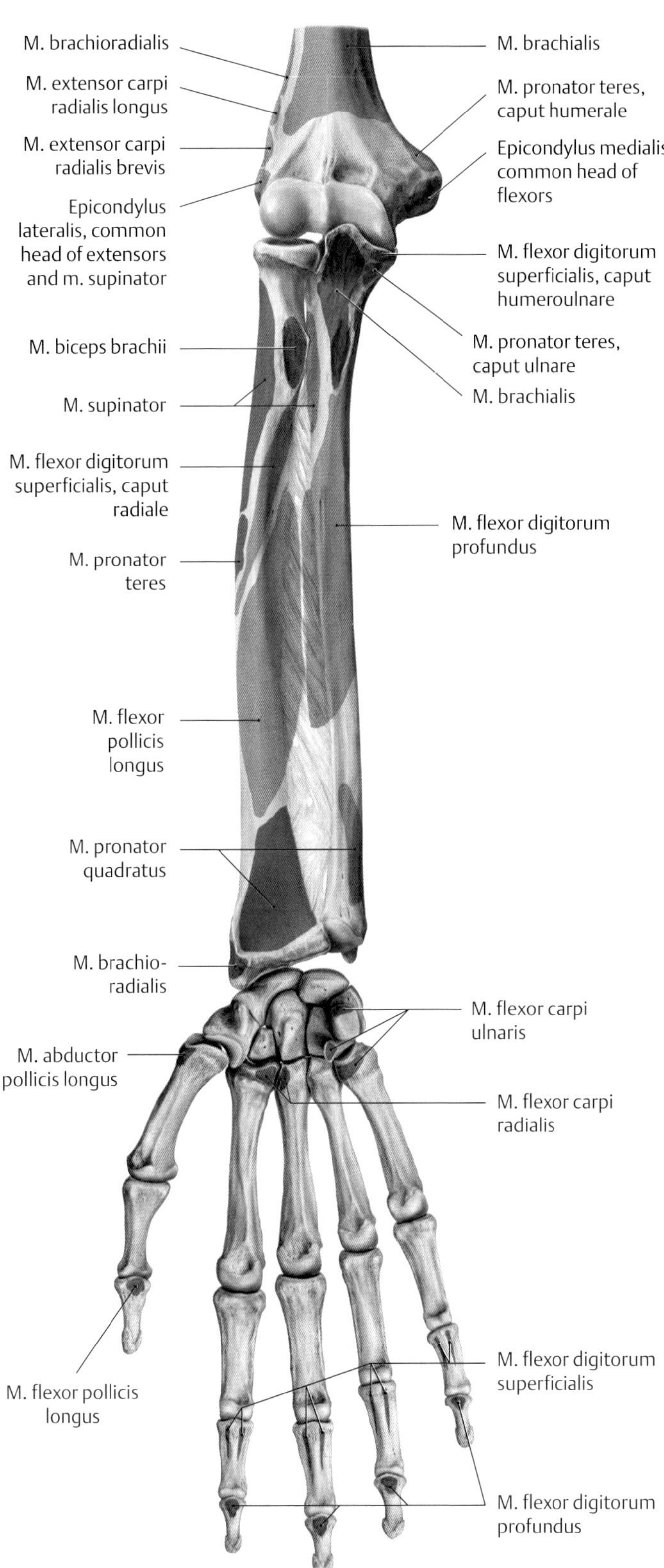
M. brachioradialis
M. brachialis
M. extensor carpi radialis longus
M. pronator teres, caput humerale
M. extensor carpi radialis brevis
Epicondylus medialis, common head of flexors
Epicondylus lateralis, common head of extensors and m. supinator
M. flexor digitorum superficialis, caput humeroulnare
M. pronator teres, caput ulnare
M. biceps brachii
M. brachialis
M. supinator
M. flexor digitorum superficialis, caput radiale
M. flexor digitorum profundus
M. pronator teres
M. flexor pollicis longus
M. pronator quadratus
M. brachio-radialis
M. flexor carpi ulnaris
M. abductor pollicis longus
M. flexor carpi radialis
M. flexor digitorum superficialis
M. flexor pollicis longus
M. flexor digitorum profundus

D *Removed:* M. brachialis, m. supinator, m. pronator quadratus, and deep flexors.

Muscles of the Forearm (II)

Fig. 20.12 **Posterior muscles**
Right forearm, posterior view. Muscle origins (O) are shown in red, insertions (I) in blue.

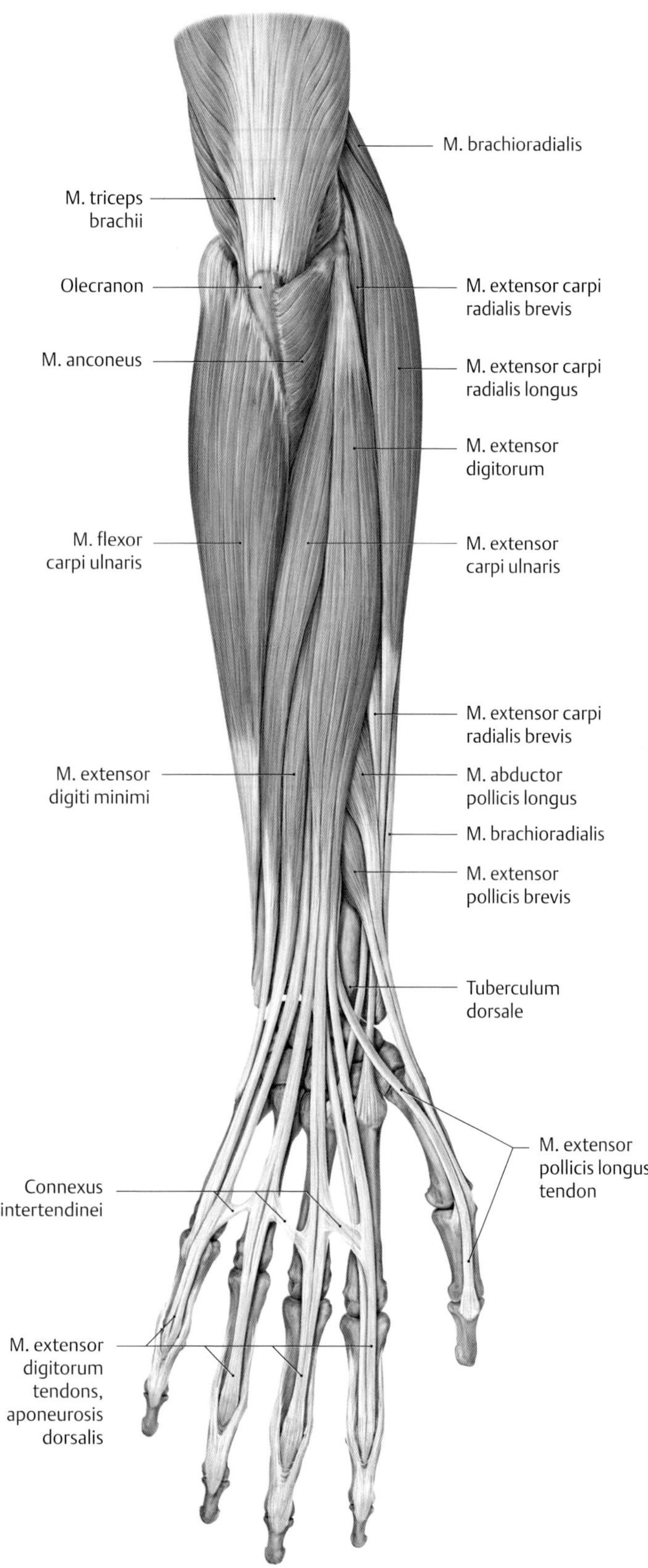
M. brachioradialis
M. triceps brachii
Olecranon
M. extensor carpi radialis brevis
M. anconeus
M. extensor carpi radialis longus
M. extensor digitorum
M. flexor carpi ulnaris
M. extensor carpi ulnaris
M. extensor carpi radialis brevis
M. extensor digiti minimi
M. abductor pollicis longus
M. brachioradialis
M. extensor pollicis brevis
Tuberculum dorsale
M. extensor pollicis longus tendon
Connexus intertendinei
M. extensor digitorum tendons, aponeurosis dorsalis

A Superficial extensors and radialis group.

M. brachioradialis
M. triceps brachii
Epicondylus medialis, common head of flexors (O)
M. extensor carpi radialis longus
M. anconeus (O and I)
M. extensor carpi radialis brevis
M. flexor digitorum profundus
M. supinator
M. flexor carpi ulnaris (O)
M. abductor pollicis longus
M. extensor pollicis longus
M. brachioradialis
M. extensor pollicis brevis
M. extensor carpi ulnaris (O and I)
M. extensor indicis
M. extensor carpi radialis brevis tendon
M. extensor carpi radialis longus tendon
M. extensor digiti minimi (I)
M. extensor digitorum (I)

B *Removed:* M. triceps brachii, m. anconeus, m. flexor carpi ulnaris, m. extensor carpi ulnaris, and m. extensor digitorum.

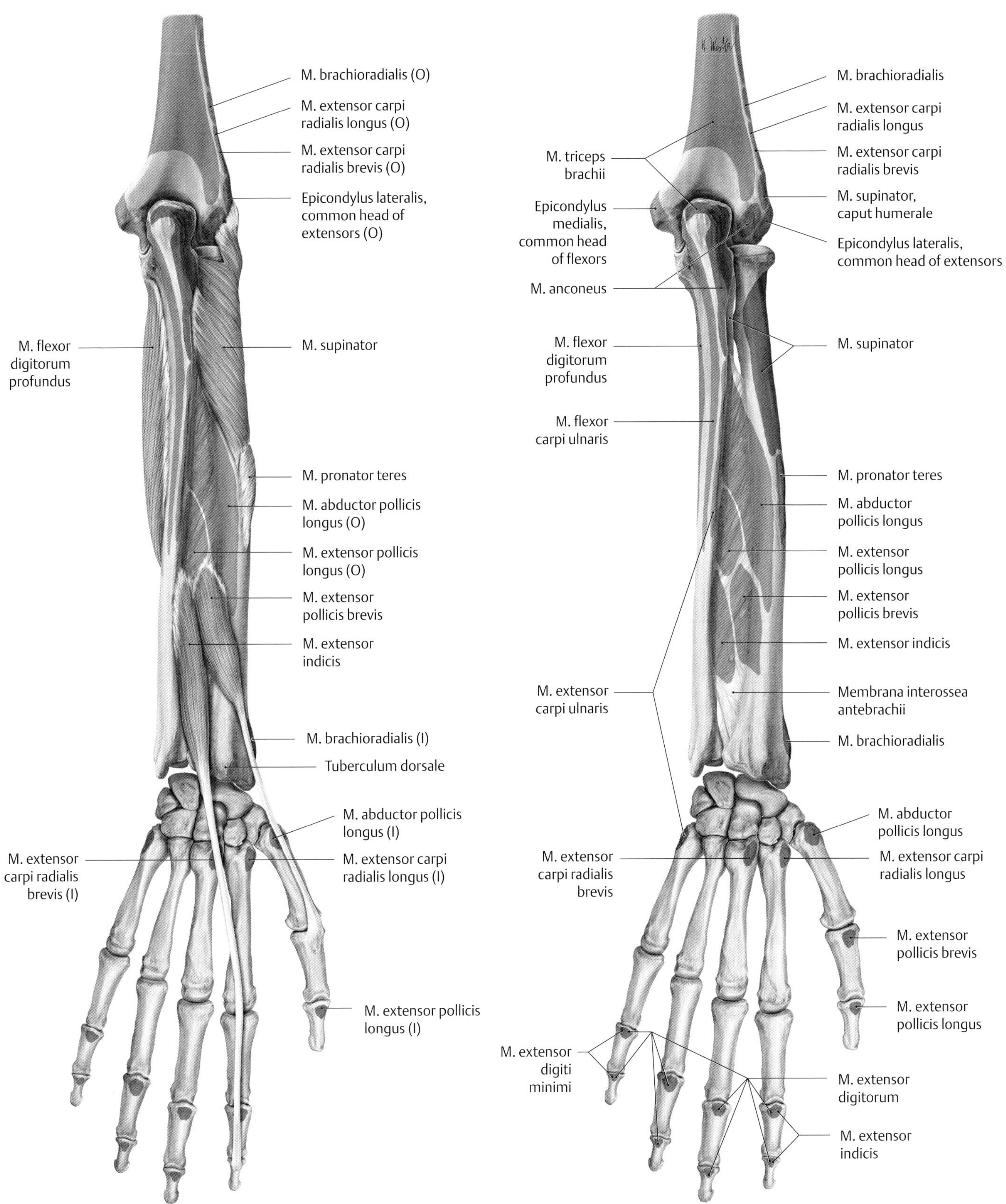

M. brachioradialis (O)
M. extensor carpi radialis longus (O)
M. extensor carpi radialis brevis (O)
Epicondylus lateralis, common head of extensors (O)
M. flexor digitorum profundus
M. supinator
M. pronator teres
M. abductor pollicis longus (O)
M. extensor pollicis longus (O)
M. extensor pollicis brevis
M. extensor indicis
M. brachioradialis (I)
Tuberculum dorsale
M. abductor pollicis longus (I)
M. extensor carpi radialis brevis (I)
M. extensor carpi radialis longus (I)
M. extensor pollicis longus (I)
M. brachioradialis
M. extensor carpi radialis longus
M. triceps brachii
M. extensor carpi radialis brevis
Epicondylus medialis, common head of flexors
M. supinator, caput humerale
Epicondylus lateralis, common head of extensors
M. anconeus
M. flexor digitorum profundus
M. supinator
M. flexor carpi ulnaris
M. pronator teres
M. abductor pollicis longus
M. extensor pollicis longus
M. extensor pollicis brevis
M. extensor indicis
M. extensor carpi ulnaris
Membrana interossea antebrachii
M. brachioradialis
M. abductor pollicis longus
M. extensor carpi radialis brevis
M. extensor carpi radialis longus
M. extensor pollicis brevis
M. extensor pollicis longus
M. extensor digiti minimi
M. extensor digitorum
M. extensor indicis

C *Removed:* M. abductor pollicis longus, m. extensor pollicis longus, and radialis group.

D *Removed:* M. flexor digitorum profundus, m. supinator, m. extensor pollicis brevis, and m. extensor indicis.

Muscle Facts (I)

Fig. 20.13 **Anterior compartment**
Right forearm, anterior view.

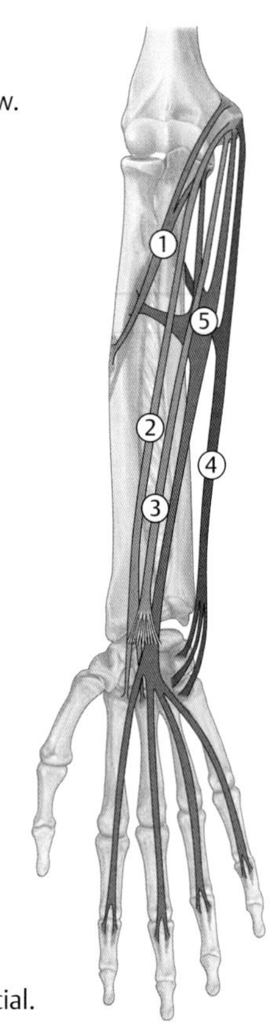

①
②
③
④
⑤

A Superficial.

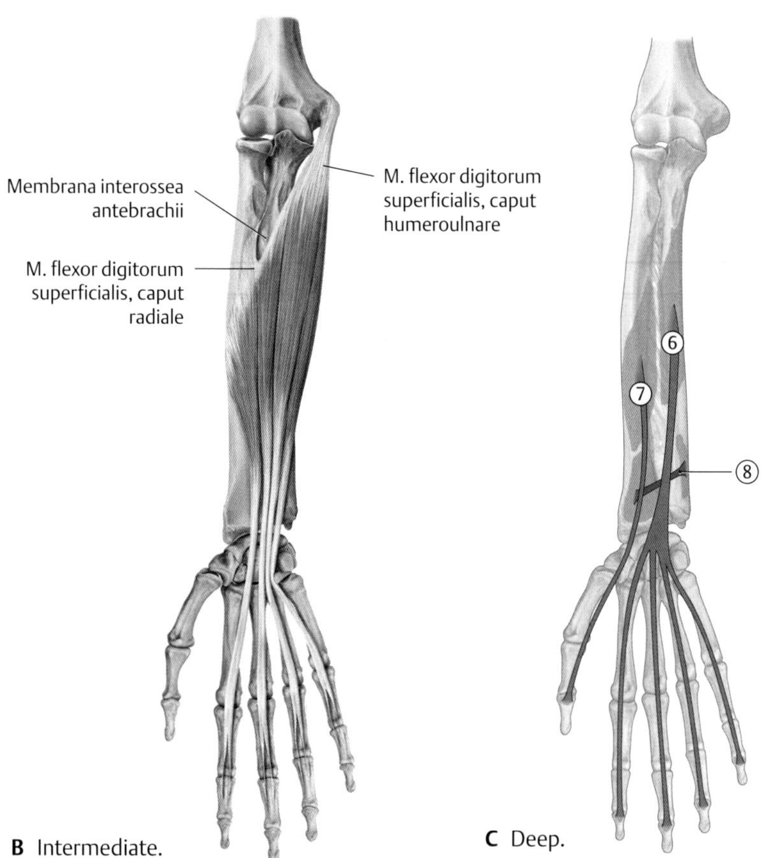

Membrana interossea antebrachii
M. flexor digitorum superficialis, caput radiale
M. flexor digitorum superficialis, caput humeroulnare
⑥
⑦
⑧

B Intermediate.

C Deep.

Table 20.2 **Anterior compartment of the forearm**

Muscle	Origin	Insertion	Innervation	Action
Superficial group				
① M. pronator teres	Caput humerale: Epicondylus medialis humeri Caput ulnare: Proc. coronoideus ulnae	Lateral radius (distal to supinator insertion)	N. medianus (C6, C7)	Art. cubiti: weak flexor Forearm: pronation
② M. flexor carpi radialis	Epicondylus medialis humeri	Base of os metacarpale II (variance: base of os metacarpale III)		Wrist: flexion and abduction (radial deviation) of hand
③ M. palmaris longus		Aponeurosis palmaris	N. medianus (C7, C8)	Art. cubiti: weak flexion Wrist: flexion tightens aponeurosis palmaris
④ M. flexor carpi ulnaris	Caput humerale: Epicondylus medialis humeri Caput ulnare: olecranon	Os pisiforme; hook of Os hamatum; base of 5th os metacarpale	N. ulnaris (C7–T1)	Wrist: flexion and adduction (ulnar deviation) of hand
Intermediate group				
⑤ M. flexor digitorum superficialis	Caput humerale: Epicondylus medialis humeri Caput ulnare: Processus coronoideus	Sides of phalanges mediales of digitus II to V	N. medianus (C8, T1)	Art. cubiti: weak flexor Wrist, art. metacarpophalangealis, and art. interphalangelais proximalis of digitus II to V: flexion
Deep group				
⑥ M. flexor digitorum profundis	Ulna (two thirds of flexor surface) and membrana interosseous antebrachii	Phalanges distales of digitus II to V (palmar surface)	N. medianus (C8, T1) N. ulnaris (C8, T1)	Wrist, art. metacarpophalangealis, and art. interphalangealis proximalis of digitus II to V: flexion
⑦ M. flexor pollicis longus	Radius (midanterior surface) and adjacent membrana interossea antebrachii	Phalanx distalis pollicis (palmar surface)	N. medianus (C7, C8)	Wrist: flexion and abduction (radial deviation) of hand Art. carpometacarpalis pollicis: flexion Art. metacarpophalangealis pollicis and art. interphalangelis pollicis: flexion
⑧ M. pronator quadratus	Distal quarter of ulna (anterior surface)	Distal quarter of radius (anterior surface)		Hand: pronation Art. radioulnaris distalis: stabilization

DIP = distal interphalangeal; IP = interphalangeal; MCP = metacarpophalangeal; PIP = proximal interphalangeal.

Fig. 20.14 Superficial and intermediate groups
Right forearm, anterior view.

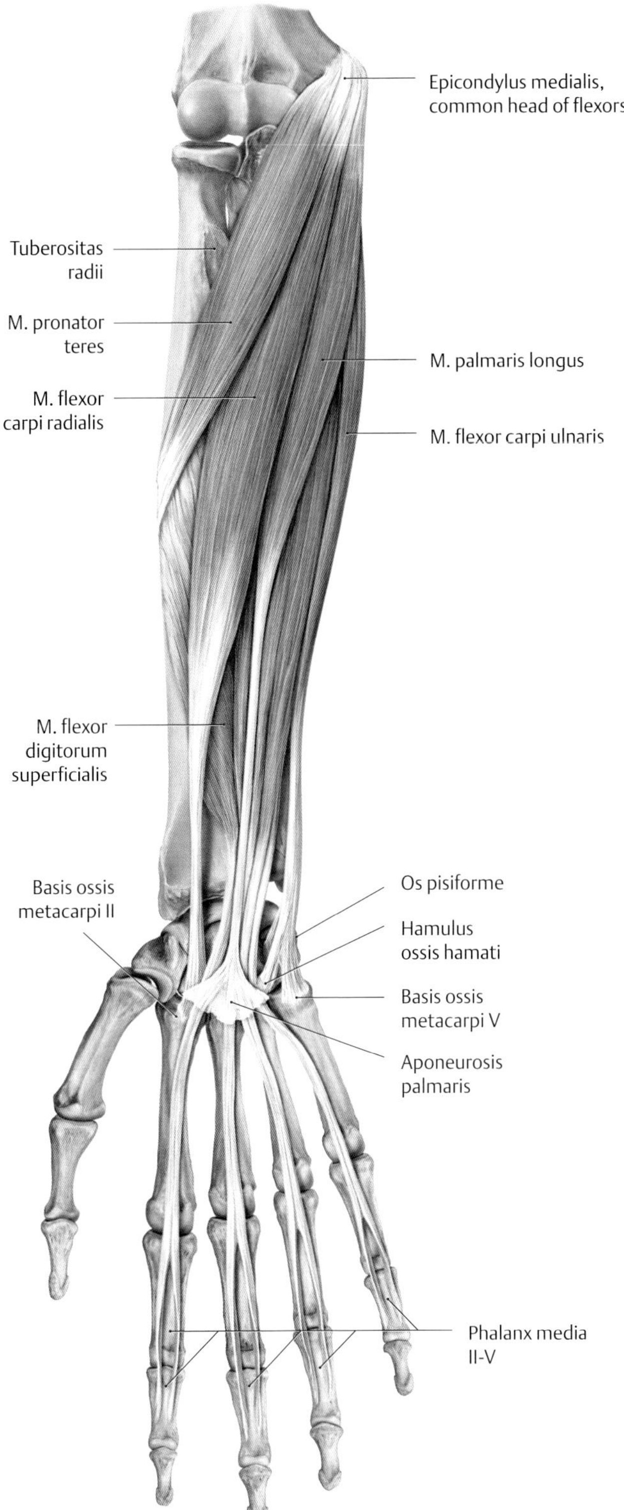
Epicondylus medialis, common head of flexors
Tuberositas radii
M. pronator teres
M. palmaris longus
M. flexor carpi radialis
M. flexor carpi ulnaris
M. flexor digitorum superficialis
Basis ossis metacarpi II
Os pisiforme
Hamulus ossis hamati
Basis ossis metacarpi V
Aponeurosis palmaris
Phalanx media II-V

Fig. 20.15 Deep group
Right forearm, anterior view.

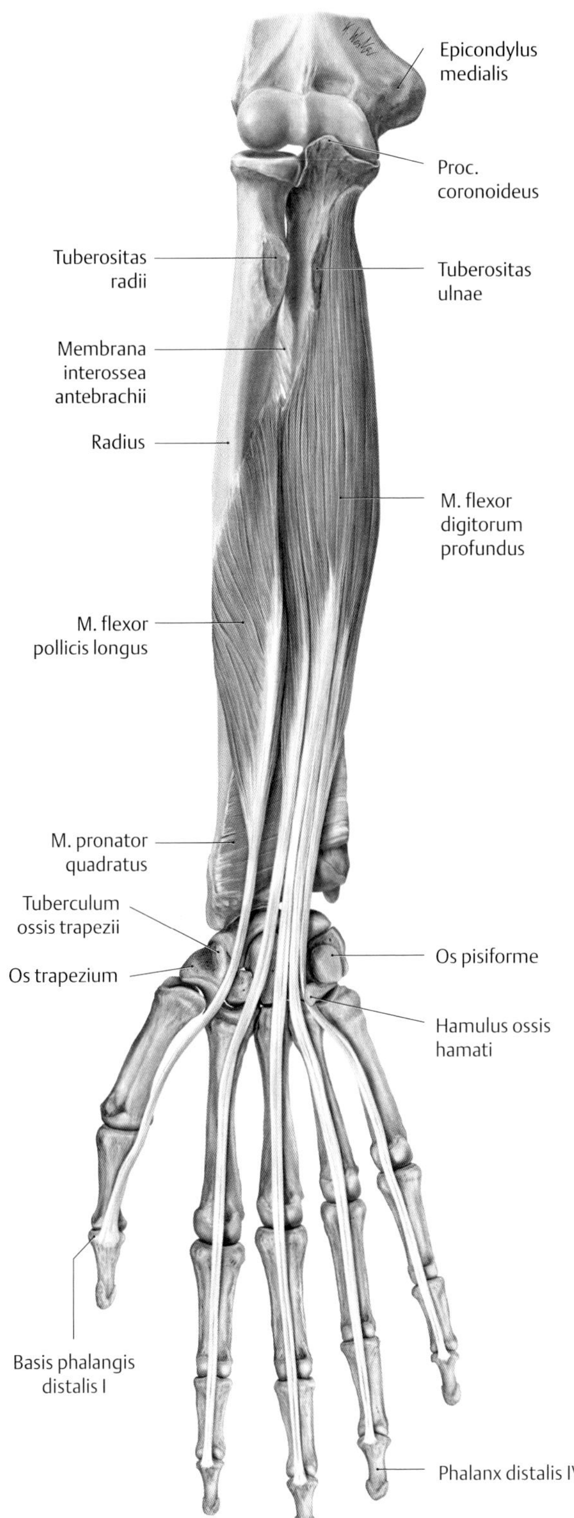
Epicondylus medialis
Proc. coronoideus
Tuberositas radii
Tuberositas ulnae
Membrana interossea antebrachii
Radius
M. flexor digitorum profundus
M. flexor pollicis longus
M. pronator quadratus
Tuberculum ossis trapezii
Os pisiforme
Os trapezium
Hamulus ossis hamati
Basis phalangis distalis I
Phalanx distalis IV

Muscle Facts (II)

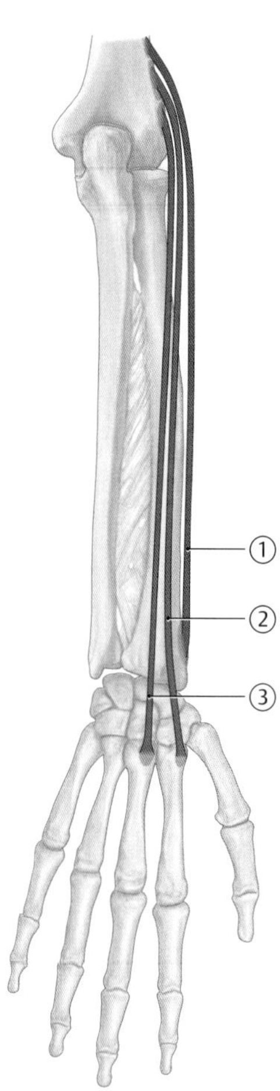
①
②
③

Fig. 20.16 **Radialis group**
Right forearm, posterior view.

Table 20.3 Posterior compartment of the forearm: Radialis muscles

Muscle	Origin	Insertion	Innervation	Action
① M. brachioradialis	Crista supra(epi)condylaris lateralis humeris, septum intermusculare laterale	Proc. styloideus radii	N. radialis (C5, C6)	Art. cubiti: flexion Forearm: semipronation
② M. extensor carpi radialis longus	Crista supra(epi)condylaris lateralis humeris, septum intermusculare laterale	Os metacarpale II	N. radialis (C6, C7)	Art. cubiti: weak flexion Wrist: extension and abduction
③ M. extensor carpi radialis brevis	Epicondylus lateralis humeri	Os metacarpale III	N. radialis (C7, C8)	

Fig. 20.17 **Radialis muscles of the forearm**
Right forearm.

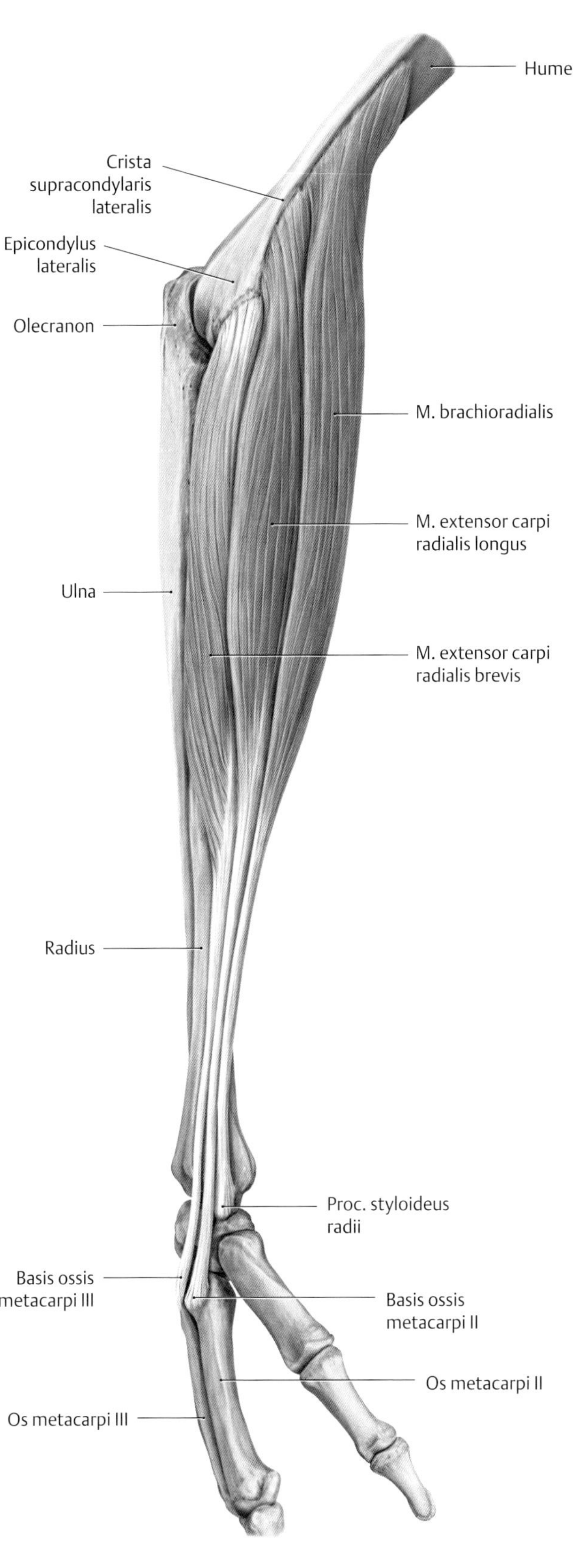
Humerus
Crista supracondylaris lateralis
Epicondylus lateralis
Olecranon
M. brachioradialis
M. extensor carpi radialis longus
Ulna
M. extensor carpi radialis brevis
Radius
Proc. styloideus radii
Basis ossis metacarpi III
Basis ossis metacarpi II
Os metacarpi II
Os metacarpi III

A Lateral (radial) view.

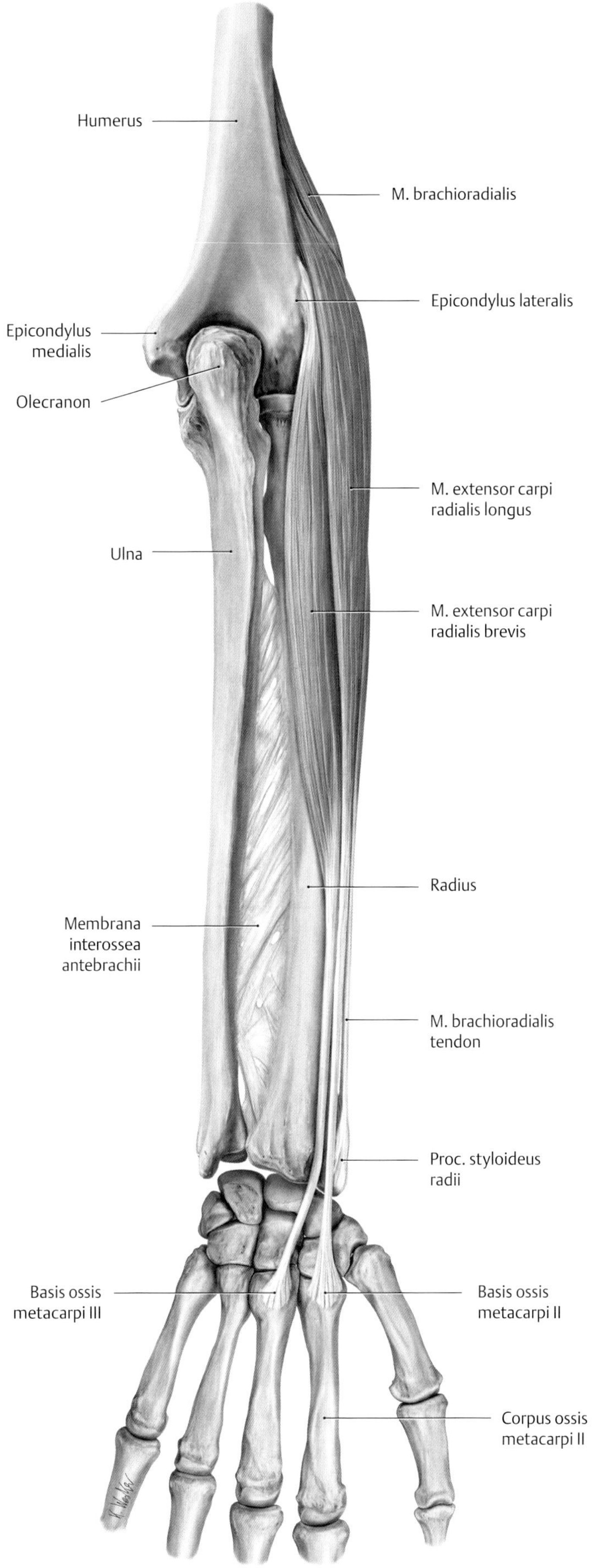

Humerus
M. brachioradialis
Epicondylus lateralis
Epicondylus medialis
Olecranon
M. extensor carpi radialis longus
Ulna
M. extensor carpi radialis brevis
Radius
Membrana interossea antebrachii
M. brachioradialis tendon
Proc. styloideus radii
Basis ossis metacarpi III
Basis ossis metacarpi II
Corpus ossis metacarpi II

B Posterior view.

Muscle Facts (III)

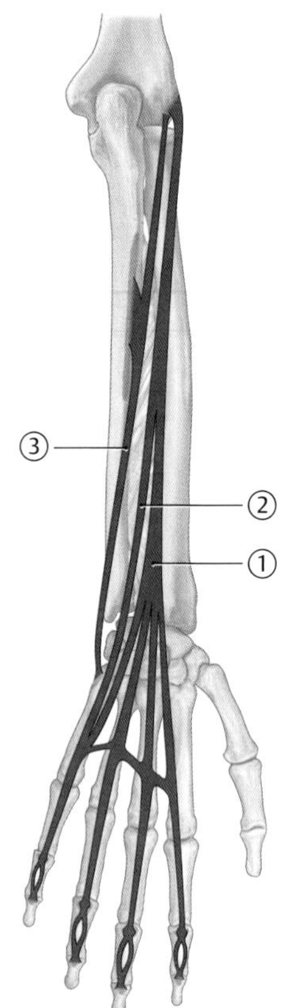
③
②
①

Fig. 20.18 **Superficial group**
Right forearm, posterior view.

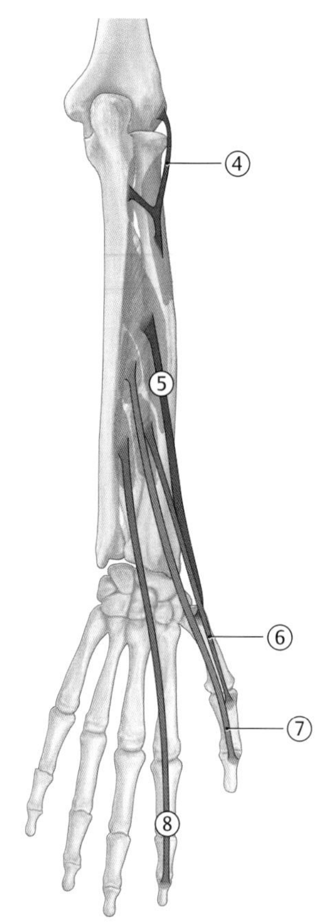
④
⑤
⑥
⑦
⑧

Fig. 20.19 **Deep group**
Right forearm, posterior view.

Table 20.4 **Posterior compartment of the forearm**

Muscle	Origin	Insertion	Innervation	Action
Superficial group				
① M. extensor digitorum	Epicondylus lateralis humeri	Aponeurosis palmaris digitus II–V	N. radialis (C7, C8)	Wrist: extension MCP, PIP, and DIP of digitus II–V: extension/ abduction of fingers
② M. extensor digiti minimi		Aponeurosis palmaris		Wrist: extension, ulnar abduction of hand MCP, PIP, and DIP of digitus V: extension and abduction of digitus V
③ M. extensor carpi ulnaris	Caput humerale: Epicondylus lat. humeri Caput ulnare: Ulnar	Os metacarpale V		Wrist: extension, adduction (ulnar deviation) of hand
Deep group				
④ M. supinator	Olecranon, Epicondylus lateralis humeri, Lig. collaterale radiale, Lig. anulare radii	Radius (tuberositas radii and insertion of M. pronator teres)	N. radialis (C6, C7)	Articulatio radioulnaris : supination
⑤ M. abductor pollicis longus	Facies dorsalis ulnae et radii, membrana interossea antebrachii	Base of Os metacarpale pollicis	N. radialis (C7, C8)	Articulatio radioulnaris: abduction of the hand Articulatio carpometacarpale pollicis: abduction
⑥ M. extensor pollicis brevis	Facies dorsalis radii and membrana interossea antebrachii	Base of Phalanx proximalis pollicis		Articulatio radiocarpale: abduction (radial deviation) of hand Art. carpometacarpale and art. metacarpophangealis pollicis : extension
⑦ M. extensor pollicis longus	Facies dorsalis ulnae and membrana interossea antebrachii	Base of Phalanx proximalis pollicis		Wrist: extension and abduction (radial deviation) of hand Art. carpometacarpale pollicis : adduction MCP and IP of thumb: extension
⑧ M. extensor indicis	Facies dorsalis ulnae, Membrana interossea antebrachii	Posterior digital extension of digitus II		Wrist: extension MCP, PIP, and DIP of digitus II: extension

DIP = distal interphalangeal; IP = interphalangeal; MCP = metacarpophalangeal; PIP = proximal interphalangeal.

Fig. 20.20 Muscles of the posterior forearm

Right forearm, posterior view.

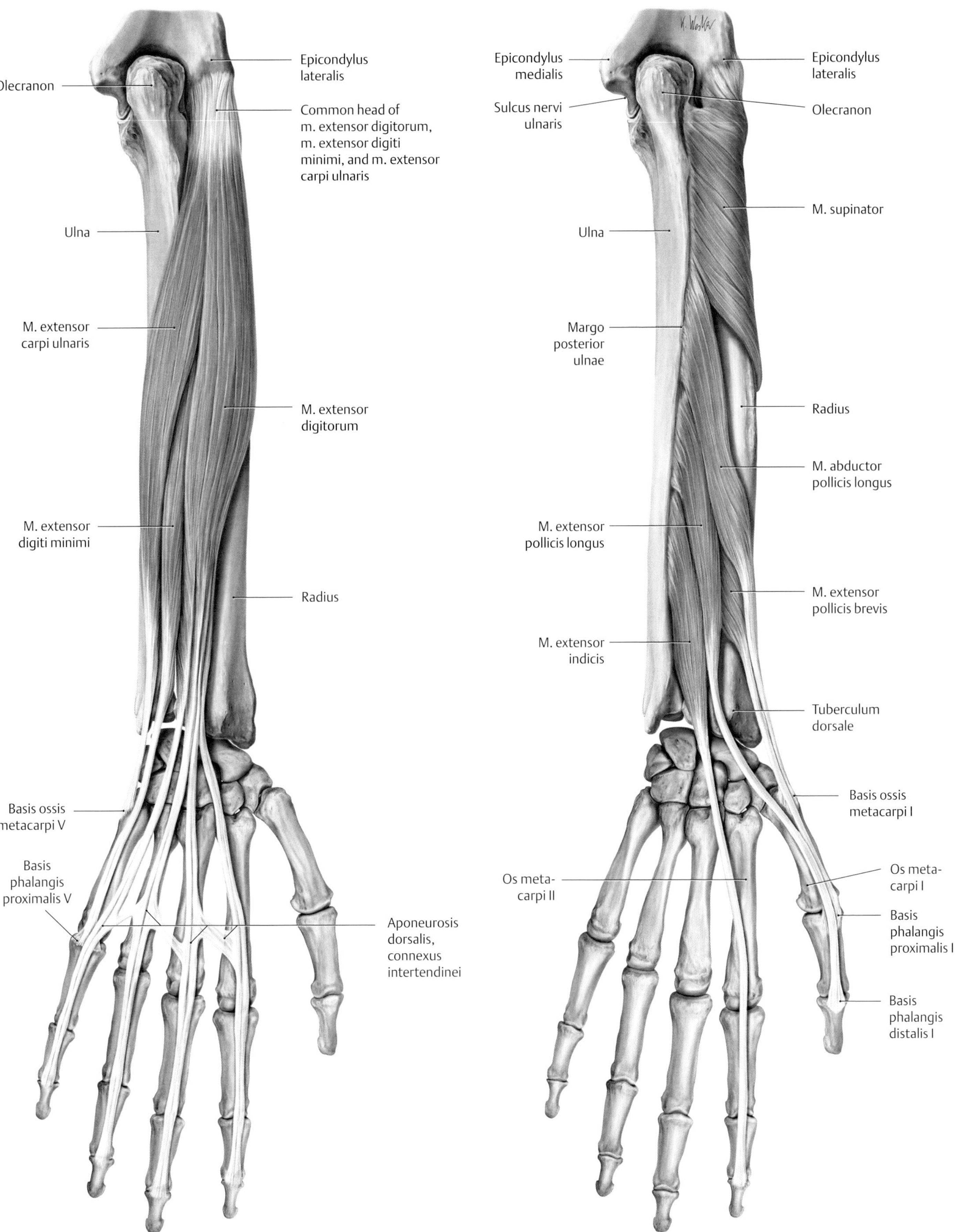
Olecranon
Epicondylus lateralis
Common head of m. extensor digitorum, m. extensor digiti minimi, and m. extensor carpi ulnaris
Ulna
M. extensor carpi ulnaris
M. extensor digitorum
M. extensor digiti minimi
Radius
Basis ossis metacarpi V
Basis phalangis proximalis V
Aponeurosis dorsalis, connexus intertendinei
Epicondylus medialis
Epicondylus lateralis
Sulcus nervi ulnaris
Olecranon
M. supinator
Ulna
Margo posterior ulnae
Radius
M. abductor pollicis longus
M. extensor pollicis longus
M. extensor pollicis brevis
M. extensor indicis
Tuberculum dorsale
Basis ossis metacarpi I
Os metacarpi II
Os metacarpi I
Basis phalangis proximalis I
Basis phalangis distalis I

A Superficial extensors.

B Deep extensors with m. supinator.

Bones of the Wrist & Hand

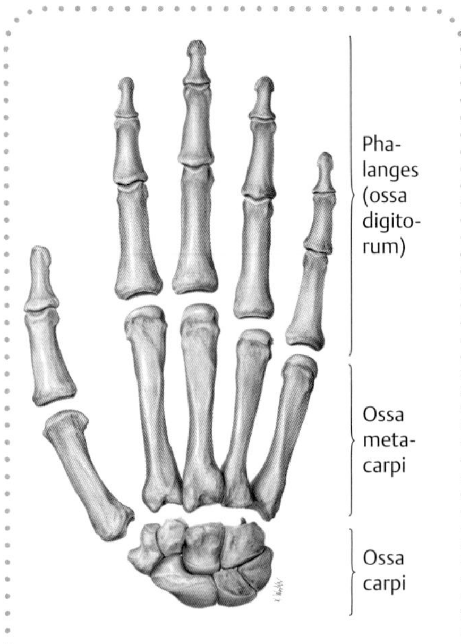
Phalanges (ossa digitorum)
Ossa metacarpi
Ossa carpi

Table 21.1	Bones of the wrist and hand	
Ossa digitorum manus	Phalanges proximales I–V	
	Phalanges mediales II–V*	
	Phalanges distales I–V	
Ossa metacarpi	Ossa metacarpalia I–V	
Ossa carpi	Os trapezium	Os scaphoideum
	Os trapezoideum	Os lunatum
	Os capitatum	Os triquetrum
	Os hamatum	

*There are only four middle phalanges (the thumb has only a proximal and a distal phalanx).

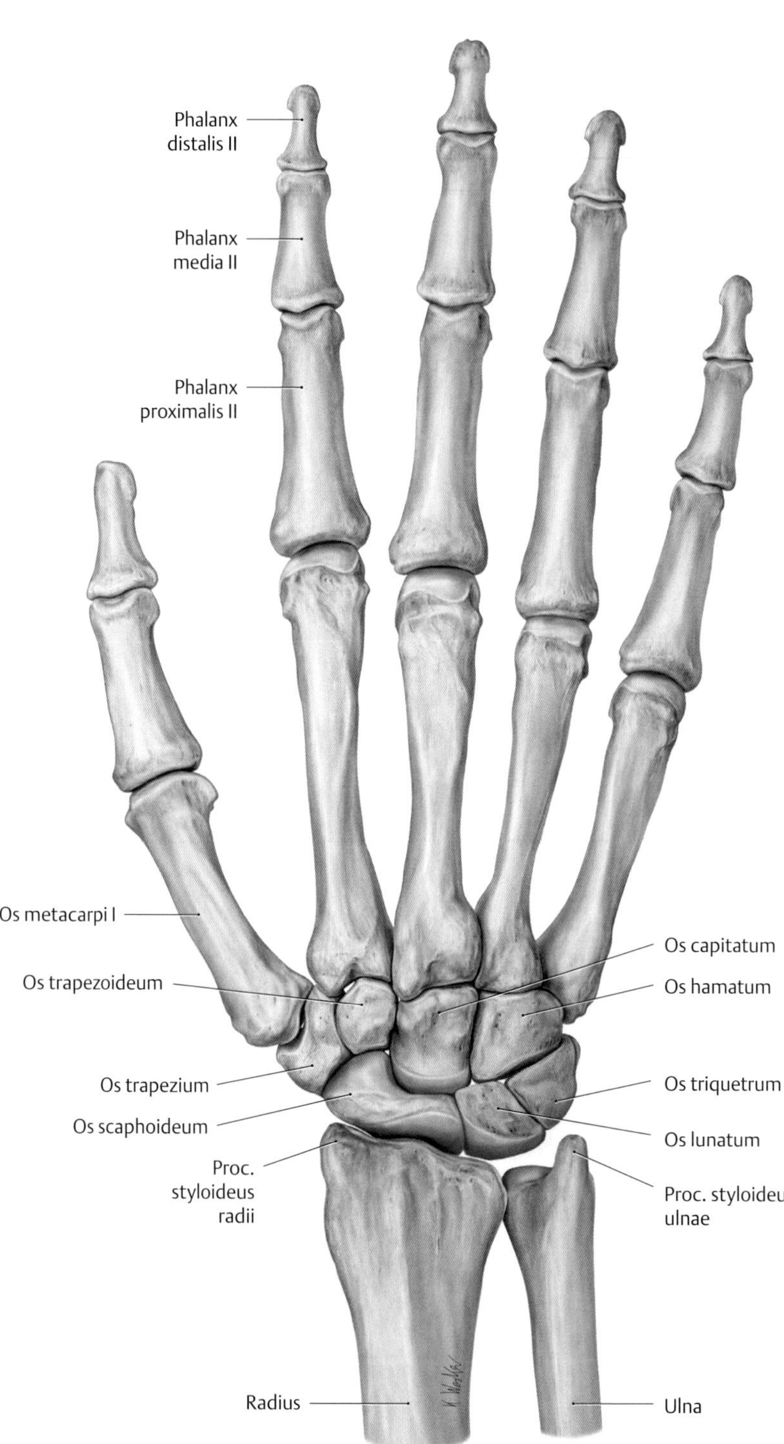
Phalanx distalis II
Phalanx media II
Phalanx proximalis II
Os metacarpi I
Os trapezoideum
Os trapezium
Os scaphoideum
Proc. styloideus radii
Radius
Os capitatum
Os hamatum
Os triquetrum
Os lunatum
Proc. styloideus ulnae
Ulna

Fig. 21.1 **Dorsal view**
Right hand.

Fig. 21.2 **Palmar view**
Right hand.

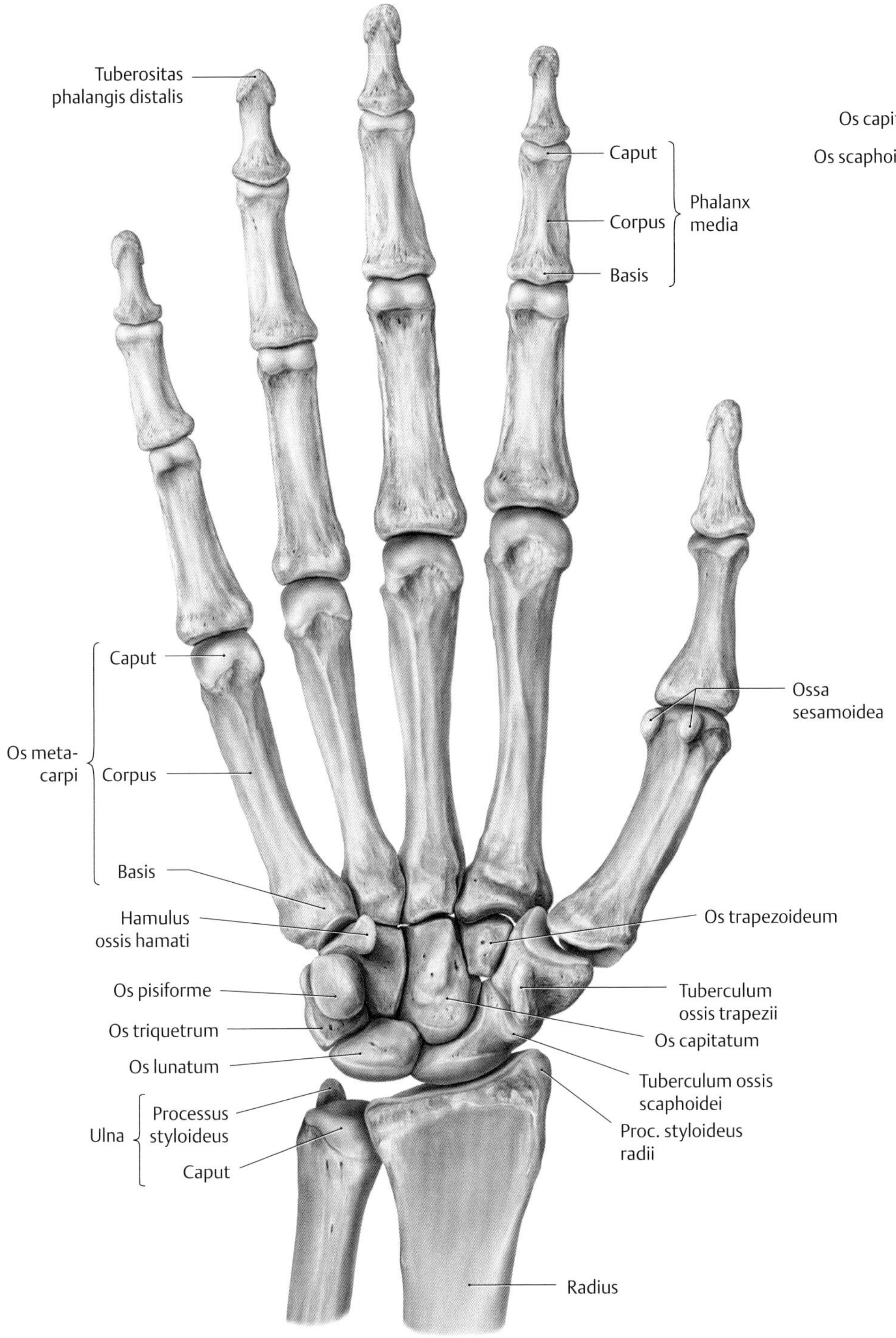

Tuberositas phalangis distalis
Caput
Corpus
Basis
Phalanx media
Os meta-carpi
Caput
Corpus
Basis
Ossa sesamoidea
Hamulus ossis hamati
Os pisiforme
Os triquetrum
Os lunatum
Ulna
Processus styloideus
Caput
Os trapezoideum
Tuberculum ossis trapezii
Os capitatum
Tuberculum ossis scaphoidei
Proc. styloideus radii
Radius

Fig. 21.3 **Radiograph of the wrist**
Anteroposterior view of left limb.

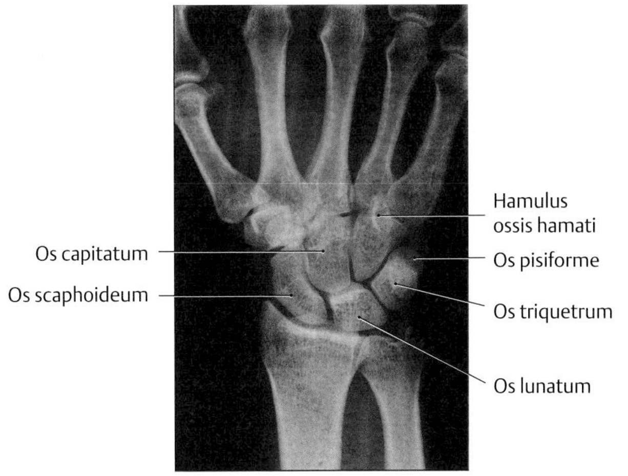

Os capitatum
Os scaphoideum
Hamulus ossis hamati
Os pisiforme
Os triquetrum
Os lunatum

Clinical

Fractures of os scaphoideum

Fractures of os scaphoideum are the most common carpal bone fractures, generally occurring at the narrowed waist between the proximal and distal poles (**A**, right scaphoid). Because blood supply to os scaphoideum is transmitted via the distal segment, fractures at the waist can compromise the supply to the proximal segment, often resulting in nonunion and avascular necrosis.

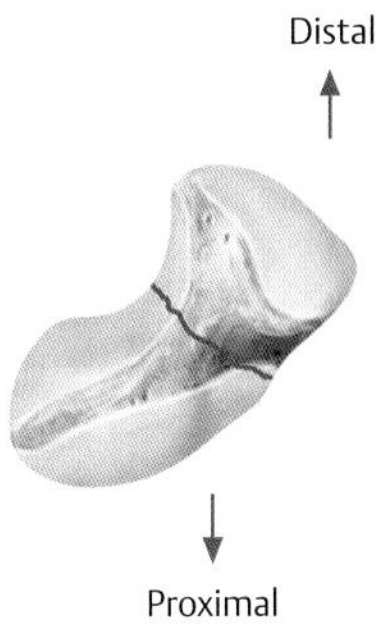

Distal
Proximal
A
B

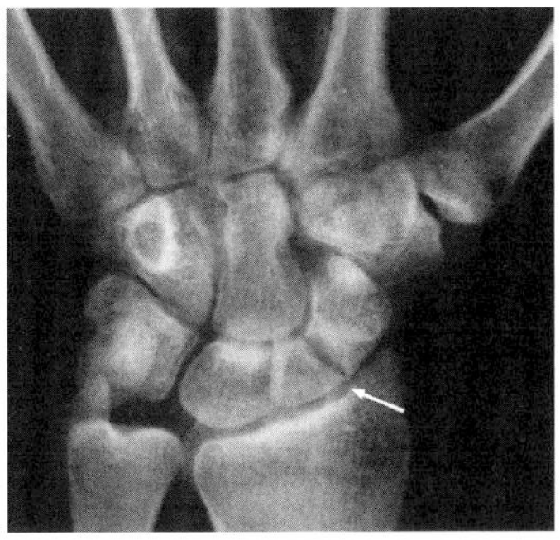

Joints of the Wrist & Hand

***Fig. 21.4* Joints of the wrist and hand**

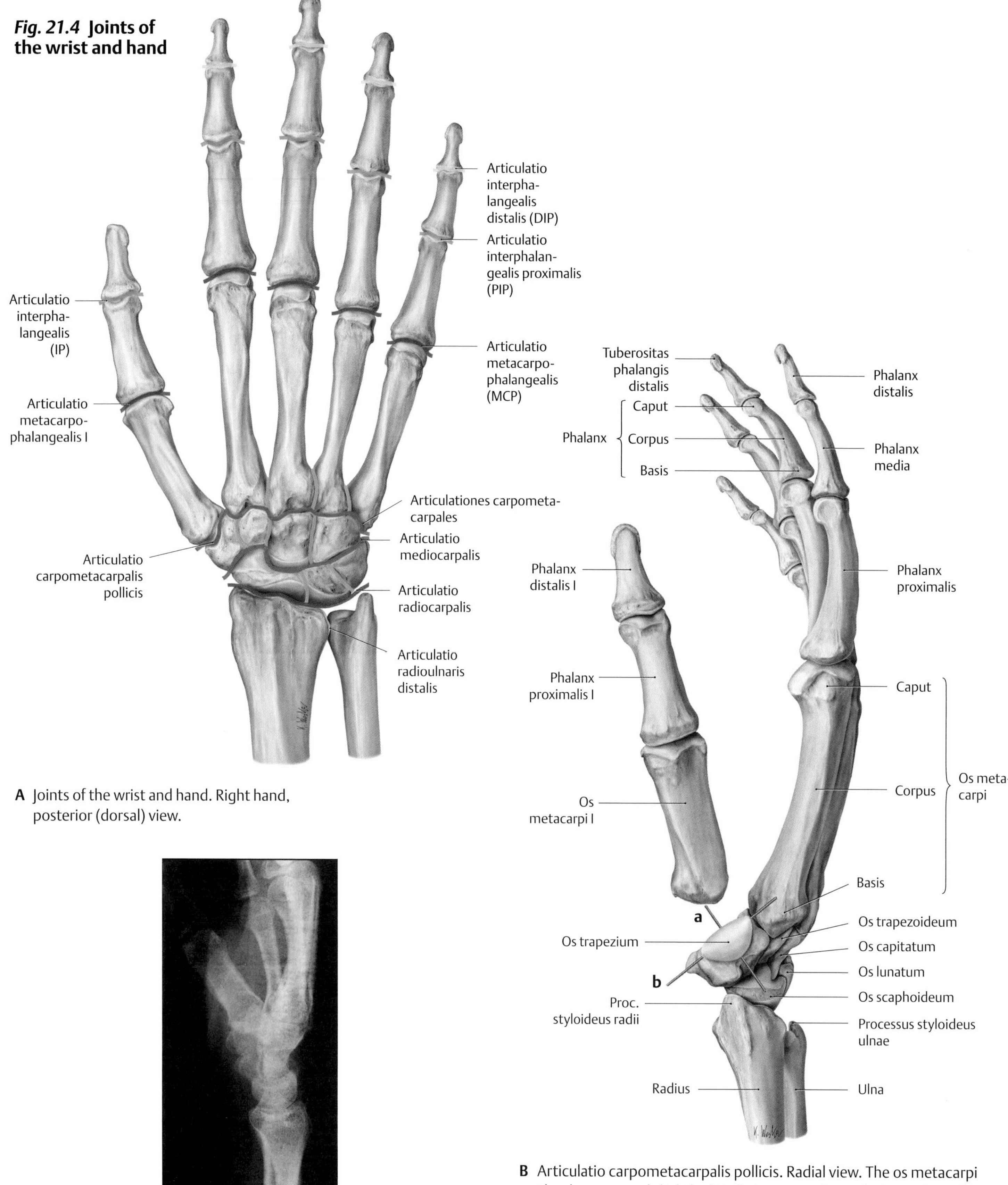
Articulatio interphalangealis distalis (DIP)
Articulatio interphalangealis proximalis (PIP)
Articulatio metacarpophalangealis (MCP)
Articulatio interphalangealis (IP)
Articulatio metacarpophalangealis I
Articulationes carpometacarpales
Articulatio mediocarpalis
Articulatio carpometacarpalis pollicis
Articulatio radiocarpalis
Articulatio radioulnaris distalis
Tuberositas phalangis distalis
Phalanx
Caput
Corpus
Basis
Phalanx distalis
Phalanx media
Phalanx proximalis
Phalanx distalis I
Phalanx proximalis I
Caput
Corpus
Os metacarpi
Os metacarpi I
Basis
a
Os trapezium
b
Os trapezoideum
Os capitatum
Os lunatum
Os scaphoideum
Proc. styloideus radii
Processus styloideus ulnae
Radius
Ulna

A Joints of the wrist and hand. Right hand, posterior (dorsal) view.

B Articulatio carpometacarpalis pollicis. Radial view. The os metacarpi I has been moved slightly distally to expose the articular surface of os trapezium. Two cardinal axes of motion are shown here: (**a**) flexion/extension and (**b**) abduction/adduction.

C Radiograph of wrist. Radial view.

Fig. 21.5 Wrist and hand: Coronal section
Right hand.

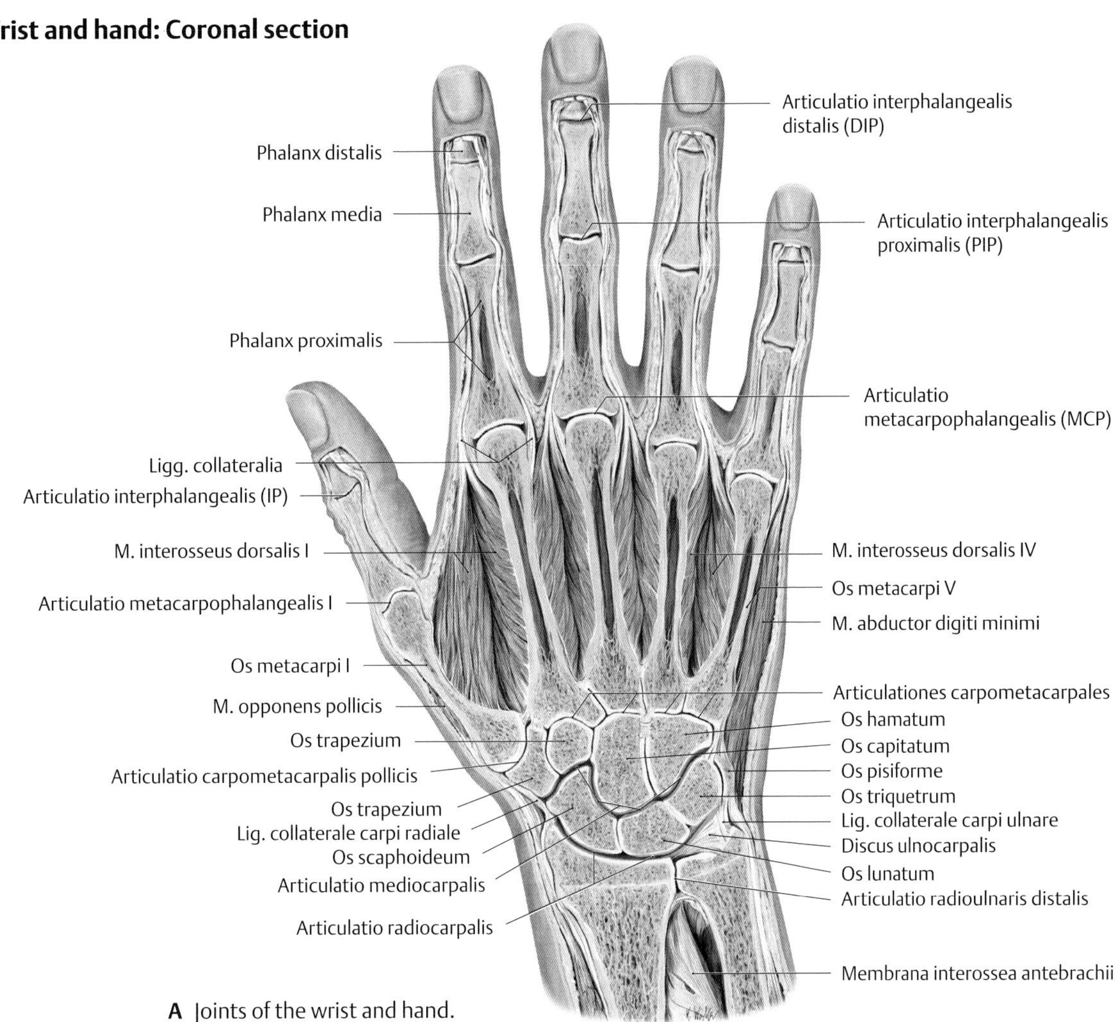
Phalanx distalis
Phalanx media
Phalanx proximalis
Ligg. collateralia
Articulatio interphalangealis (IP)
M. interosseus dorsalis I
Articulatio metacarpophalangealis I
Os metacarpi I
M. opponens pollicis
Os trapezium
Articulatio carpometacarpalis pollicis
Os trapezium
Lig. collaterale carpi radiale
Os scaphoideum
Articulatio mediocarpalis
Articulatio radiocarpalis
Articulatio interphalangealis distalis (DIP)
Articulatio interphalangealis proximalis (PIP)
Articulatio metacarpophalangealis (MCP)
M. interosseus dorsalis IV
Os metacarpi V
M. abductor digiti minimi
Articulationes carpometacarpales
Os hamatum
Os capitatum
Os pisiforme
Os triquetrum
Lig. collaterale carpi ulnare
Discus ulnocarpalis
Os lunatum
Articulatio radioulnaris distalis
Membrana interossea antebrachii

A Joints of the wrist and hand.

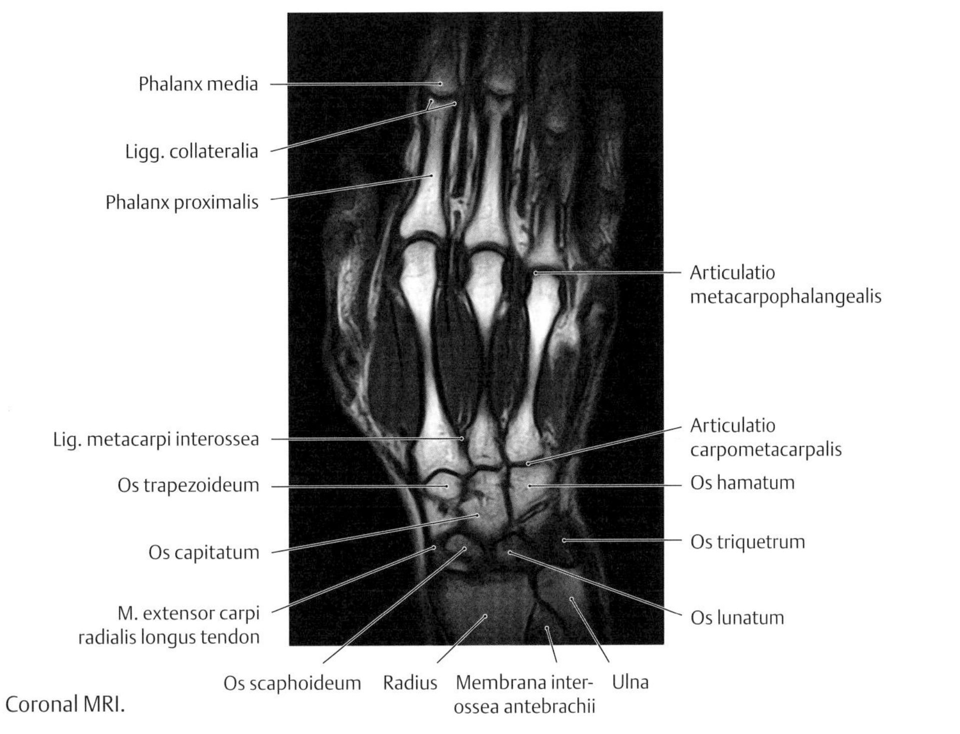
Phalanx media
Ligg. collateralia
Phalanx proximalis
Lig. metacarpi interossea
Os trapezoideum
Os capitatum
M. extensor carpi radialis longus tendon
Os scaphoideum
Radius
Membrana interossea antebrachii
Ulna
Articulatio metacarpophalangealis
Articulatio carpometacarpalis
Os hamatum
Os triquetrum
Os lunatum

B Coronal MRI.

Ligaments of the Wrist & Hand

Fig. 21.6 **Ligaments of the hand**
Right hand.

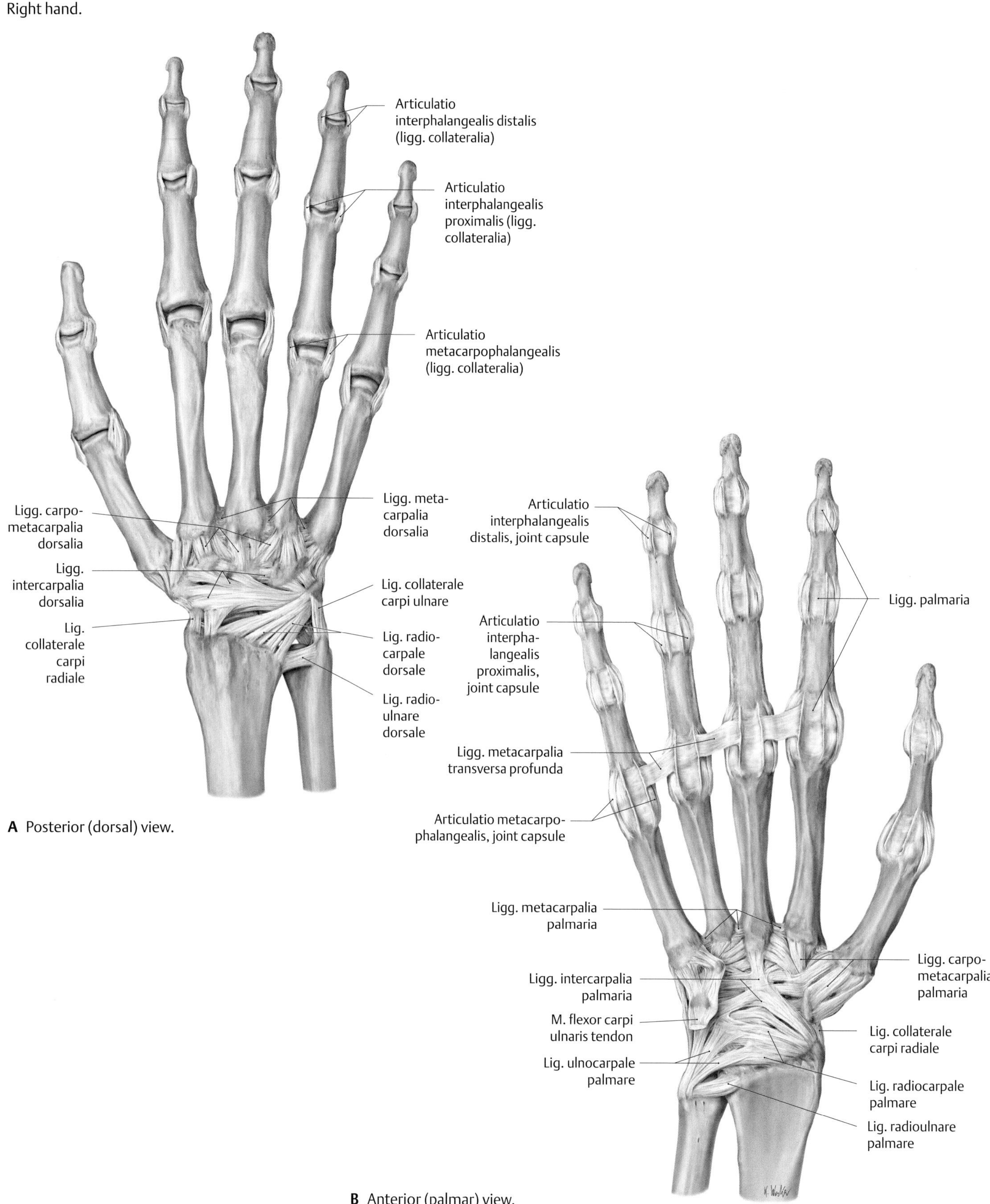
Articulatio
interphalangealis distalis
(ligg. collateralia)
Articulatio
interphalangealis
proximalis (ligg.
collateralia)
Articulatio
metacarpophalangealis
(ligg. collateralia)
Ligg. carpo-
metacarpalia
dorsalia
Ligg. meta-
carpalia
dorsalia
Ligg.
intercarpalia
dorsalia
Lig. collaterale
carpi ulnare
Lig.
collaterale
carpi
radiale
Lig. radio-
carpale
dorsale
Lig. radio-
ulnare
dorsale
Articulatio
interphalangealis
distalis, joint capsule
Ligg. palmaria
Articulatio
interpha-
langealis
proximalis,
joint capsule
Ligg. metacarpalia
transversa profunda
Articulatio metacarpo-
phalangealis, joint capsule
Ligg. metacarpalia
palmaria
Ligg. intercarpalia
palmaria
Ligg. carpo-
metacarpalia
palmaria
M. flexor carpi
ulnaris tendon
Lig. collaterale
carpi radiale
Lig. ulnocarpale
palmare
Lig. radiocarpale
palmare
Lig. radioulnare
palmare

A Posterior (dorsal) view.

B Anterior (palmar) view.

Fig. 21.7 Ligaments of canalis carpi
Right hand, anterior view.

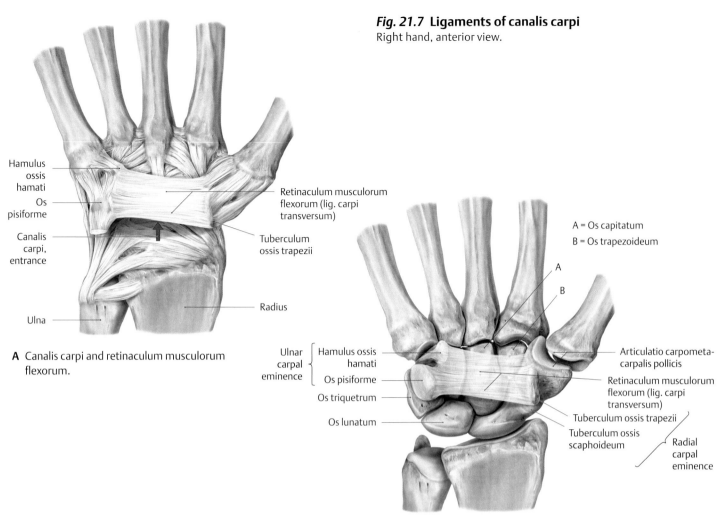

Hamulus ossis hamati
Os pisiforme
Canalis carpi, entrance
Ulna
Retinaculum musculorum flexorum (lig. carpi transversum)
Tuberculum ossis trapezii
Radius

A Canalis carpi and retinaculum musculorum flexorum.

A = Os capitatum
B = Os trapezoideum
A
B
Ulnar carpal eminence
Hamulus ossis hamati
Os pisiforme
Os triquetrum
Os lunatum
Articulatio carpometacarpalis pollicis
Retinaculum musculorum flexorum (lig. carpi transversum)
Tuberculum ossis trapezii
Tuberculum ossis scaphoideum
Radial carpal eminence

B Bony boundaries of canalis carpi.

Fig. 21.8 Canalis carpi
Transverse section. The contents of canalis carpi are discussed on p. 342. See p. 343 for canalis ulnaris and lig. carpi palmare.

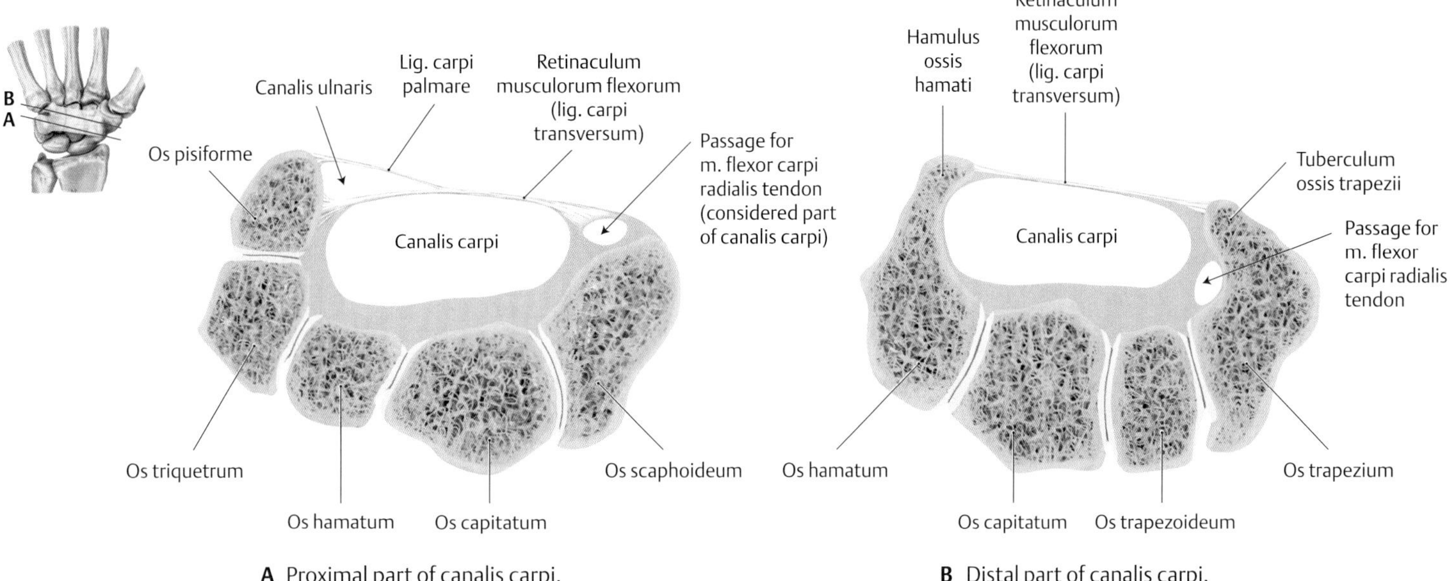
B
A
Os pisiforme
Canalis ulnaris
Lig. carpi palmare
Retinaculum musculorum flexorum (lig. carpi transversum)
Passage for m. flexor carpi radialis tendon (considered part of canalis carpi)
Canalis carpi
Os triquetrum
Os hamatum
Os capitatum
Os scaphoideum
Hamulus ossis hamati
Retinaculum musculorum flexorum (lig. carpi transversum)
Tuberculum ossis trapezii
Passage for m. flexor carpi radialis tendon
Canalis carpi
Os hamatum
Os capitatum
Os trapezoideum
Os trapezium

A Proximal part of canalis carpi.

B Distal part of canalis carpi.

Ligaments of the Fingers

Fig. 21.9 **Ligaments of the fingers: Lateral view**
Right middle finger. The outer fibrous layer of the tendon sheaths (stratum fibrosum) is strengthened by ligg. anularia and ligg. obliqua, which also bind the sheaths to the palmar surface of the phalanx and prevent palmar deviation of the sheaths during flexion.

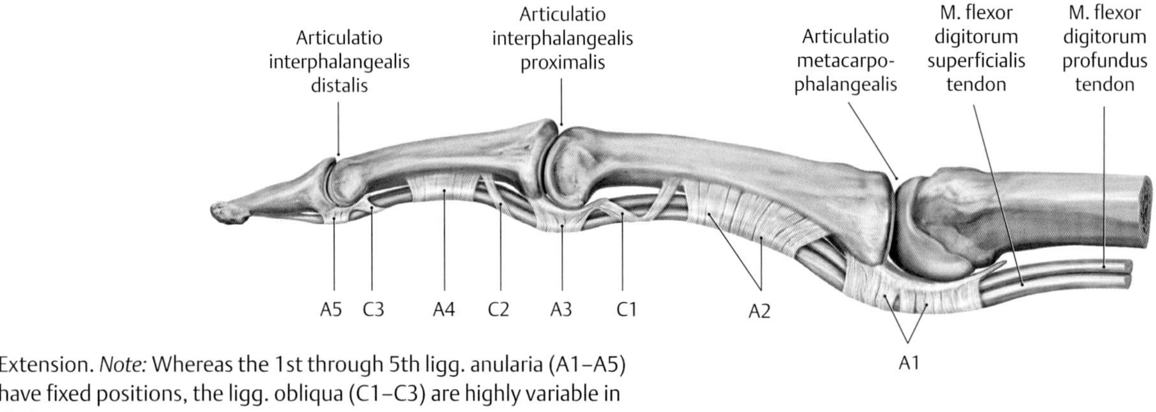

Articulatio interphalangealis distalis
Articulatio interphalangealis proximalis
Articulatio metacarpo-phalangealis
M. flexor digitorum superficialis tendon
M. flexor digitorum profundus tendon
A5
C3
A4
C2
A3
C1
A2
A1

A Extension. *Note:* Whereas the 1st through 5th ligg. anularia (A1–A5) have fixed positions, the ligg. obliqua (C1–C3) are highly variable in their course.

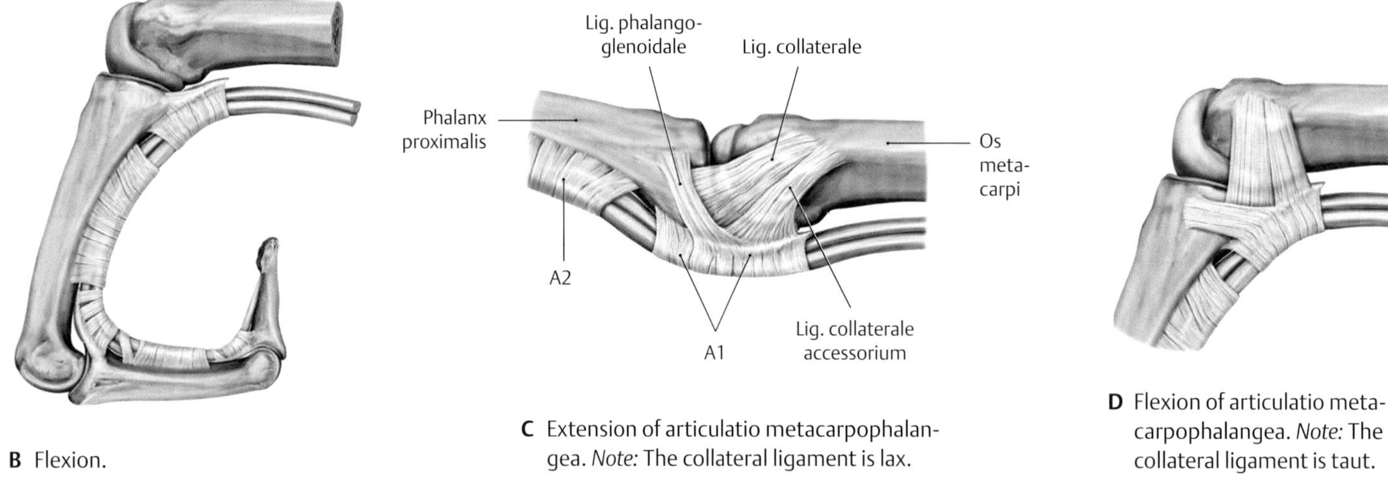

Lig. phalango-glenoidale
Lig. collaterale
Phalanx proximalis
Os meta-carpi
A2
A1
Lig. collaterale accessorium

B Flexion.

C Extension of articulatio metacarpophalangea. *Note:* The collateral ligament is lax.

D Flexion of articulatio metacarpophalangea. *Note:* The collateral ligament is taut.

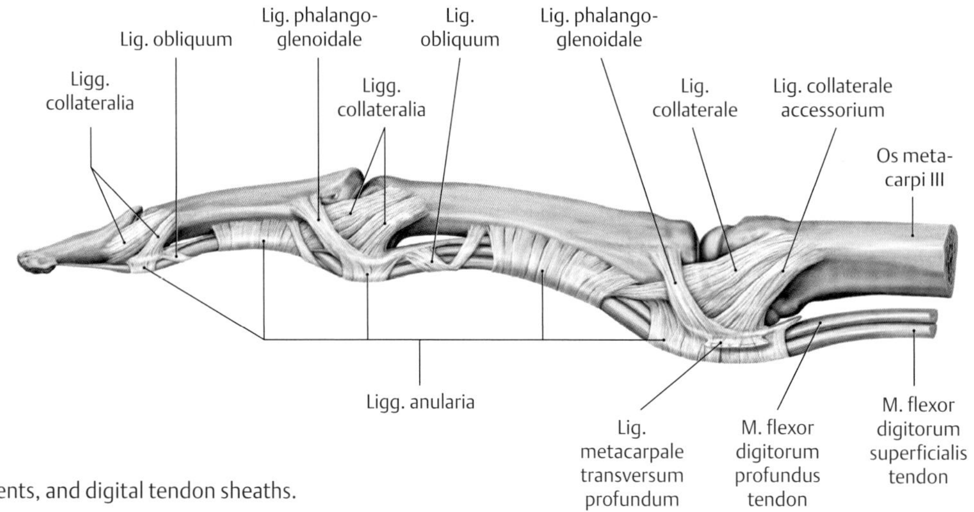

Lig. obliquum
Lig. phalango-glenoidale
Lig. obliquum
Lig. phalango-glenoidale
Ligg. collateralia
Ligg. collateralia
Lig. collaterale
Lig. collaterale accessorium
Os meta-carpi III
Ligg. anularia
Lig. metacarpale transversum profundum
M. flexor digitorum profundus tendon
M. flexor digitorum superficialis tendon

E Joint capsules, ligaments, and digital tendon sheaths.

Fig. 21.10 Anterior view

Right middle finger, palmar view.

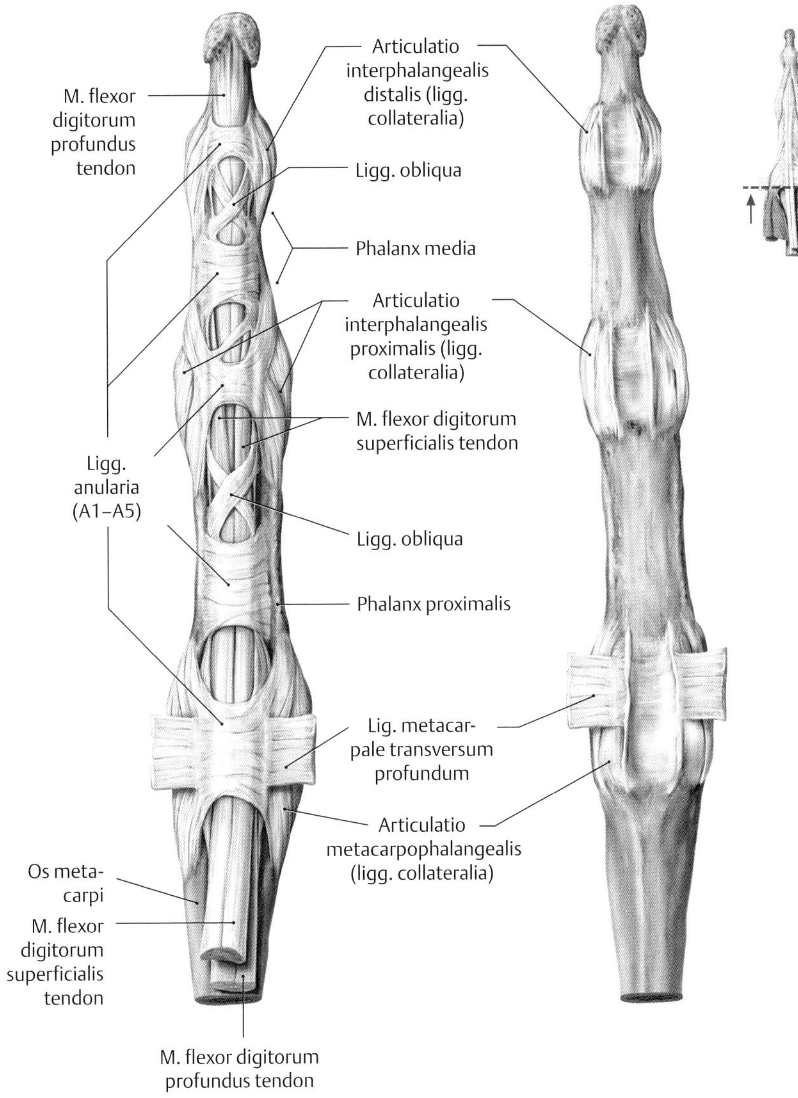

M. flexor digitorum profundus tendon
Articulatio interphalangealis distalis (ligg. collateralia)
Ligg. obliqua
Phalanx media
Articulatio interphalangealis proximalis (ligg. collateralia)
M. flexor digitorum superficialis tendon
Ligg. anularia (A1–A5)
Ligg. obliqua
Phalanx proximalis
Lig. metacarpale transversum profundum
Articulatio metacarpophalangealis (ligg. collateralia)
Os metacarpi
M. flexor digitorum superficialis tendon
M. flexor digitorum profundus tendon

A Superficial ligaments.

B Deep ligaments with digital tendon sheath removed.

Fig. 21.11 Os metacarpi III: Transverse section

Proximal view.

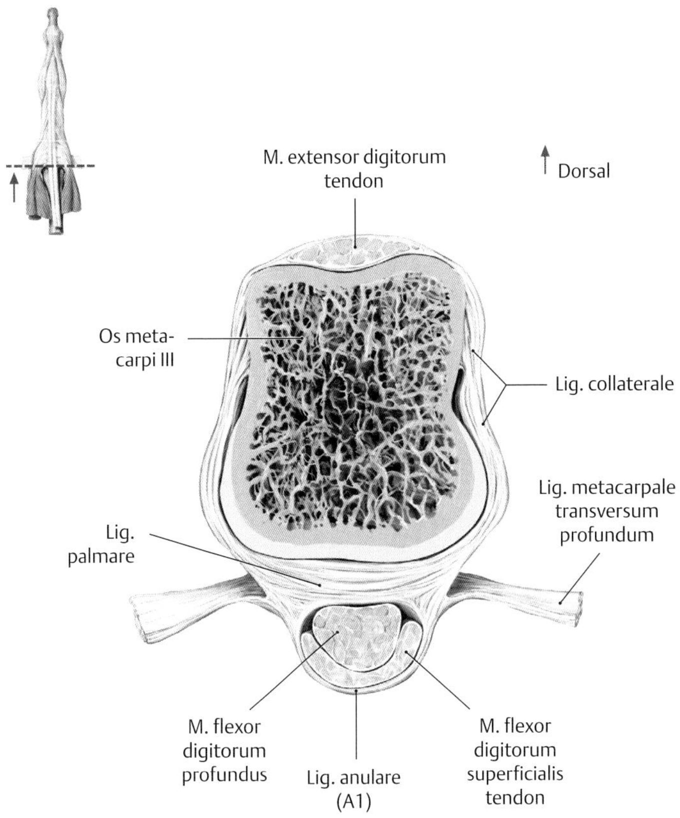

M. extensor digitorum tendon
Dorsal
Os metacarpi III
Lig. collaterale
Lig. metacarpale transversum profundum
Lig. palmare
M. flexor digitorum profundus
Lig. anulare (A1)
M. flexor digitorum superficialis tendon

Fig. 21.12 Fingertip: Longitudinal section

The palmar articular surfaces of the phalanges are enlarged proximally at the joints by the lig. palmare. This fibrocartilaginous plate, also known as the volar plate, forms the floor of the digital tendon sheaths.

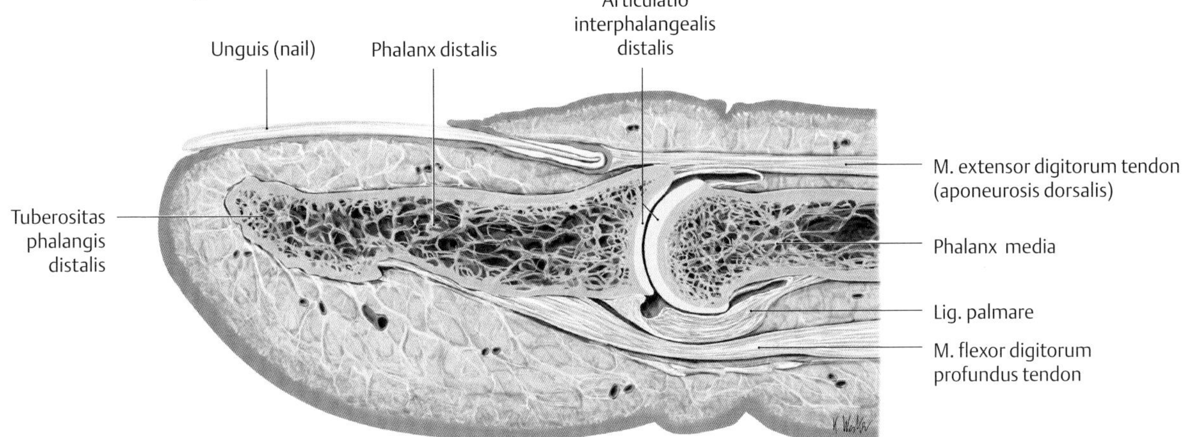
Unguis (nail)
Phalanx distalis
Articulatio interphalangealis distalis
M. extensor digitorum tendon (aponeurosis dorsalis)
Tuberositas phalangis distalis
Phalanx media
Lig. palmare
M. flexor digitorum profundus tendon

Muscles of the Hand: Superficial & Middle Layers

Fig. 21.13 Intrinsic muscles of the hand: Superficial and middle layers
Right hand, palmar surface.

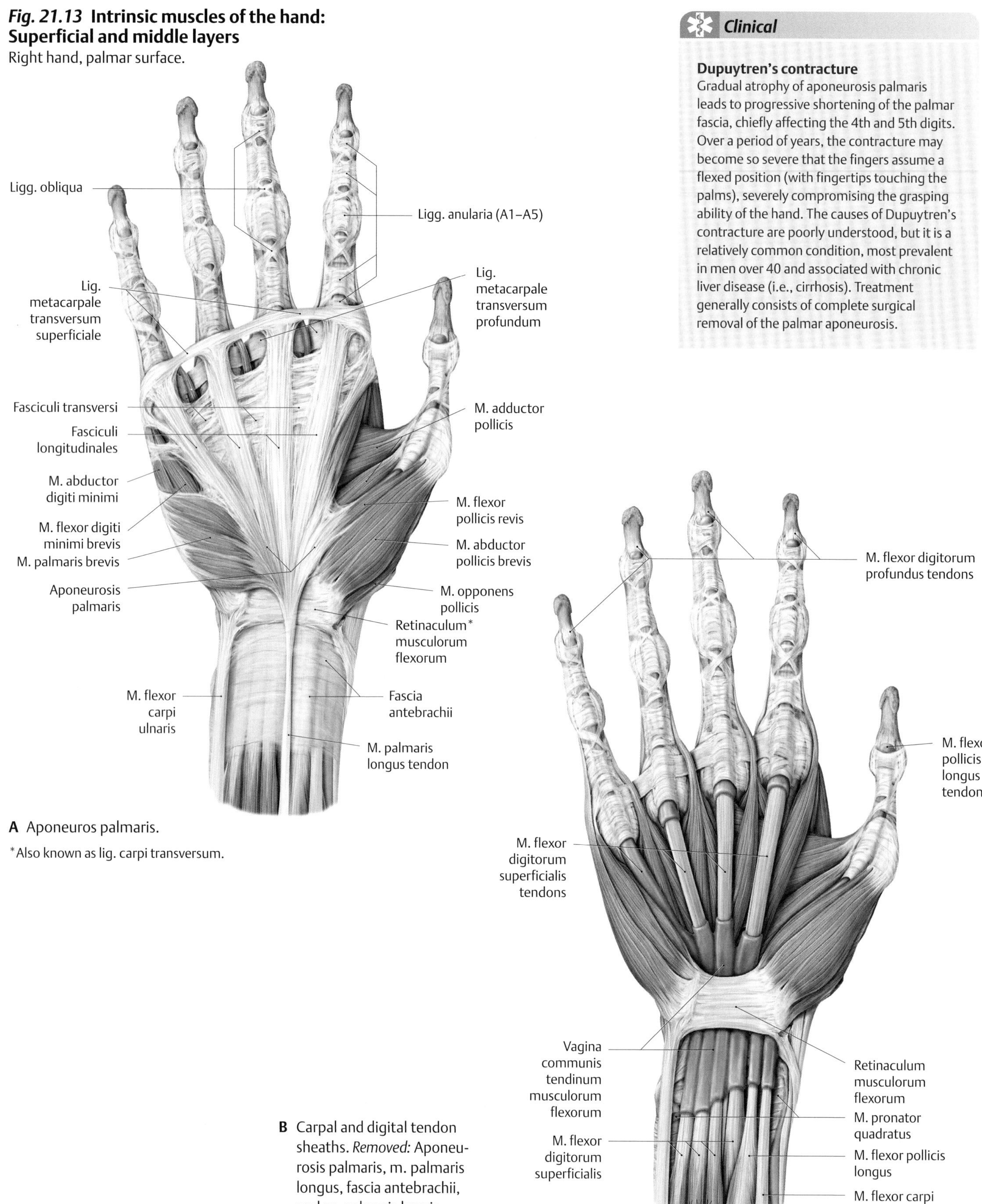

Ligg. obliqua
Ligg. anularia (A1–A5)
Lig. metacarpale transversum superficiale
Lig. metacarpale transversum profundum
Fasciculi transversi
Fasciculi longitudinales
M. adductor pollicis
M. abductor digiti minimi
M. flexor digiti minimi brevis
M. palmaris brevis
M. flexor pollicis revis
M. abductor pollicis brevis
Aponeurosis palmaris
M. opponens pollicis
Retinaculum* musculorum flexorum
M. flexor carpi ulnaris
Fascia antebrachii
M. palmaris longus tendon
M. flexor digitorum profundus tendons
M. flexor pollicis longus tendon
M. flexor digitorum superficialis tendons
Vagina communis tendinum musculorum flexorum
Retinaculum musculorum flexorum
M. pronator quadratus
M. flexor digitorum superficialis
M. flexor pollicis longus
M. flexor carpi radialis

A Aponeuros palmaris.

*Also known as lig. carpi transversum.

B Carpal and digital tendon sheaths. *Removed:* Aponeurosis palmaris, m. palmaris longus, fascia antebrachii, and m. palmaris brevis.

Clinical

Dupuytren's contracture
Gradual atrophy of aponeurosis palmaris leads to progressive shortening of the palmar fascia, chiefly affecting the 4th and 5th digits. Over a period of years, the contracture may become so severe that the fingers assume a flexed position (with fingertips touching the palms), severely compromising the grasping ability of the hand. The causes of Dupuytren's contracture are poorly understood, but it is a relatively common condition, most prevalent in men over 40 and associated with chronic liver disease (i.e., cirrhosis). Treatment generally consists of complete surgical removal of the palmar aponeurosis.

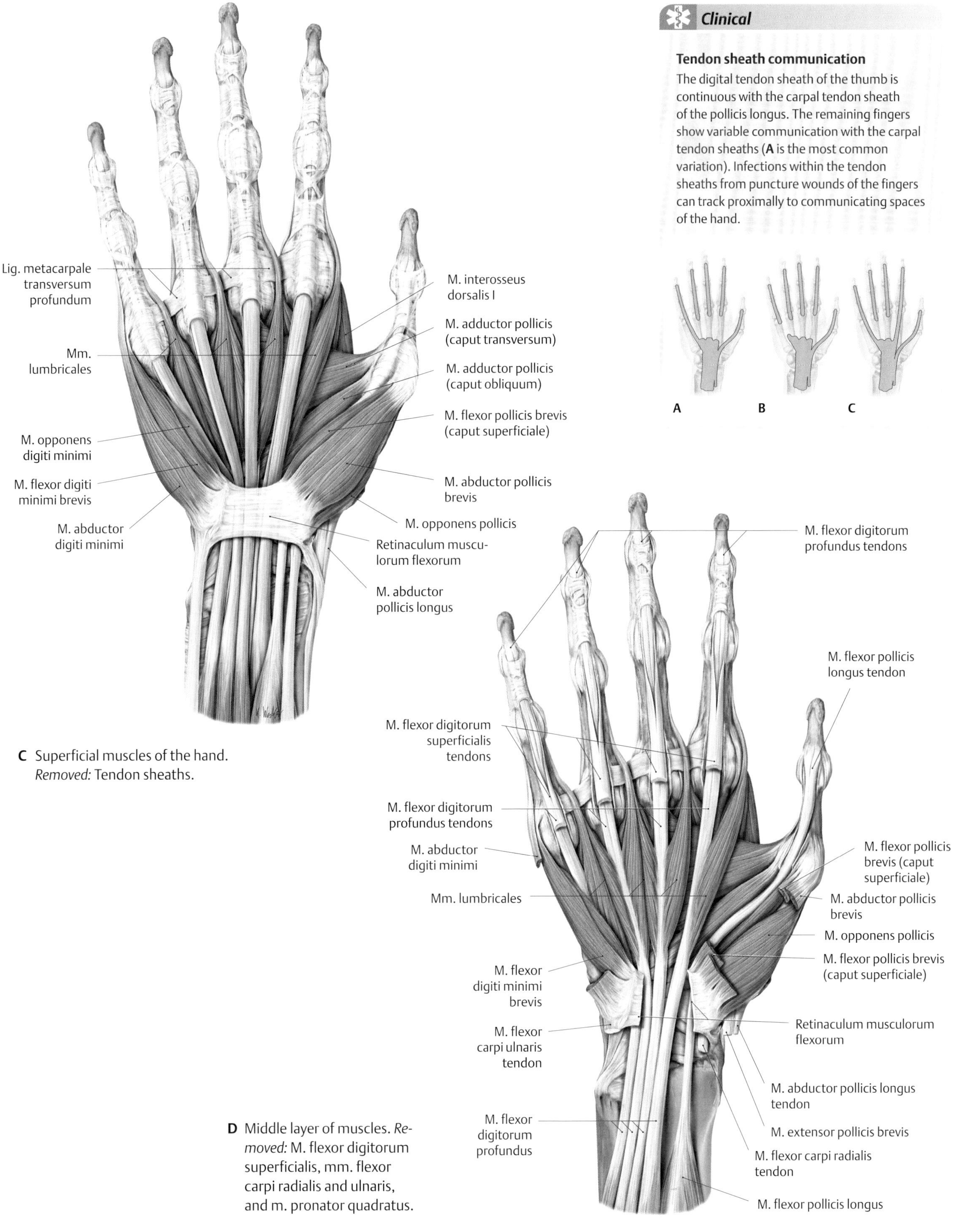
Lig. metacarpale transversum profundum
Mm. lumbricales
M. opponens digiti minimi
M. flexor digiti minimi brevis
M. abductor digiti minimi
M. interosseus dorsalis I
M. adductor pollicis (caput transversum)
M. adductor pollicis (caput obliquum)
M. flexor pollicis brevis (caput superficiale)
M. abductor pollicis brevis
M. opponens pollicis
Retinaculum musculorum flexorum
M. abductor pollicis longus
A
B
C
M. flexor digitorum profundus tendons
M. flexor pollicis longus tendon
M. flexor digitorum superficialis tendons
M. flexor digitorum profundus tendons
M. abductor digiti minimi
Mm. lumbricales
M. flexor pollicis brevis (caput superficiale)
M. abductor pollicis brevis
M. opponens pollicis
M. flexor pollicis brevis (caput superficiale)
M. flexor digiti minimi brevis
M. flexor carpi ulnaris tendon
Retinaculum musculorum flexorum
M. abductor pollicis longus tendon
M. extensor pollicis brevis
M. flexor carpi radialis tendon
M. flexor digitorum profundus
M. flexor pollicis longus

Clinical

Tendon sheath communication

The digital tendon sheath of the thumb is continuous with the carpal tendon sheath of the pollicis longus. The remaining fingers show variable communication with the carpal tendon sheaths (**A** is the most common variation). Infections within the tendon sheaths from puncture wounds of the fingers can track proximally to communicating spaces of the hand.

C Superficial muscles of the hand. *Removed:* Tendon sheaths.

D Middle layer of muscles. *Removed:* M. flexor digitorum superficialis, mm. flexor carpi radialis and ulnaris, and m. pronator quadratus.

Muscles of the Hand: Middle & Deep Layers

Fig. 21.14 **Intrinsic muscles: Middle and deep layers**
Right hand, palmar surface.

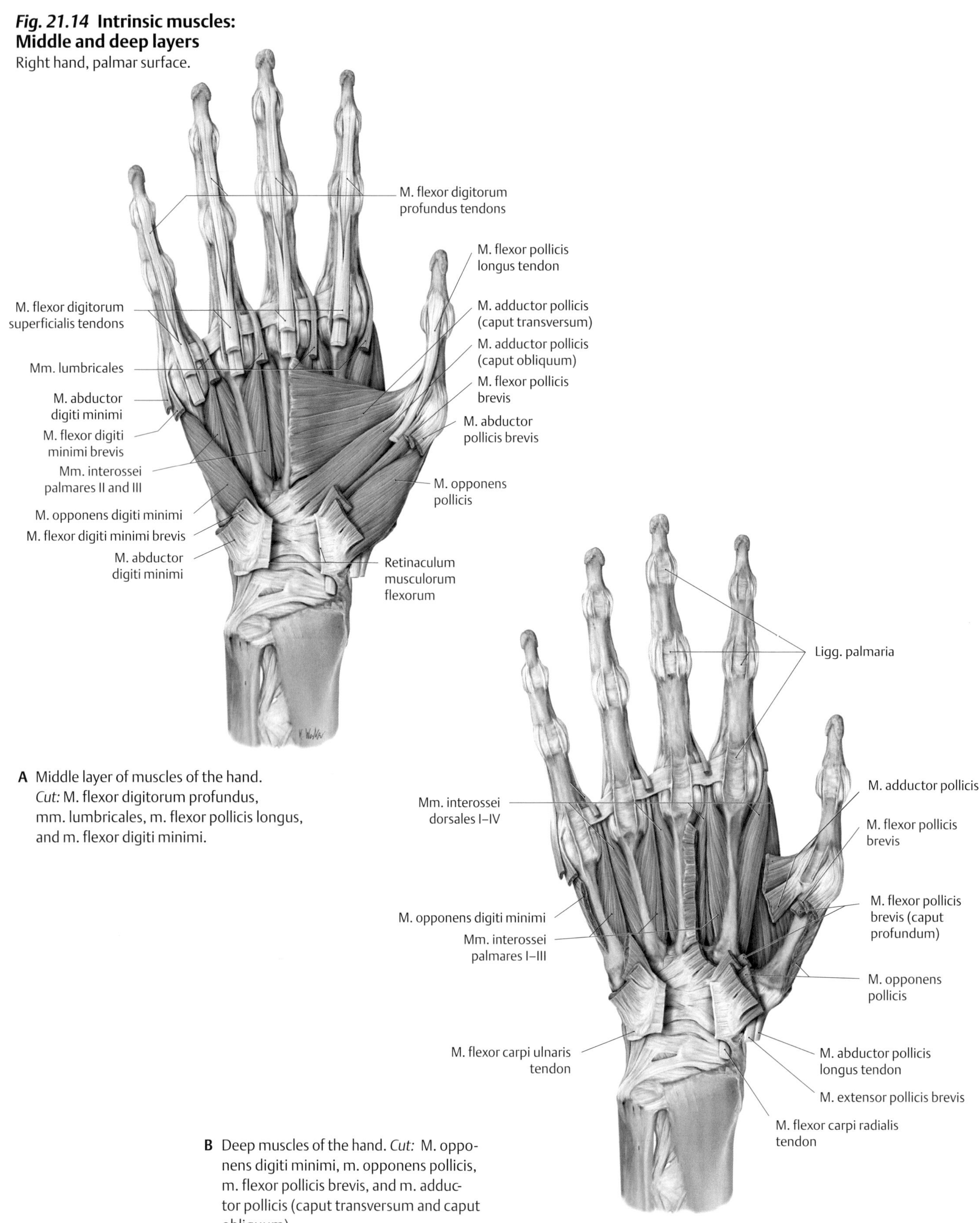
M. flexor digitorum profundus tendons
M. flexor pollicis longus tendon
M. flexor digitorum superficialis tendons
M. adductor pollicis (caput transversum)
M. adductor pollicis (caput obliquum)
Mm. lumbricales
M. flexor pollicis brevis
M. abductor digiti minimi
M. abductor pollicis brevis
M. flexor digiti minimi brevis
Mm. interossei palmares II and III
M. opponens pollicis
M. opponens digiti minimi
M. flexor digiti minimi brevis
M. abductor digiti minimi
Retinaculum musculorum flexorum
Ligg. palmaria
M. adductor pollicis
Mm. interossei dorsales I–IV
M. flexor pollicis brevis
M. flexor pollicis brevis (caput profundum)
M. opponens digiti minimi
Mm. interossei palmares I–III
M. opponens pollicis
M. flexor carpi ulnaris tendon
M. abductor pollicis longus tendon
M. extensor pollicis brevis
M. flexor carpi radialis tendon

A Middle layer of muscles of the hand. *Cut:* M. flexor digitorum profundus, mm. lumbricales, m. flexor pollicis longus, and m. flexor digiti minimi.

B Deep muscles of the hand. *Cut:* M. opponens digiti minimi, m. opponens pollicis, m. flexor pollicis brevis, and m. adductor pollicis (caput transversum and caput obliquum).

Fig. 21.15 **Origins and insertions**
Right hand. Muscle origins shown in red, insertions in blue.

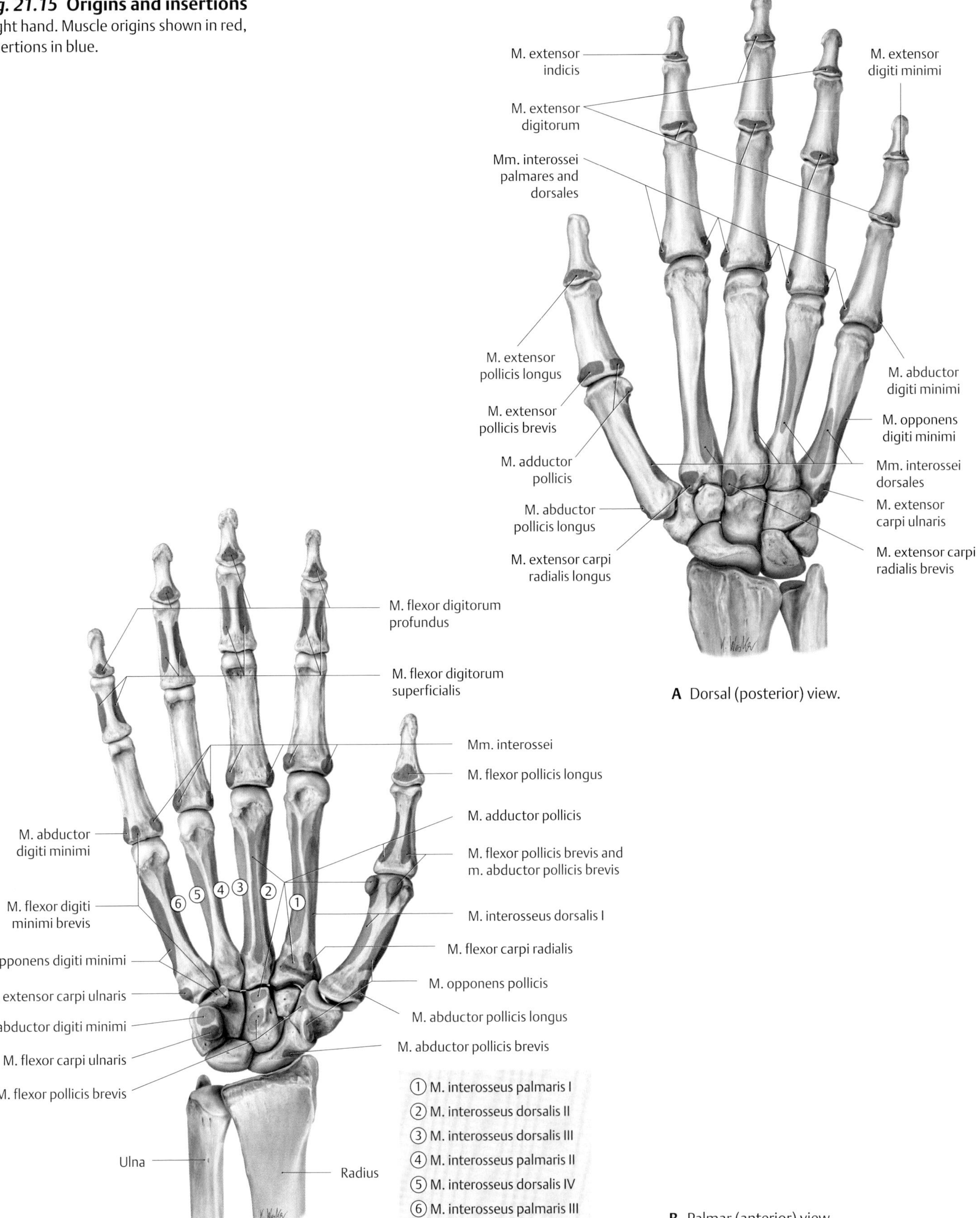

M. extensor indicis
M. extensor digitorum
Mm. interossei palmares and dorsales
M. extensor digiti minimi
M. extensor pollicis longus
M. extensor pollicis brevis
M. adductor pollicis
M. abductor pollicis longus
M. extensor carpi radialis longus
M. abductor digiti minimi
M. opponens digiti minimi
Mm. interossei dorsales
M. extensor carpi ulnaris
M. extensor carpi radialis brevis
M. flexor digitorum profundus
M. flexor digitorum superficialis
Mm. interossei
M. flexor pollicis longus
M. adductor pollicis
M. flexor pollicis brevis and m. abductor pollicis brevis
M. interosseus dorsalis I
M. flexor carpi radialis
M. opponens pollicis
M. abductor pollicis longus
M. abductor pollicis brevis
M. abductor digiti minimi
M. flexor digiti minimi brevis
M. opponens digiti minimi
M. extensor carpi ulnaris
M. abductor digiti minimi
M. flexor carpi ulnaris
M. flexor pollicis brevis
Ulna
Radius
6
5
4
3
2
1
① M. interosseus palmaris I
② M. interosseus dorsalis II
③ M. interosseus dorsalis III
④ M. interosseus palmaris II
⑤ M. interosseus dorsalis IV
⑥ M. interosseus palmaris III

A Dorsal (posterior) view.

B Palmar (anterior) view.

Dorsum of the Hand

Fig. 21.16 Retinaculum musculorum extensorum and dorsal carpal tendon sheaths

Right hand, posterior (dorsal) view.

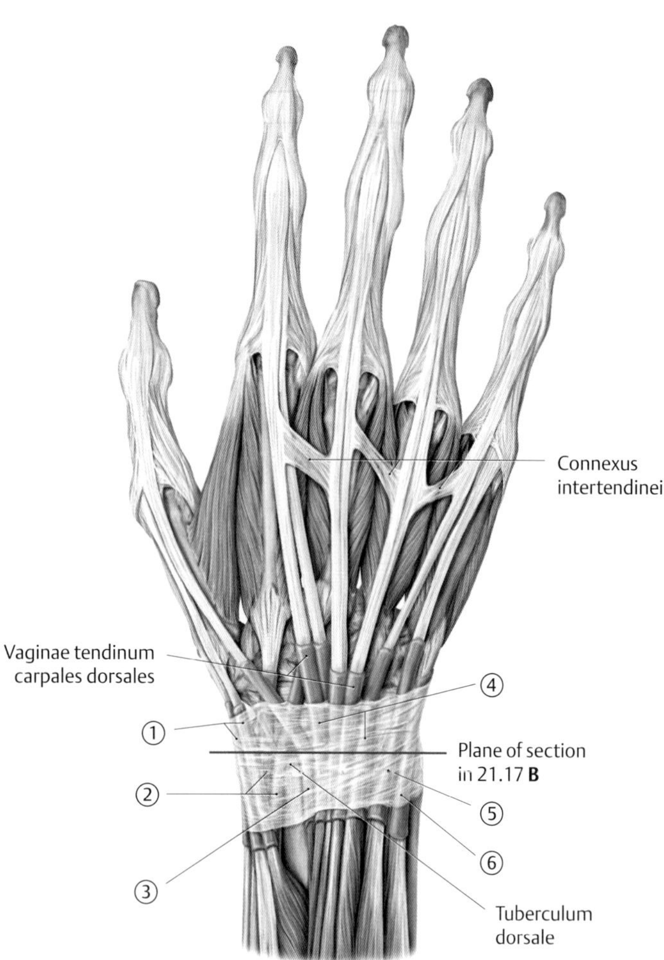

Connexus intertendinei
Vaginae tendinum carpales dorsales
①
②
③
④
⑤
⑥
Plane of section in 21.17 B
Tuberculum dorsale

Table 21.2	Dorsal compartments for extensor tendons
①	M. abductor pollicis longus
	M. extensor pollicis brevis
②	M. extensor carpi radialis longus
	M. extensor carpi radialis brevis
③	M. extensor pollicis longus
④	M. extensor digitorum
	M. extensor indicis
⑤	M. extensor digiti minimi
⑥	M. extensor carpi ulnaris

Fig. 21.17 Muscles and tendons of the dorsum

Right hand.

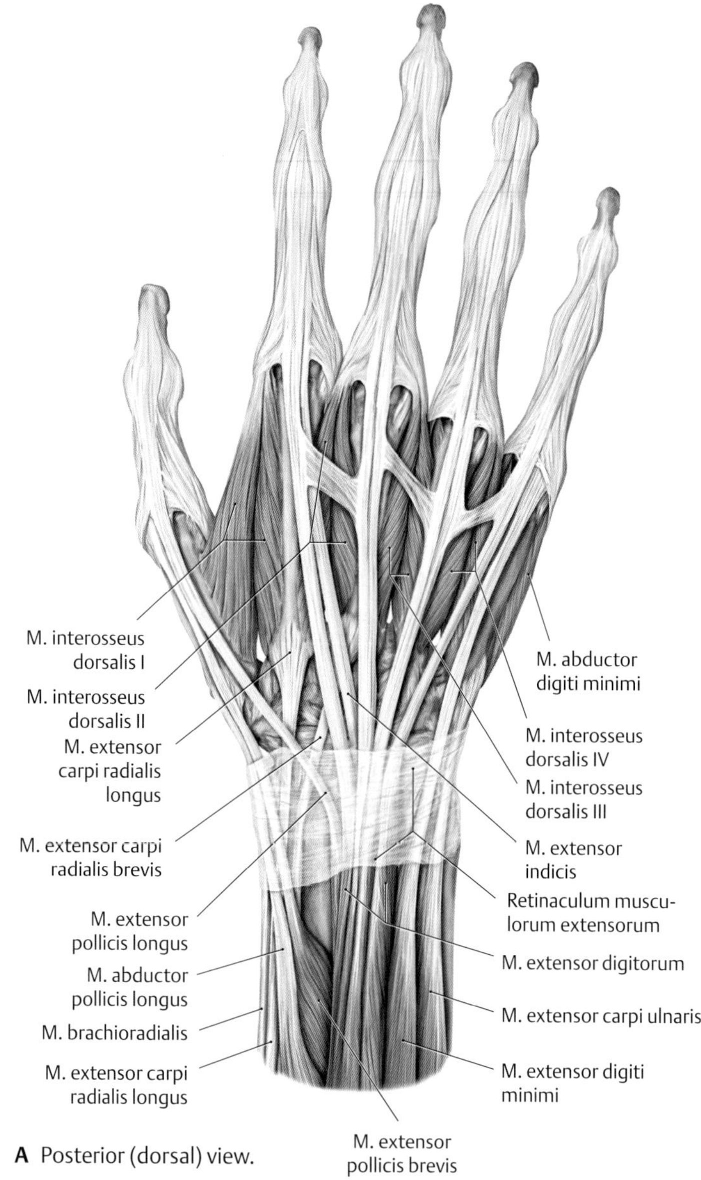

M. interosseus dorsalis I
M. interosseus dorsalis II
M. extensor carpi radialis longus
M. extensor carpi radialis brevis
M. extensor pollicis longus
M. abductor pollicis longus
M. brachioradialis
M. extensor carpi radialis longus
M. abductor digiti minimi
M. interosseus dorsalis IV
M. interosseus dorsalis III
M. extensor indicis
Retinaculum musculorum extensorum
M. extensor digitorum
M. extensor carpi ulnaris
M. extensor digiti minimi
M. extensor pollicis brevis

A Posterior (dorsal) view.

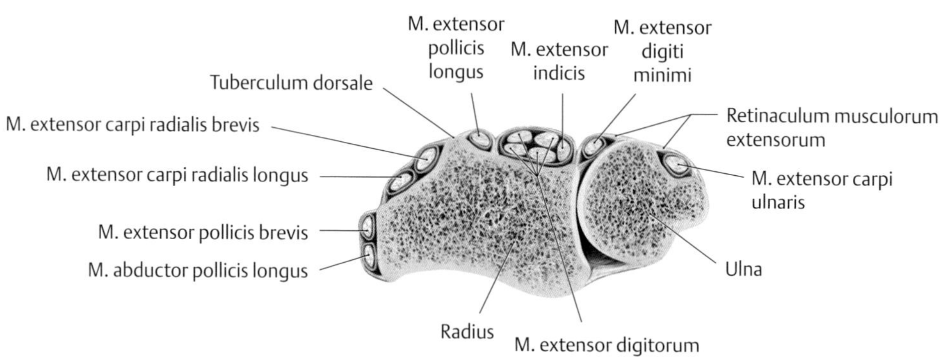

M. extensor pollicis longus
M. extensor indicis
M. extensor digiti minimi
Tuberculum dorsale
M. extensor carpi radialis brevis
Retinaculum musculorum extensorum
M. extensor carpi radialis longus
M. extensor carpi ulnaris
M. extensor pollicis brevis
M. abductor pollicis longus
Ulna
Radius
M. extensor digitorum

B Dorsal compartments, proximal view of section in Fig. 21.16.

Fig. 21.18 **Aponeurosis dorsalis**

Right hand, middle finger. The aponeuroses dorsales permits the long digital flexors and the short muscles of the hand to act on all three finger joints.

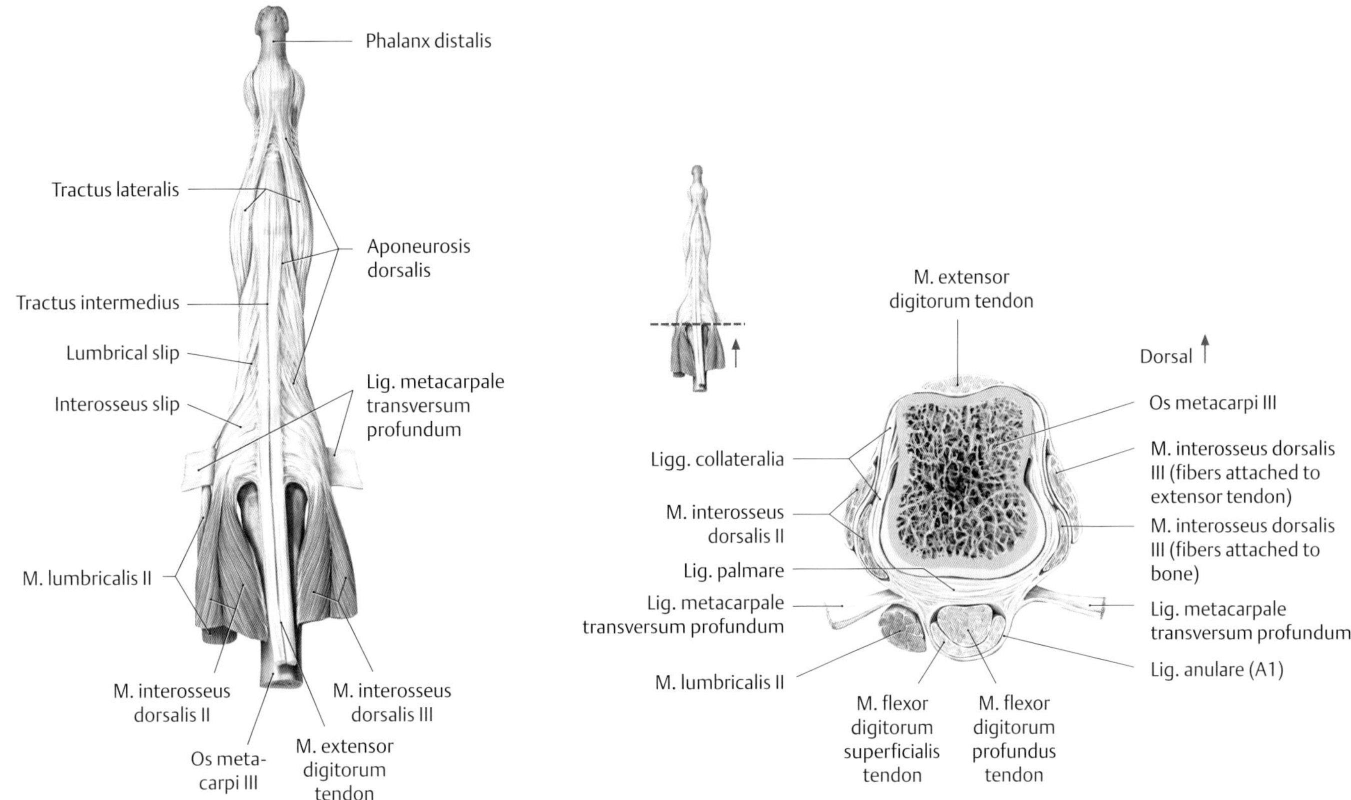
Phalanx distalis
Tractus lateralis
Aponeurosis dorsalis
Tractus intermedius
Lumbrical slip
Interosseus slip
Lig. metacarpale transversum profundum
M. lumbricalis II
M. interosseus dorsalis II
M. interosseus dorsalis III
Os metacarpi III
M. extensor digitorum tendon
M. extensor digitorum tendon
Dorsal
Os metacarpi III
Ligg. collateralia
M. interosseus dorsalis II
Lig. palmare
Lig. metacarpale transversum profundum
M. lumbricalis II
M. interosseus dorsalis III (fibers attached to extensor tendon)
M. interosseus dorsalis III (fibers attached to bone)
Lig. metacarpale transversum profundum
Lig. anulare (A1)
M. flexor digitorum superficialis tendon
M. flexor digitorum profundus tendon

A Posterior view.

B Cross section through caput os metacarpi III, proximal view.

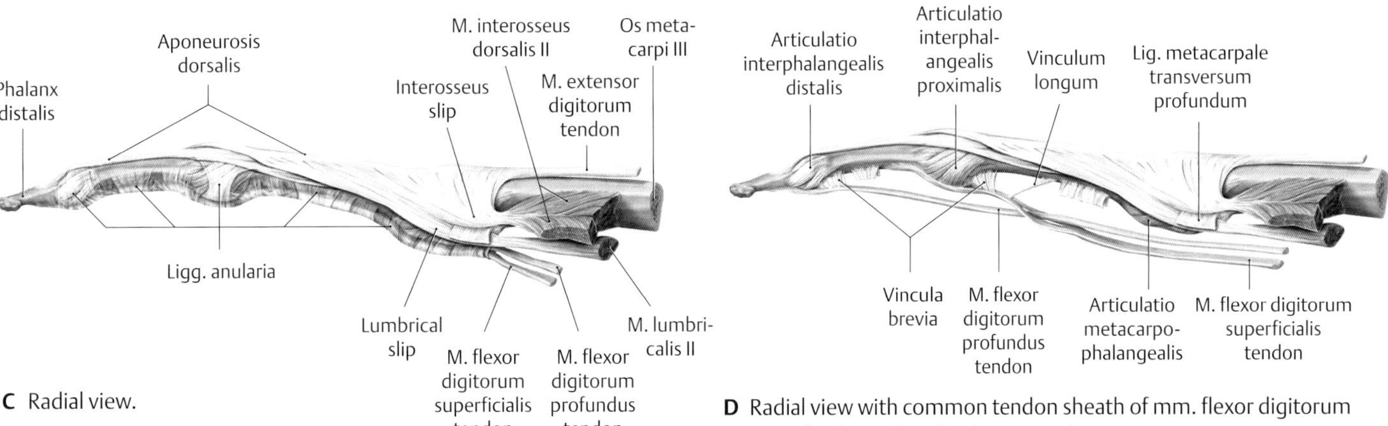
Phalanx distalis
Aponeurosis dorsalis
Interosseus slip
M. interosseus dorsalis II
Os metacarpi III
M. extensor digitorum tendon
Ligg. anularia
Lumbrical slip
M. flexor digitorum superficialis tendon
M. flexor digitorum profundus tendon
M. lumbricalis II
Articulatio interphalangealis distalis
Articulatio interphalangealis proximalis
Vinculum longum
Lig. metacarpale transversum profundum
Vincula brevia
M. flexor digitorum profundus tendon
Articulatio metacarpophalangealis
M. flexor digitorum superficialis tendon

C Radial view.

D Radial view with common tendon sheath of mm. flexor digitorum superficialis and profundus opened.

Muscle Facts (I)

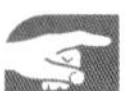

The intrinsic muscles of the hand are divided into three groups: the thenar, hypothenar, and metacarpal muscles (see p. 314). The thenar muscles are responsible for movement of the thumb, while the hypothenar muscles move the 5th digit.

Table 21.3 Mm. thenares

Muscle	Origin	Insertion		Innervation		Action
① M. adductor pollicis	Caput transversum: Os metacarpale III (facies palmaris)	Thumb (base of phalanx proximalis)	Via os sesamoid-eum ulnaris	N. ulnaris	C8, T1	Art. carpometacarpalis pollicis: adduction Art. metacarpophangealis pollicis : flexion
	Caput obliquum: Os capitatum, os metacarpale II and III					
② M. abductor pollicis brevis	Os scaphoideum and os trapezium, retinaculum flexorum		Via os sesa-moideus m. radialis	N. medianus		Art. carpometacarpalis pollicis: abduction
③ M. flexor pollicis brevis	Caput superficiale: Retinaculum flexorum			Caput superficiale: N. medianus		Art. carpometacarpalis pollicis: flexion
	Caput profundum: Os capitatum, Os trapezium			Caput profundum: N. ulnaris		
④ M. opponens pollicis	Os trapezium	Os metacarpale I (Facies radialis)		N. medianus		Art. carpometacarpalis pollicis: opposition
CMC = carpometacarpal; MCP = metacarpophalangeal.						

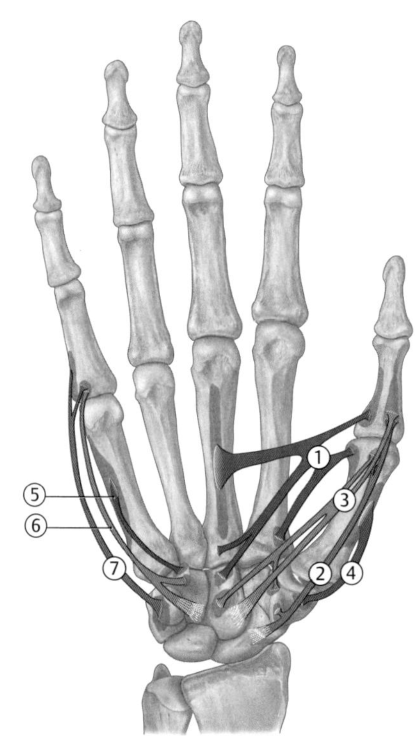

1
2
3
4
5
6
7

Fig. 21.19 **Thenar and hypothenar muscles**
Right hand, palmar (anterior) view.

Table 21.4 Mm. hypothenares

Muscle	Origin	Insertion	Innervation	Action
⑤ M. opponens digiti minimi	Hook of os hamatum, retinaculum flexorum	Os metacarpale V (facies ulnaris)	N. ulnaris (C8, T1)	Draws metacarpal in palmar direction (opposition)
⑥ M. flexor digiti minimi		Phalanx proximalis V (base)		Art. metcarpophalangealis digitus minimus: flexion
⑦ M. abductor digiti minimi	Os pisiforme	Phalanx proximalis (ulnar base) and dorsal digital expansion of digitus V		C digitus minimus: flexion and abduction of little finger Art. interphalangealis proximalis (PIP) and art. interphalangealis distalis (DIP) of digitus minimus: extension
M. palmaris brevis	Aponeurosis palmaris (facies ulnaris)	Aponeurosis palmaris		Tightens the aponeurosis palmaris (protective function)
DIP = distal interphalangeal; MCP = metacarpophalangeal; PIP = proximal interphalangeal.				

Fig. 21.20 Thenar and hypothenar muscles
Right hand, palmar (anterior) view.

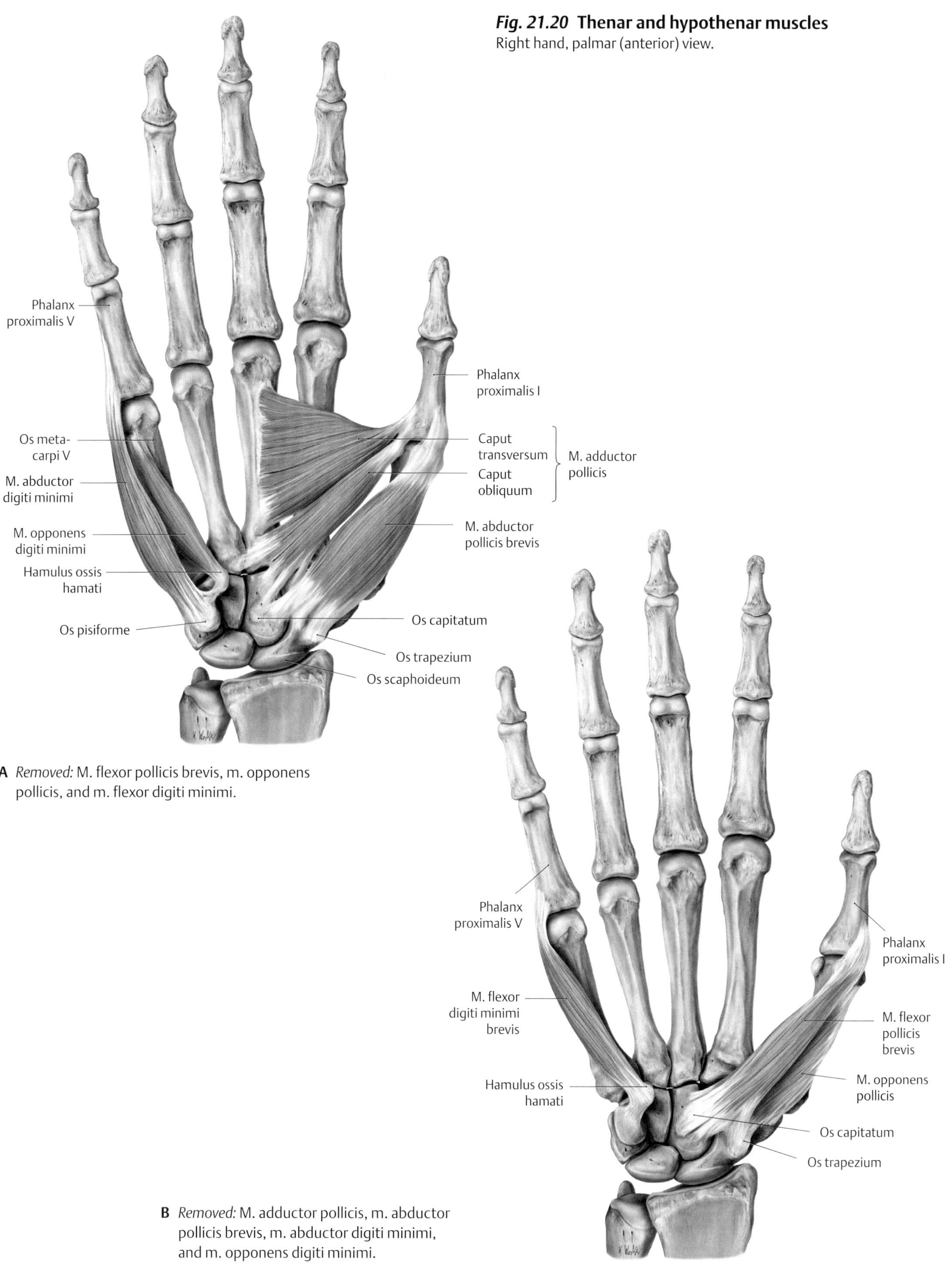
Phalanx proximalis V
Os meta-carpi V
M. abductor digiti minimi
M. opponens digiti minimi
Hamulus ossis hamati
Os pisiforme
Phalanx proximalis I
Caput transversum
Caput obliquum
M. adductor pollicis
M. abductor pollicis brevis
Os capitatum
Os trapezium
Os scaphoideum
Phalanx proximalis V
M. flexor digiti minimi brevis
Hamulus ossis hamati
Phalanx proximalis I
M. flexor pollicis brevis
M. opponens pollicis
Os capitatum
Os trapezium

A *Removed:* M. flexor pollicis brevis, m. opponens pollicis, and m. flexor digiti minimi.

B *Removed:* M. adductor pollicis, m. abductor pollicis brevis, m. abductor digiti minimi, and m. opponens digiti minimi.

Muscle Facts (II)

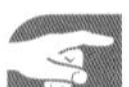

The metacarpal muscles of the hand consist of mm. lumbricales and interossei. They are responsible for the movement of the digits (with the hypothenars, which act on the 5th digit).

Fig. 21.21 Mm. lumbricales
Right hand, palmar view.

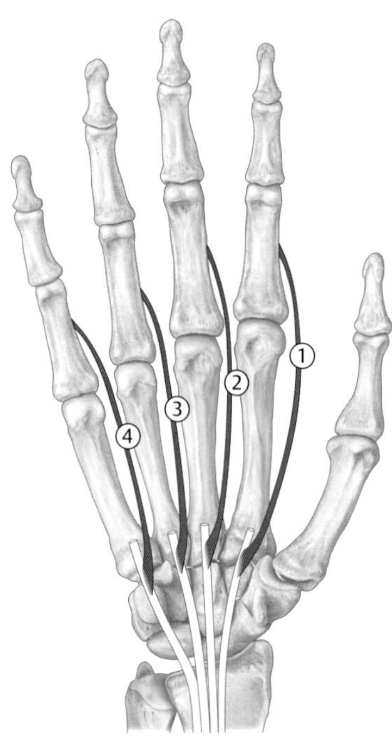
①
②
③
④

Fig. 21.22 Mm. interossei dorsales
Right hand, palmar view.

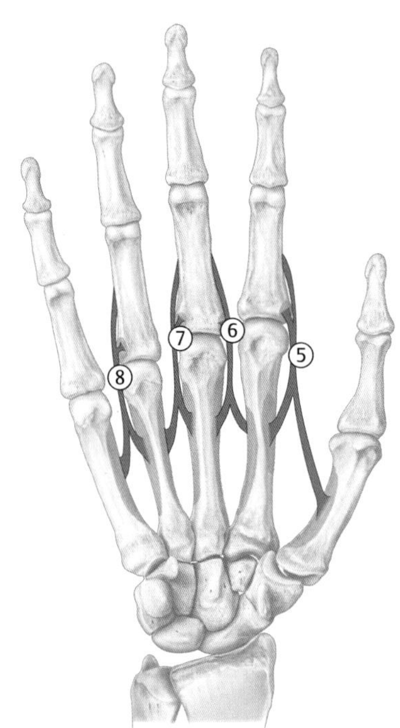
⑤
⑥
⑦
⑧

Fig. 21.23 Mm. interossei palmares
Right hand, palmar view.

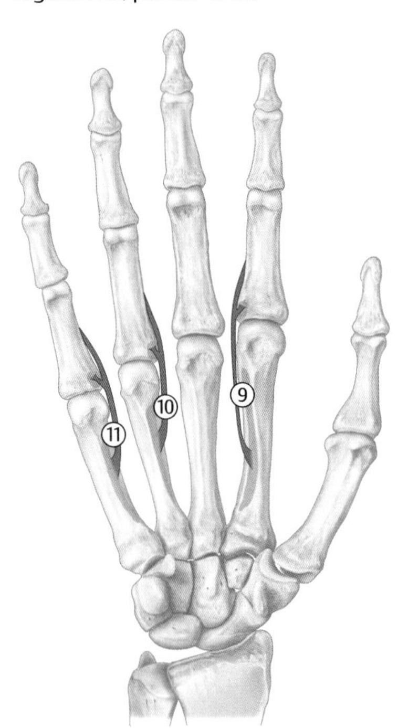
⑨
⑩
⑪

Table 21.5 Mm. metacarpales

Muscle group	Muscle	Origin	Insertion	Innervation	Action
Mm. lumbricales	① 1st	Tendo m. flexor digitorum profundus (radial sides)	Aponeurosis dorsalis digitus II	N. medianus (C8, T1)	Digitus II–V: • Art. metcarpophalangealis: flexion • Articulationes interphalangeles proximalis et distales: extension
	② 2nd		Aponeurosis dorsalis digitus III		
	③ 3rd	Tendo m. flexor digitorum profundus (bipennate from medial and lateral sides)	Aponeurosis dorsalis digitus IV	N. ulnaris (C8, T1)	
	④ 4th		Aponeurosis dorsalis digitus V		
Mm. interossei dorsales	⑤ 1st	Ossa metacarpales I and II (adjacent sides, two heads)	Aponeurosis dorsalis digitus II, phalanx proximalis II (facies radialis)		Digitus II–IV: • Art. metcarpophalangealis: flexion • Articulationes interphalangeles proximalis et distales: extension and abduction from digitus III
	⑥ 2nd	Os metacarpales II and III (adjacent sides, two heads)	Aponeurosis dorsalis digitus III, phalanx proximalis III (facies radialis)		
	⑦ 3rd	Os metacarpales III and IV (adjacent sides, two heads)	Aponeurosis dorsalis digitus III, phalanx proximalis III (facies ulnaris)		
	⑧ 4th	Os metacarpales IV and V (adjacent sides, two heads)	Aponeurosis dorsalis digitus IV, phalanx proximalis IV (facies ulnaris)		
Mm. interossei palmares	⑨ 1st	Os metacarpale II (facies ulnaris)	Aponeurosis dorsalis digitus II, phalanx proximalis II (base)		Digitus II, IV and V : • Art. metcarpophalangealis: flexion • Articulationes interphalangeles proximalis et distales: extension and adduction toward digitus III
	⑩ 2nd	Os metacarpale IV (facies radialis)	Aponeurosis dorsalis digitus IV, phalanx proximalis IV (base)		
	⑪ 3rd	Os metacarpale V (facies radialis	Aponeurosis dorsalis digitus V phalanx proximalis V (base)		

dde = dorsal digital expansion; IP = interphalangeal; MCP = metacarpophalangeal.

Fig. 21.24 **Metacarpal muscles**
Right hand, palmar (anterior) view.

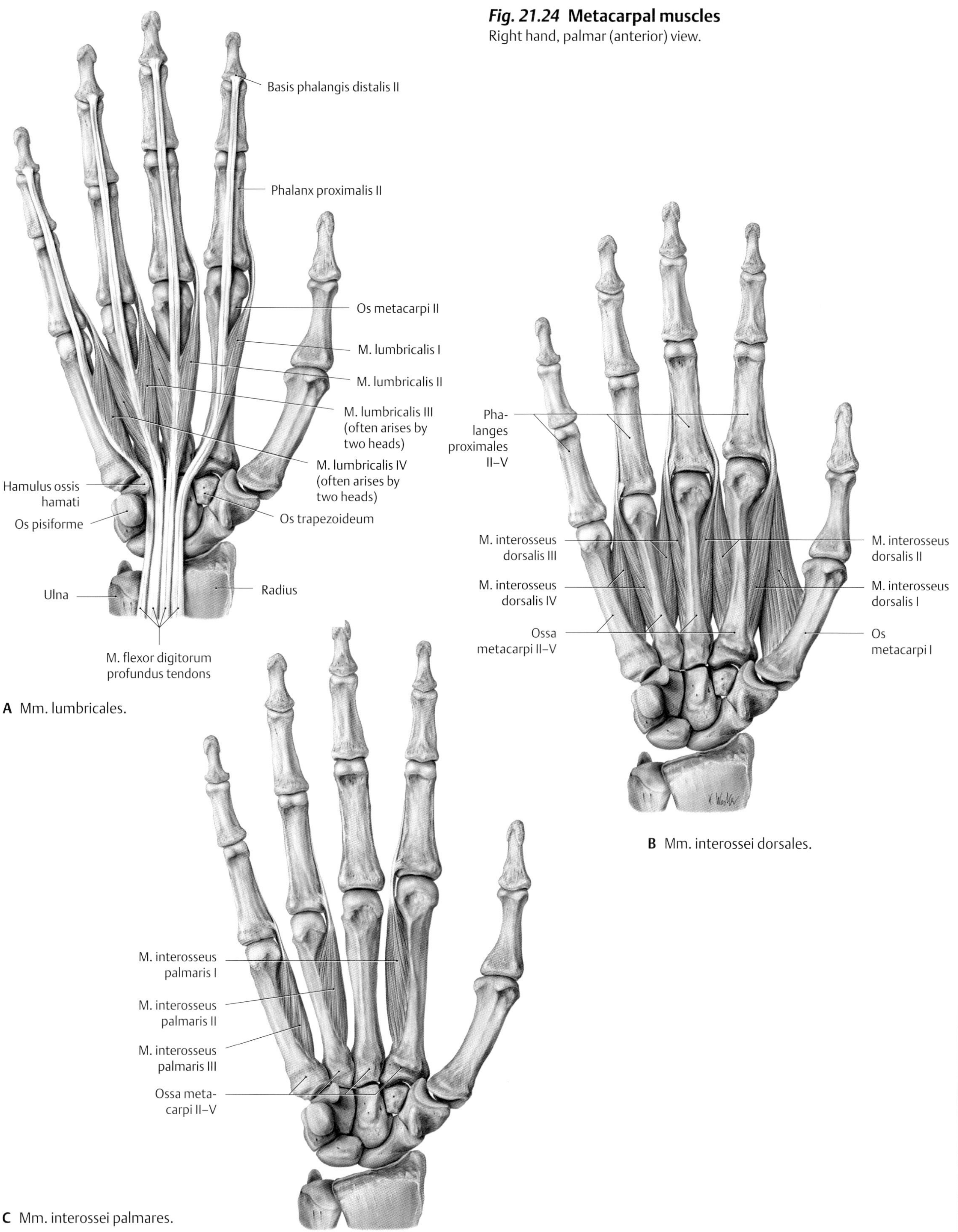
Basis phalangis distalis II
Phalanx proximalis II
Os metacarpi II
M. lumbricalis I
M. lumbricalis II
M. lumbricalis III (often arises by two heads)
M. lumbricalis IV (often arises by two heads)
Hamulus ossis hamati
Os pisiforme
Os trapezoideum
Ulna
Radius
M. flexor digitorum profundus tendons
Phalanges proximales II–V
M. interosseus dorsalis III
M. interosseus dorsalis IV
Ossa metacarpi II–V
M. interosseus dorsalis II
M. interosseus dorsalis I
Os metacarpi I
M. interosseus palmaris I
M. interosseus palmaris II
M. interosseus palmaris III
Ossa metacarpi II–V

A Mm. lumbricales.

B Mm. interossei dorsales.

C Mm. interossei palmares.

Arteries of the Upper Limb

Fig. 22.1 **Arteries of the upper limb**
Right limb, anterior view.

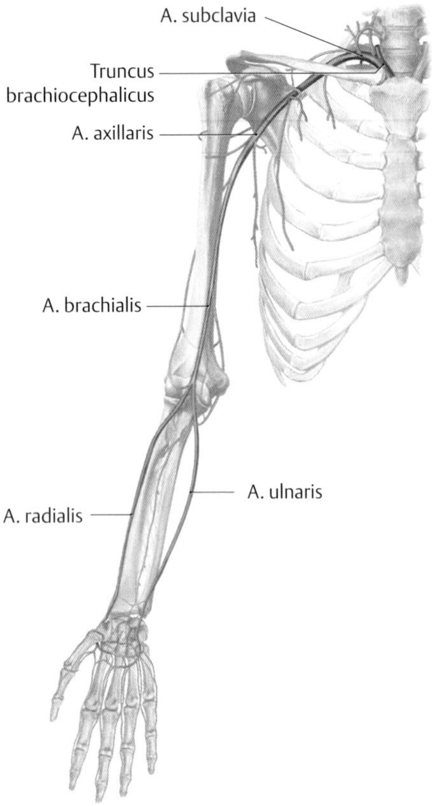

A. subclavia
Truncus brachiocephalicus
A. axillaris
A. brachialis
A. ulnaris
A. radialis

A Main arterial segments.

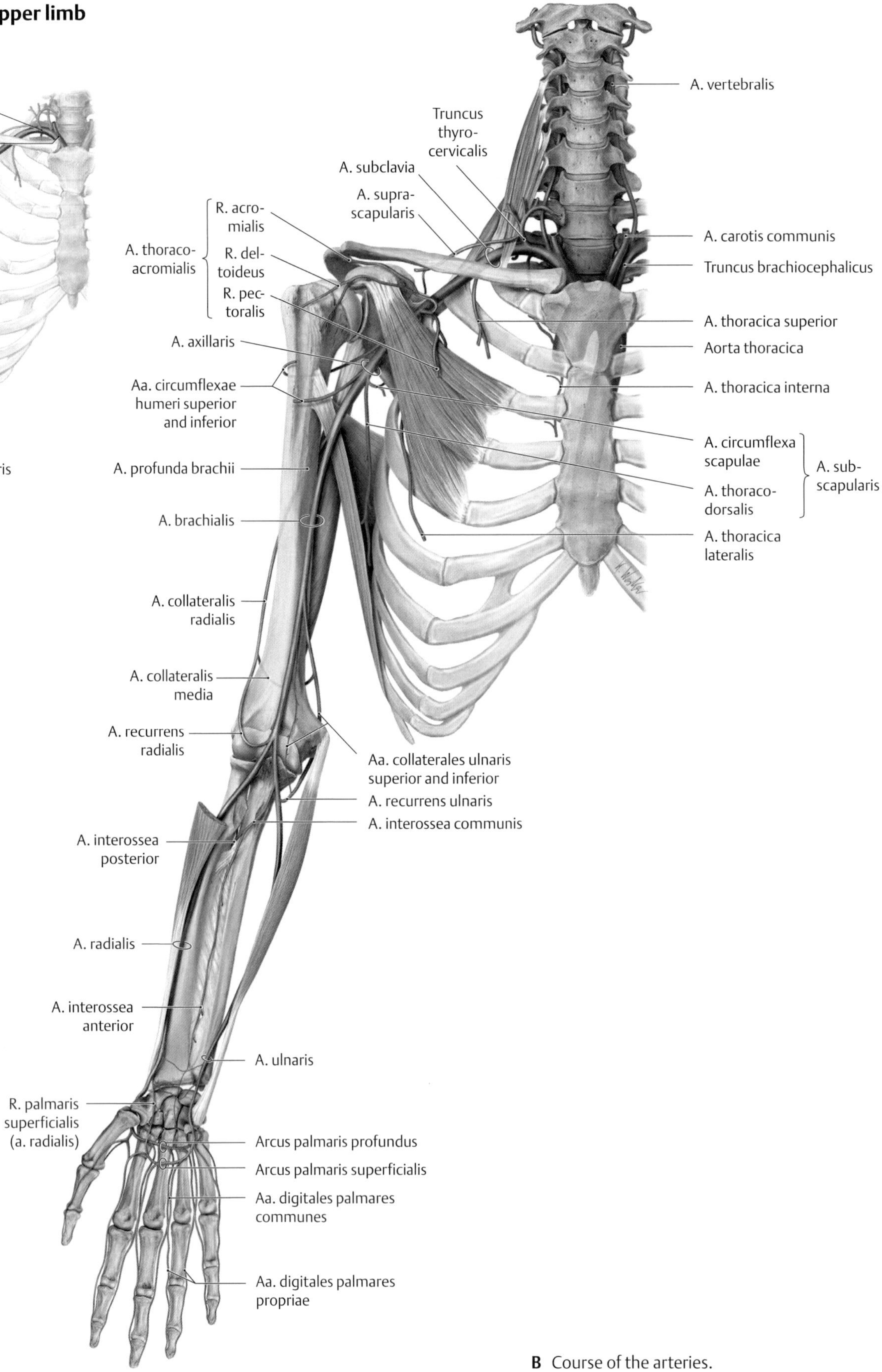

A. vertebralis
Truncus thyro-cervicalis
A. subclavia
A. supra-scapularis
A. thoraco-acromialis
R. acro-mialis
R. del-toideus
R. pec-toralis
A. carotis communis
Truncus brachiocephalicus
A. thoracica superior
A. axillaris
Aorta thoracica
Aa. circumflexae humeri superior and inferior
A. thoracica interna
A. sub-scapularis
A. circumflexa scapulae
A. thoraco-dorsalis
A. profunda brachii
A. thoracica lateralis
A. brachialis
A. collateralis radialis
A. collateralis media
A. recurrens radialis
Aa. collaterales ulnaris superior and inferior
A. recurrens ulnaris
A. interossea communis
A. interossea posterior
A. radialis
A. interossea anterior
A. ulnaris
R. palmaris superficialis (a. radialis)
Arcus palmaris profundus
Arcus palmaris superficialis
Aa. digitales palmares communes
Aa. digitales palmares propriae

B Course of the arteries.

Fig. 22.2 Branches of a. subclavia

Right side, anterior view.

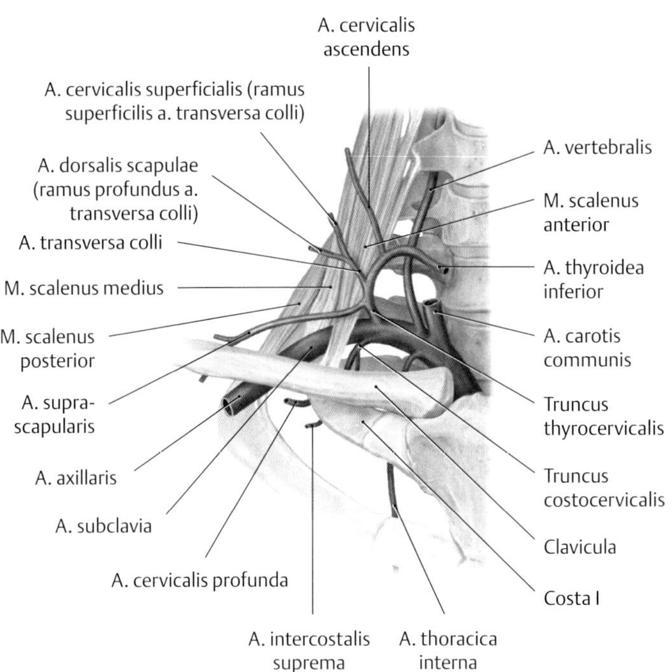
A. cervicalis ascendens
A. cervicalis superficialis (ramus superficilis a. transversa colli)
A. dorsalis scapulae (ramus profundus a. transversa colli)
A. transversa colli
M. scalenus medius
M. scalenus posterior
A. supra-scapularis
A. axillaris
A. subclavia
A. cervicalis profunda
A. intercostalis suprema
A. thoracica interna
A. vertebralis
M. scalenus anterior
A. thyroidea inferior
A. carotis communis
Truncus thyrocervicalis
Truncus costocervicalis
Clavicula
Costa I

Fig. 22.3 Scapular arcade

Right side, posterior view.

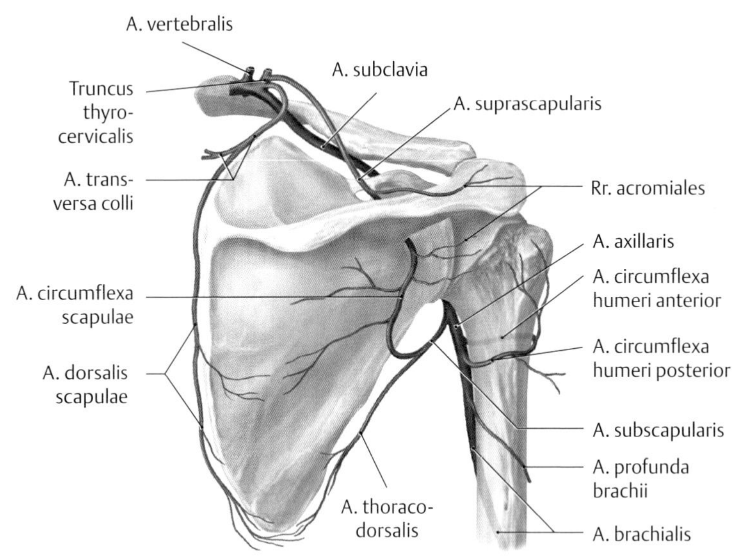
A. vertebralis
Truncus thyro-cervicalis
A. trans-versa colli
A. circumflexa scapulae
A. dorsalis scapulae
A. subclavia
A. suprascapularis
Rr. acromiales
A. axillaris
A. circumflexa humeri anterior
A. circumflexa humeri posterior
A. subscapularis
A. profunda brachii
A. brachialis
A. thoraco-dorsalis

Fig. 22.4 Arteries of the forearm and hand

Right limb. A. ulnaris and a. radialis are interconnected by the arcus palmaris superficialis and arcus palmaris profundus, the rr. perforantes, and the dorsal carpal network.

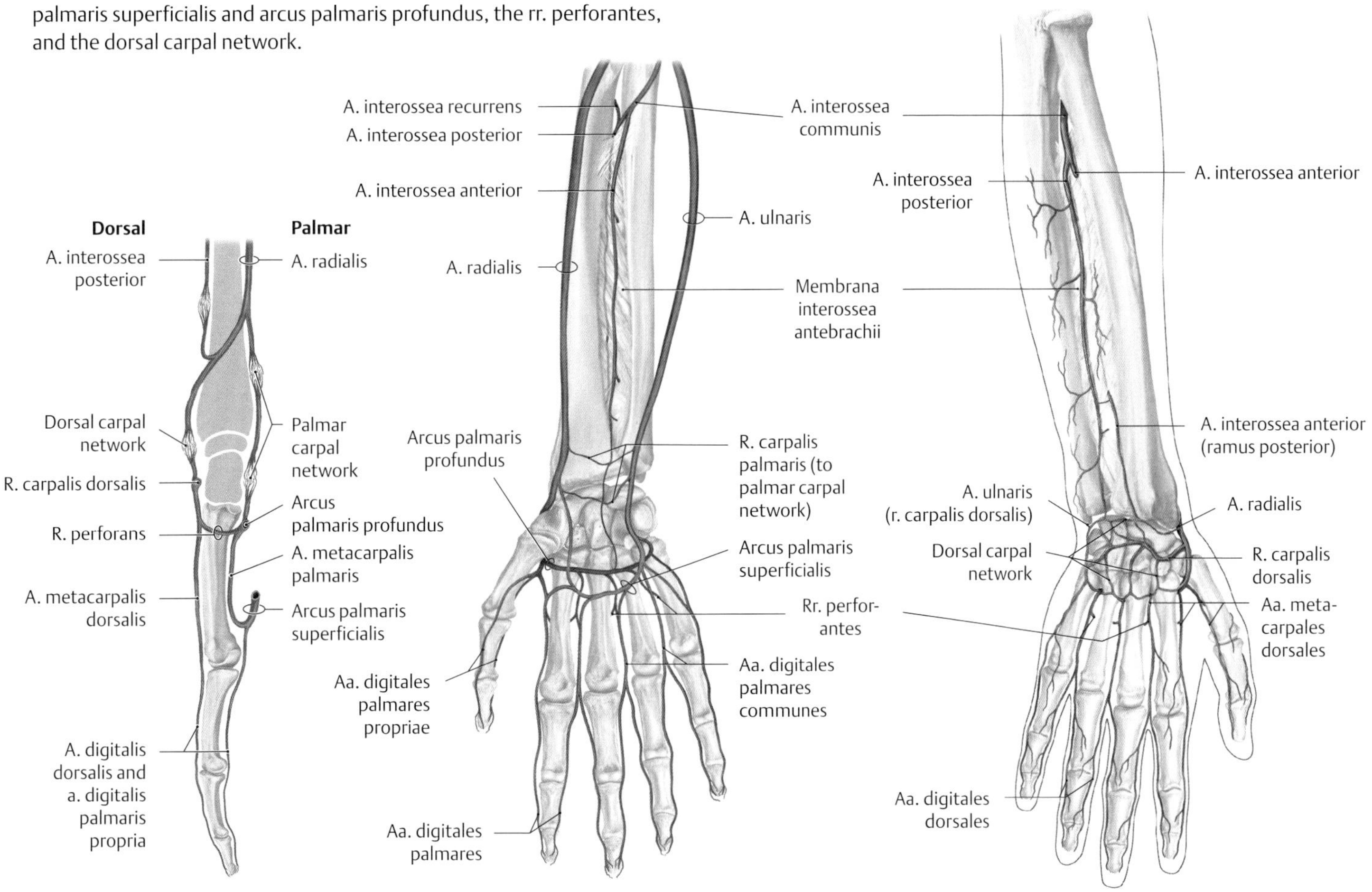

Dorsal
A. interossea posterior
Dorsal carpal network
R. carpalis dorsalis
R. perforans
A. metacarpalis dorsalis
A. digitalis dorsalis and a. digitalis palmaris propria

Palmar
A. radialis
Palmar carpal network
Arcus palmaris profundus
A. metacarpalis palmaris
Arcus palmaris superficialis

A Right middle finger, lateral view.

A. interossea recurrens
A. interossea posterior
A. interossea anterior
A. radialis
Arcus palmaris profundus
Aa. digitales palmares propriae
Aa. digitales palmares
A. interossea communis
A. ulnaris
Membrana interossea antebrachii
R. carpalis palmaris (to palmar carpal network)
Arcus palmaris superficialis
Rr. perforantes
Aa. digitales palmares communes

B Anterior (palmar) view.

A. interossea posterior
A. interossea anterior
A. interossea anterior (ramus posterior)
A. ulnaris (r. carpalis dorsalis)
A. radialis
Dorsal carpal network
R. carpalis dorsalis
Aa. metacarpales dorsales
Aa. digitales dorsales

C Posterior (dorsal) view.

Veins & Lymphatics of the Upper Limb

Fig. 22.5 Veins of the upper limb

Right limb, anterior view.

Sulcus deltoideopectoralis
V. cephalica
Basilic hiatus
V. basilica
V. mediana cubiti
V. mediana antebrachii
V. cephalica
V. mediana basilica
Vv. perforantes
Arcus venosus palmaris superficialis
Vv. intercapitulares

A Superficial veins.

V. subclavia
V. axillaris
V. thoraco-epigastricae
V. thoraco-dorsalis
Vv. brachiales
Vv. interosseae anteriores
Vv. radiales
Vv. ulnares
Arcus venosus palmaris profundus
Vv. meta-carpales palmares
Vv. digitales palmares

B Deep veins.

Fig. 22.6 Veins of the dorsum

Right hand, posterior view.

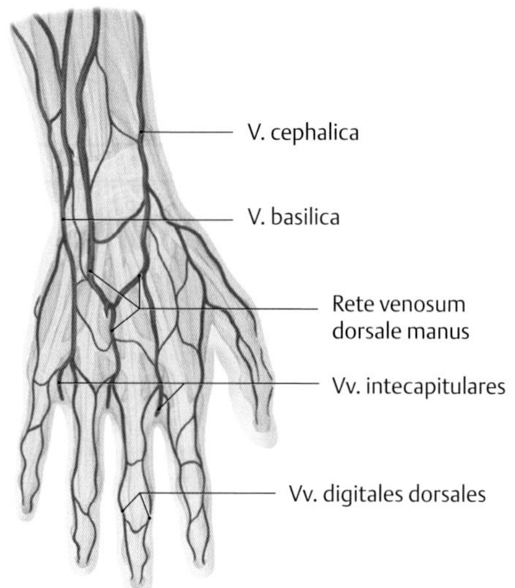
V. cephalica
V. basilica
Rete venosum dorsale manus
Vv. intecapitulares
Vv. digitales dorsales

Clinical

Venipuncture

The veins of fossa cubitalis are frequently used when drawing blood. In preparation, a tourniquet is applied. This allows arterial blood to flow, but blocks the return of venous blood. The resulting swelling makes the veins more visible and palpable.

Fig. 22.7 Fossa cubitalis

Right limb, anterior view. The subcutaneous veins of fossa cubitalis have a highly variable course.

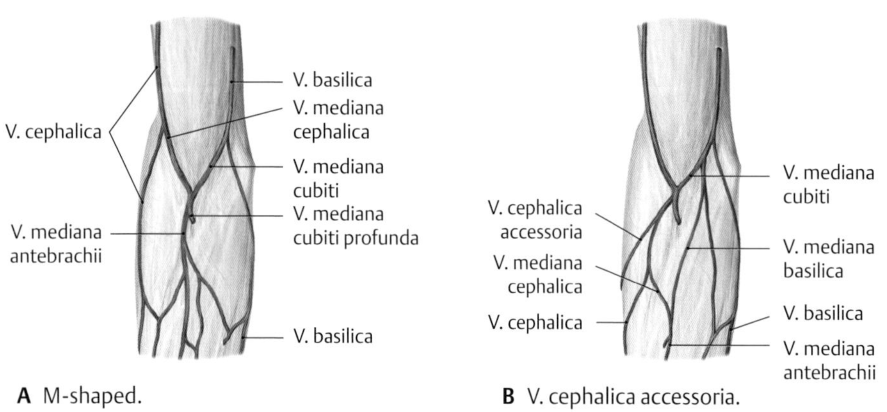
V. basilica
V. mediana cephalica
V. cephalica
V. mediana cubiti
V. mediana cubiti profunda
V. mediana antebrachii
V. basilica

A M-shaped.

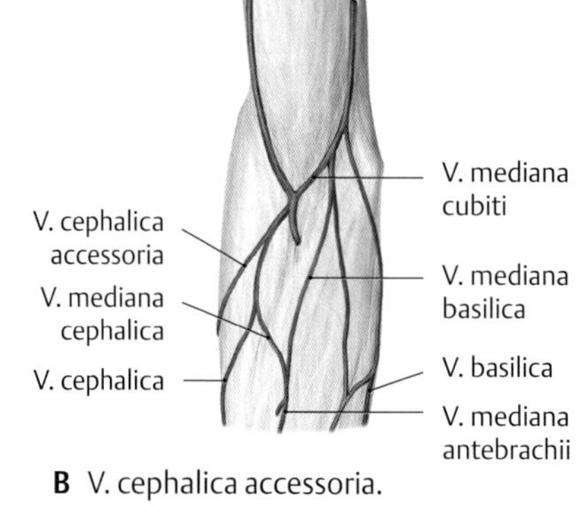
V. mediana cubiti
V. cephalica accessoria
V. mediana basilica
V. mediana cephalica
V. cephalica
V. basilica
V. mediana antebrachii

B V. cephalica accessoria.

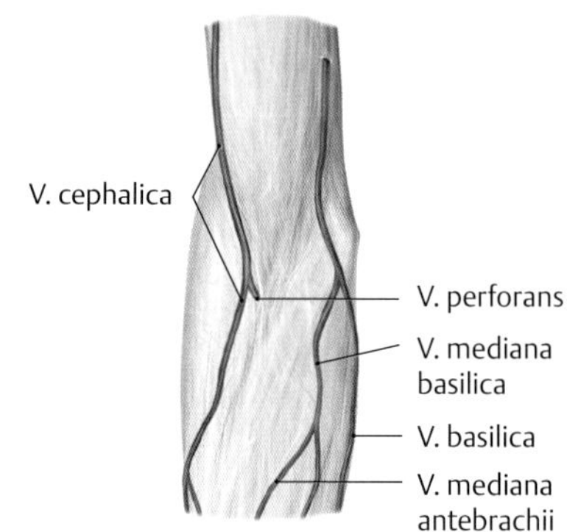
V. cephalica
V. perforans
V. mediana basilica
V. basilica
V. mediana antebrachii

C Absent v. mediana cubiti.

Lymph from the upper limb and breast drains to nll. axillares. The superficial lymphatics of the upper limb lie in the subcutaneous tissue, while the deep lymphatics accompany the arteries and deep veins. Numerous anastomoses exist between the two systems.

Fig. 22.8 **Lymph vessels of the upper limb**
Right limb.

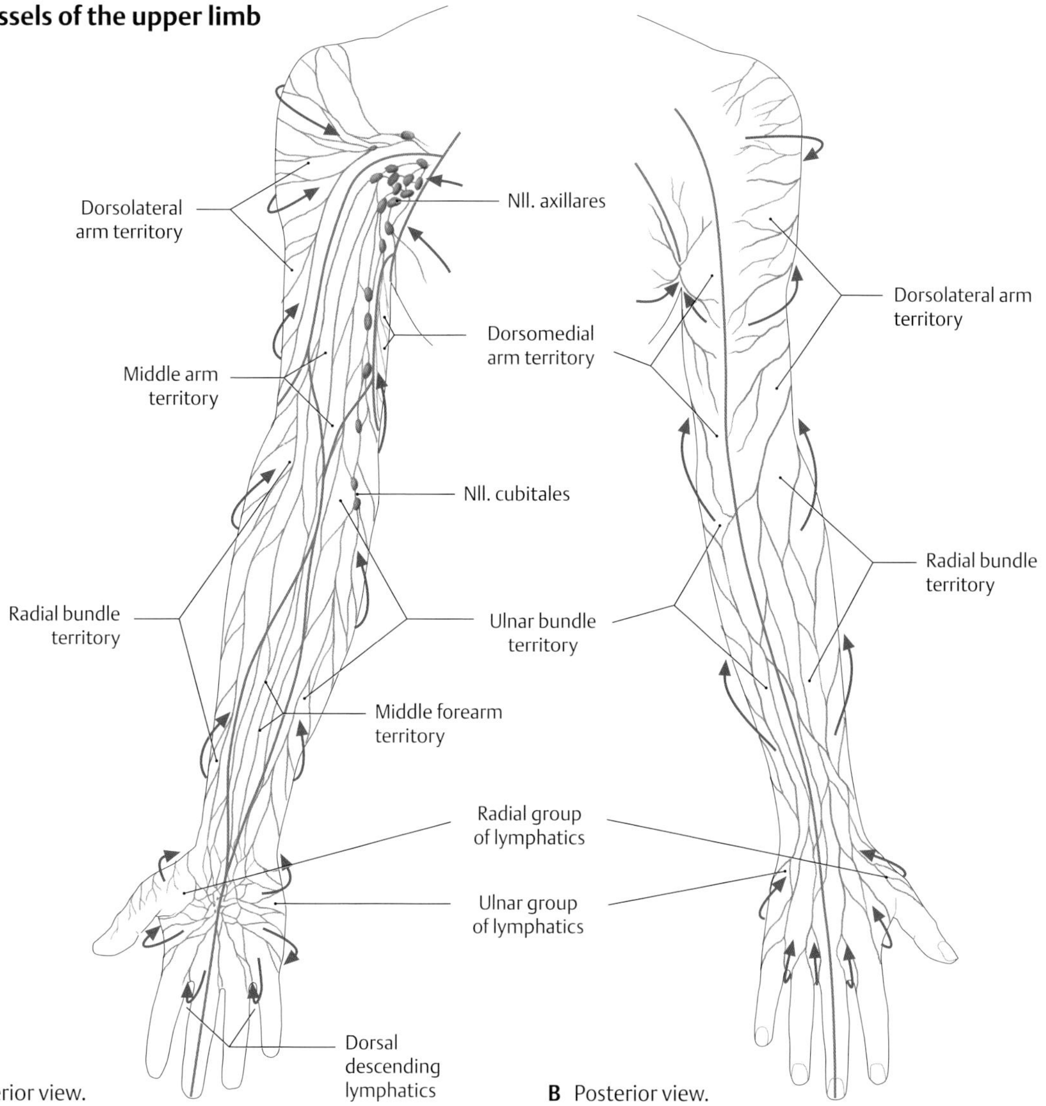

Dorsolateral arm territory
Nll. axillares
Dorsomedial arm territory
Middle arm territory
Nll. cubitales
Radial bundle territory
Ulnar bundle territory
Middle forearm territory
Radial group of lymphatics
Ulnar group of lymphatics
Dorsal descending lymphatics
Dorsolateral arm territory
Radial bundle territory

A Anterior view.

B Posterior view.

Fig. 22.9 **Lymphatic drainage of the hand**
Right hand, radial view. Most of the hand drains to nll. axillares via nll. cubitales. However, the thumb, index finger, and dorsum of the hand drain directly.

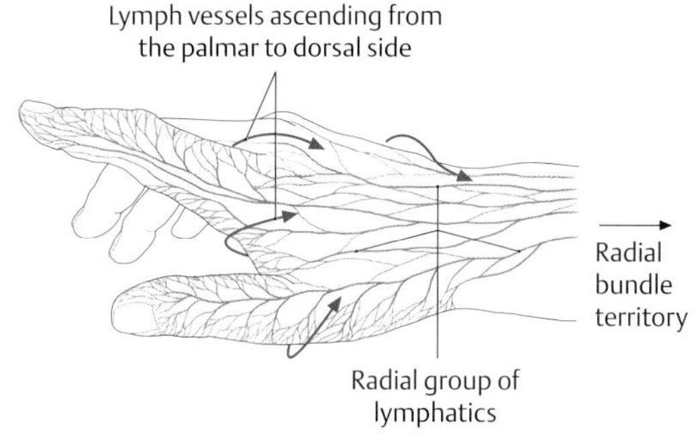
Lymph vessels ascending from the palmar to dorsal side
Radial bundle territory
Radial group of lymphatics

Fig. 22.10 **Axillary lymph nodes**
Right side, anterior view. Nll. axillares are divided into three levels with respect to m. pectoralis minor. They have major clinical importance in breast cancer (see p. 65).

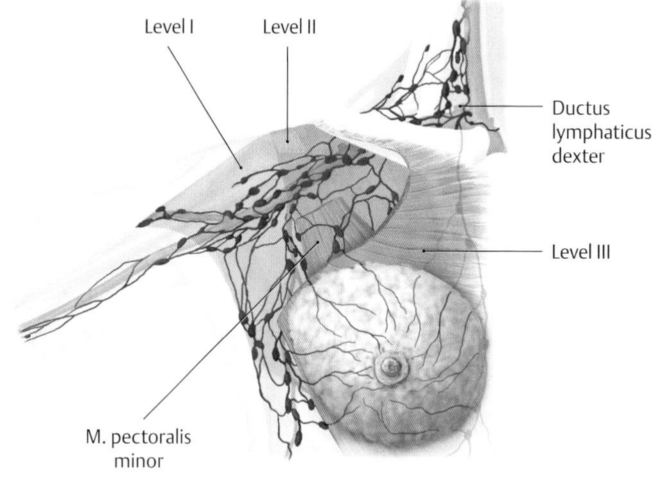
Level I
Level II
Ductus lymphaticus dexter
Level III
M. pectoralis minor

Nerves of Plexus Brachialis

Almost all muscles in the upper limb are innervated by plexus brachialis, which arises from spinal cord segments C5 to T1. The anterior rami of the spinal nerves give off direct branches (pars supraclavicularis of plexus brachialis) and merge to form three trunci, six divisiones (three anterior and three posterior), and three fasciculi. The pars infraclavicularis of plexus brachialis consists of short branches that arise directly from the fasciculi and long (terminal) branches that traverse the limb.

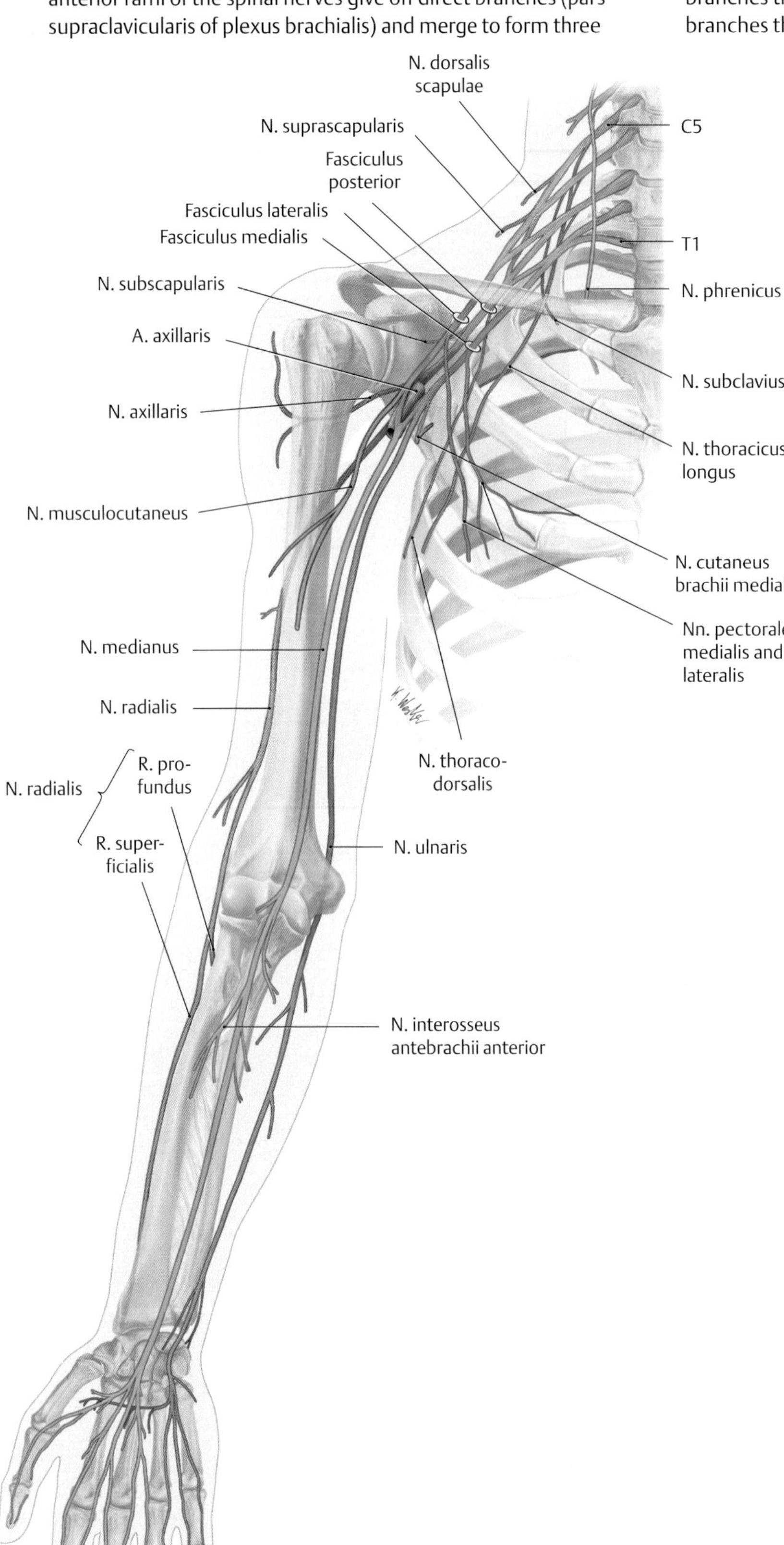
N. dorsalis scapulae
N. suprascapularis
Fasciculus posterior
Fasciculus lateralis
Fasciculus medialis
N. subscapularis
A. axillaris
N. axillaris
N. musculocutaneus
N. medianus
N. radialis
N. radialis
R. profundus
R. superficialis
N. thoracodorsalis
N. ulnaris
N. interosseus antebrachii anterior
C5
T1
N. phrenicus
N. subclavius
N. thoracicus longus
N. cutaneus brachii medialis
Nn. pectorales medialis and lateralis

Table 22.1 Nerves of the plexus brachiales

Pars supraclavicularis			
Direct branches from the rr. anteriores or trunci plexus brachialis			
●		N. dorsalis scapulae	C4–C5
		N. suprascapularis	C4–C6
		N. subclavius	C5–C6
		N. thoracicus longus	C5–C7
Pars infraclavicularis			
Short and long branches from the plexus cords			
●	**Fasciculus lateralis**	N. pectoralis lateralis	C5–C7
		N. musculocutaneus	
●		N. medianus: Radix lateralis	C6–C7
	Fasciculus medialis	N. medianus: Radix medialis	C8–T1
●		N. pectoralis medialis	
		N. cutaneus antebrachii medialis	
		N. cutaneus brachii medialis	T1
		N. ulnaris	C7–T1
●	**Fasciculus posterior**	N. subscapular superior	C5–C6
		N. thoracodorsalis	C6–C8
		N. subscapularis inferior	C5–C6
		N. axillaris	
		N. radialis	C5–T1

Fig. 22.11 **Plexus brachialis**
Right side, anterior view.

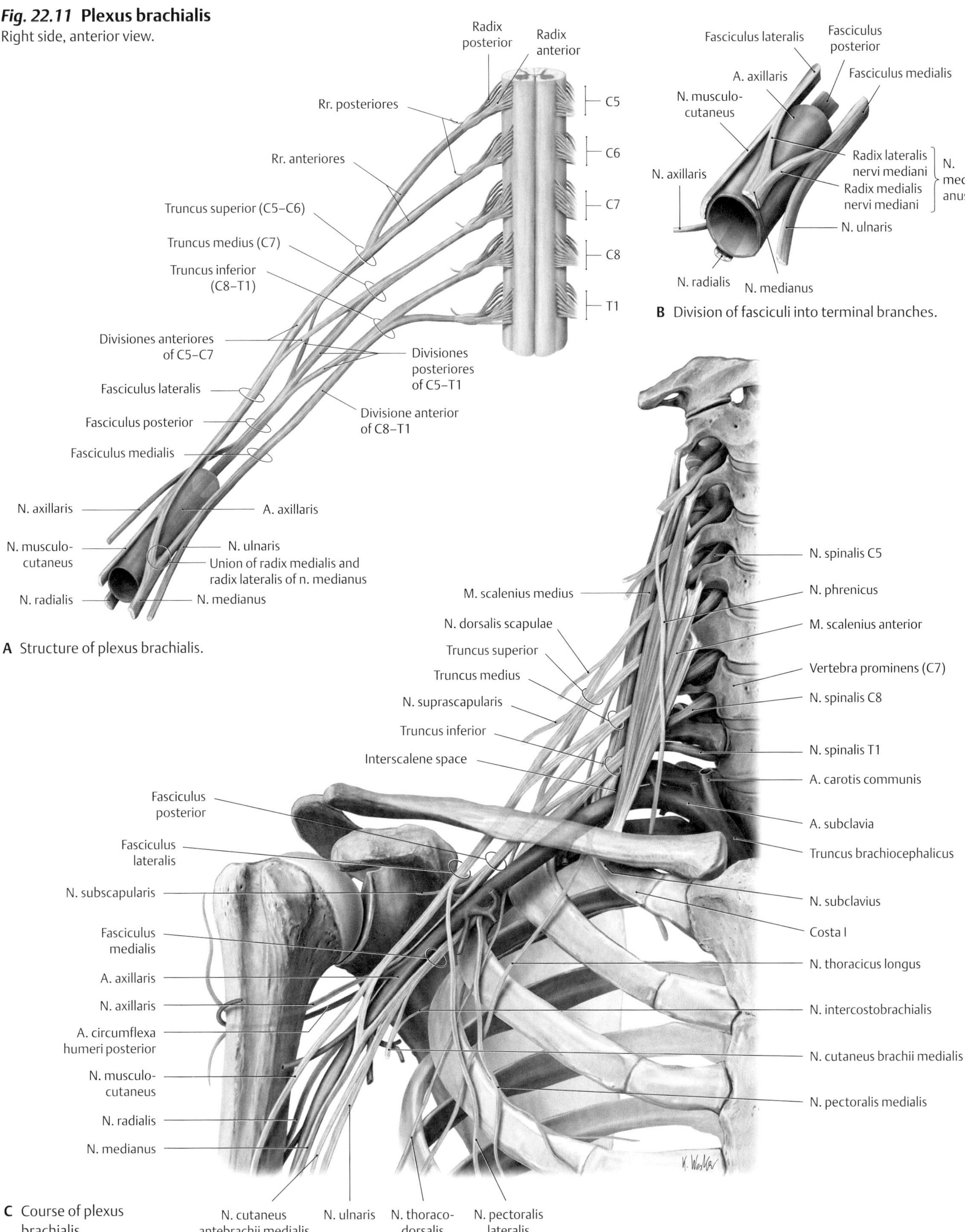
Radix posterior
Radix anterior
Rr. posteriores
Rr. anteriores
C5
C6
C7
C8
T1
Truncus superior (C5–C6)
Truncus medius (C7)
Truncus inferior (C8–T1)
Divisiones anteriores of C5–C7
Divisiones posteriores of C5–T1
Fasciculus lateralis
Fasciculus posterior
Fasciculus medialis
Divisione anterior of C8–T1
N. axillaris
A. axillaris
N. musculo-cutaneus
N. ulnaris
Union of radix medialis and radix lateralis of n. medianus
N. radialis
N. medianus
Fasciculus lateralis
Fasciculus posterior
A. axillaris
Fasciculus medialis
N. musculo-cutaneus
Radix lateralis nervi mediani
Radix medialis nervi mediani
N. medianus
N. axillaris
N. ulnaris
N. radialis
N. medianus
N. spinalis C5
M. scalenius medius
N. phrenicus
N. dorsalis scapulae
M. scalenius anterior
Truncus superior
Vertebra prominens (C7)
Truncus medius
N. suprascapularis
N. spinalis C8
Truncus inferior
N. spinalis T1
Interscalene space
A. carotis communis
Fasciculus posterior
A. subclavia
Fasciculus lateralis
Truncus brachiocephalicus
N. subscapularis
N. subclavius
Costa I
Fasciculus medialis
N. thoracicus longus
A. axillaris
N. axillaris
N. intercostobrachialis
A. circumflexa humeri posterior
N. cutaneus brachii medialis
N. musculo-cutaneus
N. pectoralis medialis
N. radialis
N. medianus
N. cutaneus antebrachii medialis
N. ulnaris
N. thoraco-dorsalis
N. pectoralis lateralis

A Structure of plexus brachialis.

B Division of fasciculi into terminal branches.

C Course of plexus brachialis.

Supraclavicular Branches & Fasciculus Posterior

Fig. 22.12 Supraclavicular branches
Right shoulder.

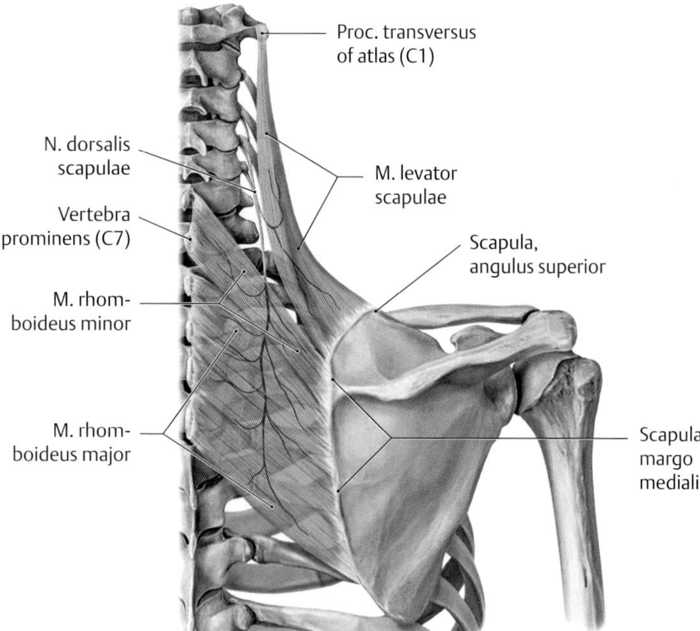
Proc. transversus of atlas (C1)
N. dorsalis scapulae
M. levator scapulae
Vertebra prominens (C7)
Scapula, angulus superior
M. rhom-boideus minor
M. rhom-boideus major
Scapula, margo medialis

A N. dorsalis scapulae. Posterior view.

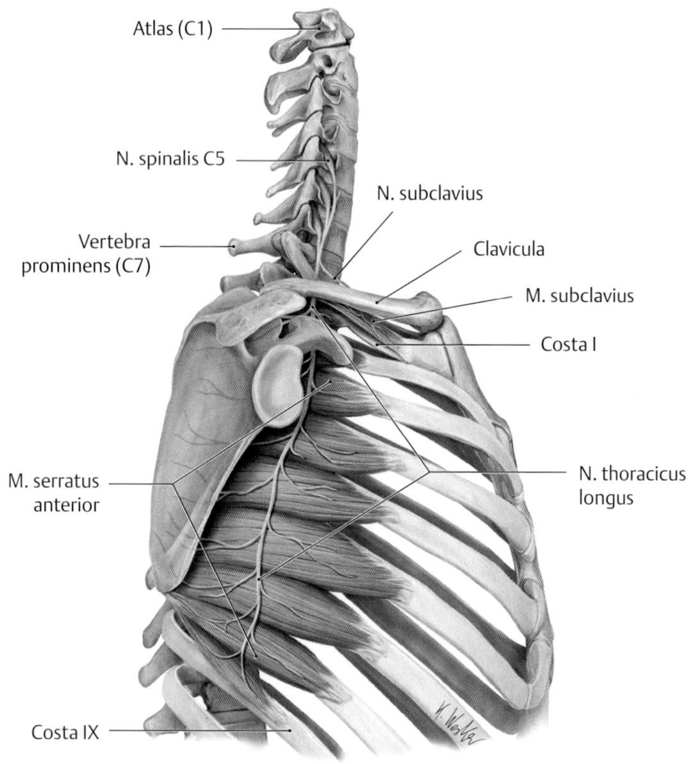
Atlas (C1)
N. spinalis C5
N. subclavius
Vertebra prominens (C7)
Clavicula
M. subclavius
Costa I
M. serratus anterior
N. thoracicus longus
Costa IX

C N. thoracicus longus and n. subclavius. Right lateral view.

The supraclavicular branches of plexus brachialis arise directly from the plexus roots (anterior rami of the spinal nerves) or from the trunci in the lateral cervical triangle.

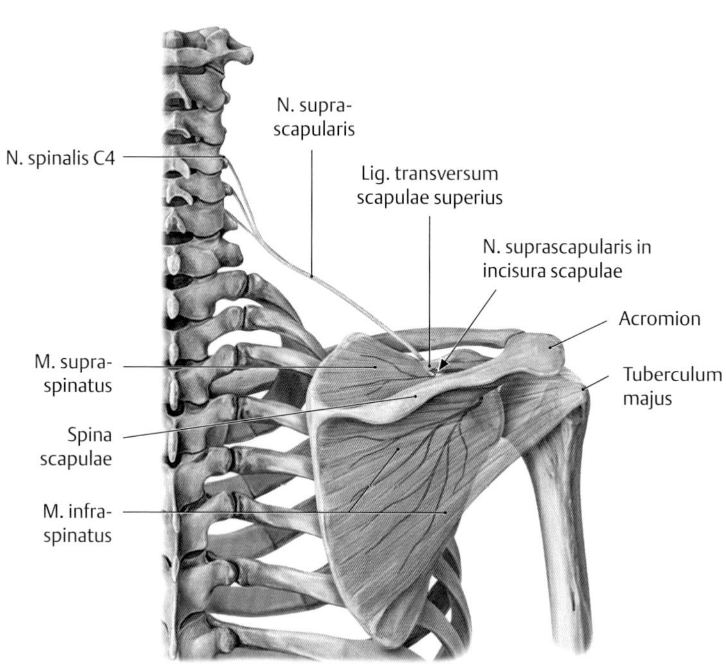
N. supra-scapularis
N. spinalis C4
Lig. transversum scapulae superius
N. suprascapularis in incisura scapulae
Acromion
M. supra-spinatus
Tuberculum majus
Spina scapulae
M. infra-spinatus

B N. suprascapularis. Posterior view.

Table 22.2 Pars supraclavicularis

Nerve	Level	Innervated muscle
N. dorsalis scapulae	C4–C5	M. levator scapulae M. rhomboideus major and minor
N. suprascapularis	C4–C6	M. supraspinatus M. infraspinatus
N. subclavius	C5–C6	M. subclavius Intercostobrachial nn.
N. thoracicus longus	C5–C7	M. serratus anterior

Fig. 22.13 Fasciculus posterior: Short branches

Right shoulder.

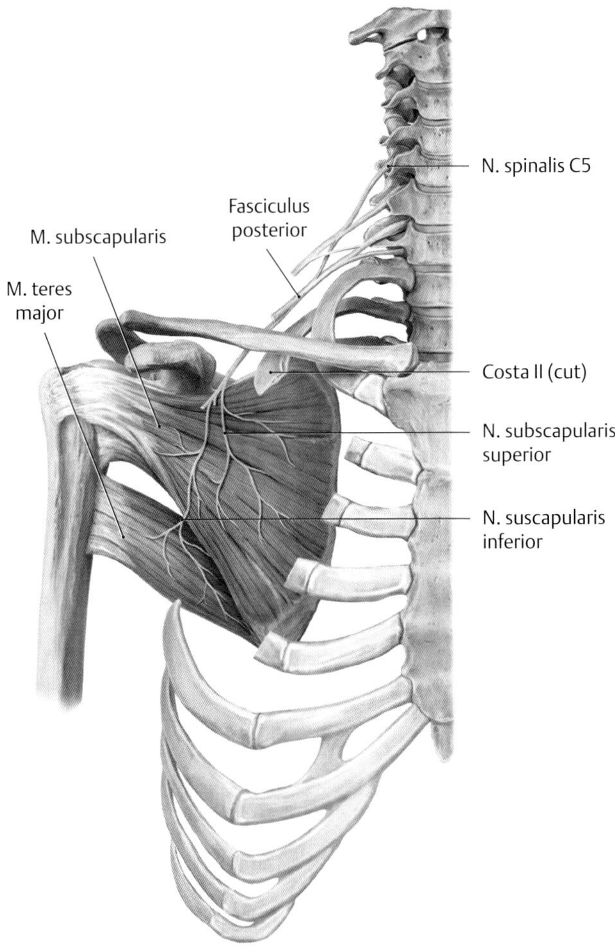
N. spinalis C5
Fasciculus posterior
M. subscapularis
M. teres major
Costa II (cut)
N. subscapularis superior
N. suscapularis inferior

A Nn. subscapulares. Anterior view.

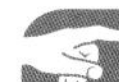

The fasciculus posterior gives off three short branches (arising at the level of the plexus cords) and two long branches (terminal nerves, see pp. 324–325).

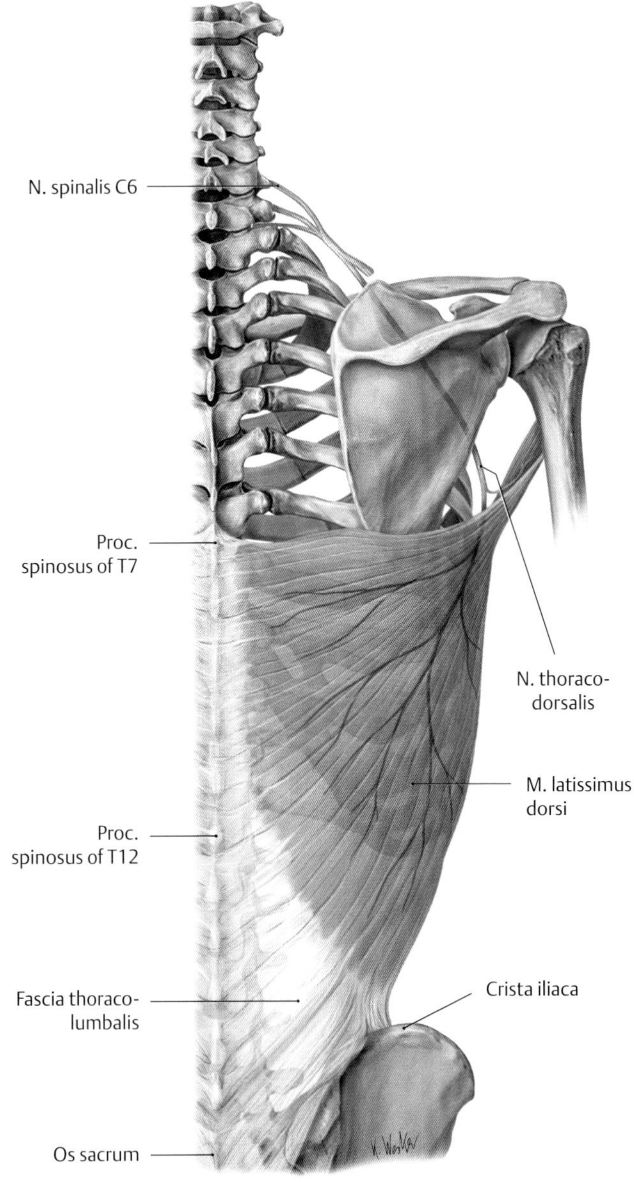
N. spinalis C6
Proc. spinosus of T7
N. thoraco-dorsalis
M. latissimus dorsi
Proc. spinosus of T12
Crista iliaca
Fascia thoraco-lumbalis
Os sacrum

B N. thoracodorsalis. Posterior view.

Table 22.3 Branches of the fasciculus posterior

Nerve	Level	Innervated muscle
Short branches		
N. subscapularis inferior	C5–C6	M. subscapularis
N. subscapularis superior		M. subscapularis M. teres major
N. thoracodorsalis	C6–C8	M. latissimus dorsi
Long (terminal) branches		
N. axillaris	C5–C6	See p. 324
N. radialis	C5–T1	See p. 325

Fasciculus Posterior: N. Axillaris & N. Radialis

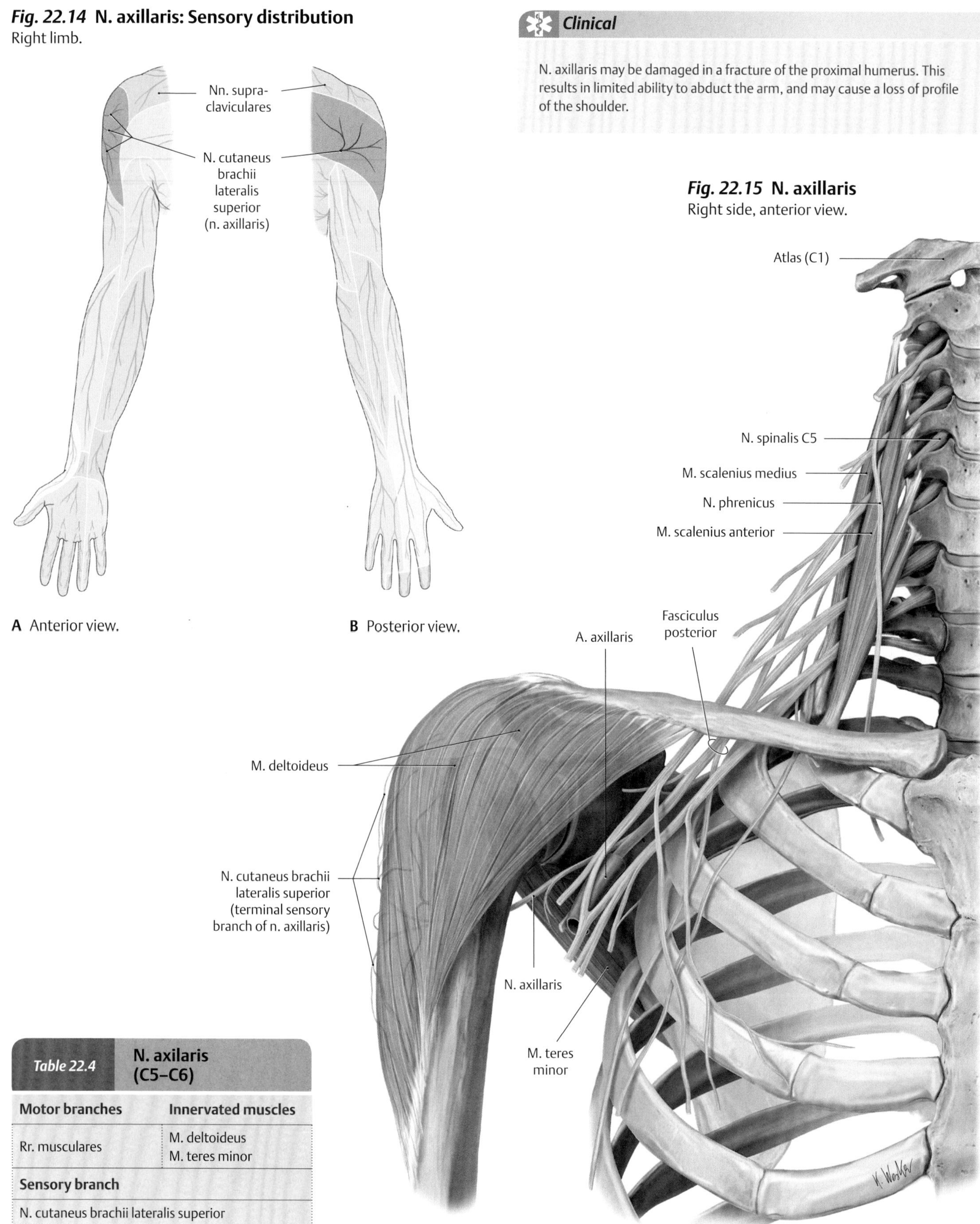
Nn. supra-
claviculares
N. cutaneus
brachii
lateralis
superior
(n. axillaris)
Atlas (C1)
N. spinalis C5
M. scalenius medius
N. phrenicus
M. scalenius anterior
Fasciculus
posterior
A. axillaris
M. deltoideus
N. cutaneus brachii
lateralis superior
(terminal sensory
branch of n. axillaris)
N. axillaris
M. teres
minor

Fig. 22.14 **N. axillaris: Sensory distribution**
Right limb.

A Anterior view.

B Posterior view.

Fig. 22.15 **N. axillaris**
Right side, anterior view.

Clinical

N. axillaris may be damaged in a fracture of the proximal humerus. This results in limited ability to abduct the arm, and may cause a loss of profile of the shoulder.

Table 22.4	**N. axilaris (C5–C6)**
Motor branches	**Innervated muscles**
Rr. musculares	M. deltoideus M. teres minor
Sensory branch	
N. cutaneus brachii lateralis superior	

Fig. 22.16 N. radialis: Sensory distribution

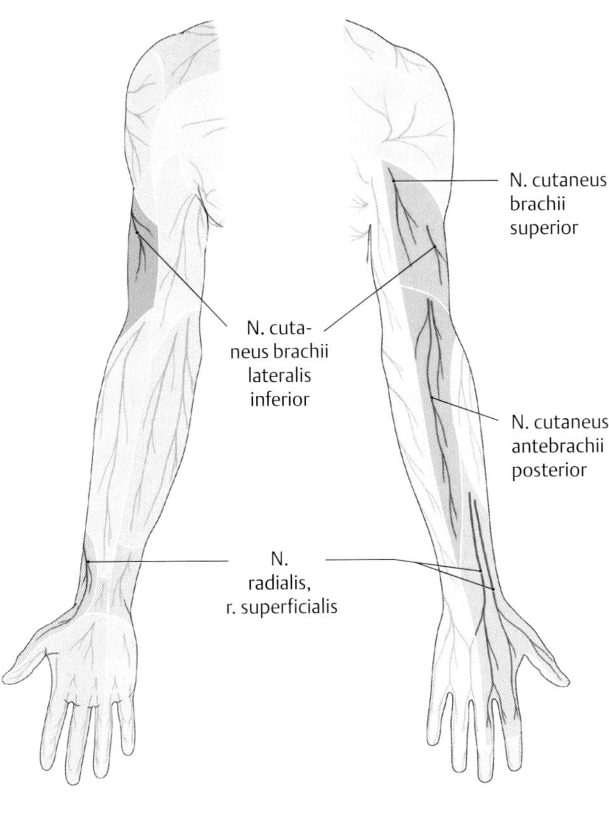

N. cutaneus brachii superior
N. cuta-neus brachii lateralis inferior
N. cutaneus antebrachii posterior
N. radialis, r. superficialis

A Anterior view. **B** Posterior view.

Table 22.5	N. radialis (C5–T1)
Motor branches	**Innervated muscles**
Rr. musculares	M. brachialis (partial)
	M. triceps brachii
	M. anconeus
	M. brachioradialis
	M. extensors carpi radialis longus and brevis
R. profundus (terminal branch : N. interosseus posterior)	M. supinator
	M. extensor digitorum
	M. extensor digiti minimi
	M. extensor carpi ulnaris
	M. extensors pollicis brevis and longus
	M. extensor indicis
	M. abductor pollicis longus
Sensory branches	
Rr. articulationes n. radialis : Capsula art. humeri	
Rr. articulationes n. interosseus posterior: Capsula art. carpalis and four articulationes metacarpophalangeales radials	
N. cutaneus brachii posterior	
N. cutaneus brachii lateralis inferior	
N. cutaneus antebrachii posterior	
Rr. superficiales	Nn. digitales dorsales
	R. ulnaris communicans

Fig. 22.17 N. radialis

Right limb, anterior view with forearm pronated.

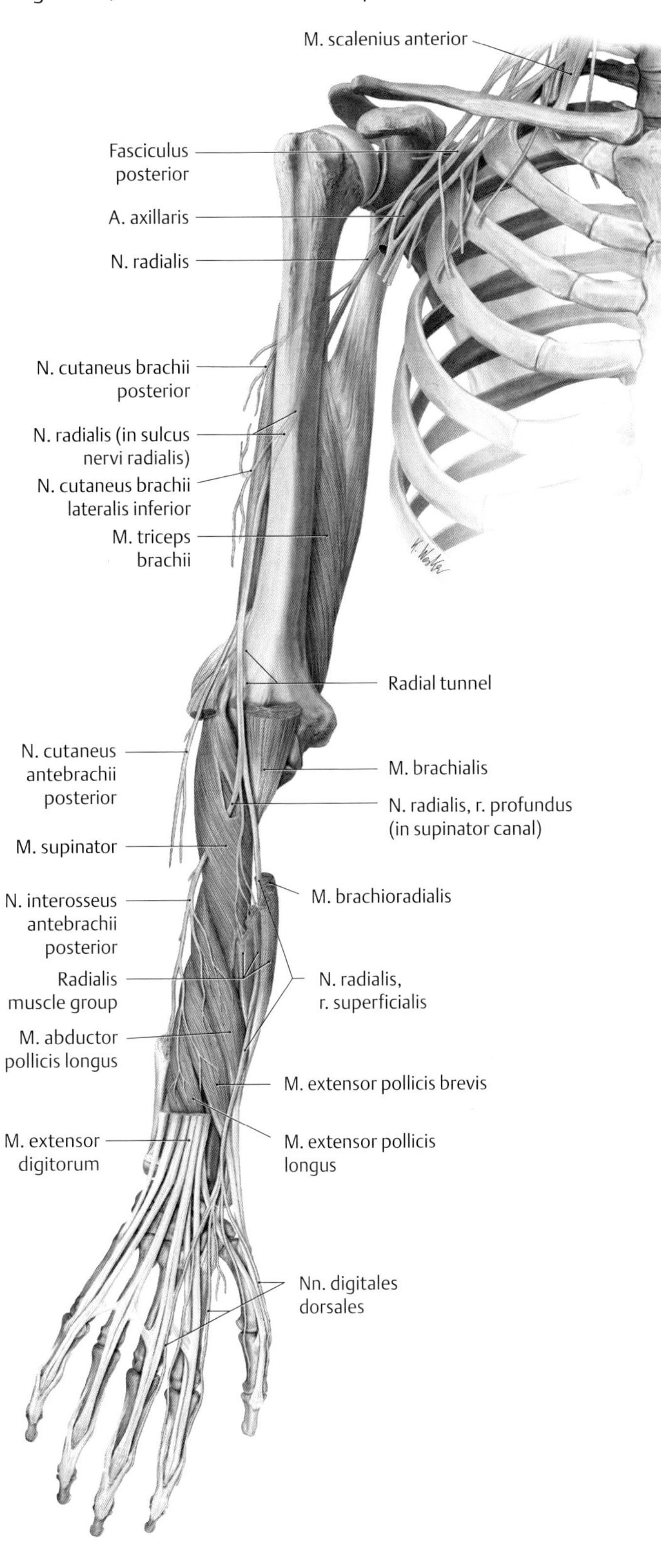

M. scalenius anterior
Fasciculus posterior
A. axillaris
N. radialis
N. cutaneus brachii posterior
N. radialis (in sulcus nervi radialis)
N. cutaneus brachii lateralis inferior
M. triceps brachii
Radial tunnel
N. cutaneus antebrachii posterior
M. brachialis
N. radialis, r. profundus (in supinator canal)
M. supinator
M. brachioradialis
N. interosseus antebrachii posterior
Radialis muscle group
N. radialis, r. superficialis
M. abductor pollicis longus
M. extensor pollicis brevis
M. extensor digitorum
M. extensor pollicis longus
Nn. digitales dorsales

Clinical

Chronic compression of n. radialis in the axilla (e.g., due to extended/improper crutch use) may cause loss of sensation or motor function in the hand, forearm, and posterior arm. More distal injuries (e.g., during anesthesia) affect fewer muscles, potentially resulting in wrist drop with intact function of m. triceps brachii.

Fasciculus Medialis & Fasciculus Lateralis

The fasciculi medialis and lateralis give off four short branches. The nn. intercostobrachiales are included with the short branches of plexus brachialis, although they are actually the cutaneous branches of the 2nd and 3rd nn. intercostales.

Table 22.6 Rr. fasciculus lateralis and medialis

Nerve	Level	Cord	Innervated muscle
Short branches			
N. pectoralis lateralis	C5–C7	Fasciculus lateralis	M. pectoralis major
N. pectoralis medialis	C8–T1	Fasciculus medialis	M. pectoralis major and minor
N. cutaneus brachii medialis	T1		— (sensory branches)
N. cutaneus antebrachii medialis	C8–T1		
Nn. Intercostobrachialis	T2–T3		
Long (terminal) branches			
N. musculocutaneus	C5–C7	Fasciculus lateralis	M. coracobrachialis M. biceps brachii M. brachialis
N. medianus	C6–T1	Fasciculus medialis	See p. 328
N. ulnaris	C7–T1		See p. 329

Fig. 22.18 **Fasciculi medialis and lateralis: Short branches**
Right side, anterior view.

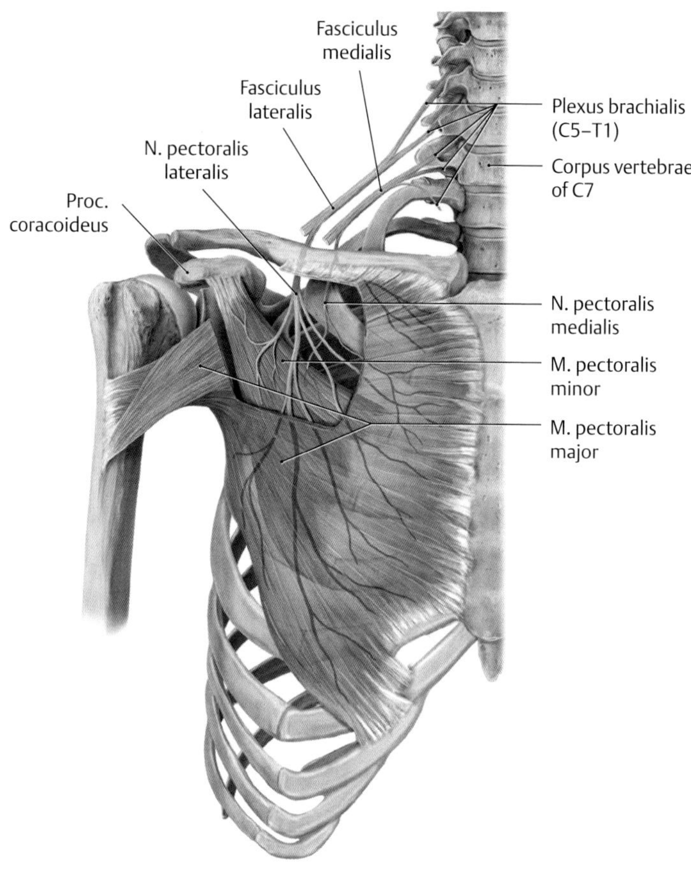
Fasciculus medialis
Fasciculus lateralis
N. pectoralis lateralis
Proc. coracoideus
Plexus brachialis (C5–T1)
Corpus vertebrae of C7
N. pectoralis medialis
M. pectoralis minor
M. pectoralis major

A Nn. pectorales medialis and lateralis.

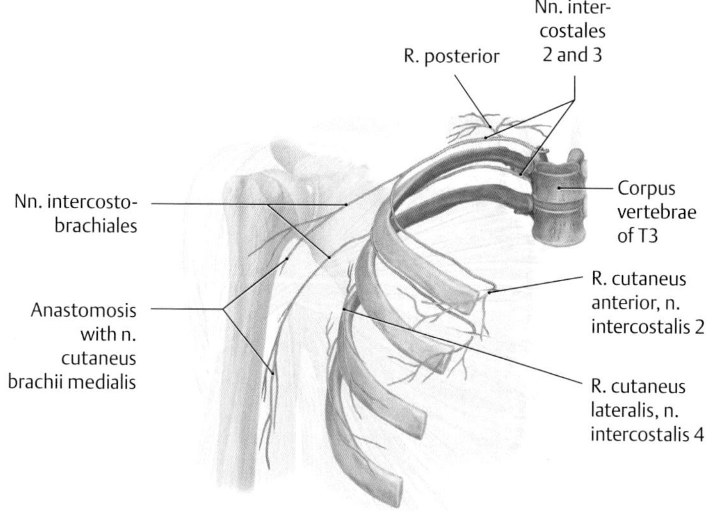
R. posterior
Nn. intercostales 2 and 3
Nn. intercosto-brachiales
Corpus vertebrae of T3
R. cutaneus anterior, n. intercostalis 2
Anastomosis with n. cutaneus brachii medialis
R. cutaneus lateralis, n. intercostalis 4

B Nn. intercostobrachiales.

Fig. 22.19 **Short branches: Sensory distribution**

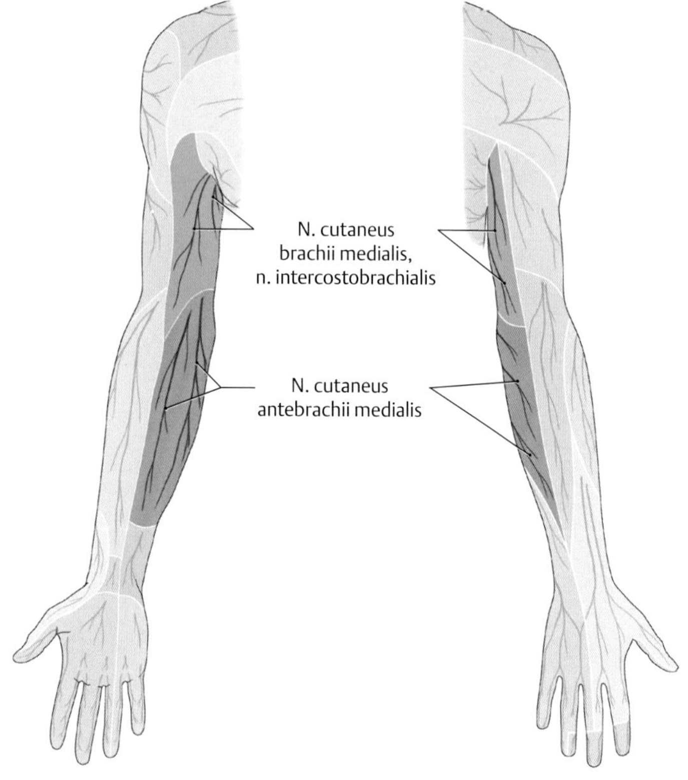
N. cutaneus brachii medialis, n. intercostobrachialis
N. cutaneus antebrachii medialis

A Anterior view.

B Posterior view.

Fig. 22.20 N. musculocutaneus
Right limb, anterior view.

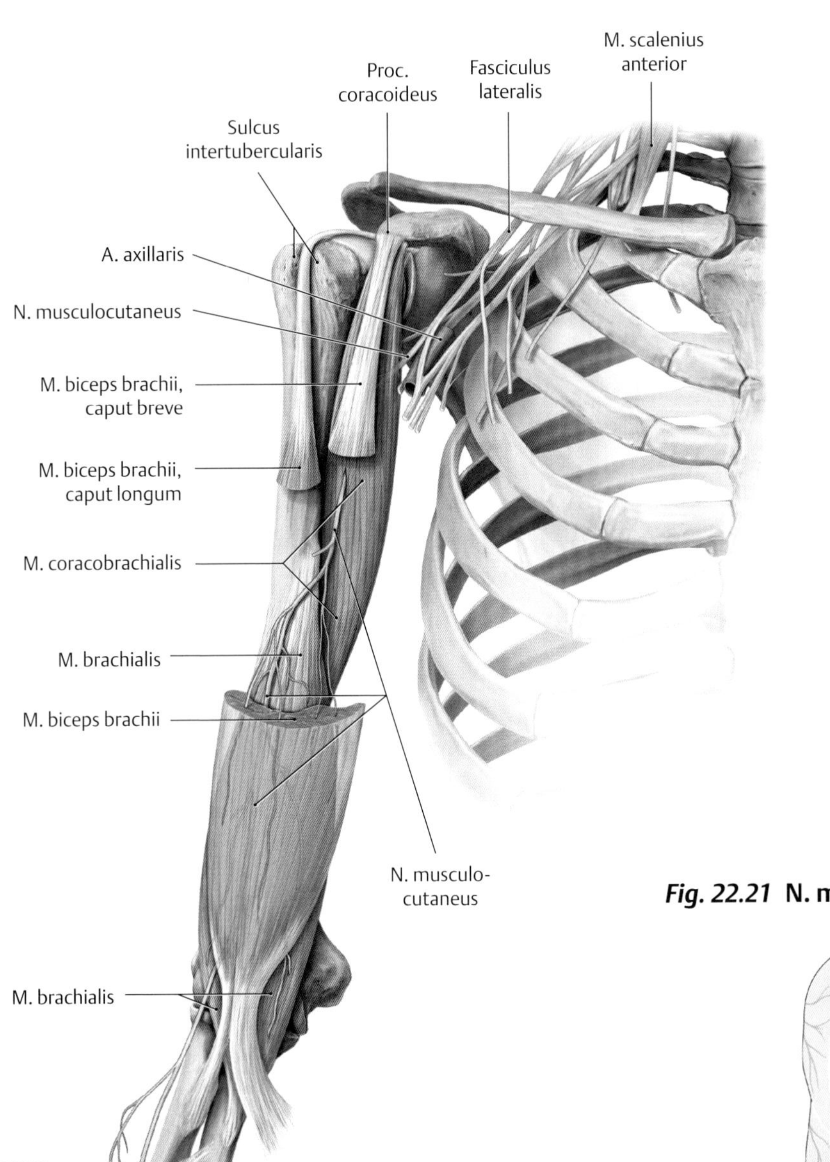
M. scalenius anterior
Proc. coracoideus
Fasciculus lateralis
Sulcus intertubercularis
A. axillaris
N. musculocutaneus
M. biceps brachii, caput breve
M. biceps brachii, caput longum
M. coracobrachialis
M. brachialis
M. biceps brachii
N. musculo-cutaneus
M. brachialis
N. cutaneus antebrachii lateralis
Ulna
Radius

Table 22.7	N. musculocutaneus (C5–C7)
Motor branches	**Innervated muscles**
Rr. musculares	M. coracobrachialis
	M. biceps brachii
	M. brachialis
Sensory branches	
M. cutaneus antebrachii lateralis	
Rr. articulationes : Capsula art. cubiti (anterior part)	
Note: N. musculocutaneus nerve innervation of the arm is purely motor; innervation of the forearm is purely sensory.	

Fig. 22.21 N. musculocutaneus: Sensory distribution

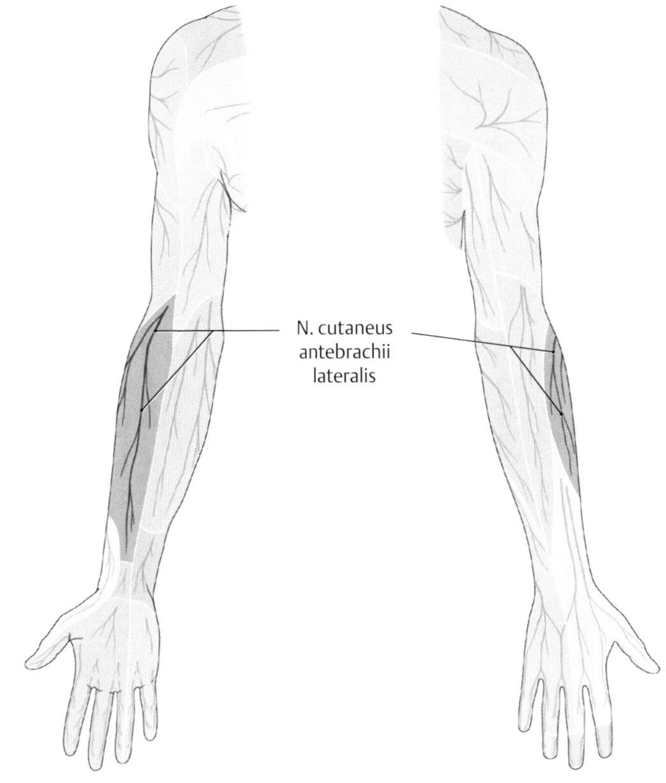
N. cutaneus antebrachii lateralis

A Anterior view. **B** Posterior view.

N. Medianus & N. Ulnaris

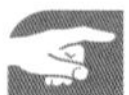

The n. medianus is a terminal branch arising from both fasciculus medialis and lateralis. The n. ulnaris arises exclusively from fasciculus medialis.

Fig. 22.22 **N. medianus**
Right limb, anterior view.

M. scalenius anterior
Fasciculus lateralis
Fasciculus medialis
A. axillaris
N. medianus
Radix lateralis
Radix medialis
N. medianus
Humerus, epicondylus medialis
R. articularis
M. pronator teres, caput humerale
M. flexor carpi radialis
M. pronator teres, caput ulnare
M. palmaris longus
M. flexor digitorum superficialis
N. interosseus antebrachii anterior
M. flexor digitorum profundus
M. flexor pollicis longus
R. muscularis thenaris
M. pronator quadratus
R. palmaris, n. medianus
Retinaculum musculorum flexorum
Nn. digitales palmares communes
Mm. lumbricales I and II
Nn. digitales palmares proprii

Fig. 22.23 **N. medianus: Sensory distribution**

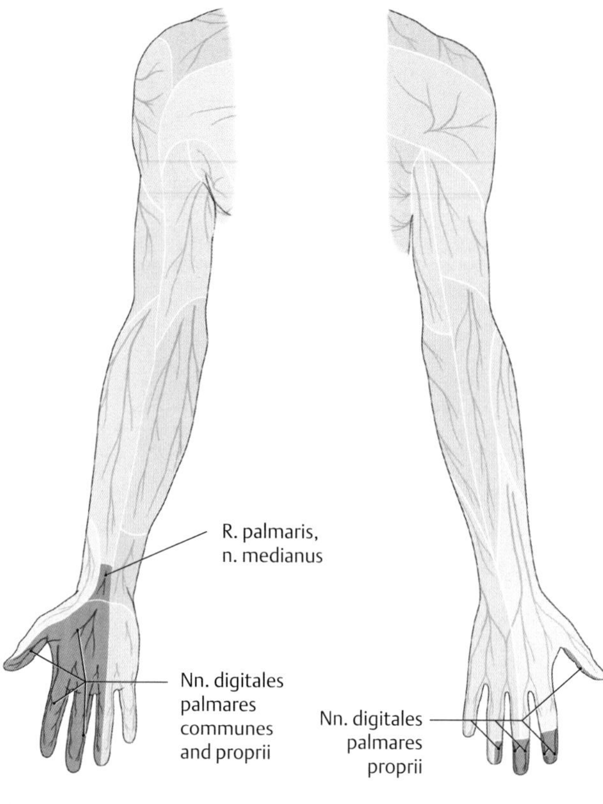

R. palmaris, n. medianus
Nn. digitales palmares communes and proprii
Nn. digitales palmares proprii

A Anterior view.

B Posterior view.

Table 22.8	**N. medianus (C6–T1)**
Motor branches	**Innervated muscles**
Rr. musculares	M. pronator teres
	M. flexor carpi radialis
	M. palmaris longus
	M. flexor digitorum superficialis
Rr. musculares branches from N. interosseus antebrachii anterior	M. pronator quadratus
	M. flexor pollicis longus
	M. flexor digitorum profundus (radial half)
Thenar muscular branch	M. abductor pollicis brevis
	M. flexor pollicis brevis (Caput superficialis)
	M. opponens pollicis
Rr. musculares nn. digitales palmares communis	1st and 2nd lumbricals
Sensory branches	
Rr. articulations: Capsula art. cubiti and capsula art. carpalis	
R. palmaris n. medianus (thenar eminence)	
Communicating branch to ulnar n.	
Nn. digitales palmares communis	

Clinical

Injury of n. medianus caused by fracture/dislocation of the elbow joint may result in compromised grasping ability and sensory loss in the fingertips (see Fig. 22.23 for territories). See also carpal tunnel syndrome (p. 343).

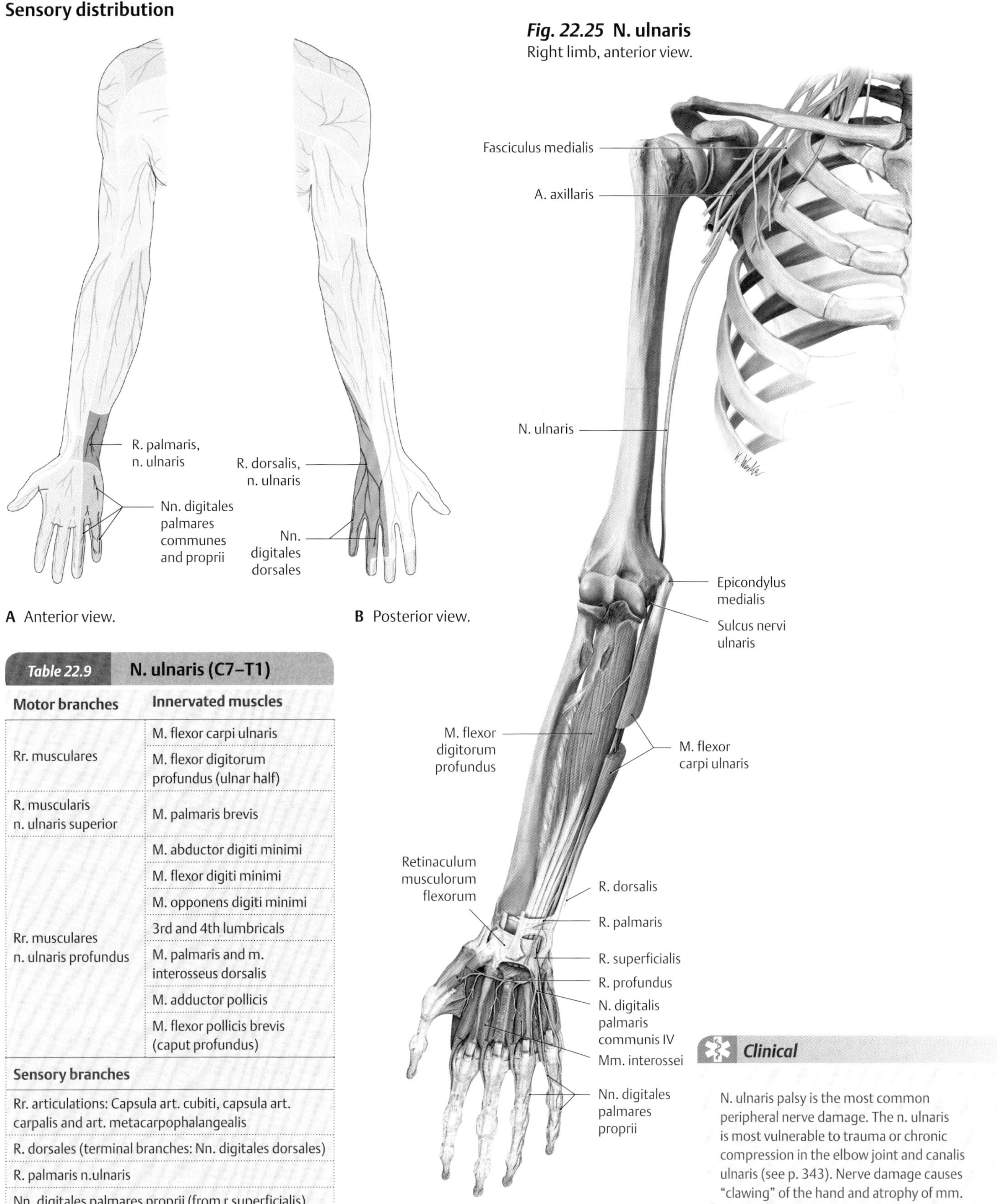
R. palmaris,
n. ulnaris
Nn. digitales
palmares
communes
and proprii
R. dorsalis,
n. ulnaris
Nn.
digitales
dorsales
Fasciculus medialis
A. axillaris
N. ulnaris
Epicondylus
medialis
Sulcus nervi
ulnaris
M. flexor
digitorum
profundus
M. flexor
carpi ulnaris
Retinaculum
musculorum
flexorum
R. dorsalis
R. palmaris
R. superficialis
R. profundus
N. digitalis
palmaris
communis IV
Mm. interossei
Nn. digitales
palmares
proprii

Fig. 22.24 **N. ulnaris: Sensory distribution**

A Anterior view.

B Posterior view.

Fig. 22.25 **N. ulnaris**
Right limb, anterior view.

Table 22.9 N. ulnaris (C7–T1)

Motor branches	Innervated muscles
Rr. musculares	M. flexor carpi ulnaris
	M. flexor digitorum profundus (ulnar half)
R. muscularis n. ulnaris superior	M. palmaris brevis
Rr. musculares n. ulnaris profundus	M. abductor digiti minimi
	M. flexor digiti minimi
	M. opponens digiti minimi
	3rd and 4th lumbricals
	M. palmaris and m. interosseus dorsalis
	M. adductor pollicis
	M. flexor pollicis brevis (caput profundus)
Sensory branches	
Rr. articulations: Capsula art. cubiti, capsula art. carpalis and art. metacarpophalangealis	
R. dorsales (terminal branches: Nn. digitales dorsales)	
R. palmaris n.ulnaris	
Nn. digitales palmares proprii (from r.superficialis)	
N. digitalis palmaris communis (from r. superficialis; terminal branches: Nn. digitales palmaris proprii)	

Clinical

N. ulnaris palsy is the most common peripheral nerve damage. The n. ulnaris is most vulnerable to trauma or chronic compression in the elbow joint and canalis ulnaris (see p. 343). Nerve damage causes "clawing" of the hand and atrophy of mm. interossei. Sensory losses are often limited to the 5th digit.

Superficial Veins & Nerves of the Upper Limb

Fig. 22.26 Cutaneous innervation of the upper limb: Anterior view

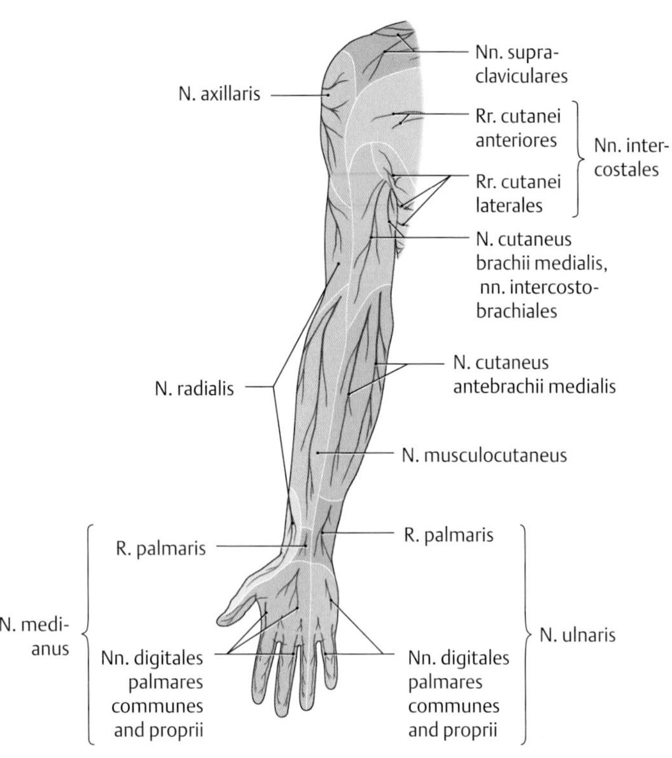
Nn. supra-
claviculares
N. axillaris
Rr. cutanei
anteriores
Rr. cutanei
laterales
Nn. inter-
costales
N. cutaneus
brachii medialis,
nn. intercosto-
brachiales
N. radialis
N. cutaneus
antebrachii medialis
N. musculocutaneus
R. palmaris
R. palmaris
N. medi-
anus
Nn. digitales
palmares
communes
and proprii
Nn. digitales
palmares
communes
and proprii
N. ulnaris

A Peripheral sensory cutaneous innervation.

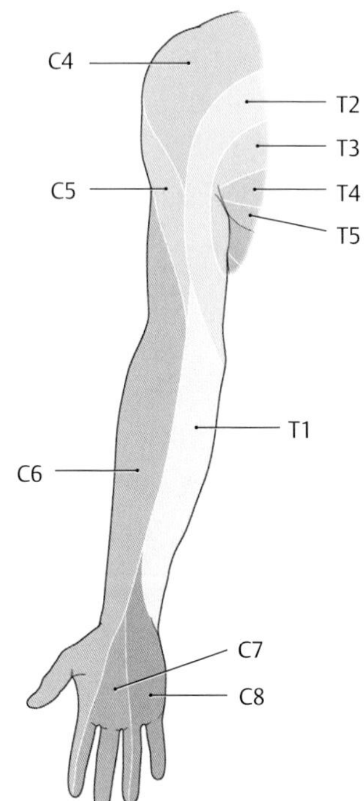
C4
T2
T3
C5
T4
T5
T1
C6
C7
C8

B Segmental, radicular cutaneous innervation (dermatomes).

Fig. 22.27 Superficial cutaneous veins and nerves of the upper limb

N. cutaneus brachii lateralis superior (n. axillaris)
Nn. supra-claviculares
Nn. inter-costales, rr. cutanei anteriores
N. intercosto-brachialis
V. cephalica
N. cutaneus brachii lateralis inferior (n. radialis)
N. cutaneus brachii medialis
Basilic hiatus
V. basilica
N. cutaneus antebrachii medialis
N. cutaneus antebrachii lateralis (n. musculo-cutaneus)
V. mediana cubiti
V. cephalica
V. mediana antebrachii
Vv. per-forantes
N. cutaneus antebrachii medialis
N. radialis, r. super-ficialis
N. ulnaris, r. palmaris
N. medianus, r. palmaris
Aponeurosis palmaris

A Anterior view. See p. 344 for nerves of the palm.

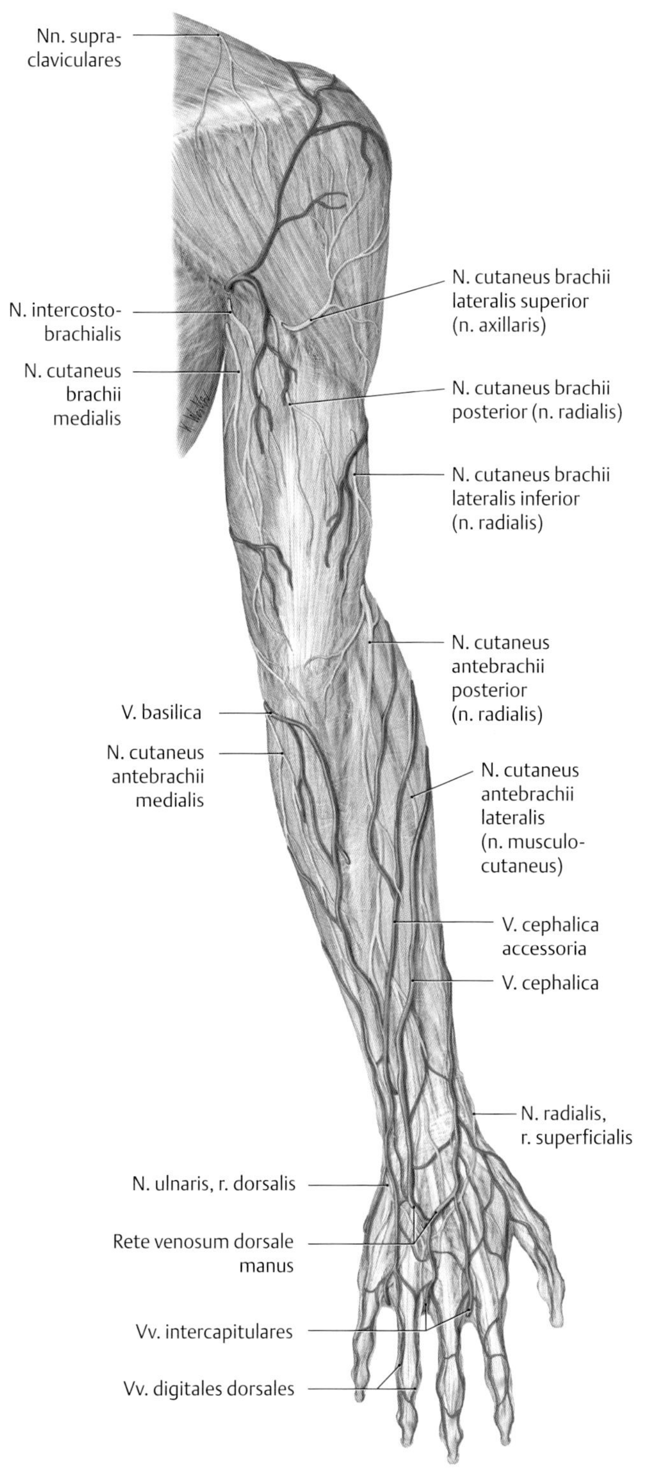
Nn. supra-
claviculares
N. intercosto-
brachialis
N. cutaneus
brachii
medialis
N. cutaneus brachii
lateralis superior
(n. axillaris)
N. cutaneus brachii
posterior (n. radialis)
N. cutaneus brachii
lateralis inferior
(n. radialis)
N. cutaneus
antebrachii
posterior
(n. radialis)
V. basilica
N. cutaneus
antebrachii
medialis
N. cutaneus
antebrachii
lateralis
(n. musculo-
cutaneus)
V. cephalica
accessoria
V. cephalica
N. radialis,
r. superficialis
N. ulnaris, r. dorsalis
Rete venosum dorsale
manus
Vv. intercapitulares
Vv. digitales dorsales

B Posterior view. See p. 346 for nerves of the dorsum.

Fig. 22.28 Cutaneous innervation of the upper limb: Posterior view

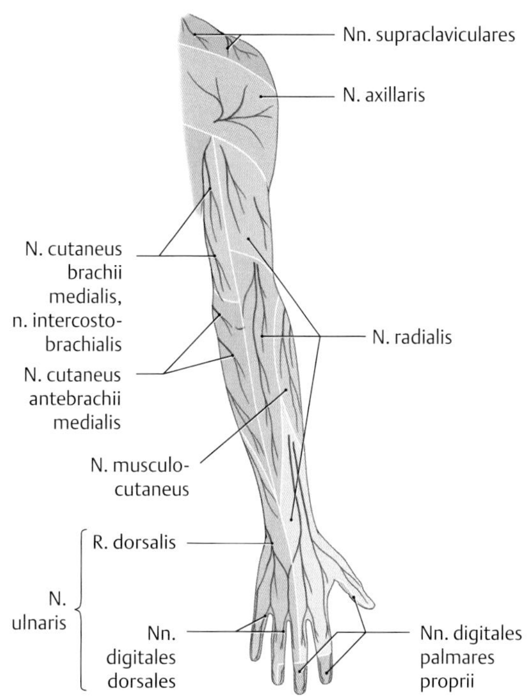
Nn. supraclaviculares
N. axillaris
N. cutaneus
brachii
medialis,
n. intercosto-
brachialis
N. radialis
N. cutaneus
antebrachii
medialis
N. musculo-
cutaneus
R. dorsalis
N.
ulnaris
Nn.
digitales
dorsales
Nn. digitales
palmares
proprii

A Peripheral sensory cutaneous innervation.

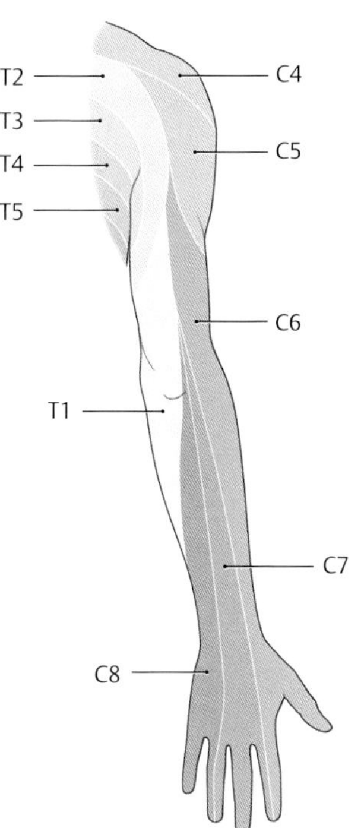
T2
T3
T4
T5
C4
C5
C6
T1
C7
C8

B Segmental, radicular cutaneous innervation (dermatomes).

Posterior Shoulder & Axilla

Fig. 22.29 **Posterior shoulder**
Right shoulder, posterior view. *Raised:* M. trapezius (pars transversa). *Windowed:* M. supraspinatus. *Revealed:* Suprascapular region.

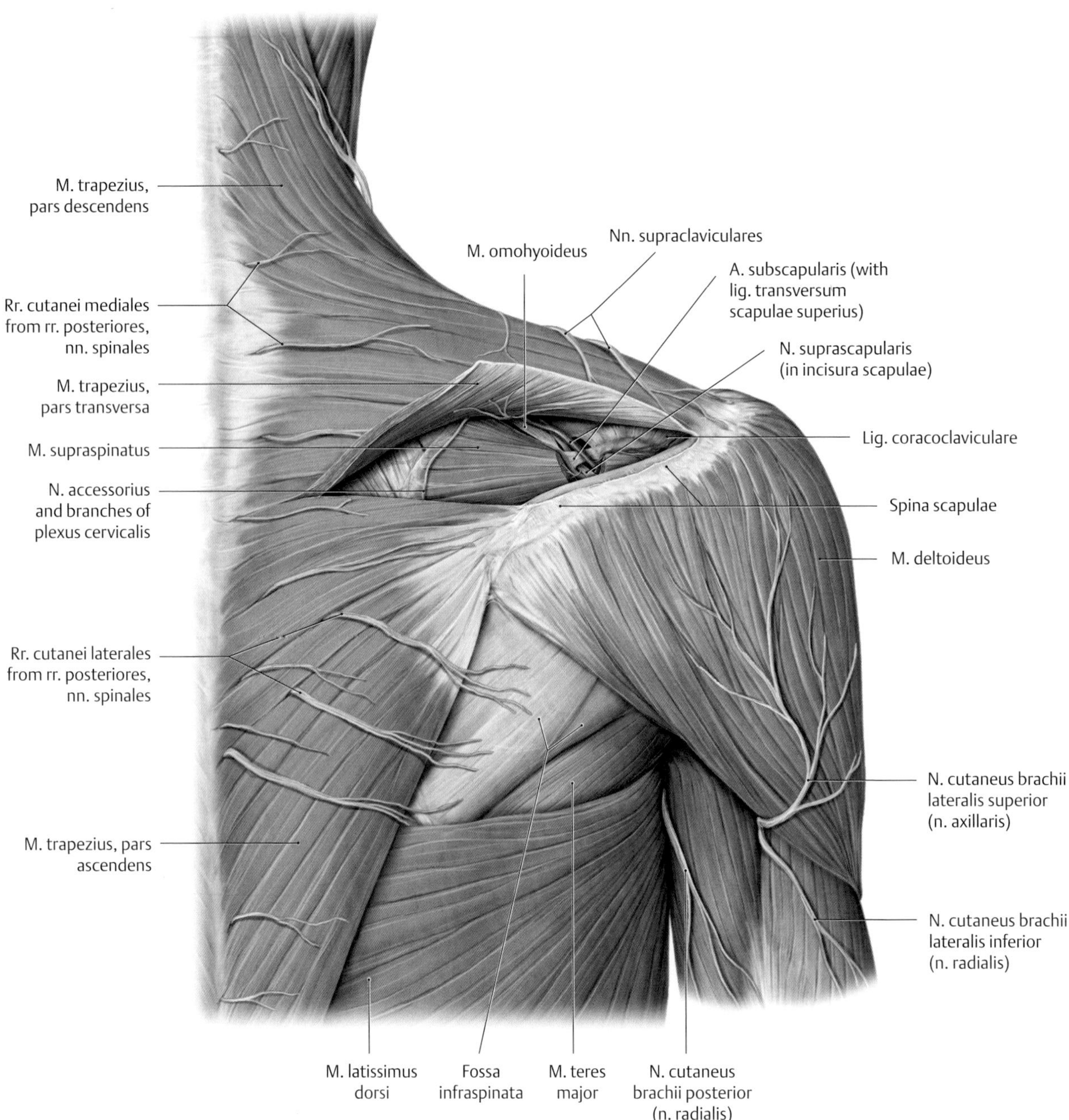
M. trapezius, pars descendens
Rr. cutanei mediales from rr. posteriores, nn. spinales
M. trapezius, pars transversa
M. supraspinatus
N. accessorius and branches of plexus cervicalis
Rr. cutanei laterales from rr. posteriores, nn. spinales
M. trapezius, pars ascendens
M. omohyoideus
Nn. supraclaviculares
A. subscapularis (with lig. transversum scapulae superius)
N. suprascapularis (in incisura scapulae)
Lig. coracoclaviculare
Spina scapulae
M. deltoideus
N. cutaneus brachii lateralis superior (n. axillaris)
N. cutaneus brachii lateralis inferior (n. radialis)
M. latissimus dorsi
Fossa infraspinata
M. teres major
N. cutaneus brachii posterior (n. radialis)

Table 22.10 Neurovascular tracts of the scapula

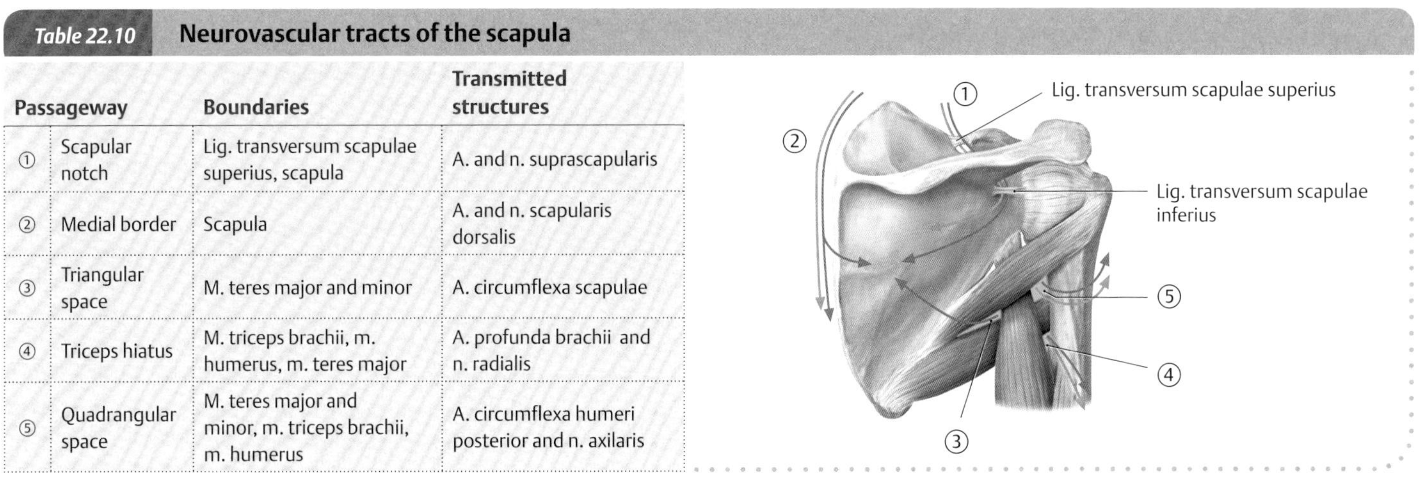
①
Lig. transversum scapulae superius
②
Lig. transversum scapulae inferius
⑤
④
③

	Passageway	Boundaries	Transmitted structures
①	Scapular notch	Lig. transversum scapulae superius, scapula	A. and n. suprascapularis
②	Medial border	Scapula	A. and n. scapularis dorsalis
③	Triangular space	M. teres major and minor	A. circumflexa scapulae
④	Triceps hiatus	M. triceps brachii, m. humerus, m. teres major	A. profunda brachii and n. radialis
⑤	Quadrangular space	M. teres major and minor, m. triceps brachii, m. humerus	A. circumflexa humeri posterior and n. axilaris

Fig. 22.30 **Axilla: Spatium axillare mediale and laterale**
Right shoulder, posterior view.

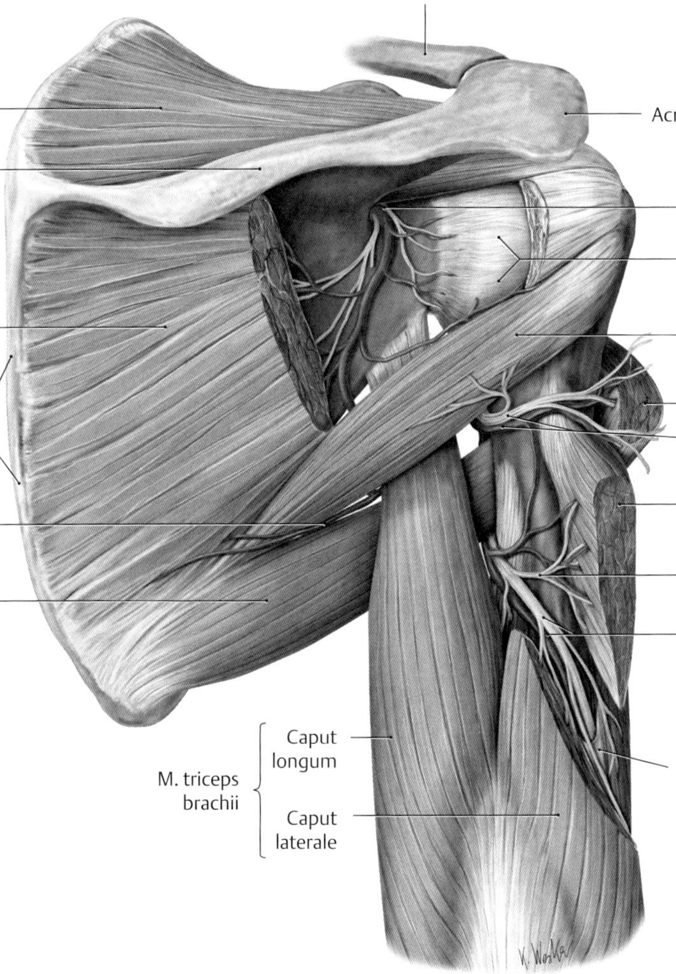

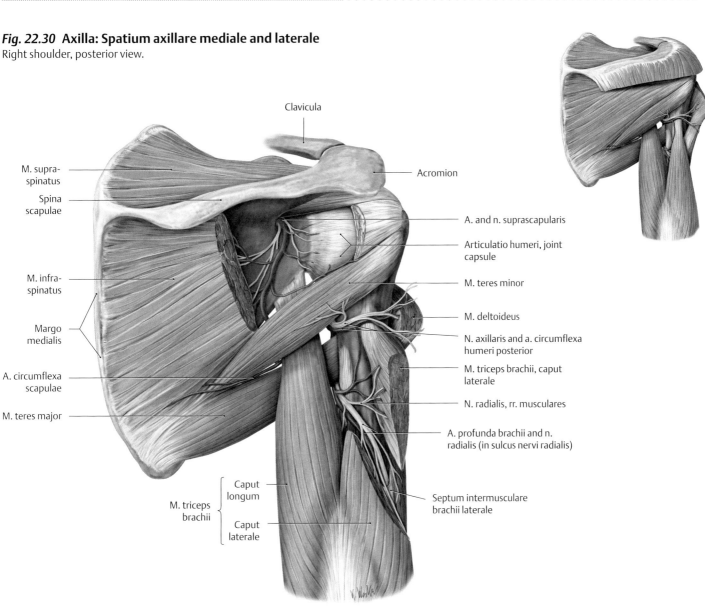

Clavicula
M. supra-spinatus
Spina scapulae
Acromion
A. and n. suprascapularis
Articulatio humeri, joint capsule
M. infra-spinatus
M. teres minor
M. deltoideus
Margo medialis
N. axillaris and a. circumflexa humeri posterior
M. triceps brachii, caput laterale
A. circumflexa scapulae
N. radialis, rr. musculares
M. teres major
A. profunda brachii and n. radialis (in sulcus nervi radialis)
M. triceps brachii
Caput longum
Caput laterale
Septum intermusculare brachii laterale

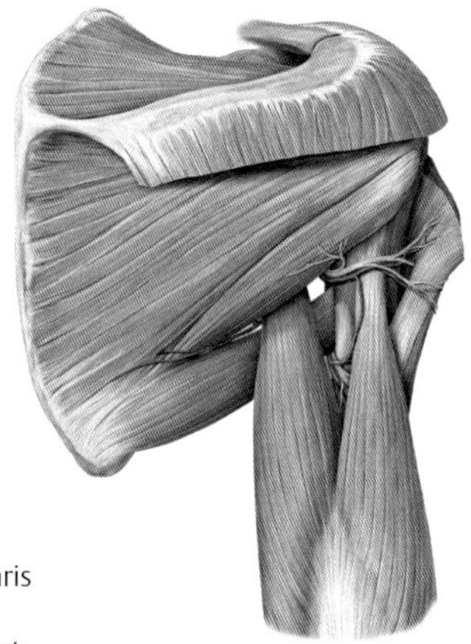

Anterior Shoulder

Fig. 22.31 Anterior shoulder: Superficial dissection
Right shoulder.

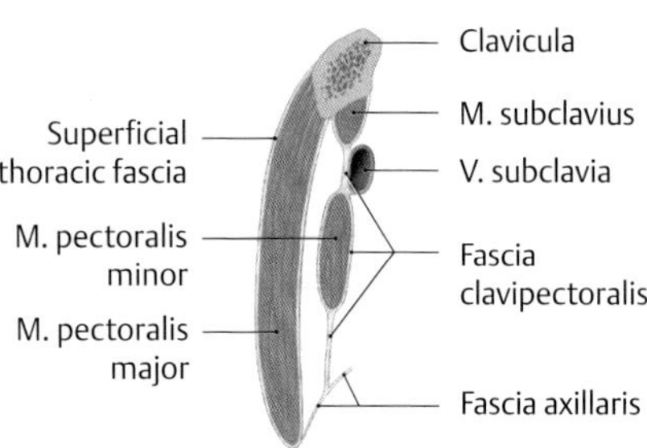
Clavicula
M. subclavius
V. subclavia
Superficial thoracic fascia
M. pectoralis minor
Fascia clavipectoralis
M. pectoralis major
Fascia axillaris

A Sagittal section through anterior wall.

V. jugularis externa
N. auricularis magnus
Nn. supraclaviculares
M. trapezius
Fossa infraclavicularis
N. transversus colli
M. sternocleidomastoideus
M. deltoideus
V. transversa colli
V. subclavia
V. cephalica (in sulcus deltoideopectoralis)
M. pectoralis major, pars clavicularis
A. thoracoacromialis
Fascia clavipectoralis
Nn. pectorales medialis and lateralis
M. pectoralis major, pars sternocostalis
M. biceps brachii
Fascia brachii
M. latissimus dorsi

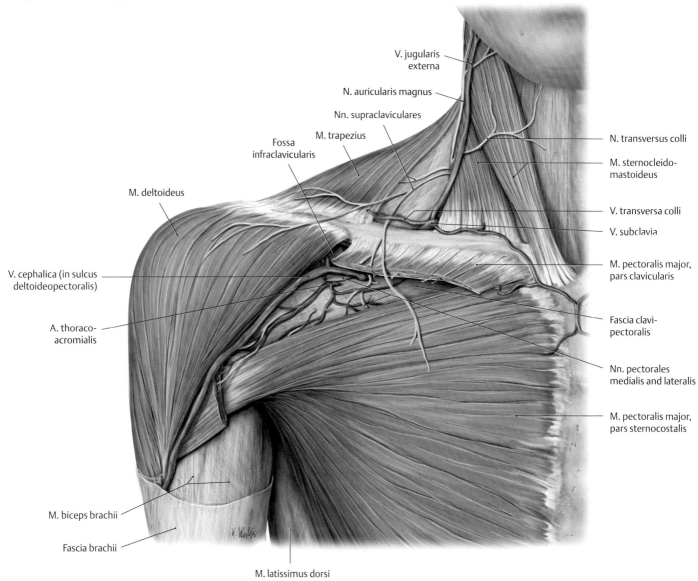

B Anterior view. *Removed:* Platysma, muscle fasciae, superficial layer of fascia cervicalis, and m. pectoralis major (clavicular part). *Revealed:* Trigonum clavipectorale (deltopectorale).

Fig. 22.32 Shoulder: Transverse section

Right shoulder, inferior view.

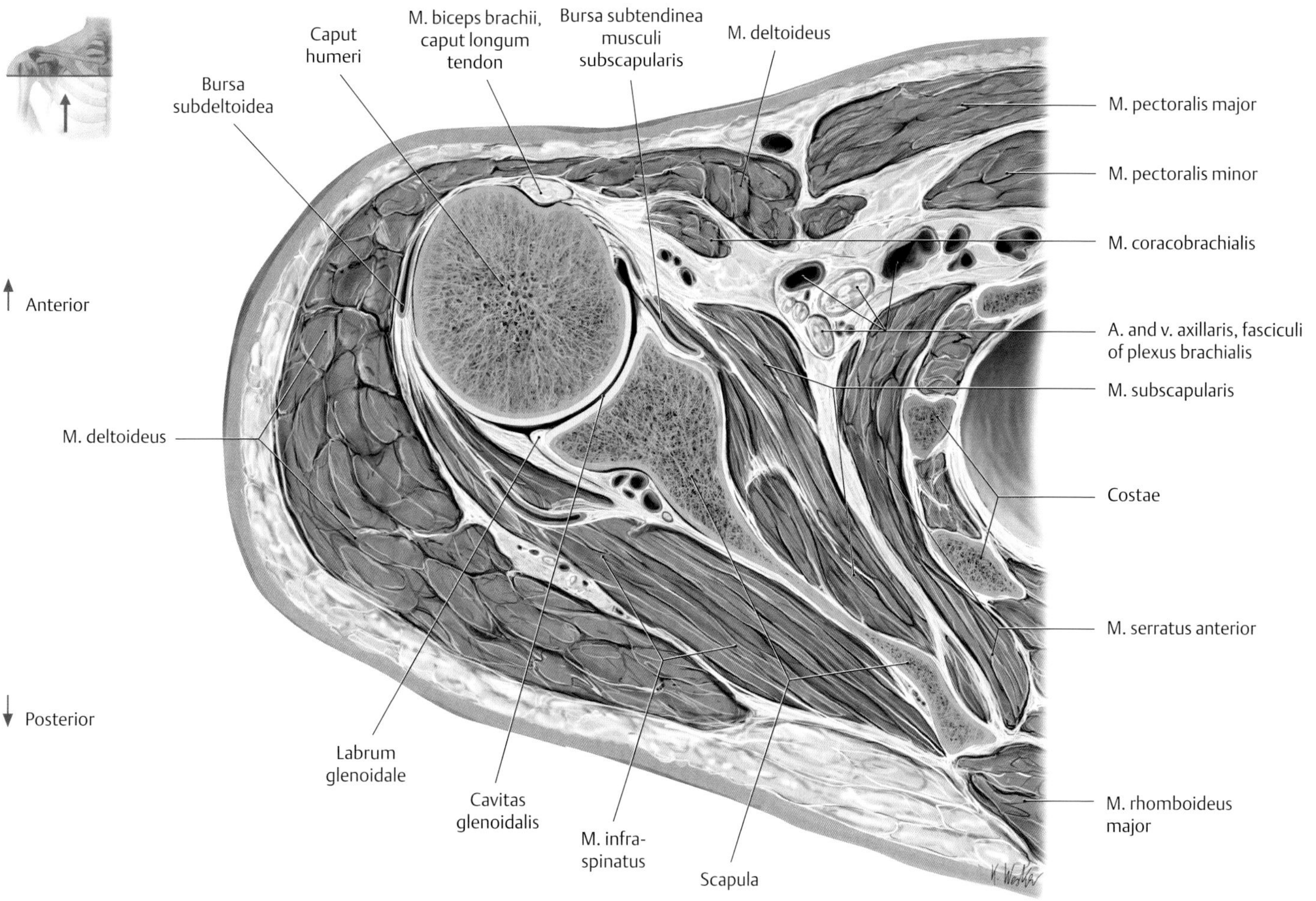

Caput humeri
M. biceps brachii, caput longum tendon
Bursa subtendinea musculi subscapularis
M. deltoideus
Bursa subdeltoidea
M. pectoralis major
M. pectoralis minor
M. coracobrachialis
Anterior
A. and v. axillaris, fasciculi of plexus brachialis
M. subscapularis
M. deltoideus
Costae
M. serratus anterior
Posterior
Labrum glenoidale
Cavitas glenoidalis
M. infra-spinatus
Scapula
M. rhomboideus major

Fig. 22.33 Anterior shoulder: Deep dissection

Right limb, anterior view. *Removed:* M. sternocleidomastoideus, m. omohyoideus, and m. pectoralis major. This dissection reveals the neurovascular contents of the lateral cervical triangle (see pp. 580–581) and axilla (see pp. 336–337).

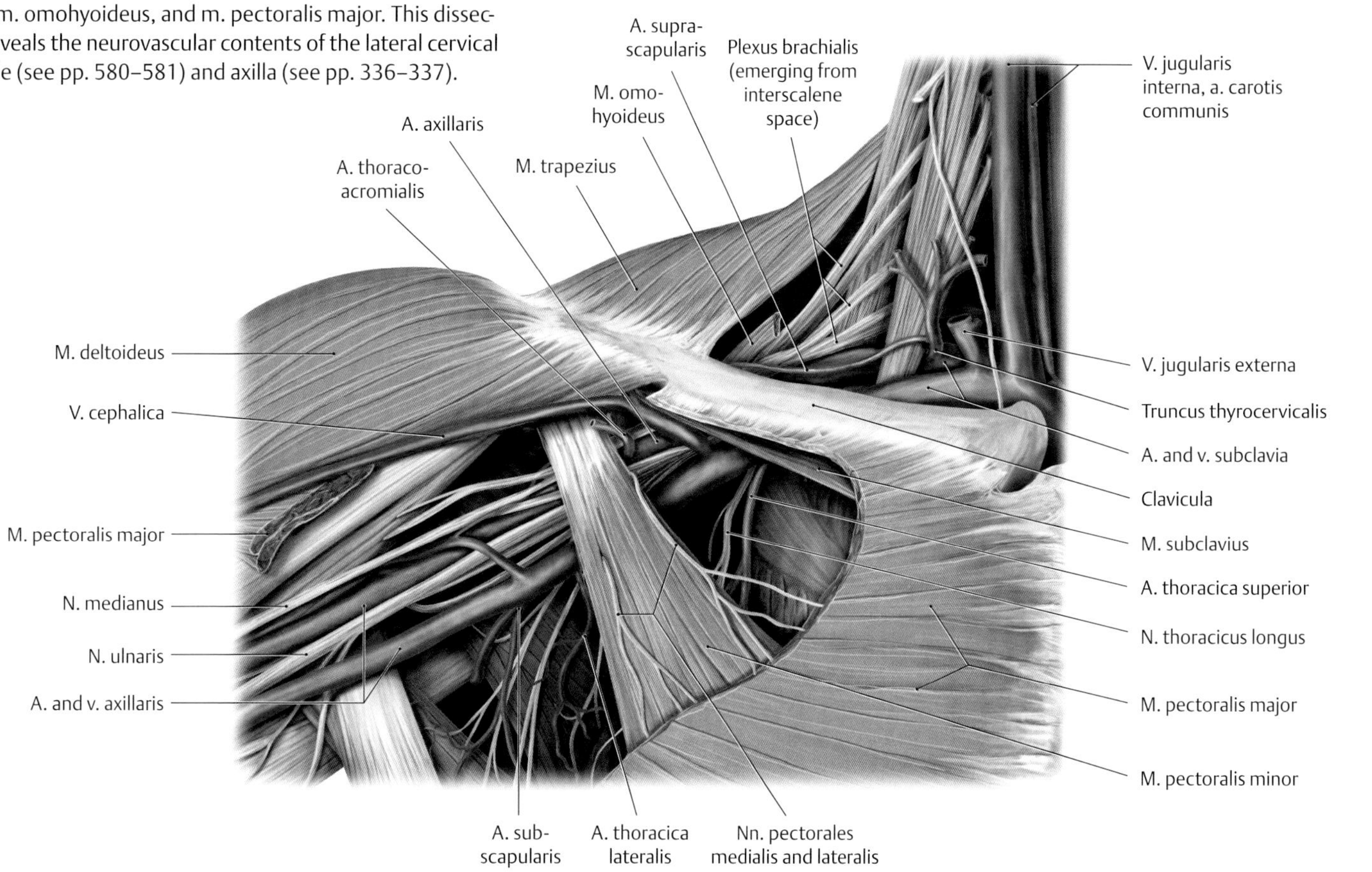

A. supra-scapularis
Plexus brachialis (emerging from interscalene space)
V. jugularis interna, a. carotis communis
M. omo-hyoideus
A. axillaris
A. thoraco-acromialis
M. trapezius
M. deltoideus
V. cephalica
M. pectoralis major
N. medianus
N. ulnaris
A. and v. axillaris
V. jugularis externa
Truncus thyrocervicalis
A. and v. subclavia
Clavicula
M. subclavius
A. thoracica superior
N. thoracicus longus
M. pectoralis major
M. pectoralis minor
A. sub-scapularis
A. thoracica lateralis
Nn. pectorales medialis and lateralis

Topography of the Axilla

Fig. 22.34 **Dissection of the axilla**
Right shoulder, anterior view.

Radix medialis and radix lateralis nervi mediani
N. musculocutaneus
A. thoracoacromialis
Fasciculus lateralis
A. and v. axillaris
V. brachialis
M. subclavius
N. thoracicus longus and a. thoracica superior
M. deltoideus
V. cephalica
M. pectoralis major
Nn. pectorales medialis and lateralis
A. thoracica lateralis
M. biceps brachii
N. medianus
N. ulnaris
M. pectoralis major
A. circumflexa scapulae
A. and v. brachialis
N. subscapularis inferior
A. and n. thoracodorsalis
N. thoracicus longus

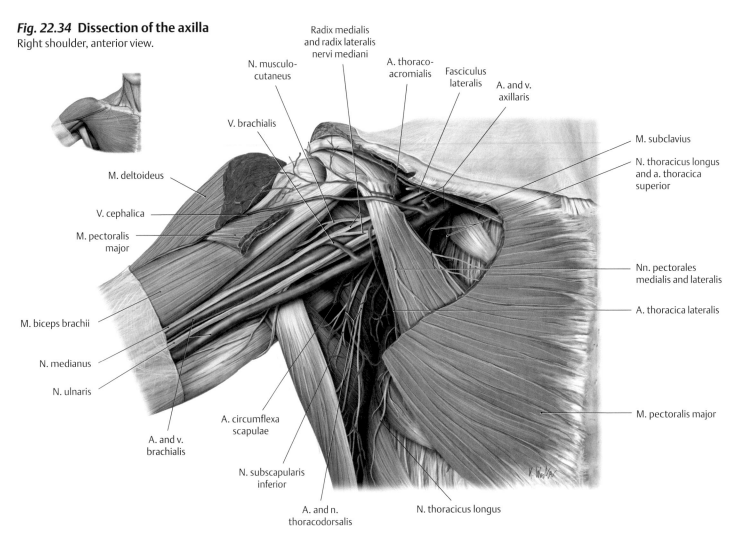

A *Removed:* M. pectoralis major and fascia clavipectoralis.

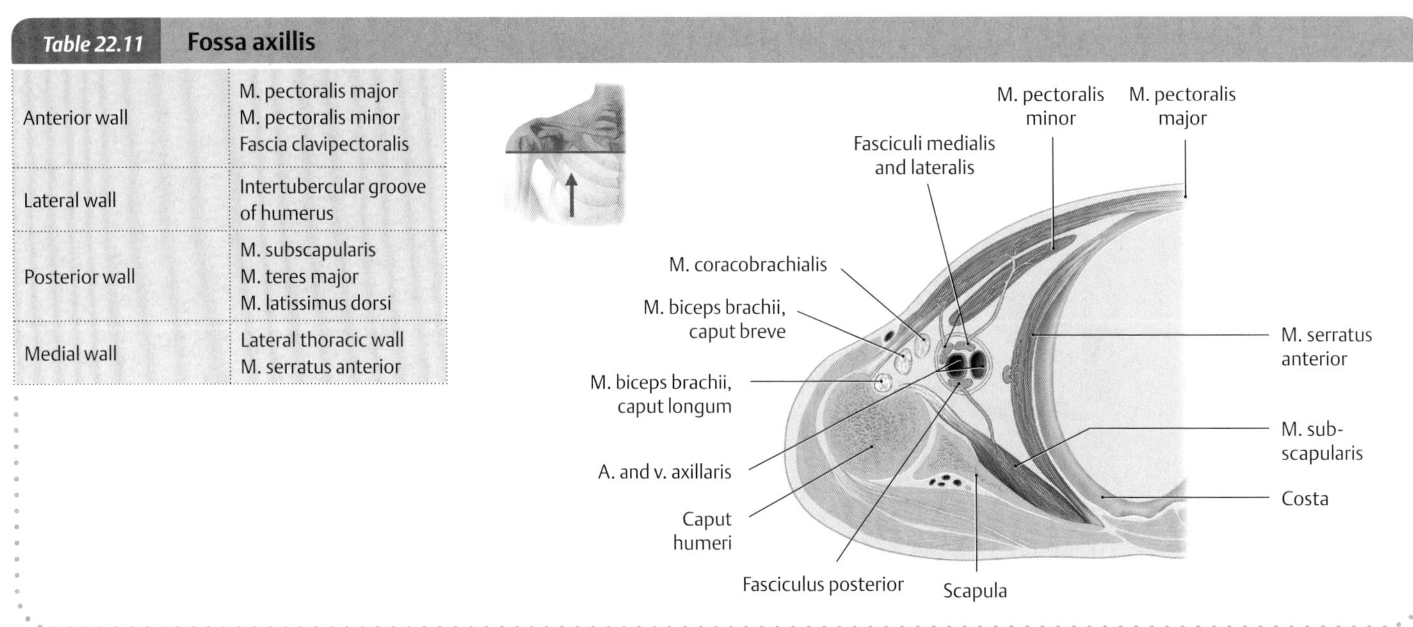

Table 22.11	**Fossa axillis**
Anterior wall	M. pectoralis major M. pectoralis minor Fascia clavipectoralis
Lateral wall	Intertubercular groove of humerus
Posterior wall	M. subscapularis M. teres major M. latissimus dorsi
Medial wall	Lateral thoracic wall M. serratus anterior

M. pectoralis minor
M. pectoralis major
Fasciculi medialis and lateralis
M. coracobrachialis
M. biceps brachii, caput breve
M. biceps brachii, caput longum
A. and v. axillaris
Caput humeri
Fasciculus posterior
Scapula
M. serratus anterior
M. subscapularis
Costa

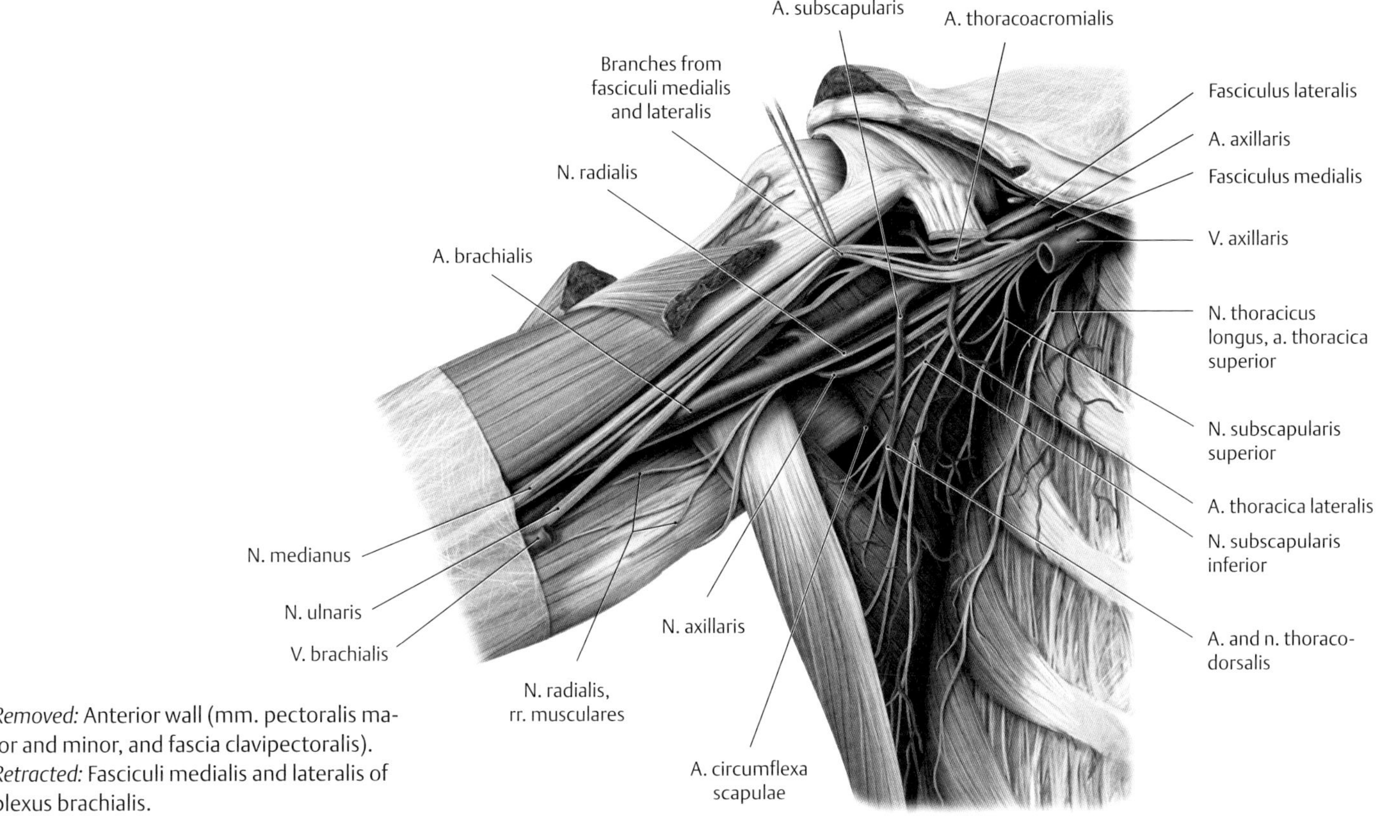
A. subscapularis
A. thoracoacromialis
Branches from fasciculi medialis and lateralis
N. radialis
A. brachialis
Fasciculus lateralis
A. axillaris
Fasciculus medialis
V. axillaris
N. thoracicus longus, a. thoracica superior
N. subscapularis superior
A. thoracica lateralis
N. subscapularis inferior
A. and n. thoraco-dorsalis
N. medianus
N. ulnaris
V. brachialis
N. axillaris
N. radialis, rr. musculares
A. circumflexa scapulae

B *Removed:* Anterior wall (mm. pectoralis major and minor, and fascia clavipectoralis). *Retracted:* Fasciculi medialis and lateralis of plexus brachialis.

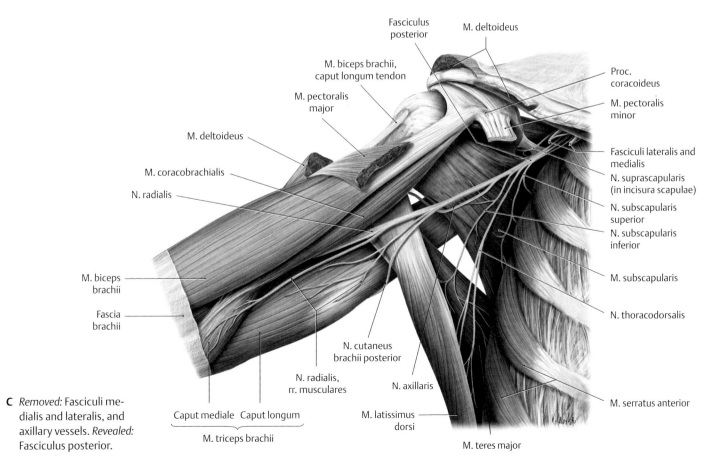

Fasciculus posterior
M. deltoideus
M. biceps brachii, caput longum tendon
M. pectoralis major
M. deltoideus
M. coracobrachialis
N. radialis
Proc. coracoideus
M. pectoralis minor
Fasciculi lateralis and medialis
N. suprascapularis (in incisura scapulae)
N. subscapularis superior
N. subscapularis inferior
M. subscapularis
N. thoracodorsalis
M. biceps brachii
Fascia brachii
N. cutaneus brachii posterior
N. radialis, rr. musculares
N. axillaris
M. serratus anterior
Caput mediale
Caput longum
M. triceps brachii
M. latissimus dorsi
M. teres major

C *Removed:* Fasciculi medialis and lateralis, and axillary vessels. *Revealed:* Fasciculus posterior.

Topography of the Brachial & Cubital Regions

Fig. 22.35 **Brachial region**
Right arm, anterior view. *Removed:* M. deltoideus, mm. pectoralis major and minor. *Revealed:* Sulcus bicipitalis medialis.

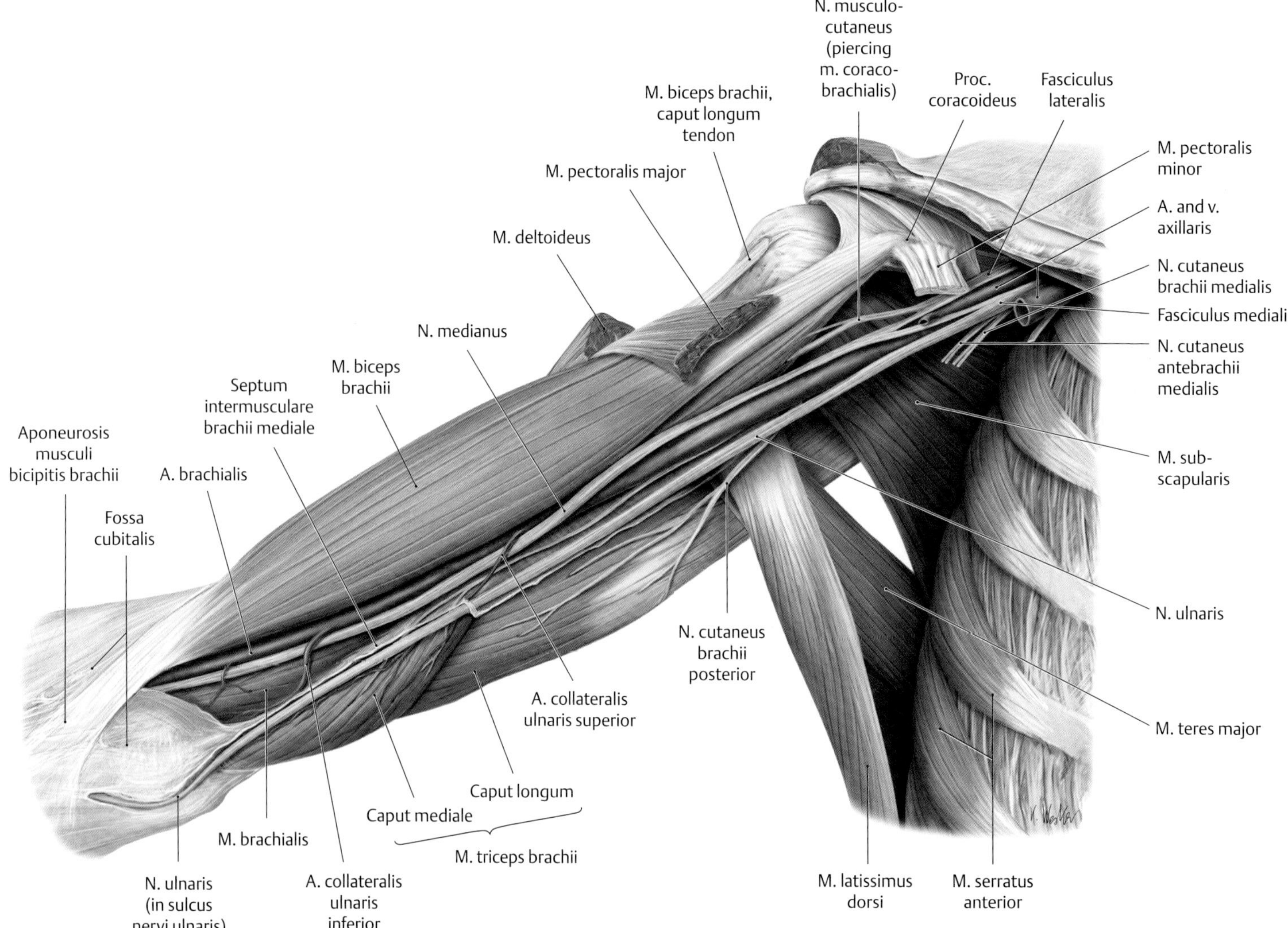
N. musculo-cutaneus (piercing m. coraco-brachialis)
Proc. coracoideus
Fasciculus lateralis
M. biceps brachii, caput longum tendon
M. pectoralis major
M. pectoralis minor
A. and v. axillaris
M. deltoideus
N. cutaneus brachii medialis
Fasciculus medialis
N. medianus
N. cutaneus antebrachii medialis
M. biceps brachii
Septum intermusculare brachii mediale
Aponeurosis musculi bicipitis brachii
A. brachialis
M. sub-scapularis
Fossa cubitalis
N. ulnaris
N. cutaneus brachii posterior
A. collateralis ulnaris superior
M. teres major
Caput longum
Caput mediale
M. triceps brachii
M. brachialis
N. ulnaris (in sulcus nervi ulnaris)
A. collateralis ulnaris inferior
M. latissimus dorsi
M. serratus anterior

***Fig. 22.36* Fossa cubitalis**
Right elbow, anterior view.

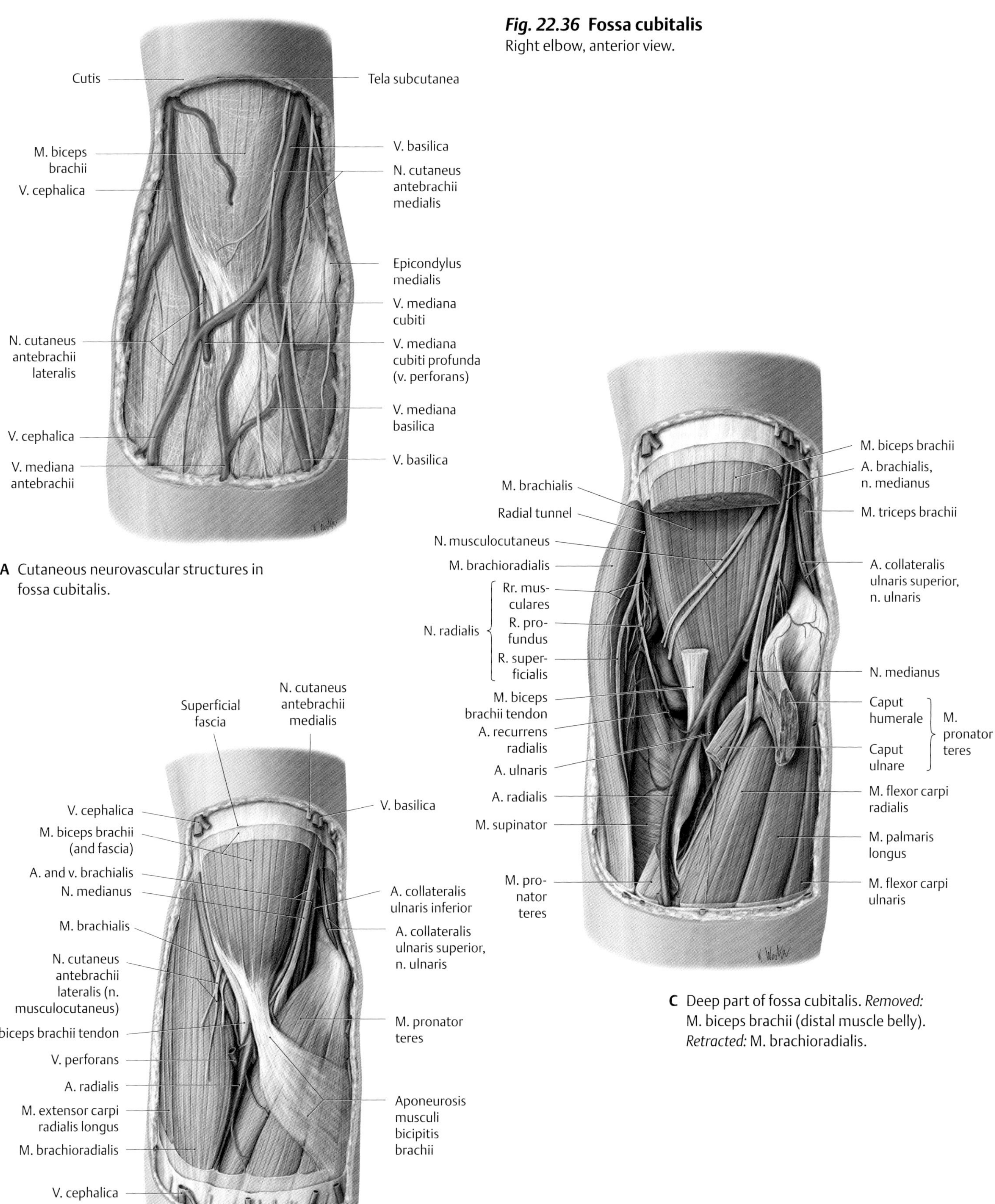
Cutis
Tela subcutanea
M. biceps brachii
V. cephalica
V. basilica
N. cutaneus antebrachii medialis
Epicondylus medialis
V. mediana cubiti
N. cutaneus antebrachii lateralis
V. mediana cubiti profunda (v. perforans)
V. mediana basilica
V. cephalica
V. mediana antebrachii
V. basilica
Superficial fascia
N. cutaneus antebrachii medialis
V. cephalica
V. basilica
M. biceps brachii (and fascia)
A. and v. brachialis
N. medianus
A. collateralis ulnaris inferior
M. brachialis
A. collateralis ulnaris superior, n. ulnaris
N. cutaneus antebrachii lateralis (n. musculocutaneus)
M. biceps brachii tendon
M. pronator teres
V. perforans
A. radialis
Aponeurosis musculi bicipitis brachii
M. extensor carpi radialis longus
M. brachioradialis
V. cephalica
V. mediana antebrachii
M. biceps brachii
A. brachialis, n. medianus
M. brachialis
Radial tunnel
M. triceps brachii
N. musculocutaneus
M. brachioradialis
A. collateralis ulnaris superior, n. ulnaris
N. radialis
Rr. musculares
R. profundus
R. superficialis
N. medianus
M. biceps brachii tendon
A. recurrens radialis
Caput humerale
Caput ulnare
M. pronator teres
A. ulnaris
A. radialis
M. flexor carpi radialis
M. supinator
M. palmaris longus
M. pronator teres
M. flexor carpi ulnaris

A Cutaneous neurovascular structures in fossa cubitalis.

B Superficial part of fossa cubitalis. *Removed:* Fasciae and epifascial neurovascular structures.

C Deep part of fossa cubitalis. *Removed:* M. biceps brachii (distal muscle belly). *Retracted:* M. brachioradialis.

Topography of the Forearm

Fig. 22.37 **Anterior forearm**

Right forearm, anterior view.

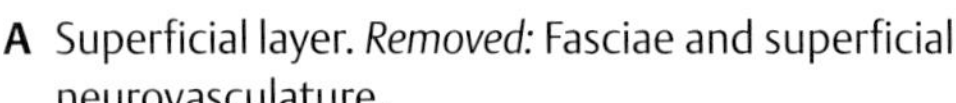

N. medianus
M. triceps brachii
M. biceps brachii
A. collateralis ulnaris inferior
A. collateralis ulnaris superior, n. ulnaris
M. brachialis
Epicondylus medialis
A. brachialis
M. biceps brachii tendon
M. pronator teres
A. radialis
M. flexor carpi radialis
M. brachio-radialis
Aponeurosis musculi bicipitis brachii
M. palmaris longus
M. extensor carpi radialis brevis
M. flexor carpi ulnaris
M. extensor carpi radialis longus
M. flexor carpi radialis
M. abductor pollicis longus
M. flexor digitorum superficialis
A. radialis
M. palmaris longus tendon
A. ulnaris
M. flexor pollicis longus
N. medianus
N. ulnaris (in canalis ulnaris)
Hypothenar muscles
Thenar muscles
Aponeurosis palmaris

A Superficial layer. *Removed:* Fasciae and superficial neurovasculature.

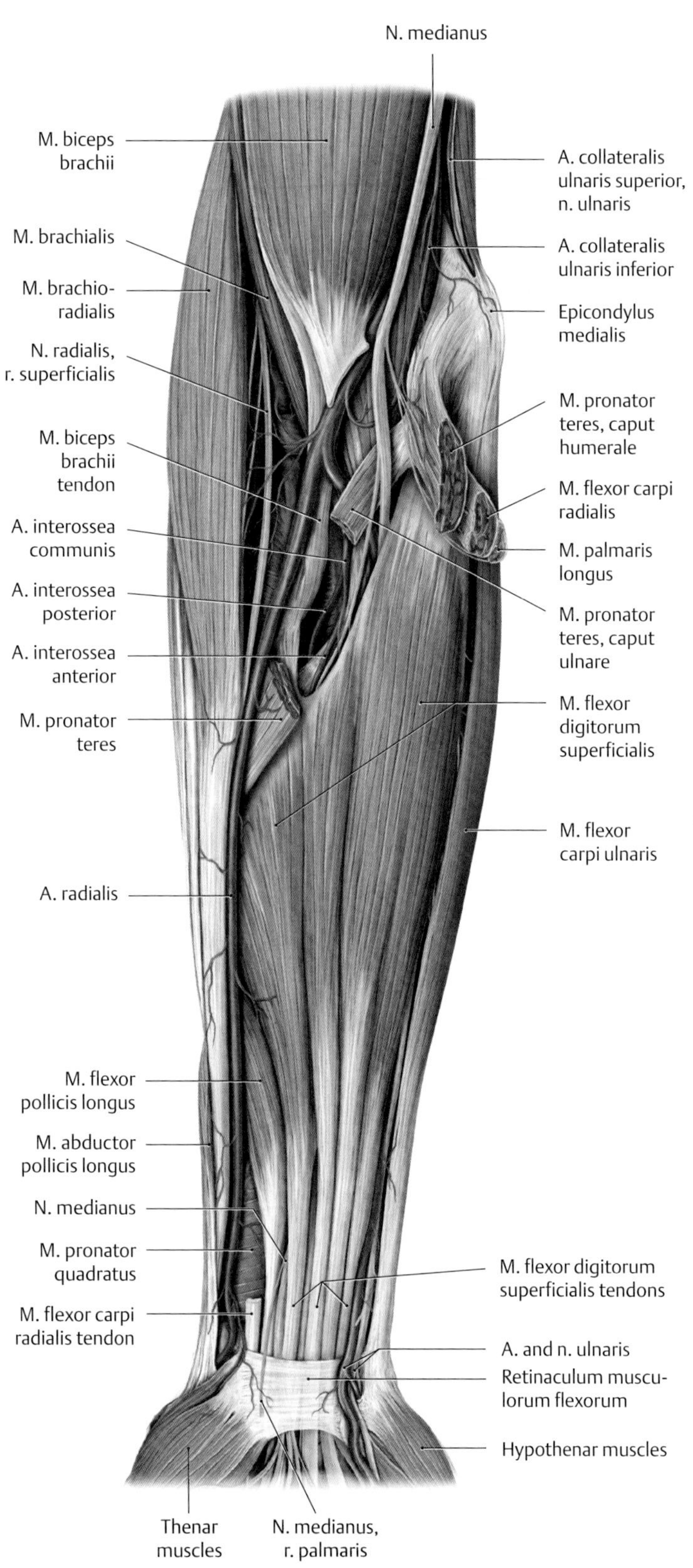

N. medianus
M. biceps brachii
A. collateralis ulnaris superior, n. ulnaris
M. brachialis
A. collateralis ulnaris inferior
M. brachio-radialis
Epicondylus medialis
N. radialis, r. superficialis
M. pronator teres, caput humerale
M. biceps brachii tendon
M. flexor carpi radialis
A. interossea communis
M. palmaris longus
A. interossea posterior
M. pronator teres, caput ulnare
A. interossea anterior
M. flexor digitorum superficialis
M. pronator teres
M. flexor carpi ulnaris
A. radialis
M. flexor pollicis longus
M. abductor pollicis longus
N. medianus
M. pronator quadratus
M. flexor digitorum superficialis tendons
M. flexor carpi radialis tendon
A. and n. ulnaris
Retinaculum musculorum flexorum
Hypothenar muscles
Thenar muscles
N. medianus, r. palmaris

B Middle layer. *Partially removed:* Superficial flexors (m. pronator teres, m. palmaris longus, and m. flexor carpi radialis).

Fig. 22.38 Posterior forearm

Right forearm, anterior view during pronation. *Reflected:* M. anconeus and m. triceps brachii. *Resected:* M. extensor carpi ulnaris and m. extensor digitorum.

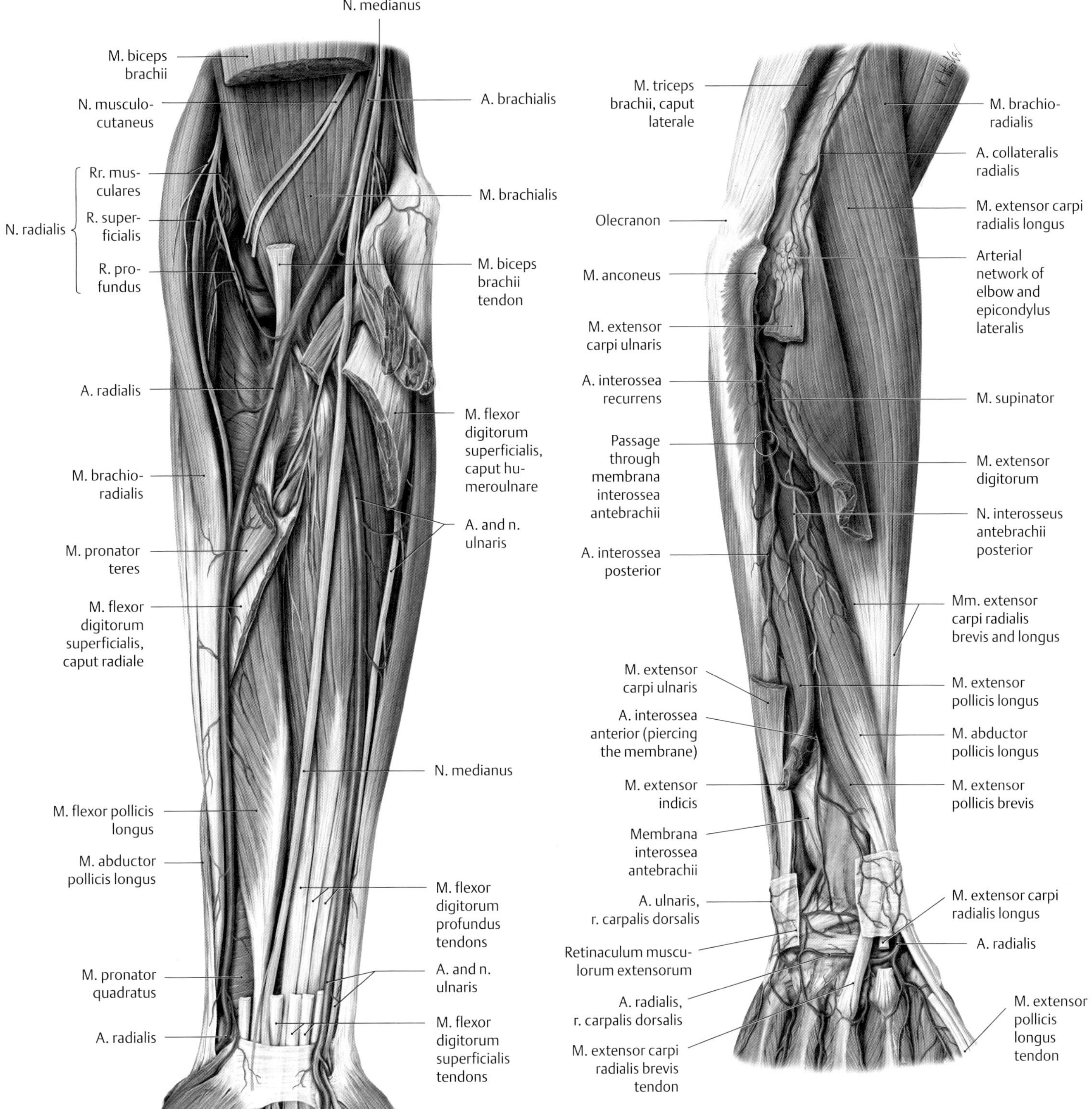
N. medianus
M. biceps brachii
N. musculo-cutaneus
A. brachialis
N. radialis
Rr. mus-culares
R. super-ficialis
R. pro-fundus
M. brachialis
M. biceps brachii tendon
A. radialis
M. flexor digitorum superficialis, caput hu-meroulnare
M. brachio-radialis
A. and n. ulnaris
M. pronator teres
M. flexor digitorum superficialis, caput radiale
N. medianus
M. flexor pollicis longus
M. abductor pollicis longus
M. flexor digitorum profundus tendons
M. pronator quadratus
A. and n. ulnaris
A. radialis
M. flexor digitorum superficialis tendons
M. triceps brachii, caput laterale
M. brachio-radialis
A. collateralis radialis
Olecranon
M. extensor carpi radialis longus
M. anconeus
Arterial network of elbow and epicondylus lateralis
M. extensor carpi ulnaris
A. interossea recurrens
M. supinator
Passage through membrana interossea antebrachii
M. extensor digitorum
N. interosseus antebrachii posterior
A. interossea posterior
Mm. extensor carpi radialis brevis and longus
M. extensor carpi ulnaris
M. extensor pollicis longus
A. interossea anterior (piercing the membrane)
M. abductor pollicis longus
M. extensor indicis
M. extensor pollicis brevis
Membrana interossea antebrachii
A. ulnaris, r. carpalis dorsalis
M. extensor carpi radialis longus
Retinaculum muscu-lorum extensorum
A. radialis
A. radialis, r. carpalis dorsalis
M. extensor pollicis longus tendon
M. extensor carpi radialis brevis tendon

C Deep layer. *Removed:* Superficial flexors.

Topography of the Carpal Region

Fig. 22.39 Anterior carpal region
Right hand, anterior (palmar) view.

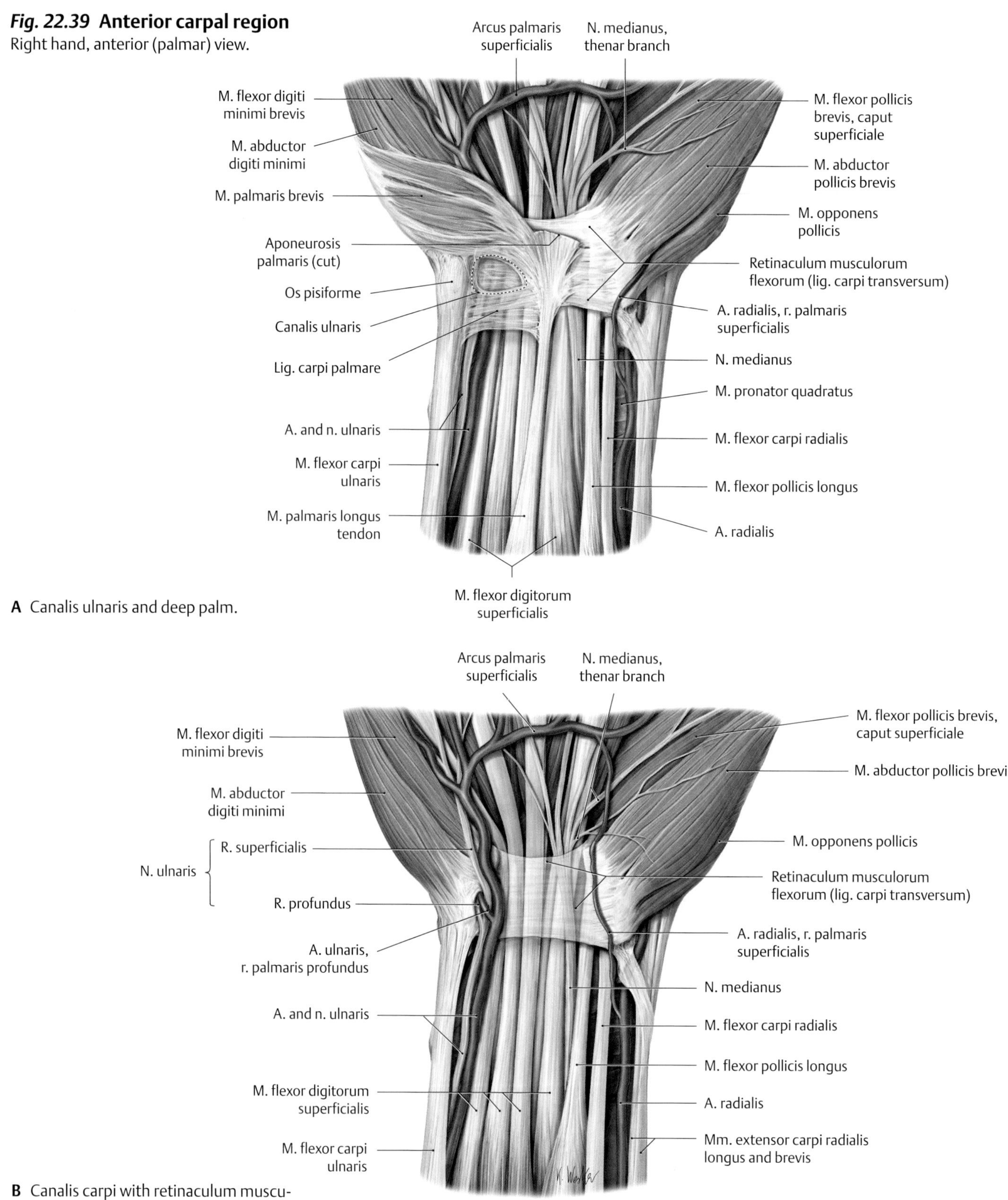
Arcus palmaris superficialis
N. medianus, thenar branch
M. flexor digiti minimi brevis
M. abductor digiti minimi
M. palmaris brevis
Aponeurosis palmaris (cut)
Os pisiforme
Canalis ulnaris
Lig. carpi palmare
A. and n. ulnaris
M. flexor carpi ulnaris
M. palmaris longus tendon
M. flexor digitorum superficialis
M. flexor pollicis brevis, caput superficiale
M. abductor pollicis brevis
M. opponens pollicis
Retinaculum musculorum flexorum (lig. carpi transversum)
A. radialis, r. palmaris superficialis
N. medianus
M. pronator quadratus
M. flexor carpi radialis
M. flexor pollicis longus
A. radialis
Arcus palmaris superficialis
N. medianus, thenar branch
M. flexor digiti minimi brevis
M. abductor digiti minimi
N. ulnaris
R. superficialis
R. profundus
A. ulnaris, r. palmaris profundus
A. and n. ulnaris
M. flexor digitorum superficialis
M. flexor carpi ulnaris
M. flexor pollicis brevis, caput superficiale
M. abductor pollicis brevis
M. opponens pollicis
Retinaculum musculorum flexorum (lig. carpi transversum)
A. radialis, r. palmaris superficialis
N. medianus
M. flexor carpi radialis
M. flexor pollicis longus
A. radialis
Mm. extensor carpi radialis longus and brevis

A Canalis ulnaris and deep palm.

B Canalis carpi with retinaculum musculorum flexorum windowed.

Fig. 22.40 Canalis ulnaris

Right hand, anterior (palmar) view.

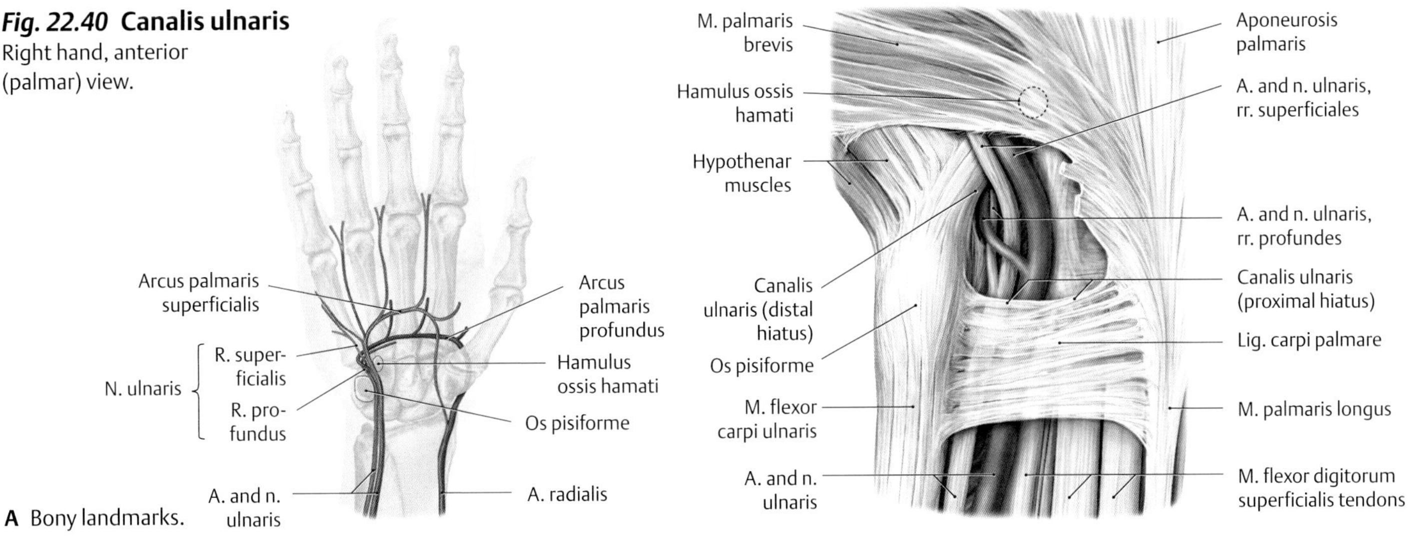
Arcus palmaris superficialis
Arcus palmaris profundus
N. ulnaris
R. superficialis
R. profundus
Hamulus ossis hamati
Os pisiforme
A. and n. ulnaris
A. radialis
M. palmaris brevis
Hamulus ossis hamati
Hypothenar muscles
Canalis ulnaris (distal hiatus)
Os pisiforme
M. flexor carpi ulnaris
A. and n. ulnaris
Aponeurosis palmaris
A. and n. ulnaris, rr. superficiales
A. and n. ulnaris, rr. profundes
Canalis ulnaris (proximal hiatus)
Lig. carpi palmare
M. palmaris longus
M. flexor digitorum superficialis tendons

A Bony landmarks.

B Apertures and walls of canalis ulnaris.

Fig. 22.41 Canalis carpi: Cross section

Right hand, proximal view. The tight fit of sensitive neurovascular structures with closely apposed, frequently moving tendons in canalis carpi often causes problems (carpal tunnel syndrome) when any of the structures swell or degenerate.

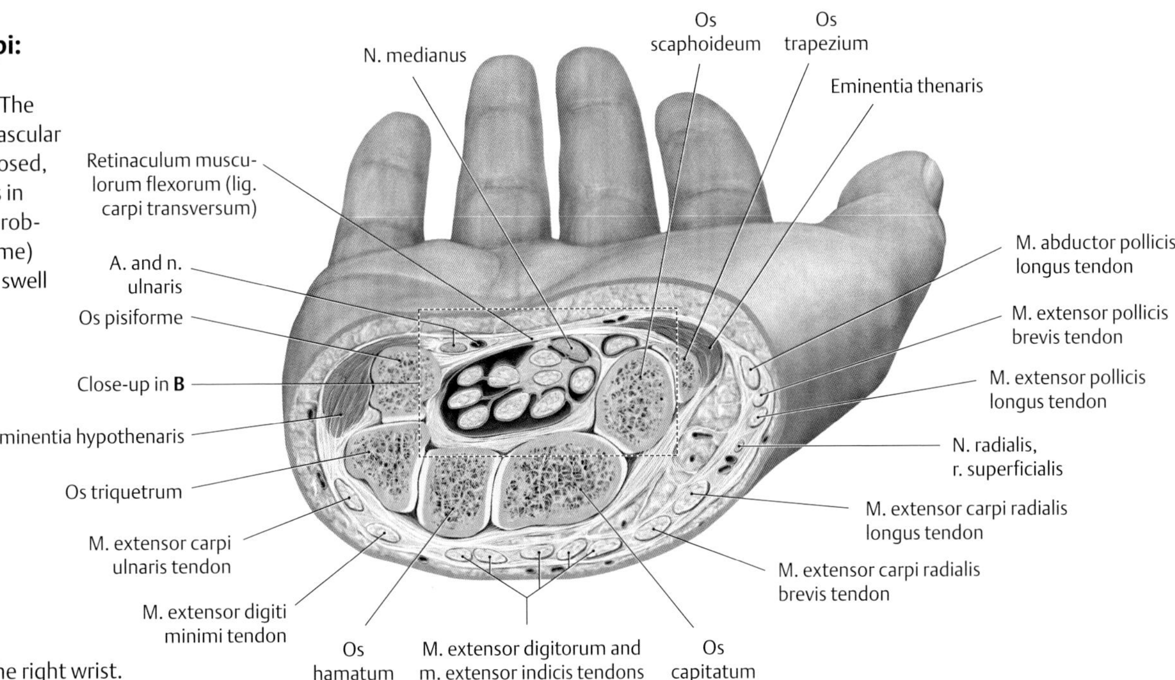
N. medianus
Os scaphoideum
Os trapezium
Eminentia thenaris
Retinaculum musculorum flexorum (lig. carpi transversum)
A. and n. ulnaris
Os pisiforme
Close-up in **B**
Eminentia hypothenaris
Os triquetrum
M. extensor carpi ulnaris tendon
M. extensor digiti minimi tendon
Os hamatum
M. extensor digitorum and m. extensor indicis tendons
Os capitatum
M. abductor pollicis longus tendon
M. extensor pollicis brevis tendon
M. extensor pollicis longus tendon
N. radialis, r. superficialis
M. extensor carpi radialis longus tendon
M. extensor carpi radialis brevis tendon

A Cross section through the right wrist.

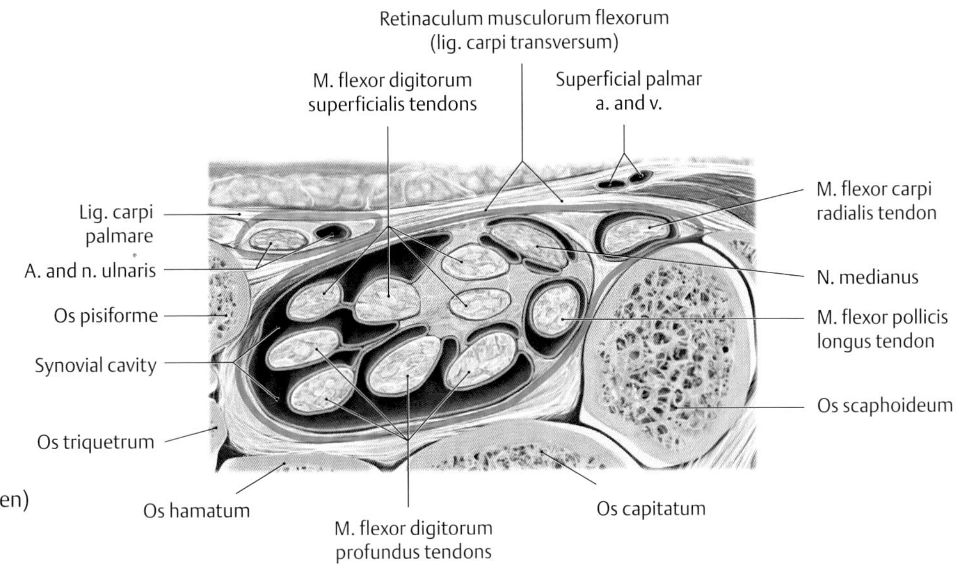
Retinaculum musculorum flexorum (lig. carpi transversum)
M. flexor digitorum superficialis tendons
Superficial palmar a. and v.
Lig. carpi palmare
A. and n. ulnaris
Os pisiforme
Synovial cavity
Os triquetrum
Os hamatum
M. flexor digitorum profundus tendons
Os capitatum
M. flexor carpi radialis tendon
N. medianus
M. flexor pollicis longus tendon
Os scaphoideum

B Structures in canalis ulnaris (green) and canalis carpi (blue).

Topography of the Palm of the Hand

Fig. 22.42 Superficial neurovascular structures of the palm

Right hand, anterior view.

Nn. digitales palmares proprii (exclusive area of n. medianus)
N. digitalis palmaris propria (exclusive area of n. ulnaris)
N. medianus, r. palmaris
N. ulnaris, r. palmaris
N. radialis, n. digitalis dorsalis

A Sensory territories. Extensive overlap exists between adjacent areas. *Exclusive* nerve territories indicated with darker shading.

Aa. digitales palmares propriae
Nn. digitales palmares proprii
Aa. digitales palmares communes
Nn. digitales palmares proprii of thumb
M. flexor digiti minimi brevis
M. adductor pollicis
M. abductor digiti minimi
M. flexor pollicis brevis, caput superficiale
Aponeurosis palmaris
M. palmaris brevis
M. abductor pollicis brevis
Retinaculum musculorum flexorum (lig. carpi transversum)
A. radialis, r. palmaris superficialis
A. and n. ulnaris
A. radialis
Canalis ulnaris
M. palmaris longus tendon
Fascia antebrachii

B Superficial arteries and nerves.

Fig. 22.43 Neurovasculature of the finger

Right middle finger, lateral view.

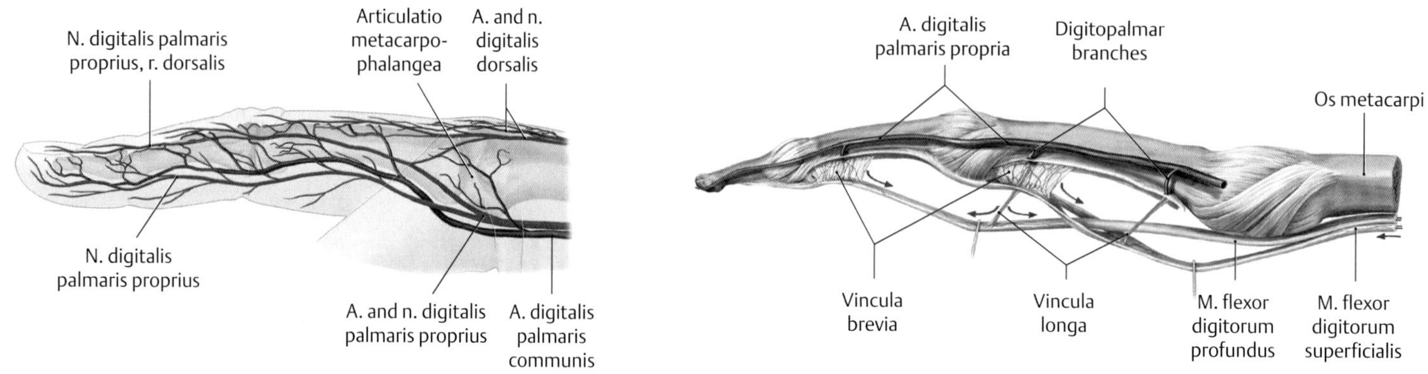
N. digitalis palmaris proprius, r. dorsalis
Articulatio metacarpo-phalangea
A. and n. digitalis dorsalis
N. digitalis palmaris proprius
A. and n. digitalis palmaris proprius
A. digitalis palmaris communis
A. digitalis palmaris propria
Digitopalmar branches
Os metacarpi
Vincula brevia
Vincula longa
M. flexor digitorum profundus
M. flexor digitorum superficialis

A Nerves and arteries.

B Blood supply to the flexor tendons in the tendon sheath.

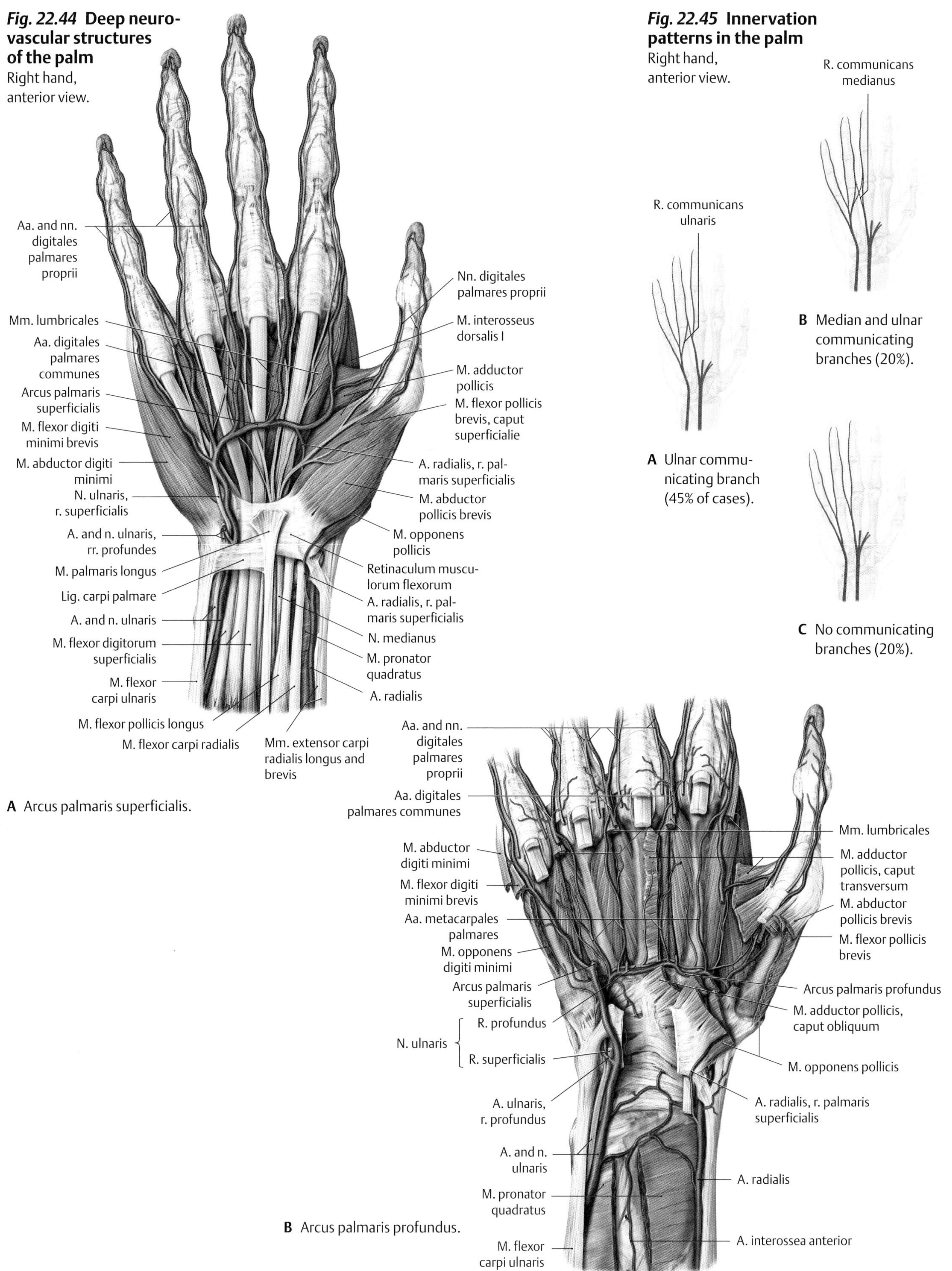
Aa. and nn. digitales palmares proprii
Mm. lumbricales
Aa. digitales palmares communes
Arcus palmaris superficialis
M. flexor digiti minimi brevis
M. abductor digiti minimi
N. ulnaris, r. superficialis
A. and n. ulnaris, rr. profundes
M. palmaris longus
Lig. carpi palmare
A. and n. ulnaris
M. flexor digitorum superficialis
M. flexor carpi ulnaris
M. flexor pollicis longus
M. flexor carpi radialis
Mm. extensor carpi radialis longus and brevis
Nn. digitales palmares proprii
M. interosseus dorsalis I
M. adductor pollicis
M. flexor pollicis brevis, caput superficialie
A. radialis, r. palmaris superficialis
M. abductor pollicis brevis
M. opponens pollicis
Retinaculum musculorum flexorum
A. radialis, r. palmaris superficialis
N. medianus
M. pronator quadratus
A. radialis
Aa. and nn. digitales palmares proprii
Aa. digitales palmares communes
M. abductor digiti minimi
M. flexor digiti minimi brevis
Aa. metacarpales palmares
M. opponens digiti minimi
Arcus palmaris superficialis
N. ulnaris
R. profundus
R. superficialis
A. ulnaris, r. profundus
A. and n. ulnaris
M. pronator quadratus
M. flexor carpi ulnaris
Mm. lumbricales
M. adductor pollicis, caput transversum
M. abductor pollicis brevis
M. flexor pollicis brevis
Arcus palmaris profundus
M. adductor pollicis, caput obliquum
M. opponens pollicis
A. radialis, r. palmaris superficialis
A. radialis
A. interossea anterior
R. communicans ulnaris
R. communicans medianus

***Fig. 22.44* Deep neurovascular structures of the palm**
Right hand, anterior view.

A Arcus palmaris superficialis.

B Arcus palmaris profundus.

***Fig. 22.45* Innervation patterns in the palm**
Right hand, anterior view.

A Ulnar communicating branch (45% of cases).

B Median and ulnar communicating branches (20%).

C No communicating branches (20%).

Topography of the Dorsum of the Hand

Fig. 22.46 Sensory innervation of the dorsum

Right hand, posterior view.

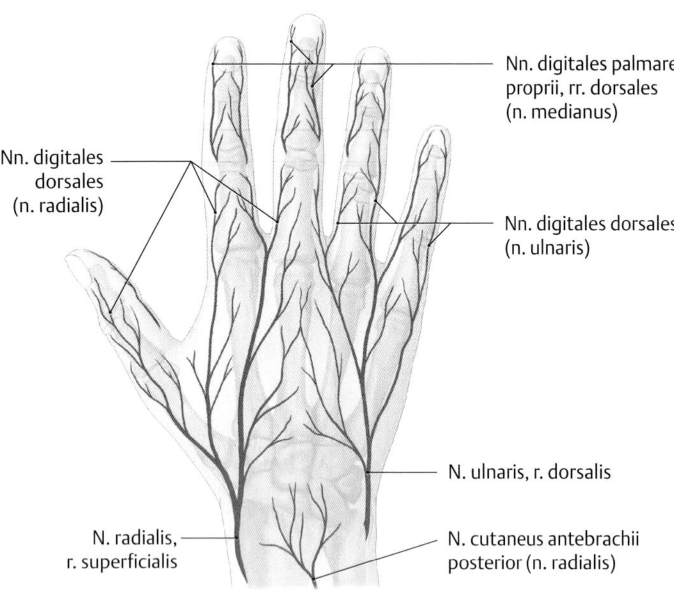

Nn. digitales palmares proprii, rr. dorsales (n. medianus)
Nn. digitales dorsales (n. radialis)
Nn. digitales dorsales (n. ulnaris)
N. ulnaris, r. dorsalis
N. radialis, r. superficialis
N. cutaneus antebrachii posterior (n. radialis)

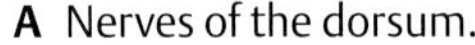

A Nerves of the dorsum.

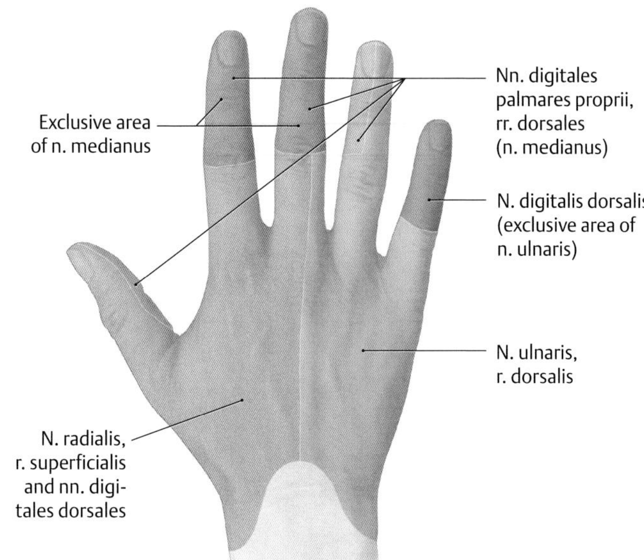

Exclusive area of n. medianus
Nn. digitales palmares proprii, rr. dorsales (n. medianus)
N. digitalis dorsalis (exclusive area of n. ulnaris)
N. ulnaris, r. dorsalis
N. radialis, r. superficialis and nn. digitales dorsales

B Sensory territories. Extensive overlap exists between adjacent areas. *Exclusive* nerve territories indicated with darker shading.

Fig. 22.47 Anatomic snuffbox

Right hand, radial view. The three-sided "anatomic snuffbox" [fovea radialis (Tabatière)] is bounded by the tendons of m. abductor pollicis longus and mm. extensors pollicis brevis and longus.

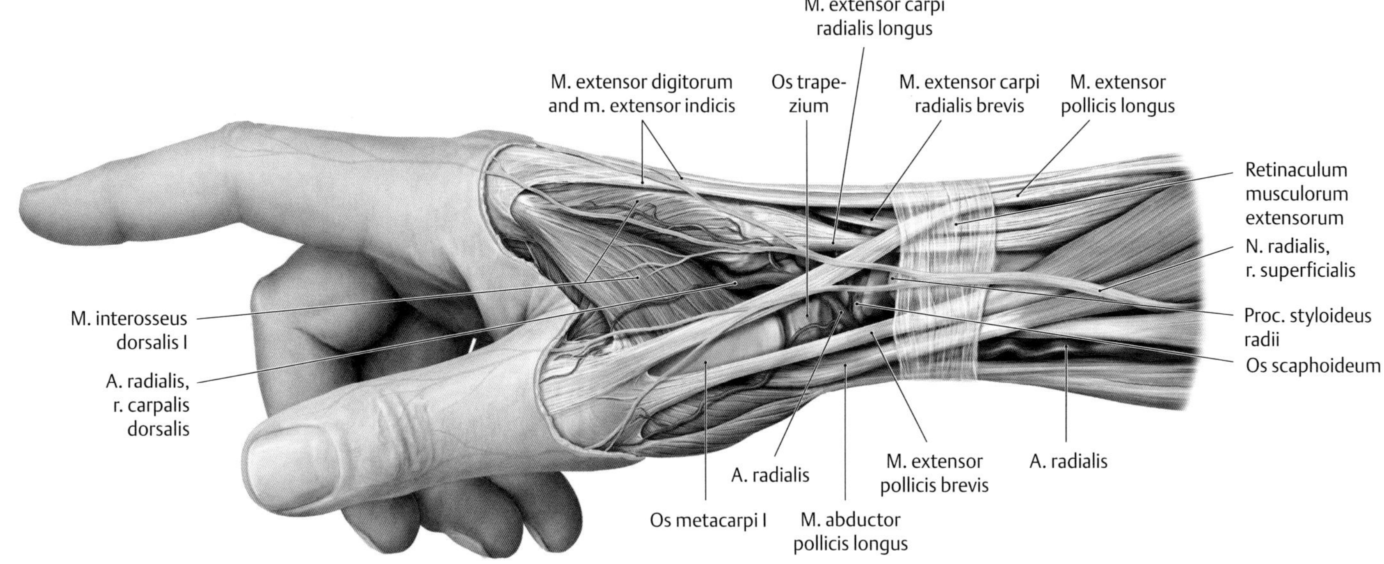

M. extensor carpi radialis longus
M. extensor digitorum and m. extensor indicis
Os trapezium
M. extensor carpi radialis brevis
M. extensor pollicis longus
Retinaculum musculorum extensorum
N. radialis, r. superficialis
Proc. styloideus radii
Os scaphoideum
M. interosseus dorsalis I
A. radialis, r. carpalis dorsalis
A. radialis
M. extensor pollicis brevis
A. radialis
Os metacarpi I
M. abductor pollicis longus

Fig. 22.48 **Neurovascular structures of the dorsum**

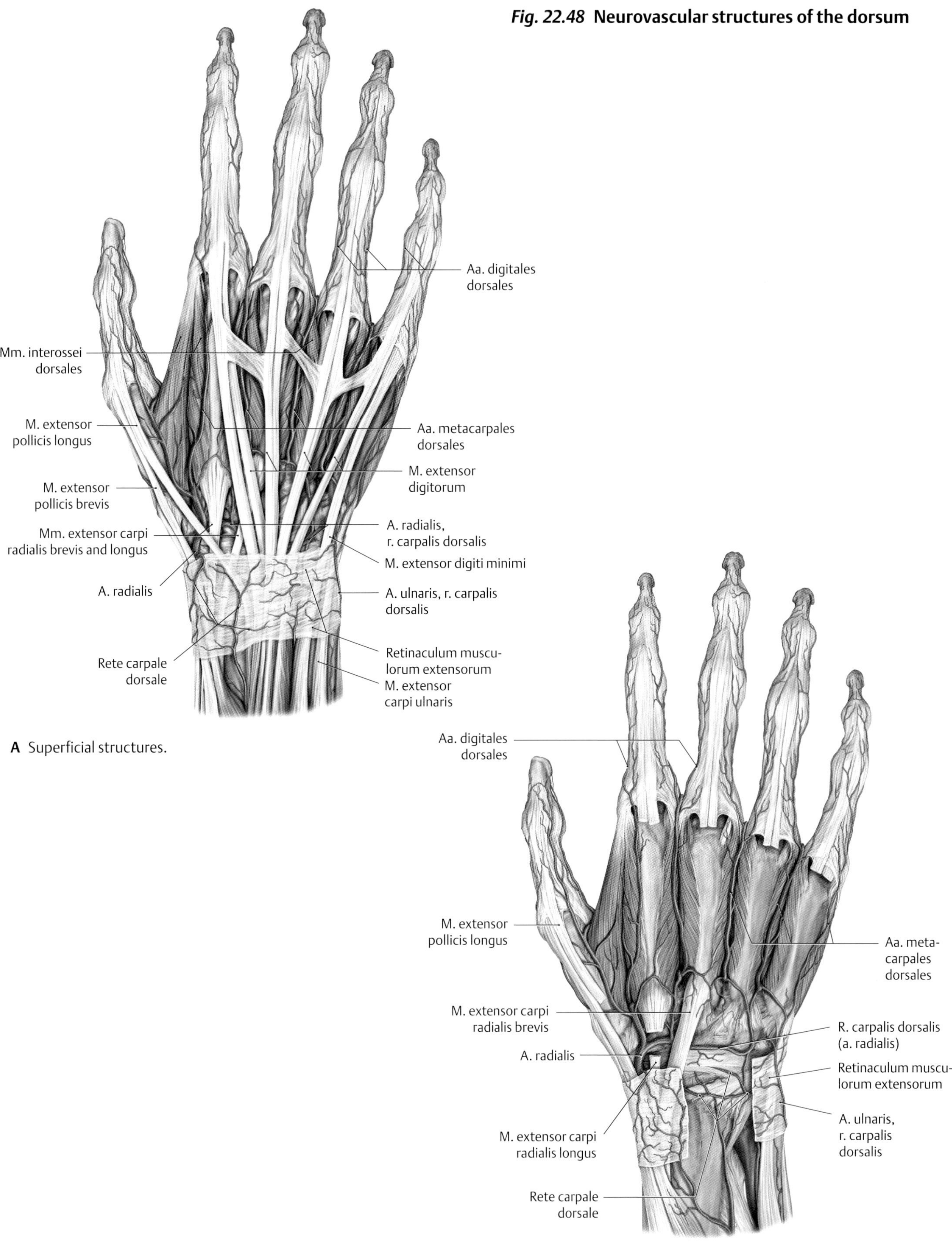
Aa. digitales dorsales
Mm. interossei dorsales
M. extensor pollicis longus
Aa. metacarpales dorsales
M. extensor digitorum
M. extensor pollicis brevis
A. radialis, r. carpalis dorsalis
Mm. extensor carpi radialis brevis and longus
M. extensor digiti minimi
A. radialis
A. ulnaris, r. carpalis dorsalis
Retinaculum musculorum extensorum
Rete carpale dorsale
M. extensor carpi ulnaris
Aa. digitales dorsales
M. extensor pollicis longus
Aa. metacarpales dorsales
M. extensor carpi radialis brevis
R. carpalis dorsalis (a. radialis)
A. radialis
Retinaculum musculorum extensorum
A. ulnaris, r. carpalis dorsalis
M. extensor carpi radialis longus
Rete carpale dorsale

A Superficial structures.

B Deep structures.

Transverse Sections

Fig. 22.49 Windowed dissection
Right limb, anterior view.

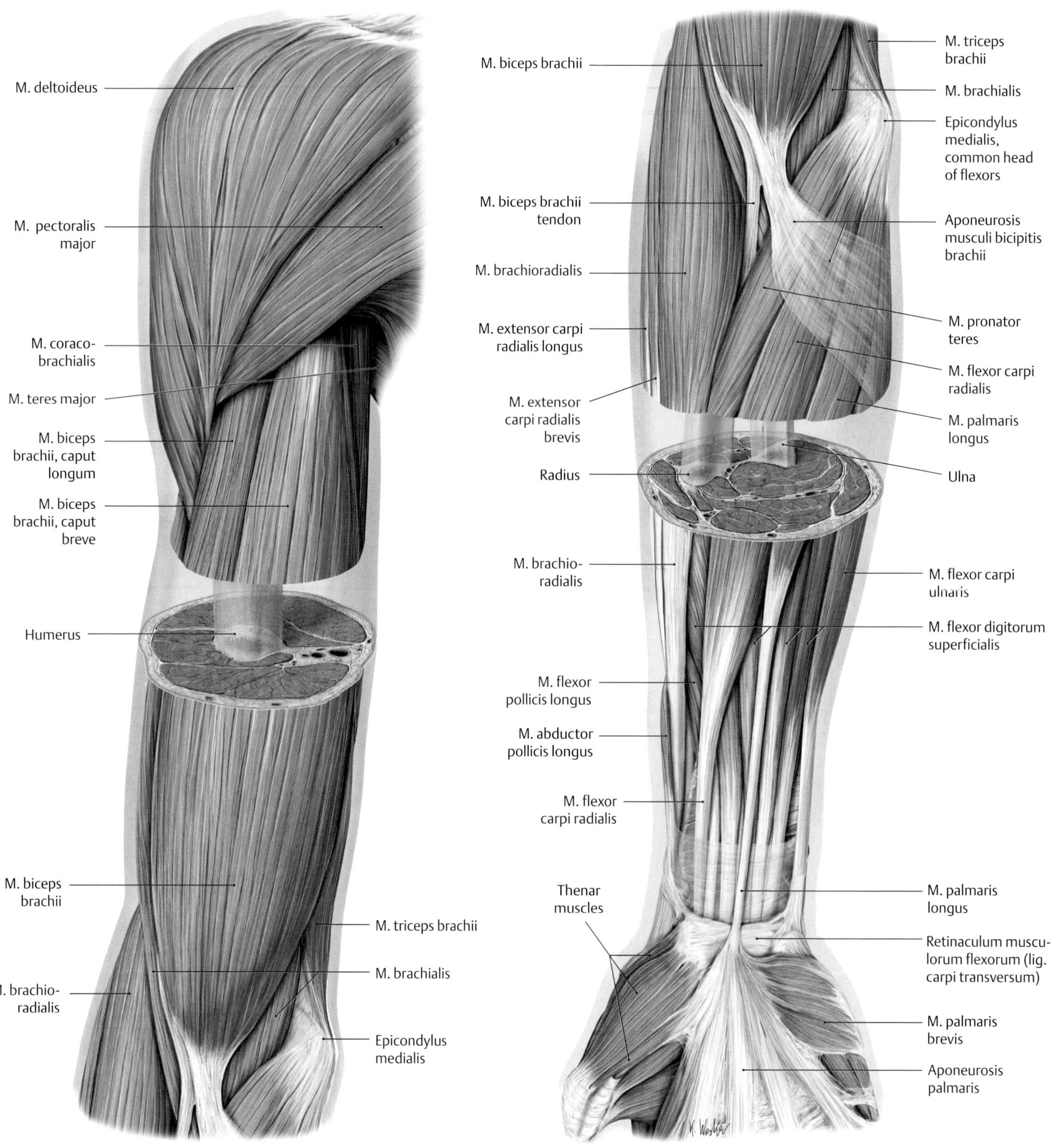
M. deltoideus
M. pectoralis major
M. coraco-brachialis
M. teres major
M. biceps brachii, caput longum
M. biceps brachii, caput breve
Humerus
M. biceps brachii
M. brachio-radialis
M. triceps brachii
M. brachialis
Epicondylus medialis
M. biceps brachii
M. biceps brachii tendon
M. brachioradialis
M. extensor carpi radialis longus
M. extensor carpi radialis brevis
Radius
M. brachio-radialis
M. flexor pollicis longus
M. abductor pollicis longus
M. flexor carpi radialis
Thenar muscles
M. triceps brachii
M. brachialis
Epicondylus medialis, common head of flexors
Aponeurosis musculi bicipitis brachii
M. pronator teres
M. flexor carpi radialis
M. palmaris longus
Ulna
M. flexor carpi ulnaris
M. flexor digitorum superficialis
M. palmaris longus
Retinaculum musculorum flexorum (lig. carpi transversum)
M. palmaris brevis
Aponeurosis palmaris

A Dissection of the arm.

B Dissection of the forearm.

Fig. 22.50 **Transverse sections**
Right limb, proximal (superior) view.

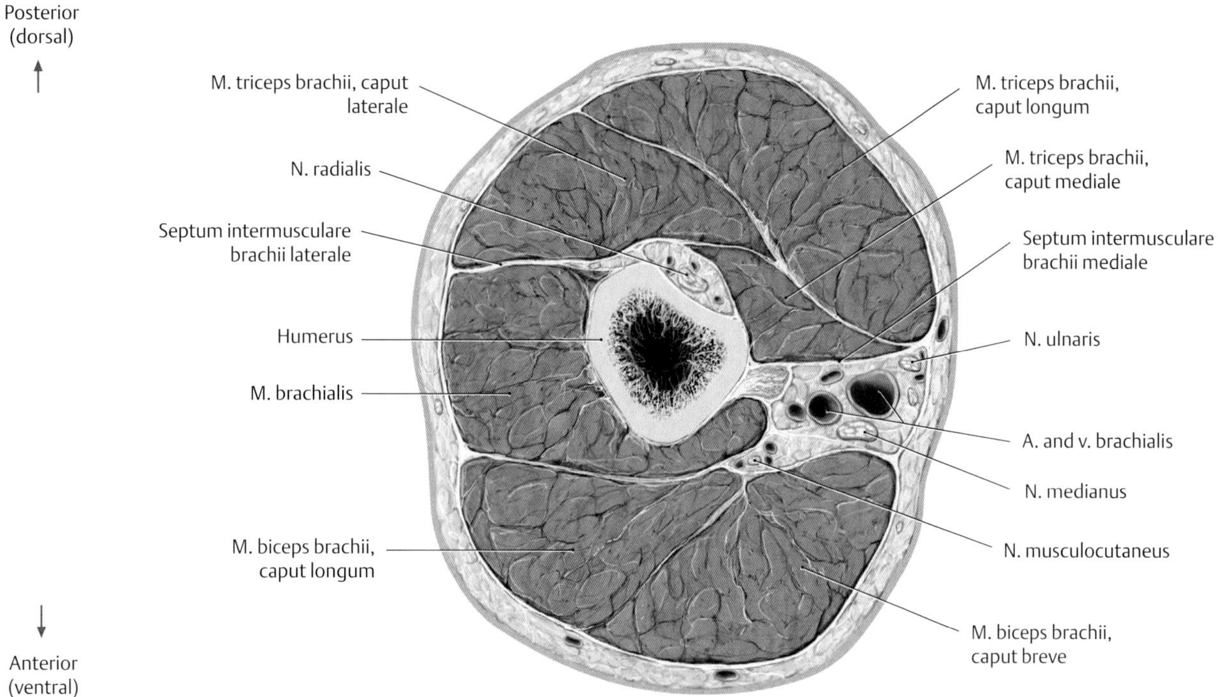
Posterior (dorsal)
Anterior (ventral)
M. triceps brachii, caput laterale
N. radialis
Septum intermusculare brachii laterale
Humerus
M. brachialis
M. biceps brachii, caput longum
M. triceps brachii, caput longum
M. triceps brachii, caput mediale
Septum intermusculare brachii mediale
N. ulnaris
A. and v. brachialis
N. medianus
N. musculocutaneus
M. biceps brachii, caput breve

A Arm (plane of section in Fig. 22.49A).

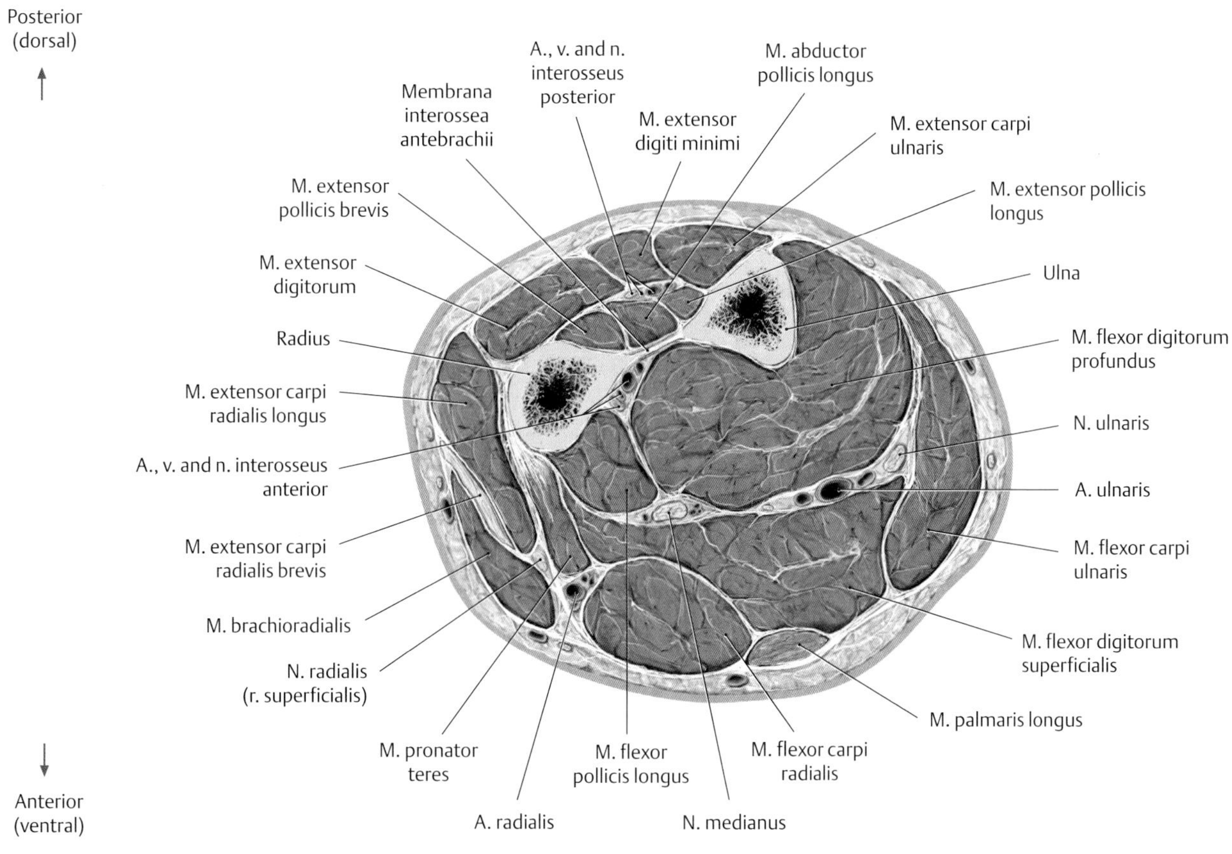
Posterior (dorsal)
Anterior (ventral)
Membrana interossea antebrachii
A., v. and n. interosseus posterior
M. extensor digiti minimi
M. abductor pollicis longus
M. extensor carpi ulnaris
M. extensor pollicis longus
Ulna
M. flexor digitorum profundus
N. ulnaris
A. ulnaris
M. flexor carpi ulnaris
M. flexor digitorum superficialis
M. palmaris longus
M. extensor pollicis brevis
M. extensor digitorum
Radius
M. extensor carpi radialis longus
A., v. and n. interosseus anterior
M. extensor carpi radialis brevis
M. brachioradialis
N. radialis (r. superficialis)
M. pronator teres
A. radialis
M. flexor pollicis longus
N. medianus
M. flexor carpi radialis

B Forearm (plane of section in Fig. 22.49B).

Surface Anatomy (I)

Fig. 23.1 Upper limb: Anterior view

Fig. 23.2 Palpable bony prominences
Right limb.

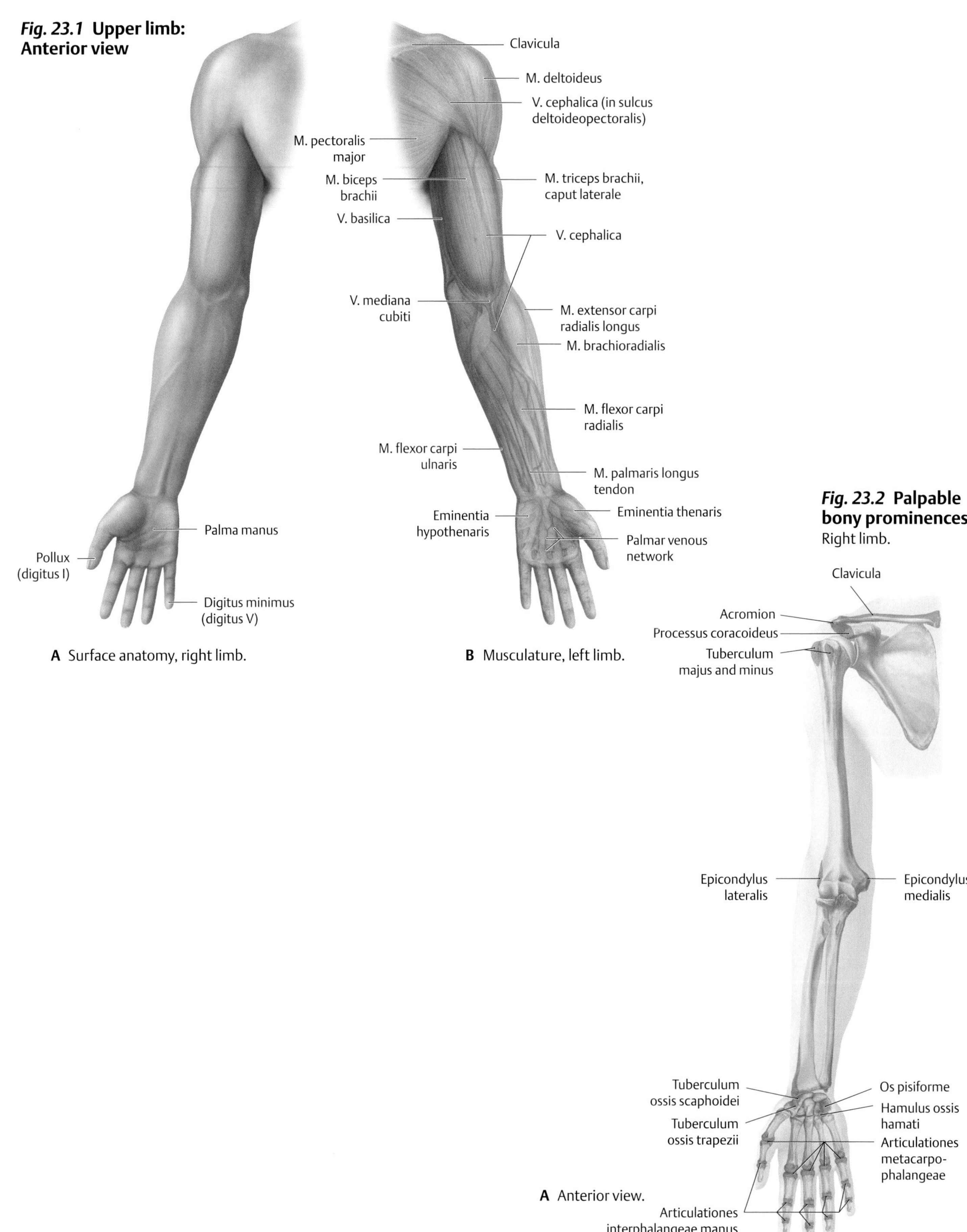
Clavicula
M. deltoideus
V. cephalica (in sulcus deltoideopectoralis)
M. pectoralis major
M. biceps brachii
M. triceps brachii, caput laterale
V. basilica
V. cephalica
V. mediana cubiti
M. extensor carpi radialis longus
M. brachioradialis
M. flexor carpi radialis
M. flexor carpi ulnaris
M. palmaris longus tendon
Eminentia hypothenaris
Eminentia thenaris
Palma manus
Palmar venous network
Pollux (digitus I)
Digitus minimus (digitus V)
Clavicula
Acromion
Processus coracoideus
Tuberculum majus and minus
Epicondylus lateralis
Epicondylus medialis
Tuberculum ossis scaphoidei
Os pisiforme
Hamulus ossis hamati
Tuberculum ossis trapezii
Articulationes metacarpo-phalangeae
Articulationes interphalangeae manus

A Surface anatomy, right limb.

B Musculature, left limb.

A Anterior view.

Q1: Which cutaneous nerves are most vulnerable during intravenous punctures (e.g., drawing blood, injections)?

Fig. 23.3 Upper limb: Posterior view

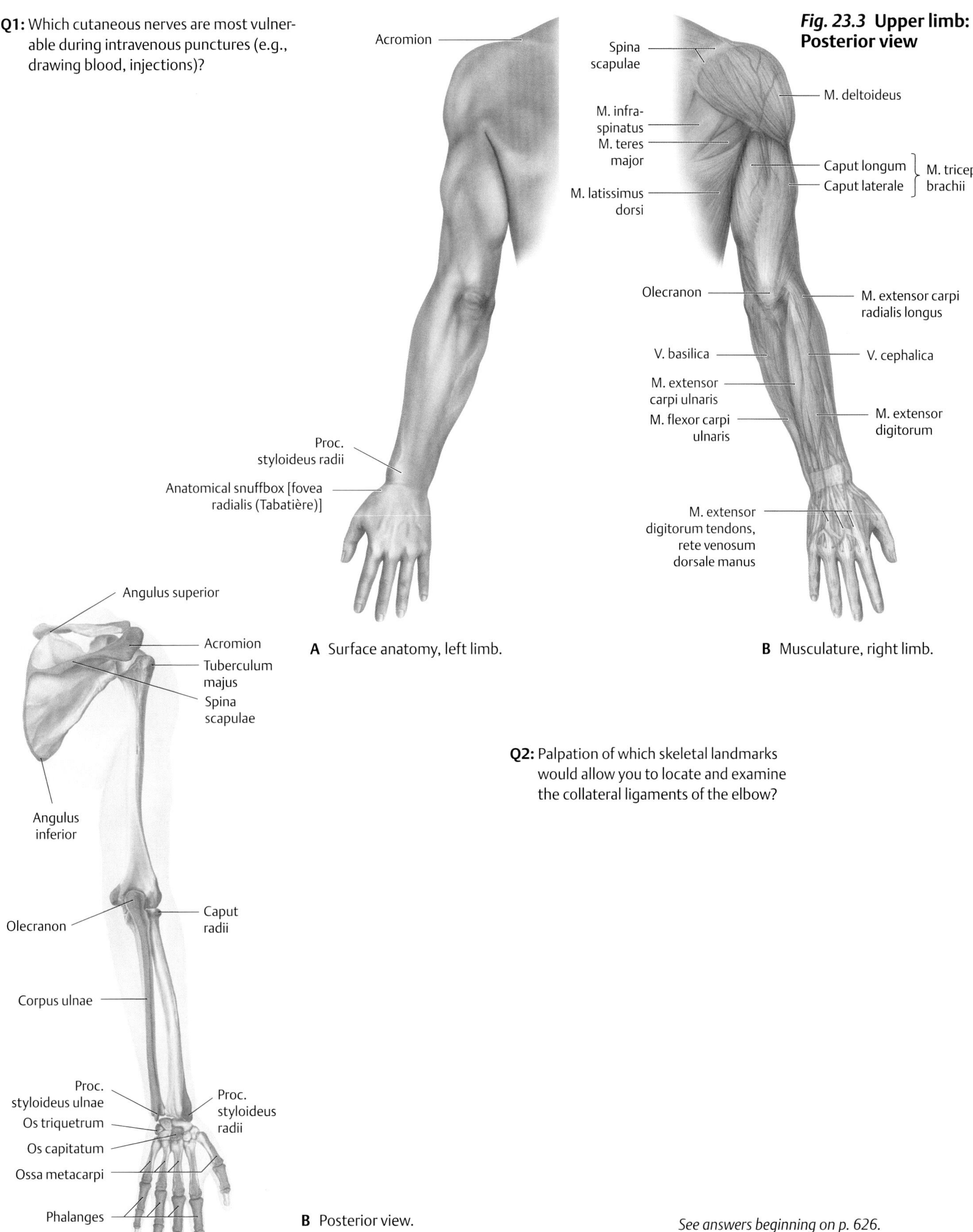
Acromion
Proc. styloideus radii
Anatomical snuffbox [fovea radialis (Tabatière)]
Spina scapulae
M. infra-spinatus
M. teres major
M. latissimus dorsi
M. deltoideus
Caput longum
Caput laterale
M. triceps brachii
Olecranon
M. extensor carpi radialis longus
V. basilica
V. cephalica
M. extensor carpi ulnaris
M. flexor carpi ulnaris
M. extensor digitorum
M. extensor digitorum tendons, rete venosum dorsale manus
Angulus superior
Acromion
Tuberculum majus
Spina scapulae
Angulus inferior
Olecranon
Caput radii
Corpus ulnae
Proc. styloideus ulnae
Os triquetrum
Os capitatum
Ossa metacarpi
Phalanges
Proc. styloideus radii

A Surface anatomy, left limb.

B Musculature, right limb.

B Posterior view.

Q2: Palpation of which skeletal landmarks would allow you to locate and examine the collateral ligaments of the elbow?

See answers beginning on p. 626.

Surface Anatomy (II)

Fig. 23.4 **Palpable bony structures**
Left hand.

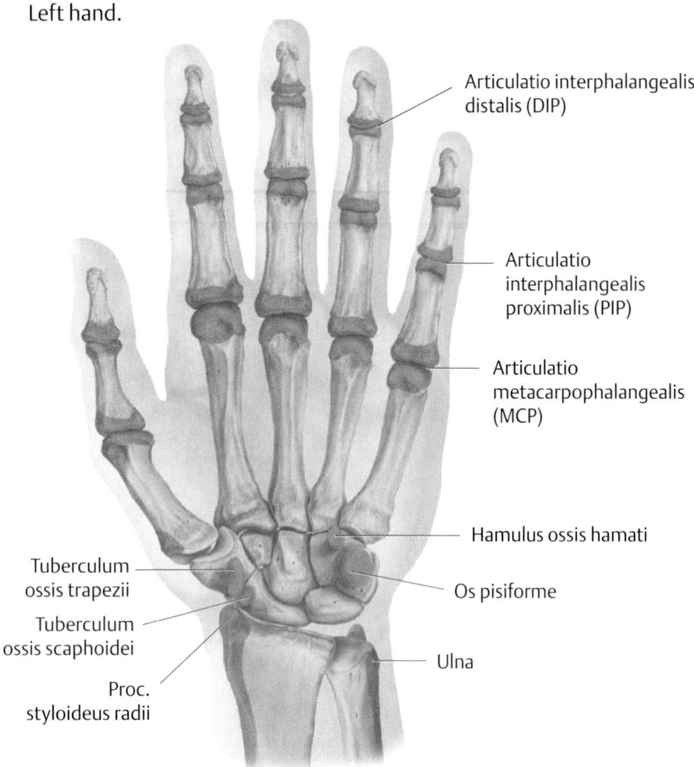
Articulatio interphalangealis distalis (DIP)
Articulatio interphalangealis proximalis (PIP)
Articulatio metacarpophalangealis (MCP)
Hamulus ossis hamati
Tuberculum ossis trapezii
Os pisiforme
Tuberculum ossis scaphoidei
Ulna
Proc. styloideus radii

A Anterior (palmar) view.

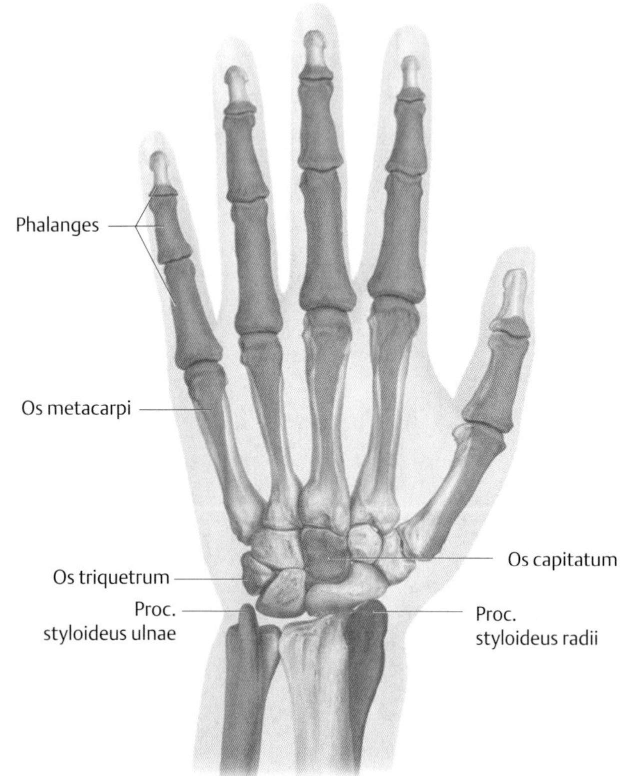
Phalanges
Os metacarpi
Os capitatum
Os triquetrum
Proc. styloideus ulnae
Proc. styloideus radii

B Posterior (dorsal) view.

Fig. 23.5 **Surface anatomy of the wrist**
Left wrist, oblique anterolateral view.

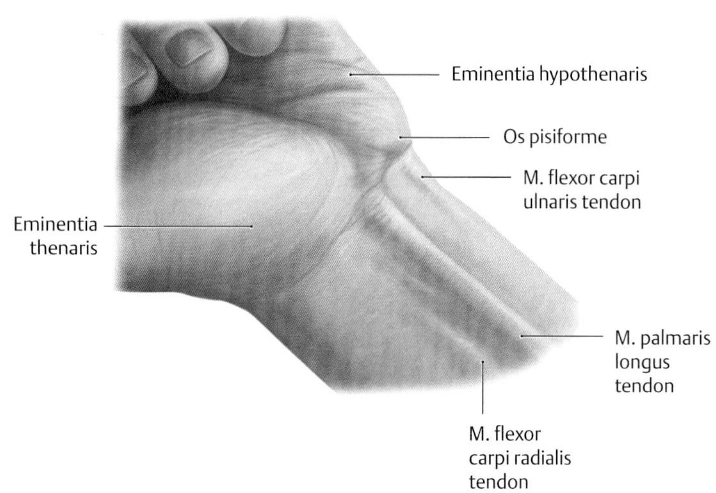
Eminentia hypothenaris
Os pisiforme
M. flexor carpi ulnaris tendon
Eminentia thenaris
M. palmaris longus tendon
M. flexor carpi radialis tendon

Q3: How can the palpable tendons in the wrist be used to determine the location of key arteries and nerves?

Fig. 23.6 **Anatomic snuffbox [fovea radialis (Tabatière)]**
Left hand, oblique posterolateral view.

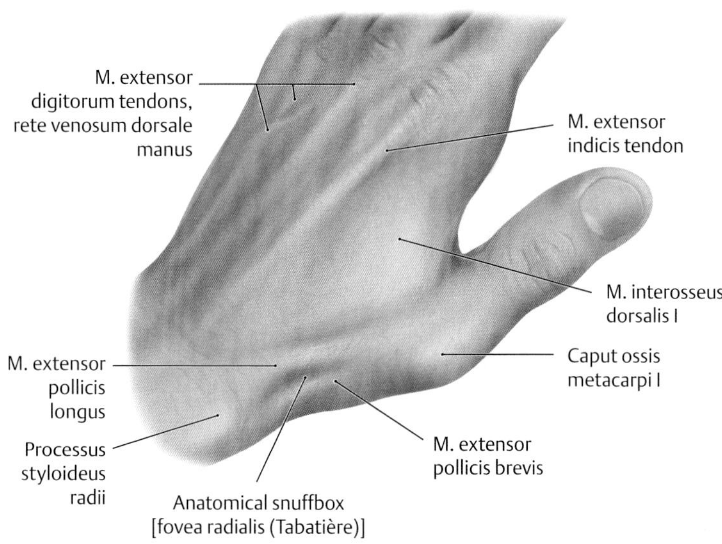
M. extensor digitorum tendons, rete venosum dorsale manus
M. extensor indicis tendon
M. interosseus dorsalis I
Caput ossis metacarpi I
M. extensor pollicis longus
Processus styloideus radii
M. extensor pollicis brevis
Anatomical snuffbox [fovea radialis (Tabatière)]

Q4: Tenderness in the base of the anatomic snuffbox can suggest a fracture of which of the carpal bones?

See answers beginning on p. 626.

Fig. 23.7 Palm

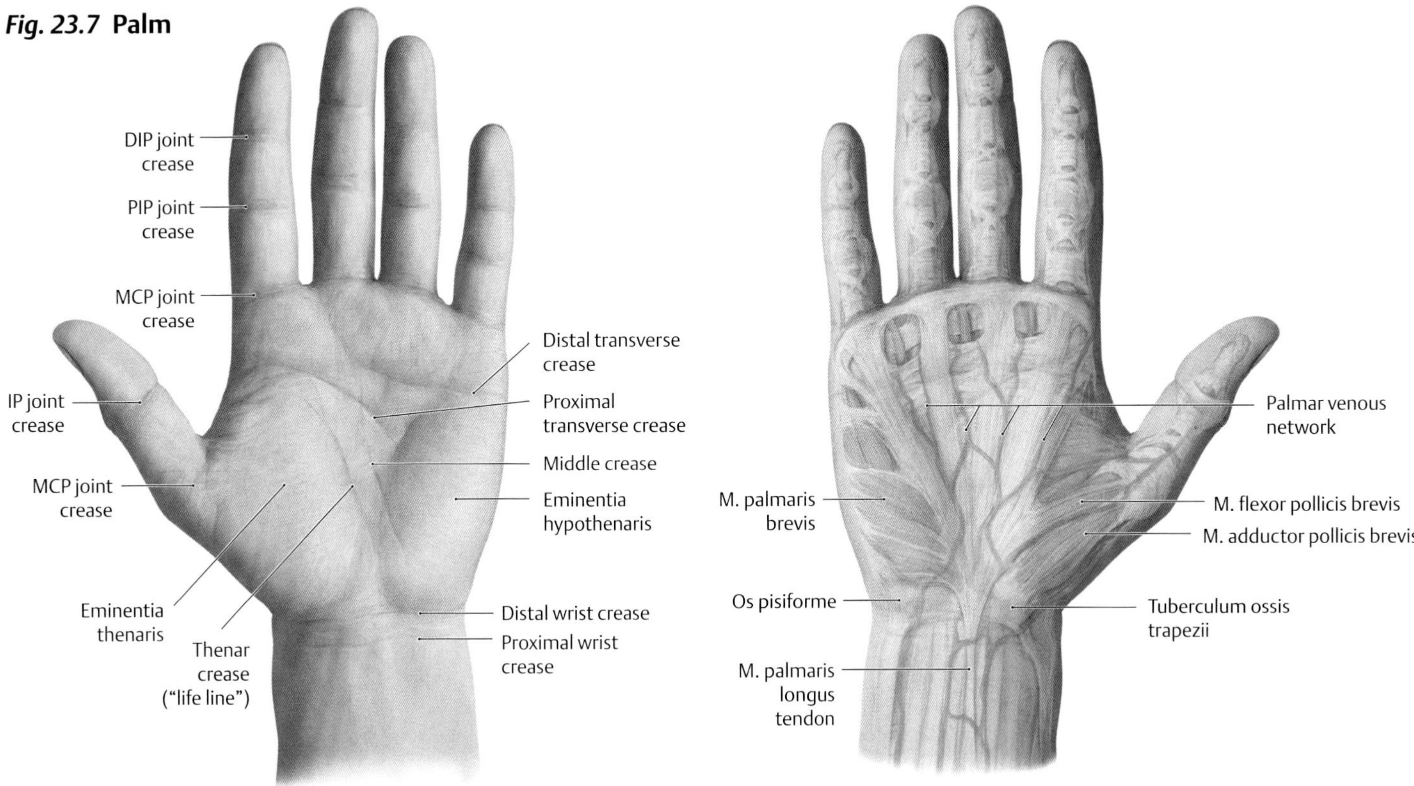
DIP joint crease
PIP joint crease
MCP joint crease
IP joint crease
MCP joint crease
Eminentia thenaris
Thenar crease ("life line")
Distal transverse crease
Proximal transverse crease
Middle crease
Eminentia hypothenaris
Distal wrist crease
Proximal wrist crease
Palmar venous network
M. palmaris brevis
M. flexor pollicis brevis
M. adductor pollicis brevis
Os pisiforme
Tuberculum ossis trapezii
M. palmaris longus tendon

A Surface anatomy, left palm.

B Musculature, right palm.

Fig. 23.8 Dorsum

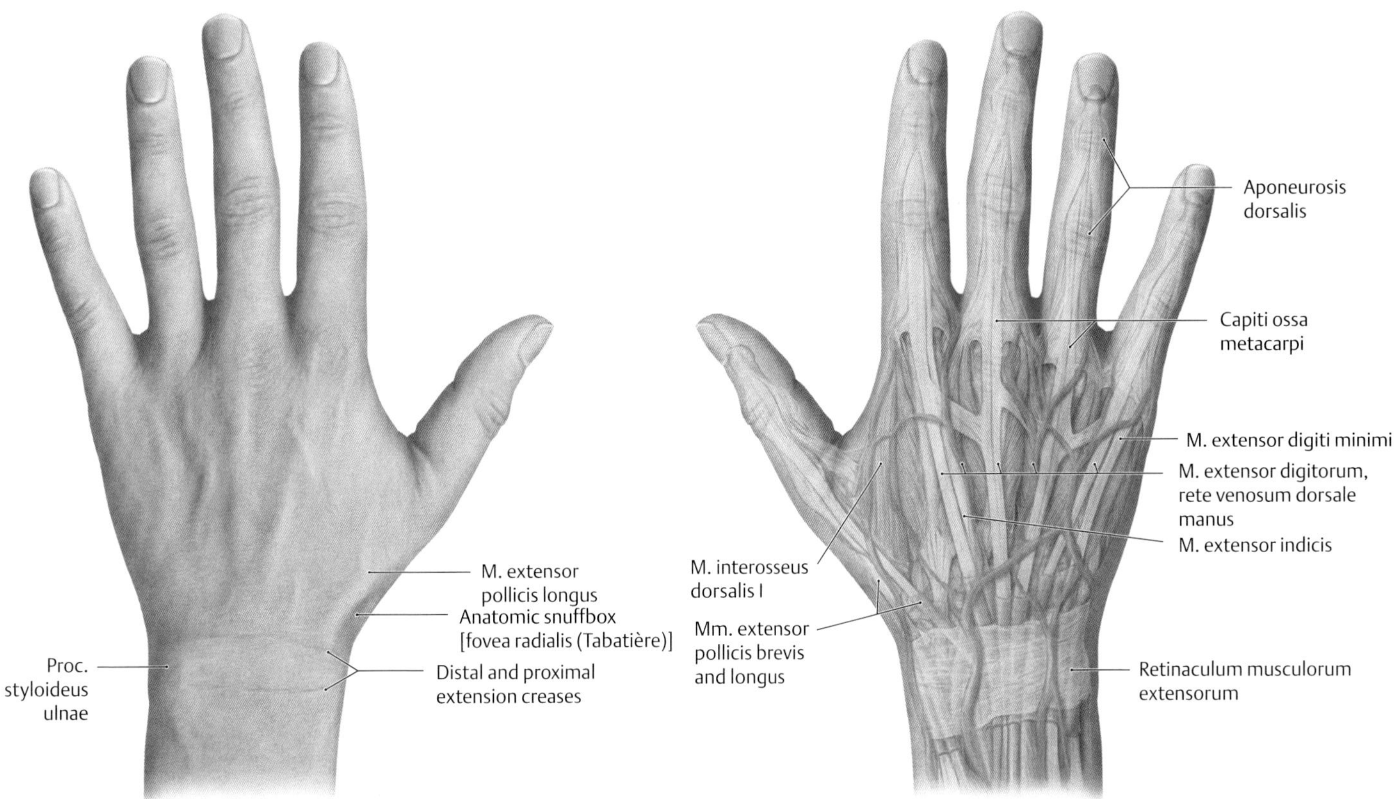
M. extensor pollicis longus
Anatomic snuffbox [fovea radialis (Tabatière)]
Proc. styloideus ulnae
Distal and proximal extension creases
Aponeurosis dorsalis
Capiti ossa metacarpi
M. extensor digiti minimi
M. extensor digitorum, rete venosum dorsale manus
M. extensor indicis
M. interosseus dorsalis I
Mm. extensor pollicis brevis and longus
Retinaculum musculorum extensorum

A Surface anatomy, left hand.

B Musculature, right hand.

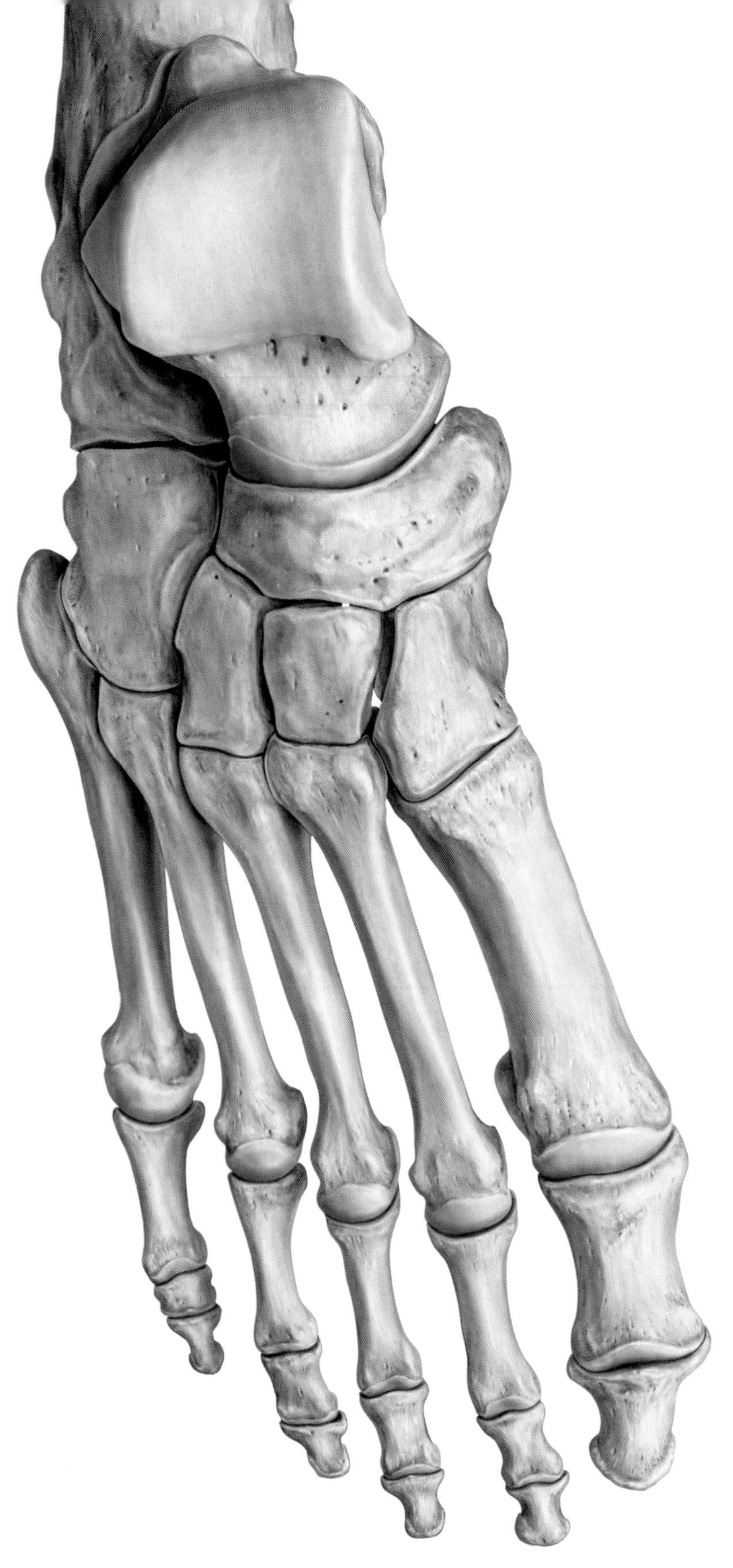

Lower Limb

24 Hip & Thigh

Bones of the Lower Limb 356
Pelvic Girdle & Os Coxae 358
Femur 360
Articulatio Coxae: Overview 362
Articulatio Coxae: Ligaments & Capsule 364
Anterior Muscles of the Thigh, Hip & Regio Glutealis (I) 366
Anterior Muscles of the Thigh, Hip & Regio Glutealis (II) 368
Posterior Muscles of the Thigh, Hip & Regio Glutealis (I) 370
Posterior Muscles of the Thigh, Hip & Regio Glutealis (II) 372
Muscle Facts (I) 374
Muscle Facts (II) 376
Muscle Facts (III) 378

25 Knee & Leg

Tibia & Fibula 380
Articulatio Genus: Overview 382
Articulatio Genus: Capsule, Ligaments & Bursae 384
Articulatio Genus: Ligaments & Menisci 386
Ligamenta Cruciata 388
Articulatio Genus Cavitas Articularis 390
Muscles of the Leg: Anterior & Lateral Views 392
Muscles of the Leg: Posterior View 394
Muscle Facts (I) 396
Muscle Facts (II) 398

26 Ankle & Foot

Ossa Pedis 400
Articulationes Pedis (I) 402
Articulationes Pedis (II) 404
Articulationes Pedis (III) 406
Ligaments of the Ankle & Foot 408
Plantar Vault & Arches of the Foot 410
Muscles of the Sole of the Foot 412
Muscles & Tendon Sheaths of the Foot 414
Muscle Facts (I) 416
Muscle Facts (II) 418

27 Neurovasculature

Arteries of the Lower Limb 420
Veins & Lymphatics of the Lower Limb 422
Plexus Lumbosacralis 424
Nerves of Plexus Lumbalis 426
Nerves of Plexus Lumbalis: N. Obturatoris & N. Femoralis 428
Nerves of Plexus Sacralis 430
Nerves of Plexus Sacralis: N. Ischiadicus 432
Superficial Nerves & Vessels of the Lower Limb 434
Topography of Regio Inguinalis 436
Topography of Regio Glutealis 438
Topography of the Anterior & Posterior Thigh 440
Topography of the Posterior & Medial Leg 442
Topography of the Lateral & Anterior Leg 444
Topography of Planta Pedis 446
Transverse Sections of the Thigh & Leg 448

28 Surface Anatomy

Surface Anatomy 450

Bones of the Lower Limb

Fig. 24.1 Bones of the lower limb

Right limb. The skeleton of the lower limb consists of a pelvic girdle (cingulum pelvicum; os coxae and os sacrum) and an attached free limb. The free limb is divided into the thigh (femur), leg (tibia and fibula), and foot. It is connected to the pelvic girdle by the articulatio coxae.

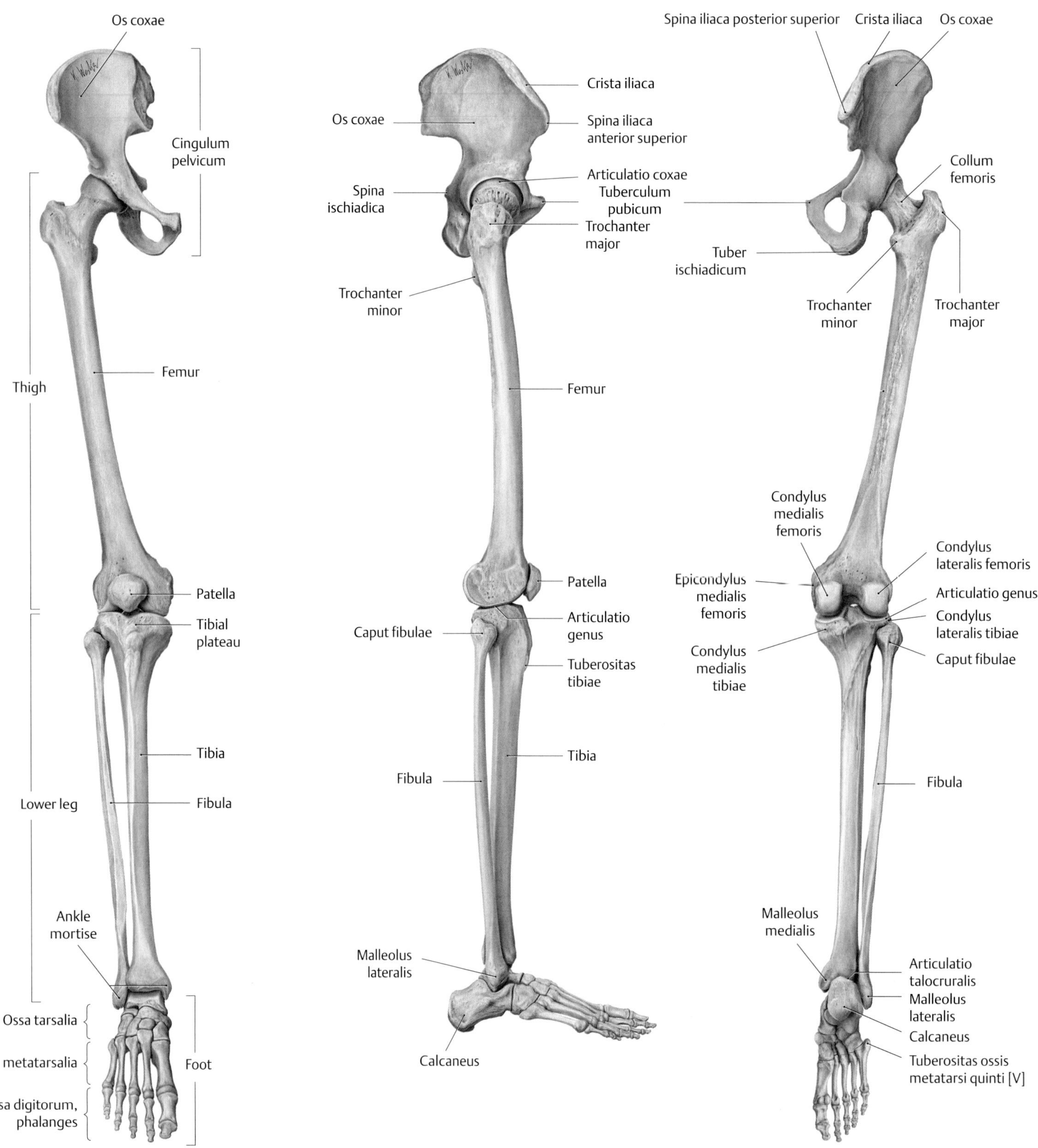

Os coxae
Cingulum pelvicum
Thigh
Femur
Patella
Tibial plateau
Tibia
Lower leg
Fibula
Ankle mortise
Ossa tarsalia
Ossa metatarsalia
Foot
Ossa digitorum, phalanges
Crista iliaca
Os coxae
Spina iliaca anterior superior
Articulatio coxae
Spina ischiadica
Tuberculum pubicum
Trochanter major
Trochanter minor
Femur
Patella
Articulatio genus
Caput fibulae
Tuberositas tibiae
Tibia
Fibula
Malleolus lateralis
Calcaneus
Spina iliaca posterior superior
Crista iliaca
Os coxae
Collum femoris
Tuber ischiadicum
Trochanter minor
Trochanter major
Condylus medialis femoris
Condylus lateralis femoris
Epicondylus medialis femoris
Articulatio genus
Condylus lateralis tibiae
Condylus medialis tibiae
Caput fibulae
Fibula
Malleolus medialis
Articulatio talocruralis
Malleolus lateralis
Calcaneus
Tuberositas ossis metatarsi quinti [V]

A Anterior view.

B Right lateral view.

C Posterior view.

Fig. 24.2 Line of gravity
Right lateral view. The line of gravity runs vertically from the whole-body center of gravity to the ground with characteristic points of intersection.

Fig. 24.3 Palpable bony prominences in the lower limb
Most skeletal elements of the lower limb have bony prominences, margins, or surfaces (e.g., medial or tibial surfaces) that can be palpated through the skin and soft tissues.

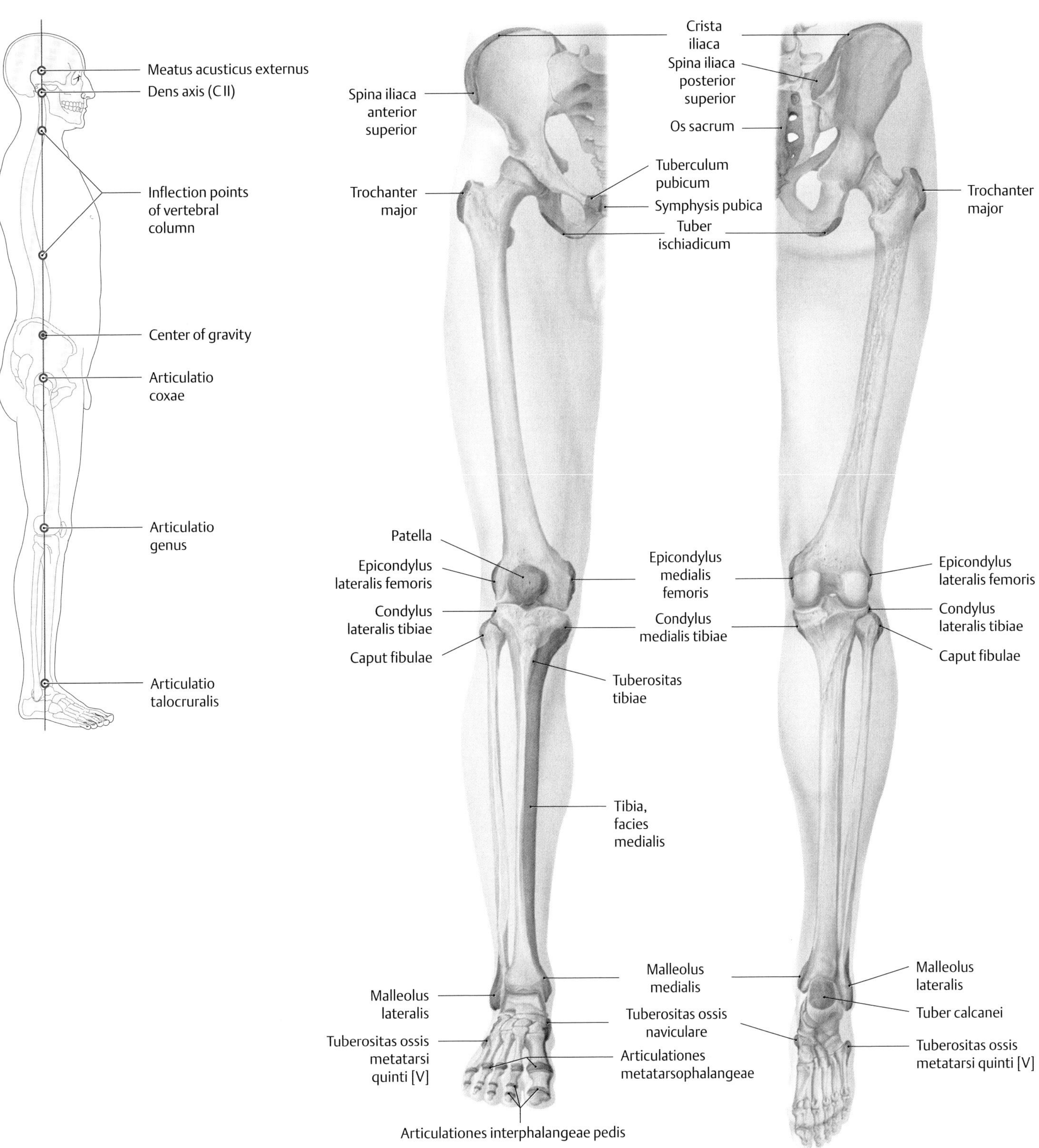
Meatus acusticus externus
Dens axis (C II)
Inflection points of vertebral column
Center of gravity
Articulatio coxae
Articulatio genus
Articulatio talocruralis
Crista iliaca
Spina iliaca anterior superior
Spina iliaca posterior superior
Os sacrum
Tuberculum pubicum
Symphysis pubica
Tuber ischiadicum
Trochanter major
Trochanter major
Patella
Epicondylus lateralis femoris
Epicondylus medialis femoris
Epicondylus lateralis femoris
Condylus lateralis tibiae
Condylus medialis tibiae
Condylus lateralis tibiae
Caput fibulae
Caput fibulae
Tuberositas tibiae
Tibia, facies medialis
Malleolus lateralis
Malleolus medialis
Malleolus lateralis
Tuber calcanei
Tuberositas ossis metatarsi quinti [V]
Tuberositas ossis naviculare
Tuberositas ossis metatarsi quinti [V]
Articulationes metatarsophalangeae
Articulationes interphalangeae pedis

A Anterior view.

B Posterior view.

Pelvic Girdle & Os Coxae

***Fig. 24.4* Pelvic girdle**
Anterior view. Pelvic ring in red.

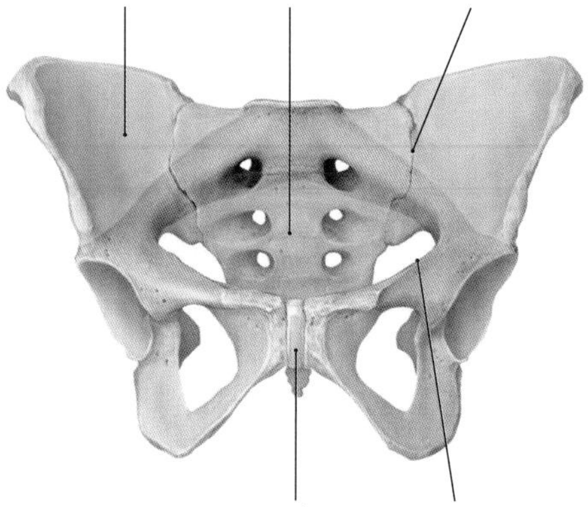

Os coxae
Os sacrum
Articulatio sacroiliaca
Symphysis pubica
Linea arcuata

Each pelvic girdle consists of a hip bone (os coxae), which articulates with caput femoris. Unlike the shoulder girdle, the pelvic girdle is firmly integrated into the axial skeleton: the paired hip bones are connected to each other at the cartilaginous symphysis pubica and to os sacrum via the articulationes sacroiliacae. These attachments create the bony pelvic ring (red), permitting very little motion. This stability is an important prerequisite for the transfer of trunk loads to the lower limb (necessary for normal gait).

***Fig. 24.5* Right hip bone**

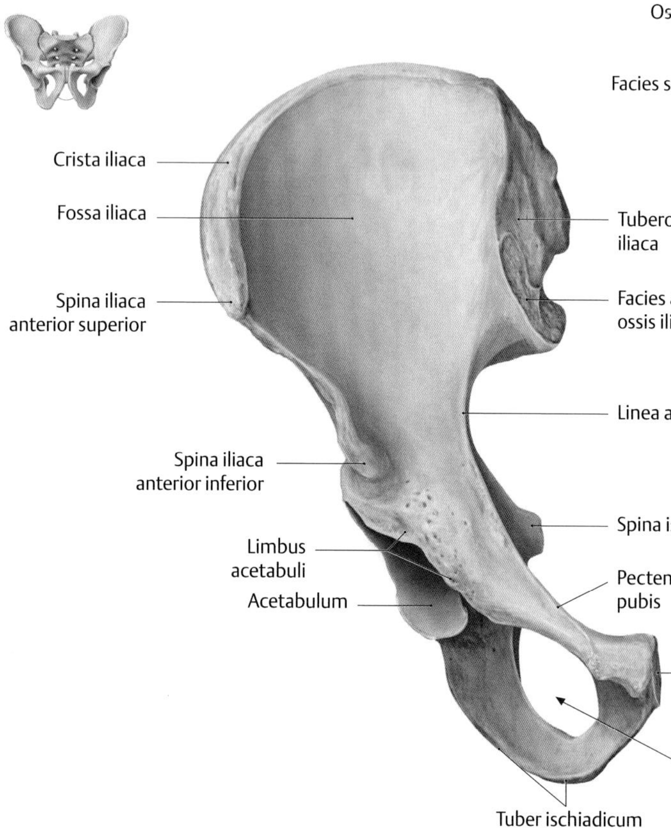

Crista iliaca
Fossa iliaca
Spina iliaca anterior superior
Spina iliaca anterior inferior
Limbus acetabuli
Acetabulum
Tuberositas iliaca
Facies auricularis ossis ilii
Linea arcuata
Spina ischiadica
Pecten ossis pubis
Facies symphysialis
Foramen obturatum
Tuber ischiadicum

A Anterior view.

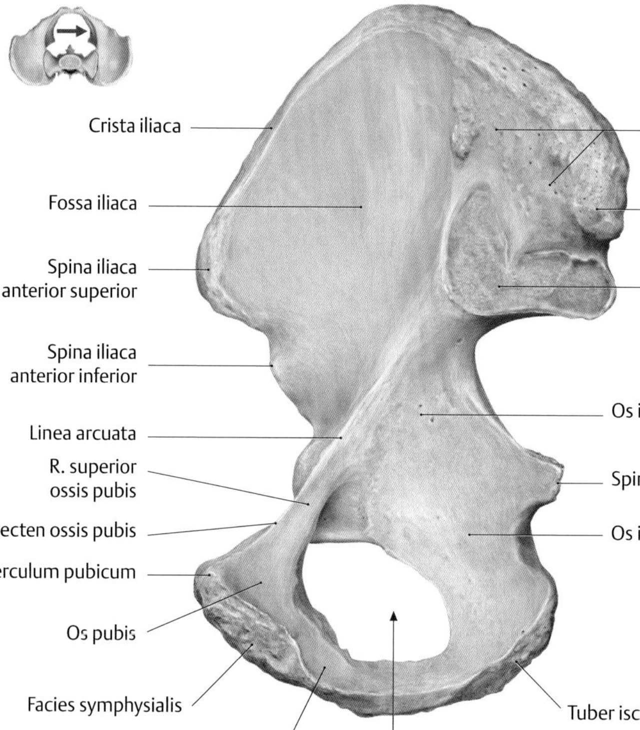

Crista iliaca
Fossa iliaca
Spina iliaca anterior superior
Spina iliaca anterior inferior
Linea arcuata
R. superior ossis pubis
Pecten ossis pubis
Tuberculum pubicum
Os pubis
Facies symphysialis
R. inferior ossis pubis
Foramen obturatum
Tuberositas iliaca
Spina iliaca posterior superior
Facies auricularis ossis ilii
Os ilium, corpus
Spina ischiadica
Os ischii, corpus
Tuber ischiadicum

B Medial view.

Fig. 24.6 **Components of os coxae**
Right os coxae. The three bony elements of os coxae (os ilium, os ischium, and os pubis) come together at the acetabulum. Definitive fusion of the Y-shaped growth plate (triradiate cartilage) occurs between the 14th and 16th years of life.

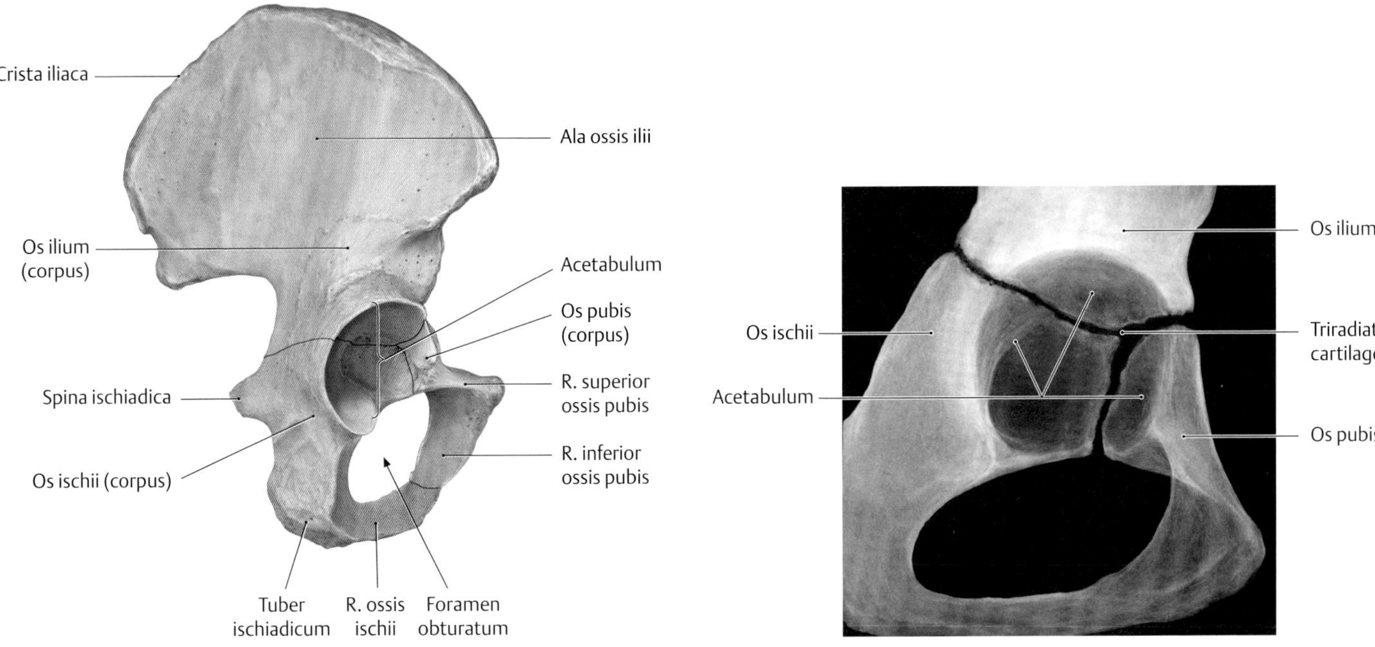
Crista iliaca
Ala ossis ilii
Os ilium (corpus)
Acetabulum
Os pubis (corpus)
R. superior ossis pubis
Spina ischiadica
R. inferior ossis pubis
Os ischii (corpus)
Tuber ischiadicum
R. ossis ischii
Foramen obturatum
Os ilium
Os ischii
Triradiate cartilage
Acetabulum
Os pubis

A Triradiate cartilage of os coxae. Lateral view.

B Radiograph of right acetabulum of a child.

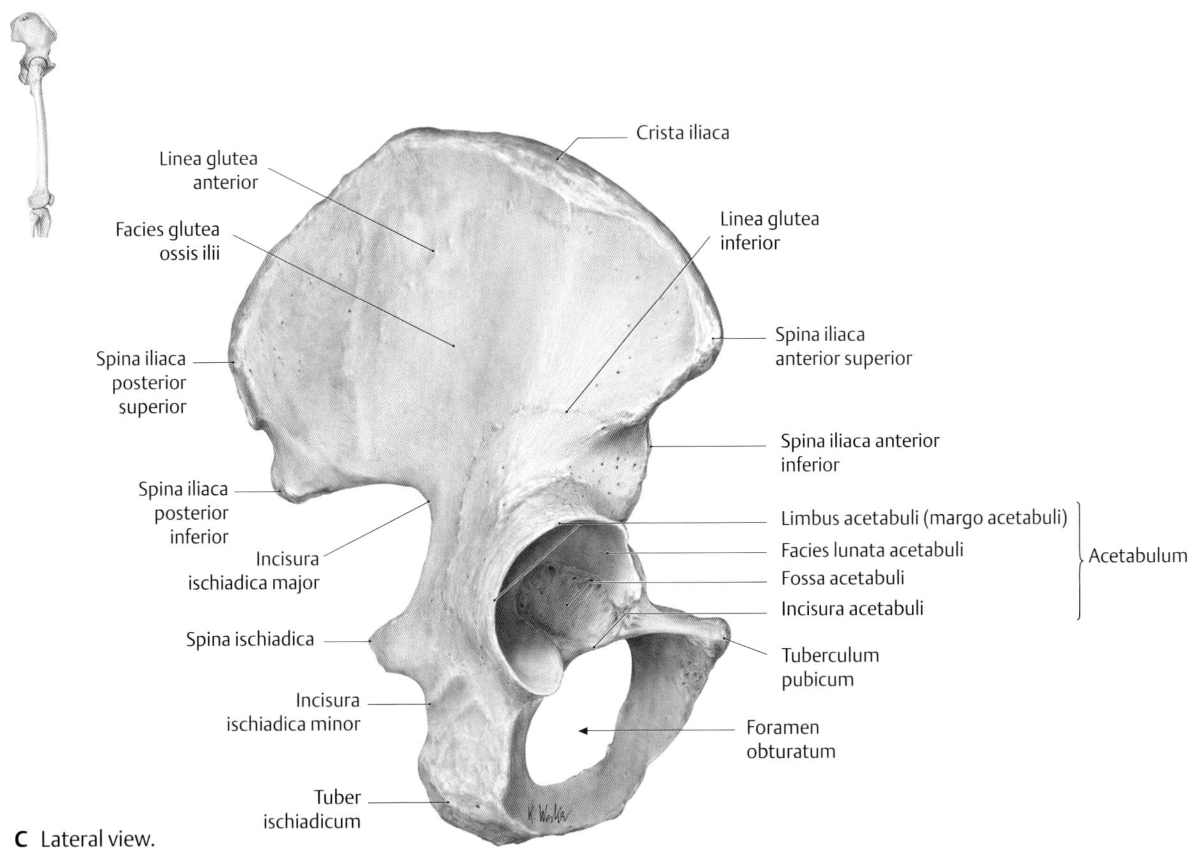
Crista iliaca
Linea glutea anterior
Facies glutea ossis ilii
Linea glutea inferior
Spina iliaca anterior superior
Spina iliaca posterior superior
Spina iliaca anterior inferior
Spina iliaca posterior inferior
Incisura ischiadica major
Limbus acetabuli (margo acetabuli)
Facies lunata acetabuli
Fossa acetabuli
Incisura acetabuli
Acetabulum
Spina ischiadica
Tuberculum pubicum
Incisura ischiadica minor
Foramen obturatum
Tuber ischiadicum

C Lateral view.

Femur

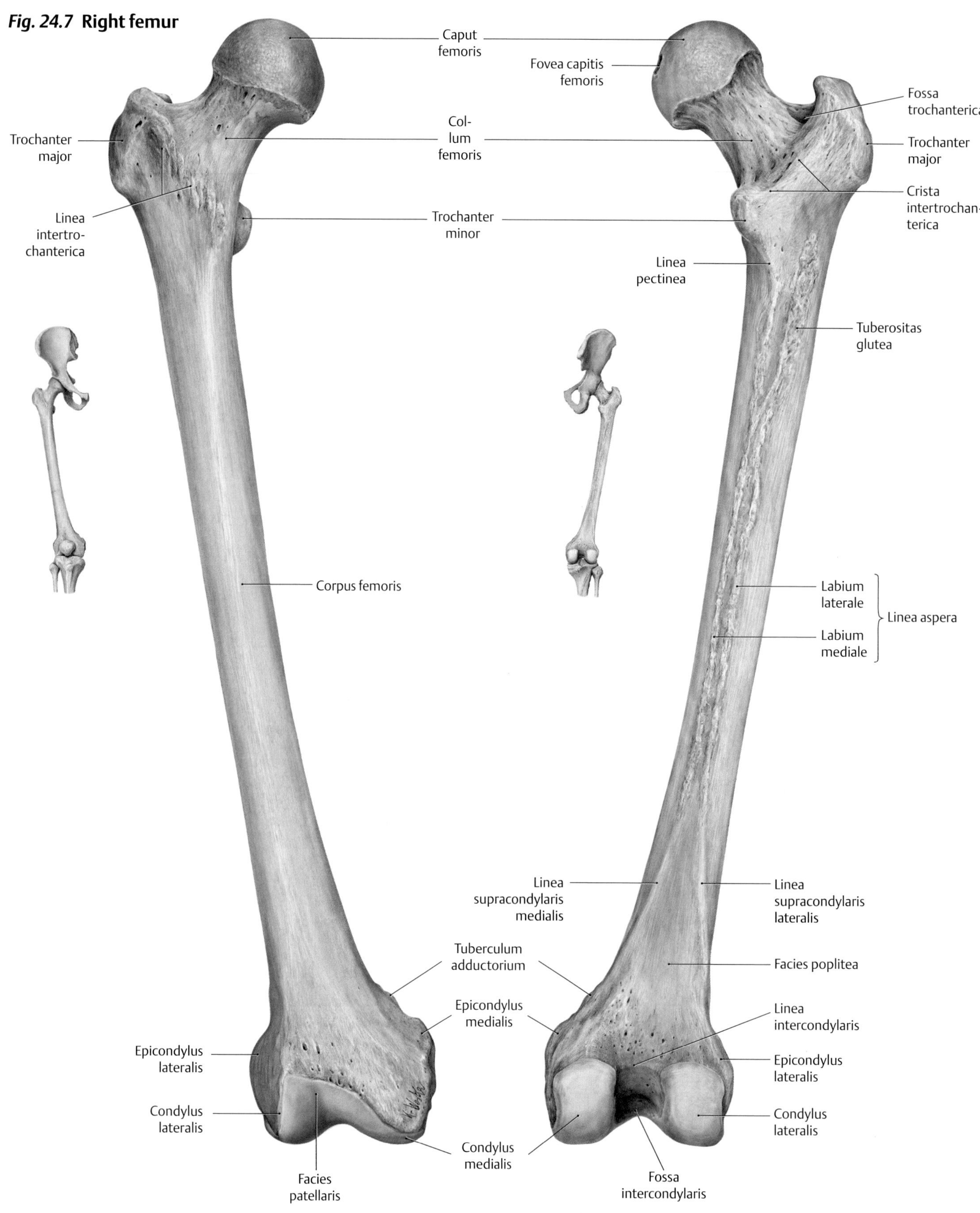
Caput
femoris
Fovea capitis
femoris
Fossa
trochanterica
Col-
lum
femoris
Trochanter
major
Trochanter
major
Crista
intertrochan-
terica
Linea
intertro-
chanterica
Trochanter
minor
Linea
pectinea
Tuberositas
glutea
Corpus femoris
Labium
laterale
Labium
mediale
Linea aspera
Linea
supracondylaris
medialis
Linea
supracondylaris
lateralis
Tuberculum
adductorium
Facies poplitea
Epicondylus
medialis
Linea
intercondylaris
Epicondylus
lateralis
Epicondylus
lateralis
Condylus
lateralis
Condylus
lateralis
Condylus
medialis
Facies
patellaris
Fossa
intercondylaris

Fig. 24.7 **Right femur**

A Anterior view.

B Posterior view.

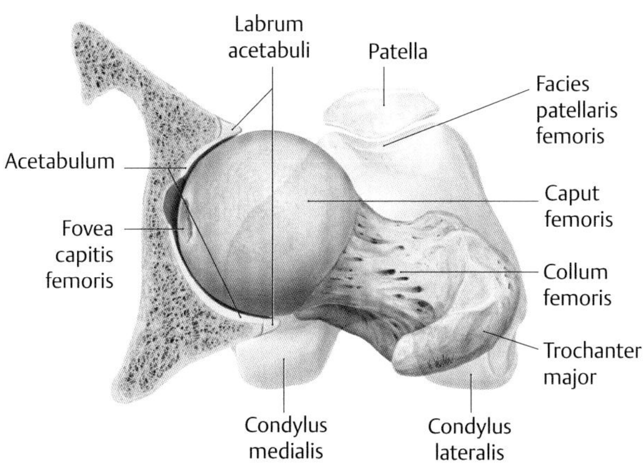
Labrum acetabuli
Patella
Facies patellaris femoris
Acetabulum
Caput femoris
Fovea capitis femoris
Collum femoris
Trochanter major
Condylus medialis
Condylus lateralis

C Proximal view. The acetabulum has been sectioned in the horizontal plane.

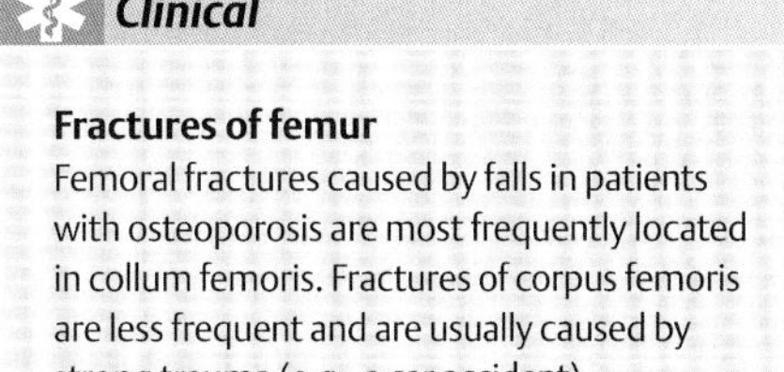

Clinical

Fractures of femur

Femoral fractures caused by falls in patients with osteoporosis are most frequently located in collum femoris. Fractures of corpus femoris are less frequent and are usually caused by strong trauma (e.g., a car accident).

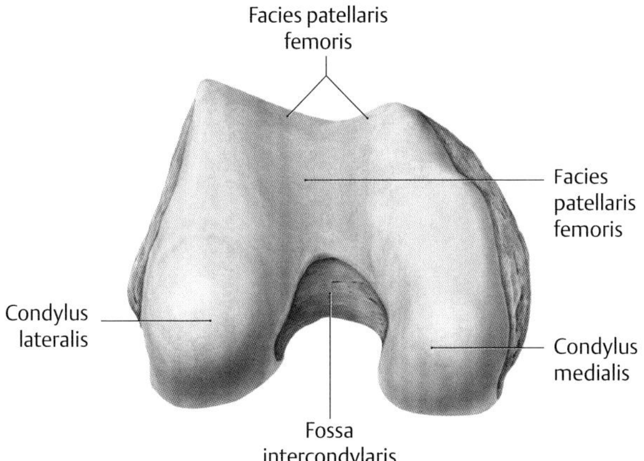
Facies patellaris femoris
Facies patellaris femoris
Condylus lateralis
Condylus medialis
Fossa intercondylaris

D Distal view. See pp. 382–383 for articulatio genus.

Fig. 24.8 **Caput femoris in articulatio coxae**
Right articulatio coxae, superior view.

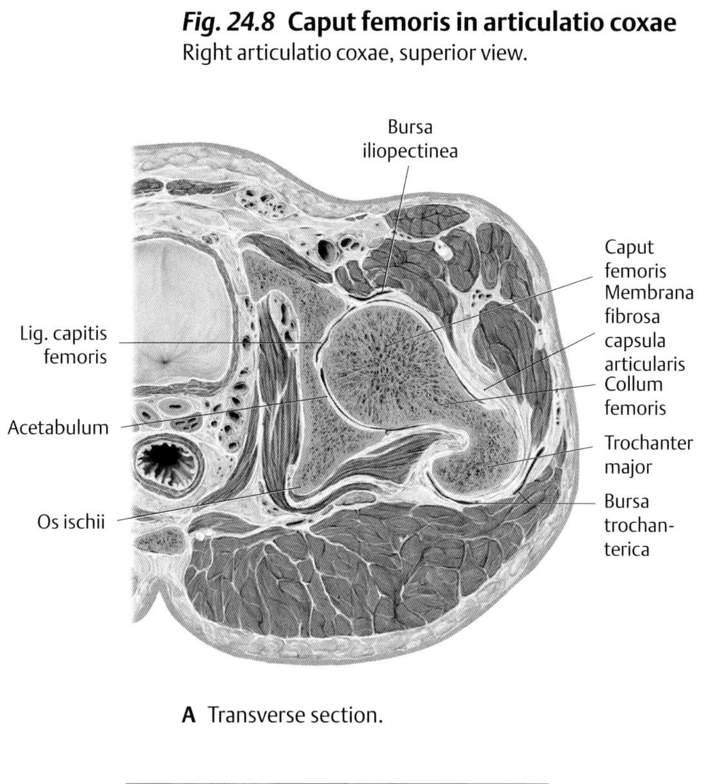
Bursa iliopectinea
Caput femoris
Membrana fibrosa capsula articularis
Lig. capitis femoris
Collum femoris
Acetabulum
Trochanter major
Bursa trochan-terica
Os ischii

A Transverse section.

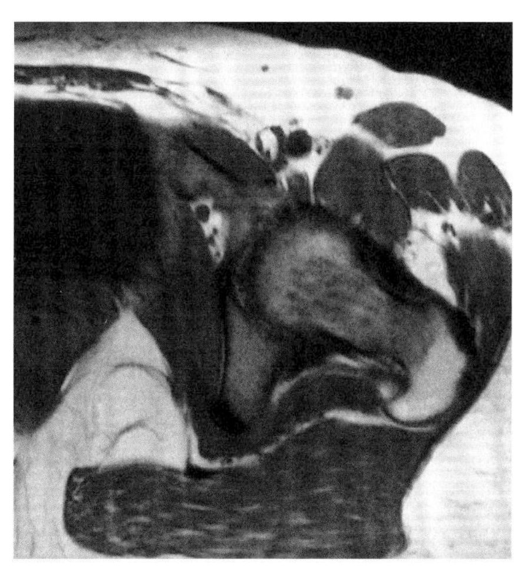

B T1-weighted MRI.

Articulatio coxae: Overview

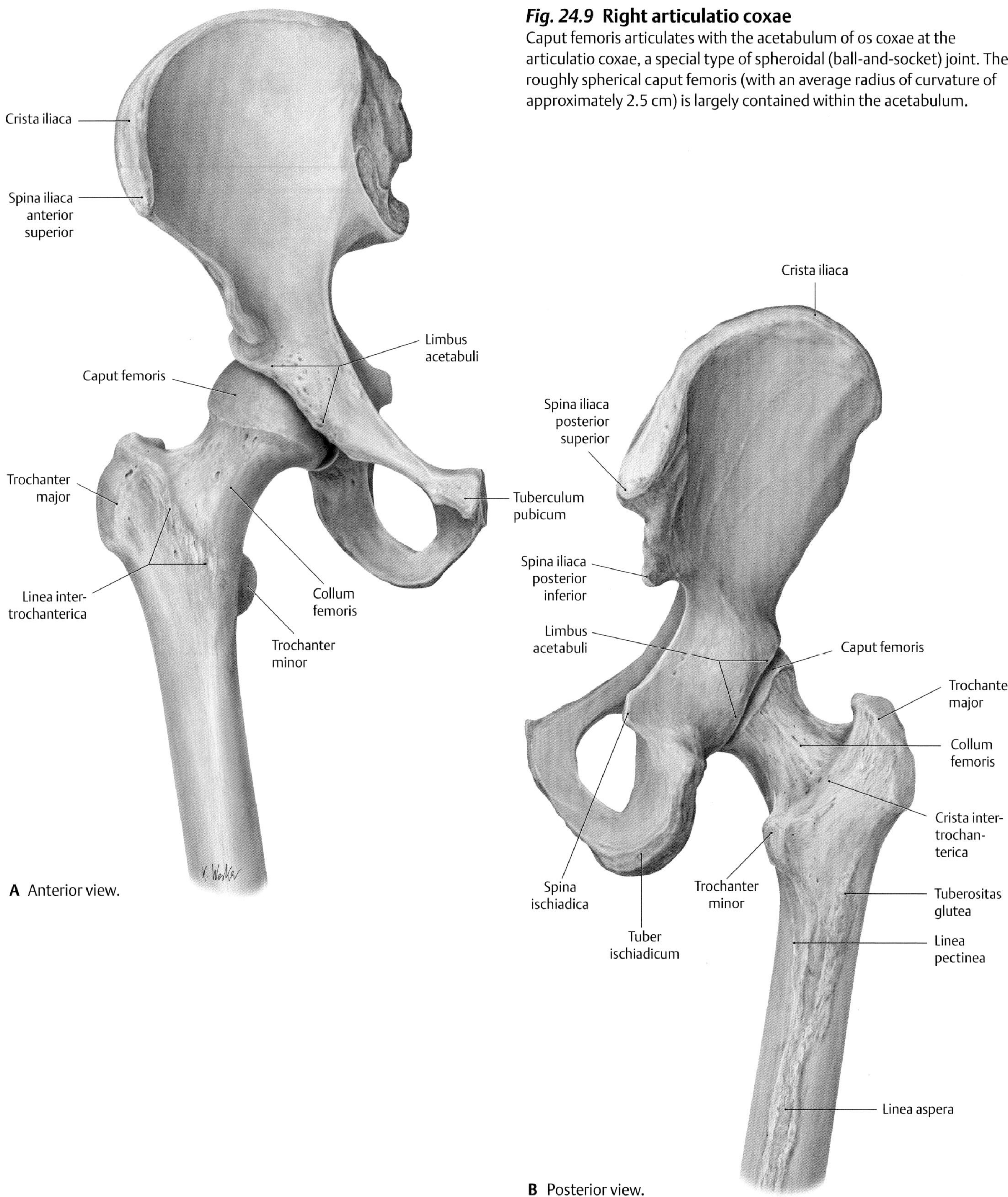
Crista iliaca
Spina iliaca anterior superior
Limbus acetabuli
Caput femoris
Trochanter major
Tuberculum pubicum
Linea inter-trochanterica
Collum femoris
Trochanter minor
Crista iliaca
Spina iliaca posterior superior
Spina iliaca posterior inferior
Limbus acetabuli
Caput femoris
Trochanter major
Collum femoris
Crista inter-trochan-terica
Spina ischiadica
Trochanter minor
Tuberositas glutea
Tuber ischiadicum
Linea pectinea
Linea aspera

Fig. 24.9 **Right articulatio coxae**

Caput femoris articulates with the acetabulum of os coxae at the articulatio coxae, a special type of spheroidal (ball-and-socket) joint. The roughly spherical caput femoris (with an average radius of curvature of approximately 2.5 cm) is largely contained within the acetabulum.

A Anterior view.

B Posterior view.

Fig. 24.10 Articulatio coxae: Coronal section
Right articulatio coxae, anterior view.

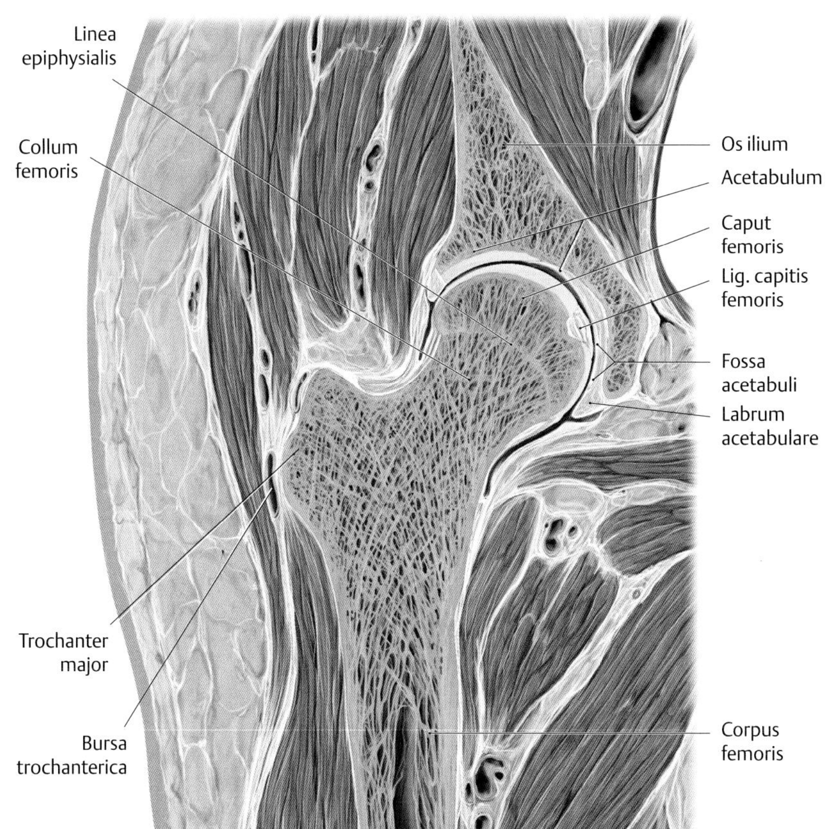
Linea epiphysialis
Collum femoris
Trochanter major
Bursa trochanterica
Os ilium
Acetabulum
Caput femoris
Lig. capitis femoris
Fossa acetabuli
Labrum acetabulare
Corpus femoris

A Coronal section.

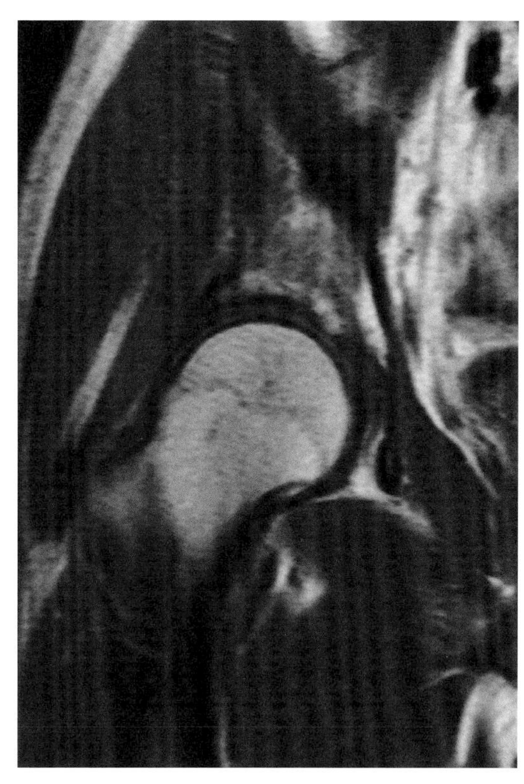

B T1-weighted MRI.

Clinical

Diagnosing hip dysplasia and dislocation

Ultrasonography, the most important imaging method for screening the infant hip, is used to identify morphological changes such as hip dysplasia and dislocation. Clinically, hip dislocation presents itself with instability and limited abduction of articulatio coxae, and leg shortening with asymmetry of the gluteal folds.

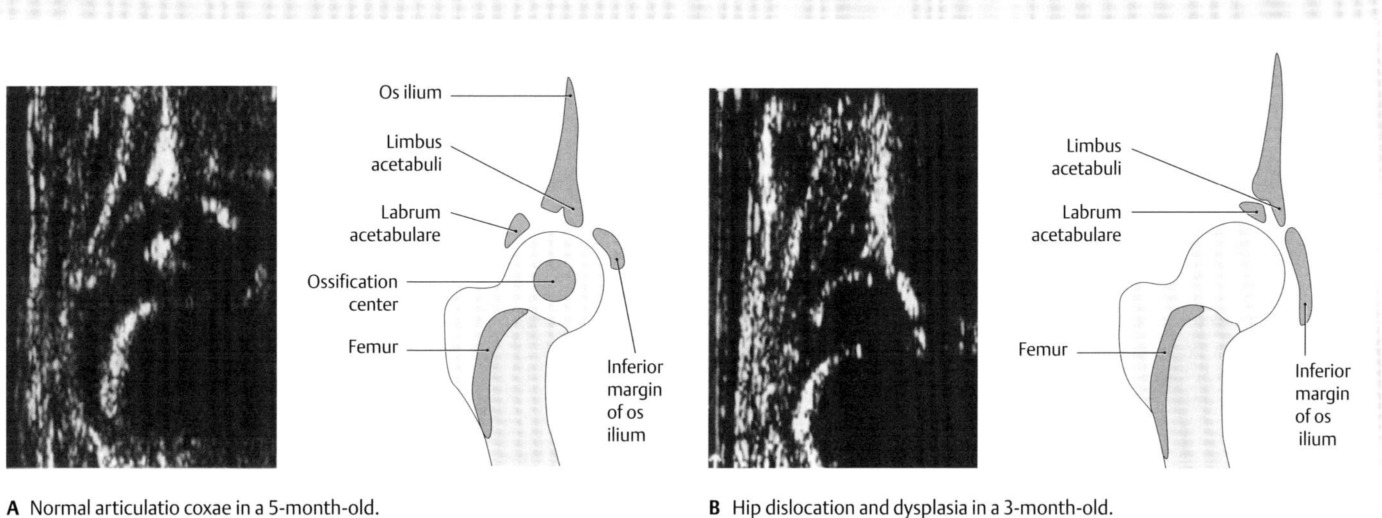
Os ilium
Limbus acetabuli
Labrum acetabulare
Ossification center
Femur
Inferior margin of os ilium
Limbus acetabuli
Labrum acetabulare
Femur
Inferior margin of os ilium

A Normal articulatio coxae in a 5-month-old.

B Hip dislocation and dysplasia in a 3-month-old.

Articulatio Coxae: Ligaments & Capsule

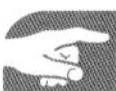

The articulatio coxae has three major ligaments: lig. iliofemorale, lig. pubofemorale, and lig. ischiofemorale. The zona orbicularis (annular ligament) is not visible externally and encircles collum femoris like a buttonhole.

Fig. 24.11 **Articulatio coxae: Lateral view**

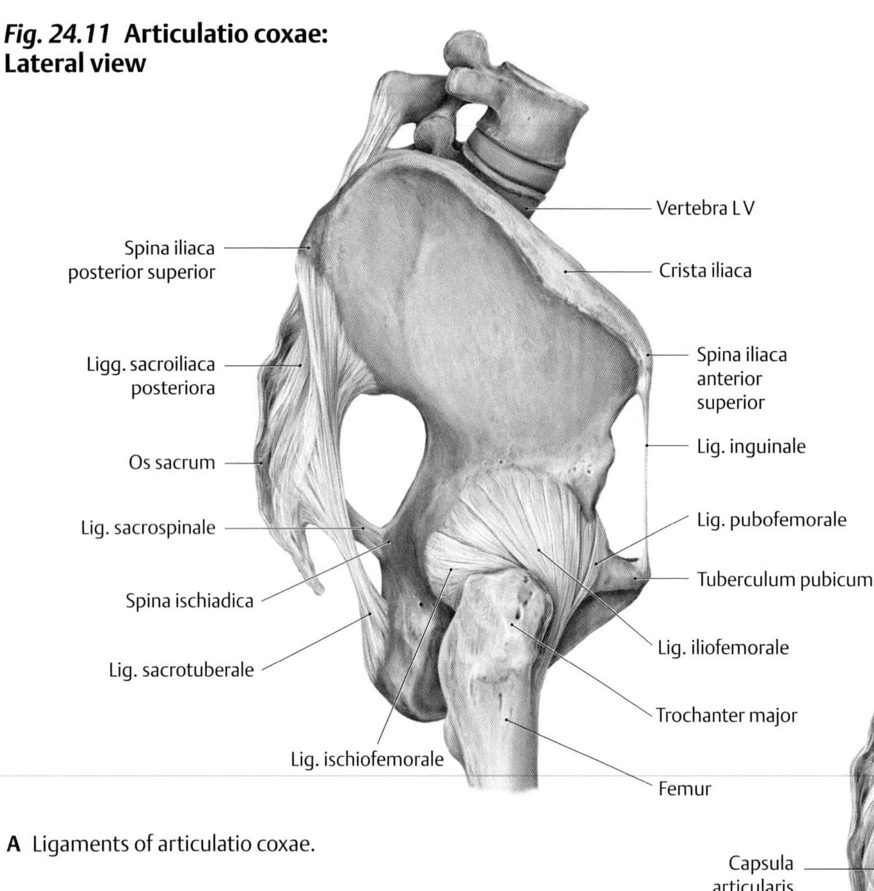
Vertebra L V
Spina iliaca posterior superior
Crista iliaca
Ligg. sacroiliaca posteriora
Spina iliaca anterior superior
Lig. inguinale
Os sacrum
Lig. pubofemorale
Lig. sacrospinale
Tuberculum pubicum
Spina ischiadica
Lig. iliofemorale
Lig. sacrotuberale
Trochanter major
Lig. ischiofemorale
Femur

A Ligaments of articulatio coxae.

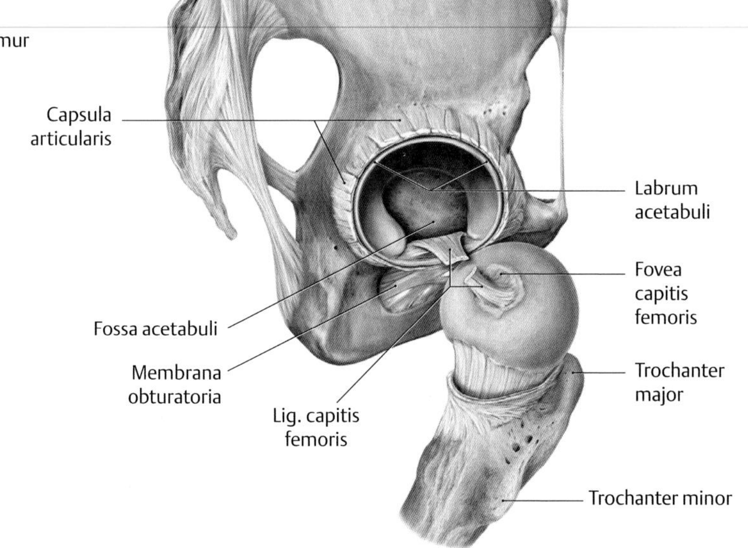
Capsula articularis
Labrum acetabuli
Fovea capitis femoris
Fossa acetabuli
Membrana obturatoria
Trochanter major
Lig. capitis femoris
Trochanter minor

B Capsula articularis. The capsule has been divided and caput femoris dislocated to expose the cut lig. capitis femoris.

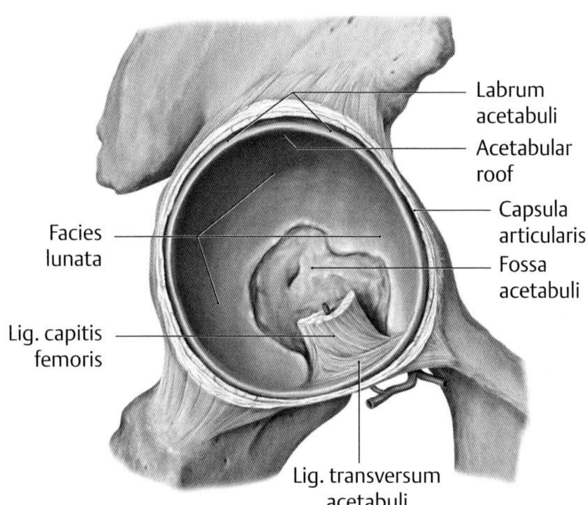
Labrum acetabuli
Acetabular roof
Capsula articularis
Facies lunata
Fossa acetabuli
Lig. capitis femoris
Lig. transversum acetabuli

C Acetabulum of right articulatio coxae. *Note:* Lig. capitis femoris (cut) transmits branches from a. obturatoria that nourish the caput femoris (see p. 421).

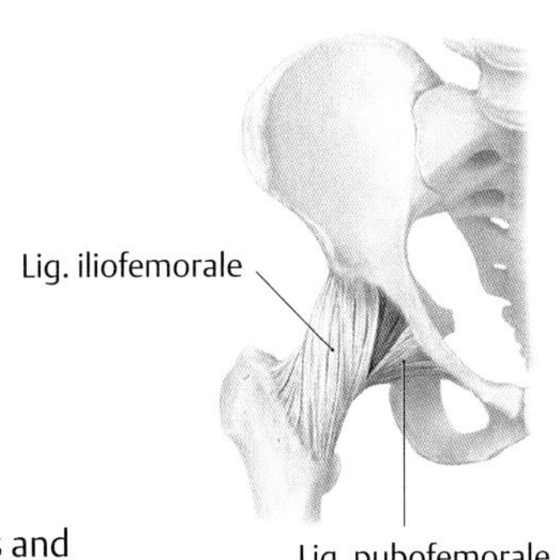
Lig. iliofemorale
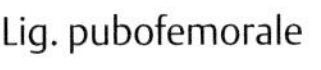
Lig. pubofemorale

A Ligaments and weak spot (red).

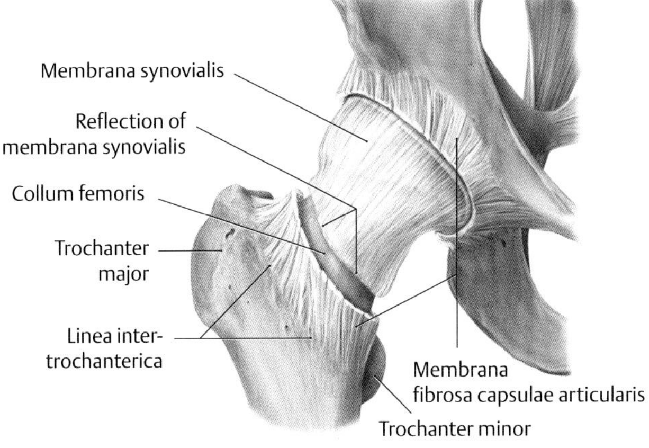
Membrana synovialis
Reflection of membrana synovialis
Collum femoris
Trochanter major
Linea inter-trochanterica
Membrana fibrosa capsulae articularis
Trochanter minor

C Capsula articularis. *Removed:* Membrana fibrosa (at level of femoral neck). *Exposed:* Membrana synovialis.

Fig. 24.12 Articulatio coxae: Anterior view

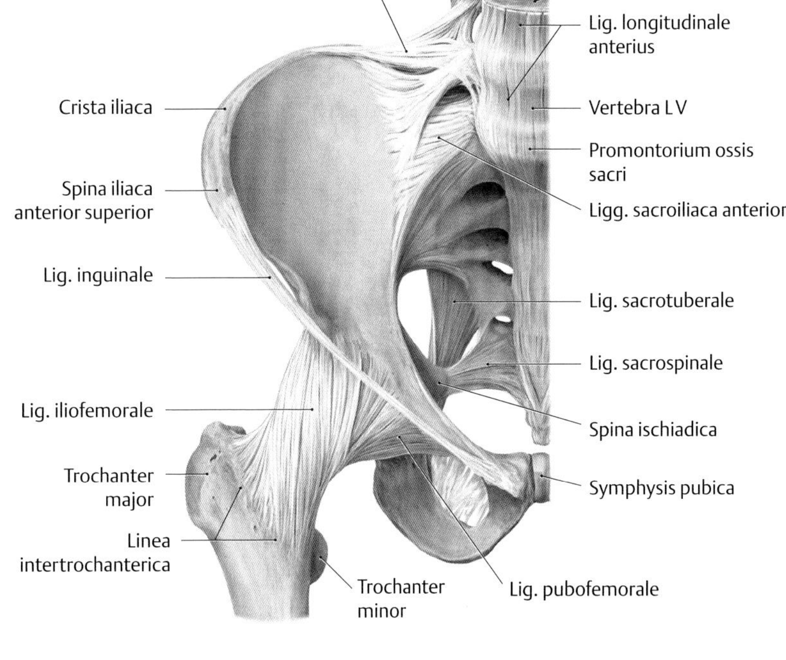
Lig. iliolumbale
Vertebra L IV
Lig. longitudinale anterius
Crista iliaca
Vertebra L V
Promontorium ossis sacri
Spina iliaca anterior superior
Ligg. sacroiliaca anteriora
Lig. inguinale
Lig. sacrotuberale
Lig. sacrospinale
Lig. iliofemorale
Spina ischiadica
Trochanter major
Symphysis pubica
Linea intertrochanterica
Trochanter minor
Lig. pubofemorale

B Ligaments of articulatio coxae.

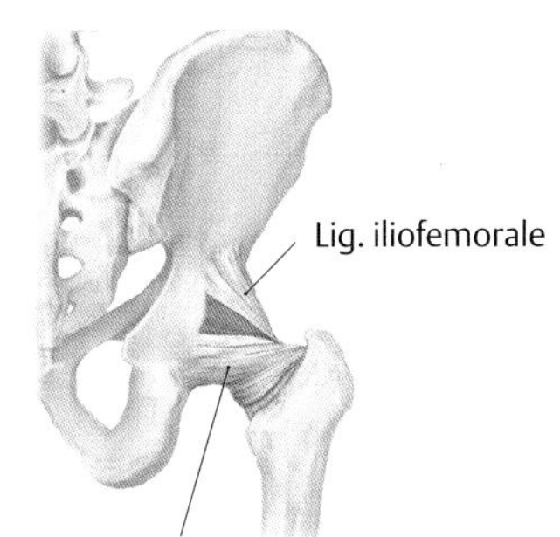
Lig. iliofemorale
Lig. ischiofemorale

A Ligaments and weak spot (red).

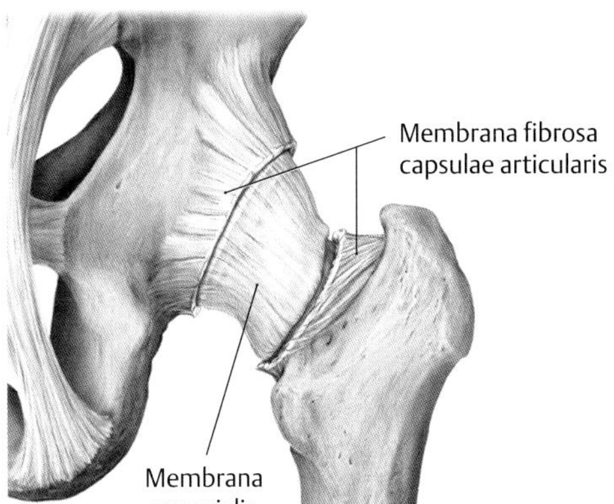
Membrana fibrosa capsulae articularis
Membrana synovialis

C Joint capsule.

Fig. 24.13 Articulatio coxae: Posterior view

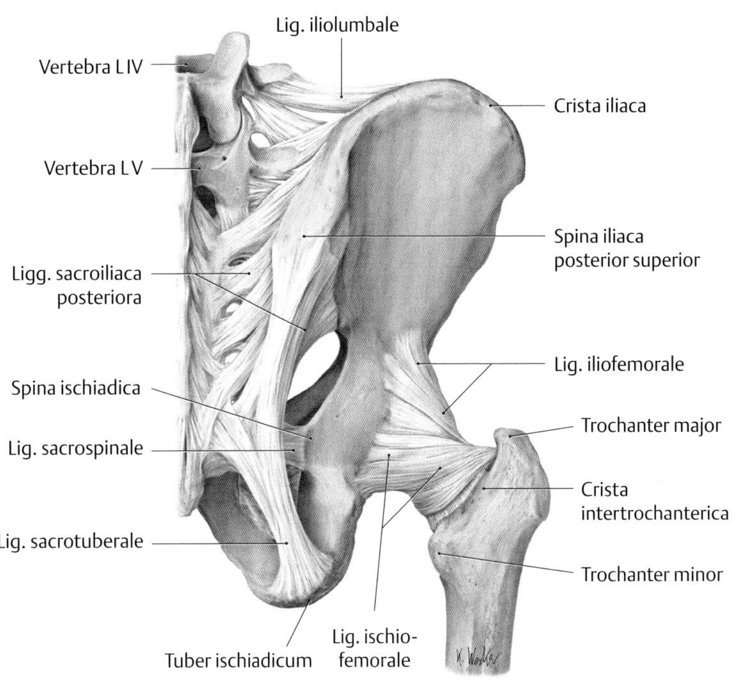
Lig. iliolumbale
Vertebra L IV
Crista iliaca
Vertebra L V
Spina iliaca posterior superior
Ligg. sacroiliaca posteriora
Lig. iliofemorale
Spina ischiadica
Trochanter major
Lig. sacrospinale
Crista intertrochanterica
Lig. sacrotuberale
Trochanter minor
Tuber ischiadicum
Lig. ischio-femorale

B Ligaments of the articulatio coxae.

Anterior Muscles of the Thigh, Hip & Regio Glutealis (I)

Fig. 24.14 **Muscles of the hip and thigh: Anterior view (I)**
Right limb. Muscle origins (O) are shown in red, insertions (I) in blue.

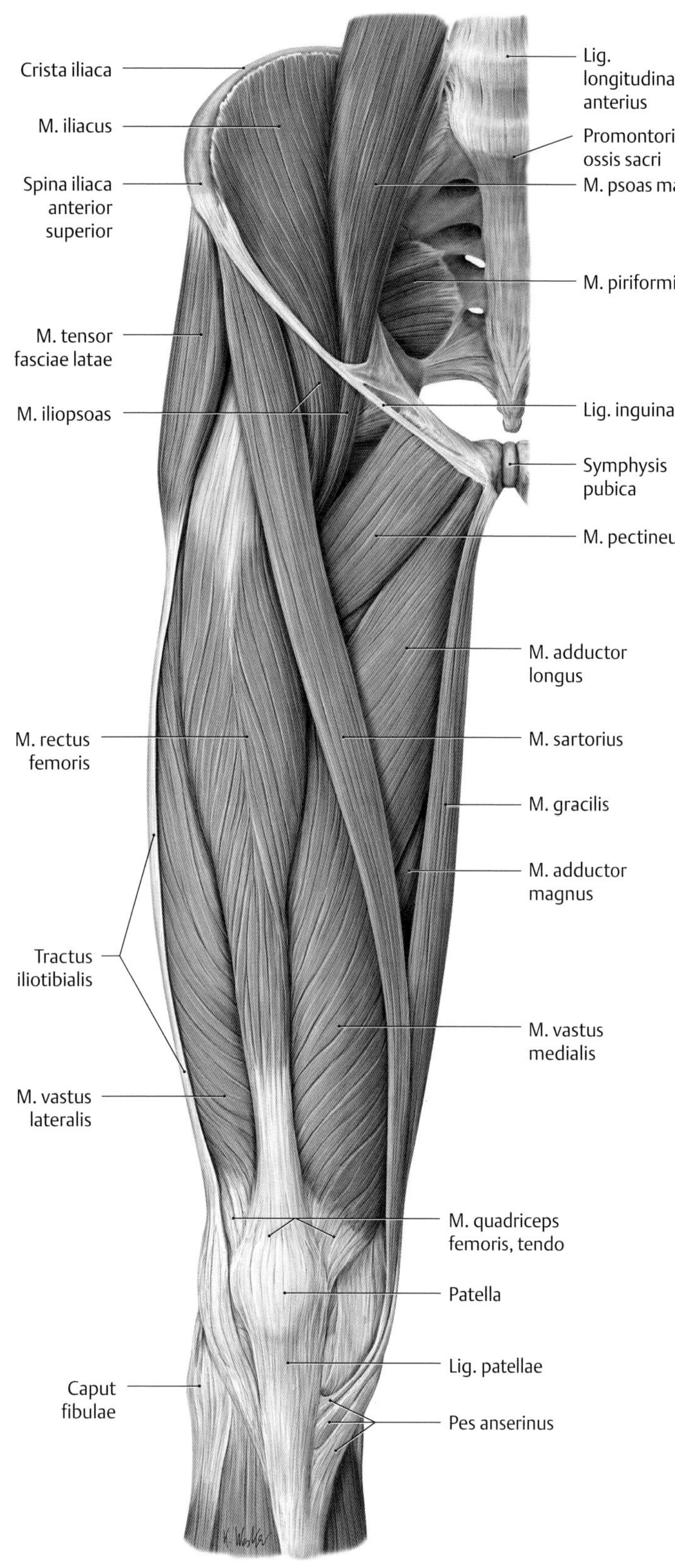
Crista iliaca
M. iliacus
Spina iliaca anterior superior
M. tensor fasciae latae
M. iliopsoas
M. rectus femoris
Tractus iliotibialis
M. vastus lateralis
Caput fibulae
Lig. longitudinale anterius
Promontorium ossis sacri
M. psoas major
M. piriformis
Lig. inguinale
Symphysis pubica
M. pectineus
M. adductor longus
M. sartorius
M. gracilis
M. adductor magnus
M. vastus medialis
M. quadriceps femoris, tendo
Patella
Lig. patellae
Pes anserinus

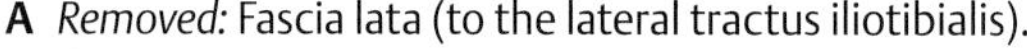

A *Removed:* Fascia lata (to the lateral tractus iliotibialis).

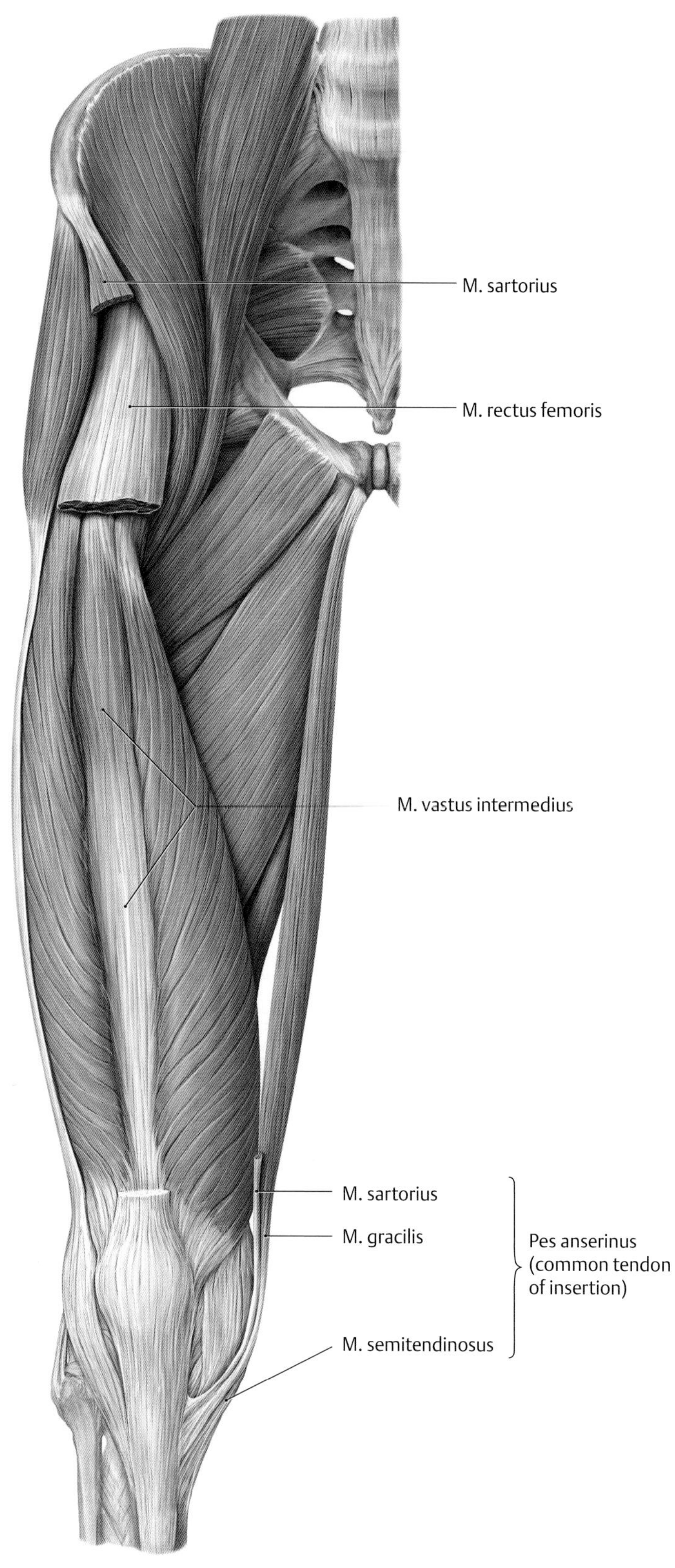
M. sartorius
M. rectus femoris
M. vastus intermedius
M. sartorius
M. gracilis
M. semitendinosus
Pes anserinus (common tendon of insertion)

B *Removed:* M. sartorius and m. rectus femoris.

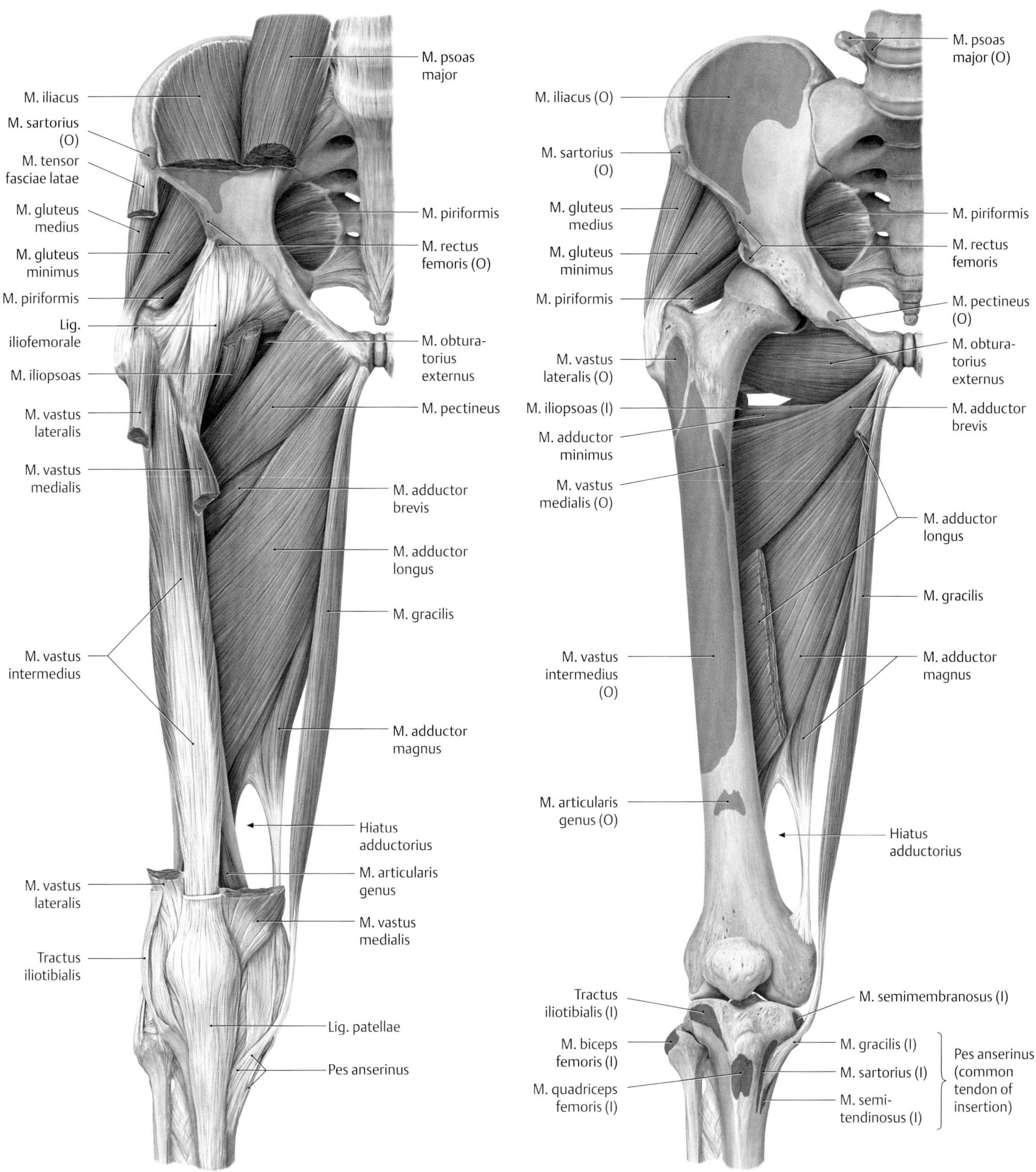
M. psoas major
M. iliacus
M. sartorius (O)
M. tensor fasciae latae
M. gluteus medius
M. gluteus minimus
M. piriformis
Lig. iliofemorale
M. iliopsoas
M. vastus lateralis
M. vastus medialis
M. vastus intermedius
M. piriformis
M. rectus femoris (O)
M. obturatorius externus
M. pectineus
M. adductor brevis
M. adductor longus
M. gracilis
M. adductor magnus
Hiatus adductorius
M. articularis genus
M. vastus lateralis
M. vastus medialis
Tractus iliotibialis
Lig. patellae
Pes anserinus
M. psoas major (O)
M. iliacus (O)
M. sartorius (O)
M. gluteus medius
M. gluteus minimus
M. piriformis
M. vastus lateralis (O)
M. iliopsoas (I)
M. adductor minimus
M. vastus medialis (O)
M. vastus intermedius (O)
M. articularis genus (O)
M. piriformis
M. rectus femoris
M. pectineus (O)
M. obturatorius externus
M. adductor brevis
M. adductor longus
M. gracilis
M. adductor magnus
Hiatus adductorius
Tractus iliotibialis (I)
M. biceps femoris (I)
M. quadriceps femoris (I)
M. semimembranosus (I)
M. gracilis (I)
M. sartorius (I)
M. semitendinosus (I)
Pes anserinus (common tendon of insertion)

C *Removed:* M. rectus femoris (completely), m. vastus lateralis, m. vastus medialis, m. iliopsoas, and m. tensor fasciae latae.

D *Removed:* M. quadriceps femoris (m. rectus femoris, m. vastus lateralis, m. vastus medialis, m. vastus intermedius), m. iliopsoas, m. tensor fasciae latae, m. pectineus, and midportion of m. adductor longus.

Anterior Muscles of the Thigh, Hip & Regio Glutealis (II)

Fig. 24.15 **Muscles of the hip and thigh: Anterior view (II)**
Right limb. Muscle origins (O) are shown in red, insertions (I) in blue.

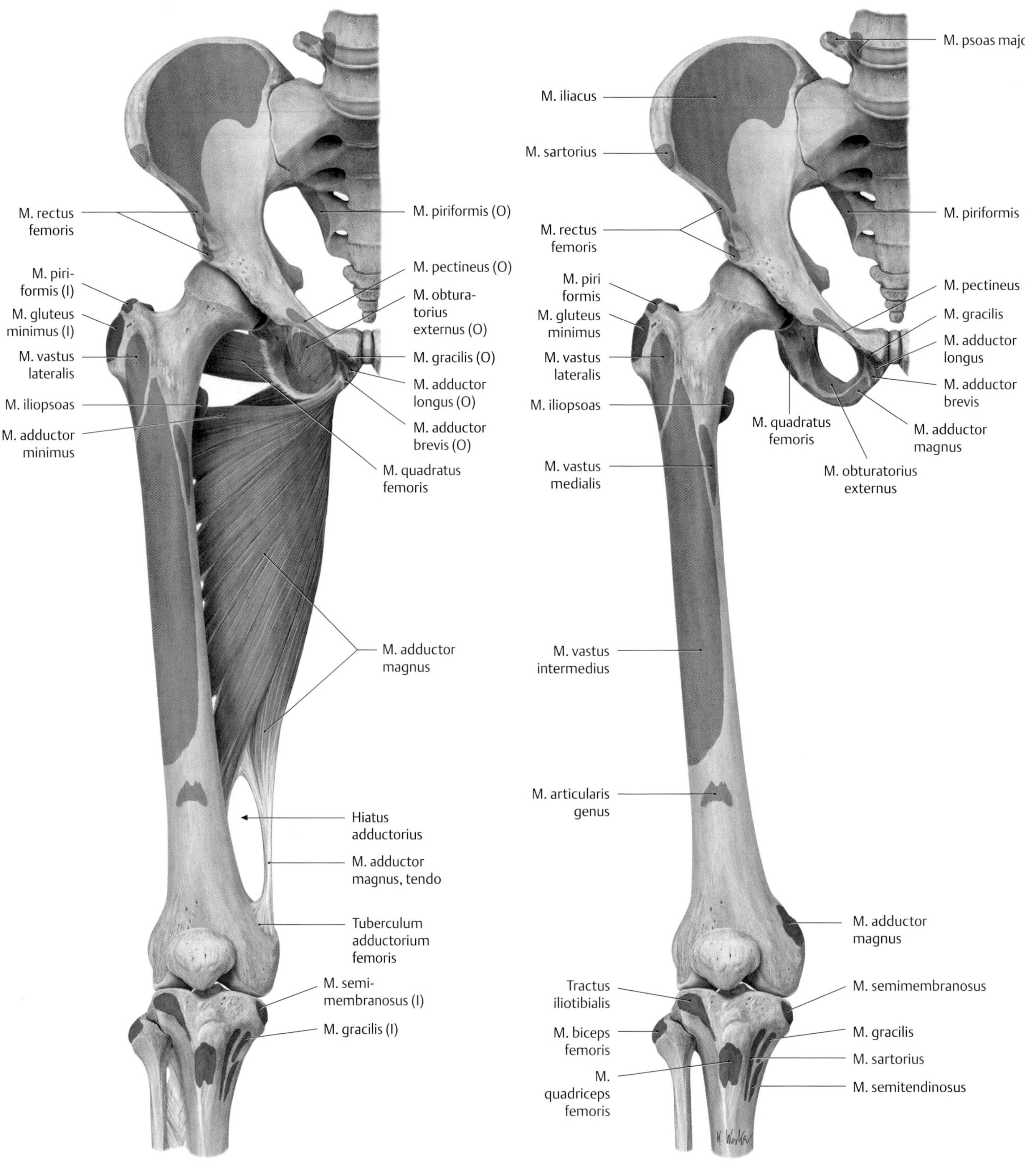
M. rectus femoris
M. piri-formis (I)
M. gluteus minimus (I)
M. vastus lateralis
M. iliopsoas
M. adductor minimus
M. piriformis (O)
M. pectineus (O)
M. obtura-torius externus (O)
M. gracilis (O)
M. adductor longus (O)
M. adductor brevis (O)
M. quadratus femoris
M. adductor magnus
Hiatus adductorius
M. adductor magnus, tendo
Tuberculum adductorium femoris
M. semi-membranosus (I)
M. gracilis (I)
M. psoas major
M. iliacus
M. sartorius
M. piriformis
M. rectus femoris
M. piri formis
M. gluteus minimus
M. vastus lateralis
M. iliopsoas
M. vastus medialis
M. pectineus
M. gracilis
M. adductor longus
M. adductor brevis
M. quadratus femoris
M. adductor magnus
M. obturatorius externus
M. vastus intermedius
M. articularis genus
M. adductor magnus
Tractus iliotibialis
M. semimembranosus
M. biceps femoris
M. gracilis
M. sartorius
M. quadriceps femoris
M. semitendinosus

A *Removed:* M. gluteus medius and minimus, m. piriformis, m. obturatorius externus, m. adductor brevis and longus, and m. gracilis.

B *Removed:* All muscles.

Fig. 24.16 **Muscles of the hip, thigh, and regio glutealis: Medial view**
Midsagittal section.

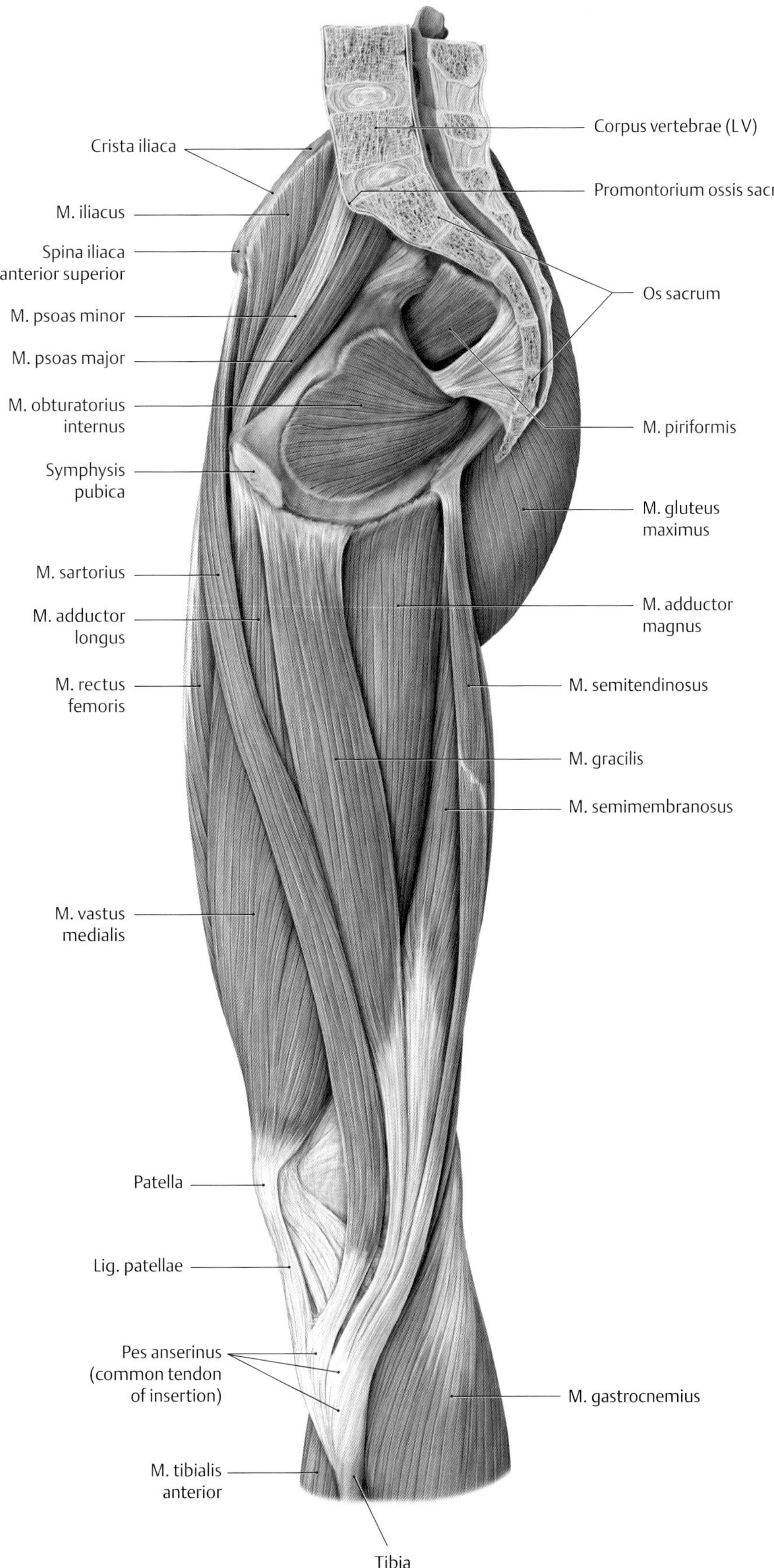
Crista iliaca
M. iliacus
Spina iliaca anterior superior
M. psoas minor
M. psoas major
M. obturatorius internus
Symphysis pubica
M. sartorius
M. adductor longus
M. rectus femoris
M. vastus medialis
Patella
Lig. patellae
Pes anserinus (common tendon of insertion)
M. tibialis anterior
Tibia
Corpus vertebrae (LV)
Promontorium ossis sacri
Os sacrum
M. piriformis
M. gluteus maximus
M. adductor magnus
M. semitendinosus
M. gracilis
M. semimembranosus
M. gastrocnemius

Posterior Muscles of the Thigh, Hip & Regio Glutealis (I)

***Fig. 24.17* Muscles of the hip, thigh, and regio glutealis: Posterior view (I)**
Right limb. Muscle origins (O) are shown in red, insertions (I) in blue.

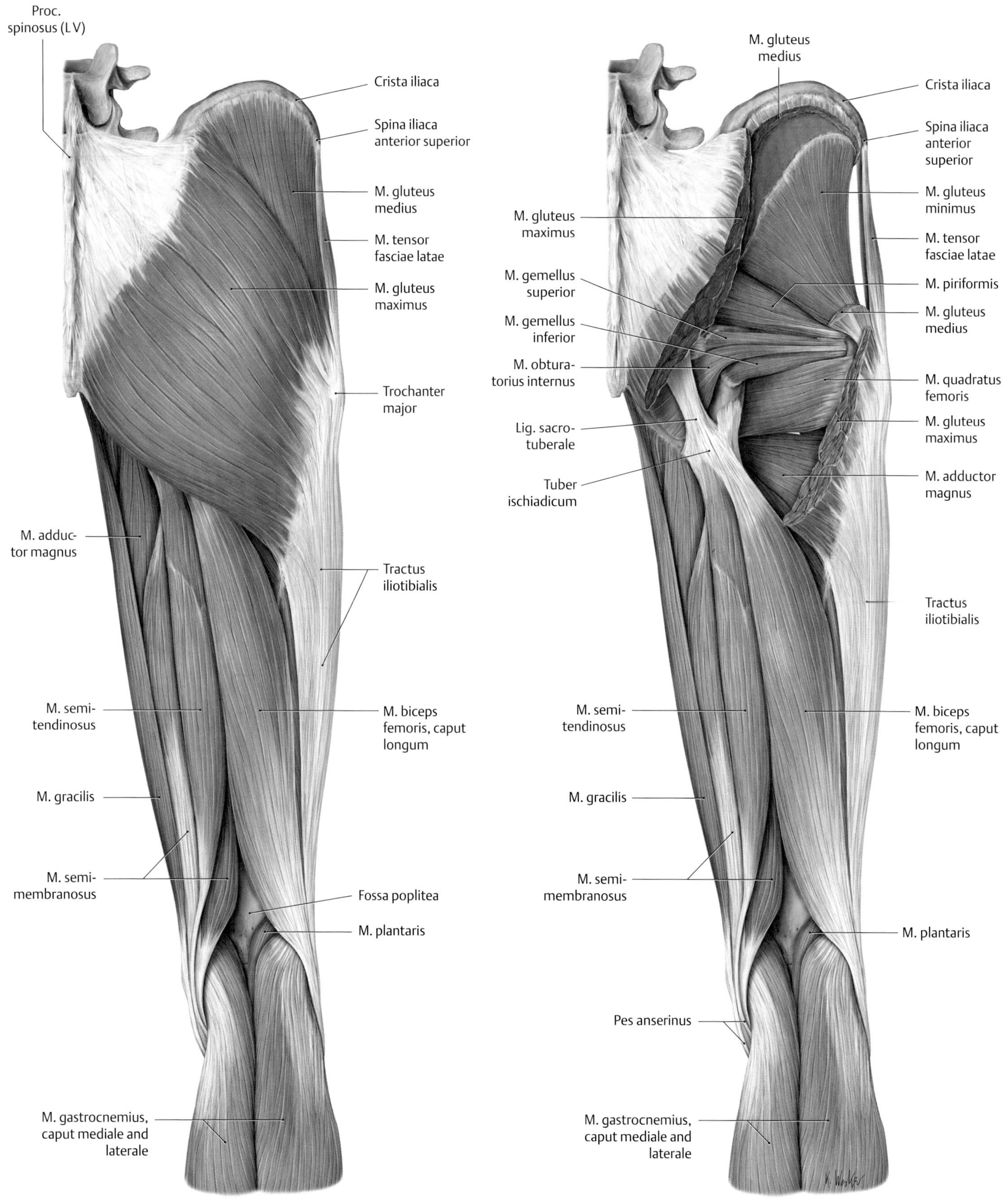
Proc. spinosus (L V)
Crista iliaca
Spina iliaca anterior superior
M. gluteus medius
M. tensor fasciae latae
M. gluteus maximus
Trochanter major
M. adductor magnus
Tractus iliotibialis
M. semitendinosus
M. biceps femoris, caput longum
M. gracilis
M. semimembranosus
Fossa poplitea
M. plantaris
M. gastrocnemius, caput mediale and laterale
M. gluteus medius
Crista iliaca
Spina iliaca anterior superior
M. gluteus minimus
M. gluteus maximus
M. tensor fasciae latae
M. gemellus superior
M. piriformis
M. gluteus medius
M. gemellus inferior
M. obturatorius internus
M. quadratus femoris
Lig. sacrotuberale
M. gluteus maximus
Tuber ischiadicum
M. adductor magnus
Tractus iliotibialis
M. semitendinosus
M. biceps femoris, caput longum
M. gracilis
M. semimembranosus
M. plantaris
Pes anserinus
M. gastrocnemius, caput mediale and laterale

A *Removed:* Fascia lata (to tractus iliotibialis).

B *Partially removed:* Mm. gluteus maximus and medius.

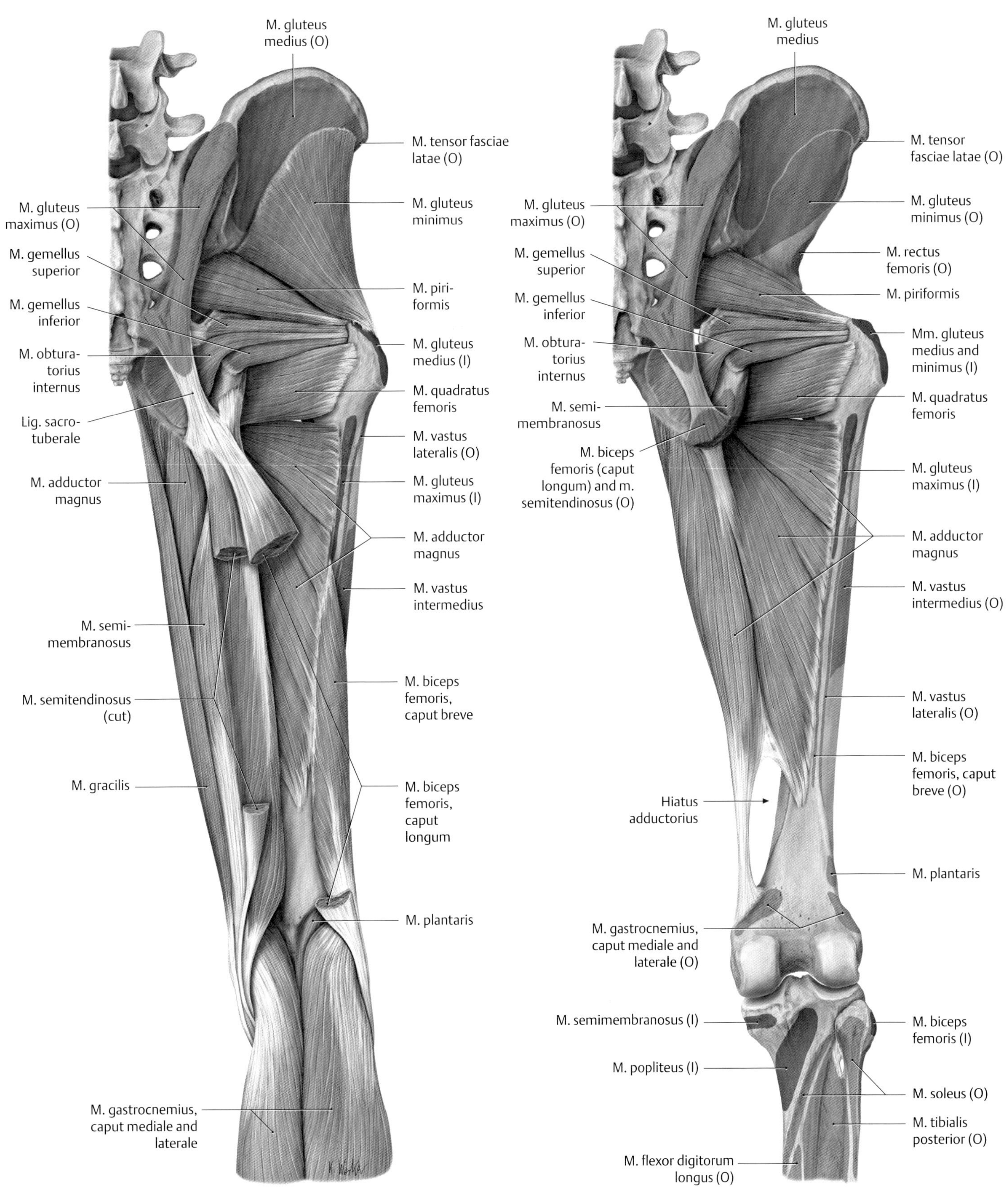
M. gluteus medius (O)
M. tensor fasciae latae (O)
M. gluteus maximus (O)
M. gluteus minimus
M. gemellus superior
M. piri-formis
M. gemellus inferior
M. gluteus medius (I)
M. obtura-torius internus
M. quadratus femoris
Lig. sacro-tuberale
M. vastus lateralis (O)
M. adductor magnus
M. gluteus maximus (I)
M. adductor magnus
M. vastus intermedius
M. semi-membranosus
M. biceps femoris, caput breve
M. semitendinosus (cut)
M. gracilis
M. biceps femoris, caput longum
M. plantaris
M. gastrocnemius, caput mediale and laterale
M. gluteus medius
M. tensor fasciae latae (O)
M. gluteus maximus (O)
M. gluteus minimus (O)
M. gemellus superior
M. rectus femoris (O)
M. piriformis
M. gemellus inferior
Mm. gluteus medius and minimus (I)
M. obtura-torius internus
M. quadratus femoris
M. semi-membranosus
M. biceps femoris (caput longum) and m. semitendinosus (O)
M. gluteus maximus (I)
M. adductor magnus
M. vastus intermedius (O)
M. vastus lateralis (O)
M. biceps femoris, caput breve (O)
Hiatus adductorius
M. plantaris
M. gastrocnemius, caput mediale and laterale (O)
M. semimembranosus (I)
M. biceps femoris (I)
M. popliteus (I)
M. soleus (O)
M. tibialis posterior (O)
M. flexor digitorum longus (O)

C *Removed:* M. semitendinosus and m. biceps femoris (partially); m. gluteus maximus and medius (completely).

D *Removed:* Hamstrings (m. semitendinosus, m. semimembranosus, and m. biceps femoris), m. gluteus minimus, m. gastrocnemius, and muscles of the leg.

Posterior Muscles of the Thigh, Hip & Regio Glutealis (II)

Fig. 24.18 **Muscles of the hip, thigh, and regio glutealis: Posterior view (II)**
Right limb. Muscle origins (O) are shown in red, insertions (I) in blue.

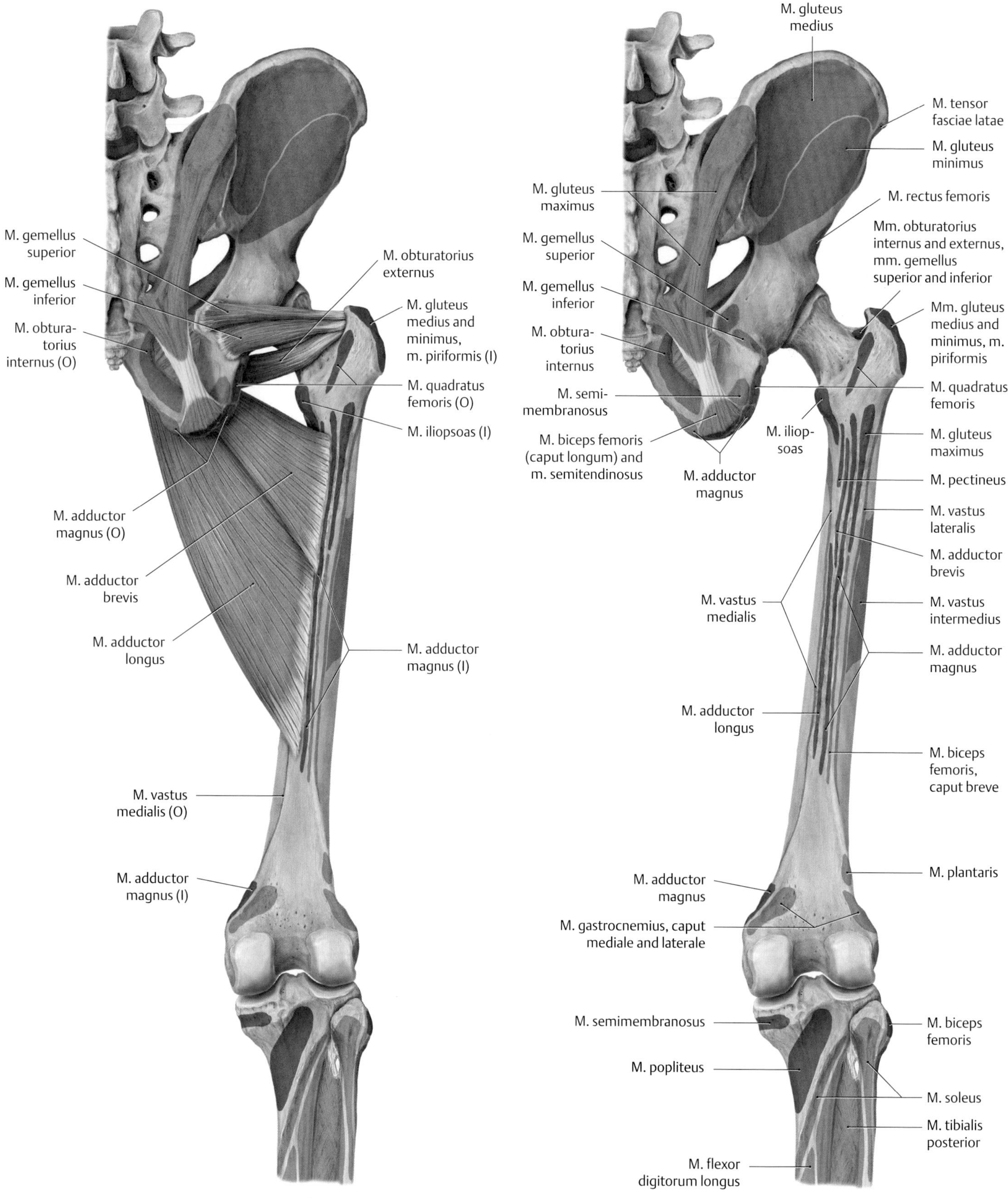

M. gemellus superior
M. gemellus inferior
M. obturatorius internus (O)
M. obturatorius externus
M. gluteus medius and minimus, m. piriformis (I)
M. quadratus femoris (O)
M. iliopsoas (I)
M. adductor magnus (O)
M. adductor brevis
M. adductor longus
M. adductor magnus (I)
M. vastus medialis (O)
M. adductor magnus (I)
M. gluteus medius
M. tensor fasciae latae
M. gluteus minimus
M. gluteus maximus
M. rectus femoris
M. gemellus superior
Mm. obturatorius internus and externus, mm. gemellus superior and inferior
M. gemellus inferior
Mm. gluteus medius and minimus, m. piriformis
M. obturatorius internus
M. semimembranosus
M. quadratus femoris
M. biceps femoris (caput longum) and m. semitendinosus
M. iliopsoas
M. gluteus maximus
M. adductor magnus
M. pectineus
M. vastus lateralis
M. adductor brevis
M. vastus medialis
M. vastus intermedius
M. adductor magnus
M. adductor longus
M. biceps femoris, caput breve
M. plantaris
M. adductor magnus
M. gastrocnemius, caput mediale and laterale
M. semimembranosus
M. biceps femoris
M. popliteus
M. soleus
M. tibialis posterior
M. flexor digitorum longus

A *Removed:* M. piriformis, m. obturatorius internus, m. quadratus femoris, and m. adductor magnus.

B *Removed:* All muscles.

Fig. 24.19 **Muscles of the hip, thigh, and gluteal region: Lateral view**
Note: Tractus iliotibialis (the thickened band of fascia lata) functions as a tension band to reduce the bending loads on the proximal femur.

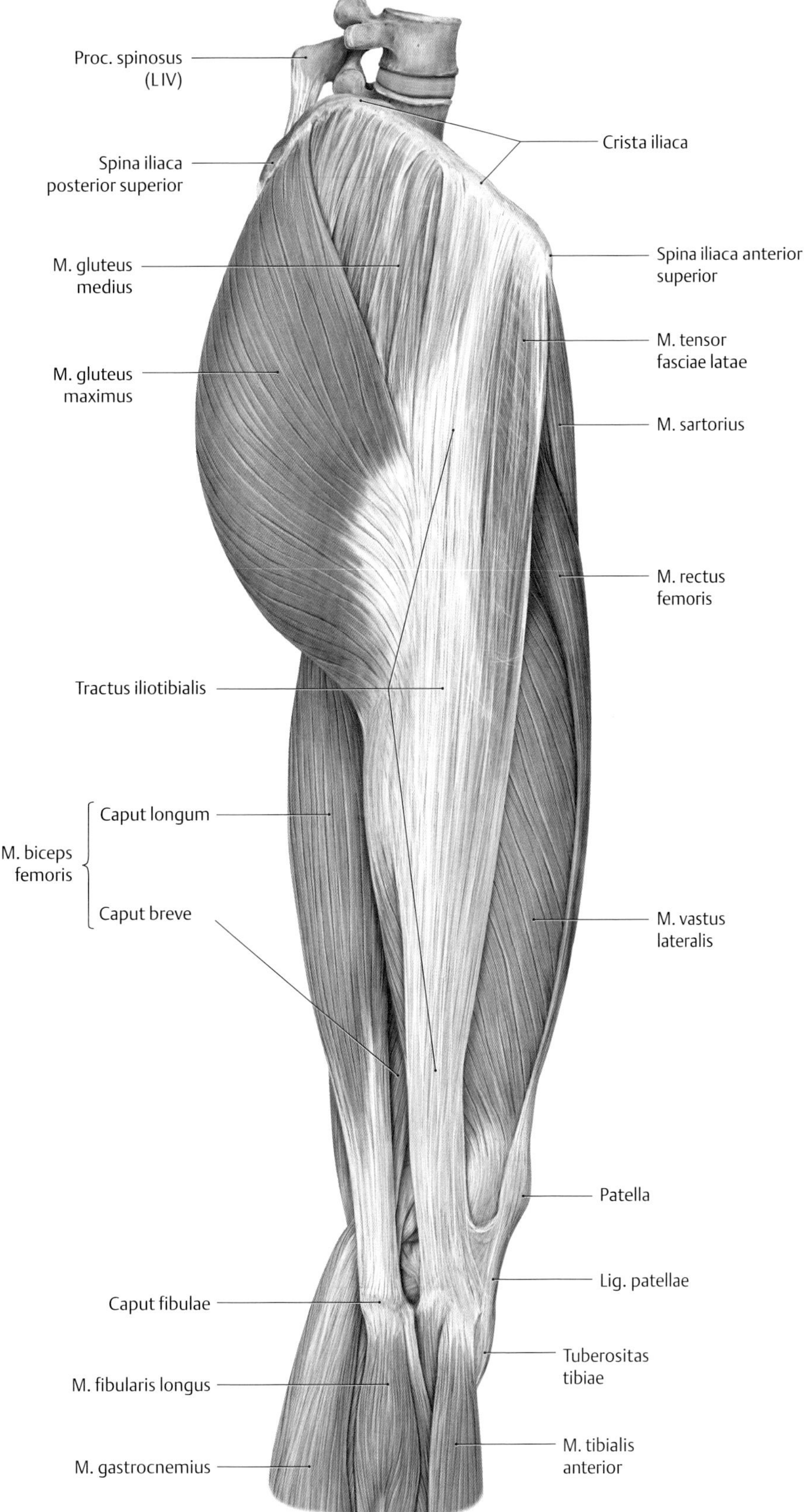
Proc. spinosus (L IV)
Crista iliaca
Spina iliaca posterior superior
Spina iliaca anterior superior
M. gluteus medius
M. tensor fasciae latae
M. gluteus maximus
M. sartorius
M. rectus femoris
Tractus iliotibialis
M. biceps femoris
Caput longum
Caput breve
M. vastus lateralis
Patella
Lig. patellae
Caput fibulae
Tuberositas tibiae
M. fibularis longus
M. tibialis anterior
M. gastrocnemius

Muscle Facts (I)

Table 24.1 Psoas and iliacus muscles

Muscles		Origin	Insertion	Innervation	Action
③ Mm. iliopsoas	M. psoas minor	Vertebrae T XII–L I (Disci intervertebrales) (lateral surfaces)	Arcus iliopectineus	Direct branches from the lumbar plexus (psoas) (L2–L4)	Assists in upward rotation of the pelvis
	① M. psoas major	*Superficial:* Vertebrae T XII–L IV (Disci intervertebrales) (lateral surfaces) *Deep:* Vertebrae L I–L V (proc. transversus)	Trochanter minor		• Articulatio coxae: flexion and external rotation • Lumbar spine: *unilateral* contraction (with the femur fixed) bends the trunk laterally to the same side; *bilateral* contraction raises the trunk from the supine position
	② M. iliacus	Fossa iliaca		N. femoralis (L2–L4)	

***Fig. 24.20* Muscles of the hip**
Right side.

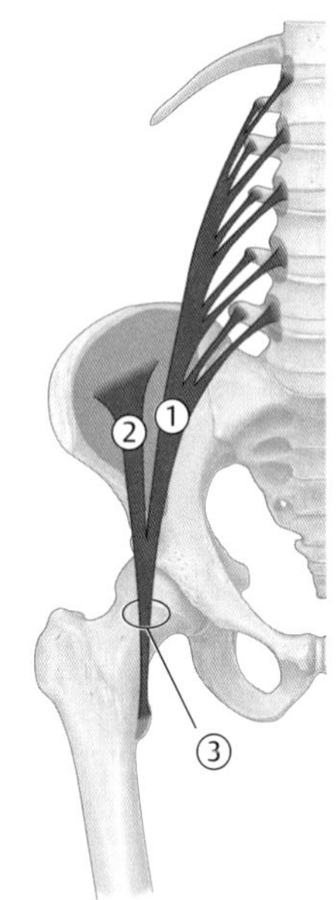
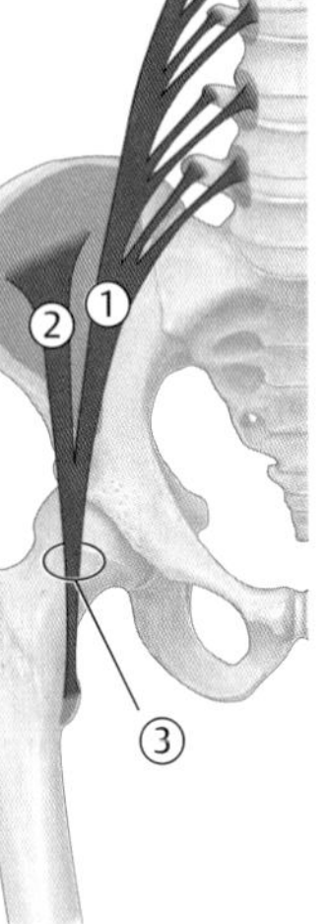
1
2
3

A M. iliopsoas, anterior view.

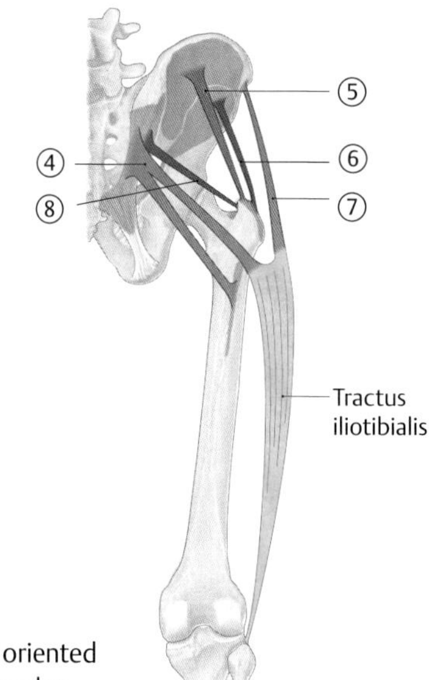
4
8
5
6
7
Tractus iliotibialis

B Vertically oriented gluteal muscles, posterior view.

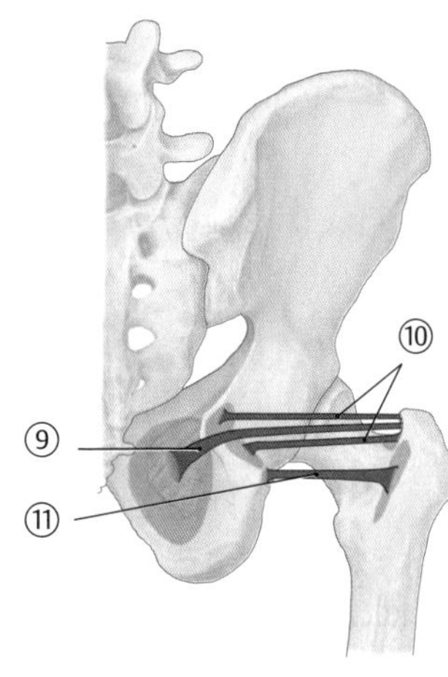
10
9
11

C Horizontally oriented gluteal muscles, posterior view.

Table 24.2 Gluteal muscles

Muscle	Origin	Insertion	Innervation	Action
④ M. gluteus maximus	Os sacrum (fascies posterior), os ilium (gluteal surface, pars posterior), fascia thoracolumbalis, lig. sacrotuberale	• Fibrae superior: tractus iliotibialis • Fibrae inferior: tuberositas glutea	N. gluteus inferios (L5–S2)	• Entire muscle: extends and externally rotates the hip in sagittal and coronal planes • Upper fibers: abduction • Lower fibers: adduction
⑤ M. gluteus medius	Os ilium (gluteal surface below the iliac crest between lineae gluteae anterior and posterior)	Trochanter major (lateral surface)	N. gluteus superior (L4–S1)	• Entire muscle: abducts the hip, stabilizes the pelvis in the coronal plane • Anterior part: flexion and internal rotation • Posterior part: extension and external rotation
⑥ M. gluteus minimus	Os ilium (gluteal surface below the origin m. gluteus medius)	Trochanter major (anterolateral surface)		
⑦ M. tensor fasciae latae	Spina iliaca anterior superior	Tractus iliotibialis		• Tenses the fascia lata • Articulatio coxae: abduction, flexion, and internal rotation
⑧ M. piriformis	Facies pelvica of os sacrum	Apex of the trochanter major	Direct branches from the plexus sacralis (S1–S2)	• External rotation, abduction, and extension of articulatio coxae • Stabilizes articulatio coxae
⑨ M. obturatorius internus	Inner surface of membrana obturatoria and its bony boundaries	Fossa trochanterica	Direct branches from the plexus sacralis (L5, S1)	External rotation, adduction, and extension of articulatio coxae (also active in abduction, depending on the joint's position)
⑩ Mm. gemelli	• M. gemellus superior: spina ischiadica • M. gemellus inferior: tuber ischiadicum	Fossa trochanterica		
⑪ M. quadratus femoris	Lateral border of the tuber ischiadicum	Crista intertrochanterica		External rotation and adduction of articulatio coxae

Fig. 24.21 Mm. psoas and m. iliacus
Right side, anterior view.

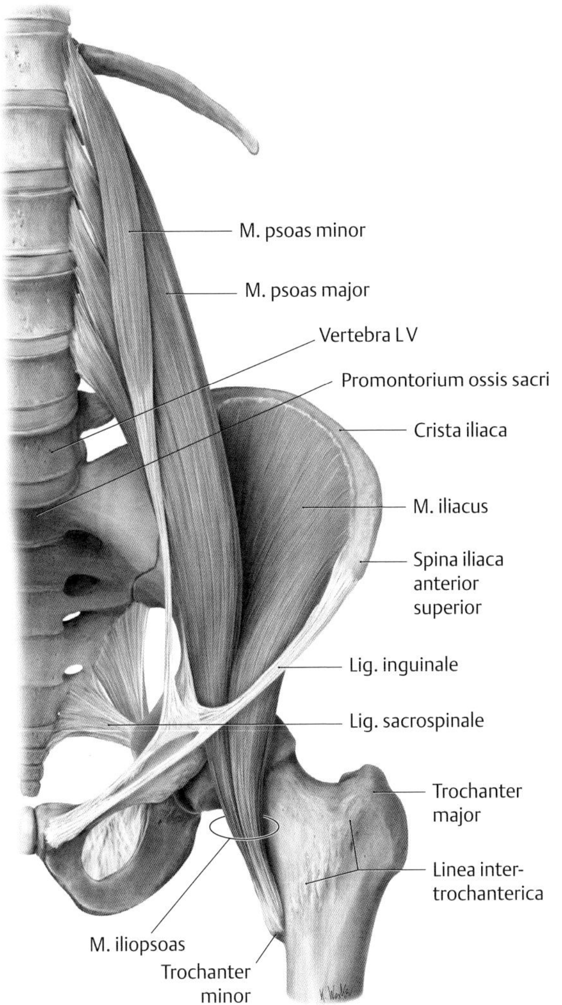
M. psoas minor
M. psoas major
Vertebra LV
Promontorium ossis sacri
Crista iliaca
M. iliacus
Spina iliaca anterior superior
Lig. inguinale
Lig. sacrospinale
Trochanter major
Linea inter-trochanterica
M. iliopsoas
Trochanter minor

Fig. 24.22 Superficial muscles of the gluteal region
Right side, posterior view.

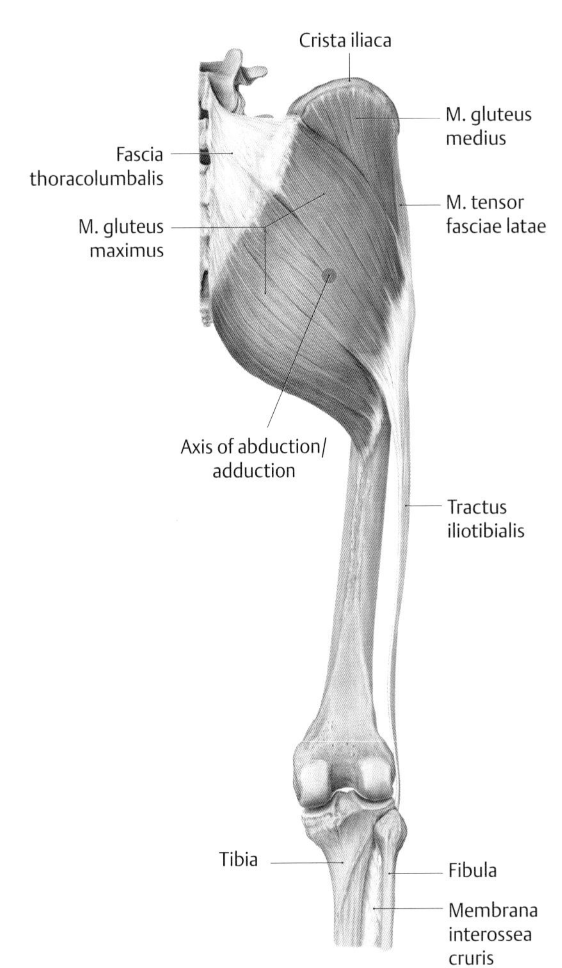
Crista iliaca
Fascia thoracolumbalis
M. gluteus maximus
M. gluteus medius
M. tensor fasciae latae
Axis of abduction/ adduction
Tractus iliotibialis
Tibia
Fibula
Membrana interossea cruris

Fig. 24.23 Deep muscles of the gluteal region

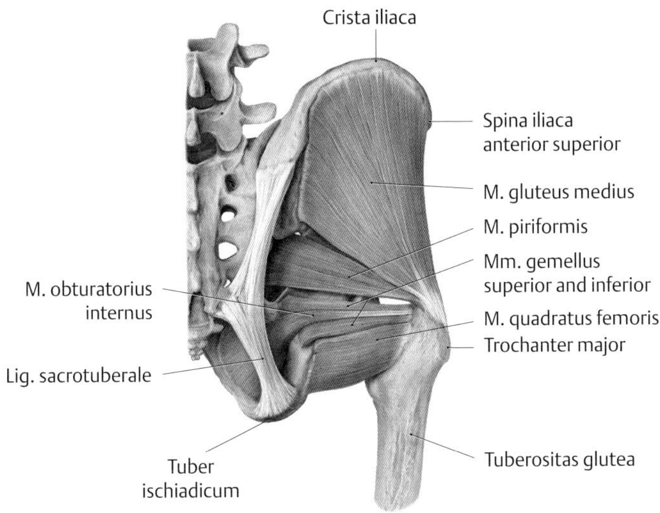
Crista iliaca
Spina iliaca anterior superior
M. gluteus medius
M. piriformis
Mm. gemellus superior and inferior
M. quadratus femoris
Trochanter major
M. obturatorius internus
Lig. sacrotuberale
Tuber ischiadicum
Tuberositas glutea

A Deep layer with m. gluteus maximus removed.

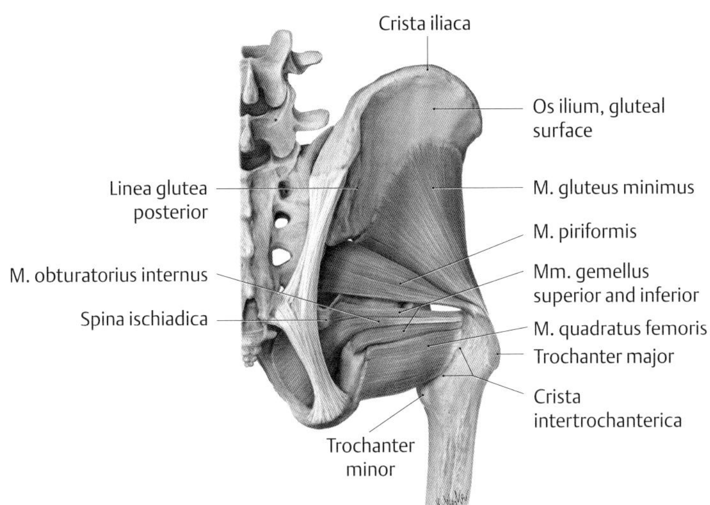
Crista iliaca
Os ilium, gluteal surface
Linea glutea posterior
M. gluteus minimus
M. piriformis
M. obturatorius internus
Mm. gemellus superior and inferior
Spina ischiadica
M. quadratus femoris
Trochanter major
Crista intertrochanterica
Trochanter minor

B Deep layer with m. gluteus medius removed.

Muscle Facts (II)

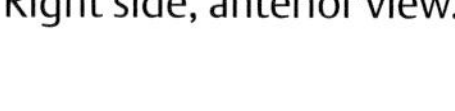

Functionally, the medial thigh muscles are considered the adductors of the hip.

Fig. 24.24 Medial group: Superficial layer
Right side, anterior view.

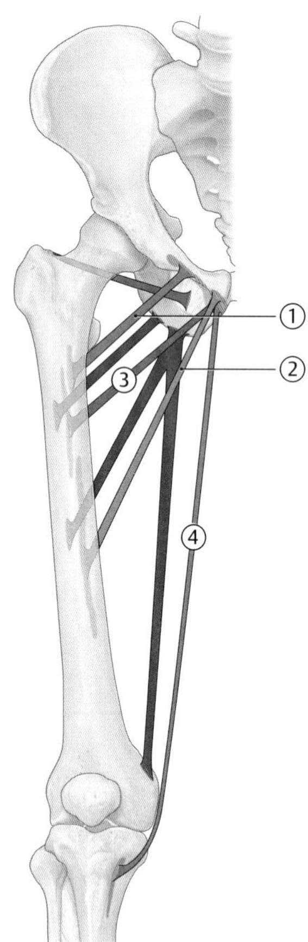

①
②
③
④

A Schematic.

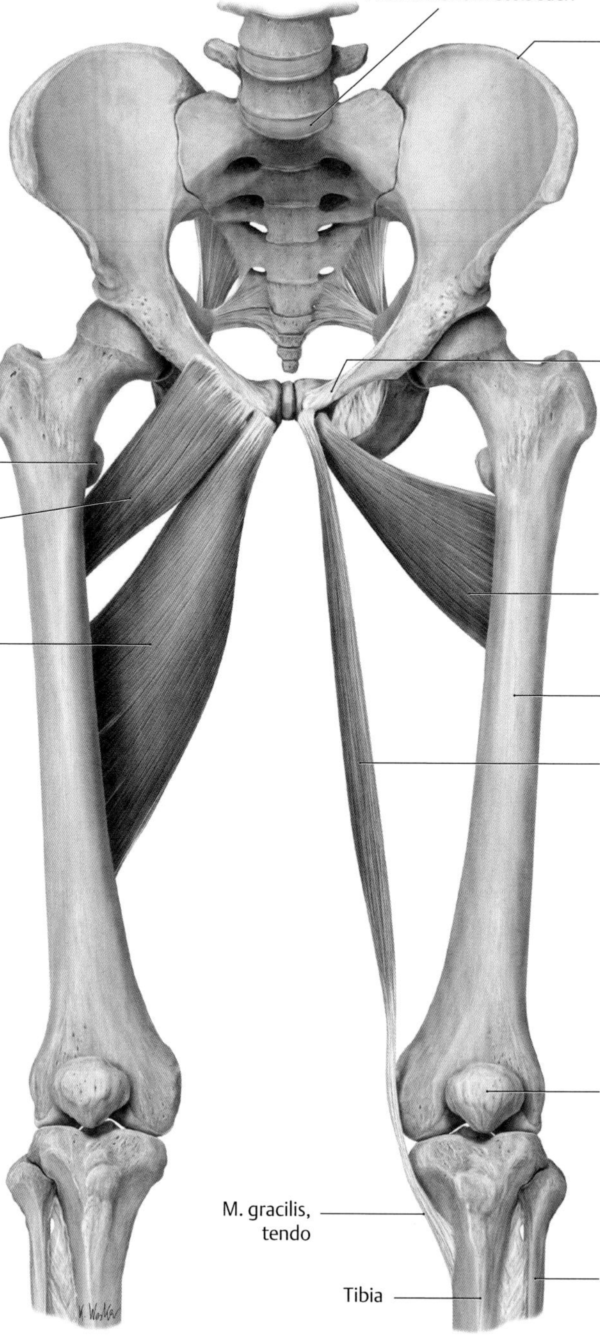

B Superficial adductor group.

Table 24.3 Medial thigh muscles: Superficial layer

Muscle	Origin	Insertion	Innervation	Action
① M. pectineus	Pecten ossis pubis	Linea pectinea	N. femoralis, N. obturatorius (L2, L3)	• Articulatio coxae: adduction, external rotation, and slight flexion • Stabilizes the pelvis in the coronal and sagittal planes
② M. adductor longus	Os pubis (superior pubic ramus and anterior side of the symphysis)	Femur (labium mediale linea aspera)	N. obturatorius (L2–L4)	• Articulatio coxae: adduction and flexion (up to 70 degrees); extension (past 80 degrees of flexion) • Stabilizes the pelvis in the coronal and sagittal planes
③ M. adductor brevis	R. inferior ossis pubis		N. obturatorius (L2, L3)	
④ M. gracilis	R. inferior ossis pubis	Tibia (medial border of the tuberositas tibiae, along with the tendons of m. sartorius and m. semitendinosus)		• Articulatio coxae: adduction and flexion • Articulatio genus: flexion and internal rotation

Fig. 24.25 **Medial group: Deep layer**
Right side, anterior view.

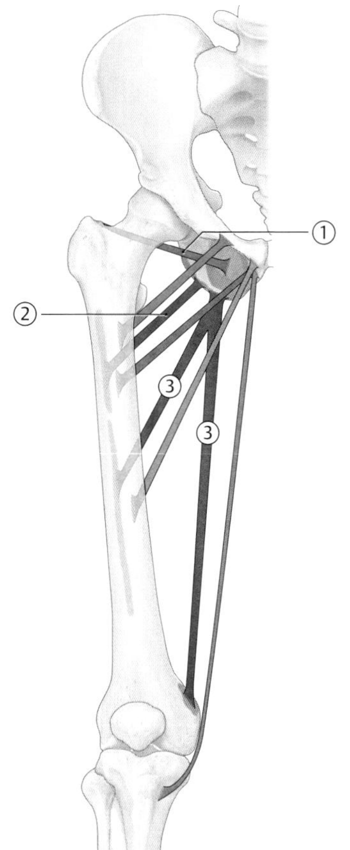

①
②
③
③

A Schematic.

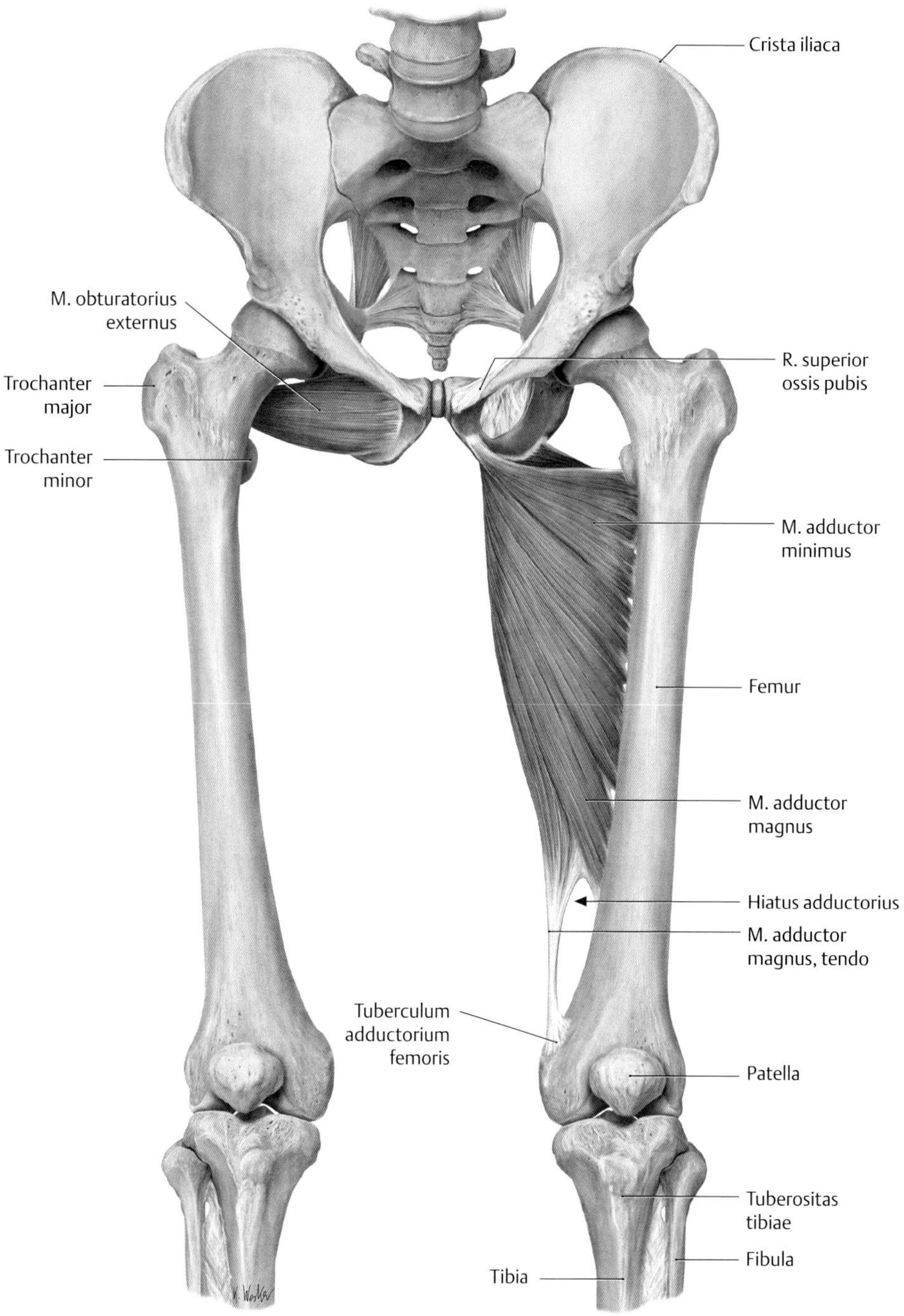

Crista iliaca
M. obturatorius externus
Trochanter major
Trochanter minor
R. superior ossis pubis
M. adductor minimus
Femur
M. adductor magnus
Hiatus adductorius
M. adductor magnus, tendo
Tuberculum adductorium femoris
Patella
Tuberositas tibiae
Fibula
Tibia

B Deep adductor group.

Table 24.4 **Medial thigh muscles: Deep layer**

Muscle	Origin	Insertion	Innervation	Action
① M. obturatorius externus	Outer surface of membrana obturatoria and its bony boundaries	Fossa trochanterica	N. obturatorius (L3, L4)	• Articulatio coxae: adduction and external rotation • Stabilizes the pelvis in the sagittal plane
② M. adductor minimus	R. inferior ossis pubis	Labium mediale of linea aspera	N. obturatorius (L2–L4)	Articulatio coxae: adduction extension, and slight flexion of the hip joint
③ M. adductor magnus	R. inferior ossis pubis, r. ossis ischii, tuber ischiadicum	• Pars profunda ("fleshy insertion"): labium mediale of linea aspera • Pars superficiale ("tendinous insertion"): tuberculum adductorium	• Pars profundus: N. obturatorius (L2–L4) • Pars superficiale: N. tibialis (L4)	• Articulatio coxae: adduction, extention, and slight flexion (the tendinous insertion is also active in internal rotation) • Stabilizes the pelvis in the coronal and sagittal plane

Muscle Facts (III)

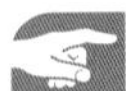

The anterior and posterior muscles of the thigh can be classified as extensors and flexors, respectively, with regard to the knee joint.

Fig. 24.26 Anterior thigh muscles

Right side, anterior view.

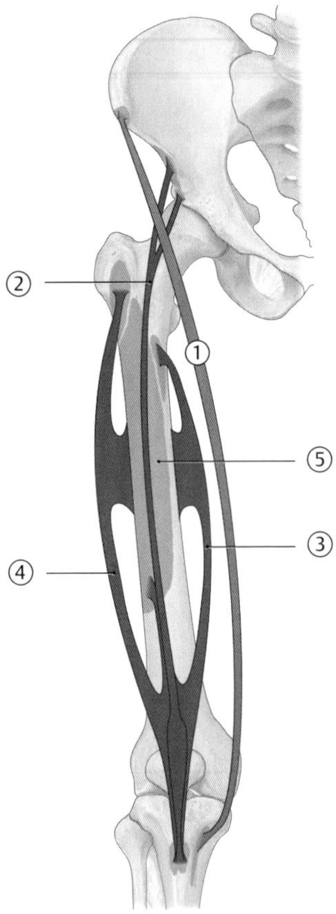

②
①
⑤
③
④ sartorius

A Schematic.

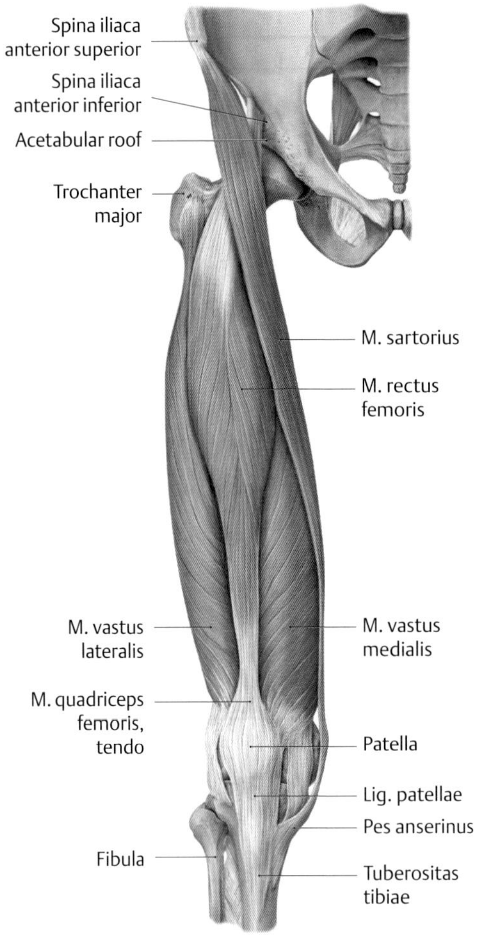

Spina iliaca anterior superior
Spina iliaca anterior inferior
Acetabular roof
Trochanter major
M. sartorius
M. rectus femoris
M. vastus lateralis
M. vastus medialis
M. quadriceps femoris, tendo
Patella
Lig. patellae
Pes anserinus
Fibula
Tuberositas tibiae

B Superficial group.

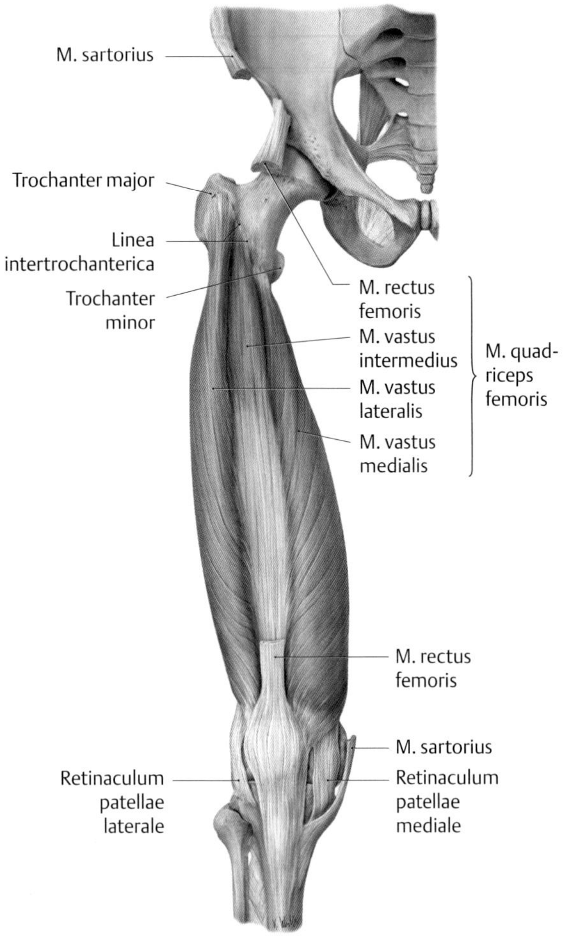

M. sartorius
Trochanter major
Linea intertrochanterica
Trochanter minor
M. rectus femoris
M. vastus intermedius
M. vastus lateralis
M. vastus medialis
M. quadriceps femoris
M. rectus femoris
M. sartorius
Retinaculum patellae laterale
Retinaculum patellae mediale

C Deep group. *Removed:* M. sartorius and m. rectus femoris.

Table 24.5 Anterior thigh muscles

Muscle		Origin	Insertion	Innervation	Action
① M. sartorius		Spina iliaca anterior superior	Medial to tuberositas tibiae (together with m. gracilis and m. semitendinosus)	N. femoralis (L2, L3)	• Articulatio coxae: flexion, abduction, and external rotation • Articulatio genus: flexion and internal rotation
M. quadriceps femoris*	② M. rectus femoris	Spina iliaca anterior inferior, acetabular roof of articulatio coxae	Tuberositas tibiae (via lig. patellae)	N. femoralis (L2–L4)	• Articulatio coxae: flexion • Articulatio genus: extension
	③ M. vastus medialis	Labium mediale of linea aspera, linea intertrochanterica	Both sides of tuberositas tibiae on the condylus medialis and lateralis (via the medial and longitudinal retinacula patellae)		Articulatio genus: extension
	④ M. vastus lateralis	Labium laterale of linea aspera, trochanter major (lateral surface)			
	⑤ M. vastus intermedius	fascies anterior of femur	Tuberositas tibiae (via lig. patellae)		
	M. articularis genus	Fascies anterior of femoral shaft at level of the recessus suprapatellaris	Recessus suprapatellares of knee joint capsule		Articulatio genus: extension; prevents entrapment of capsule

*The entire muscle inserts on the tibial tuberosity via the patellar ligament.

Fig. 24.27 Posterior thigh muscles

Right side, posterior view.

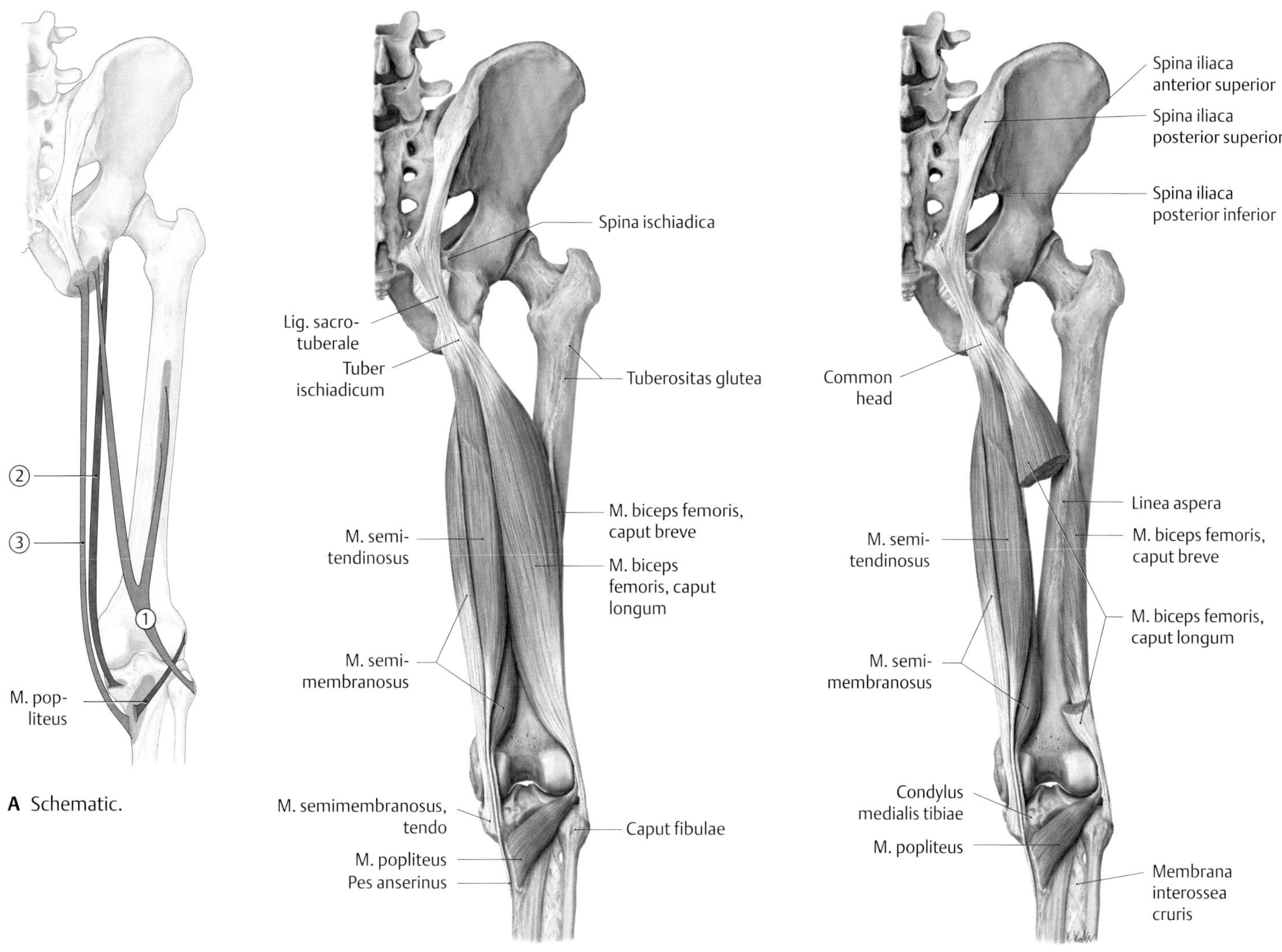

②
③
①
M. pop-liteus
Spina ischiadica
Lig. sacro-tuberale
Tuber ischiadicum
Tuberositas glutea
M. biceps femoris, caput breve
M. semi-tendinosus
M. biceps femoris, caput longum
M. semi-membranosus
M. semimembranosus, tendo
Caput fibulae
M. popliteus
Pes anserinus
Spina iliaca anterior superior
Spina iliaca posterior superior
Spina iliaca posterior inferior
Common head
Linea aspera
M. biceps femoris, caput breve
M. semi-tendinosus
M. biceps femoris, caput longum
M. semi-membranosus
Condylus medialis tibiae
M. popliteus
Membrana interossea cruris

A Schematic.

B Superficial group.

C Deep group. *Removed:* M. biceps femoris (long head) and m. semitendinosus.

Table 24.6 **Posterior thigh muscles**

Muscle	Origin	Insertion	Innervation	Action
① M. biceps femoris	Caput longum: tuber ischiadicum, lig. sacrotuberale (common head with m. semitendinosus)	Caput fibulae	N. tibialis (L5–S2)	• Articulatio coxae (long head): extends the hip, stabilizes the pelvis in the sagittal plane • Articulatio genus: flexion and external rotation
	Caput breve: labium laterale of linea aspera (in the middle third of the femur)		N. fibularis communis (L5–S2)	Articulatio genus: flexion and external rotation
② M. semimembranosus	Tuber ischiadicum	Condylus medialis of tibia, lig. popliteum obliquum, fascia poplitea	N. tibialis (L5–S2)	• Articulatio coxae: extends the hip, stabilizes the pelvis in the sagittal plane • Articulatio genus: flexion and internal rotation
③ M. semitendinosus	Tuber ischiadicum, lig. sacrotuberale (common head with long head of m. biceps femoris)	Medial to tuberositas tibiae, pes anserinus (along with the tendons of m. gracilis and m. sartorius)		
See p. 399 for m. popliteus.				

Tibia & Fibula

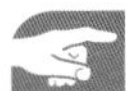

The tibia and fibula articulate at two joints, allowing limited motion (rotation). Membrana interossea cruris is a sheet of tough connective tissue that serves as an origin for several muscles in the leg. It also acts with syndesmosis tibiofibularis to stabilize articulatio talocruralis.

Fig. 25.1 **Tibia and fibula**
Right leg.

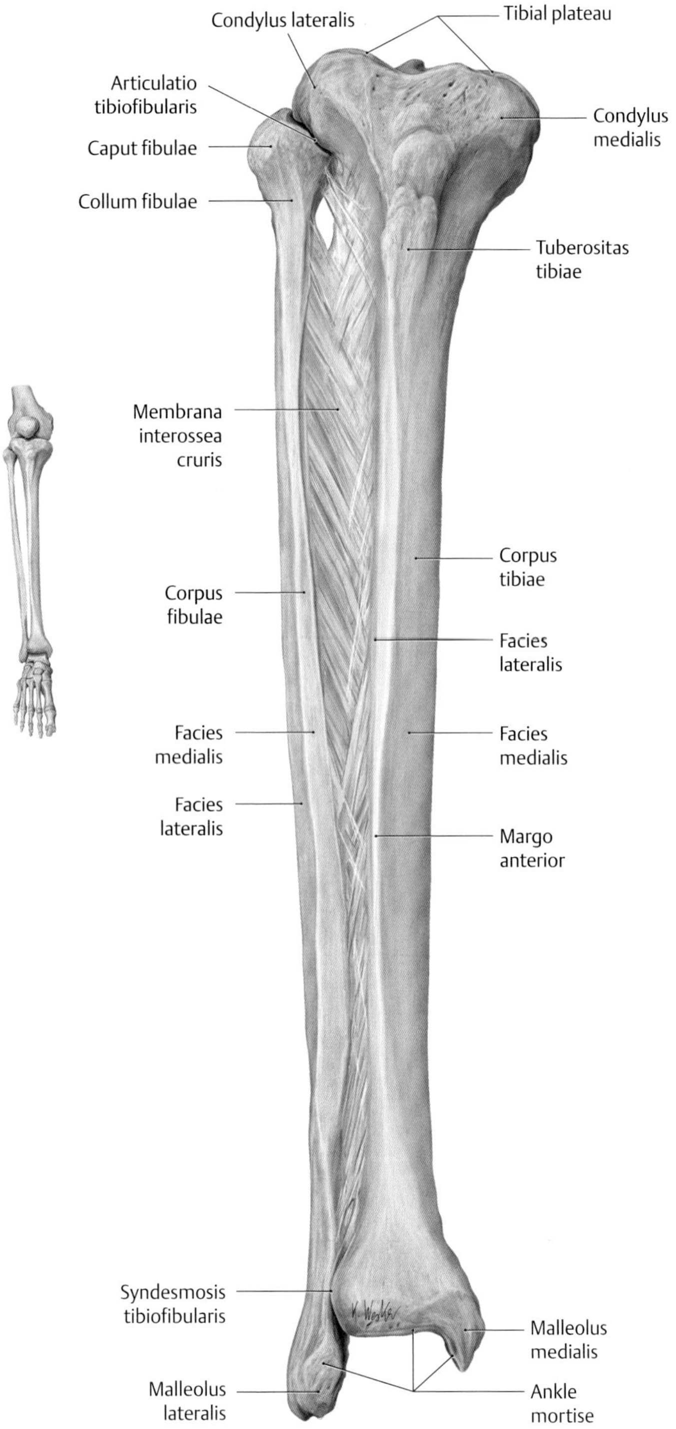

Condylus lateralis
Tibial plateau
Articulatio tibiofibularis
Condylus medialis
Caput fibulae
Collum fibulae
Tuberositas tibiae
Membrana interossea cruris
Corpus tibiae
Corpus fibulae
Facies lateralis
Facies medialis
Facies medialis
Facies lateralis
Margo anterior
Syndesmosis tibiofibularis
Malleolus medialis
Malleolus lateralis
Ankle mortise

A Anterior view.

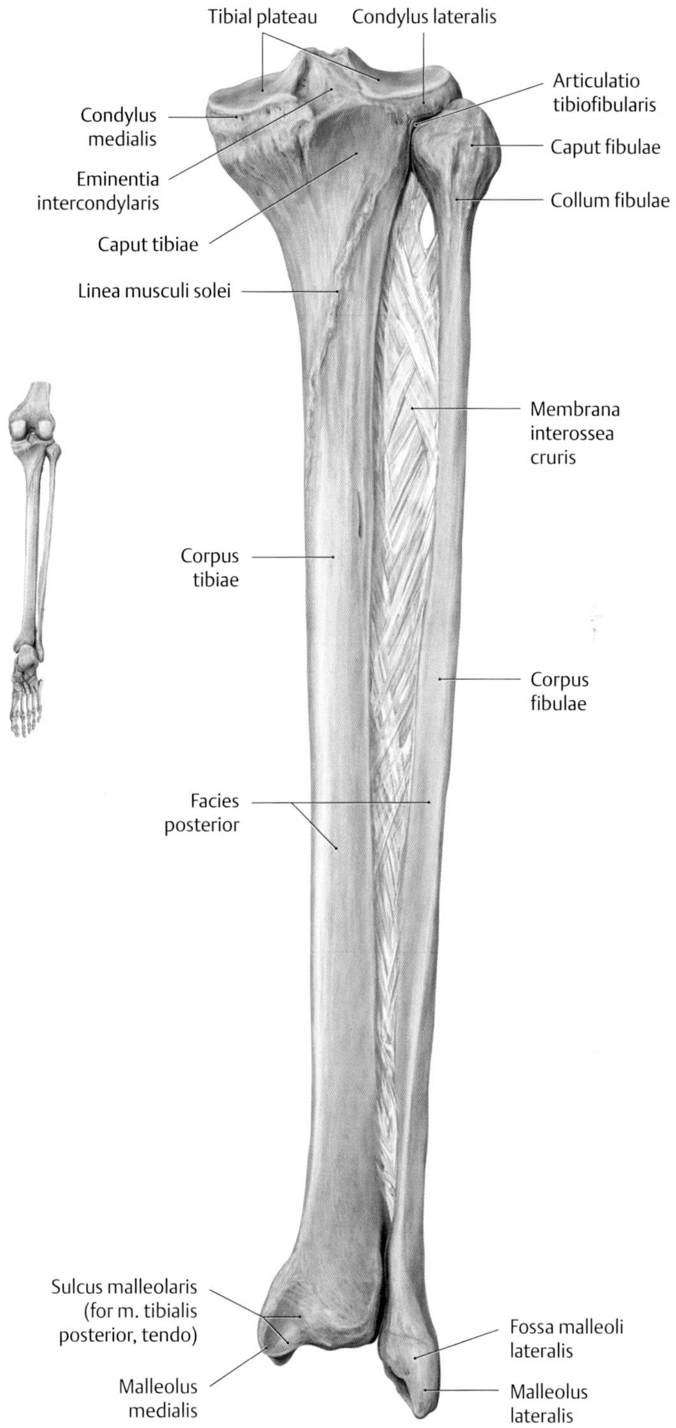

Tibial plateau
Condylus lateralis
Articulatio tibiofibularis
Condylus medialis
Caput fibulae
Eminentia intercondylaris
Collum fibulae
Caput tibiae
Linea musculi solei
Membrana interossea cruris
Corpus tibiae
Corpus fibulae
Facies posterior
Sulcus malleolaris (for m. tibialis posterior, tendo)
Fossa malleoli lateralis
Malleolus medialis
Malleolus lateralis

B Posterior view.

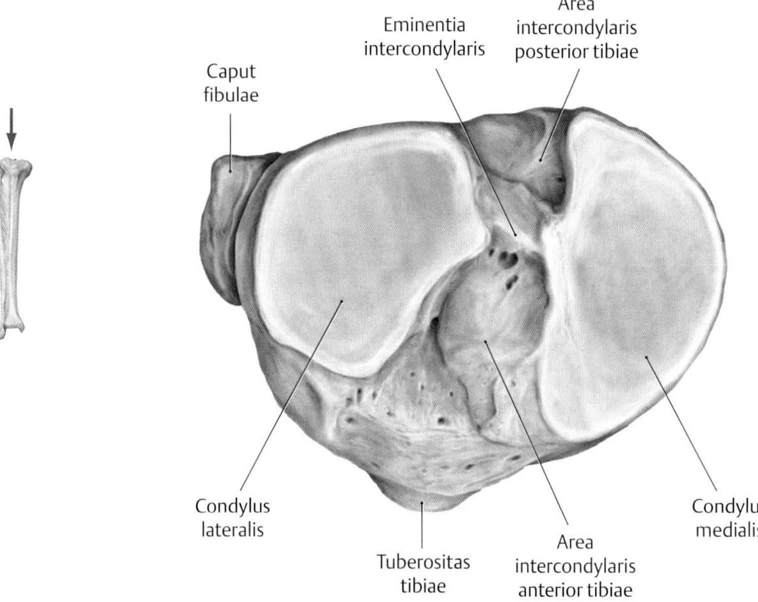
Caput
fibulae
Eminentia
intercondylaris
Area
intercondylaris
posterior tibiae
Condylus
lateralis
Tuberositas
tibiae
Area
intercondylaris
anterior tibiae
Condylus
medialis

C Proximal view.

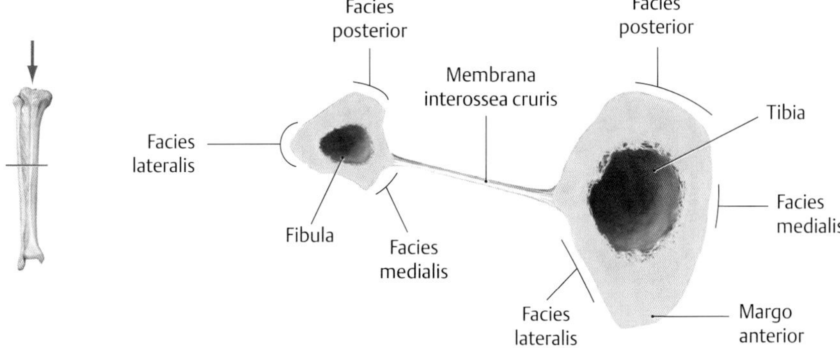
Facies
posterior
Facies
posterior
Membrana
interossea cruris
Facies
lateralis
Tibia
Fibula
Facies
medialis
Facies
medialis
Facies
lateralis
Margo
anterior

D Transverse section, superior view.

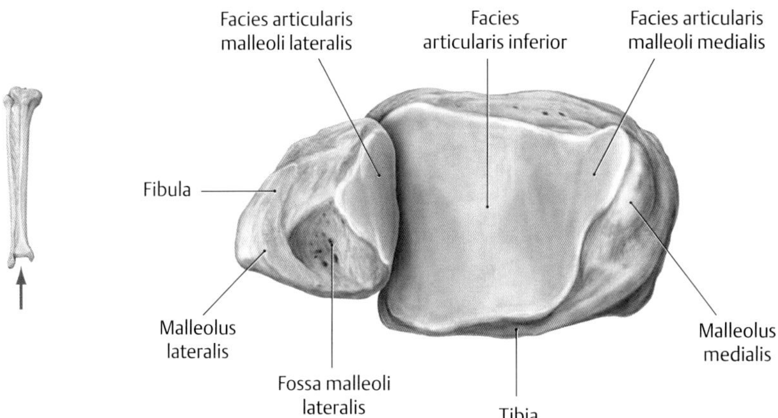
Facies articularis
malleoli lateralis
Facies
articularis inferior
Facies articularis
malleoli medialis
Fibula
Malleolus
lateralis
Fossa malleoli
lateralis
Tibia
Malleolus
medialis

E Distal view.

Clinical

Fibular fracture

When diagnosing a fibular fracture, it is important to determine whether the syndesmosis (see p. 380) is disrupted. Fibular fractures may occur distal to, level with, or proximal to the syndesmosis; the latter two frequently involve tearing of the syndesmosis.

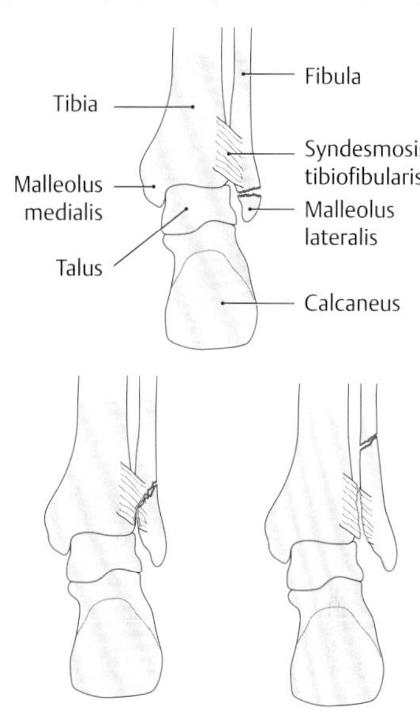
Tibia
Fibula
Syndesmosis
tibiofibularis
Malleolus
medialis
Malleolus
lateralis
Talus
Calcaneus

In this fracture, located proximal to the syndesmosis, the syndesmosis is torn, as indicated by the widened medial joint space of the articulatio talocruralis (see p. 405).

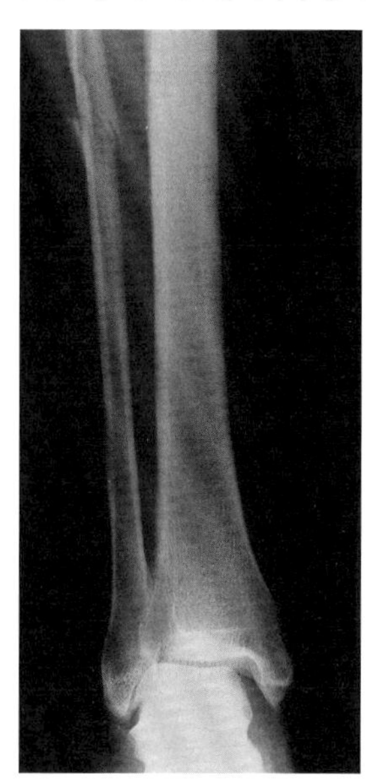

Articulatio Genus: Overview

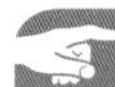

In articulatio genus, the femur articulates with the tibia and patella. Both joints are contained within a common capsule and have communicating articular cavities. *Note:* The fibula is not included in the knee joint (contrast to the humerus in the elbow; see p. 282). Instead, it forms a separate rigid articulation with the tibia.

Fig. 25.2 **Right articulatio genus**

Femur
Patella
Epicondylus lateralis
Condylus lateralis femoris
Condylus lateralis tibiae
Tibial plateau
Caput fibulae
Epicondylus medialis
Condylus medialis femoris
Condylus medialis tibiae
Tuberositas tibiae
Fibula
Tibia

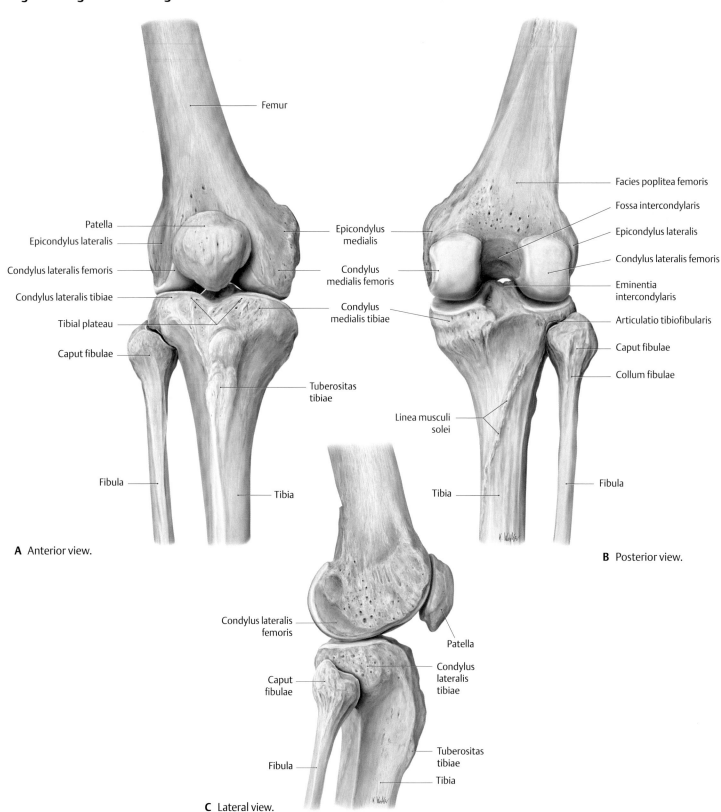

A Anterior view.

Facies poplitea femoris
Fossa intercondylaris
Epicondylus lateralis
Condylus lateralis femoris
Eminentia intercondylaris
Articulatio tibiofibularis
Caput fibulae
Collum fibulae
Linea musculi solei
Fibula
Tibia

B Posterior view.

Condylus lateralis femoris
Patella
Condylus lateralis tibiae
Caput fibulae
Tuberositas tibiae
Fibula
Tibia

C Lateral view.

Fig. 25.4 Patella

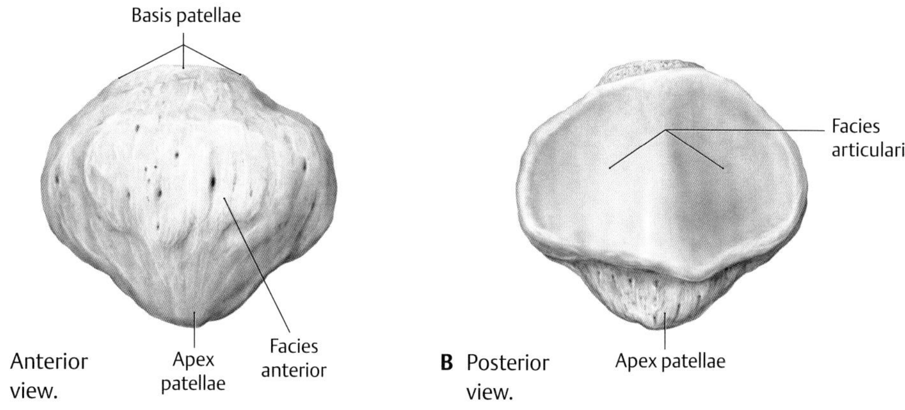
Basis patellae
Facies articularis
Apex patellae
Facies anterior
Apex patellae

A Anterior view.

B Posterior view.

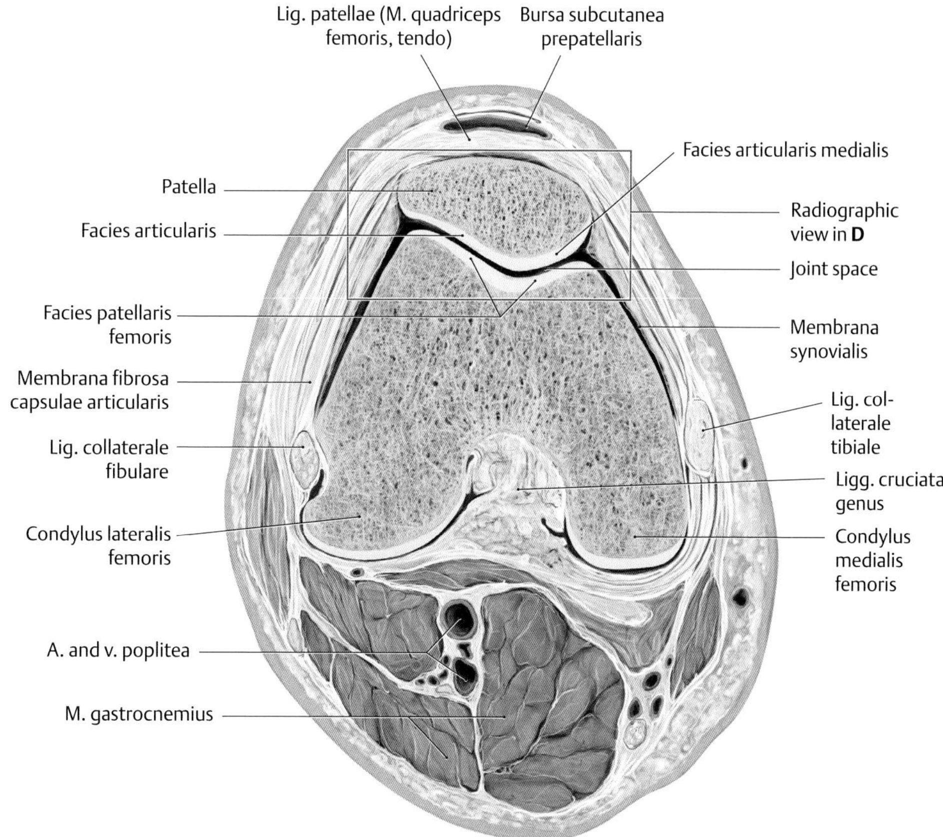
Lig. patellae (M. quadriceps femoris, tendo)
Bursa subcutanea prepatellaris
Facies articularis medialis
Patella
Radiographic view in D
Facies articularis
Joint space
Facies patellaris femoris
Membrana synovialis
Membrana fibrosa capsulae articularis
Lig. collaterale tibiale
Lig. collaterale fibulare
Ligg. cruciata genus
Condylus lateralis femoris
Condylus medialis femoris
A. and v. poplitea
M. gastrocnemius

C Transverse section through femoro-patellar joint. Distal view with right knee in slight flexion.

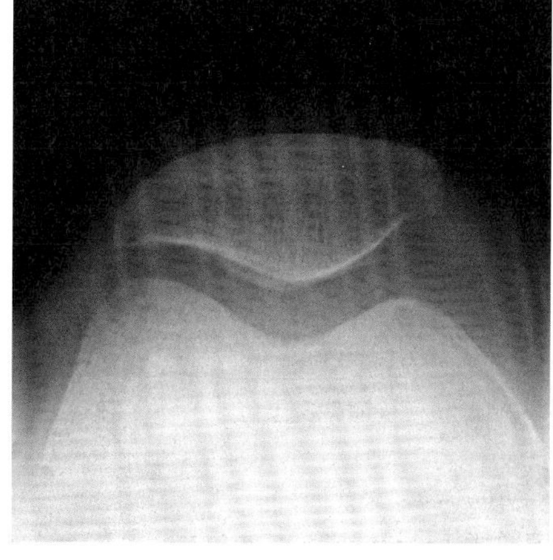

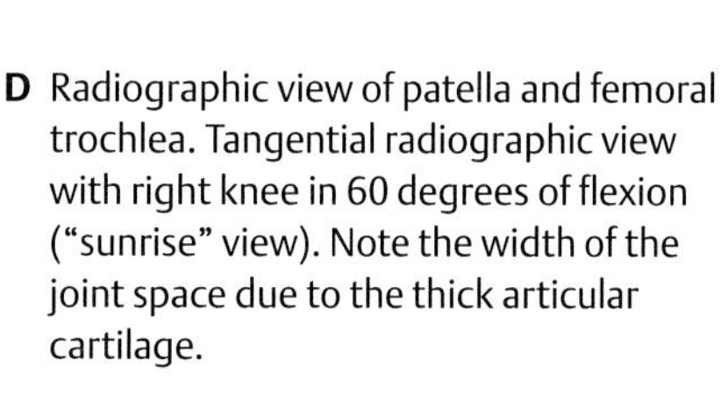

D Radiographic view of patella and femoral trochlea. Tangential radiographic view with right knee in 60 degrees of flexion ("sunrise" view). Note the width of the joint space due to the thick articular cartilage.

Fig. 25.3 Articulatio genus: Radiographs

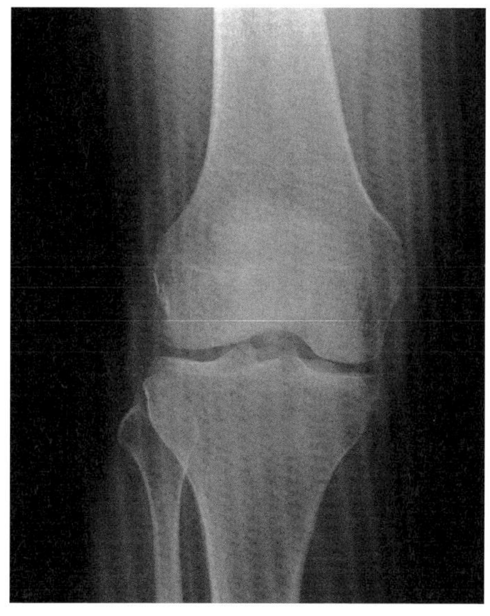

A Anteroposterior projection.

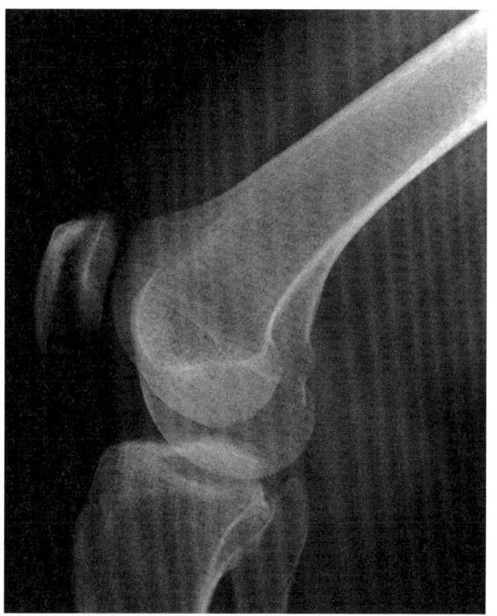

B Lateral projection.

Articulatio Genus: Capsule, Ligaments & Bursae

Table 25.1 Ligaments of the knee joint

Extrinsic ligaments	
Anterior side	Lig. patellae
	Retinaculum patellae mediale longitudinale
	Retinaculum patellae laterale longitudinale
	Retinaculum patellae mediale transversale
	Retinaculum patellae laterale transversale
Medial and lateral sides	Lig. collaterale tibiale
	Lig. collaterale fibulare
Posterior side	Lig. popliteum obliquum
	Lig. popliteum arcuatum
Intrinsic ligaments	
Lig. cruciatum anterius	
Lig. cruciatum posterius	
Lig. transversum genus	
Lig. meniscofemorale posterius	

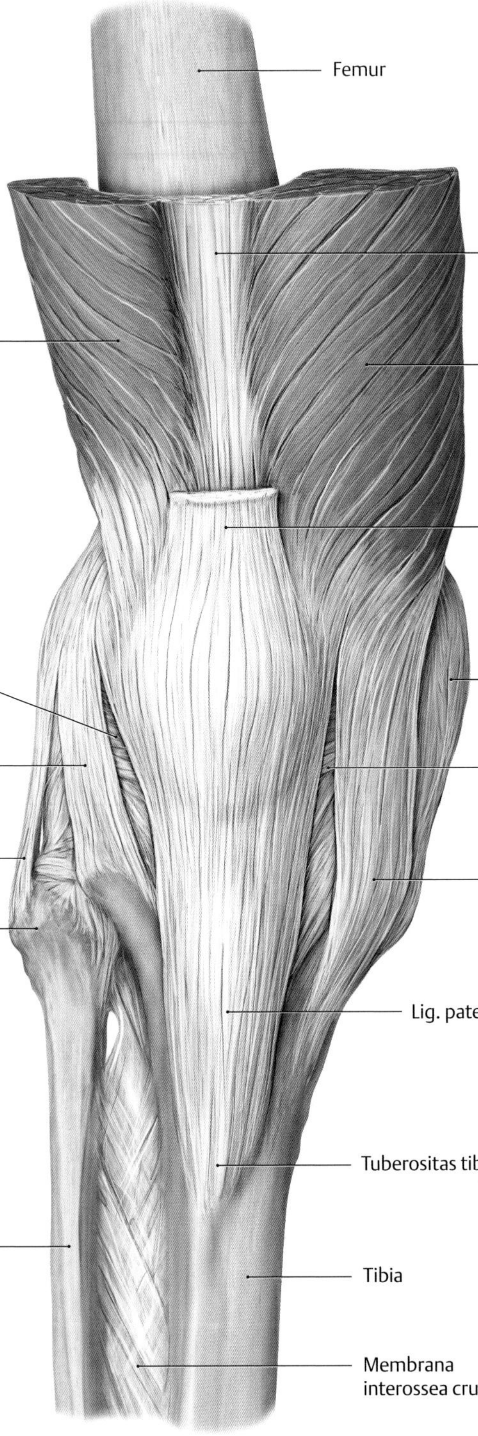

Fig. 25.5 **Ligaments of articulatio genus**
Anterior view of right knee.

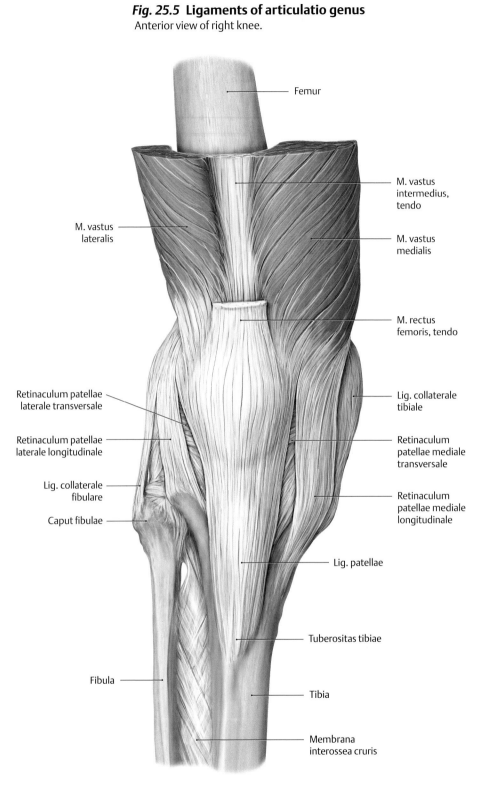

Femur
M. vastus intermedius, tendo
M. vastus lateralis
M. vastus medialis
M. rectus femoris, tendo
Retinaculum patellae laterale transversale
Lig. collaterale tibiale
Retinaculum patellae laterale longitudinale
Retinaculum patellae mediale transversale
Lig. collaterale fibulare
Retinaculum patellae mediale longitudinale
Caput fibulae
Lig. patellae
Tuberositas tibiae
Fibula
Tibia
Membrana interossea cruris

Fig. 25.6 Capsule, ligaments, and periarticular bursae

Posterior view of right knee. The joint cavity communicates with periarticular bursae at the subpopliteal recess, semimembranosus bursa, and medial subtendinous bursa of m. gastrocnemius.

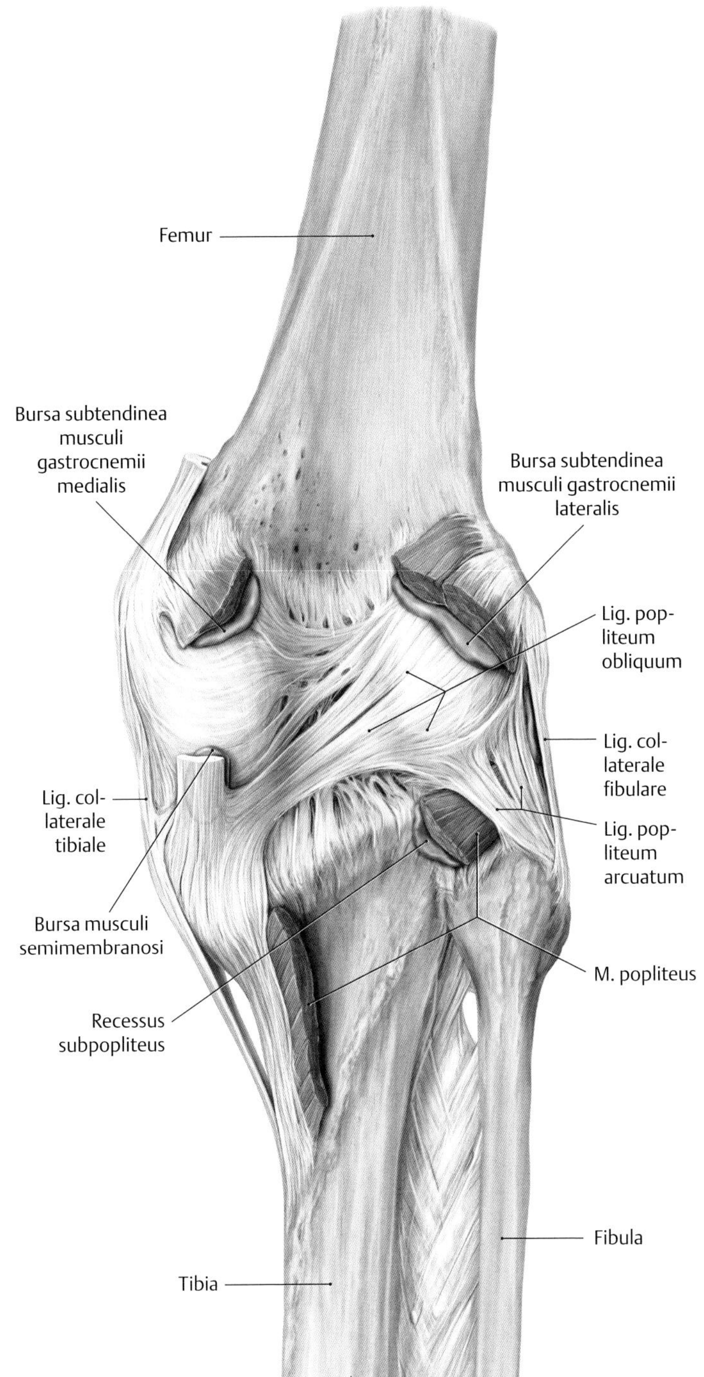

Femur
Bursa subtendinea musculi gastrocnemii medialis
Bursa subtendinea musculi gastrocnemii lateralis
Lig. popliteum obliquum
Lig. collaterale fibulare
Lig. collaterale tibiale
Lig. popliteum arcuatum
Bursa musculi semimembranosi
M. popliteus
Recessus subpopliteus
Fibula
Tibia

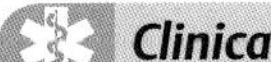

Clinical

Gastrocnemio-semimembranosus bursa (Baker's cyst)

Painful swelling behind the knee may be caused by a cystic outpouching of the joint capsule (synovial popliteal cyst). This frequently results from a rise in intra-articular pressure (e.g., in rheumatoid arthritis).

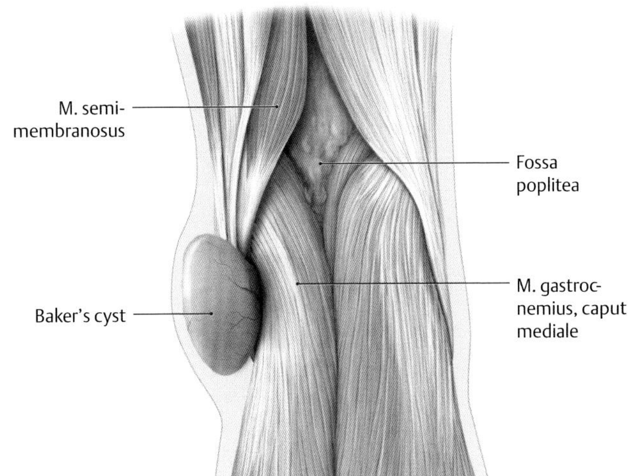

M. semimembranosus
Fossa poplitea
M. gastrocnemius, caput mediale
Baker's cyst

A Baker's cyst in the right fossa poplitea. Baker's cysts often occur in the medial part of fossa poplitea between m. semimembranosus tendon and caput mediale of m. gastrocnemius at the level of the posteromedial condylus femoris.

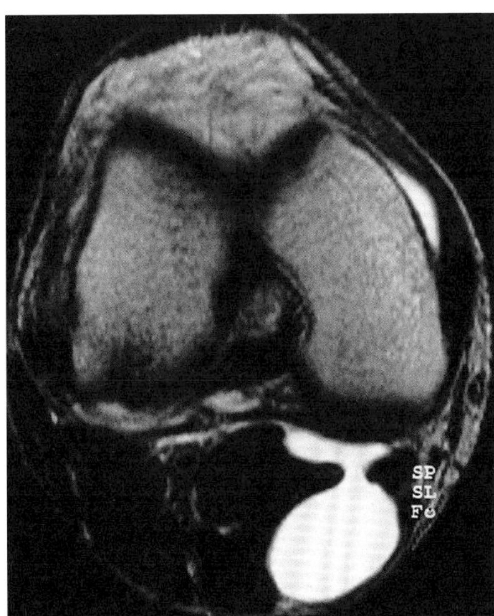

SP
SI
Fe

B Axial magnetic resonance imaging (MRI) of a Baker's cyst in fossa poplitea, inferior view.

Articulatio Genus: Ligaments & Menisci

Fig. 25.7 **Collateral and patellar ligaments of articulatio genus**
Right articulatio genus. Each articulatio genus has medial and lateral collateral ligaments. The medial collateral ligament (lig. collaterale tibiale) is attached to both the capsule and meniscus medialis, whereas the lig. collateral fibulare has no direct contact with either the capsule or the lateral meniscus. Both collateral ligaments are taut when the knee is in extension and stabilize the joint in the coronal plane.

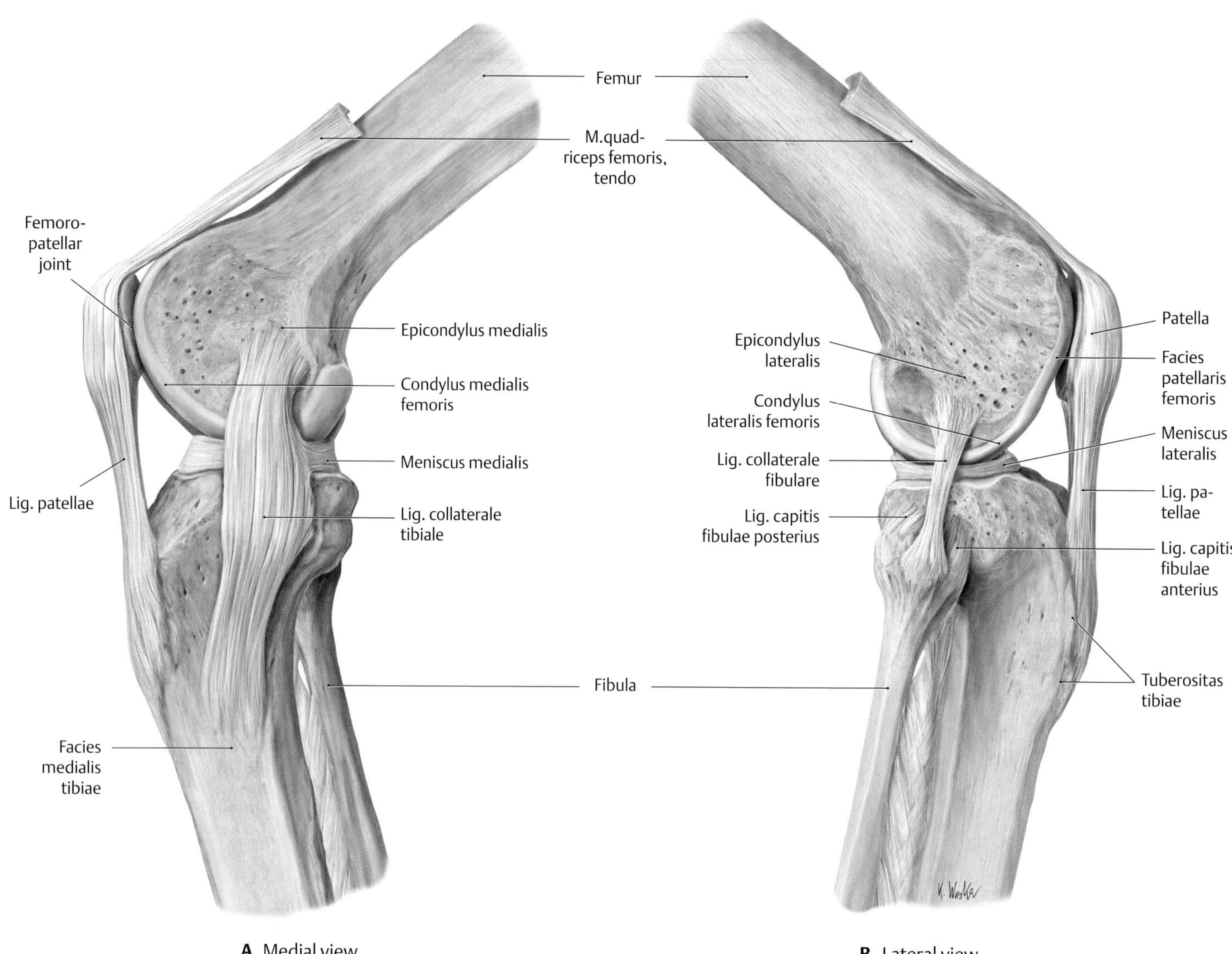
Femur
M.quadriceps femoris, tendo
Femoro-patellar joint
Epicondylus medialis
Condylus medialis femoris
Meniscus medialis
Lig. patellae
Lig. collaterale tibiale
Fibula
Facies medialis tibiae
Patella
Epicondylus lateralis
Facies patellaris femoris
Condylus lateralis femoris
Meniscus lateralis
Lig. collaterale fibulare
Lig. patellae
Lig. capitis fibulae posterius
Lig. capitis fibulae anterius
Tuberositas tibiae

A Medial view.

B Lateral view.

Fig. 25.8 Menisci in articulatio genus
Right tibial plateau, proximal view.

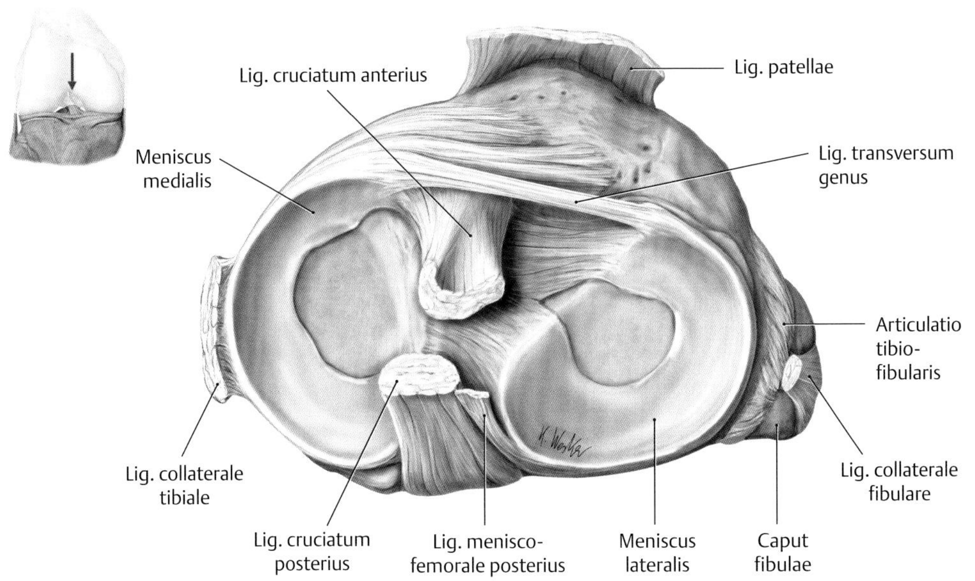
Lig. cruciatum anterius
Lig. patellae
Meniscus medialis
Lig. transversum genus
Articulatio tibio-fibularis
Lig. collaterale tibiale
Lig. collaterale fibulare
Lig. cruciatum posterius
Lig. menisco-femorale posterius
Meniscus lateralis
Caput fibulae

A Right tibial plateau with ligg. cruciata, lig. patellae, and ligg. collaterale tibiale and fibulare divided.

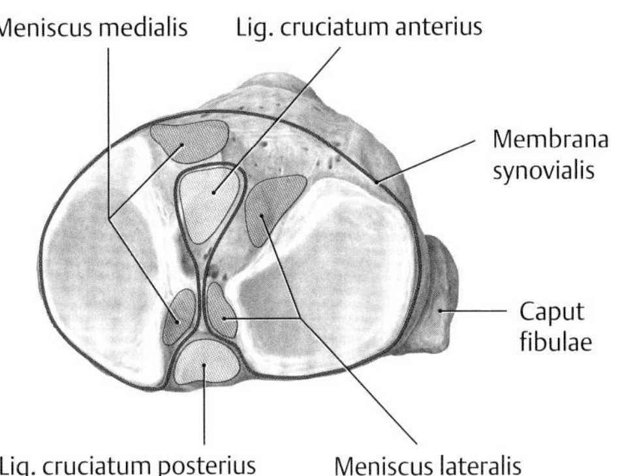
Meniscus medialis
Lig. cruciatum anterius
Membrana synovialis
Caput fibulae
Lig. cruciatum posterius
Meniscus lateralis

B Attachment sites of menisci and ligg. cruciata. Red line indicates the tibial attachment of membrana synovialis that covers ligg. cruciata. The ligg. cruciata lie in the subsynovial connective tissue.

Clinical

Injury of the menisci
The less mobile meniscus medialis is more susceptible to injury than meniscus lateralis. Trauma generally results from sudden extension or rotation of the flexed knee while the leg is fixed.

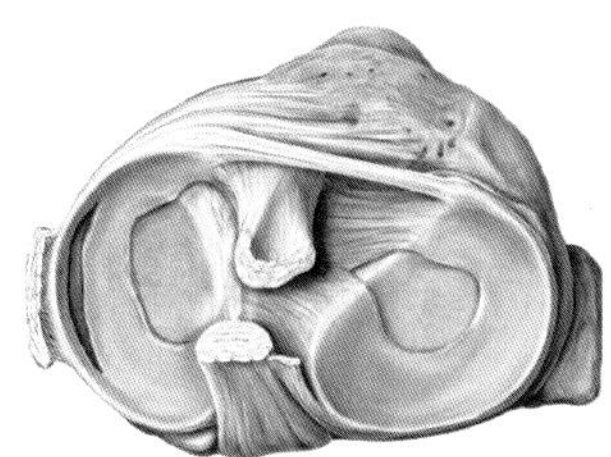

A Bucket-handle tear.

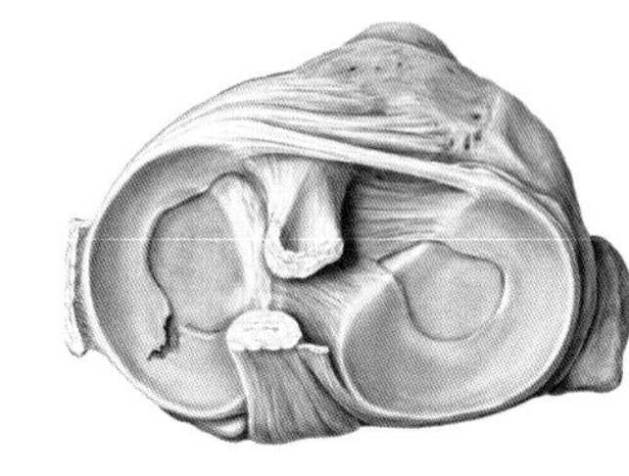

B Radial tear of posterior horn.

Fig. 25.9 Movements of the menisci
Right knee joint.

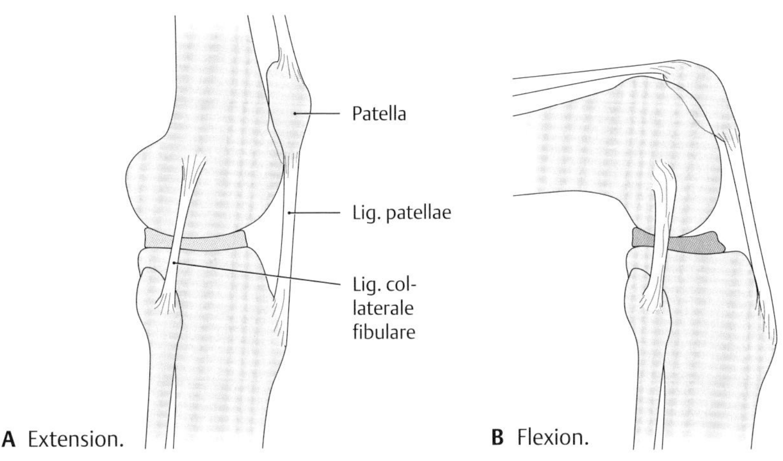
Patella
Lig. patellae
Lig. col-laterale fibulare

A Extension.

B Flexion.

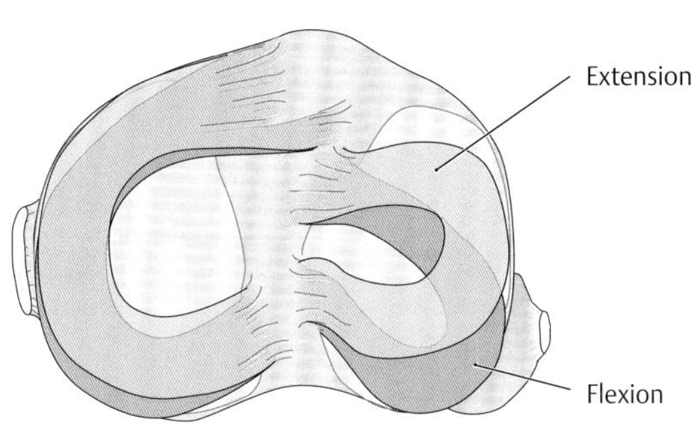
Extension
Flexion

C Tibial plateau, proximal view.

Ligamenta Cruciata

Fig. 25.10 Ligg. cruciata and collateralia

Right articulatio genus. Ligg. cruciata keep the articular surfaces of the femur and tibia in contact, while stabilizing the knee joint primarily in the sagittal plane. Portions of ligg. cruciata are taut in every joint position.

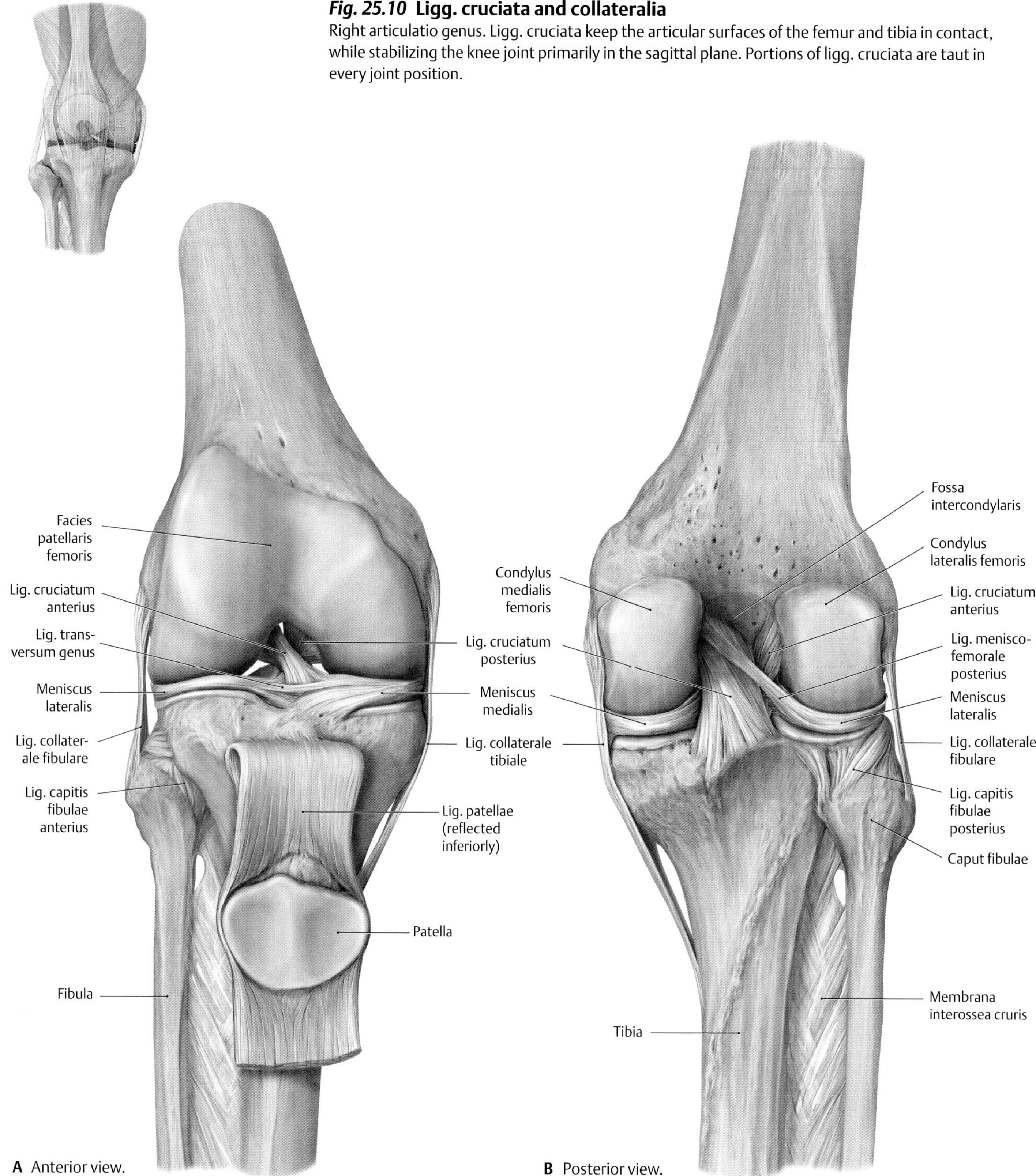
Facies patellaris femoris
Lig. cruciatum anterius
Lig. transversum genus
Meniscus lateralis
Lig. collaterale fibulare
Lig. capitis fibulae anterius
Fibula
Lig. cruciatum posterius
Meniscus medialis
Lig. collaterale tibiale
Lig. patellae (reflected inferiorly)
Patella
Condylus medialis femoris
Lig. cruciatum posterius
Meniscus medialis
Lig. collaterale tibiale
Tibia
Fossa intercondylaris
Condylus lateralis femoris
Lig. cruciatum anterius
Lig. meniscofemorale posterius
Meniscus lateralis
Lig. collaterale fibulare
Lig. capitis fibulae posterius
Caput fibulae
Membrana interossea cruris

A Anterior view.

B Posterior view.

Fig. 25.11 Right articulatio genus in flexion

Anterior view with capsula articularis and patella removed.

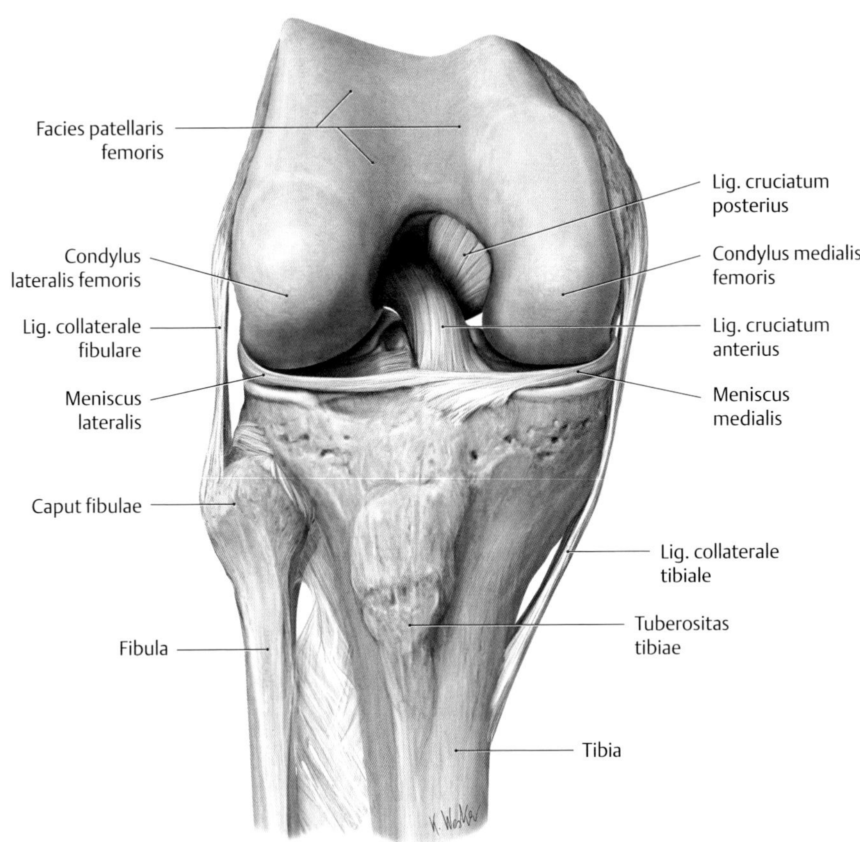
Facies patellaris femoris
Condylus lateralis femoris
Lig. collaterale fibulare
Meniscus lateralis
Caput fibulae
Fibula
Lig. cruciatum posterius
Condylus medialis femoris
Lig. cruciatum anterius
Meniscus medialis
Lig. collaterale tibiale
Tuberositas tibiae
Tibia

Fig. 25.12 Ligg. cruciata and collateralia in flexion and extension

Right knee, anterior view. Taut ligament fibers in red.

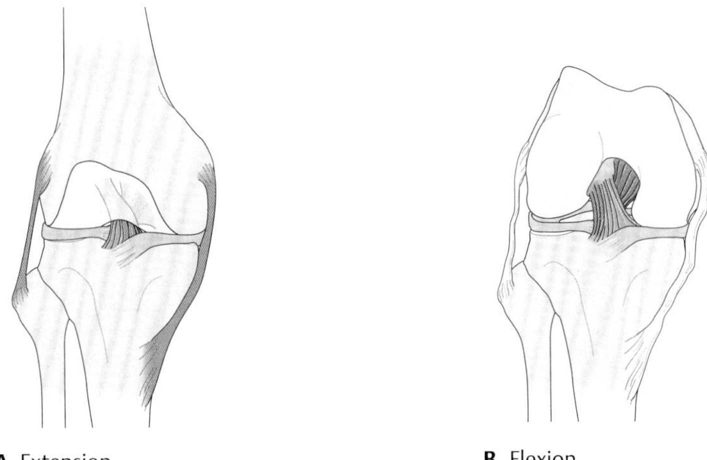

A Extension.

B Flexion.

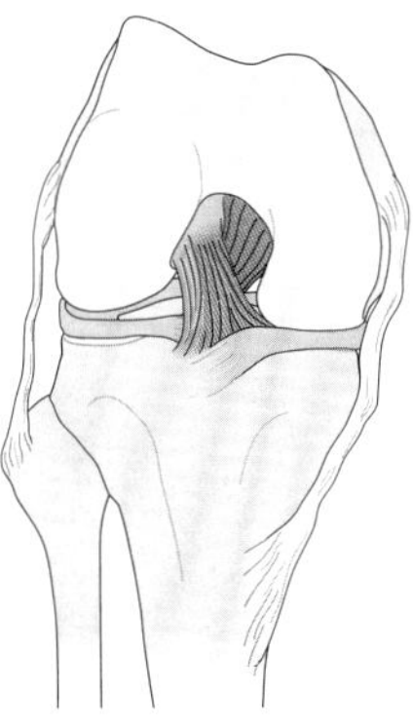

C Flexion and internal rotation.

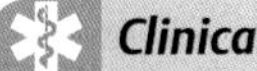

Clinical

Rupture of ligg. cruciata

Rupture of ligg. cruciata destabilizes the knee joint, allowing the tibia to move forward (anterior "drawer sign") or backward (posterior "drawer sign") relative to the femur. Lig. cruciata anterius ruptures are approximately 10 times more common than posterior ligament ruptures. The most common mechanism of injury is an internal rotation trauma with the leg fixed. A lateral blow to the fully extended knee with the foot planted tends to cause concomitant rupture of lig. cruciatum anterius and lig. collaterale tibiale, as well as tearing of the attached meniscus medialis.

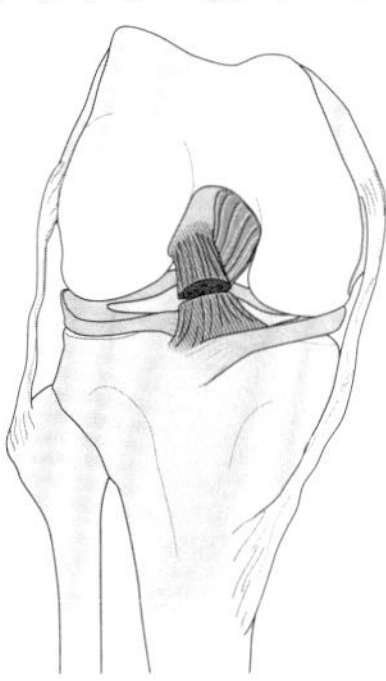

A Rupture of lig. cruciatum anterius. Anterior view.

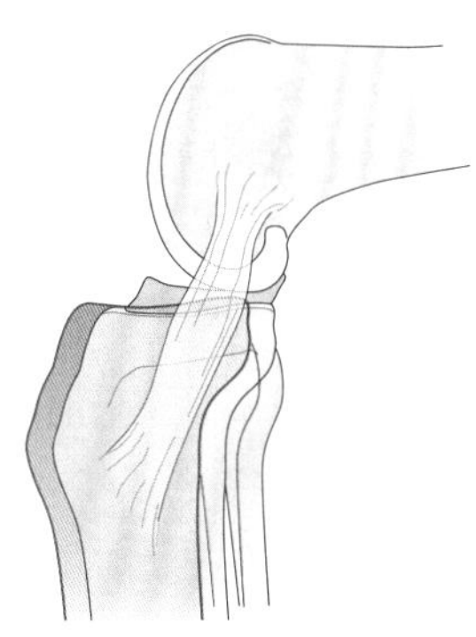

B "Anterior drawer sign." Medial view.

Right knee joint in flexion.

Articulatio Genus Cavitas Articularis

Fig. 25.13 Cavitas articularis

Right knee, lateral view. Cavitas articularis was demonstrated by injecting liquid plastic into the knee joint and later removing the capsule.

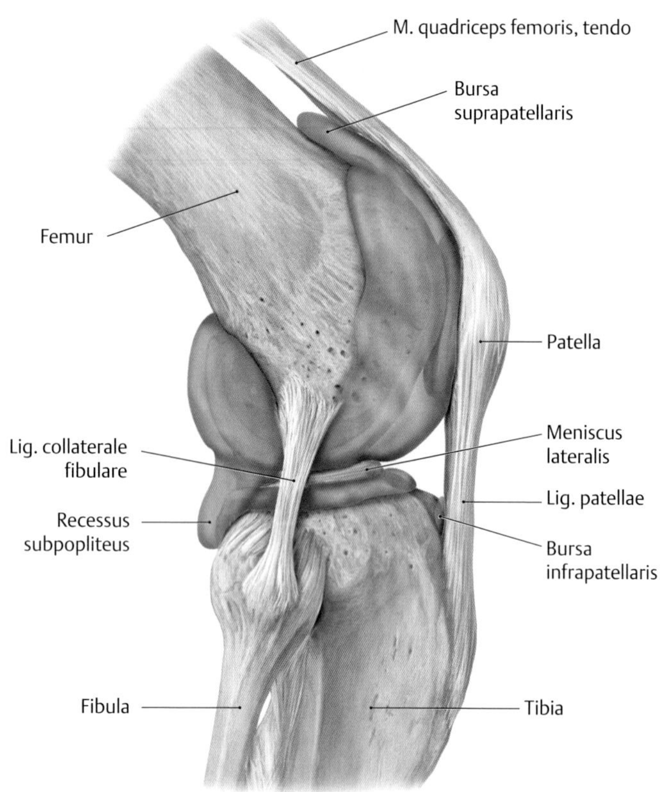
M. quadriceps femoris, tendo
Bursa suprapatellaris
Femur
Patella
Lig. collaterale fibulare
Meniscus lateralis
Lig. patellae
Recessus subpopliteus
Bursa infrapatellaris
Fibula
Tibia

Fig. 25.14 Opened capsula articularis

Right knee, anterior view with patella reflected downward.

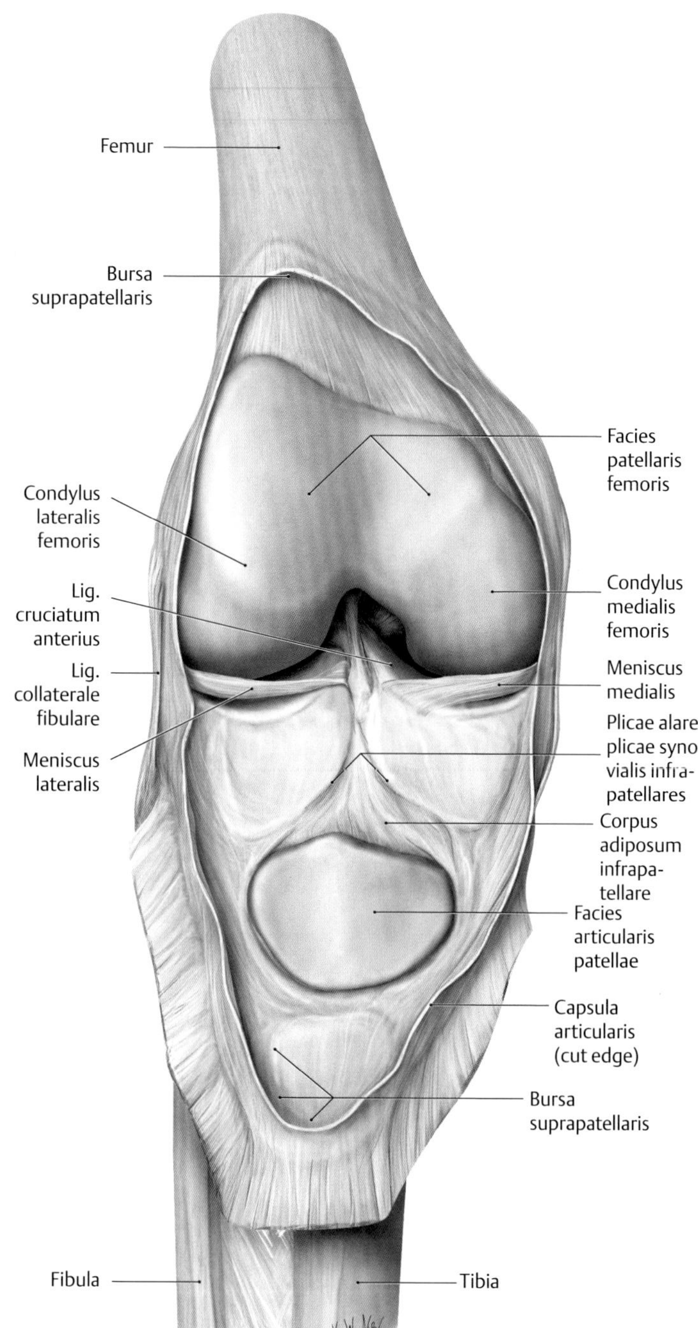
Femur
Bursa suprapatellaris
Facies patellaris femoris
Condylus lateralis femoris
Condylus medialis femoris
Lig. cruciatum anterius
Lig. collaterale fibulare
Meniscus medialis
Plicae alares, plicae synovialis infrapatellares
Meniscus lateralis
Corpus adiposum infrapatellare
Facies articularis patellae
Capsula articularis (cut edge)
Bursa suprapatellaris
Fibula
Tibia

Fig. 25.15 Attachments of capsula articularis

Right knee joint, anterior view.

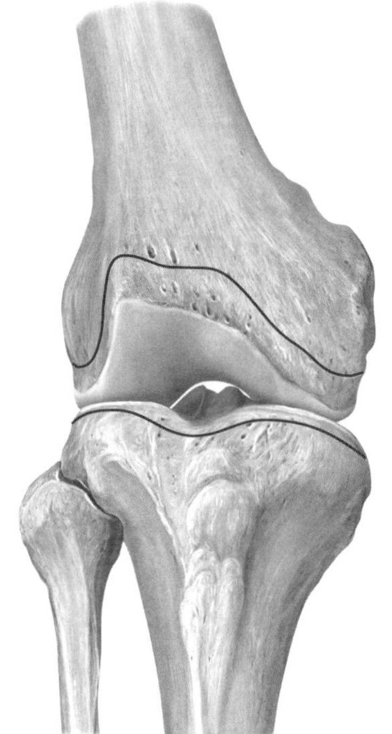

Fig. 25.16 Bursa suprapatellaris during flexion

Right knee joint, medial view.

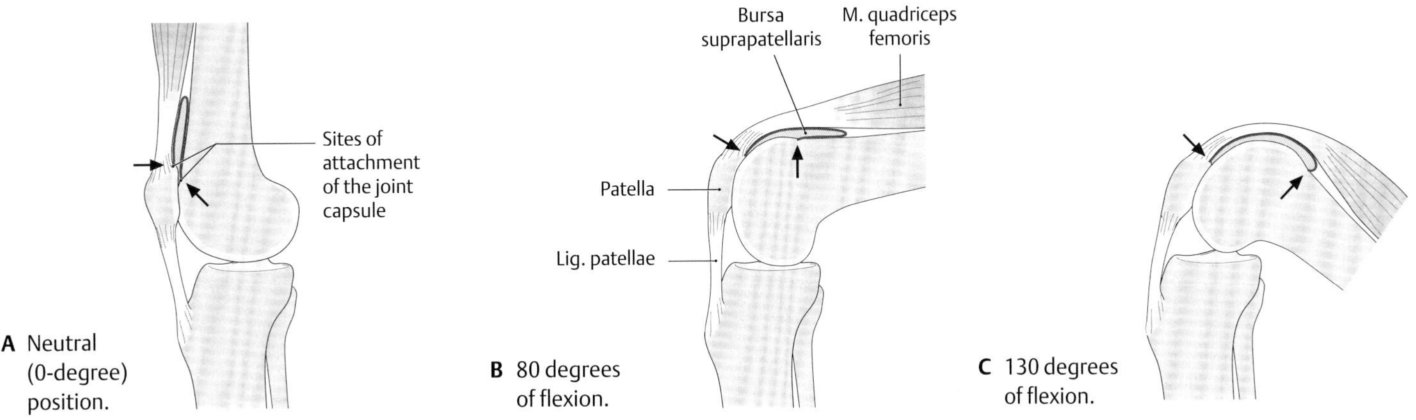

Sites of attachment of the joint capsule
Bursa suprapatellaris
M. quadriceps femoris
Patella
Lig. patellae

A Neutral (0-degree) position.

B 80 degrees of flexion.

C 130 degrees of flexion.

Fig. 25.17 Right knee joint: Midsagittal section

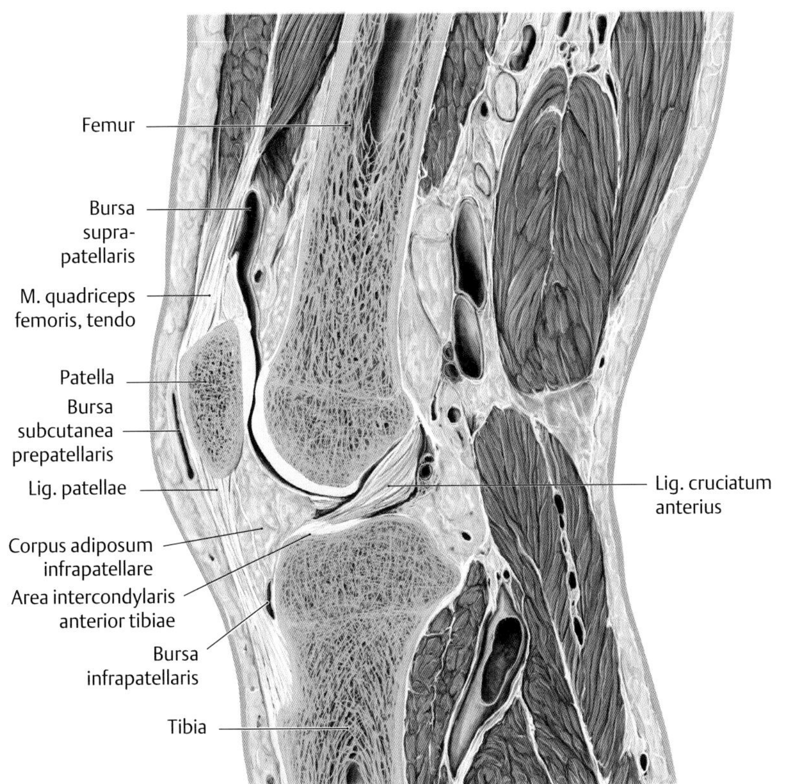

Femur
Bursa supra-patellaris
M. quadriceps femoris, tendo
Patella
Bursa subcutanea prepatellaris
Lig. patellae
Corpus adiposum infrapatellare
Area intercondylaris anterior tibiae
Bursa infrapatellaris
Tibia
Lig. cruciatum anterius

Fig. 25.18 MRI of articulatio genus

Sagittal T2-weighted MRI.

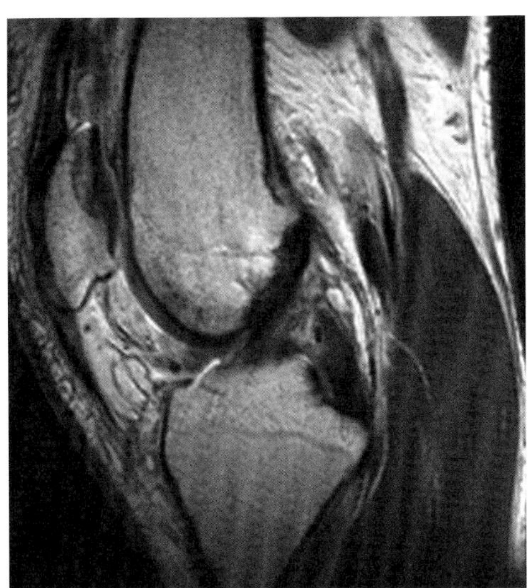

Muscles of the Leg: Anterior & Lateral Views

Fig. 25.19 Muscles of the leg: Anterior view
Right leg. Muscle origins (O) shown in red, insertions (I) in blue.

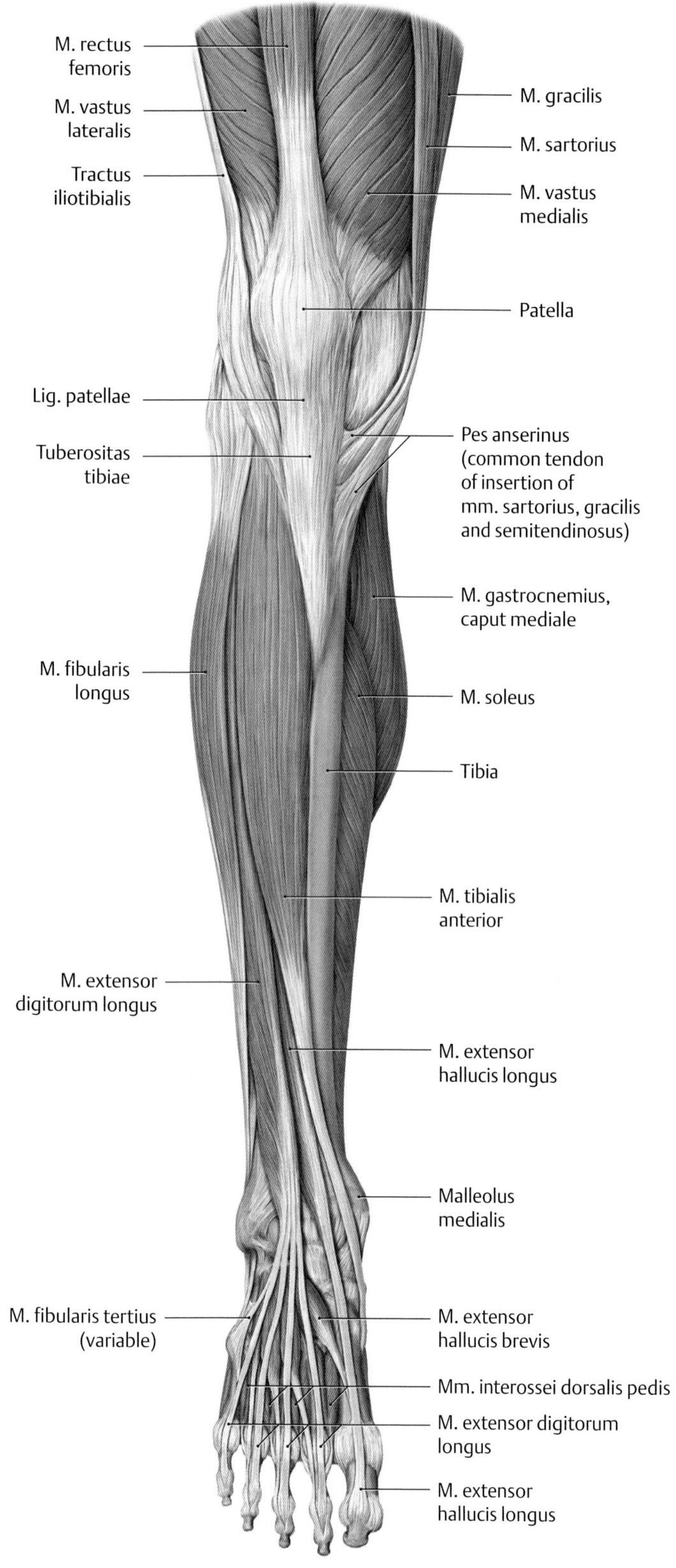
M. rectus femoris
M. vastus lateralis
Tractus iliotibialis
M. gracilis
M. sartorius
M. vastus medialis
Patella
Lig. patellae
Tuberositas tibiae
Pes anserinus (common tendon of insertion of mm. sartorius, gracilis and semitendinosus)
M. gastrocnemius, caput mediale
M. fibularis longus
M. soleus
Tibia
M. tibialis anterior
M. extensor digitorum longus
M. extensor hallucis longus
Malleolus medialis
M. fibularis tertius (variable)
M. extensor hallucis brevis
Mm. interossei dorsalis pedis
M. extensor digitorum longus
M. extensor hallucis longus

A All muscles shown.

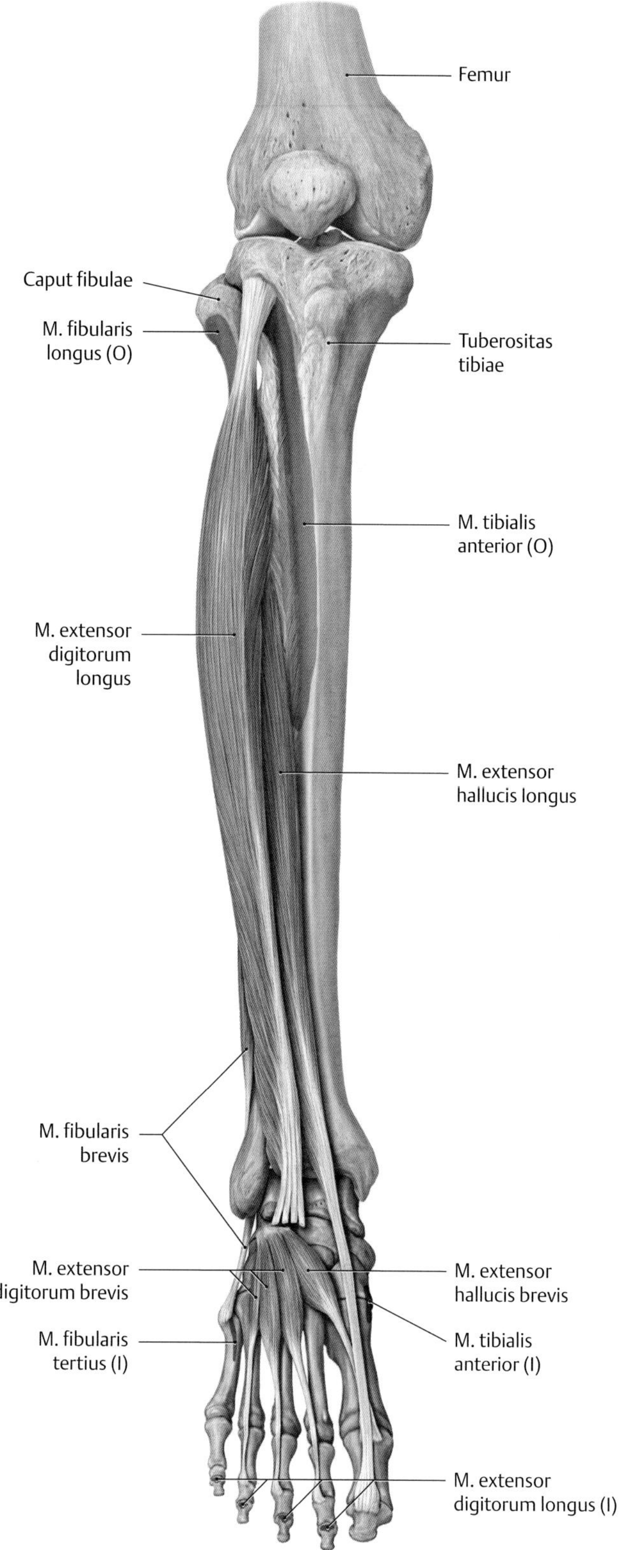
Femur
Caput fibulae
M. fibularis longus (O)
Tuberositas tibiae
M. tibialis anterior (O)
M. extensor digitorum longus
M. extensor hallucis longus
M. fibularis brevis
M. extensor digitorum brevis
M. extensor hallucis brevis
M. fibularis tertius (I)
M. tibialis anterior (I)
M. extensor digitorum longus (I)

B *Removed:* M. tibialis anterior and m. fibularis longus; m. extensor digitorum longus tendons (distal portions). *Note*: M. fibularis tertius is a division of m. extensor digitorum longus.

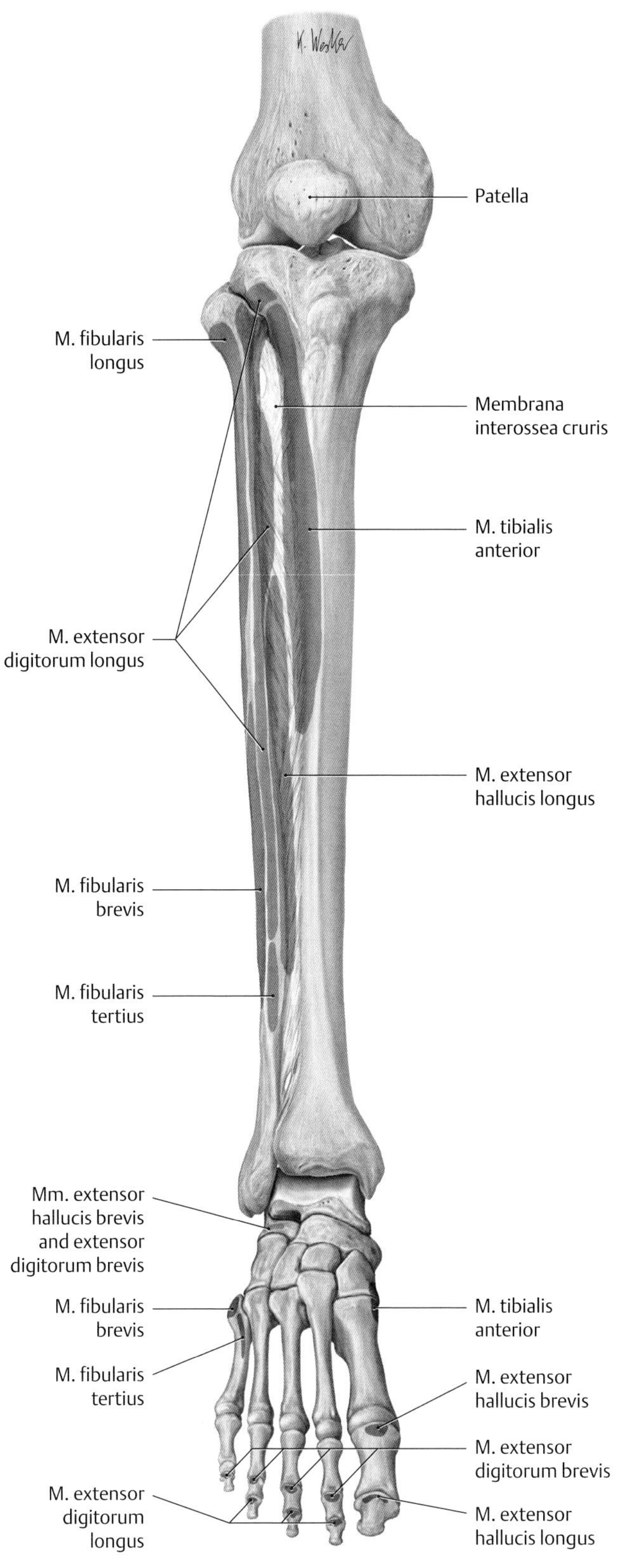
Patella
M. fibularis longus
Membrana interossea cruris
M. tibialis anterior
M. extensor digitorum longus
M. extensor hallucis longus
M. fibularis brevis
M. fibularis tertius
Mm. extensor hallucis brevis and extensor digitorum brevis
M. fibularis brevis
M. tibialis anterior
M. fibularis tertius
M. extensor hallucis brevis
M. extensor digitorum brevis
M. extensor digitorum longus
M. extensor hallucis longus

C *Removed:* All muscles.

Fig. 25.20 Muscles of the leg: Lateral view

Right leg.

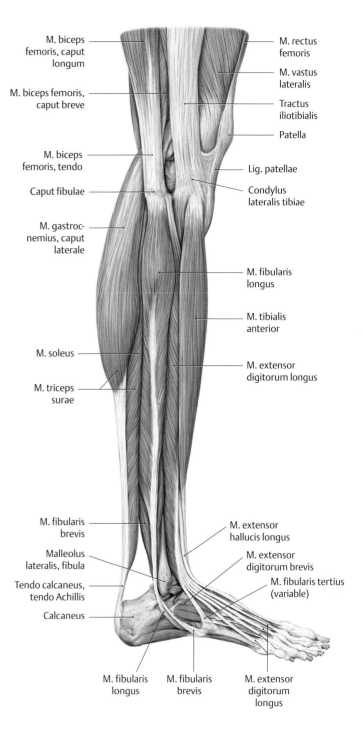

M. biceps femoris, caput longum
M. rectus femoris
M. vastus lateralis
M. biceps femoris, caput breve
Tractus iliotibialis
Patella
M. biceps femoris, tendo
Lig. patellae
Caput fibulae
Condylus lateralis tibiae
M. gastrocnemius, caput laterale
M. fibularis longus
M. tibialis anterior
M. soleus
M. extensor digitorum longus
M. triceps surae
M. fibularis brevis
M. extensor hallucis longus
Malleolus lateralis, fibula
M. extensor digitorum brevis
Tendo calcaneus, tendo Achillis
M. fibularis tertius (variable)
Calcaneus
M. fibularis longus
M. fibularis brevis
M. extensor digitorum longus

Muscles of the Leg: Posterior View

Fig. 25.21 **Muscles of the leg: Posterior view**
Right leg. Muscle origins (O) shown in red, insertions (I) in blue.

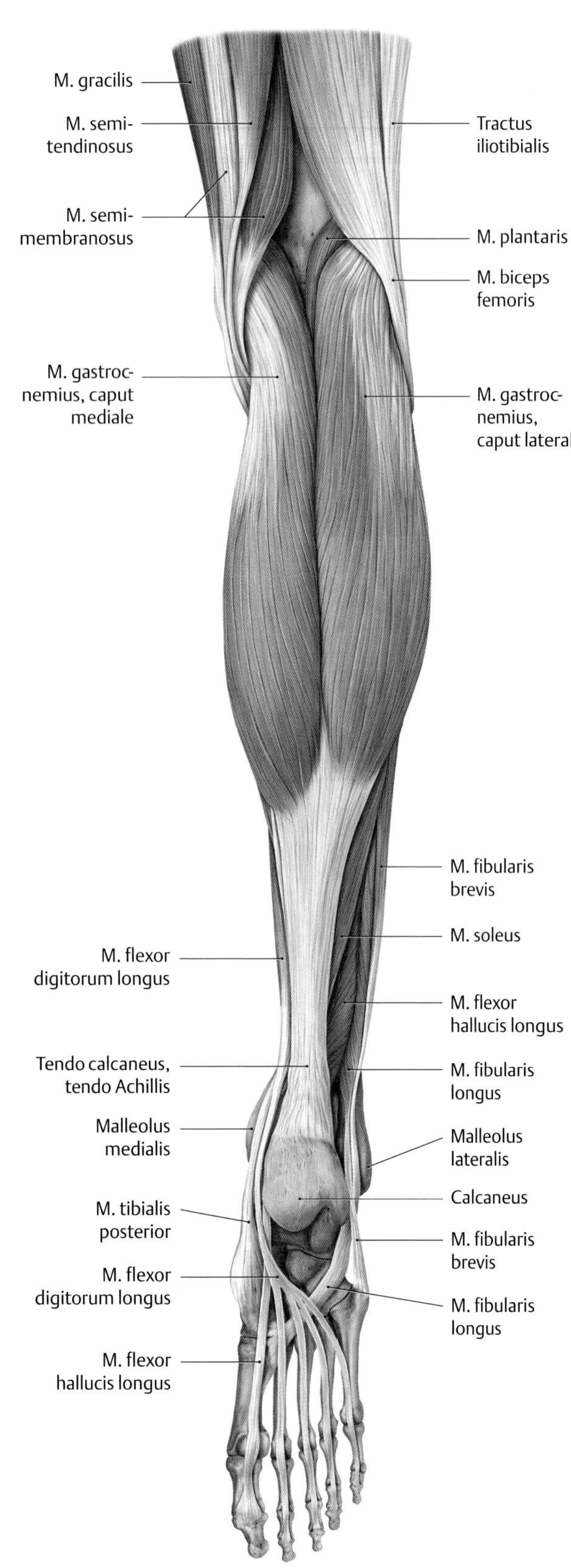
M. gracilis
M. semi-tendinosus
M. semi-membranosus
M. gastroc-nemius, caput mediale
Tractus iliotibialis
M. plantaris
M. biceps femoris
M. gastroc-nemius, caput laterale
M. fibularis brevis
M. soleus
M. flexor digitorum longus
M. flexor hallucis longus
Tendo calcaneus, tendo Achillis
M. fibularis longus
Malleolus medialis
Malleolus lateralis
Calcaneus
M. tibialis posterior
M. fibularis brevis
M. flexor digitorum longus
M. fibularis longus
M. flexor hallucis longus

A *Note:* The bulge of the calf is produced mainly by m. triceps surae (m. soleus and the two heads of m. gastrocnemius).

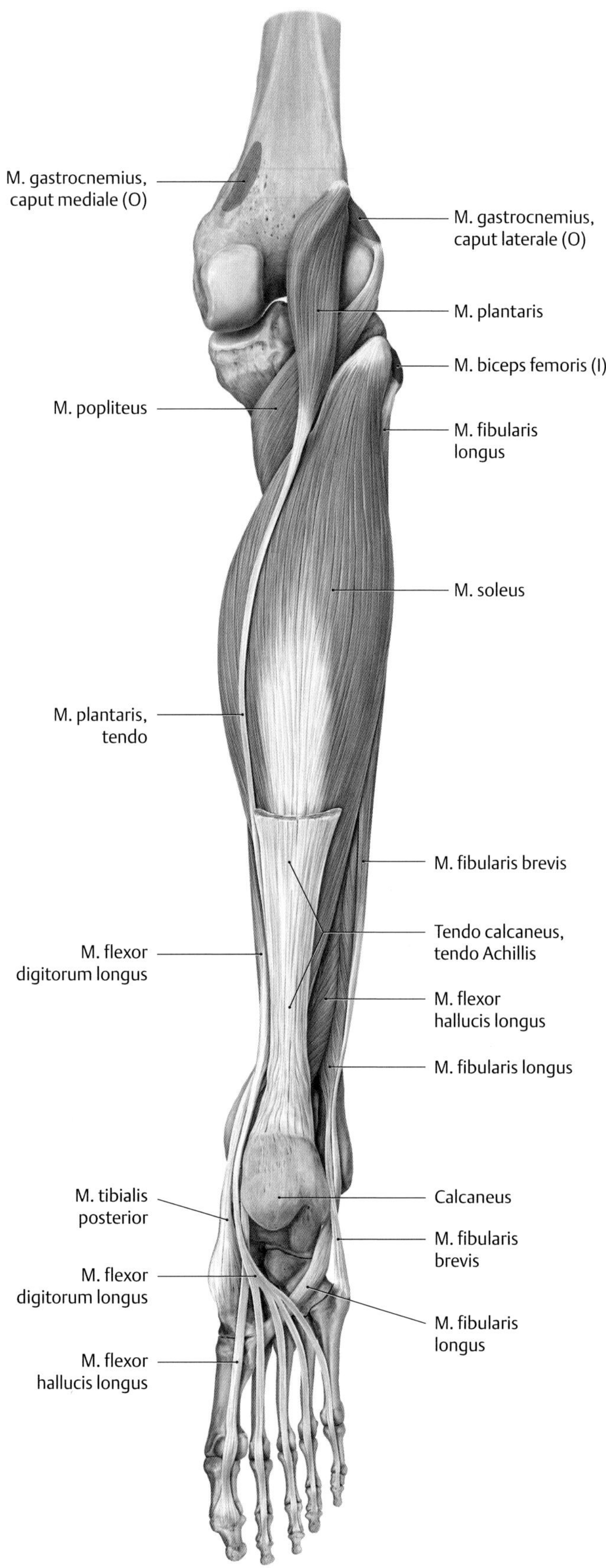
M. gastrocnemius, caput mediale (O)
M. gastrocnemius, caput laterale (O)
M. plantaris
M. biceps femoris (I)
M. popliteus
M. fibularis longus
M. soleus
M. plantaris, tendo
M. fibularis brevis
Tendo calcaneus, tendo Achillis
M. flexor digitorum longus
M. flexor hallucis longus
M. fibularis longus
M. tibialis posterior
Calcaneus
M. fibularis brevis
M. flexor digitorum longus
M. fibularis longus
M. flexor hallucis longus

B *Removed:* M. gastrocnemius (both heads).

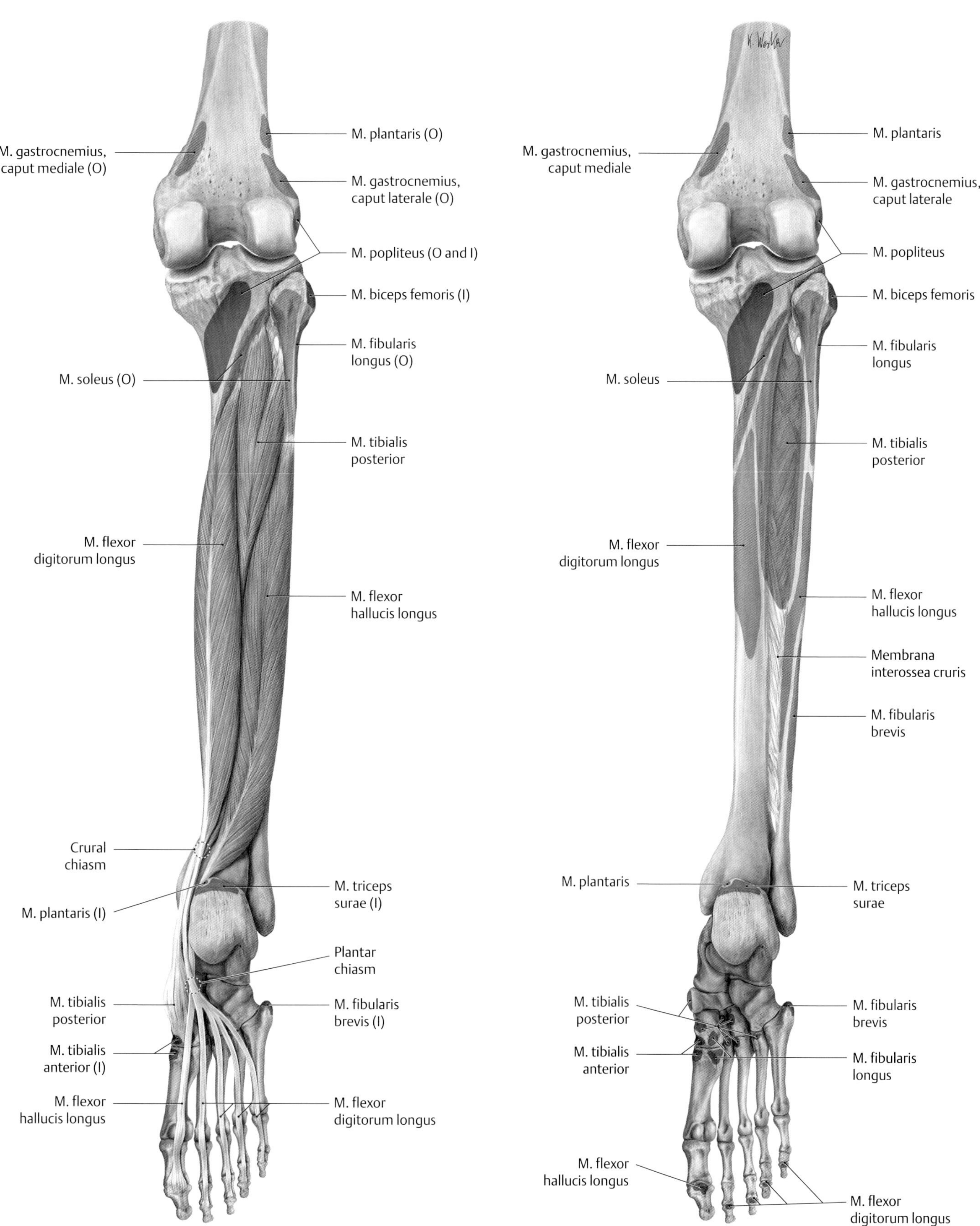
M. gastrocnemius, caput mediale (O)
M. plantaris (O)
M. gastrocnemius, caput laterale (O)
M. popliteus (O and I)
M. biceps femoris (I)
M. fibularis longus (O)
M. soleus (O)
M. tibialis posterior
M. flexor digitorum longus
M. flexor hallucis longus
Crural chiasm
M. plantaris (I)
M. triceps surae (I)
Plantar chiasm
M. tibialis posterior
M. fibularis brevis (I)
M. tibialis anterior (I)
M. flexor hallucis longus
M. flexor digitorum longus
M. gastrocnemius, caput mediale
M. plantaris
M. gastrocnemius, caput laterale
M. popliteus
M. biceps femoris
M. fibularis longus
M. soleus
M. tibialis posterior
M. flexor digitorum longus
M. flexor hallucis longus
Membrana interossea cruris
M. fibularis brevis
M. plantaris
M. triceps surae
M. tibialis posterior
M. fibularis brevis
M. tibialis anterior
M. fibularis longus
M. flexor hallucis longus
M. flexor digitorum longus

C *Removed:* M. triceps surae, m. plantaris, m. popliteus, and m. fibularis longus.

D *Removed:* All muscles.

Muscle Facts (I)

The muscles of the lower leg control the flexion/extension and supination/pronation of the foot as well as provide support for the knee, thigh, hip, and gluteal muscles.

Fig. 25.22 **Lateral compartment**
Right leg and foot.

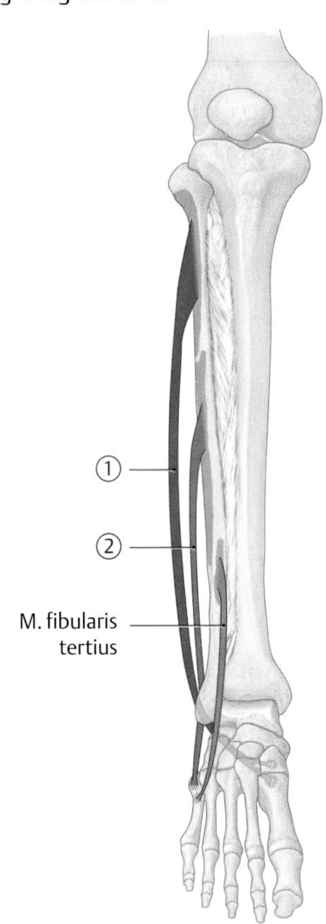
①
②
M. fibularis tertius

A Fibularis group, anterior view.

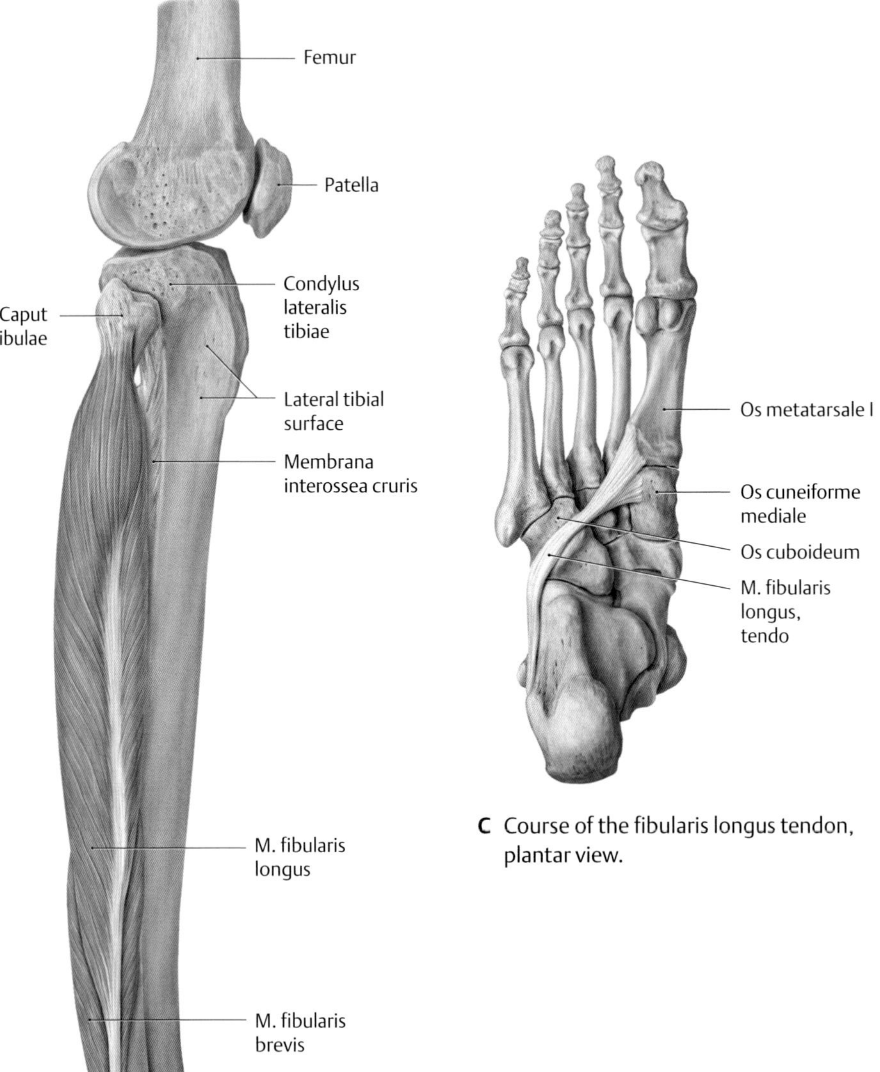
Femur
Patella
Caput fibulae
Condylus lateralis tibiae
Lateral tibial surface
Membrana interossea cruris
M. fibularis longus
M. fibularis brevis
Malleolus lateralis
Calcaneus
Os cuboideum
M. fibularis longus, tendo
M. fibularis brevis, tendo
Tuberositas ossis metatarsalis quinti [V]
Os metatarsale I
Os cuneiforme mediale
Os cuboideum
M. fibularis longus, tendo

B Lateral compartment, right lateral view.

C Course of the fibularis longus tendon, plantar view.

Table 25.2 Lateral compartment

Muscle	Origin	Insertion	Innervation	Action
① M. fibularis longus	Caput fibulae, facies lateralis and margo anterior of fibula, septa intermuscularia	Os cuneiforme intermedium (pars plantaris), tuberositas ossis metatarsi I	N. fibularis superficialis (L5, S1)	• Articulatio talocruralis: plantar flexion • Articulatio subtalaris: eversion (pronation) • Supports the transverse arch of the foot
② M. fibularis brevis	Fibula (distal half of the lateral surface), septa intermuscularia	Tuberositas ossis metatarsi V		• Articulatio talocruralis: plantar flexion • Articulatio subtalaris: eversion (pronation)

Fig. 25.23 **Anterior compartment**
Right leg, anterior view.

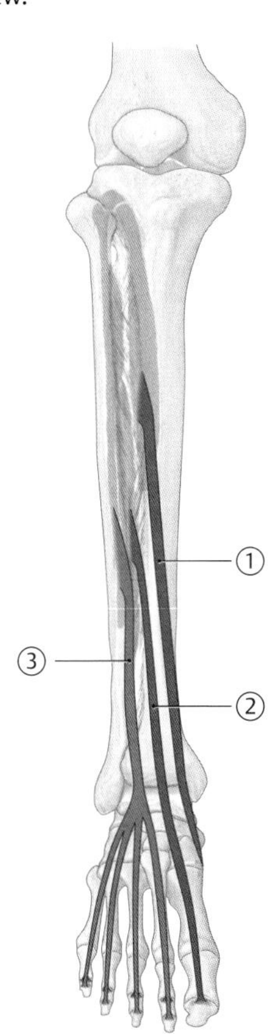
①
③
②

A Schematic.

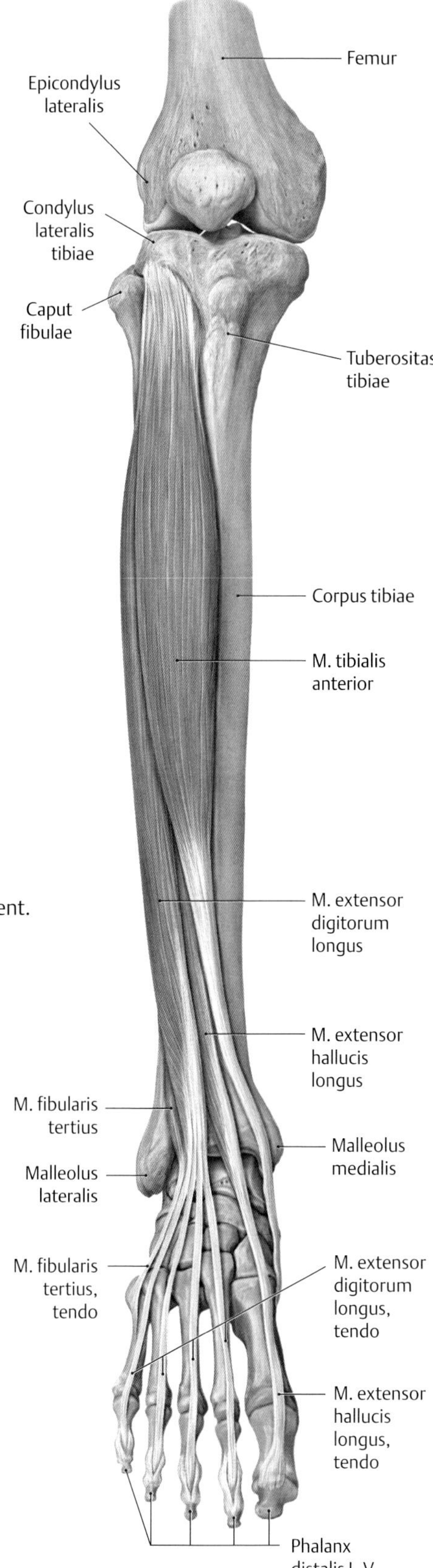
Femur
Epicondylus lateralis
Condylus lateralis tibiae
Caput fibulae
Tuberositas tibiae
Corpus tibiae
M. tibialis anterior
M. extensor digitorum longus
M. extensor hallucis longus
M. fibularis tertius
Malleolus medialis
Malleolus lateralis
M. fibularis tertius, tendo
M. extensor digitorum longus, tendo
M. extensor hallucis longus, tendo
Phalanx distalis I–V

B Anterior compartment.

Table 25.3 **Anterior compartment**

Muscle	Origin	Insertion	Innervation	Action
① M. tibialis anterior	Fascies lateralis of tibia (upper two thirds), membrana interossea, fascia cruris (highest part)	Os cuneiforme mediale (medial and plantar surface), medial base os metatarsi I	N. fibularis profundus (L4, L5)	• Articulatio talocruralis: dorsiflexion • Articulatio subtalaris: inversion (supination)
② M. extensor hallucis longus	Fascies medialis of fibula, membrana interossea	1st toe (aponeurosis dorsalis and the base of its phalanx distalis)	N. fibularis profundus (L5)	• Articulatio talocruralis: dorsiflexion • Articulatio subtalaris: active in both eversion and inversion (pronation/supination), depending on the initial position of the foot • Extends the MTP and IP joints of the big toe
③ M. extensor digitorum longus	Caput fibulae, fascies medialis of fibula, tibia (condylus lateralis), membrana interossea	2nd to 5th toes (at the aponeuroses dorsales and bases of the phalanx distalis)	N. fibularis profundus (L5, S1)	• Articulatio talocruralis: dorsiflexion • Articulatio subtalaris: eversion (pronation) • Extends the MTP and IP joints of the 2nd to 5th toes
M. fibularis tertius (see Fig. 25.22A)	Distal fibula (anterior border)	Os metatarsi I (base)	N. fibularis profundus (L5, S1)	• Articulatio talocruralis: dorsiflexion • Articulatio subtalaris: eversion (pronation)

IP = Articulationes interphalangeae pedis; MTP = Articulationes metatarsophalangeae.

Muscle Facts (II)

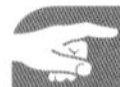

The muscles of the posterior compartment are divided into two groups: the superficial and deep flexors. These groups are separated by the transverse intermuscular septum.

Fig. 25.24 Superficial flexors

Right leg, posterior view.

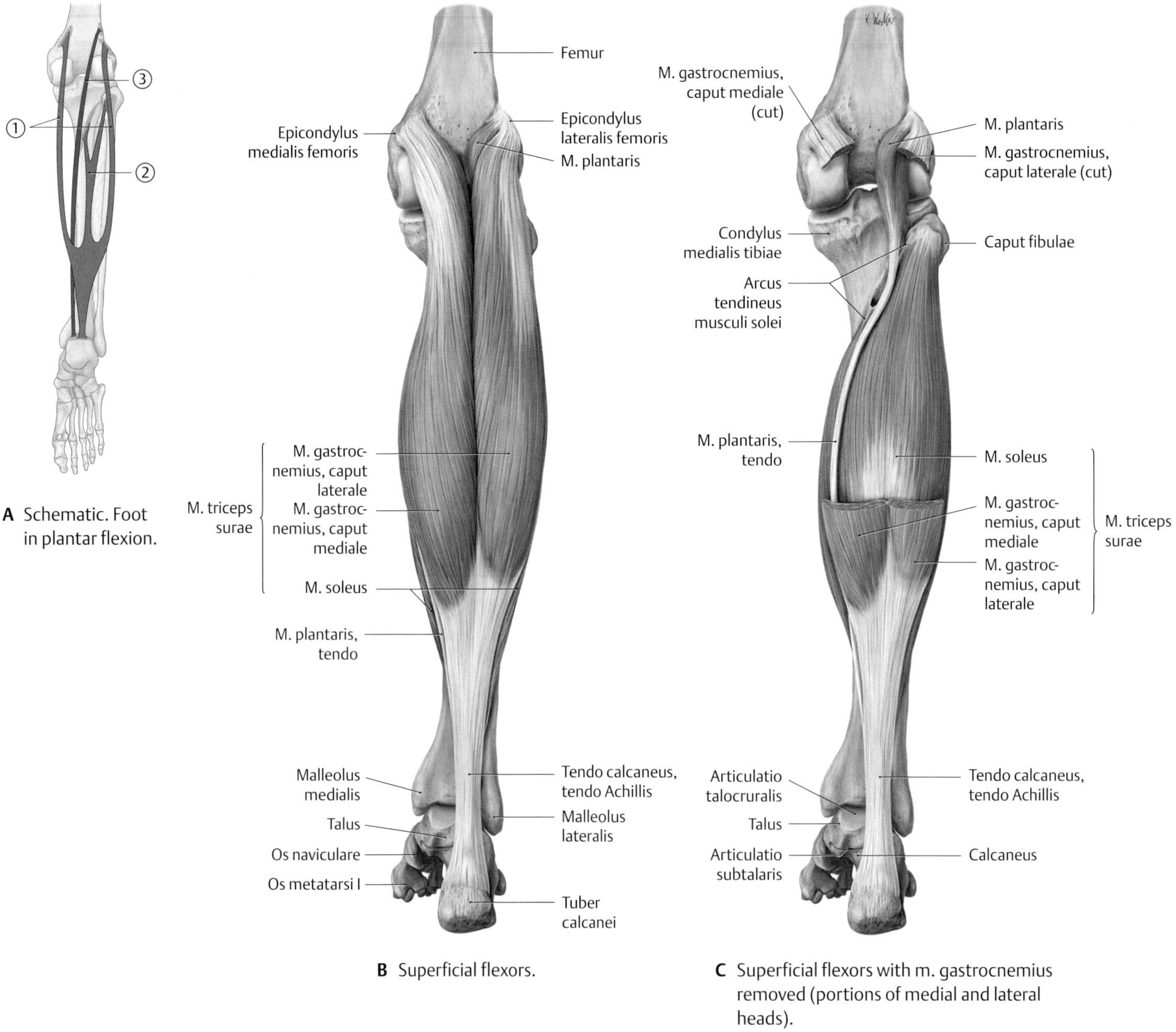

①
③
②

A Schematic. Foot in plantar flexion.

Femur
Epicondylus medialis femoris
Epicondylus lateralis femoris
M. plantaris
M. triceps surae
M. gastrocnemius, caput laterale
M. gastrocnemius, caput mediale
M. soleus
M. plantaris, tendo
Malleolus medialis
Talus
Os naviculare
Os metatarsi I
Tendo calcaneus, tendo Achillis
Malleolus lateralis
Tuber calcanei

B Superficial flexors.

M. gastrocnemius, caput mediale (cut)
M. plantaris
M. gastrocnemius, caput laterale (cut)
Condylus medialis tibiae
Caput fibulae
Arcus tendineus musculi solei
M. plantaris, tendo
M. soleus
M. gastrocnemius, caput mediale
M. gastrocnemius, caput laterale
M. triceps surae
Articulatio talocruralis
Talus
Articulatio subtalaris
Tendo calcaneus, tendo Achillis
Calcaneus

C Superficial flexors with m. gastrocnemius removed (portions of medial and lateral heads).

Table 25.4 Superficial flexors of the posterior compartment

Muscle		Origin	Insertion	Innervation	Action
M. triceps surae	① M. gastrocnemius	Femur (epicondylus medialis and lateralis)	Tuber calcanei via tendo calcaneus	N. tibialis (S1, S2)	• Articulatio talocruralis: plantar flexion • Articulatio genus: flexion (m. gastrocnemius)
	② M. soleus	Caput fibula, facies posterior and margo posterior of fibula, tibia, arcus tendineus musculi solei			
③ M. plantaris		Femur (epicondylus lateralis, proximal to caput laterale of m. gastrocnemius)			Negligible; may prevent compression of posterior leg musculature during knee flexion

Fig. 25.25 Deep flexors

Right leg with foot in plantar flexion, posterior view.

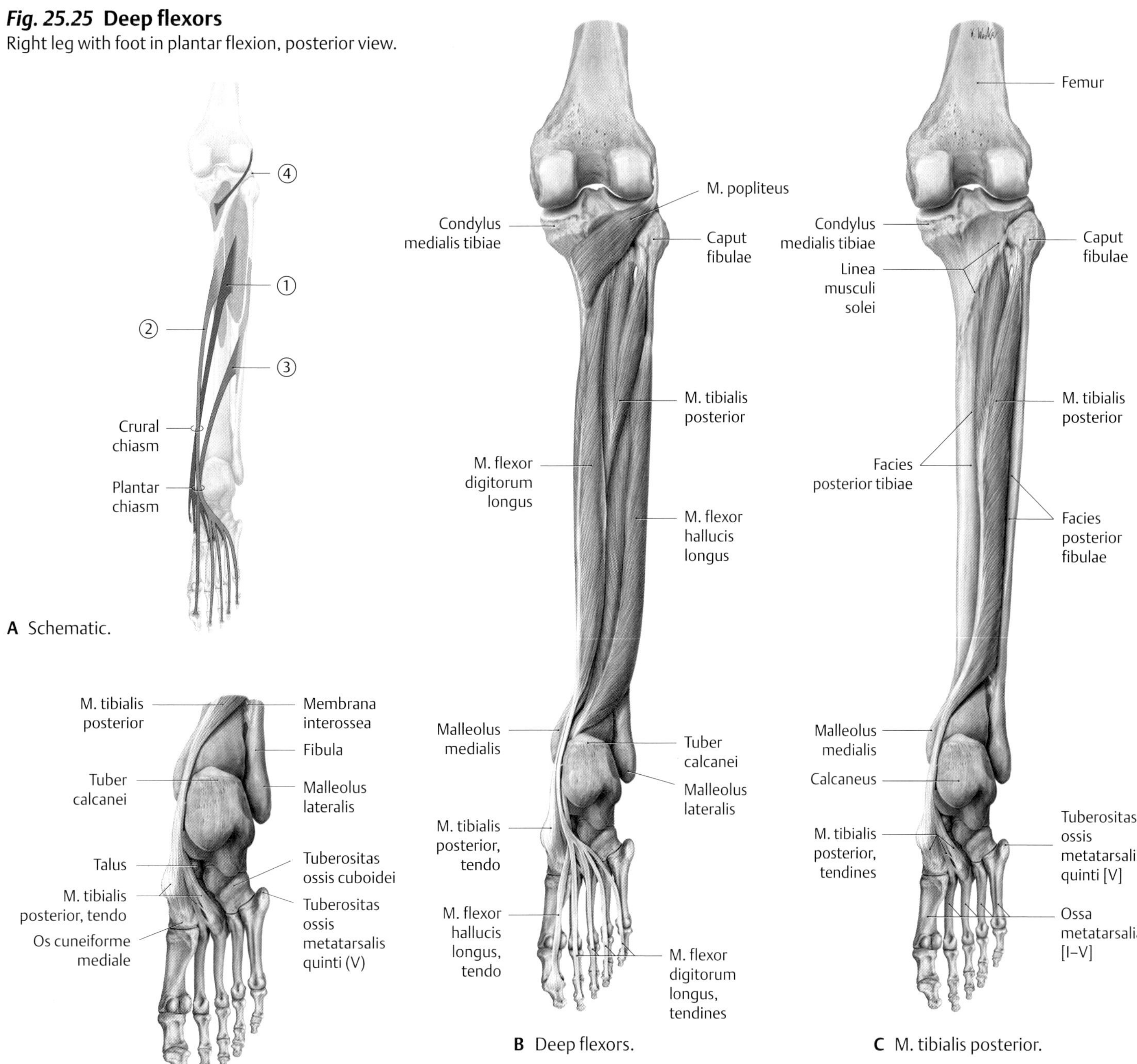
④
①
②
③
Crural chiasm
Plantar chiasm
M. popliteus
Condylus medialis tibiae
Caput fibulae
M. tibialis posterior
M. flexor digitorum longus
M. flexor hallucis longus
Malleolus medialis
Tuber calcanei
Malleolus lateralis
M. tibialis posterior, tendo
M. flexor hallucis longus, tendo
M. flexor digitorum longus, tendines
Femur
Linea musculi solei
Facies posterior tibiae
Facies posterior fibulae
Calcaneus
M. tibialis posterior, tendines
Tuberositas ossis metatarsalis quinti [V]
Ossa metatarsalia [I–V]
Membrana interossea
Fibula
Talus
Tuberositas ossis cuboidei
Os cuneiforme mediale
Tuberositas ossis metatarsalis quinti (V)

A Schematic.

B Deep flexors.

C M. tibialis posterior.

D Insertion of the m. tibialis posterior.

Table 25.5 **Deep flexors of the posterior compartment**

Muscle	Origin	Insertion	Innervation	Action
① M. tibialis posterior	Membrana interossea, fascies posterior of tibia and fibula	Tuberositas ossis navicularis; ossa cuneiforme, ossa metatarsi II–IV (bases)	N. tibialis (L4, L5)	• Articulatio talocruralis: plantar flexion • Articulatio subtalaris: inversion (supination) • Supports the longitudinal and transverse arches
② M. flexor digitorum longus	Tibia (fascies posterior)	Phalanx distalis II–V (bases)	N. tibialis (L5–S2)	• Articulatio talocruralis: plantar flexion • Articulatio subtalaris: inversion (supination) • MTP and IP joints of the 2nd to 5th toes: plantar flexion
③ M. flexor hallucis longus	Fibula (facies posterior, distal two thirds), membrana interossea	Phalanx distalis I (base)		• Articulatio talocruralis: plantar flexion • Articulatio subtalaris: inversion (supination) • MTP and IP joints of the 2nd to 5th toes: plantar flexion • Supports the medial longitudinal arch
④ M. popliteus	Epicondylus lateralis of femur, posterior horn of the meniscus lateralis	Tibia (facies posterior, above the origin at the m. soleus)	N. tibialis (L4–S1)	Articulatio genus: flexion and internal rotation (stabilizes the knee)

IP = Articulationes interphalangeae pedis; MTP = Articulationes metatarsophalangeae.

Ossa Pedis

Fig. 26.1 Subdivisions of the pedal skeleton

Right foot, dorsal view. Descriptive anatomy divides the skeletal elements of the foot into the tarsus, metatarsus, and forefoot (antetarsus). Functional and clinical criteria divide the pedal skeleton into hindfoot, midfoot, and forefoot.

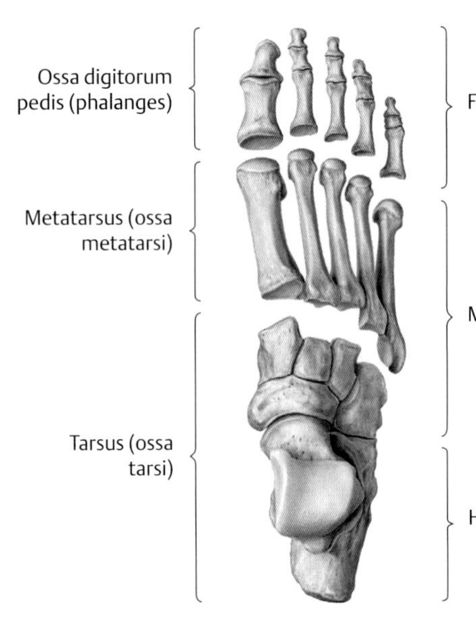
Ossa digitorum pedis (phalanges)
Metatarsus (ossa metatarsi)
Tarsus (ossa tarsi)
Forefoot
Midfoot
Hindfoot

Fig. 26.2 Ossa pedis dexter

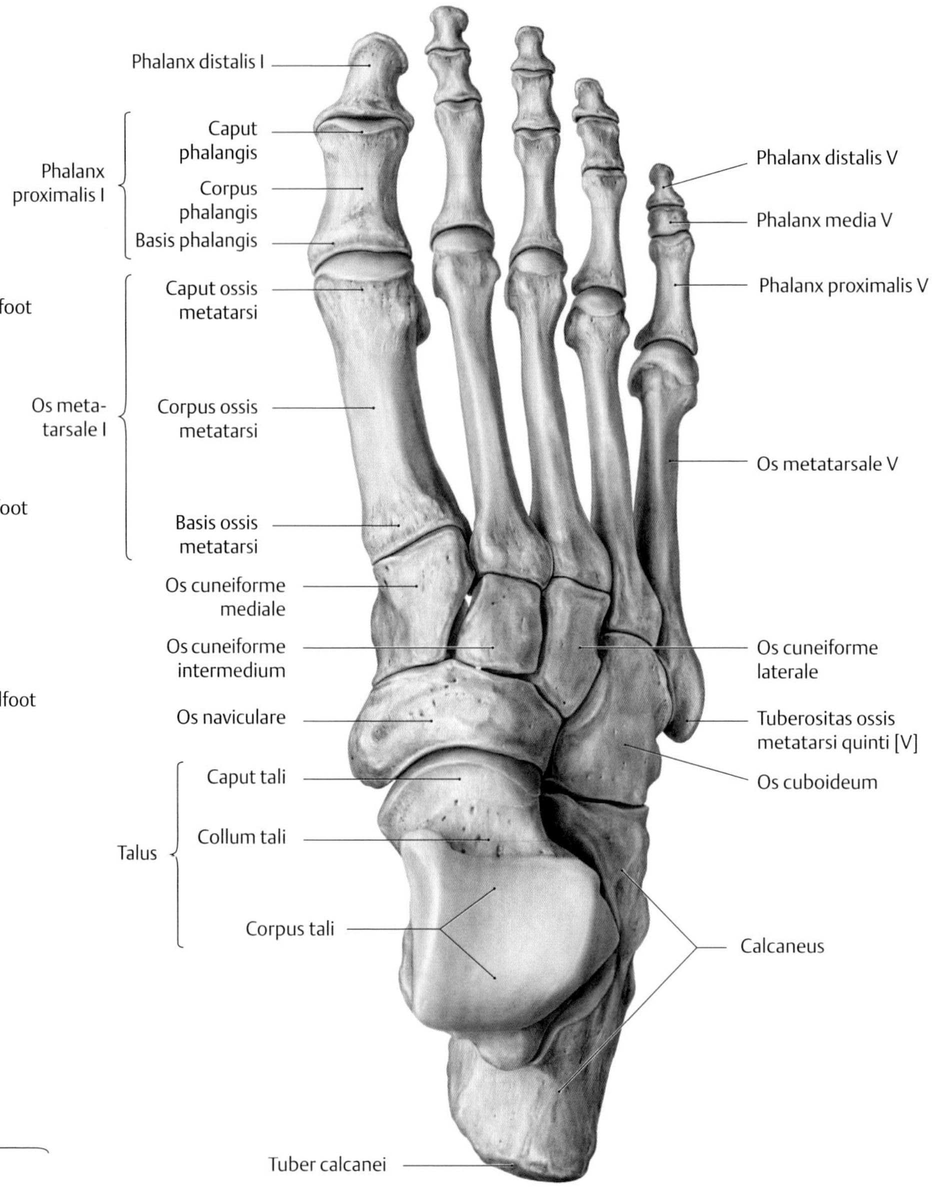

Phalanx distalis I
Phalanx proximalis I
Caput phalangis
Corpus phalangis
Basis phalangis
Os metatarsale I
Caput ossis metatarsi
Corpus ossis metatarsi
Basis ossis metatarsi
Os cuneiforme mediale
Os cuneiforme intermedium
Os naviculare
Talus
Caput tali
Collum tali
Corpus tali
Tuber calcanei
Phalanx distalis V
Phalanx media V
Phalanx proximalis V
Os metatarsale V
Os cuneiforme laterale
Tuberositas ossis metatarsi quinti [V]
Os cuboideum
Calcaneus

A Dorsal (superior) view.

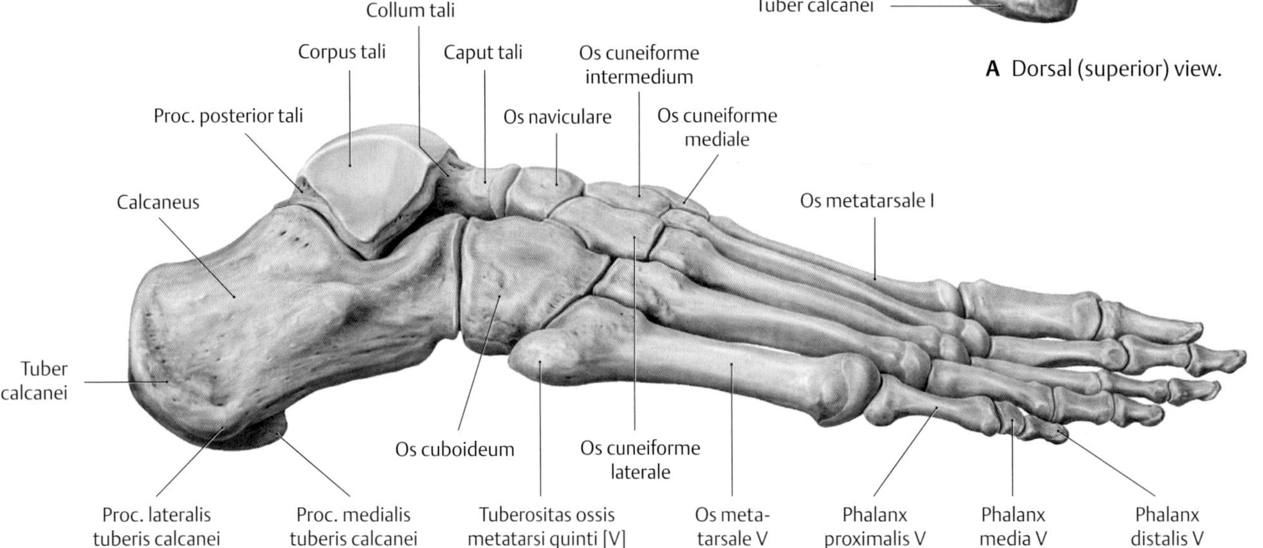
Talus
Collum tali
Corpus tali
Caput tali
Os cuneiforme intermedium
Proc. posterior tali
Os naviculare
Os cuneiforme mediale
Calcaneus
Os metatarsale I
Tuber calcanei
Os cuboideum
Os cuneiforme laterale
Proc. lateralis tuberis calcanei
Proc. medialis tuberis calcanei
Tuberositas ossis metatarsi quinti [V]
Os metatarsale V
Phalanx proximalis V
Phalanx media V
Phalanx distalis V

B Lateral view.

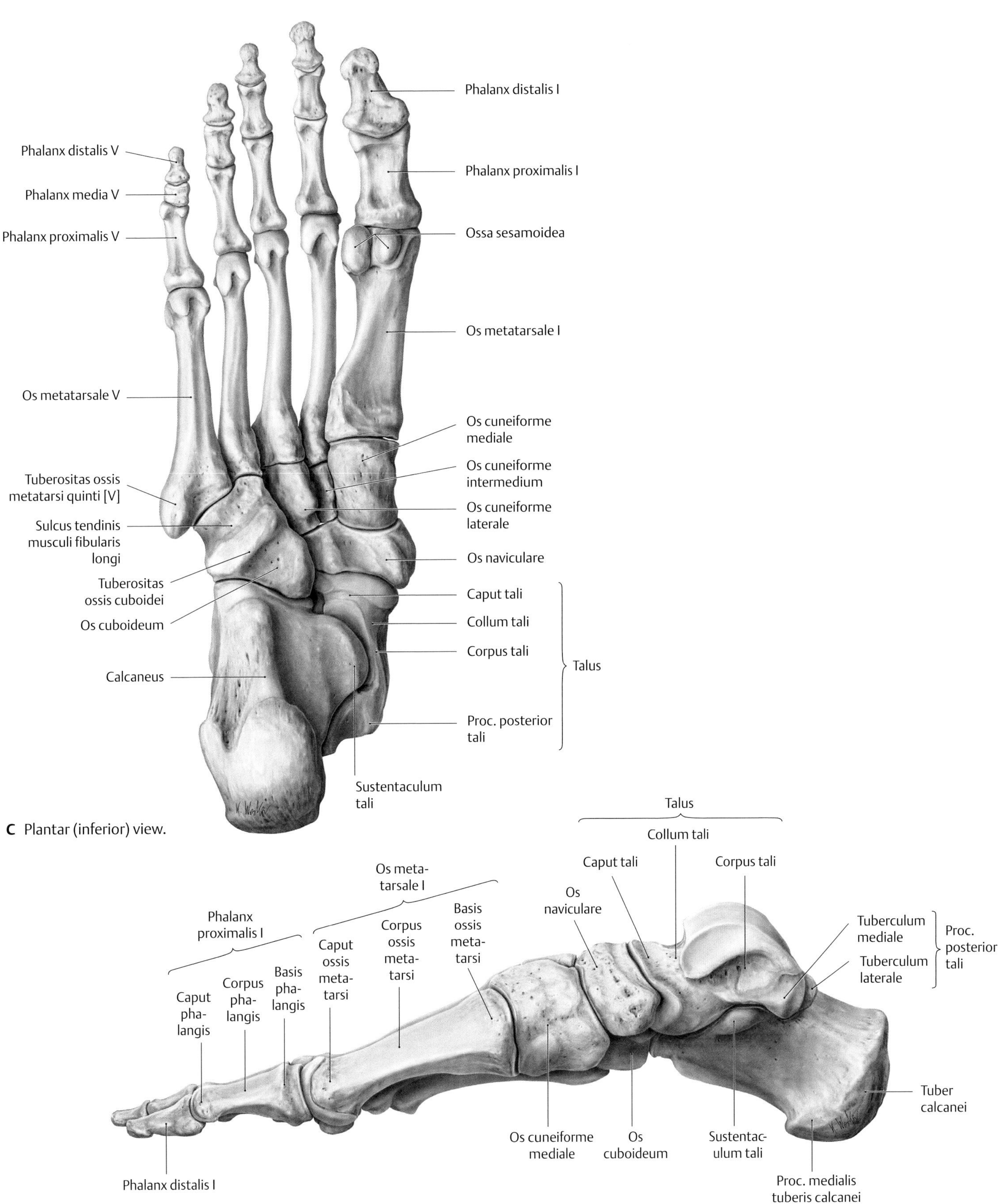

Phalanx distalis I
Phalanx proximalis I
Ossa sesamoidea
Os metatarsale I
Os cuneiforme mediale
Os cuneiforme intermedium
Os cuneiforme laterale
Os naviculare
Caput tali
Collum tali
Corpus tali
Talus
Proc. posterior tali
Sustentaculum tali
Phalanx distalis V
Phalanx media V
Phalanx proximalis V
Os metatarsale V
Tuberositas ossis metatarsi quinti [V]
Sulcus tendinis musculi fibularis longi
Tuberositas ossis cuboidei
Os cuboideum
Calcaneus

C Plantar (inferior) view.

Talus
Collum tali
Caput tali
Corpus tali
Os naviculare
Os metatarsale I
Basis ossis metatarsi
Corpus ossis metatarsi
Caput ossis metatarsi
Phalanx proximalis I
Basis phalangis
Corpus phalangis
Caput phalangis
Tuberculum mediale
Tuberculum laterale
Proc. posterior tali
Tuber calcanei
Os cuneiforme mediale
Os cuboideum
Sustentaculum tali
Proc. medialis tuberis calcanei
Phalanx distalis I

D Medial view.

Articulationes Pedis (I)

Fig. 26.3 **Joints of the foot**
Right foot with articulatio talocruralis in plantar flexion.

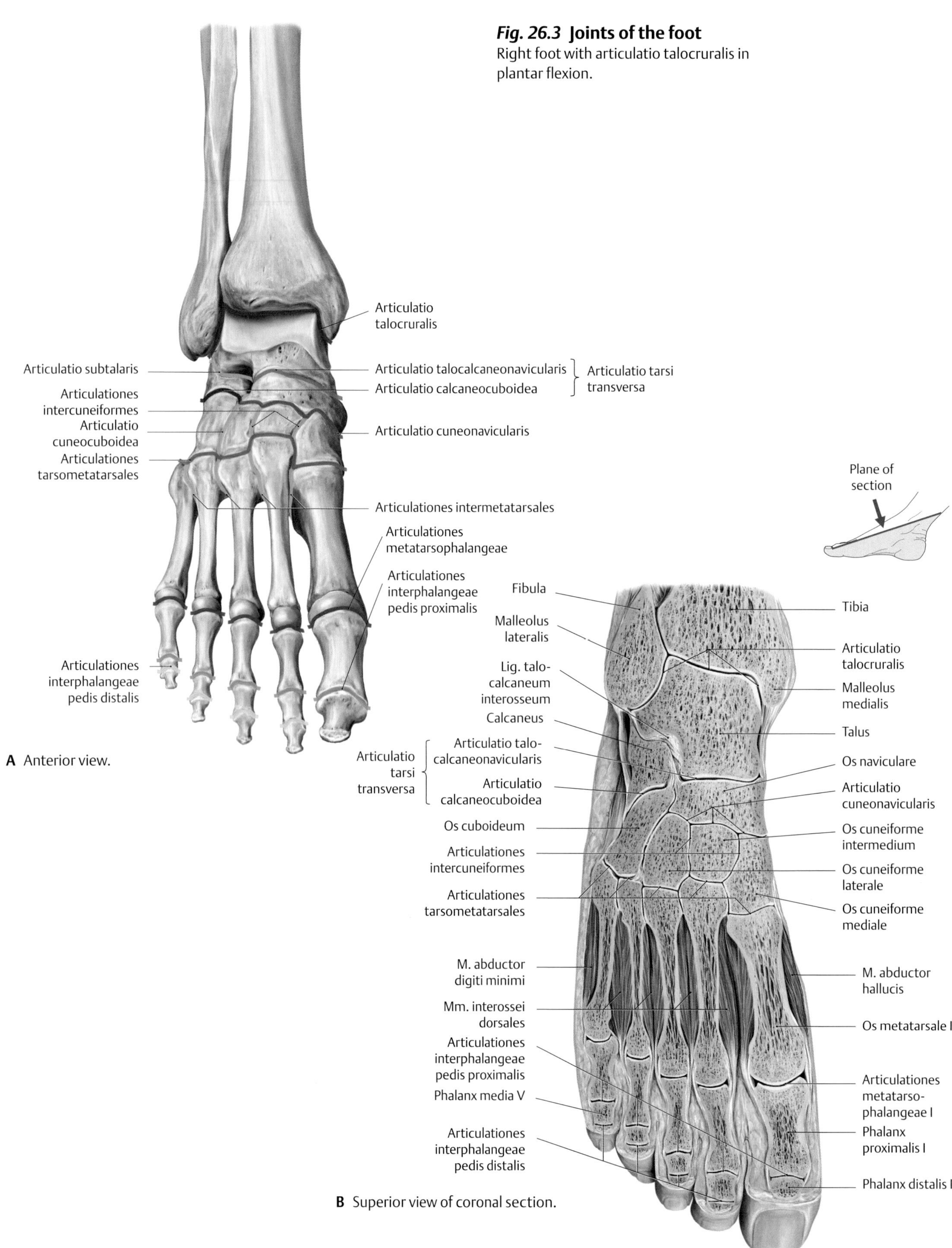
Articulatio talocruralis
Articulatio subtalaris
Articulatio talocalcaneonavicularis
Articulatio calcaneocuboidea
Articulatio tarsi transversa
Articulationes intercuneiformes
Articulatio cuneocuboidea
Articulatio cuneonavicularis
Articulationes tarsometatarsales
Articulationes intermetatarsales
Articulationes metatarsophalangeae
Articulationes interphalangeae pedis proximalis
Articulationes interphalangeae pedis distalis
Plane of section
Fibula
Tibia
Malleolus lateralis
Articulatio talocruralis
Lig. talocalcaneum interosseum
Malleolus medialis
Calcaneus
Talus
Articulatio tarsi transversa
Articulatio talocalcaneonavicularis
Os naviculare
Articulatio calcaneocuboidea
Articulatio cuneonavicularis
Os cuboideum
Os cuneiforme intermedium
Articulationes intercuneiformes
Os cuneiforme laterale
Articulationes tarsometatarsales
Os cuneiforme mediale
M. abductor digiti minimi
M. abductor hallucis
Mm. interossei dorsales
Os metatarsale I
Articulationes interphalangeae pedis proximalis
Articulationes metatarsophalangeae I
Phalanx media V
Phalanx proximalis I
Articulationes interphalangeae pedis distalis
Phalanx distalis I

A Anterior view.

B Superior view of coronal section.

Fig. 26.4 **Proximal articular surfaces**

Right foot, proximal view.

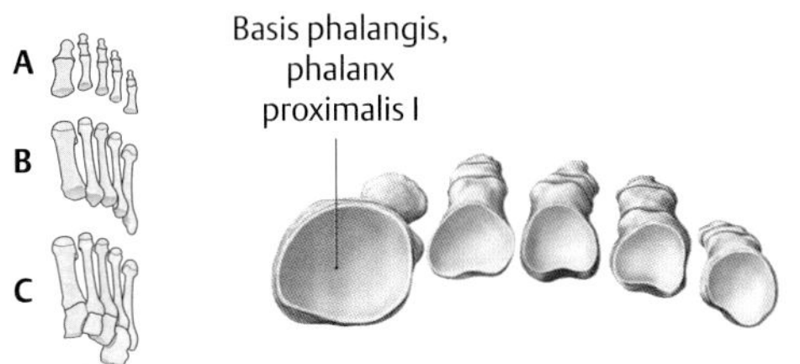
A
B
C
D
Basis phalangis, phalanx proximalis I

A Articulationes metatarsophalangea.

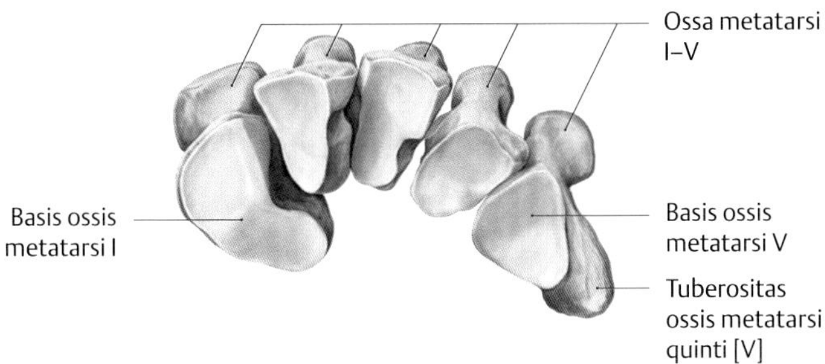
Ossa metatarsi I–V
Basis ossis metatarsi I
Basis ossis metatarsi V
Tuberositas ossis metatarsi quinti [V]

B Articulationes tarsometatarsales.

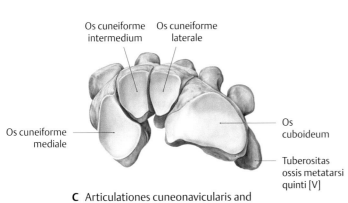

Os cuneiforme intermedium
Os cuneiforme laterale
Os cuneiforme mediale
Os cuboideum
Tuberositas ossis metatarsi quinti [V]

C Articulationes cuneonavicularis and calcaneocuboidea.

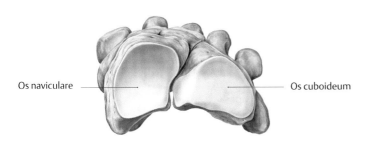

Os naviculare
Os cuboideum

D Articulationes talocalcaneonavicularis and calcaneocuboidea.

Fig. 26.5 **Distal articular surfaces**

Right foot, distal view.

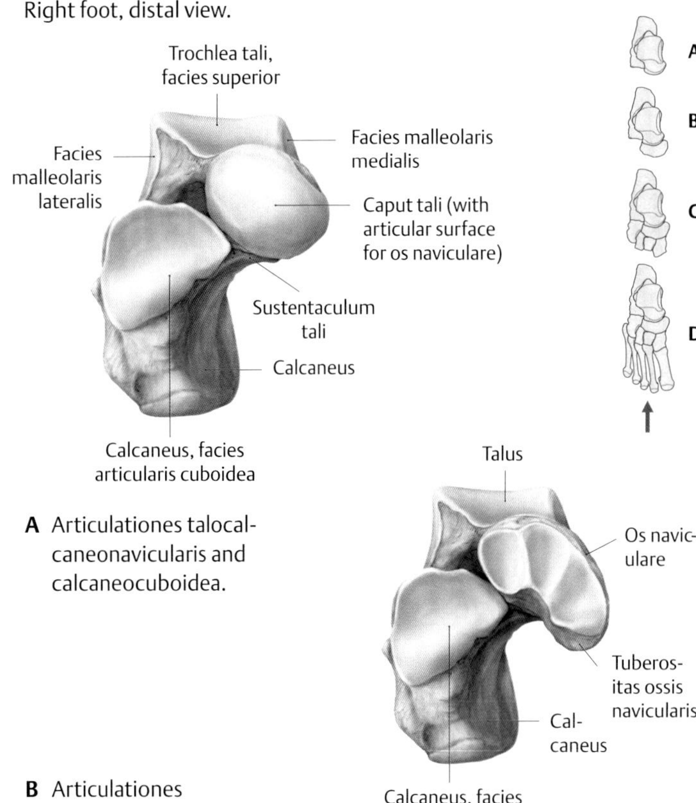
Trochlea tali, facies superior
Facies malleolaris lateralis
Facies malleolaris medialis
Caput tali (with articular surface for os naviculare)
Sustentaculum tali
Calcaneus
Calcaneus, facies articularis cuboidea
A
B
C
D
Talus
Os navicculare
Tuberositas ossis navicularis
Calcaneus
Calcaneus, facies articularis cuboidea

A Articulationes talocalcaneonavicularis and calcaneocuboidea.

B Articulationes cuneonavicularis and calcaneocuboidea.

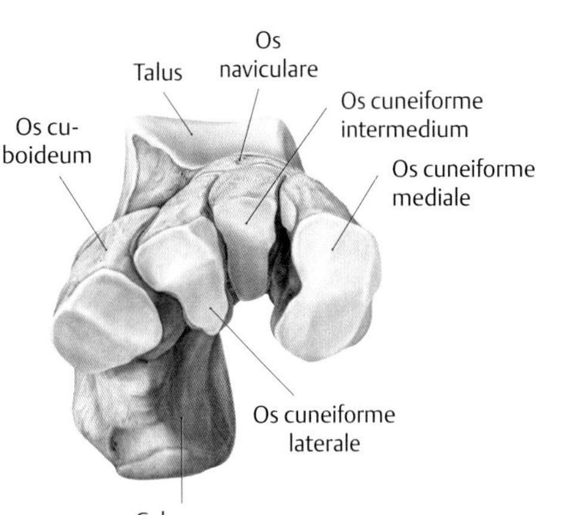
Talus
Os naviculare
Os cuneiforme intermedium
Os cuboideum
Os cuneiforme mediale
Os cuneiforme laterale
Calcaneus

C Articulationes tarsometatarsales.

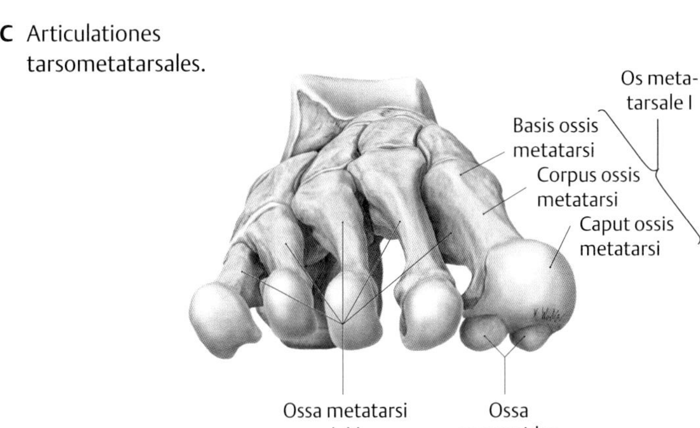
Os metatarsale I
Basis ossis metatarsi
Corpus ossis metatarsi
Caput ossis metatarsi
Ossa metatarsi I–V
Ossa sesamoidea

D Articulationes metatarsophalangeae.

Articulationes Pedis (II)

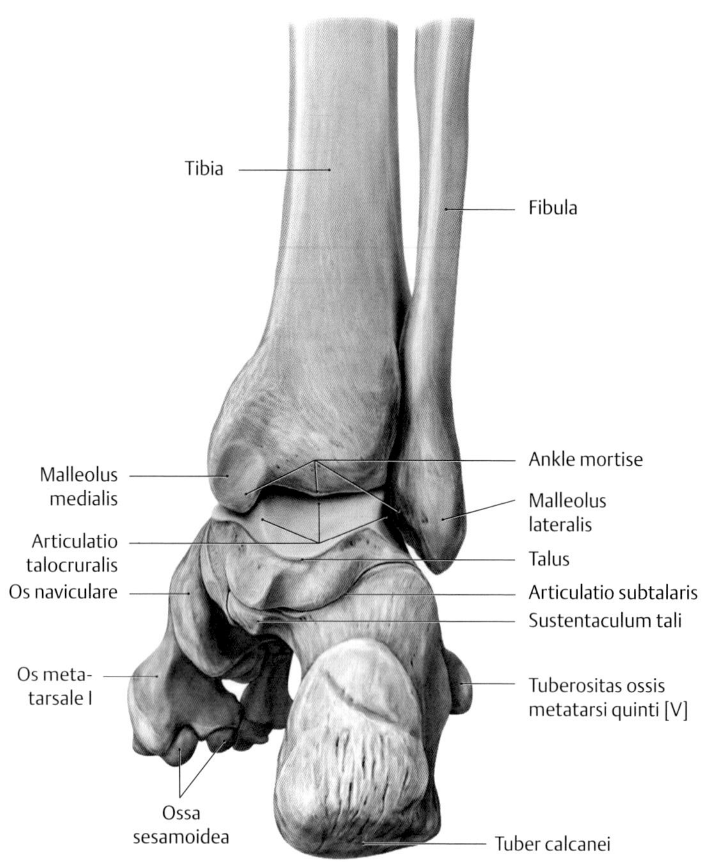
Tibia
Fibula
Malleolus medialis
Ankle mortise
Malleolus lateralis
Articulatio talocruralis
Talus
Os naviculare
Articulatio subtalaris
Sustentaculum tali
Os metatarsale I
Tuberositas ossis metatarsi quinti [V]
Ossa sesamoidea
Tuber calcanei

A Posterior view with foot in neutral (0-degree) position.

Fig. 26.6 **Articulationes talocruralis and subtalaris**
Right foot. Articulatio talocruralis (ankle) joint is formed by the distal ends of the tibia and fibula (ankle mortise) articulating with trochlea tali. The articulatio subtalaris joint consists of an anterior and a posterior compartment (the articulatio talocalcaneus and articulatio talocalcaneonavicularis, respectively) divided by the lig. talocalcaneum interosseum (see p. 409).

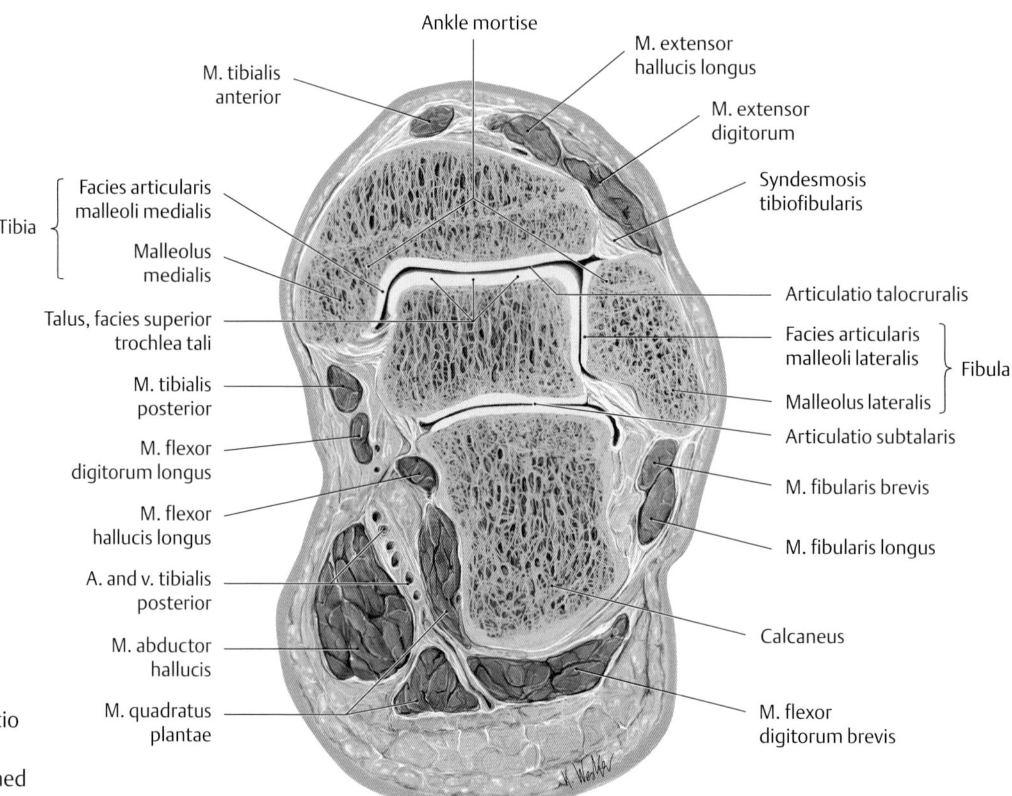
Plane of section
Ankle mortise
M. tibialis anterior
M. extensor hallucis longus
M. extensor digitorum
Syndesmosis tibiofibularis
Tibia
Facies articularis malleoli medialis
Malleolus medialis
Articulatio talocruralis
Talus, facies superior trochlea tali
Facies articularis malleoli lateralis
Fibula
Malleolus lateralis
M. tibialis posterior
Articulatio subtalaris
M. flexor digitorum longus
M. fibularis brevis
M. flexor hallucis longus
M. fibularis longus
A. and v. tibialis posterior
Calcaneus
M. abductor hallucis
M. quadratus plantae
M. flexor digitorum brevis

B Coronal section, proximal view. Articulatio talocruralis is plantar flexed, and the articulatio subtalaris joint has been sectioned through its posterior compartment.

Fig. 26.7 Articulatio talocruralis and articulatio subtalaris: Sagittal section
Right foot, medial view.

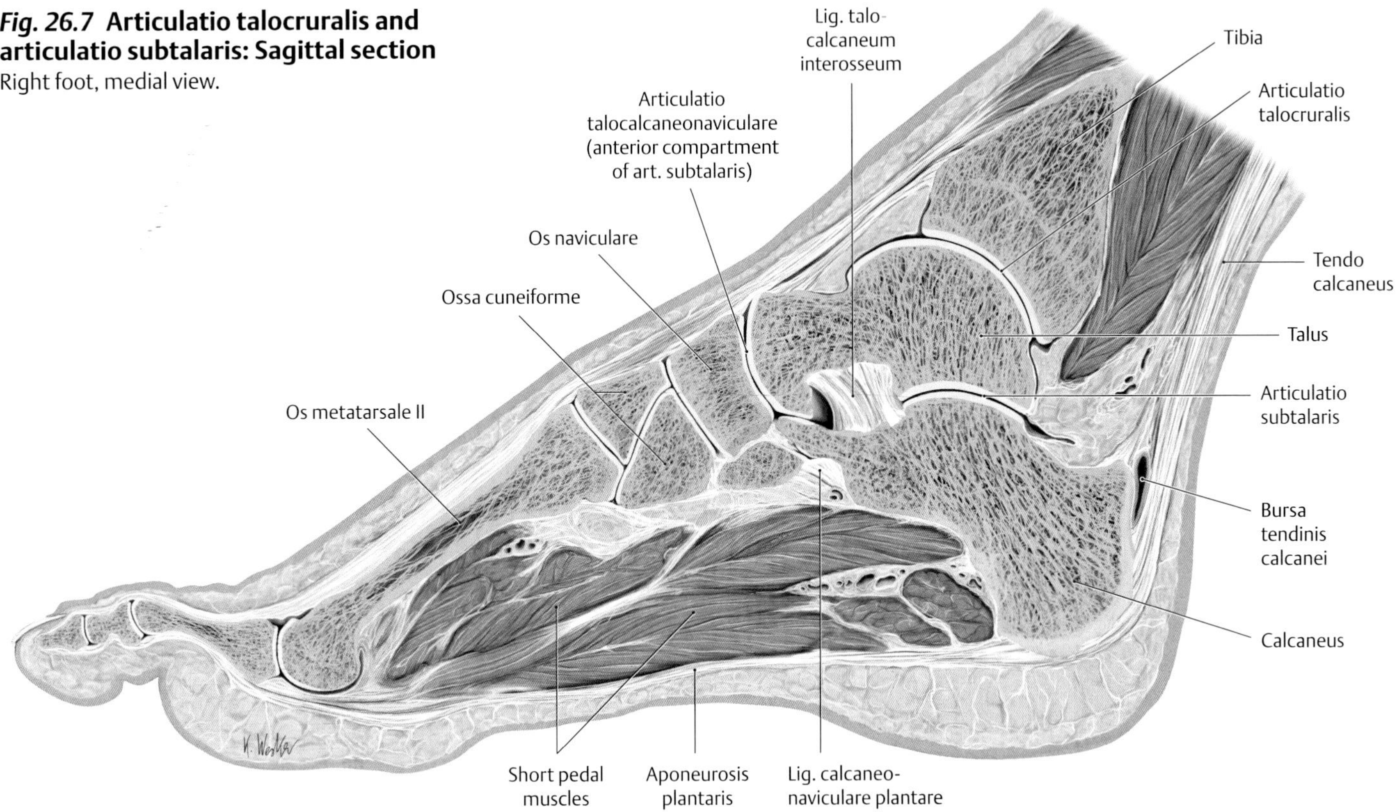
Lig. talo-
calcaneum
interosseum
Tibia
Articulatio
talocalcaneonaviculare
(anterior compartment
of art. subtalaris)
Articulatio
talocruralis
Os naviculare
Ossa cuneiforme
Tendo
calcaneus
Talus
Os metatarsale II
Articulatio
subtalaris
Bursa
tendinis
calcanei
Calcaneus
Short pedal
muscles
Aponeurosis
plantaris
Lig. calcaneo-
naviculare plantare

Fig. 26.8 Articulatio talocruralis
Right foot.

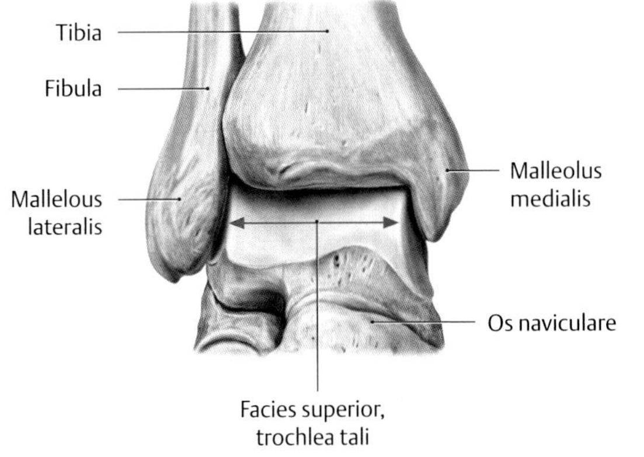
Tibia
Fibula
Malleolus
medialis
Mallelous
lateralis
Os naviculare
Facies superior,
trochlea tali

A Anterior view.

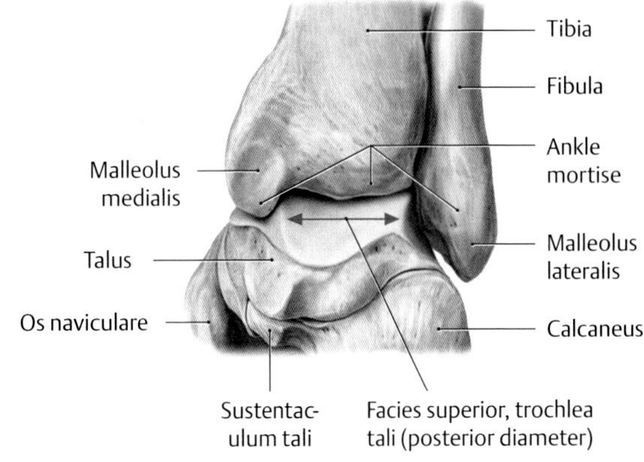
Tibia
Fibula
Ankle
mortise
Malleolus
medialis
Malleolus
lateralis
Talus
Os naviculare
Calcaneus
Sustentac-
ulum tali
Facies superior, trochlea
tali (posterior diameter)

B Posterior view.

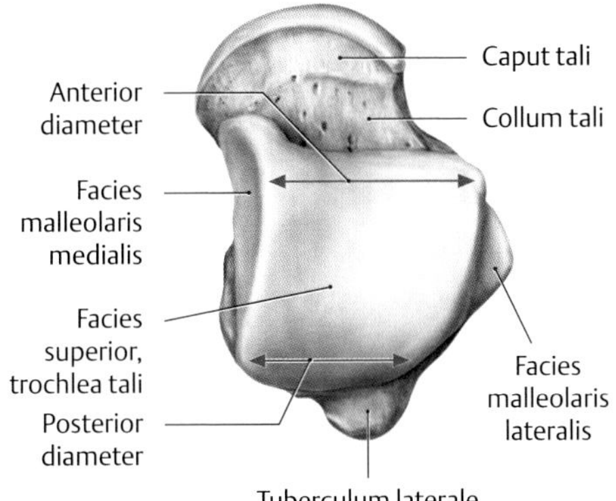
Caput tali
Anterior
diameter
Collum tali
Facies
malleolaris
medialis
Facies
superior,
trochlea tali
Facies
malleolaris
lateralis
Posterior
diameter
Tuberculum laterale

C Proximal (superior) view of talus.

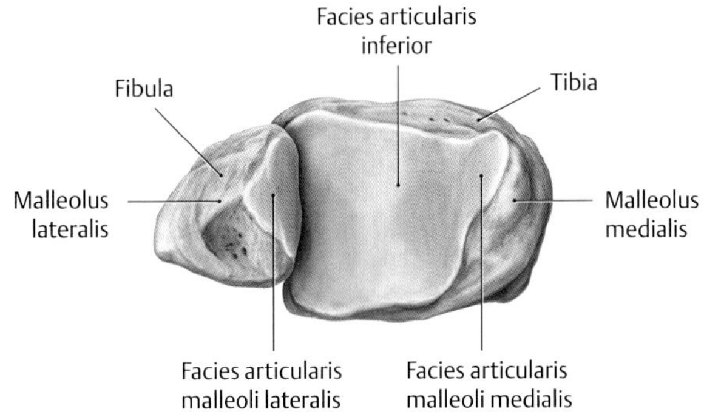
Facies articularis
inferior
Fibula
Tibia
Malleolus
lateralis
Malleolus
medialis
Facies articularis
malleoli lateralis
Facies articularis
malleoli medialis

D Distal (inferior) view of ankle mortise.

Articulationes Pedis (III)

Fig. 26.9 Articulatio subtalaris and ligaments
Right foot with opened articulatio subtalaris. The articulatio subtalaris consists of two distinct articulations separated by lig. talocalcaneus interosseum: the posterior compartment (articulatio talocalcaneus) and the anterior compartment (articulatio talocalcaneonavicularis).

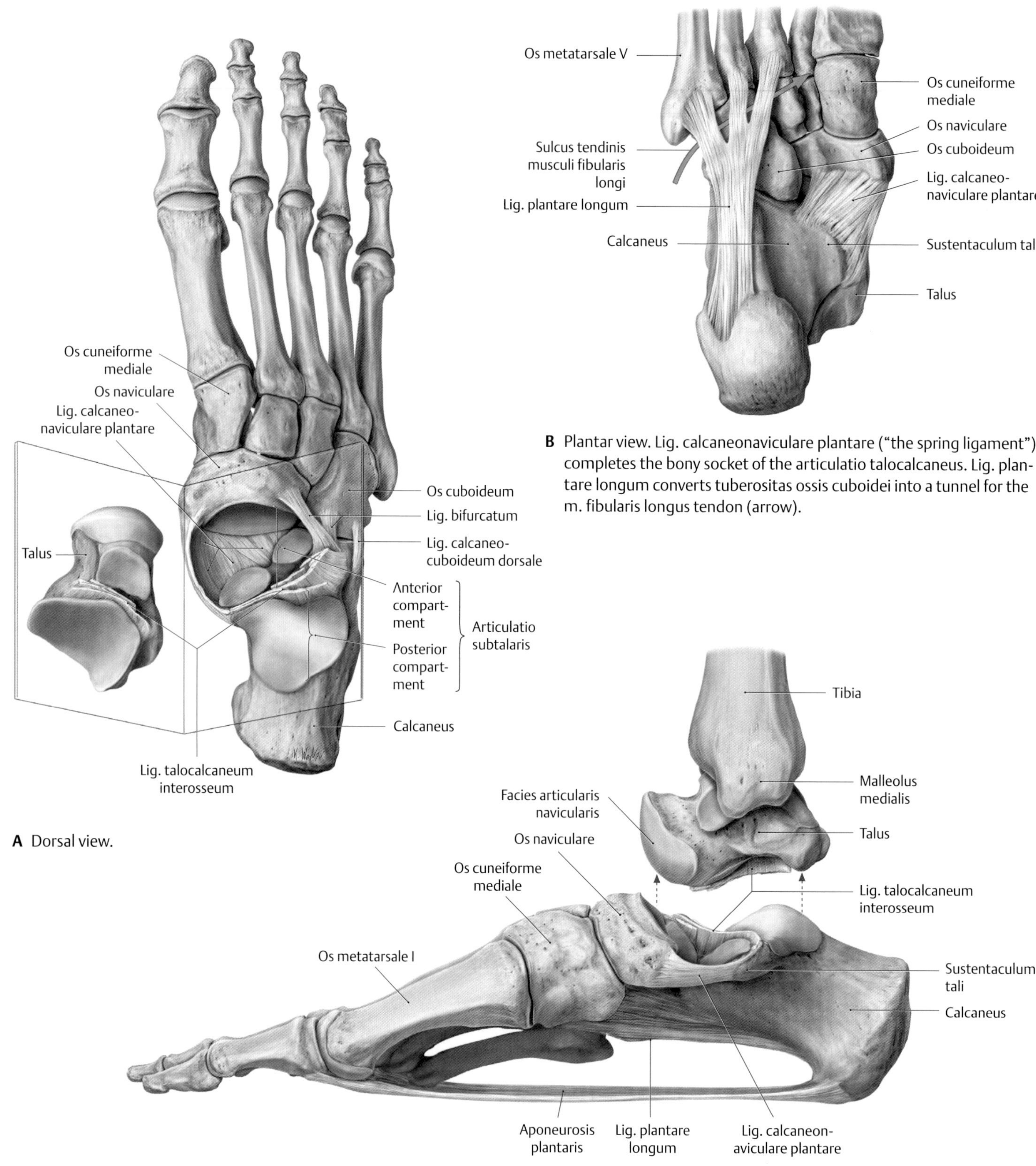

Os metatarsale V
Os cuneiforme mediale
Os naviculare
Os cuboideum
Sulcus tendinis musculi fibularis longi
Lig. calcaneo-naviculare plantare
Lig. plantare longum
Calcaneus
Sustentaculum tali
Talus
Os cuneiforme mediale
Os naviculare
Lig. calcaneo-naviculare plantare
Talus
Os cuboideum
Lig. bifurcatum
Lig. calcaneo-cuboideum dorsale
Anterior compart-ment
Posterior compart-ment
Articulatio subtalaris
Calcaneus
Lig. talocalcaneum interosseum
Tibia
Malleolus medialis
Facies articularis navicularis
Os naviculare
Talus
Os cuneiforme mediale
Lig. talocalcaneum interosseum
Os metatarsale I
Sustentaculum tali
Calcaneus
Aponeurosis plantaris
Lig. plantare longum
Lig. calcaneon-aviculare plantare

A Dorsal view.

B Plantar view. Lig. calcaneonaviculare plantare ("the spring ligament") completes the bony socket of the articulatio talocalcaneus. Lig. plantare longum converts tuberositas ossis cuboidei into a tunnel for the m. fibularis longus tendon (arrow).

C Medial view. Lig. talocalcaneum interosseum has been divided and the talus displaced upward. Note the course of lig. calcaneonaviculare plantare, which functions with lig. plantare longum and aponeurosis plantaris to support the longitudinal arch of the foot.

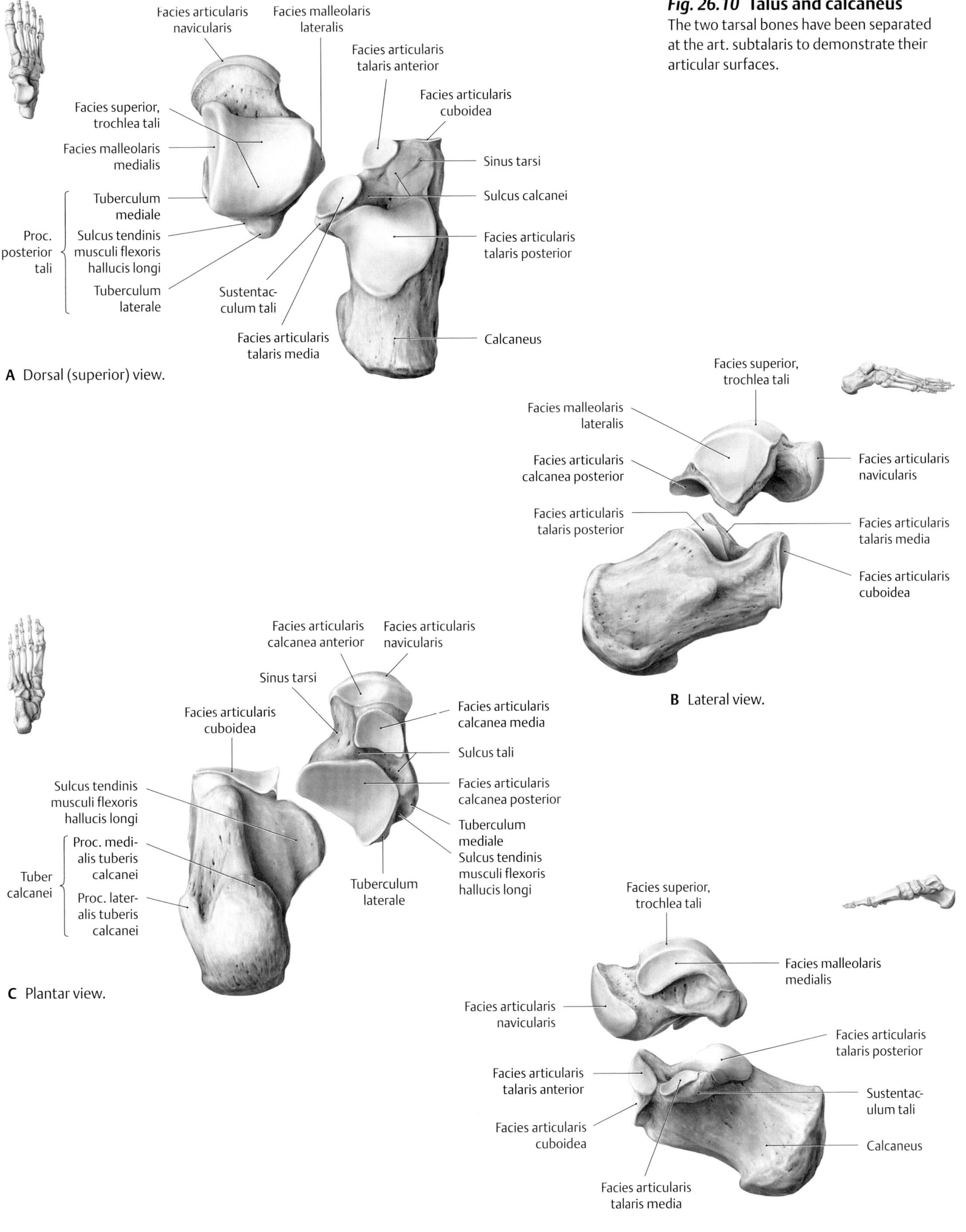

Facies articularis navicularis
Facies malleolaris lateralis
Facies articularis talaris anterior
Facies articularis cuboidea
Facies superior, trochlea tali
Facies malleolaris medialis
Sinus tarsi
Sulcus calcanei
Tuberculum mediale
Proc. posterior tali
Sulcus tendinis musculi flexoris hallucis longi
Facies articularis talaris posterior
Tuberculum laterale
Sustentaculum tali
Facies articularis talaris media
Calcaneus
A Dorsal (superior) view.
Facies superior, trochlea tali
Facies malleolaris lateralis
Facies articularis navicularis
Facies articularis calcanea posterior
Facies articularis talaris posterior
Facies articularis talaris media
Facies articularis cuboidea
B Lateral view.
Facies articularis calcanea anterior
Facies articularis navicularis
Sinus tarsi
Facies articularis cuboidea
Facies articularis calcanea media
Sulcus tali
Sulcus tendinis musculi flexoris hallucis longi
Facies articularis calcanea posterior
Proc. medialis tuberis calcanei
Tuber calcanei
Proc. lateralis tuberis calcanei
Tuberculum mediale
Sulcus tendinis musculi flexoris hallucis longi
Tuberculum laterale
C Plantar view.
Facies superior, trochlea tali
Facies malleolaris medialis
Facies articularis navicularis
Facies articularis talaris posterior
Facies articularis talaris anterior
Sustentaculum tali
Facies articularis cuboidea
Calcaneus
Facies articularis talaris media
D Medial view.

Fig. 26.10 **Talus and calcaneus**

The two tarsal bones have been separated at the art. subtalaris to demonstrate their articular surfaces.

Ligaments of the Ankle & Foot

The ligaments of the foot are classified as belonging to the articulatio talocruralis, articulatio subtalaris, metatarsus, forefoot, or sole of the foot. Lig. collaterale mediale and laterale, along with the syndesmotic ligaments, are of major importance in the stabilization of the subtalar joint.

Fig. 26.11 Ligaments of the ankle and foot
Right foot. See p. 406 for inferior view.

Fibula
Tibia
Lig. tibiofibulare anterius
Malleolus medialis
Malleolus lateralis
Talus
Lig. deltoideum
Lig. talofibularis anterior
Lig. talonaviculare
Lig. bifurcatum
Os naviculare
Os cuboideum
Ligg. tarsi dorsalia
Ligg. metatarsalia dorsalia
Os metatarsale I
Articulationes metatarsophalangeae, capsulae
Phalanx proximalis I
Phalanx distalis I

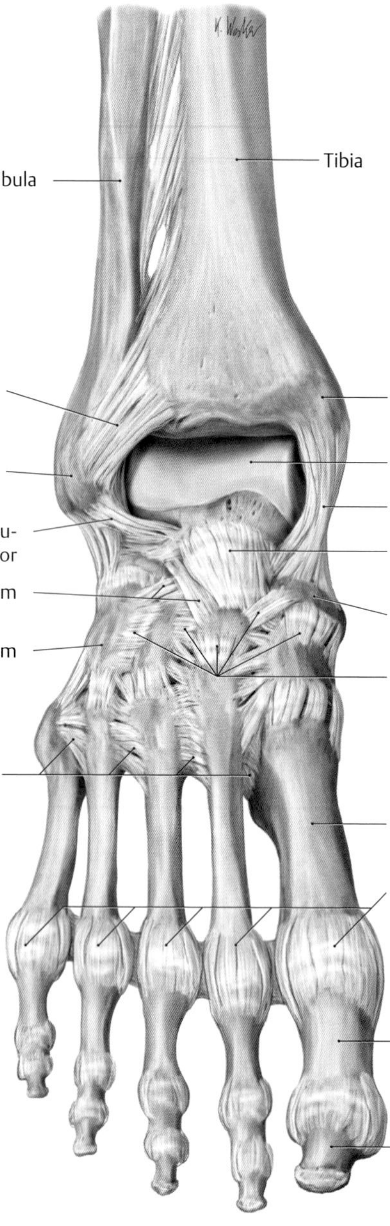

A Anterior view with articulatio talocruralis in plantar flexion.

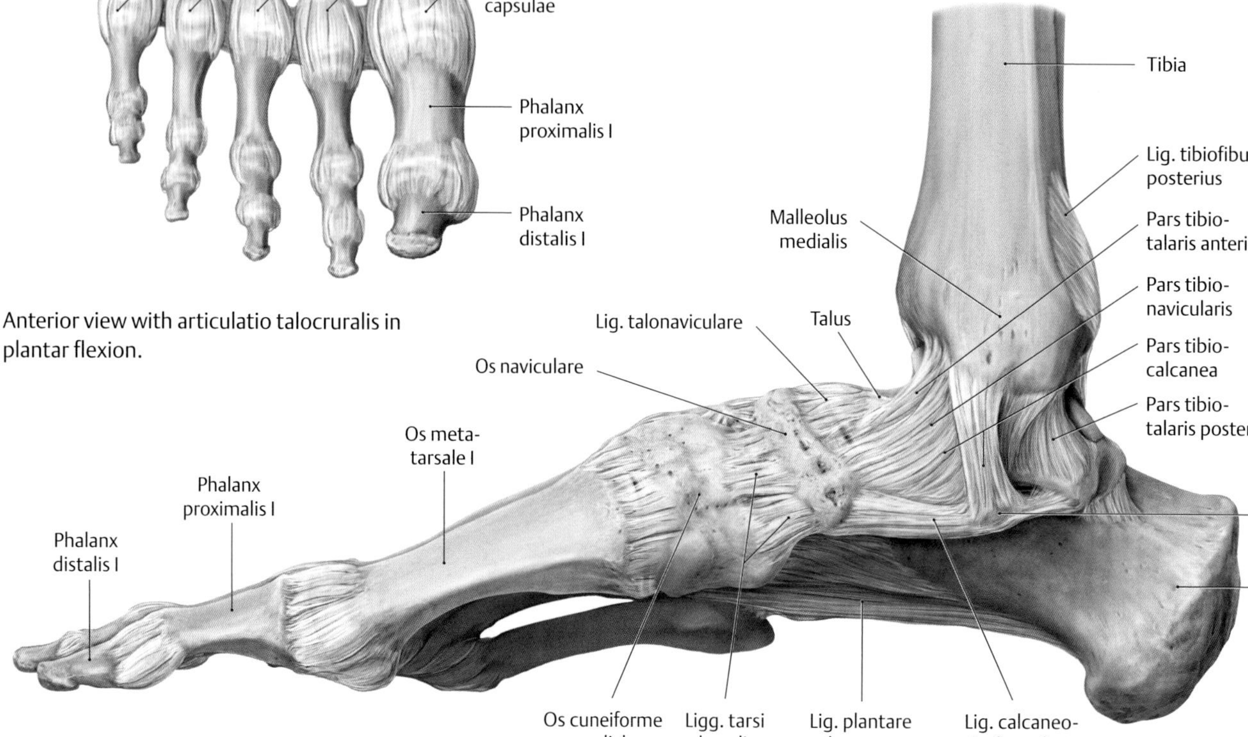

Tibia
Lig. tibiofibulare posterius
Malleolus medialis
Pars tibiotalaris anterior
Pars tibionavicularis
Lig. deltoideum
Lig. talonaviculare
Talus
Pars tibiocalcanea
Os naviculare
Pars tibiotalaris posterior
Os metatarsale I
Phalanx proximalis I
Sustentaculum tali
Phalanx distalis I
Calcaneus
Os cuneiforme mediale
Ligg. tarsi dorsalia
Lig. plantare longum
Lig. calcaneonaviculare plantare

B Medial view.

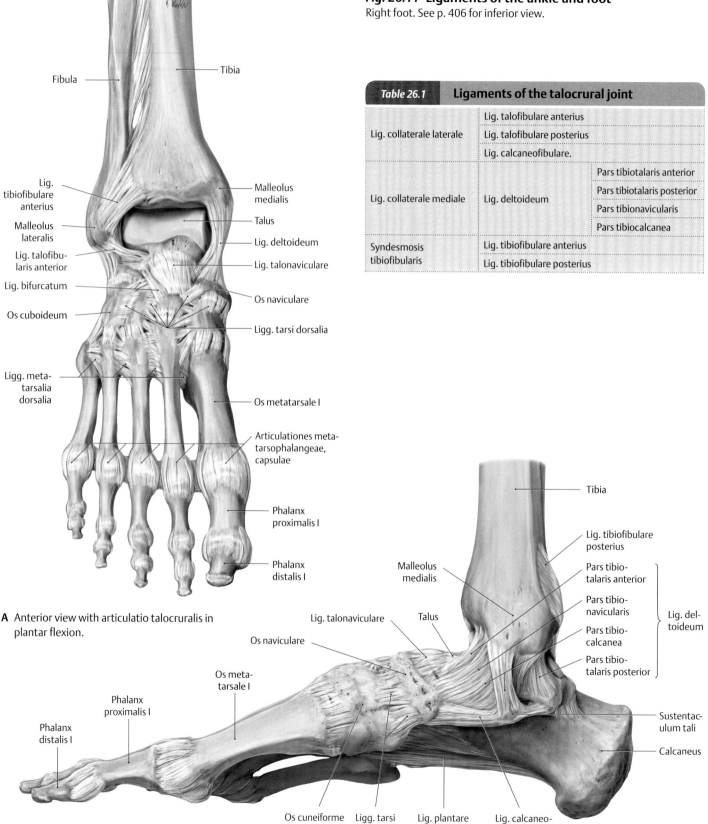

Table 26.1	**Ligaments of the talocrural joint**	
Lig. collaterale laterale	Lig. talofibulare anterius	
	Lig. talofibulare posterius	
	Lig. calcaneofibulare.	
Lig. collaterale mediale	Lig. deltoideum	Pars tibiotalaris anterior
		Pars tibiotalaris posterior
		Pars tibionavicularis
		Pars tibiocalcanea
Syndesmosis tibiofibularis	Lig. tibiofibulare anterius	
	Lig. tibiofibulare posterius	

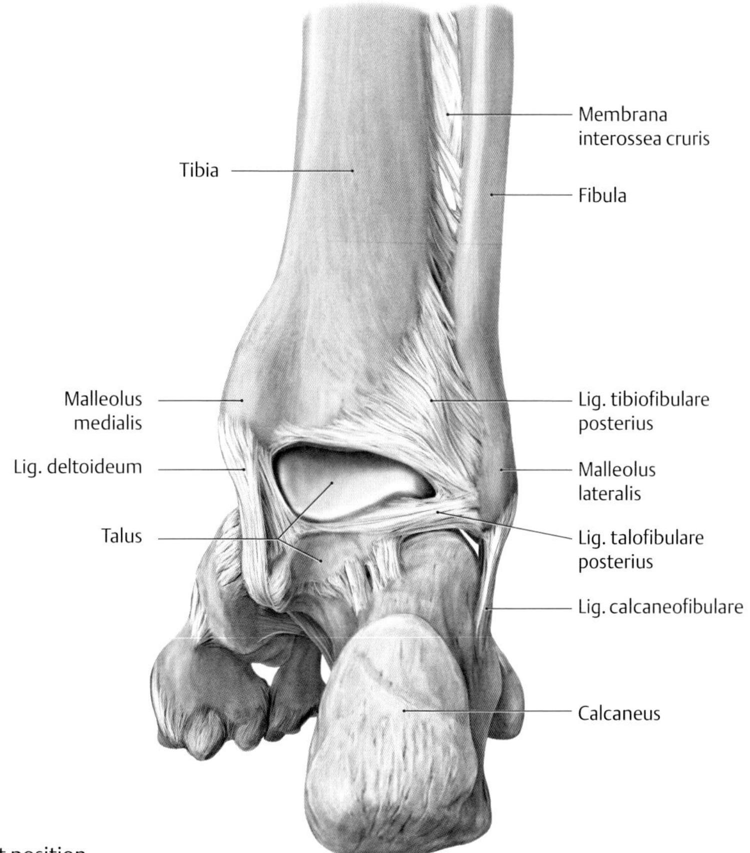
Membrana
interossea cruris
Tibia
Fibula
Malleolus
medialis
Lig. tibiofibulare
posterius
Lig. deltoideum
Malleolus
lateralis
Talus
Lig. talofibulare
posterius
Lig. calcaneofibulare
Calcaneus

C Posterior view in plantigrade foot position.

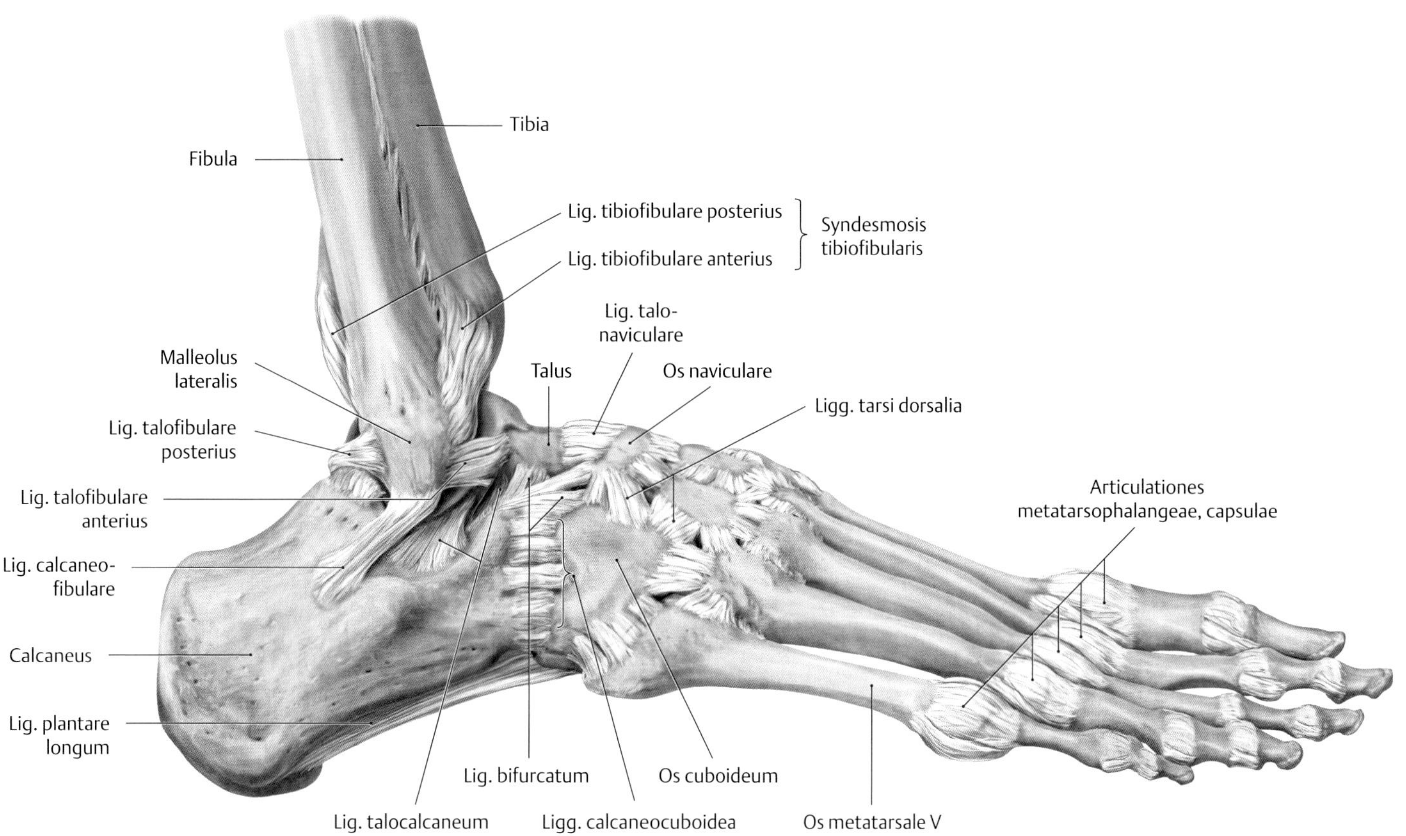
Tibia
Fibula
Lig. tibiofibulare posterius
Lig. tibiofibulare anterius
Syndesmosis
tibiofibularis
Lig. talo-
naviculare
Malleolus
lateralis
Talus
Os naviculare
Ligg. tarsi dorsalia
Lig. talofibulare
posterius
Articulationes
metatarsophalangeae, capsulae
Lig. talofibulare
anterius
Lig. calcaneo-
fibulare
Calcaneus
Lig. plantare
longum
Lig. bifurcatum
Os cuboideum
Lig. talocalcaneum
interosseum
Ligg. calcaneocuboidea
Os metatarsale V

D Lateral view.

Plantar Vault & Arches of the Foot

Fig. 26.12 Plantar vault

Right foot. The forces of the foot are distributed among two lateral (fibular) and three medial (tibial) rays. The arrangement of these rays creates a longitudinal and a transverse arch in the sole of the foot, helping the foot absorb vertical loads.

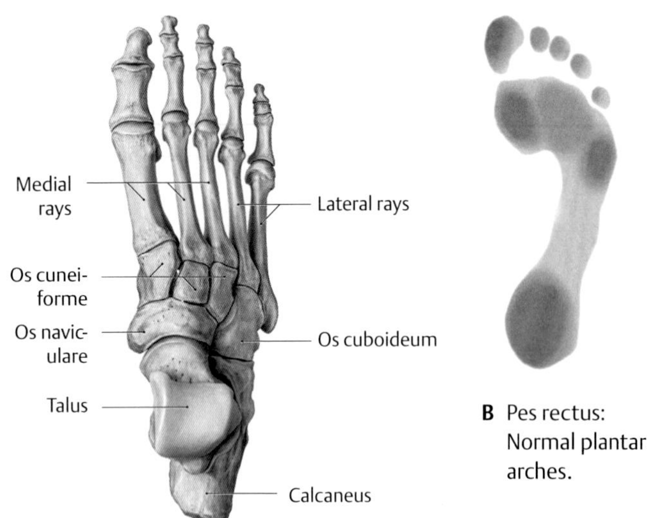

Medial rays
Lateral rays
Os cuneiforme
Os naviculare
Os cuboideum
Talus
Calcaneus

A Plantar vault, superior view. Lateral rays in green, medial rays in red.

B Pes rectus: Normal plantar arches.

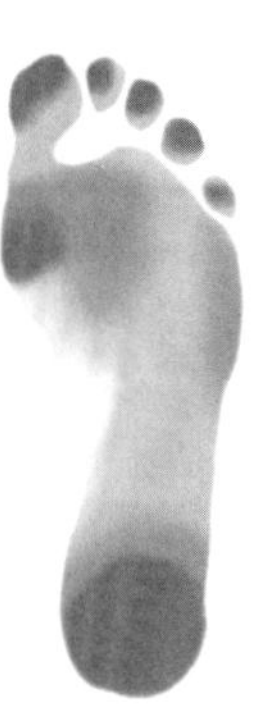

C Pes planus: Loss of longitudinal arch (flat foot).

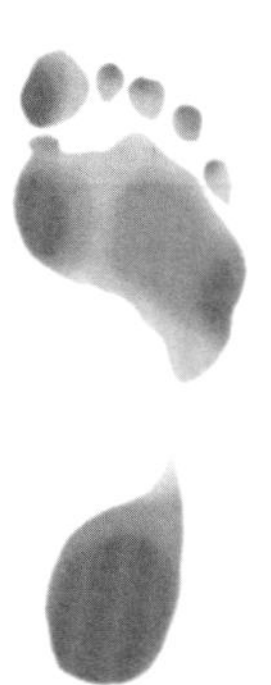

D Pes cavus: Increased height of longitudinal arch.

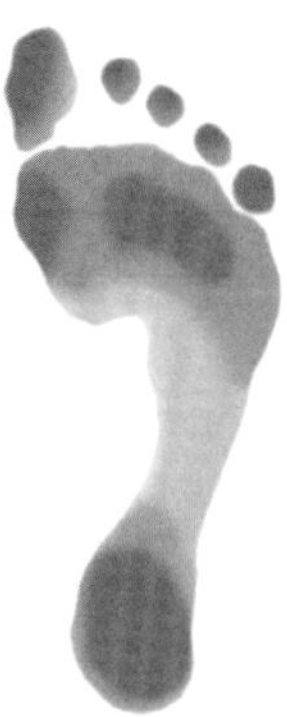

E Pes transversoplanus: Loss of transverse arch (splayfoot).

Fig. 26.13 Stabilizers of the transverse arch

Right foot. The transverse pedal arch is supported by both active and passive stabilizing structures (muscles and ligaments, respectively).

Note: The arch of the forefoot has only passive stabilizers, whereas the arches of the metatarsus and tarsus have only active stabilizers.

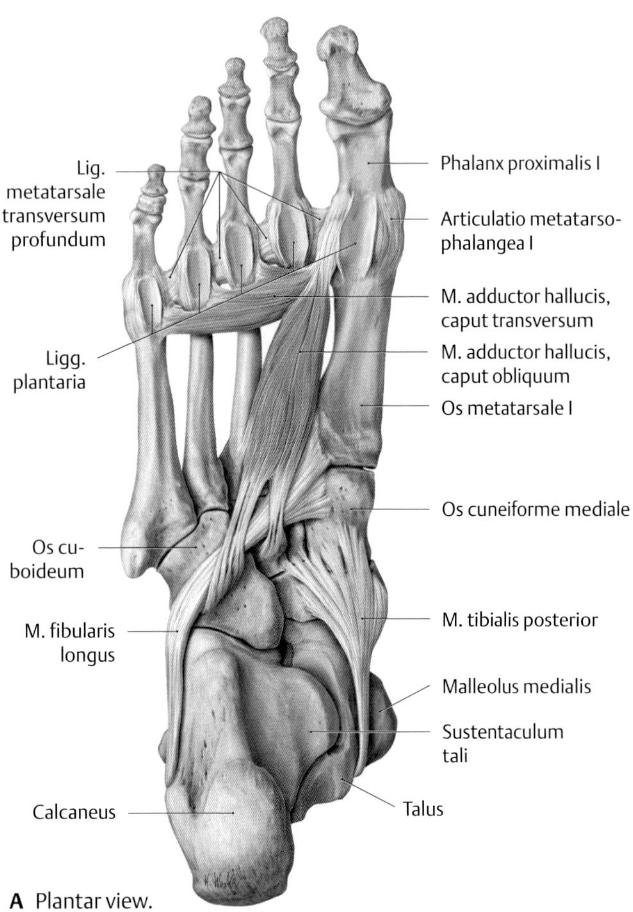

Lig. metatarsale transversum profundum
Ligg. plantaria
Os cuboideum
M. fibularis longus
Calcaneus
Phalanx proximalis I
Articulatio metatarsophalangea I
M. adductor hallucis, caput transversum
M. adductor hallucis, caput obliquum
Os metatarsale I
Os cuneiforme mediale
M. tibialis posterior
Malleolus medialis
Sustentaculum tali
Talus

A Plantar view.

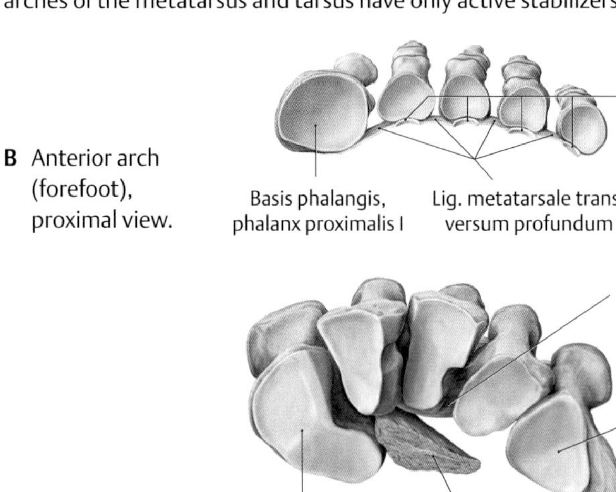

Ligg. plantaria
Basis phalangis, phalanx proximalis I
Lig. metatarsale transversum profundum
M. adductor hallucis, caput transversum
Basis ossis metatarsi V
Basis ossis metatarsi I
M. adductor hallucis, caput obliquum

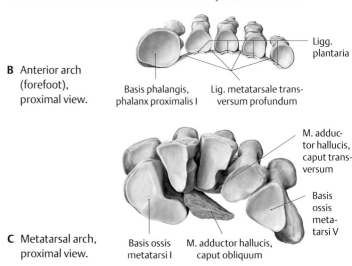

B Anterior arch (forefoot), proximal view.

C Metatarsal arch, proximal view.

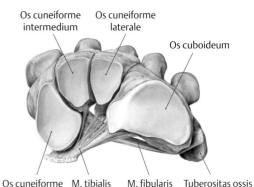

Os cuneiforme intermedium
Os cuneiforme laterale
Os cuboideum
Os cuneiforme mediale
M. tibialis posterior
M. fibularis longus
Tuberositas ossis metatarsi quinti [V]

D Tarsal region, proximal view.

Fig. 26.14 Stabilizers of the longitudinal arch
Right foot, medial view.

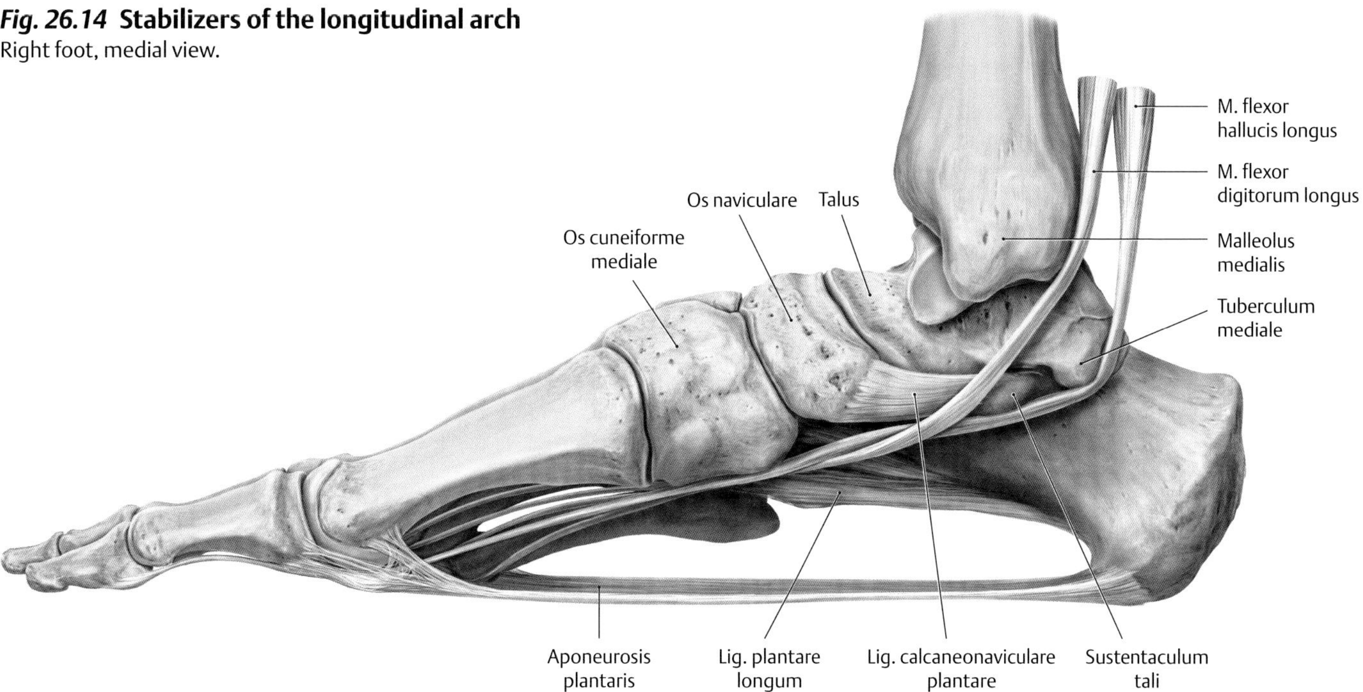
M. flexor hallucis longus
M. flexor digitorum longus
Malleolus medialis
Tuberculum mediale
Os naviculare
Talus
Os cuneiforme mediale
Aponeurosis plantaris
Lig. plantare longum
Lig. calcaneonaviculare plantare
Sustentaculum tali

A Passive stabilizers of the longitudinal arch.

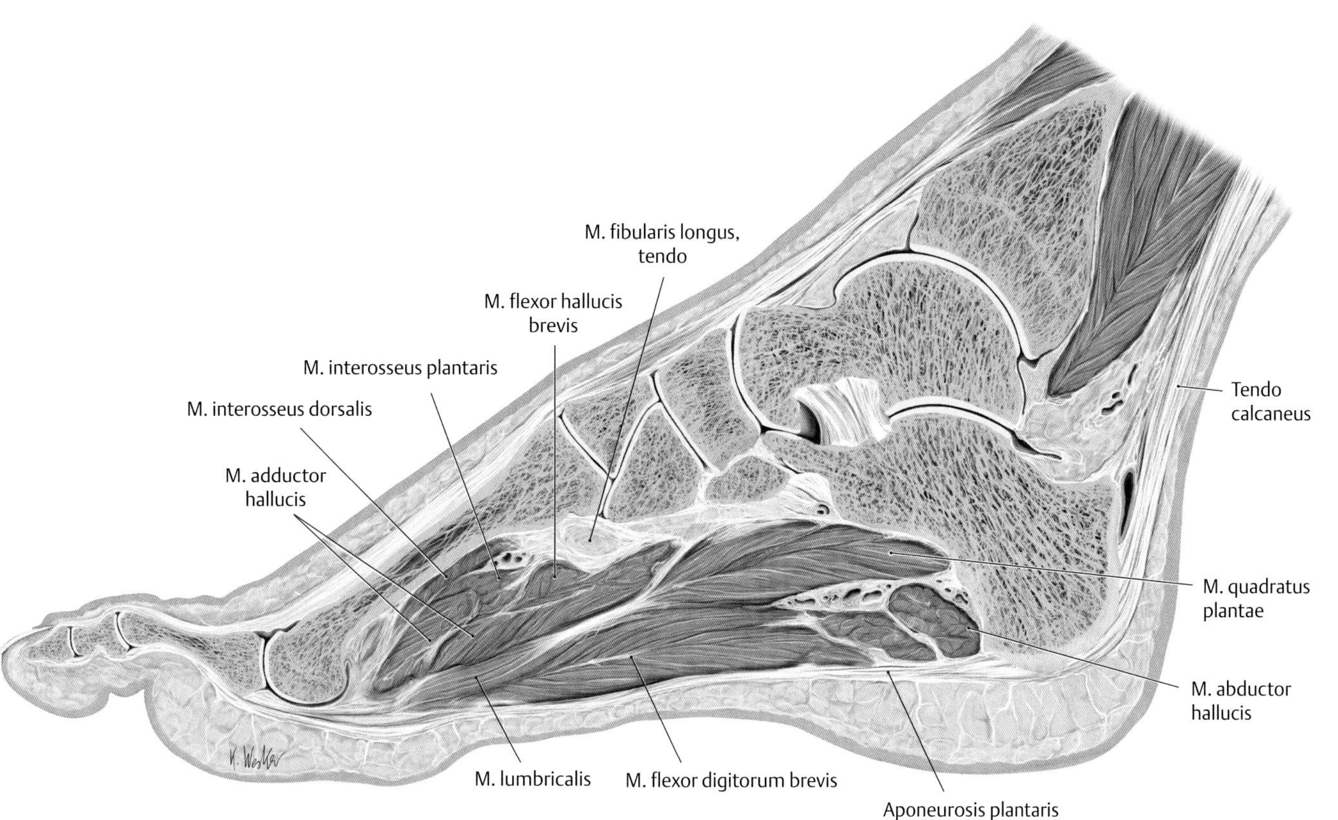
M. fibularis longus, tendo
M. flexor hallucis brevis
M. interosseus plantaris
M. interosseus dorsalis
M. adductor hallucis
Tendo calcaneus
M. quadratus plantae
M. abductor hallucis
M. lumbricalis
M. flexor digitorum brevis
Aponeurosis plantaris

B Active stabilizers of the longitudinal arch. Sagittal section at the level of the second ray. The major active stabilizers of the foot are the m. abductor hallucis, m. flexor hallucis brevis, m. flexor digitorum brevis, m. quadratus plantae, and m. abductor digiti minimi.

Muscles of the Sole of the Foot

Fig. 26.15 Aponeurosis plantaris
Right foot, plantar view. Aponeurosis plantaris is a tough aponeurotic sheet, thickest at the center, that blends with the dorsal fascia (not shown) at the borders of the foot.

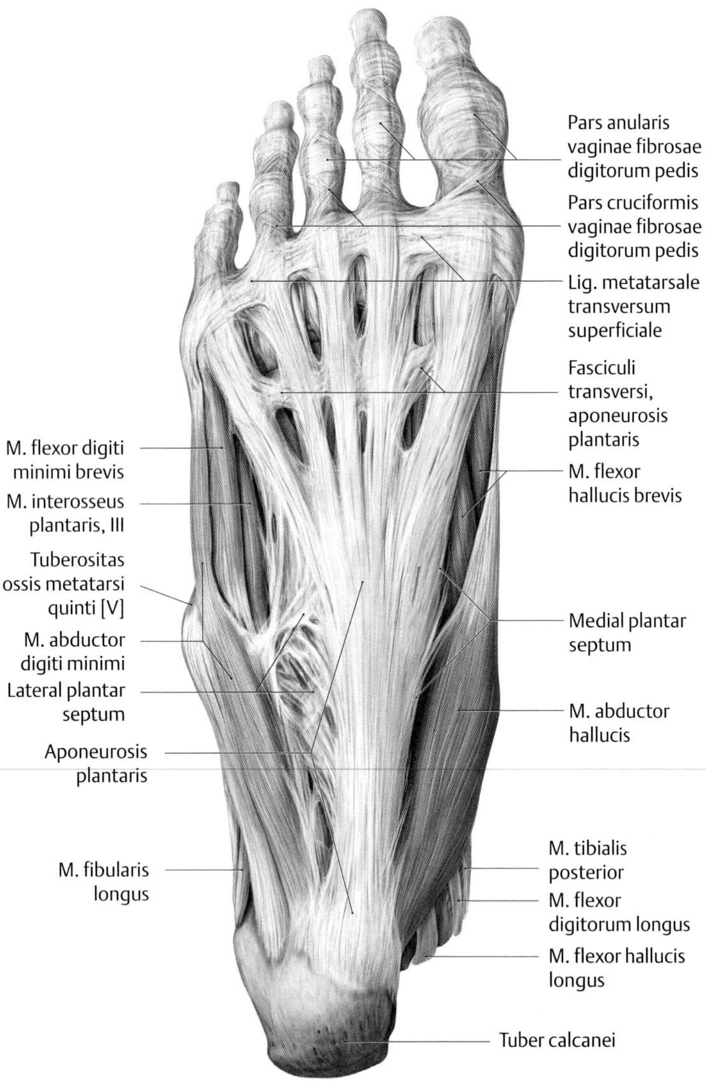
Pars anularis vaginae fibrosae digitorum pedis
Pars cruciformis vaginae fibrosae digitorum pedis
Lig. metatarsale transversum superficiale
Fasciculi transversi, aponeurosis plantaris
M. flexor hallucis brevis
Medial plantar septum
M. abductor hallucis
M. tibialis posterior
M. flexor digitorum longus
M. flexor hallucis longus
Tuber calcanei
M. flexor digiti minimi brevis
M. interosseus plantaris, III
Tuberositas ossis metatarsi quinti [V]
M. abductor digiti minimi
Lateral plantar septum
Aponeurosis plantaris
M. fibularis longus

Fig. 26.16 Intrinsic muscles
Right foot, plantar view.

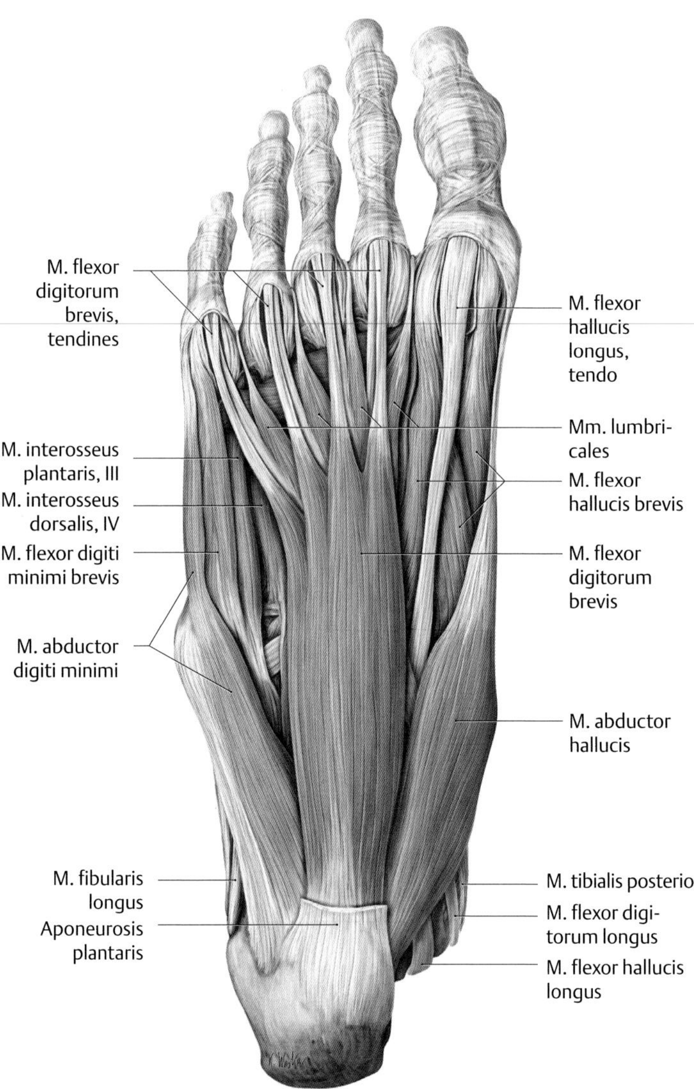
M. flexor digitorum brevis, tendines
M. interosseus plantaris, III
M. interosseus dorsalis, IV
M. flexor digiti minimi brevis
M. abductor digiti minimi
M. fibularis longus
Aponeurosis plantaris
M. flexor hallucis longus, tendo
Mm. lumbri-cales
M. flexor hallucis brevis
M. flexor digitorum brevis
M. abductor hallucis
M. tibialis posterior
M. flexor digi-torum longus
M. flexor hallucis longus

A Superficial (first) layer. *Removed:* Aponeurosis plantaris, including lig. metatarsale transversum superficiale.

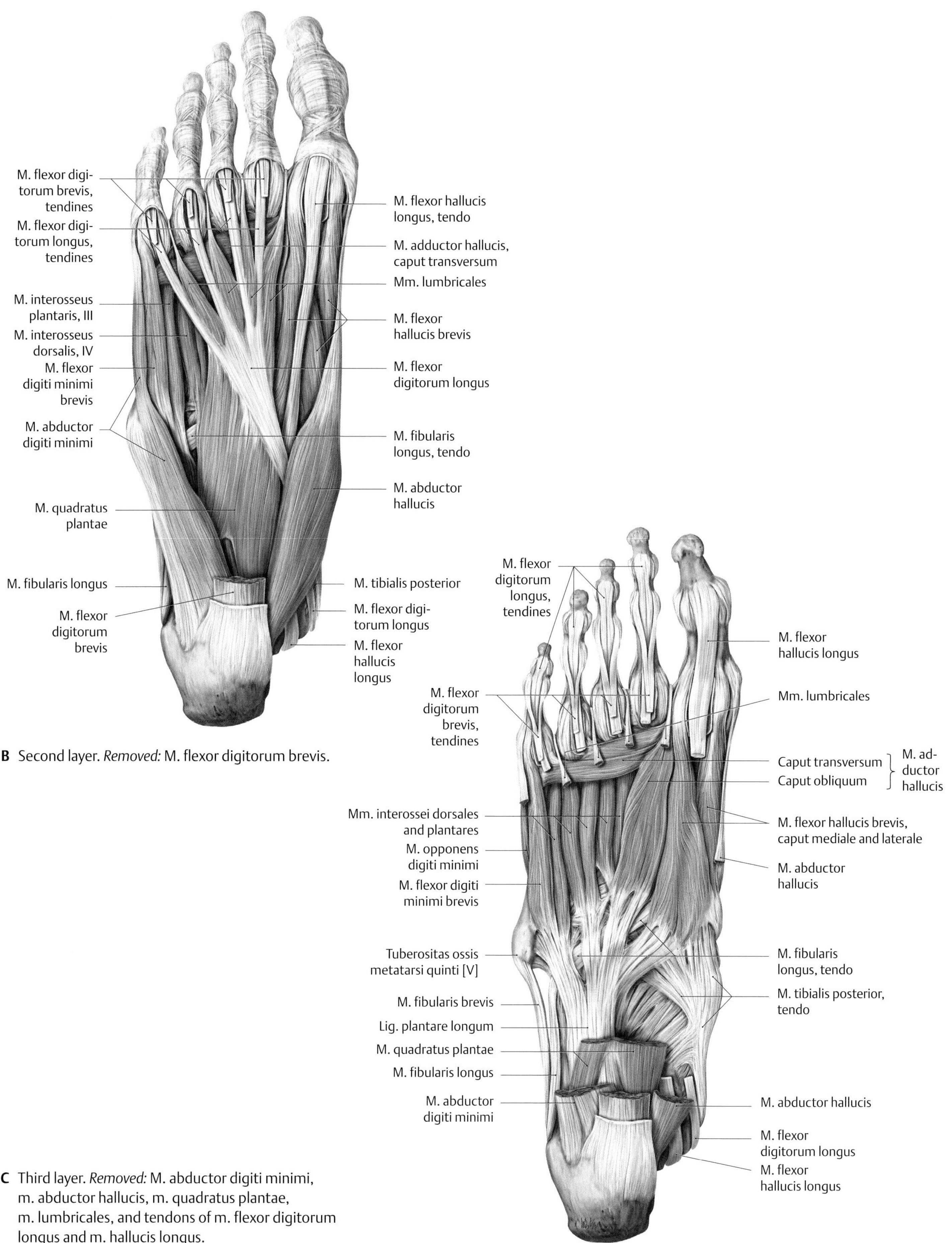
M. flexor digitorum brevis, tendines
M. flexor digitorum longus, tendines
M. interosseus plantaris, III
M. interosseus dorsalis, IV
M. flexor digiti minimi brevis
M. abductor digiti minimi
M. quadratus plantae
M. fibularis longus
M. flexor digitorum brevis
M. flexor hallucis longus, tendo
M. adductor hallucis, caput transversum
Mm. lumbricales
M. flexor hallucis brevis
M. flexor digitorum longus
M. fibularis longus, tendo
M. abductor hallucis
M. tibialis posterior
M. flexor digitorum longus
M. flexor hallucis longus
M. flexor digitorum longus, tendines
M. flexor digitorum brevis, tendines
Mm. interossei dorsales and plantares
M. opponens digiti minimi
M. flexor digiti minimi brevis
Tuberositas ossis metatarsi quinti [V]
M. fibularis brevis
Lig. plantare longum
M. quadratus plantae
M. fibularis longus
M. abductor digiti minimi
M. flexor hallucis longus
Mm. lumbricales
Caput transversum
Caput obliquum
M. adductor hallucis
M. flexor hallucis brevis, caput mediale and laterale
M. abductor hallucis
M. fibularis longus, tendo
M. tibialis posterior, tendo
M. abductor hallucis
M. flexor digitorum longus
M. flexor hallucis longus

B Second layer. *Removed:* M. flexor digitorum brevis.

C Third layer. *Removed:* M. abductor digiti minimi, m. abductor hallucis, m. quadratus plantae, m. lumbricales, and tendons of m. flexor digitorum longus and m. hallucis longus.

Muscles & Tendon Sheaths of the Foot

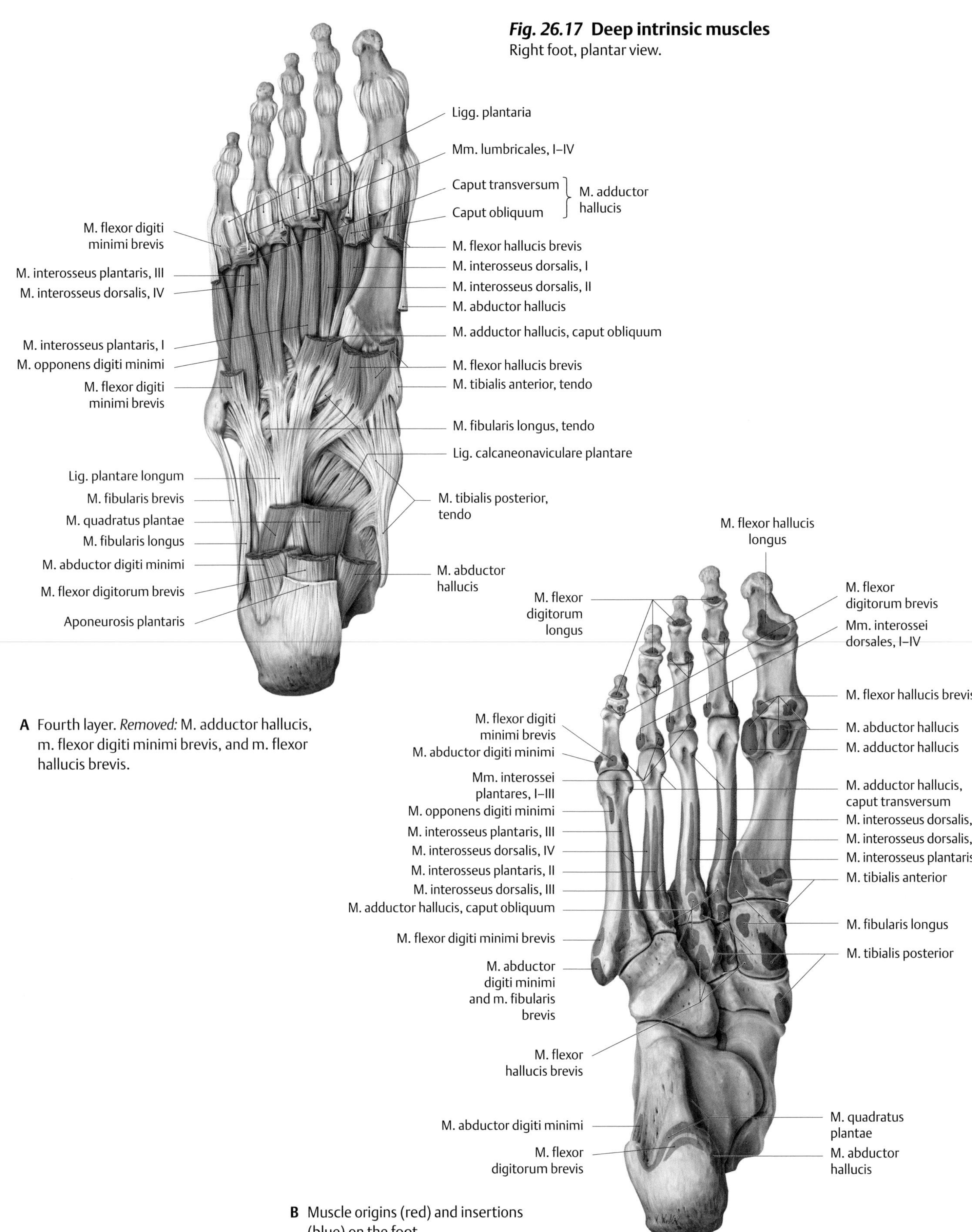
Ligg. plantaria
Mm. lumbricales, I–IV
Caput transversum
Caput obliquum
M. adductor hallucis
M. flexor digiti minimi brevis
M. flexor hallucis brevis
M. interosseus plantaris, III
M. interosseus dorsalis, I
M. interosseus dorsalis, IV
M. interosseus dorsalis, II
M. abductor hallucis
M. interosseus plantaris, I
M. adductor hallucis, caput obliquum
M. opponens digiti minimi
M. flexor hallucis brevis
M. flexor digiti minimi brevis
M. tibialis anterior, tendo
M. fibularis longus, tendo
Lig. calcaneonaviculare plantare
Lig. plantare longum
M. fibularis brevis
M. tibialis posterior, tendo
M. quadratus plantae
M. fibularis longus
M. abductor digiti minimi
M. abductor hallucis
M. flexor digitorum brevis
Aponeurosis plantaris
M. flexor hallucis longus
M. flexor digitorum longus
M. flexor digitorum brevis
Mm. interossei dorsales, I–IV
M. flexor hallucis brevis
M. flexor digiti minimi brevis
M. abductor hallucis
M. abductor digiti minimi
M. adductor hallucis
Mm. interossei plantares, I–III
M. adductor hallucis, caput transversum
M. opponens digiti minimi
M. interosseus plantaris, III
M. interosseus dorsalis, I
M. interosseus dorsalis, IV
M. interosseus dorsalis, II
M. interosseus plantaris, II
M. interosseus plantaris, I
M. interosseus dorsalis, III
M. tibialis anterior
M. adductor hallucis, caput obliquum
M. fibularis longus
M. flexor digiti minimi brevis
M. tibialis posterior
M. abductor digiti minimi and m. fibularis brevis
M. flexor hallucis brevis
M. abductor digiti minimi
M. quadratus plantae
M. flexor digitorum brevis
M. abductor hallucis

Fig. 26.17 **Deep intrinsic muscles**
Right foot, plantar view.

A Fourth layer. *Removed:* M. adductor hallucis, m. flexor digiti minimi brevis, and m. flexor hallucis brevis.

B Muscle origins (red) and insertions (blue) on the foot.

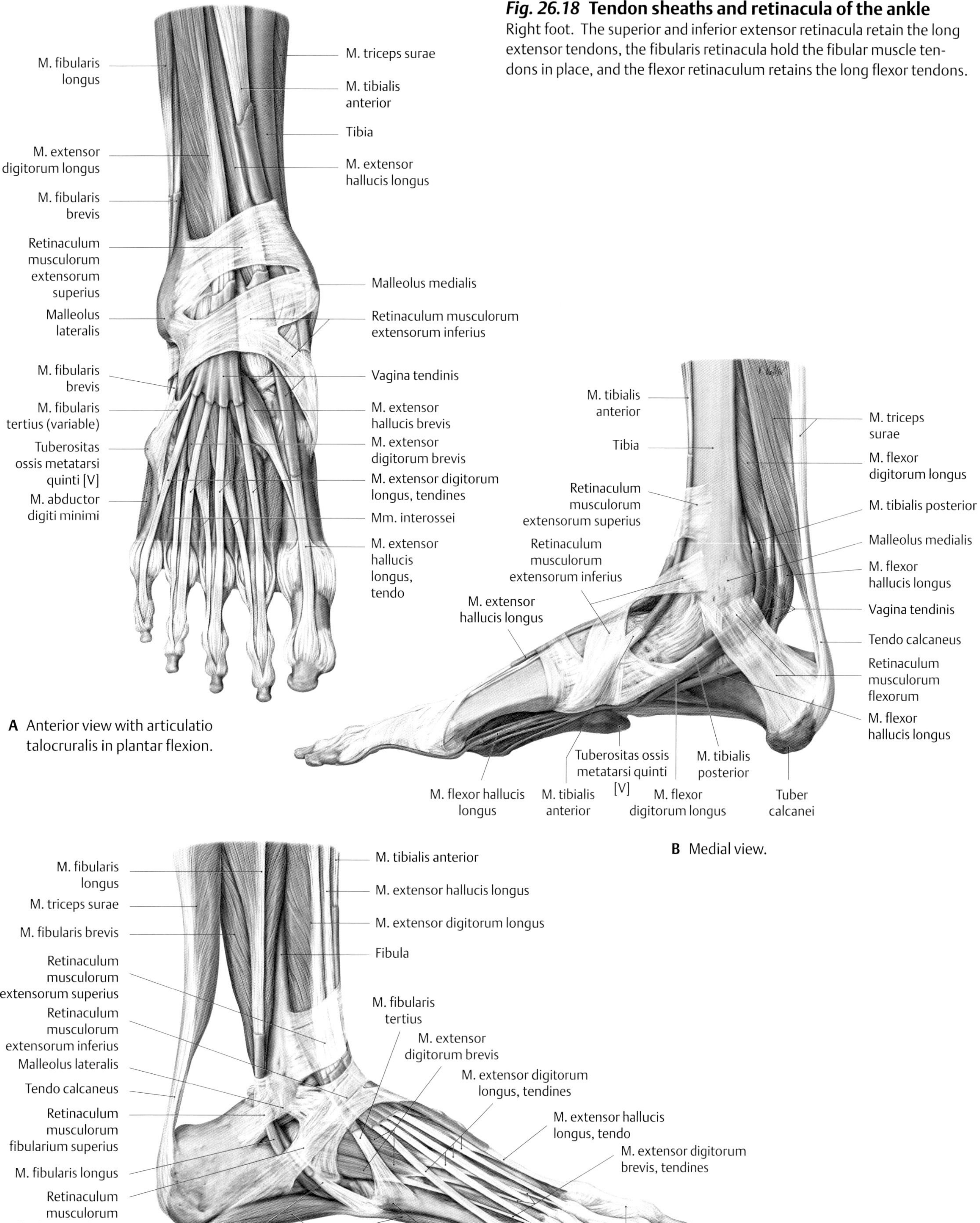
M. fibularis longus
M. triceps surae
M. tibialis anterior
Tibia
M. extensor digitorum longus
M. extensor hallucis longus
M. fibularis brevis
Retinaculum musculorum extensorum superius
Malleolus medialis
Malleolus lateralis
Retinaculum musculorum extensorum inferius
M. fibularis brevis
Vagina tendinis
M. fibularis tertius (variable)
M. extensor hallucis brevis
Tuberositas ossis metatarsi quinti [V]
M. extensor digitorum brevis
M. extensor digitorum longus, tendines
M. abductor digiti minimi
Mm. interossei
M. extensor hallucis longus, tendo
M. tibialis anterior
Tibia
M. triceps surae
M. flexor digitorum longus
Retinaculum musculorum extensorum superius
M. tibialis posterior
Malleolus medialis
Retinaculum musculorum extensorum inferius
M. flexor hallucis longus
M. extensor hallucis longus
Vagina tendinis
Tendo calcaneus
Retinaculum musculorum flexorum
M. flexor hallucis longus
Tuberositas ossis metatarsi quinti [V]
M. tibialis posterior
M. flexor hallucis longus
M. tibialis anterior
M. flexor digitorum longus
Tuber calcanei
M. fibularis longus
M. tibialis anterior
M. extensor hallucis longus
M. triceps surae
M. fibularis brevis
M. extensor digitorum longus
Fibula
Retinaculum musculorum extensorum superius
M. fibularis tertius
Retinaculum musculorum extensorum inferius
M. extensor digitorum brevis
Malleolus lateralis
M. extensor digitorum longus, tendines
Tendo calcaneus
Retinaculum musculorum fibularium superius
M. extensor hallucis longus, tendo
M. extensor digitorum brevis, tendines
M. fibularis longus
Retinaculum musculorum fibularium inferius
M. fibularis brevis
M. abductor digiti minimi
Tuberositas ossis metatarsi quinti [V]
Aponeurosis dorsalis

***Fig. 26.18* Tendon sheaths and retinacula of the ankle**
Right foot. The superior and inferior extensor retinacula retain the long extensor tendons, the fibularis retinacula hold the fibular muscle tendons in place, and the flexor retinaculum retains the long flexor tendons.

A Anterior view with articulatio talocruralis in plantar flexion.

B Medial view.

C Lateral view.

Muscle Facts (I)

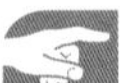

The dorsal surface (dorsum) of the foot contains only two muscles, m. extensor digitorum brevis and m. extensor hallucis brevis. The sole of the foot, however, is composed of four complex layers that maintain the arches of the foot.

Fig. 26.19 Intrinsic muscles of the dorsum
Right foot, dorsal view.

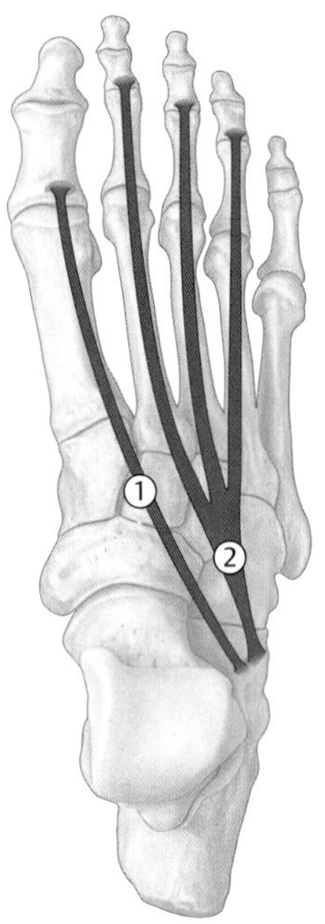

①
②

A Schematic.

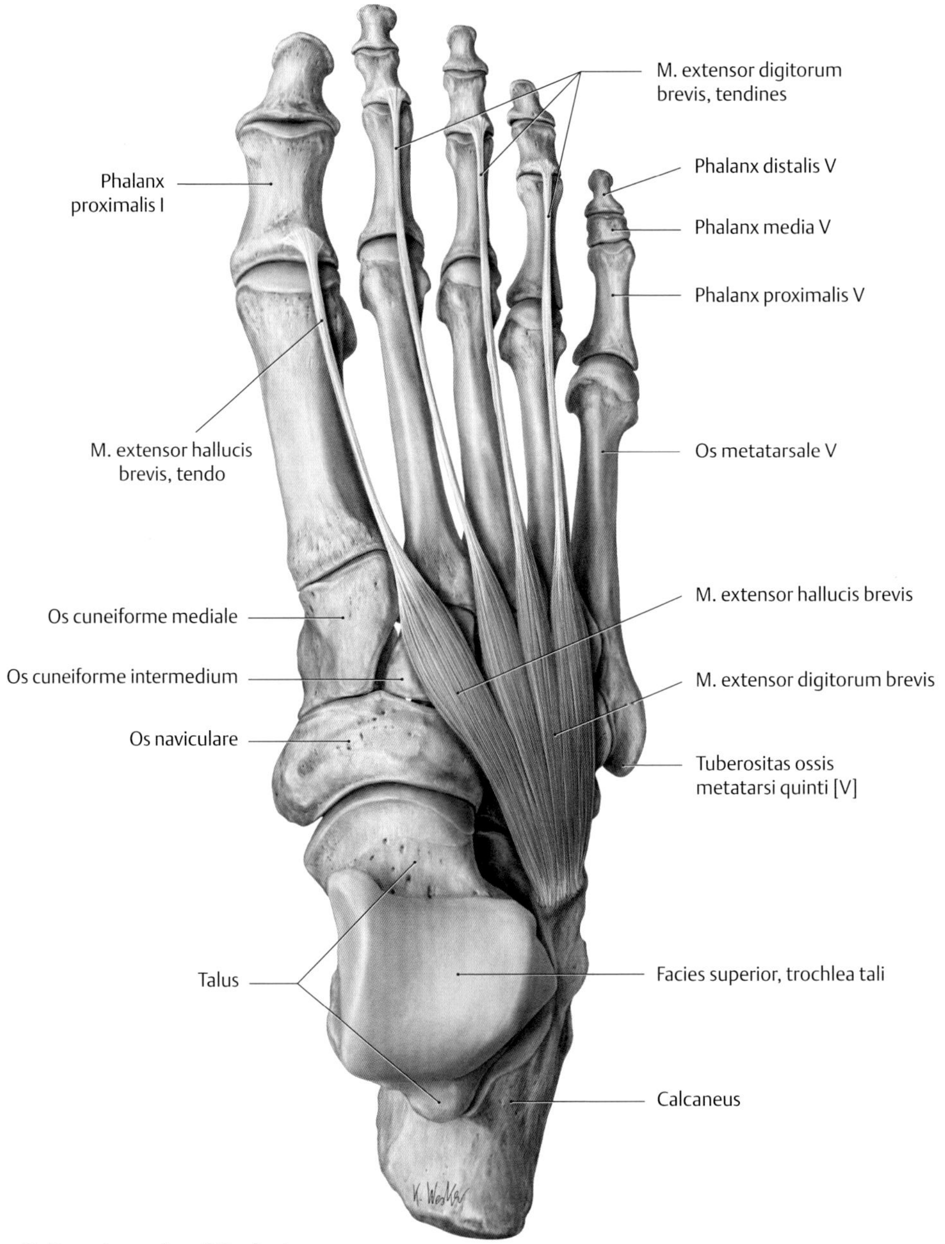

M. extensor digitorum brevis, tendines
Phalanx proximalis I
Phalanx distalis V
Phalanx media V
Phalanx proximalis V
M. extensor hallucis brevis, tendo
Os metatarsale V
M. extensor hallucis brevis
Os cuneiforme mediale
Os cuneiforme intermedium
M. extensor digitorum brevis
Os naviculare
Tuberositas ossis metatarsi quinti [V]
Talus
Facies superior, trochlea tali
Calcaneus

B Dorsal muscles of the foot.

Table 26.2 Intrinsic muscles of the dorsum

Muscle	Origin	Insertion	Innervation	Action
① M. extensor digitorum brevis	Calcaneus (fascies dorsalis)	2nd to 4th toes (aponeurosis dorsalis and bases of phalanges mediales)	N. fibularis profundus (L5, S1)	Extension of the MTP and PIP joints of the 2nd to 4th toes
② M. extensor hallucis brevis		1st toe (aponeurosis dorsalis and phalanx proximalis)		Extension of the MTP joints of the 1st toe

MTP = Articulationes metatarsophalangeae; PIP = Articulationes interphalangeae proximales.

Fig. 26.20 **Superficial intrinsic muscles of the sole**
Right foot, plantar view.

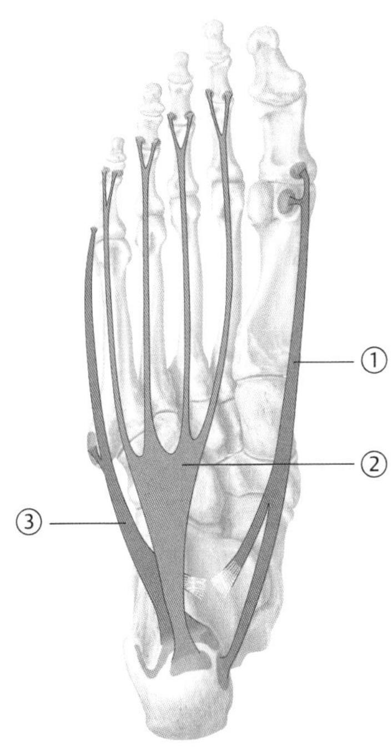
①
②
③

A First layer (schematic).

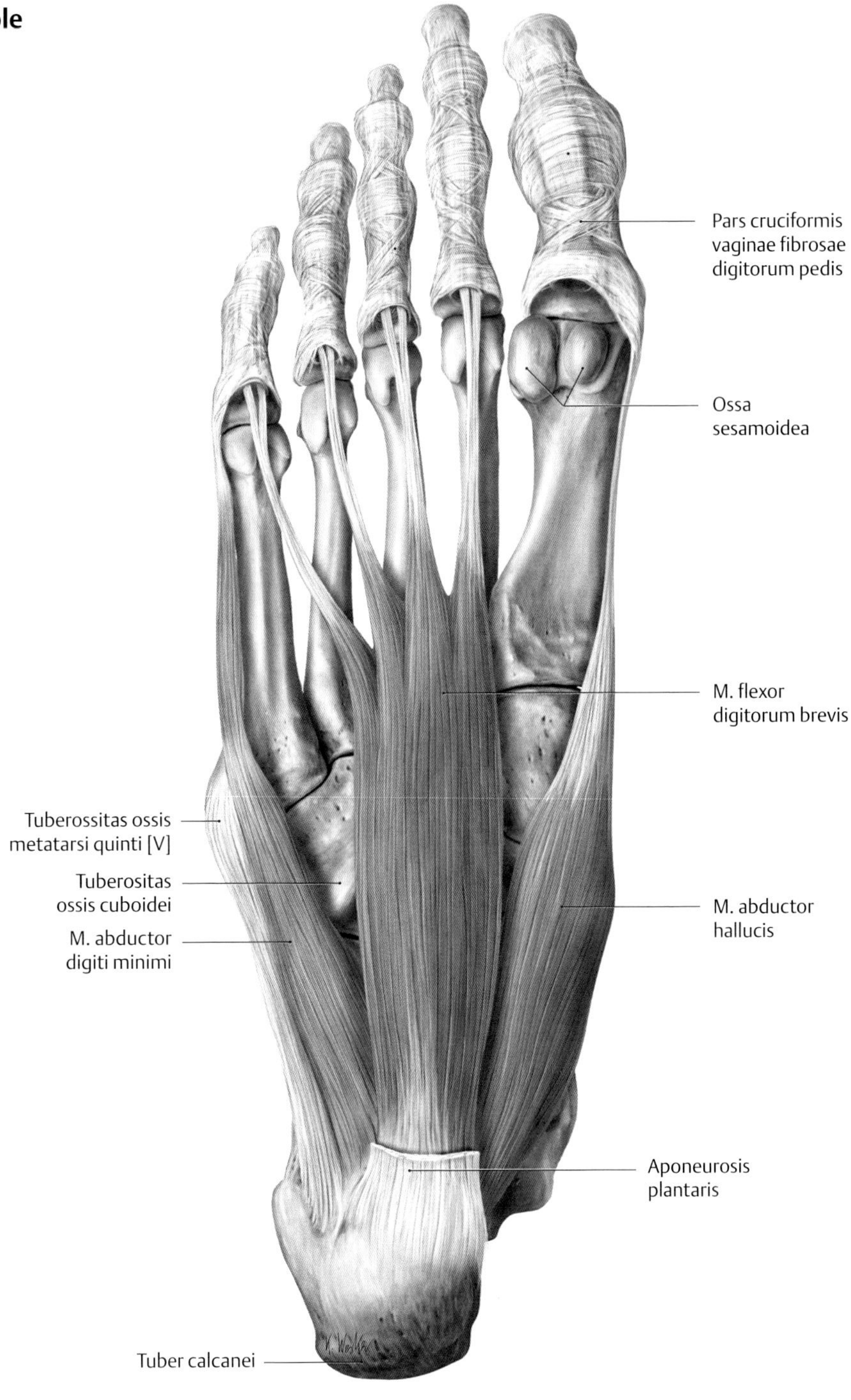

Pars cruciformis vaginae fibrosae digitorum pedis

Ossa sesamoidea

M. flexor digitorum brevis

Tuberossitas ossis metatarsi quinti [V]

Tuberositas ossis cuboidei

M. abductor digiti minimi

M. abductor hallucis

Aponeurosis plantaris

Tuber calcanei

B Intrinsic muscles of the sole, first layer.

Table 26.3 **Superficial intrinsic muscles of the sole**

Muscle	Origin	Insertion	Innervation	Action
① M. abductor hallucis	Tuber calcanei (proc. medialis)	1st toe, basis phalanx proximalis via the medial sesamoid	N. plantaris medialis (S1, S2)	• 1st MTP joint: flexion and abduction of the 1st toe • Supports the longitudinal arch
② M. flexor digitorum brevis	Tuber calcanei, aponeurosis plantaris	2nd to 5th toes, phalanx medialis		• Flexes the MTP and PIP joints of the 2nd to 5th toes • Supports the longitudinal arch
③ M. abductor digiti minimi		5th toe (basis phalanx proximalis, tuberositas ossis metatarsi V)	N. plantaris lateralis (S1–S3)	• Flexes the MTP joint of the 5th toe • Abducts the 5th toe • Supports the longitudinal arch

MTP = Articulationes metatarsophalangeae; PIP = Articulationes interphalangeae proximales.

Muscle Facts (II)

Fig. 26.21 **Deep intrinsic muscles of the sole**
Right foot, plantar view.

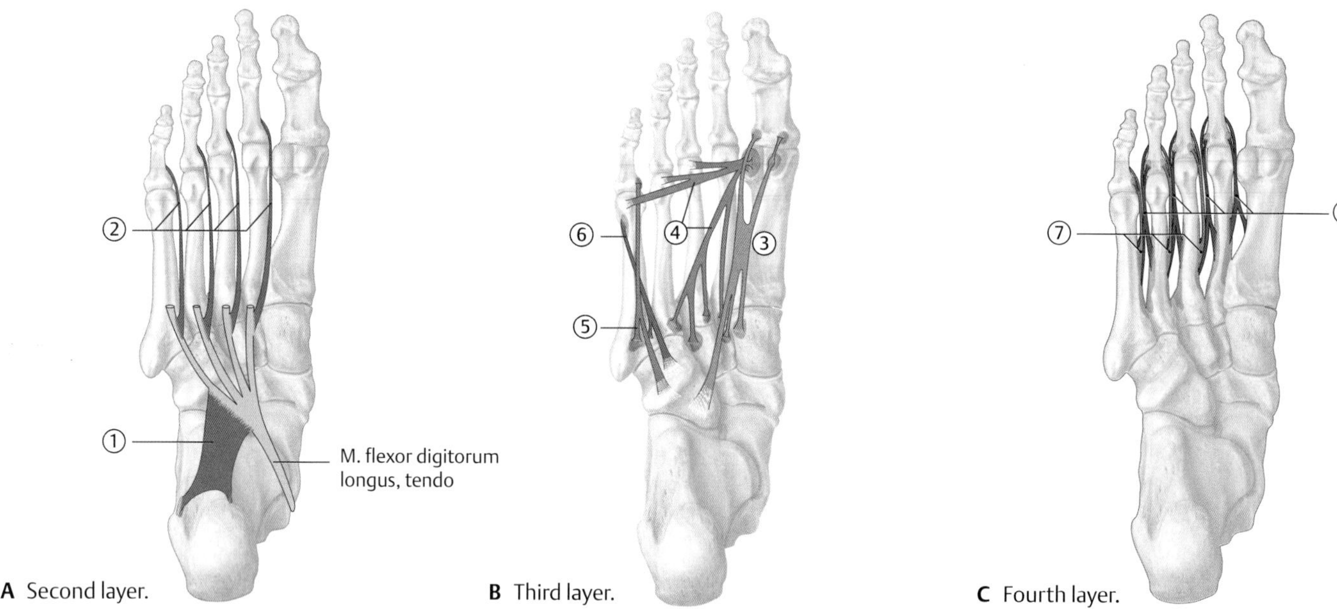
②
①
M. flexor digitorum longus, tendo
⑥
④
③
⑤
⑦
⑧

A Second layer. **B** Third layer. **C** Fourth layer.

Table 26.4 **Deep intrinsic muscles of the sole**

Muscle	Origin	Insertion	Innervation	Action
① M. quadratus plantae	Tuber calcanei (medial and plantar borders on plantar side)	M. flexor digitorum longus tendon (lateral border)	N. plantaris lateralis (S1–S3)	Redirects and augments the pull of m. flexor digitorum longus
② Mm. lumbricales pedis I–IV	M. flexor digitorum longus tendons (medial borders)	2nd to 5th toes (at aponeurosis dorsalis)	M. lumbricalis I: n. plantaris medialis (S2, S3) Mm. lumbricales II–IV: n. plantaris lateralis (S2, S3)	• Flexes the MTP joints of 2nd to 5th toes • Extension of IP joints of 2nd to 5th toes • Adducts 2nd to 5th toes toward the big toe
③ M. flexor hallucis brevis	Os cuboideum, os cuneiforme laterale and lig. calcaneocuboideum plantare	1st toe (at base of phalanx proximales via medial and lateral sesamoids)	Caput mediale: n. plantaris medialis (S1, S2) Caput laterale: n. plantaris lateralis (S1, S2)	• Flexes the first MTP joint • Supports the longitudinal arch
④ M. adductor hallucis	Caput obliquum: Ossa metatarsi II–IV (at bases) Caput transversum: MTPs of 3rd to 5th toes, lig. metatarsale transversum profundum	1st phalanx proximales (at base, by a common tendon via the lateral sesamoid)	N. plantaris lateralis, r. profundus (S2, S3)	• Flexes the first MTP joint • Adducts big toe • Caput transversum: supports transverse arch • Caput obliquum: supports longitudinal arch
⑤ M. flexor digiti minimi brevis	Os metatarsi V (base), lig. plantare longum	5th toe (base of phalanx proximales)	N. plantaris lateralis, r. superficialis (S2, S3)	Flexes the MTP joint of the little toe
⑥ M. opponens digiti minimi*	Lig. plantare longum; m. fibularis longus (at plantar tendon sheath)	Os metatarsale V		Pulls 5th metatarsal in plantar and medial direction
⑦ Mm. interossei plantares I–III	Ossa metatarsi III–V (margo mediales)	3rd to 5th toes (medial base of phalanx proximales)	N. plantaris lateralis (S2, S3)	• Flexes the MTP joints of 3rd to 5th toes • Extension of IP joints of 3rd to 5th toes • Adducts 3rd to 5th toes toward 2nd toe
⑧ Mm. interossei dorsales pedis I–IV	Ossa metatarsi I–V (by two heads on opposing sides)	M. interosseus I: phalanx proximales II (medial base) 2nd to 4th mm. interossei: 2nd to 4th phalangis proximales (lateral base), 2nd to 4th toes (at aponeurosis dorsalis)		• Flexes the MTP joints of 2nd to 4th toes • Extension of IP joints of 2nd to 4th toes • Abducts 3rd and 4th toes from 2nd toe

IP = Articulationes interphalangeae pedis; MTP = Articulationes metatarsophalangeae. *May be absent.

Fig. 26.22 **Deep intrinsic muscles of the sole**
Right foot, plantar view.

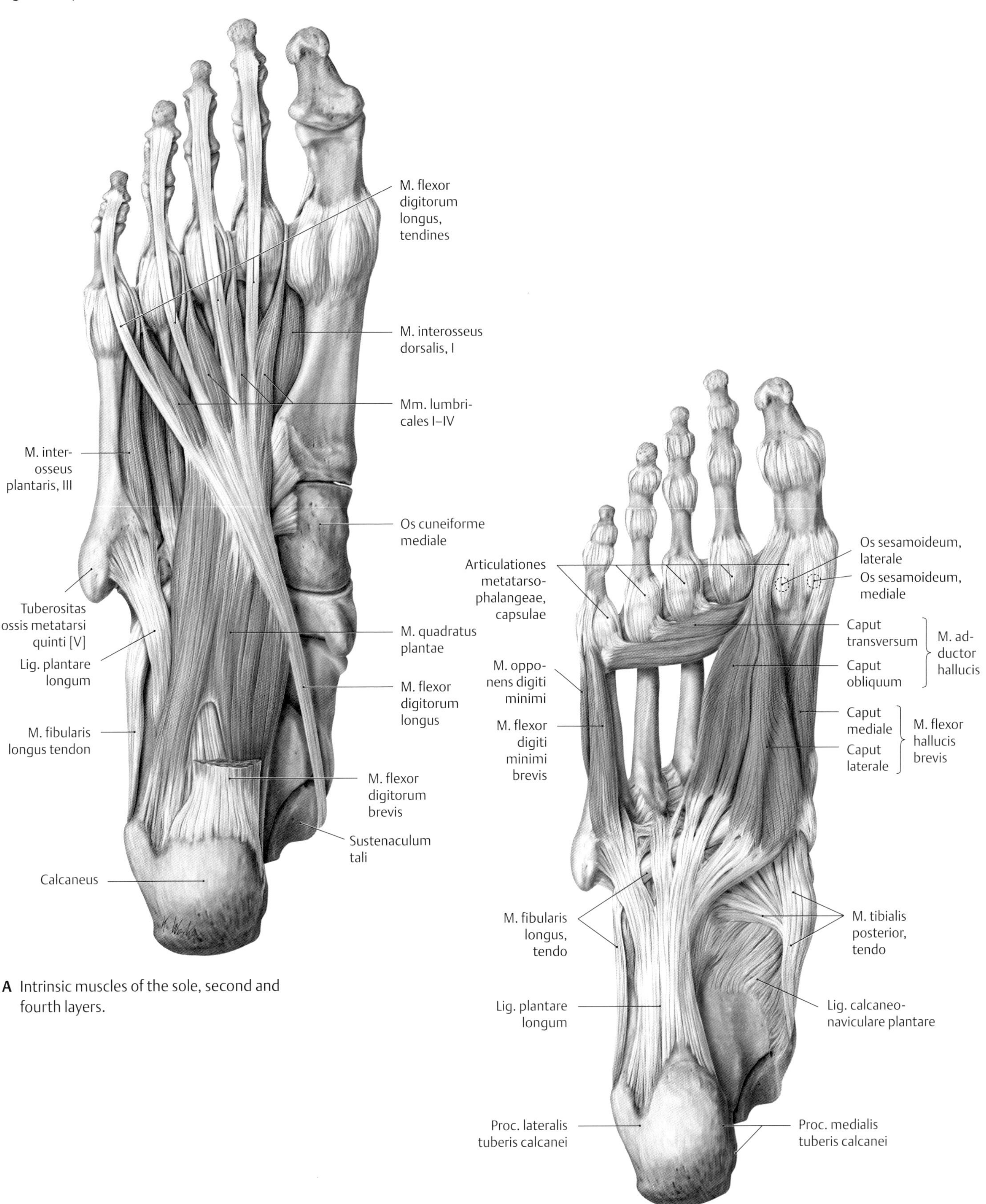
M. flexor digitorum longus, tendines
M. interosseus dorsalis, I
Mm. lumbricales I–IV
M. interosseus plantaris, III
Os cuneiforme mediale
Tuberositas ossis metatarsi quinti [V]
M. quadratus plantae
Lig. plantare longum
M. flexor digitorum longus
M. fibularis longus tendon
M. flexor digitorum brevis
Sustenaculum tali
Calcaneus
Articulationes metatarso-phalangeae, capsulae
Os sesamoideum, laterale
Os sesamoideum, mediale
Caput transversum
Caput obliquum
M. adductor hallucis
M. opponens digiti minimi
M. flexor digiti minimi brevis
Caput mediale
Caput laterale
M. flexor hallucis brevis
M. fibularis longus, tendo
M. tibialis posterior, tendo
Lig. plantare longum
Lig. calcaneo-naviculare plantare
Proc. lateralis tuberis calcanei
Proc. medialis tuberis calcanei

A Intrinsic muscles of the sole, second and fourth layers.

B Intrinsic muscles of the sole, third layer.

Arteries of the Lower Limb

Fig. 27.1 Arteries of the lower limb

Right limb, anterior (**A**) and posterior (**B**) views.

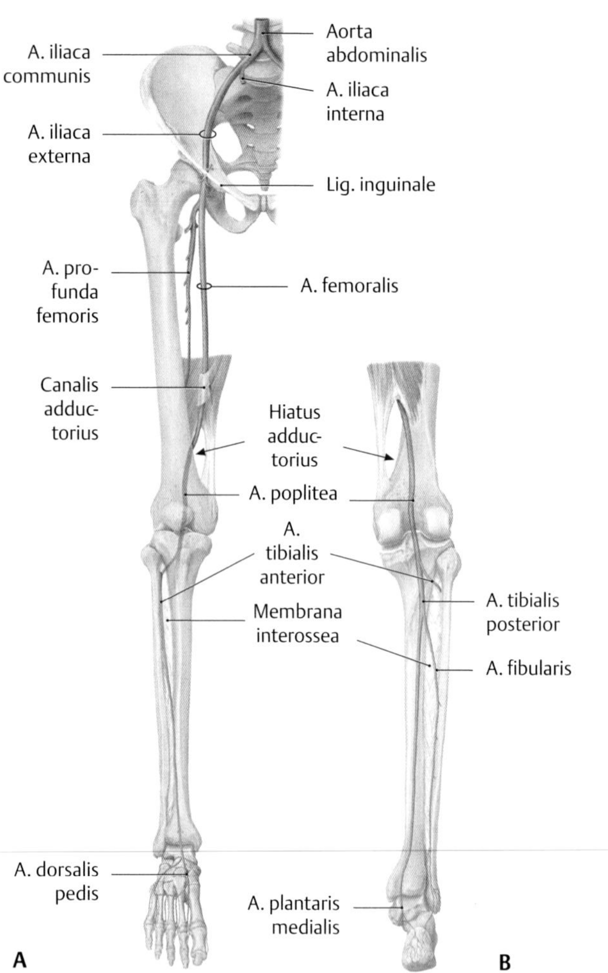

A. iliaca communis
Aorta abdominalis
A. iliaca interna
A. iliaca externa
Lig. inguinale
A. profunda femoris
A. femoralis
Canalis adductorius
Hiatus adductorius
A. poplitea
A. tibialis anterior
Membrana interossea
A. tibialis posterior
A. fibularis
A. dorsalis pedis
A. plantaris medialis
A
B

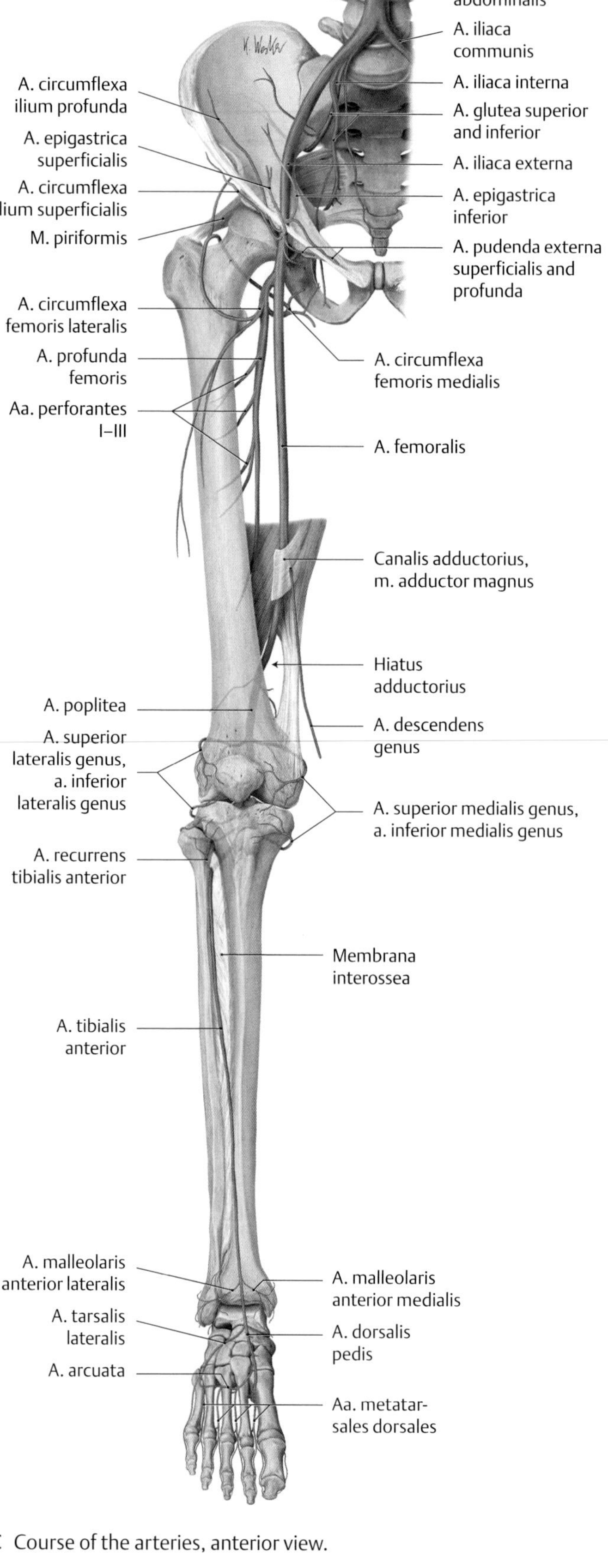

Aorta abdominalis
A. iliaca communis
A. iliaca interna
A. glutea superior and inferior
A. iliaca externa
A. epigastrica inferior
A. pudenda externa superficialis and profunda
A. circumflexa ilium profunda
A. epigastrica superficialis
A. circumflexa ilium superficialis
M. piriformis
A. circumflexa femoris lateralis
A. profunda femoris
Aa. perforantes I–III
A. circumflexa femoris medialis
A. femoralis
Canalis adductorius, m. adductor magnus
Hiatus adductorius
A. poplitea
A. descendens genus
A. superior lateralis genus, a. inferior lateralis genus
A. superior medialis genus, a. inferior medialis genus
A. recurrens tibialis anterior
Membrana interossea
A. tibialis anterior
A. malleolaris anterior lateralis
A. malleolaris anterior medialis
A. tarsalis lateralis
A. dorsalis pedis
A. arcuata
Aa. metatarsales dorsales

C Course of the arteries, anterior view.

Fig. 27.2 Arteries of the sole of the foot

Right foot, plantar view.

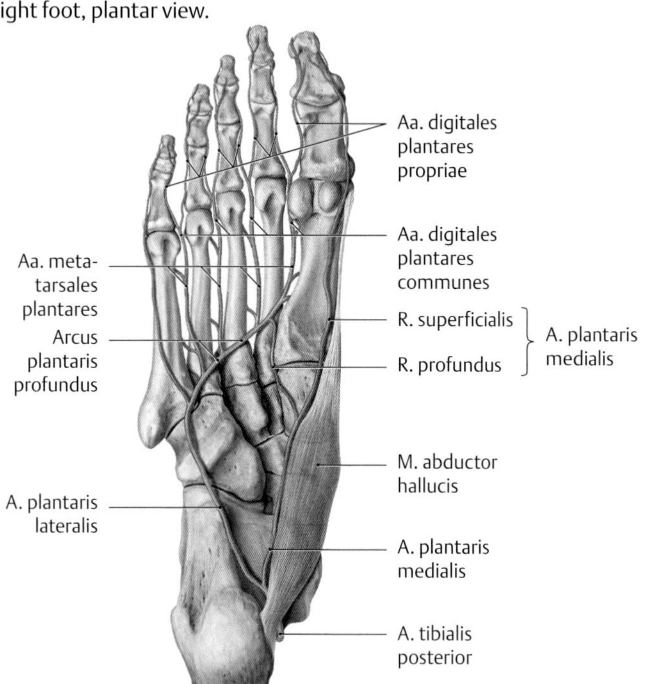

Aa. digitales plantares propriae
Aa. digitales plantares communes
Aa. metatarsales plantares
R. superficialis
R. profundus
A. plantaris medialis
Arcus plantaris profundus
M. abductor hallucis
A. plantaris lateralis
A. plantaris medialis
A. tibialis posterior

Clinical

Necrosis of caput femoris

Dislocation or fracture of caput femoris (e.g., in patients with osteoporosis) may disrupt the anastomoses between r. acetabularis and the femoral neck vessels, resulting in femoral head necrosis.

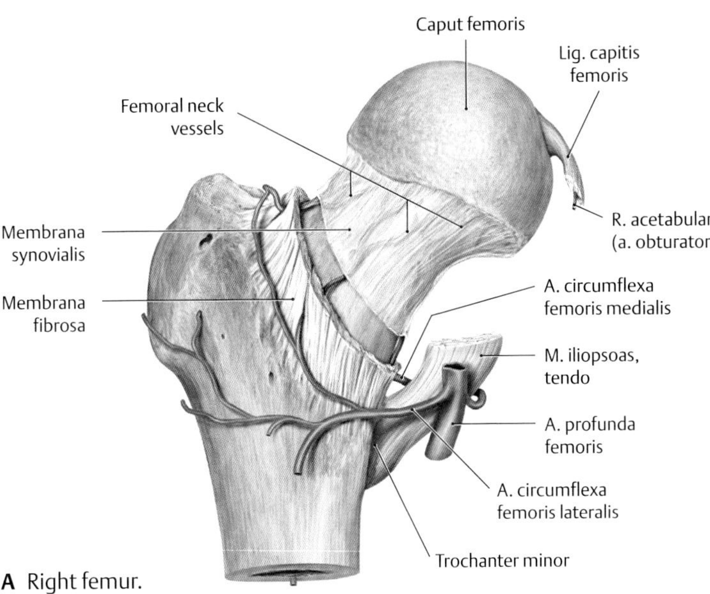

Caput femoris
Lig. capitis femoris
Femoral neck vessels
Membrana synovialis
Membrana fibrosa
R. acetabularis (a. obturatoria)
A. circumflexa femoris medialis
M. iliopsoas, tendo
A. profunda femoris
A. circumflexa femoris lateralis
Trochanter minor

A Right femur.

Fig. 27.3 Arteries of caput femoris

Right art. coxae, anterior view.

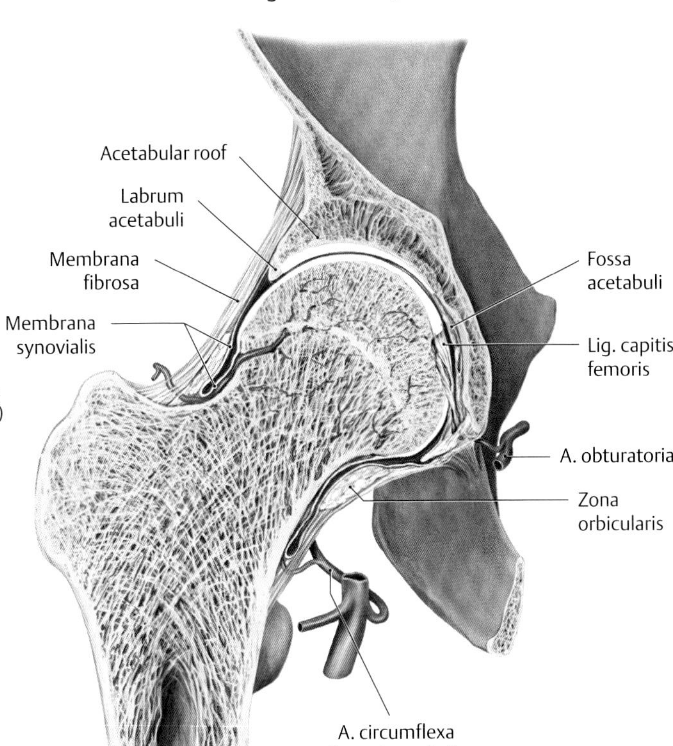

Acetabular roof
Labrum acetabuli
Membrana fibrosa
Membrana synovialis
Fossa acetabuli
Lig. capitis femoris
A. obturatoria
Zona orbicularis
A. circumflexa femoris medialis

B Coronal section.

Fig. 27.4 Arteries of the thigh and leg

Right leg.

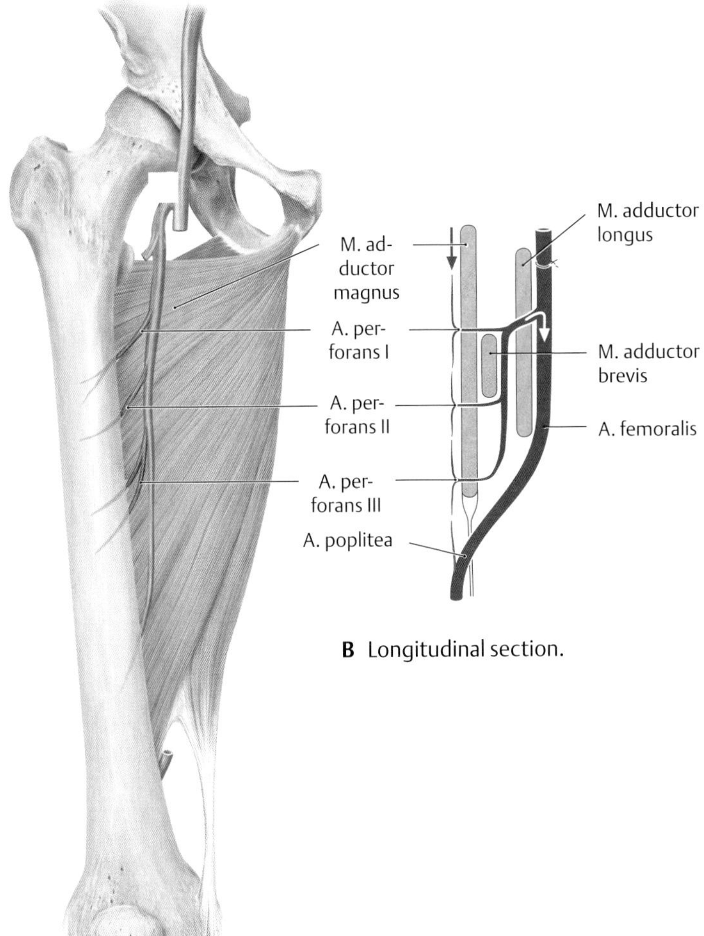

M. adductor magnus
A. perforans I
A. perforans II
A. perforans III
A. poplitea
M. adductor longus
M. adductor brevis
A. femoralis

B Longitudinal section.

A Aa. perforantes, posterior view.

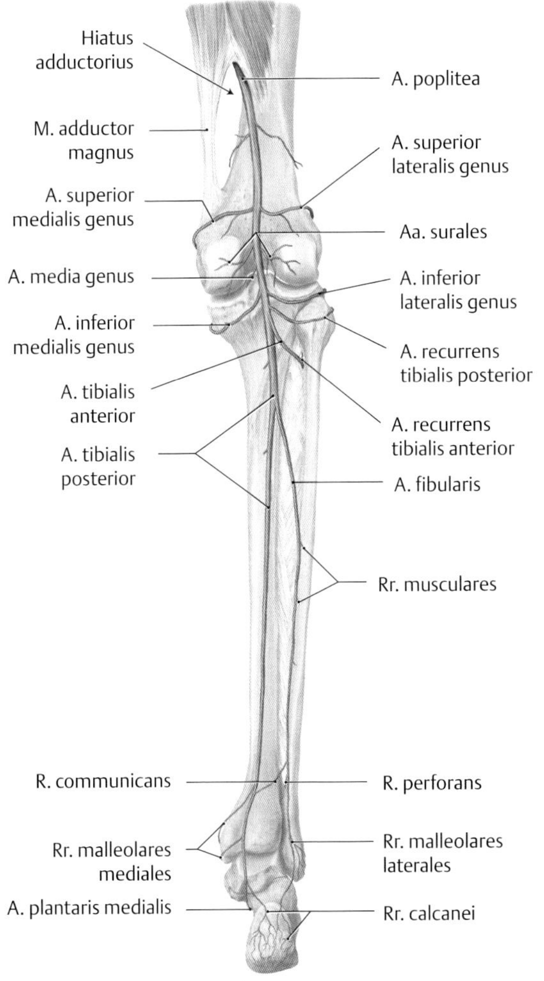

Hiatus adductorius
M. adductor magnus
A. superior medialis genus
A. media genus
A. inferior medialis genus
A. tibialis anterior
A. tibialis posterior
R. communicans
Rr. malleolares mediales
A. plantaris medialis
A. poplitea
A. superior lateralis genus
Aa. surales
A. inferior lateralis genus
A. recurrens tibialis posterior
A. recurrens tibialis anterior
A. fibularis
Rr. musculares
R. perforans
Rr. malleolares laterales
Rr. calcanei

C Arteries of the posterior leg.

Veins & Lymphatics of the Lower Limb

Fig. 27.5 Veins of the lower limb

Right limb, anterior view.

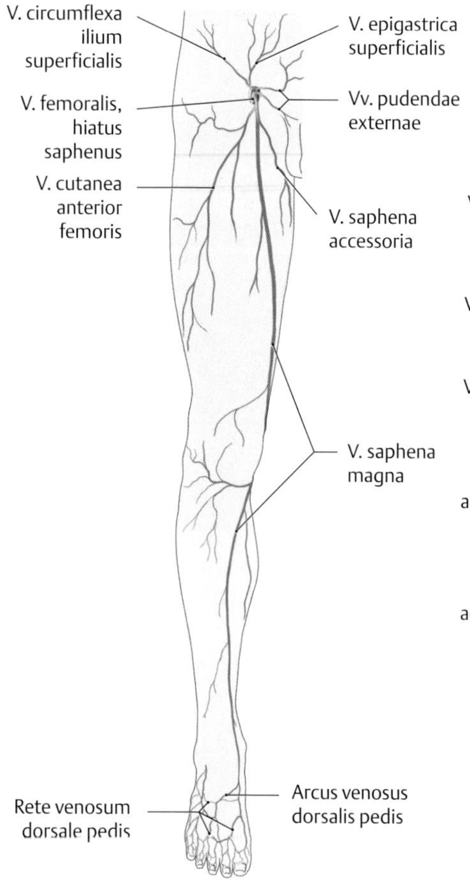

V. circumflexa ilium superficialis
V. epigastrica superficialis
V. femoralis, hiatus saphenus
Vv. pudendae externae
V. cutanea anterior femoris
V. saphena accessoria
V. saphena magna
Rete venosum dorsale pedis
Arcus venosus dorsalis pedis

A Superficial (epifascial) veins.

Lig. inguinale
V. iliaca externa
M. piriformis
Vv. circumflexae femoris laterales
Vv. circumflexa femoris mediales
V. profunda femoris
V. saphena magna
V. femoralis
V. saphena accessoria
Canalis adductorius
V. poplitea
Hiatus adductorius
M. adductor magnus
Vv. geniculares
V. saphena magna
Vv. tibiales anteriores
V. saphena parva
Rete venosum dorsale pedis

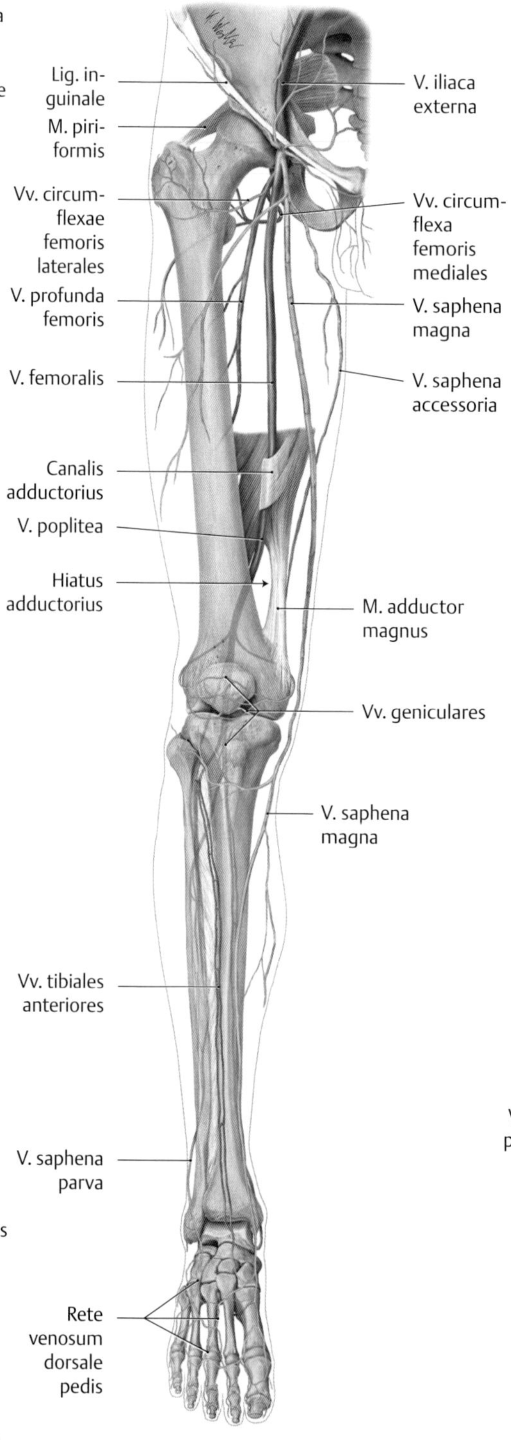

B Deep veins.

Fig. 27.6 Veins of the sole of the foot

Right foot, plantar view.

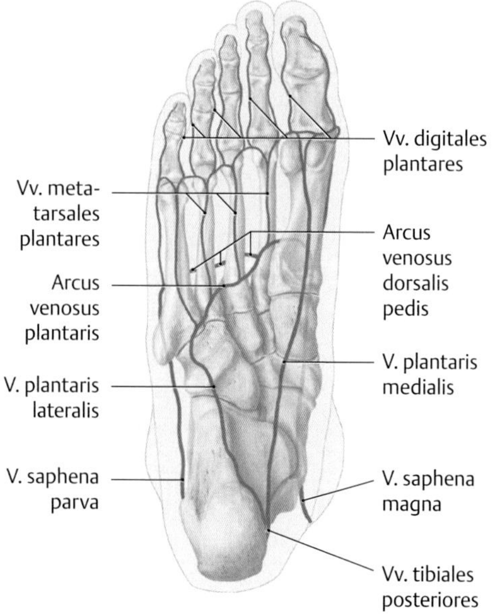

Vv. digitales plantares
Vv. metatarsales plantares
Arcus venosus dorsalis pedis
Arcus venosus plantaris
V. plantaris medialis
V. plantaris lateralis
V. saphena parva
V. saphena magna
Vv. tibiales posteriores

Fig. 27.7 Veins of the leg

Right leg, posterior view.

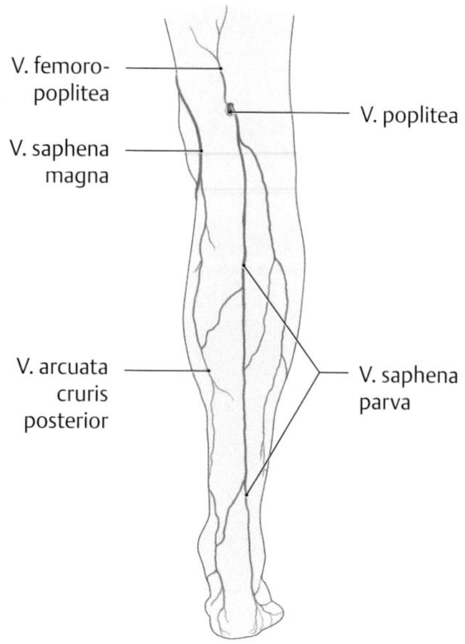

V. femoropoplitea
V. poplitea
V. saphena magna
V. arcuata cruris posterior
V. saphena parva

A Superficial (epifascial) veins.

V. poplitea
V. saphena parva
V. tibialis anterior
Vv. fibulares
Vv. tibiales posteriores
V. saphena parva
Malleolus lateralis

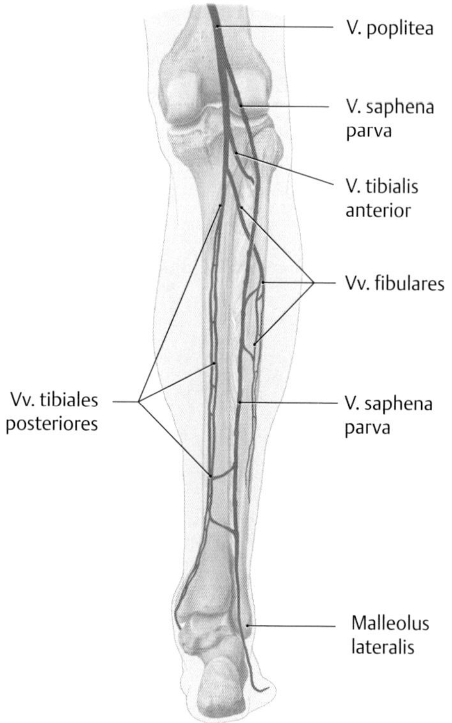

B Deep veins.

Fig. 27.8 Clinically important perforating veins

Right leg, medial view.

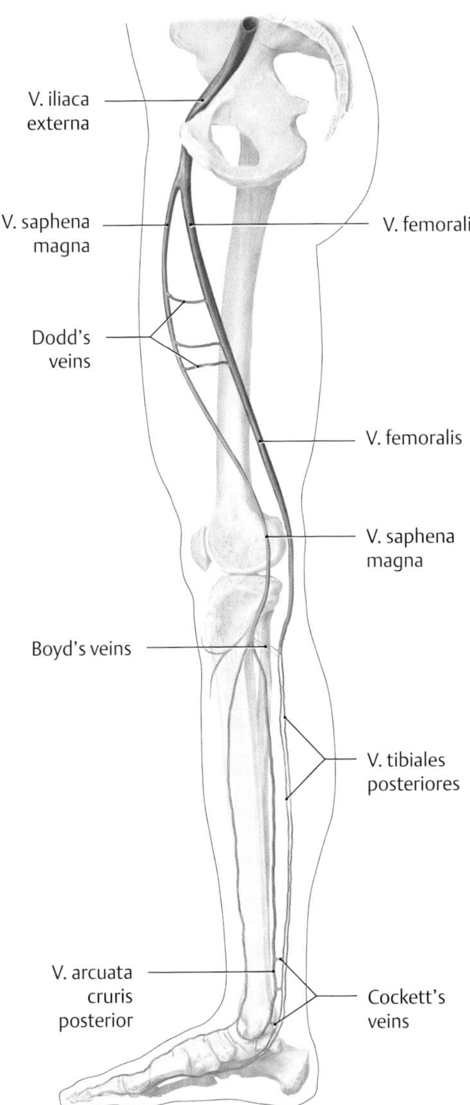
V. iliaca externa
V. saphena magna
V. femoralis
Dodd's veins
V. femoralis
V. saphena magna
Boyd's veins
V. tibiales posteriores
V. arcuata cruris posterior
Cockett's veins

Fig. 27.9 Superficial lymphatics

Right limb. Arrows indicate the main directions of lymphatic drainage.

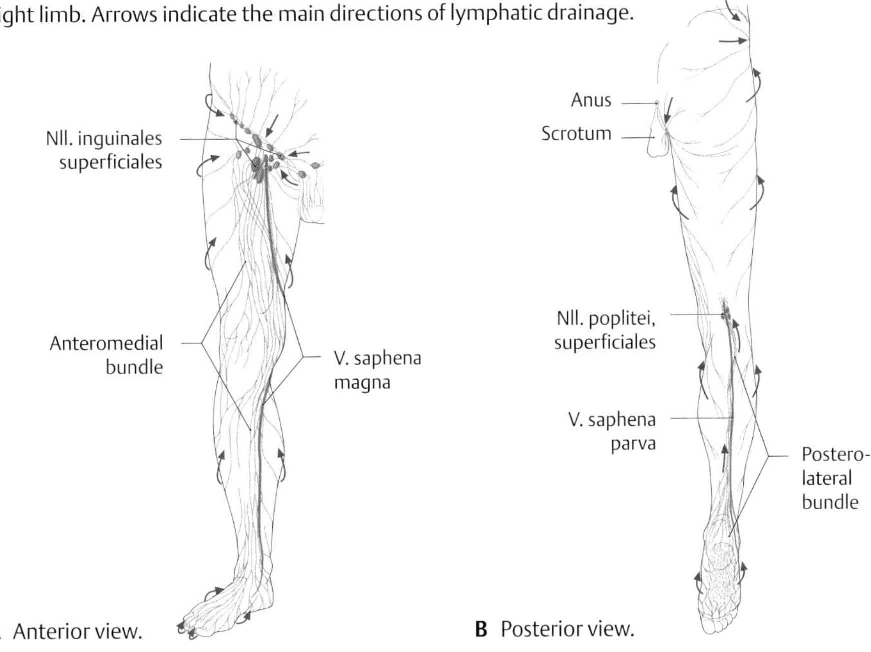
Nll. inguinales superficiales
Anteromedial bundle
V. saphena magna
Anus
Scrotum
Nll. poplitei, superficiales
V. saphena parva
Postero-lateral bundle

A Anterior view.

B Posterior view.

Fig. 27.10 Nodus lymphaticus and drainage

Right limb, anterior view.

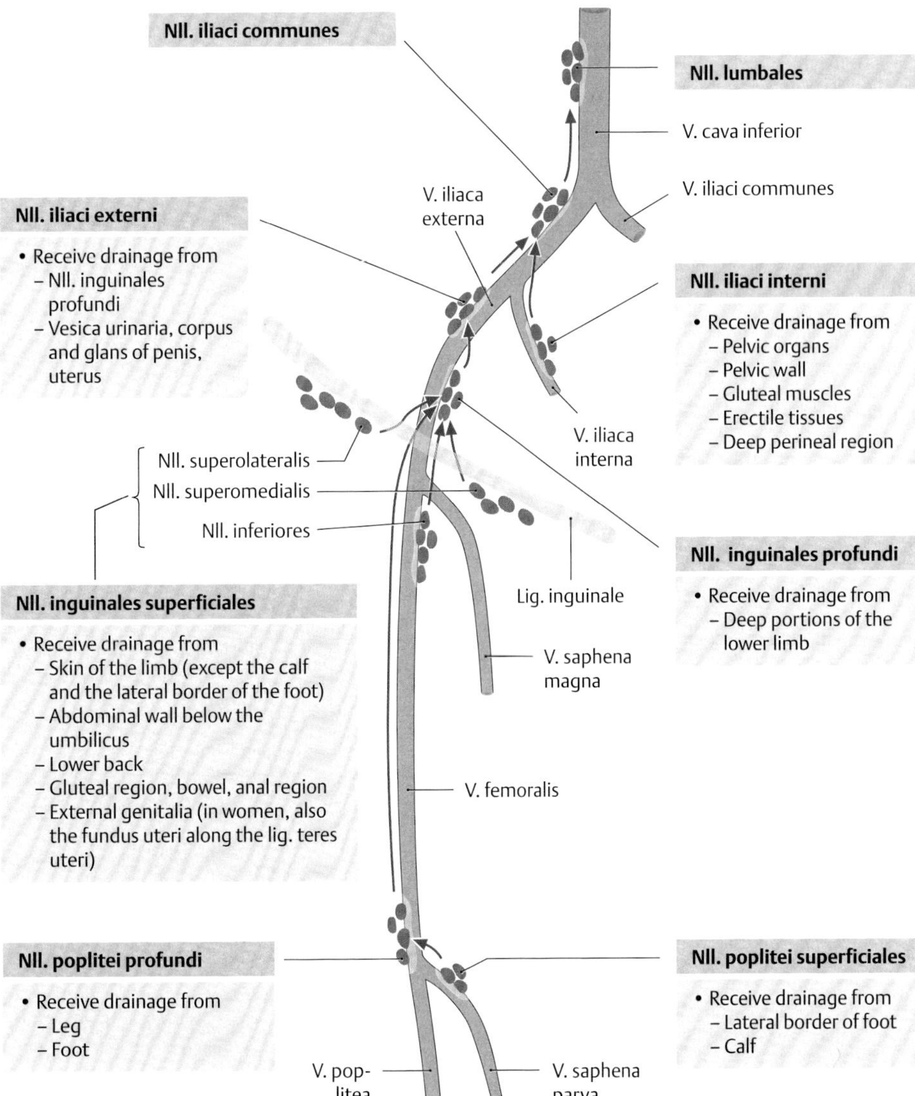
Nll. iliaci communes
Nll. lumbales
V. cava inferior
V. iliaci communes
V. iliaca externa
Nll. iliaci externi
• Receive drainage from
– Nll. inguinales profundi
– Vesica urinaria, corpus and glans of penis, uterus
Nll. iliaci interni
• Receive drainage from
– Pelvic organs
– Pelvic wall
– Gluteal muscles
– Erectile tissues
– Deep perineal region
V. iliaca interna
Nll. superolateralis
Nll. superomedialis
Nll. inferiores
Nll. inguinales profundi
• Receive drainage from
– Deep portions of the lower limb
Lig. inguinale
Nll. inguinales superficiales
• Receive drainage from
– Skin of the limb (except the calf and the lateral border of the foot)
– Abdominal wall below the umbilicus
– Lower back
– Gluteal region, bowel, anal region
– External genitalia (in women, also the fundus uteri along the lig. teres uteri)
V. saphena magna
V. femoralis
Nll. poplitei profundi
• Receive drainage from
– Leg
– Foot
Nll. poplitei superficiales
• Receive drainage from
– Lateral border of foot
– Calf
V. pop-litea
V. saphena parva

Plexus Lumbosacralis

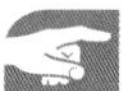

Plexus lumbosacralis supplies sensory and motor innervation to the lower limb. It is formed by the rr. anteriores of nn. lumbales and sacrales, with contributions from the n. subcostalis (T12) and n. coccygeus (Co).

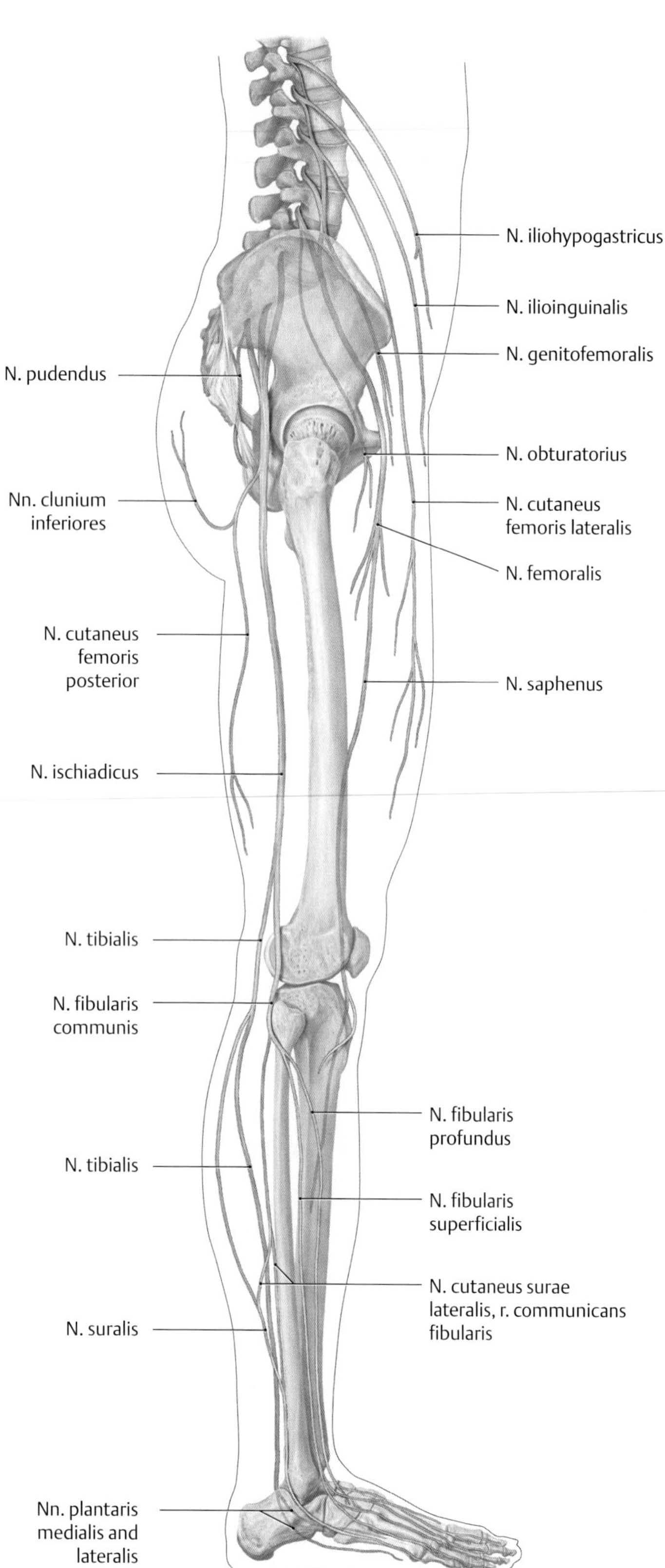
N. iliohypogastricus
N. ilioinguinalis
N. genitofemoralis
N. pudendus
N. obturatorius
Nn. clunium inferiores
N. cutaneus femoris lateralis
N. femoralis
N. cutaneus femoris posterior
N. saphenus
N. ischiadicus
N. tibialis
N. fibularis communis
N. fibularis profundus
N. tibialis
N. fibularis superficialis
N. cutaneus surae lateralis, r. communicans fibularis
N. suralis
Nn. plantaris medialis and lateralis

Table 27.1 Nerves of the lumbosacral plexus

Plexus lumbalis			
N. iliohypogastricus		L1	p. 427
N. ilioinguinalis			
N. genitofemoralis		L1–L2	
N. cutaneus femoralis lateralis		L2–L3	
N. obturatorius		L2–L4	p. 428
N. femoralis			p. 429
Plexus sacralis			
N. gluteus superior		L4–S1	p. 431
N. gluteus inferior		L5–S2	
N. cutaneus femoris posterior		S1–S3	p. 430
N. ischiadicus	N. fibularis communis	L4–S2	p. 432
	N. tibialis	L4–S3	p. 433
N. pudendus		S2–S4	pp. 194, 202

Fig. 27.11 Plexus lumbosacralis

Right side, anterior view.

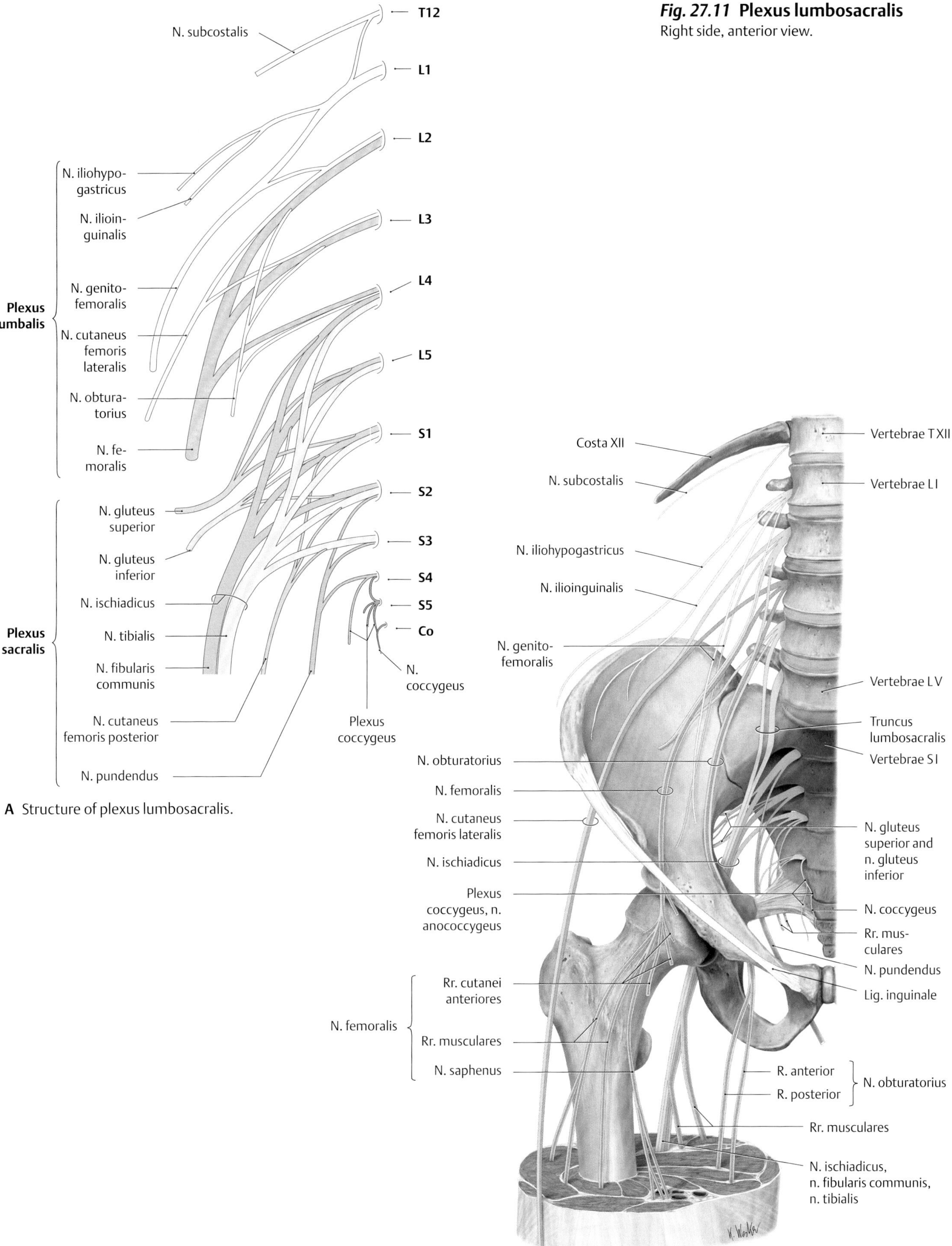
T12
L1
L2
L3
L4
L5
S1
S2
S3
S4
S5
Co
N. subcostalis
Plexus lumbalis
N. iliohypo-gastricus
N. ilioin-guinalis
N. genito-femoralis
N. cutaneus femoris lateralis
N. obtura-torius
N. fe-moralis
Plexus sacralis
N. gluteus superior
N. gluteus inferior
N. ischiadicus
N. tibialis
N. fibularis communis
N. cutaneus femoris posterior
N. pundendus
Plexus coccygeus
N. coccygeus

A Structure of plexus lumbosacralis.

Costa XII
N. subcostalis
N. iliohypogastricus
N. ilioinguinalis
N. genito-femoralis
N. obturatorius
N. femoralis
N. cutaneus femoris lateralis
N. ischiadicus
Plexus coccygeus, n. anococcygeus
N. femoralis
Rr. cutanei anteriores
Rr. musculares
N. saphenus
Vertebrae T XII
Vertebrae L I
Vertebrae L V
Truncus lumbosacralis
Vertebrae S I
N. gluteus superior and n. gluteus inferior
N. coccygeus
Rr. mus-culares
N. pundendus
Lig. inguinale
R. anterior
R. posterior
N. obturatorius
Rr. musculares
N. ischiadicus, n. fibularis communis, n. tibialis

B Course of plexus lumbosacralis.

Nerves of Plexus Lumbalis

Table 27.2 Nerves of the lumbar plexus

Nerve	Level	Innervated muscle	Cutaneous branches
N. iliohypogastricus	T12–L1	M. transversus abdominis and m. obliquus internus abdominis (inferior portions)	R. cutaneus lateralis, r.cutaneus anterior
N. ilioinguinalis	L1		Male: Nn. scrotales anteriores Female: Nn. labiales anteriores
N. genitofemoralis	L1–L2	Male: M.cremaster (r. genitalis)	R. genitalis R. femoralis
N. cutaneus femoralis lateralis	L2–L3	–	N. cutaneus femoralis lateralis
N. obturatorius	L2–L4	See p. 428	
N. femoralis	L2–L4	See p. 429	
Short, direct muscular branches	T12–L4	M. psoas major M. quadratus lumborum M. iliacus Mm. intertransversarii lumborum	–

Fig. 27.12 **Sensory innervation of the inguinal region**
Right male inguinal region, anterior view.

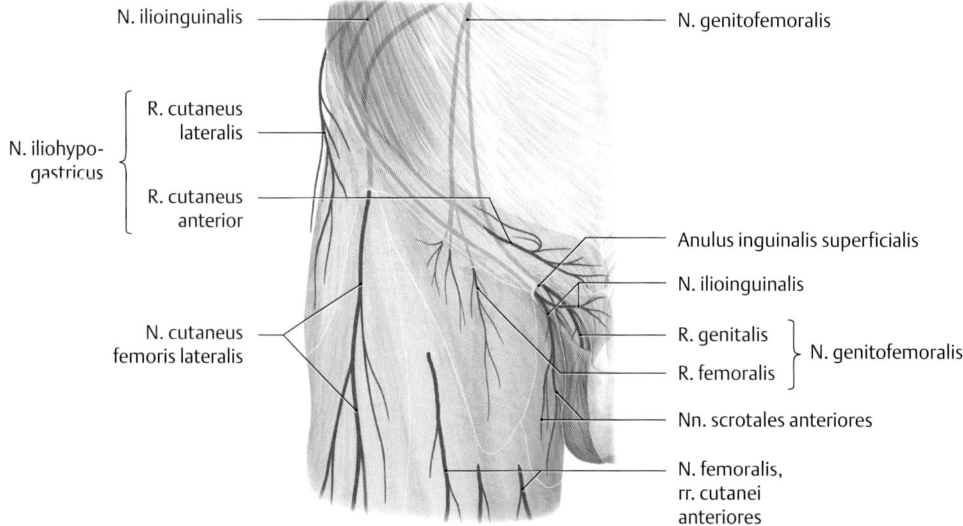
N. ilioinguinalis
N. genitofemoralis
N. iliohypo-gastricus
R. cutaneus lateralis
R. cutaneus anterior
Anulus inguinalis superficialis
N. ilioinguinalis
R. genitalis
R. femoralis
N. genitofemoralis
N. cutaneus femoris lateralis
Nn. scrotales anteriores
N. femoralis, rr. cutanei anteriores

Fig. 27.13 Nerves of plexus lumbalis

Right side, anterior view with the anterior abdominal wall removed.

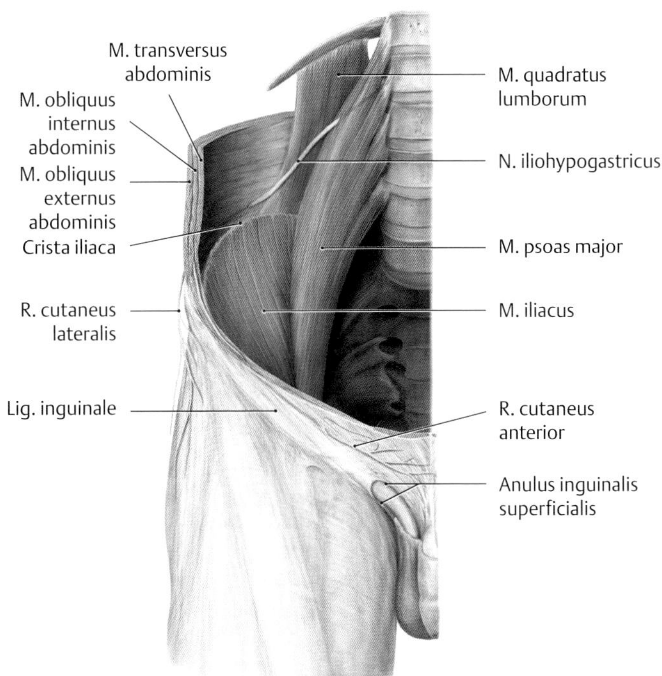
M. transversus abdominis
M. obliquus internus abdominis
M. obliquus externus abdominis
Crista iliaca
R. cutaneus lateralis
Lig. inguinale
M. quadratus lumborum
N. iliohypogastricus
M. psoas major
M. iliacus
R. cutaneus anterior
Anulus inguinalis superficialis

A N. iliohypogastricus.

M. transversus abdominis
M. obliquus internus abdominis
M. iliacus
Lig. inguinale
N. ilioinguinalis
M. quadratus lumborum
N. ilioinguinalis
M. psoas major
Anulus inguinalis superficialis
Funiculus spermaticus

B N. ilioinguinalis.

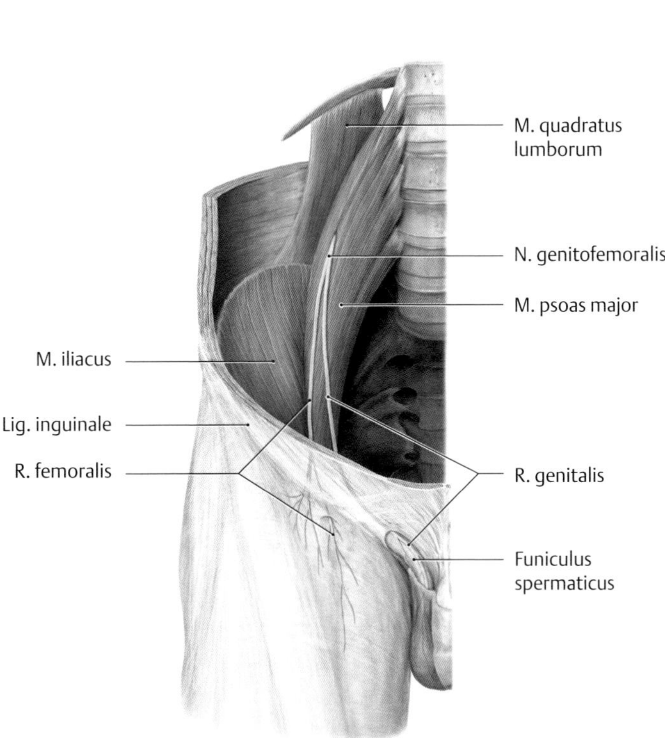
M. quadratus lumborum
N. genitofemoralis
M. psoas major
M. iliacus
Lig. inguinale
R. femoralis
R. genitalis
Funiculus spermaticus

C N. genitofemoralis.

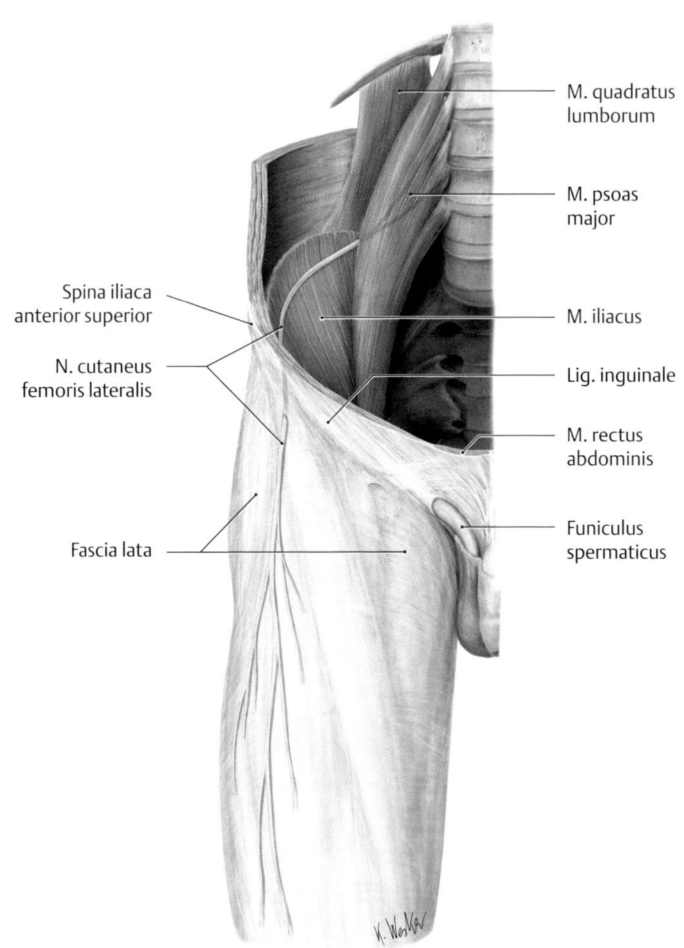
M. quadratus lumborum
M. psoas major
Spina iliaca anterior superior
M. iliacus
N. cutaneus femoris lateralis
Lig. inguinale
M. rectus abdominis
Fascia lata
Funiculus spermaticus

D N. cutaneus femoris lateralis.

Nerves of Plexus Lumbalis: N. Obturatoris & N. Femoralis

Fig. 27.15 **N. obturatorius**
Right side, anterior view.

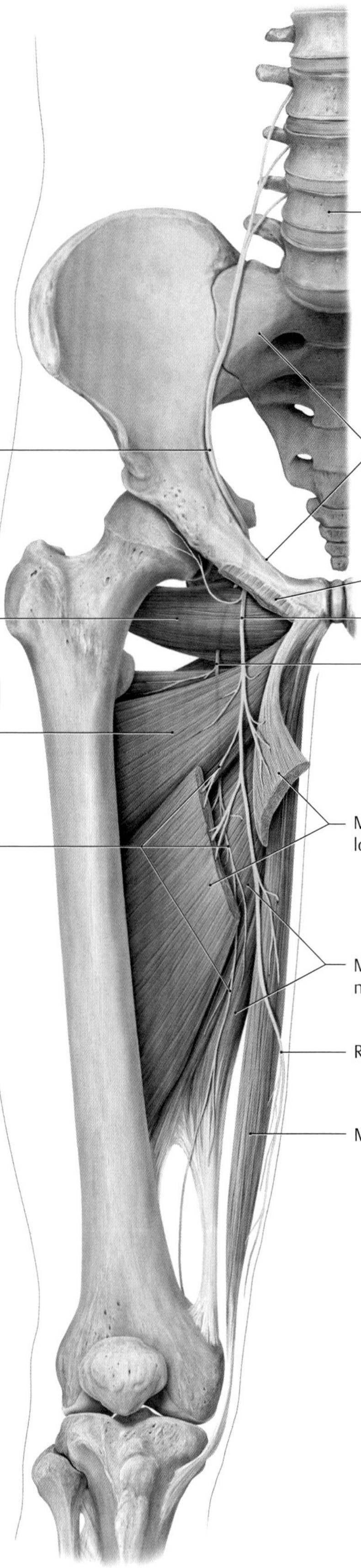

Vertebrae L IV
N. obturatorius
Linea terminalis
M. pectineus
M. obturatorius externus
R. anterior
R. posterior
M. adductor brevis
Rr. musculares
M. adductor longus
M. adductor magnus
R. cutaneus
M. gracilis

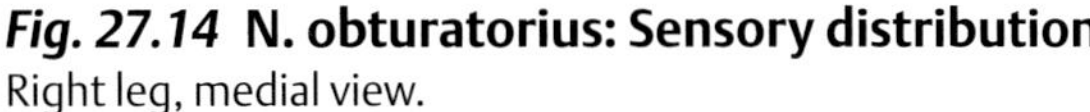

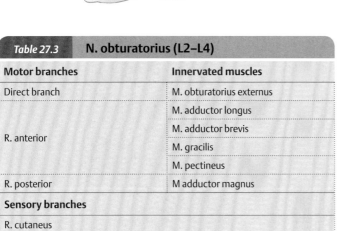

Fig. 27.14 **N. obturatorius: Sensory distribution**
Right leg, medial view.

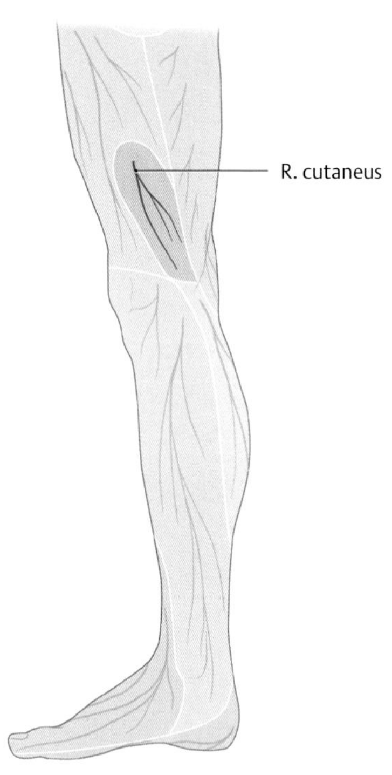
R. cutaneus

Table 27.3 N. obturatorius (L2–L4)

Motor branches	Innervated muscles
Direct branch	M. obturatorius externus
R. anterior	M. adductor longus
	M. adductor brevis
	M. gracilis
	M. pectineus
R. posterior	M adductor magnus
Sensory branches	
R. cutaneus	

Fig. 27.16 **N. femoralis**
Right side, anterior view.

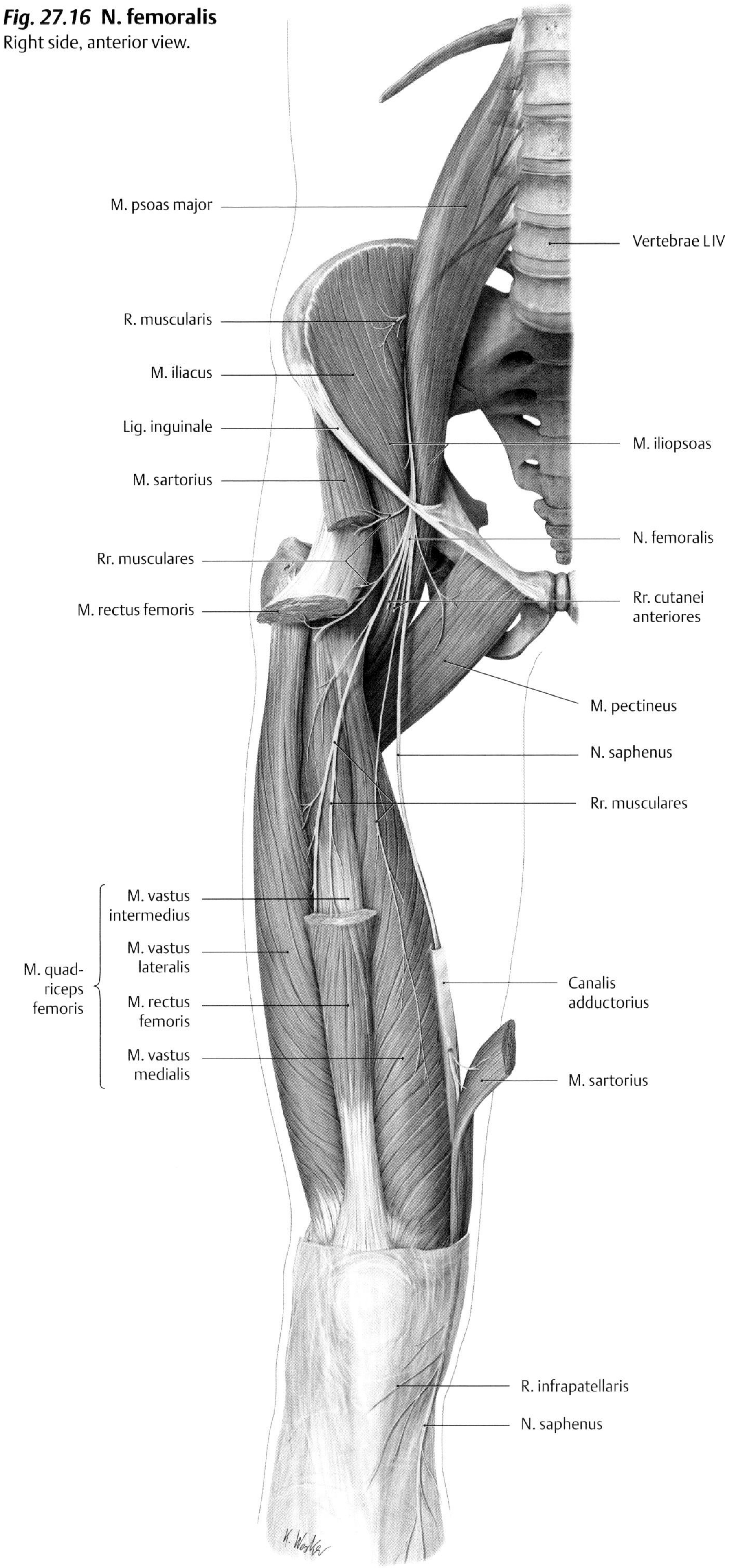

M. psoas major
Vertebrae L IV
R. muscularis
M. iliacus
Lig. inguinale
M. iliopsoas
M. sartorius
N. femoralis
Rr. musculares
M. rectus femoris
Rr. cutanei anteriores
M. pectineus
N. saphenus
Rr. musculares
M. quadriceps femoris: M. vastus intermedius, M. vastus lateralis, M. rectus femoris, M. vastus medialis
Canalis adductorius
M. sartorius
R. infrapatellaris
N. saphenus

Fig. 27.17 **N. femoralis: Sensory distribution**
Right limb, anterior view.

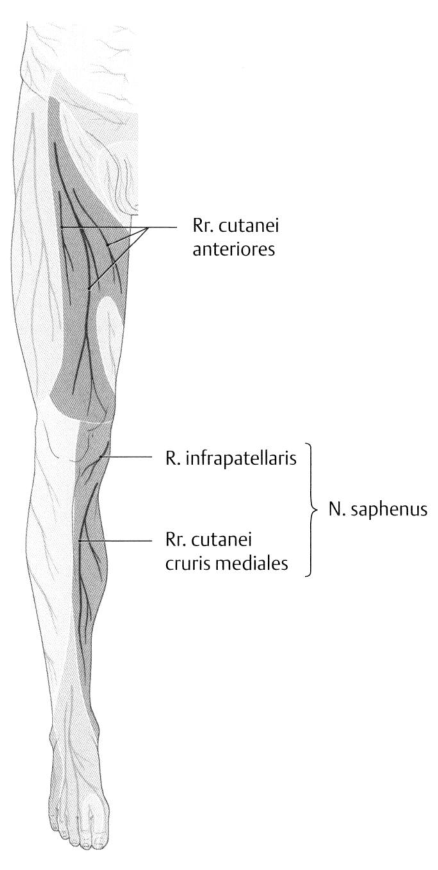
Rr. cutanei anteriores
R. infrapatellaris
Rr. cutanei cruris mediales
N. saphenus

Table 27.4	**N. femoralis (L2–L4)**
Motor branches	**Innervated muscles**
Rr. musculares	M. iliopsoas
	M. pectineus
	M. sartorius
	M. quadriceps femoris
Sensory branches	
Rr. cutanei anteriores	
N. saphenus	

Nerves of Plexus Sacralis

Table 27.5 Nerves of plexus sacralis

Nerve		Level	Innervated muscle	Cutaneous branches	
N. gluteus superior		L4–S1	M. gluteus medius M. gluteus minimus M. tensor fasciae latae	–	
N. gluteus inferior		L5–S2	M. gluteus maximus	–	
N. cutaneus femoris lateralis		S1–S3	–	N. cutaneus femoris posterior	Nn. clunium inferiores
					Rr. perineales
Direct branches	N. musculi piriformis	S1–S2	M. piriformis	–	
	N. musculi obturatorii interni	L5–S1	M. obturatorius internus Mm. gemelli	–	
	N. musculi quadrati femoris		M. quadratus femoris	–	
N. ischiadicus	N. fibularis communis	L4–S2	See p. 432		
	N. tibialis	L4–S3	See p. 433		

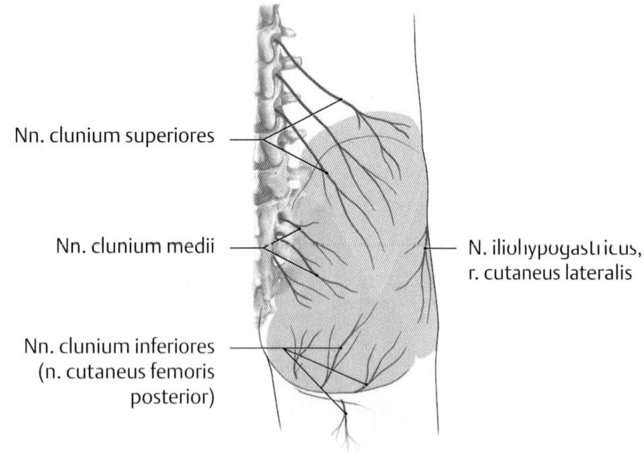
Nn. clunium superiores
Nn. clunium medii
N. iliohypogastricus,
r. cutaneus lateralis
Nn. clunium inferiores
(n. cutaneus femoris
posterior)

Fig. 27.18 **Sensory innervation of the gluteal region**
Right limb, posterior view.

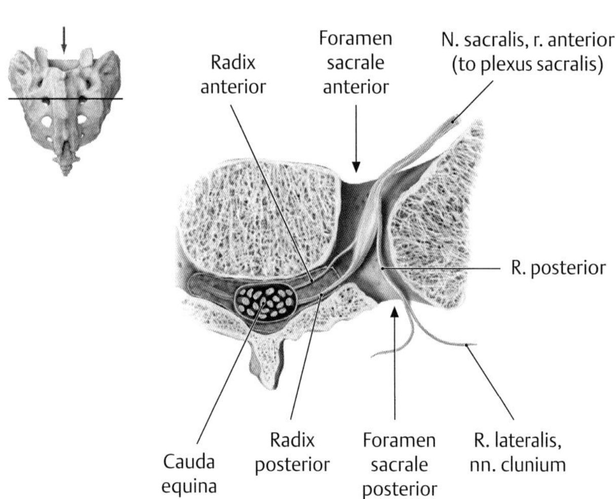
Radix
anterior
Foramen
sacrale
anterior
N. sacralis, r. anterior
(to plexus sacralis)
R. posterior
Cauda
equina
Radix
posterior
Foramen
sacrale
posterior
R. lateralis,
nn. clunium

Fig. 27.20 **Emerging n. sacralis**
Horizontal section, superior view.

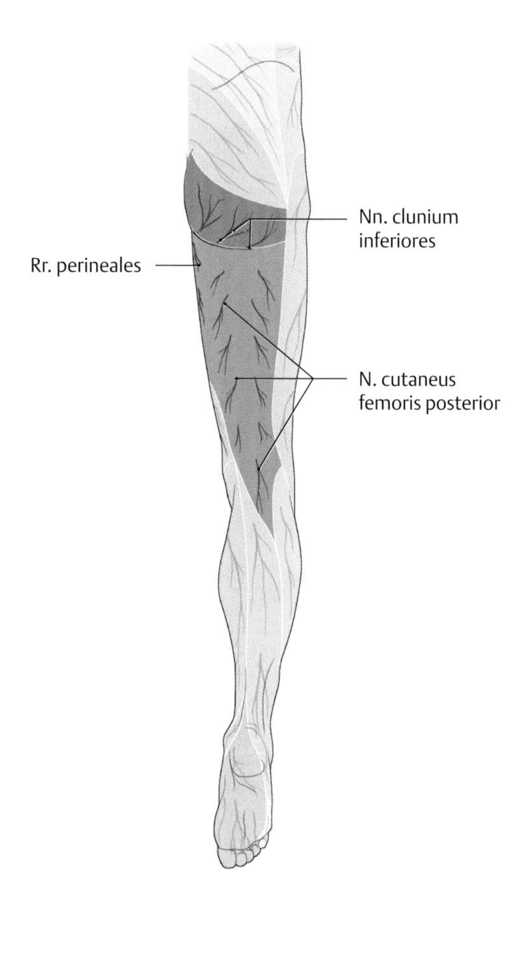
Nn. clunium
inferiores
Rr. perineales
N. cutaneus
femoris posterior

Fig. 27.19 **N. cutaneus femoris posterior: Sensory distribution**
Right limb, posterior view.

Fig. 27.21 Nerves of plexus sacralis

Right limb.

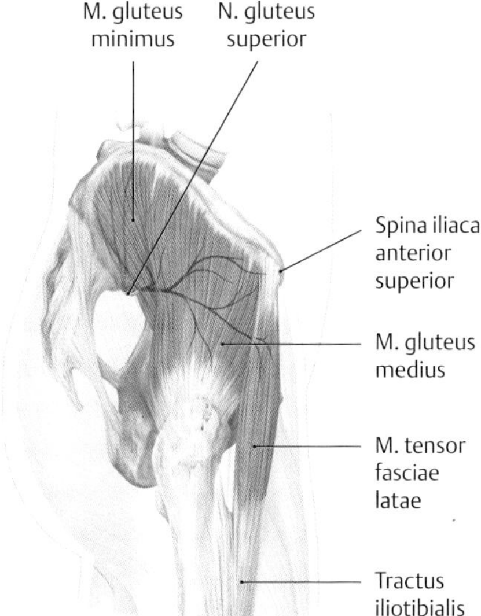
M. gluteus minimus
N. gluteus superior
Spina iliaca anterior superior
M. gluteus medius
M. tensor fasciae latae
Tractus iliotibialis

A N. gluteus superior. Lateral view.

Clinical

Small gluteal muscle weakness

The small gluteal muscles on the stance side stabilize the pelvis in the coronal plane. Weakness or paralysis of the small gluteal muscles from damage to the n. gluteus superior (e.g., due to a faulty intramuscular injection) is manifested by weak abduction of the affected hip joint.
In a positive Trendelenburg's test, the pelvis sags toward the normal, unsupported side. Tilting the upper body toward the affected side shifts the center of gravity onto the stance side, thereby elevating the pelvis on the swing side (Duchenne's limp). With bilateral loss of the small gluteals, the patient exhibits a typical waddling gait.

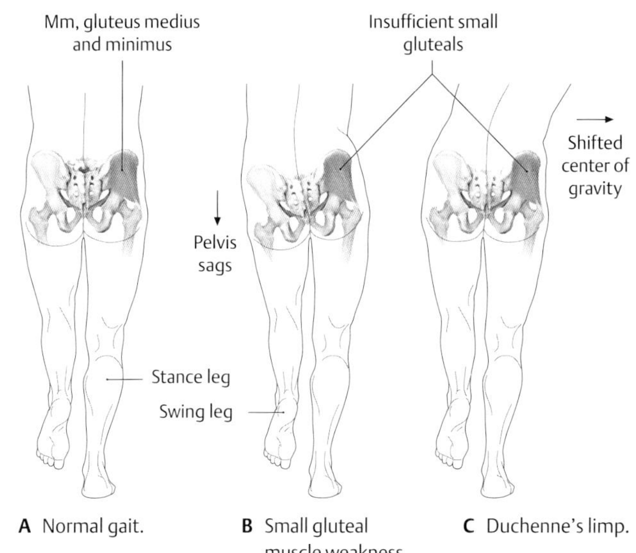
Mm, gluteus medius and minimus
Insufficient small gluteals
Shifted center of gravity
Pelvis sags
Stance leg
Swing leg

A Normal gait. **B** Small gluteal muscle weakness. **C** Duchenne's limp.

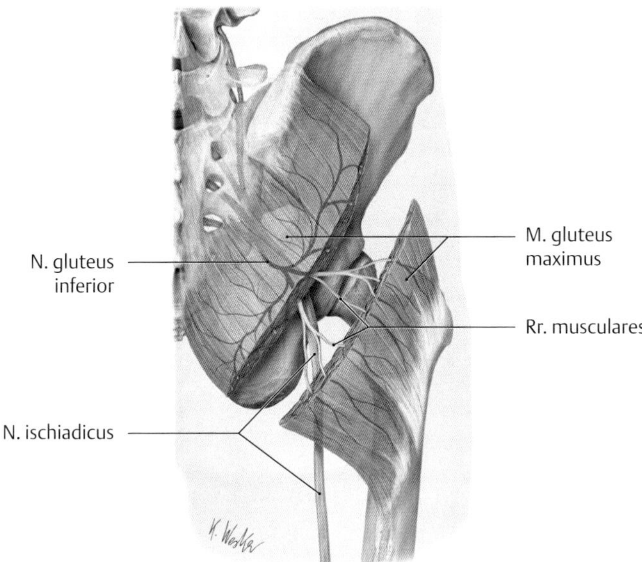
N. gluteus inferior
M. gluteus maximus
Rr. musculares
N. ischiadicus

B N. gluteus inferior. Posterior view.

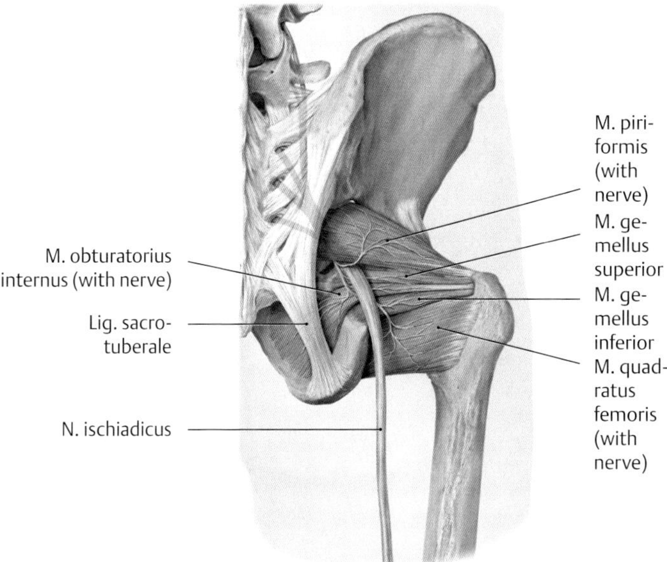
M. obturatorius internus (with nerve)
Lig. sacrotuberale
N. ischiadicus
M. piriformis (with nerve)
M. gemellus superior
M. gemellus inferior
M. quadratus femoris (with nerve)

C Direct branches. Posterior view.

Nerves of Plexus Sacralis: N. Ischiadicus

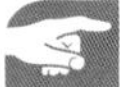

N. ischiadicus gives off several direct muscular branches before dividing into the n. tibialis and n. fibularis communis proximal to the fossa poplitea.

Fig. 27.22 N. fibularis communis: Sensory distribution

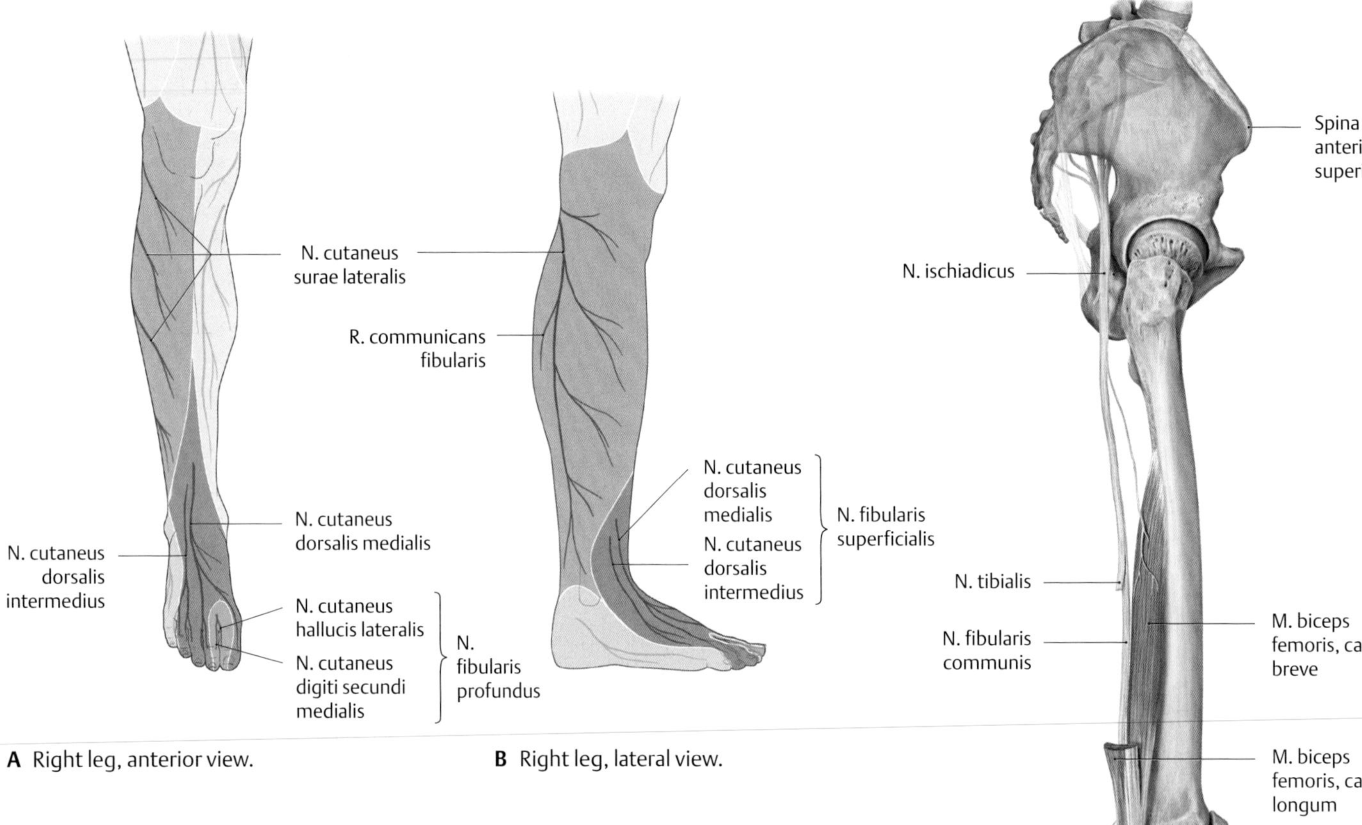

N. cutaneus surae lateralis
R. communicans fibularis
N. cutaneus dorsalis medialis
N. cutaneus dorsalis intermedius
N. cutaneus hallucis lateralis
N. cutaneus digiti secundi medialis
N. fibularis profundus
N. cutaneus dorsalis medialis
N. cutaneus dorsalis intermedius
N. fibularis superficialis

A Right leg, anterior view.

B Right leg, lateral view.

Table 27.6 N. fibularis communis (L4–S2)

Nerve	Innervated muscles	Sensory branches
Direct branches from n. ischiadicus	M. biceps femoris (caput breve)	–
N. fibularis superficialis	M. fibularis brevis and longus	N. cutaneus dorsalis medialis N. cutaneus dorsalis intermedius
N. fibularis profundus	M. tibialis anterior Mm. extensor digitorum brevis and longus Mm. extensor hallucis brevis and longus M. fibularis tertius	N. cutaneus hallucis lateralis N. cutaneus digiti secundi medialis

Fig. 27.23 N. fibularis communis
Right limb, lateral view.

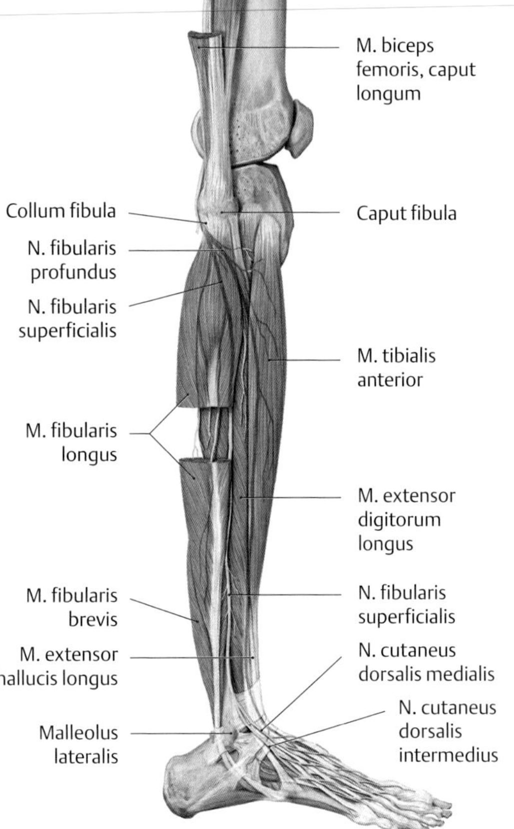

Spina iliaca anterior superior
N. ischiadicus
N. tibialis
N. fibularis communis
M. biceps femoris, caput breve
M. biceps femoris, caput longum
Collum fibula
Caput fibula
N. fibularis profundus
N. fibularis superficialis
M. tibialis anterior
M. fibularis longus
M. extensor digitorum longus
M. fibularis brevis
N. fibularis superficialis
M. extensor hallucis longus
N. cutaneus dorsalis medialis
N. cutaneus dorsalis intermedius
Malleolus lateralis

Fig. 27.24 **N. tibialis**
Right limb.

Fig. 27.25 **N. tibialis: Sensory distribution**
Right lower limb, posterior view.

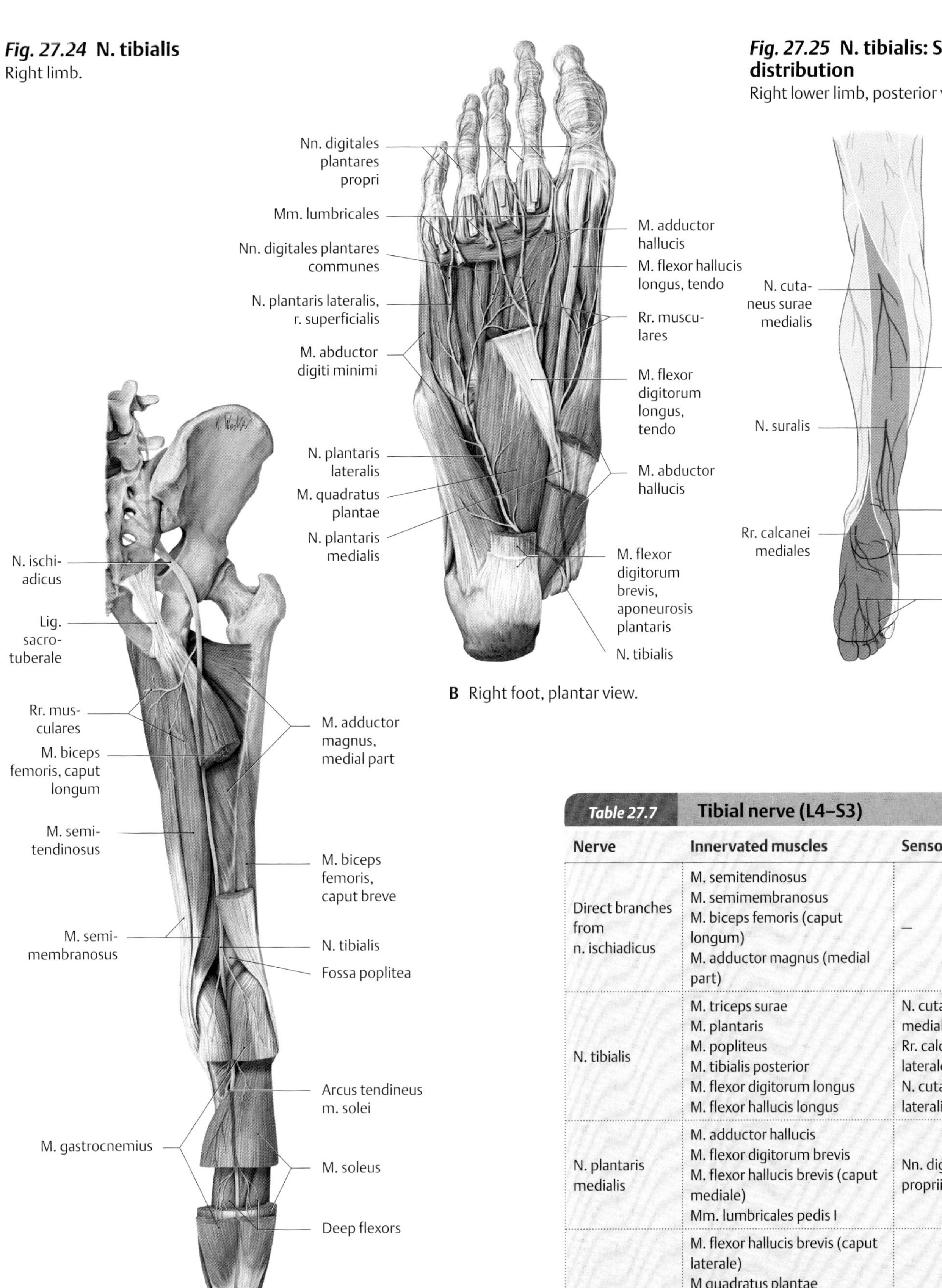
Nn. digitales plantares propri
Mm. lumbricales
Nn. digitales plantares communes
N. plantaris lateralis, r. superficialis
M. abductor digiti minimi
N. plantaris lateralis
M. quadratus plantae
N. plantaris medialis
M. adductor hallucis
M. flexor hallucis longus, tendo
Rr. musculares
M. flexor digitorum longus, tendo
M. abductor hallucis
M. flexor digitorum brevis, aponeurosis plantaris
N. tibialis
N. ischiadicus
Lig. sacrotuberale
Rr. musculares
M. biceps femoris, caput longum
M. semitendinosus
M. semimembranosus
M. gastrocnemius
Deep flexor tendons
N. tibialis (in malleolar canal)
M. adductor magnus, medial part
M. biceps femoris, caput breve
N. tibialis
Fossa poplitea
Arcus tendineus m. solei
M. soleus
Deep flexors
Malleolus lateralis
N. cutaneus surae medialis
R. communicans fibularis
N. suralis
Rr. calcanei mediales
N. cutaneus dorsalis lateralis
Rr. calcanei laterales
Nn. digitales plantares proprii

B Right foot, plantar view.

A Posterior view.

Table 27.7 **Tibial nerve (L4–S3)**

Nerve	Innervated muscles	Sensory branches
Direct branches from n. ischiadicus	M. semitendinosus M. semimembranosus M. biceps femoris (caput longum) M. adductor magnus (medial part)	–
N. tibialis	M. triceps surae M. plantaris M. popliteus M. tibialis posterior M. flexor digitorum longus M. flexor hallucis longus	N. cutaneus surae mediales Rr. calcanei mediales and laterales N. cutaneus dorsalis lateralis
N. plantaris medialis	M. adductor hallucis M. flexor digitorum brevis M. flexor hallucis brevis (caput mediale) Mm. lumbricales pedis I	Nn. digitales plantares proprii
N. plantaris lateralis	M. flexor hallucis brevis (caput laterale) M quadratus plantae M. abductor digiti minimi M. flexor digiti minimi brevis M. opponens digiti minimi Mm. lumbricales pedis II–IV Mm. interossei plantares I–III Mm. interossei dorsales I–IV M. adductor hallucis	Nn. digitales plantares proprii

Superficial Nerves & Vessels of the Lower Limb

Fig. 27.26 Cutaneous innervation: Anterior view

Right limb.

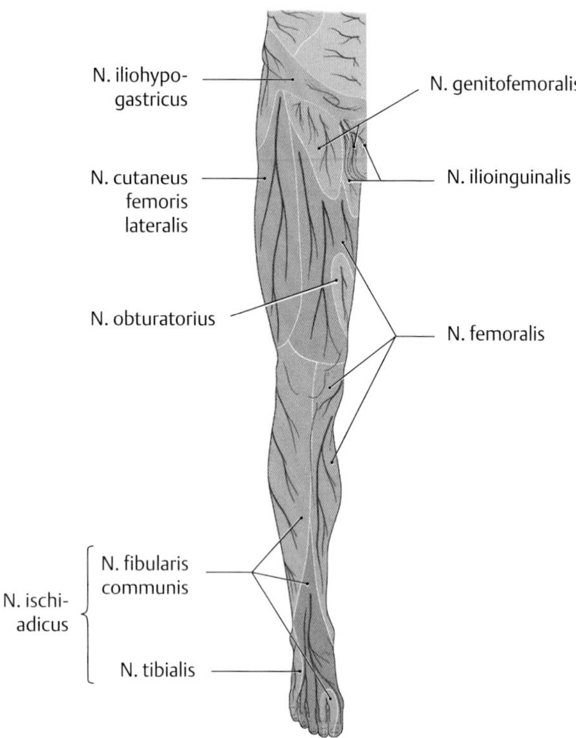

N. iliohypo-
gastricus
N. genitofemoralis
N. cutaneus
femoris
lateralis
N. ilioinguinalis
N. obturatorius
N. femoralis
N. ischi-
adicus
N. fibularis
communis
N. tibialis

A Peripheral sensory cutaneous innervation.

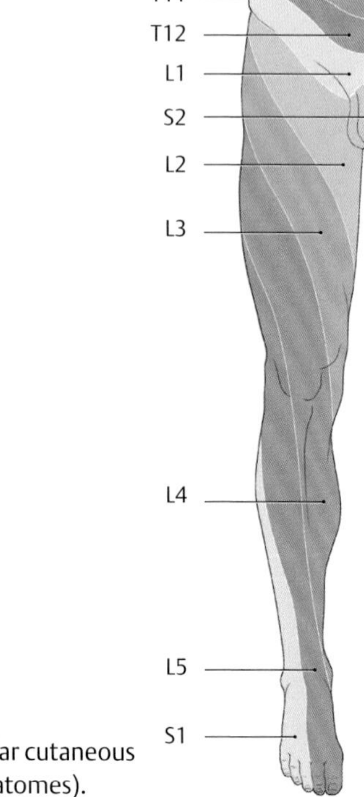

T11
T12
L1
S2
L2
L3
L4
L5
S1

B Segmental, radicular cutaneous innervation (dermatomes).

Fig. 27.27 Superficial cutaneous veins and nerves

Right limb.

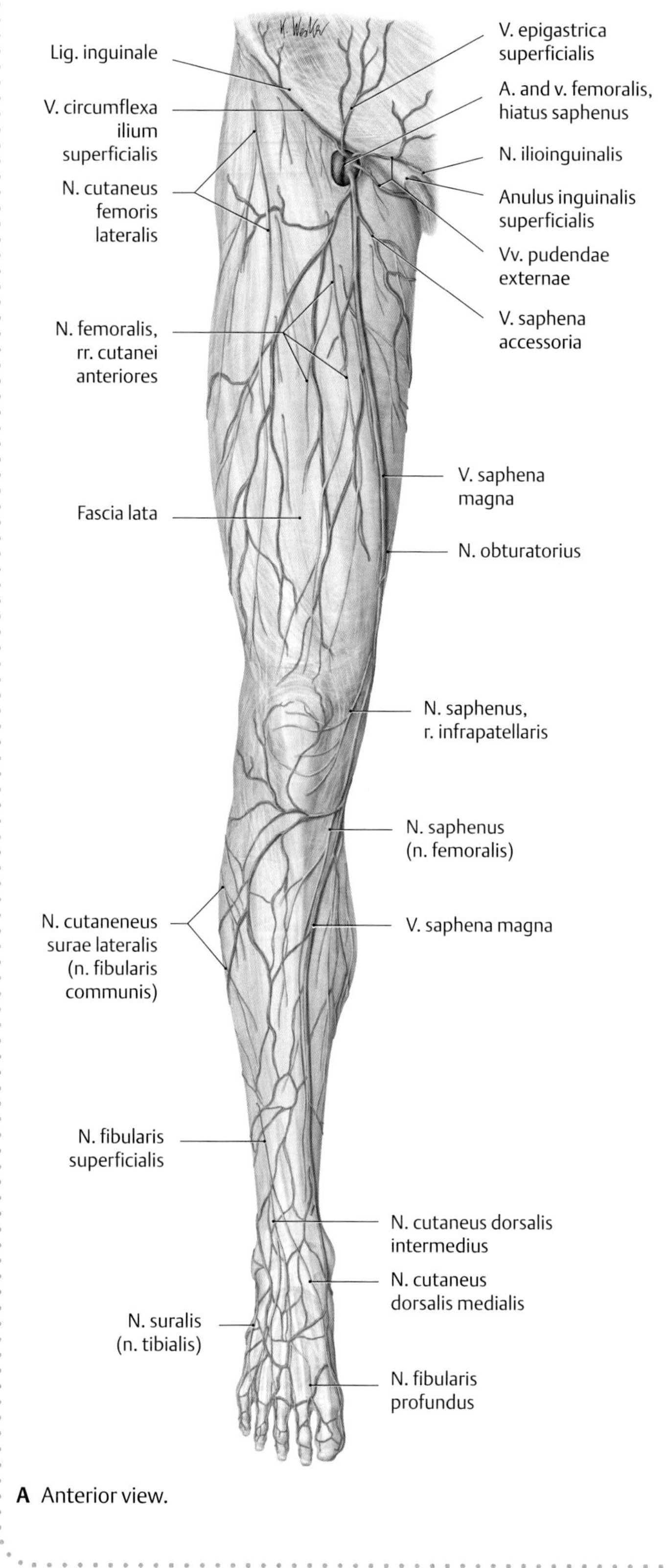

Lig. inguinale
V. circumflexa
ilium
superficialis
N. cutaneus
femoris
lateralis
N. femoralis,
rr. cutanei
anteriores
Fascia lata
N. cutaneneus
surae lateralis
(n. fibularis
communis)
N. fibularis
superficialis
N. suralis
(n. tibialis)
V. epigastrica
superficialis
A. and v. femoralis,
hiatus saphenus
N. ilioinguinalis
Anulus inguinalis
superficialis
Vv. pudendae
externae
V. saphena
accessoria
V. saphena
magna
N. obturatorius
N. saphenus,
r. infrapatellaris
N. saphenus
(n. femoralis)
V. saphena magna
N. cutaneus dorsalis
intermedius
N. cutaneus
dorsalis medialis
N. fibularis
profundus

A Anterior view.

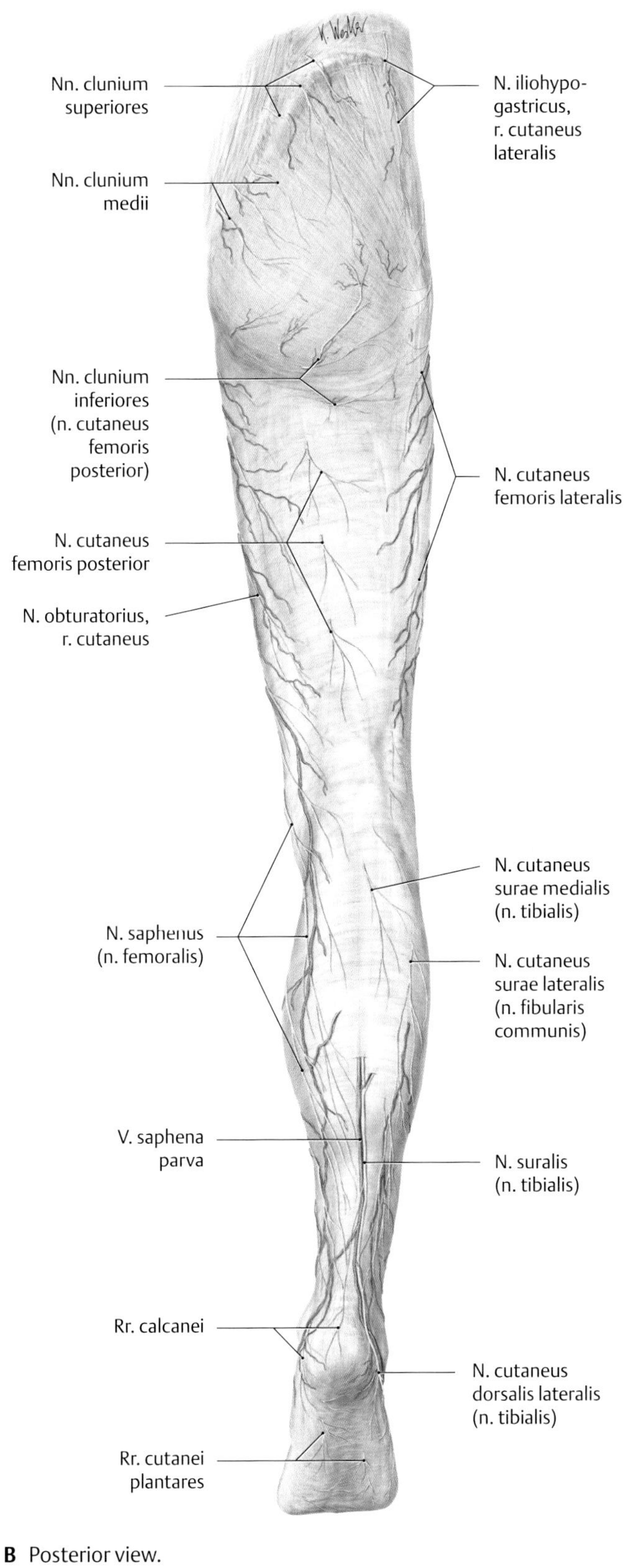
Nn. clunium superiores
N. iliohypogastricus, r. cutaneus lateralis
Nn. clunium medii
Nn. clunium inferiores (n. cutaneus femoris posterior)
N. cutaneus femoris lateralis
N. cutaneus femoris posterior
N. obturatorius, r. cutaneus
N. cutaneus surae medialis (n. tibialis)
N. saphenus (n. femoralis)
N. cutaneus surae lateralis (n. fibularis communis)
V. saphena parva
N. suralis (n. tibialis)
Rr. calcanei
N. cutaneus dorsalis lateralis (n. tibialis)
Rr. cutanei plantares

B Posterior view.

Fig. 27.28 Cutaneous innervation: Posterior view

Right limb.

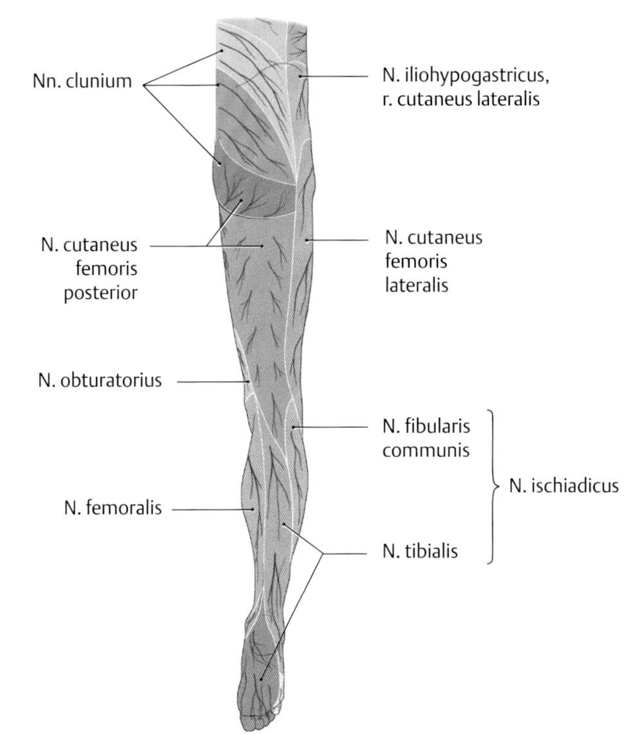
Nn. clunium
N. iliohypogastricus, r. cutaneus lateralis
N. cutaneus femoris posterior
N. cutaneus femoris lateralis
N. obturatorius
N. fibularis communis
N. ischiadicus
N. femoralis
N. tibialis

A Peripheral sensory cutaneous innervation.

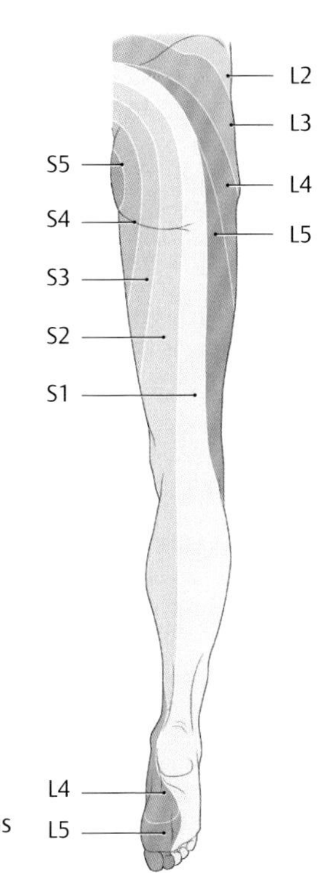
L2
L3
S5
L4
S4
L5
S3
S2
S1
L4
L5

B Segmental, radicular cutaneous innervation (dermatomes).

Topography of Regio Inguinalis

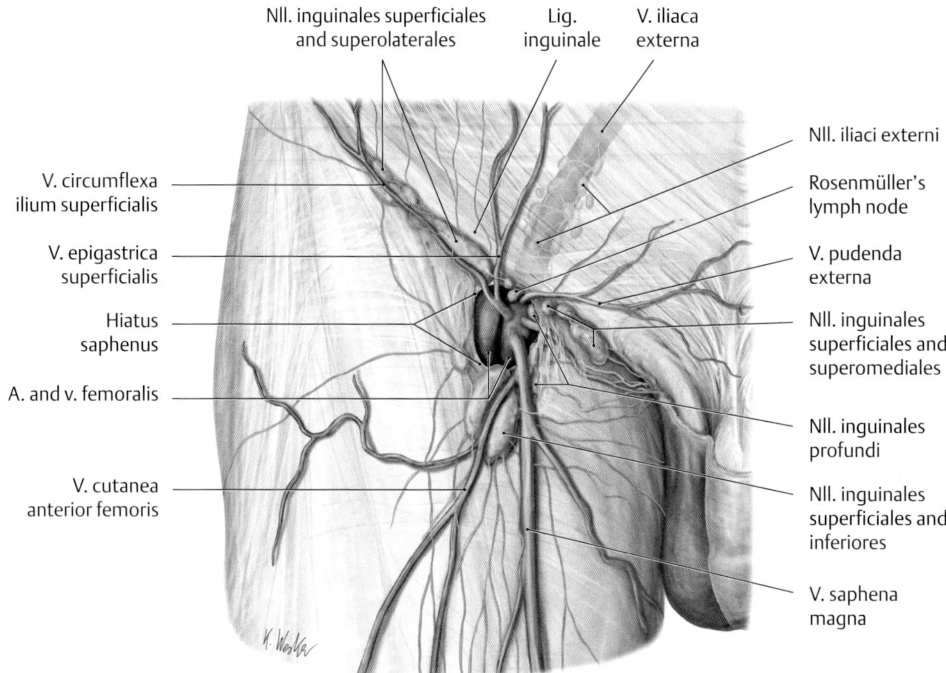
Nll. inguinales superficiales and superolaterales
Lig. inguinale
V. iliaca externa
Nll. iliaci externi
Rosenmüller's lymph node
V. pudenda externa
Nll. inguinales superficiales and superomediales
Nll. inguinales profundi
Nll. inguinales superficiales and inferiores
V. saphena magna
V. circumflexa ilium superficialis
V. epigastrica superficialis
Hiatus saphenus
A. and v. femoralis
V. cutanea anterior femoris

Fig. 27.29 **Superficial veins and lymph nodes**
Right male regio inguinales, anterior view. *Removed:* Fascia cribrosa about hiatus saphenus.

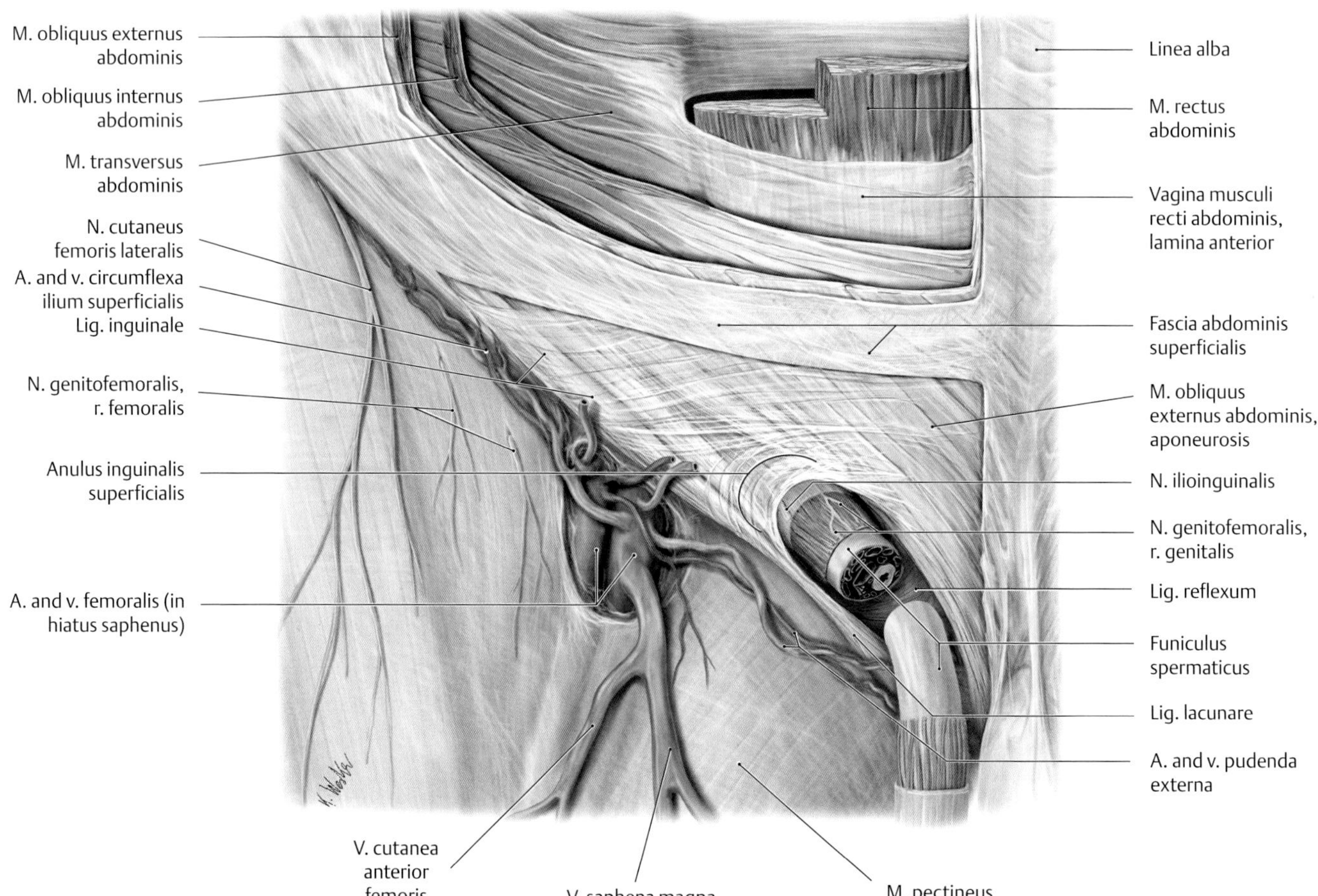
M. obliquus externus abdominis
M. obliquus internus abdominis
M. transversus abdominis
N. cutaneus femoris lateralis
A. and v. circumflexa ilium superficialis
Lig. inguinale
N. genitofemoralis, r. femoralis
Anulus inguinalis superficialis
A. and v. femoralis (in hiatus saphenus)
V. cutanea anterior femoris
V. saphena magna
M. pectineus
Linea alba
M. rectus abdominis
Vagina musculi recti abdominis, lamina anterior
Fascia abdominis superficialis
M. obliquus externus abdominis, aponeurosis
N. ilioinguinalis
N. genitofemoralis, r. genitalis
Lig. reflexum
Funiculus spermaticus
Lig. lacunare
A. and v. pudenda externa

Fig. 27.30 **Regio inguinales**
Right male regio inguinales, anterior view.

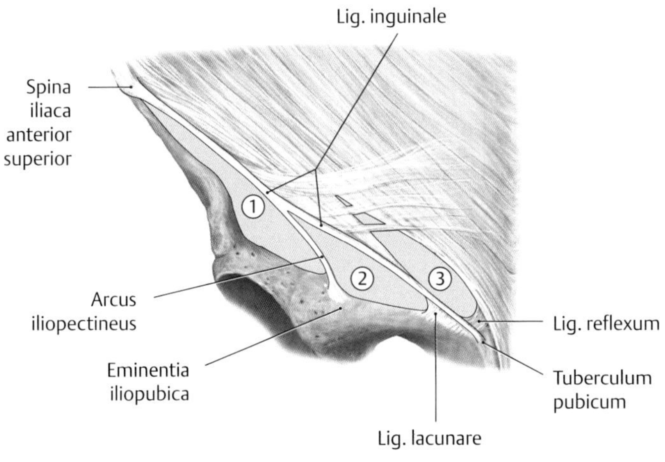
Lig. inguinale
Spina iliaca anterior superior
Arcus iliopectineus
Eminentia iliopubica
Lig. lacunare
Lig. reflexum
Tuberculum pubicum
①
②
③

Table 27.8 Structures in the inguinal region

Region	Boundaries	Contents
① Lacuna musculorum	Spina iliaca anterior superior Lig. inguinale Arcus iliopectineus	N. femoralis N. cutaneus femoris lateralis M. iliacus M. psoas major
② Lacuna vasorum	Lig. inguinale Arcus iliopectineus Lig. lacunare	A. and v. femoralis N. genitofemoralis (r. femoralis) Rosenmüller's lymph node
③ Anulus inguinalis superficialis	Crus mediale Crus laterale Lig. reflexum	N. ilioinguinalis N. genitofemoralis (r. genitalis) Funiculus spermaticus

Fig. 27.31 **Lacunae musculorum and vasorum**
Right inguinal region, anterior view.

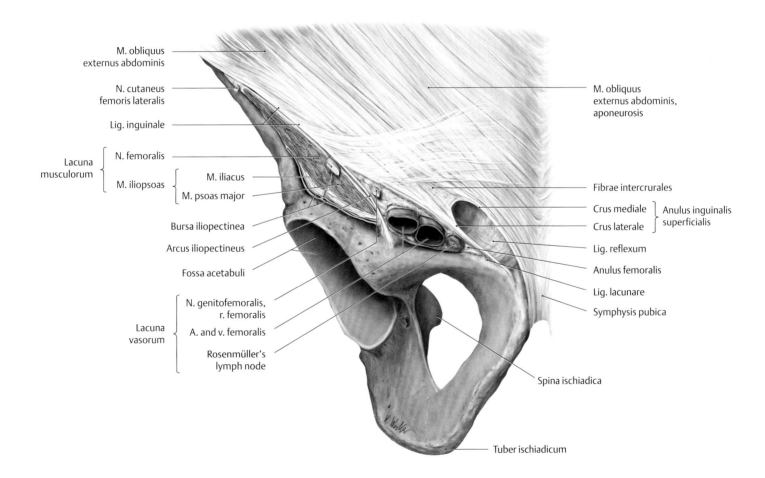

M. obliquus externus abdominis
N. cutaneus femoris lateralis
Lig. inguinale
Lacuna musculorum
N. femoralis
M. iliopsoas
M. iliacus
M. psoas major
Bursa iliopectinea
Arcus iliopectineus
Fossa acetabuli
Lacuna vasorum
N. genitofemoralis, r. femoralis
A. and v. femoralis
Rosenmüller's lymph node
M. obliquus externus abdominis, aponeurosis
Fibrae intercrurales
Crus mediale
Crus laterale
Anulus inguinalis superficialis
Lig. reflexum
Anulus femoralis
Lig. lacunare
Symphysis pubica
Spina ischiadica
Tuber ischiadicum

Topography of Regio Glutealis

Fig. 27.32 Regio glutealis
Right regio glutealis, posterior view.

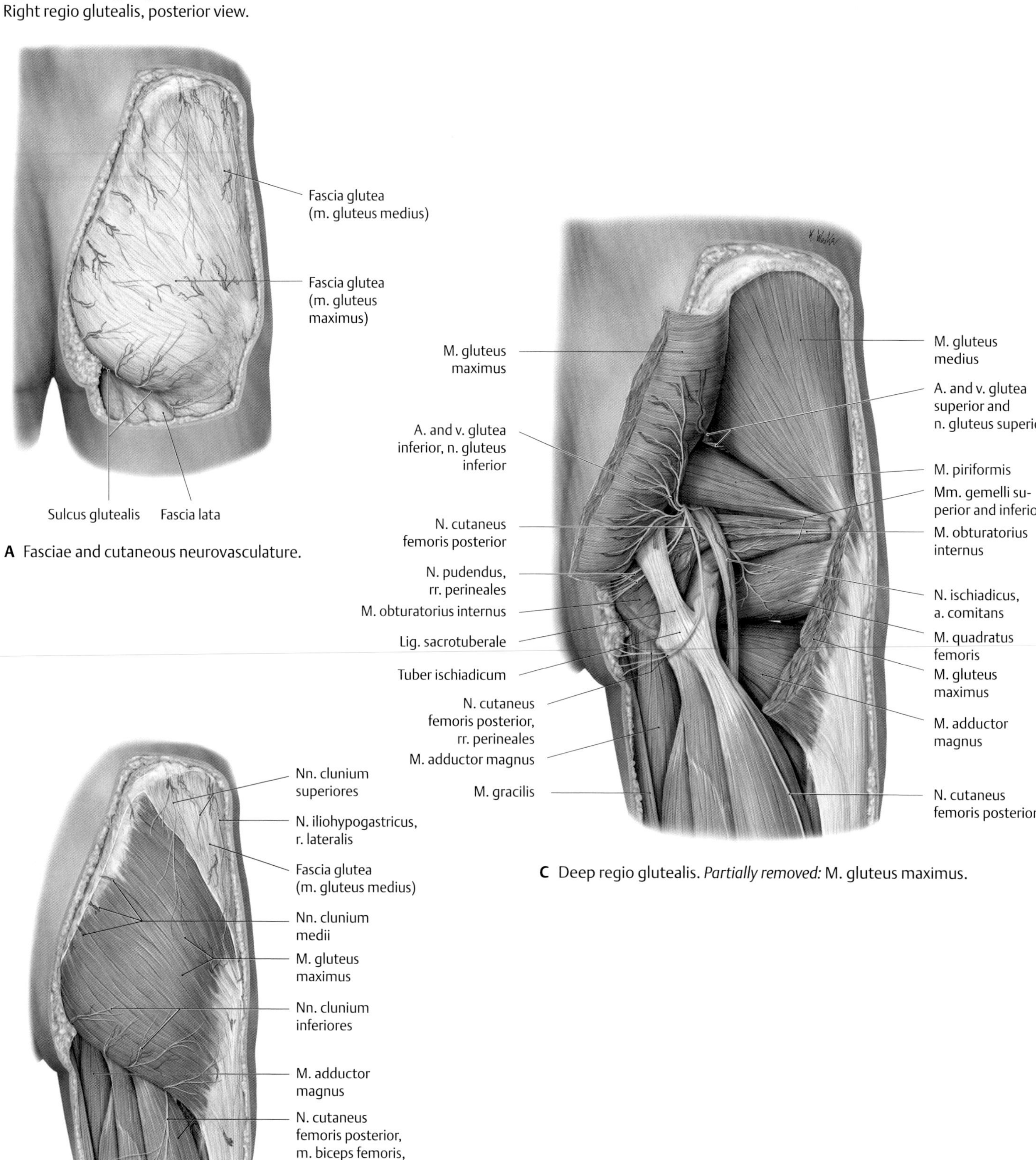
Fascia glutea (m. gluteus medius)
Fascia glutea (m. gluteus maximus)
Sulcus glutealis
Fascia lata
M. gluteus maximus
A. and v. glutea inferior, n. gluteus inferior
N. cutaneus femoris posterior
N. pudendus, rr. perineales
M. obturatorius internus
Lig. sacrotuberale
Tuber ischiadicum
N. cutaneus femoris posterior, rr. perineales
M. adductor magnus
M. gracilis
M. gluteus medius
A. and v. glutea superior and n. gluteus superior
M. piriformis
Mm. gemelli superior and inferior
M. obturatorius internus
N. ischiadicus, a. comitans
M. quadratus femoris
M. gluteus maximus
M. adductor magnus
N. cutaneus femoris posterior
Nn. clunium superiores
N. iliohypogastricus, r. lateralis
Fascia glutea (m. gluteus medius)
Nn. clunium medii
M. gluteus maximus
Nn. clunium inferiores
M. adductor magnus
N. cutaneus femoris posterior, m. biceps femoris, caput longum
M. semimembranosus
M. semitendinosus

A Fasciae and cutaneous neurovasculature.

C Deep regio glutealis. *Partially removed:* M. gluteus maximus.

B Regio glutealis. *Removed:* Fascia lata.

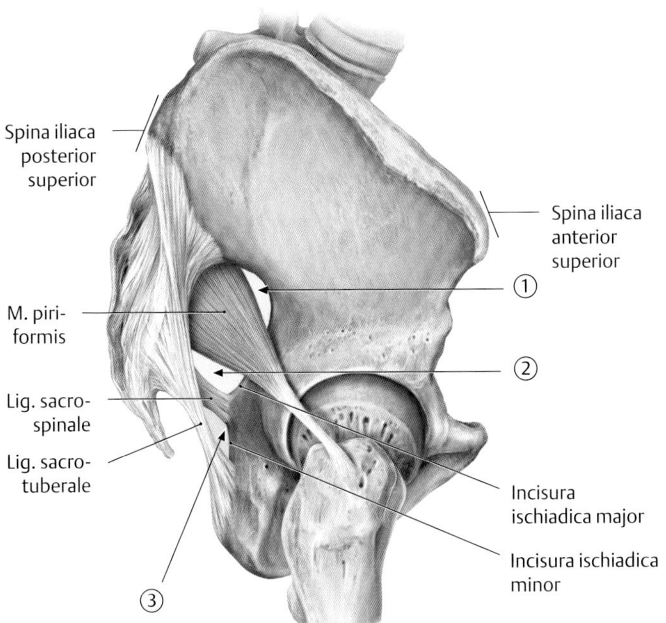

Spina iliaca posterior superior
Spina iliaca anterior superior
M. piriformis
①
②
Lig. sacrospinale
Lig. sacrotuberale
Incisura ischiadica major
Incisura ischiadica minor
③

Table 27.9 Sciatic foramina			
Foramen		**Transmitted structures**	**Boundaries**
Foramen ischiadicum majus	① Foramen suprapiriforme	A. and v. glutea superior N. gluteus superior	Incisura ischiadica major Lig. sacrospinale Os sacrum
	② Foramen infrapiriforme	A. and v. glutea inferior N. gluteus inferior A. and v. pudenda interna N. pudendus N. ischiadicus N. cutaneus femoris posterior	
③ Foramen ischiadicum minus		A. and v. pudenda interna N. pudendus M. obturatorius internus	Incisura ischiadica minor Lig. sacrospinale Lig. sacrotuberale

Fig. 27.33 **Regio glutealis and fossa ischioanalis**
Right regio glutealis, posterior view.
Removed: Mm. gluteus maximus and medius.

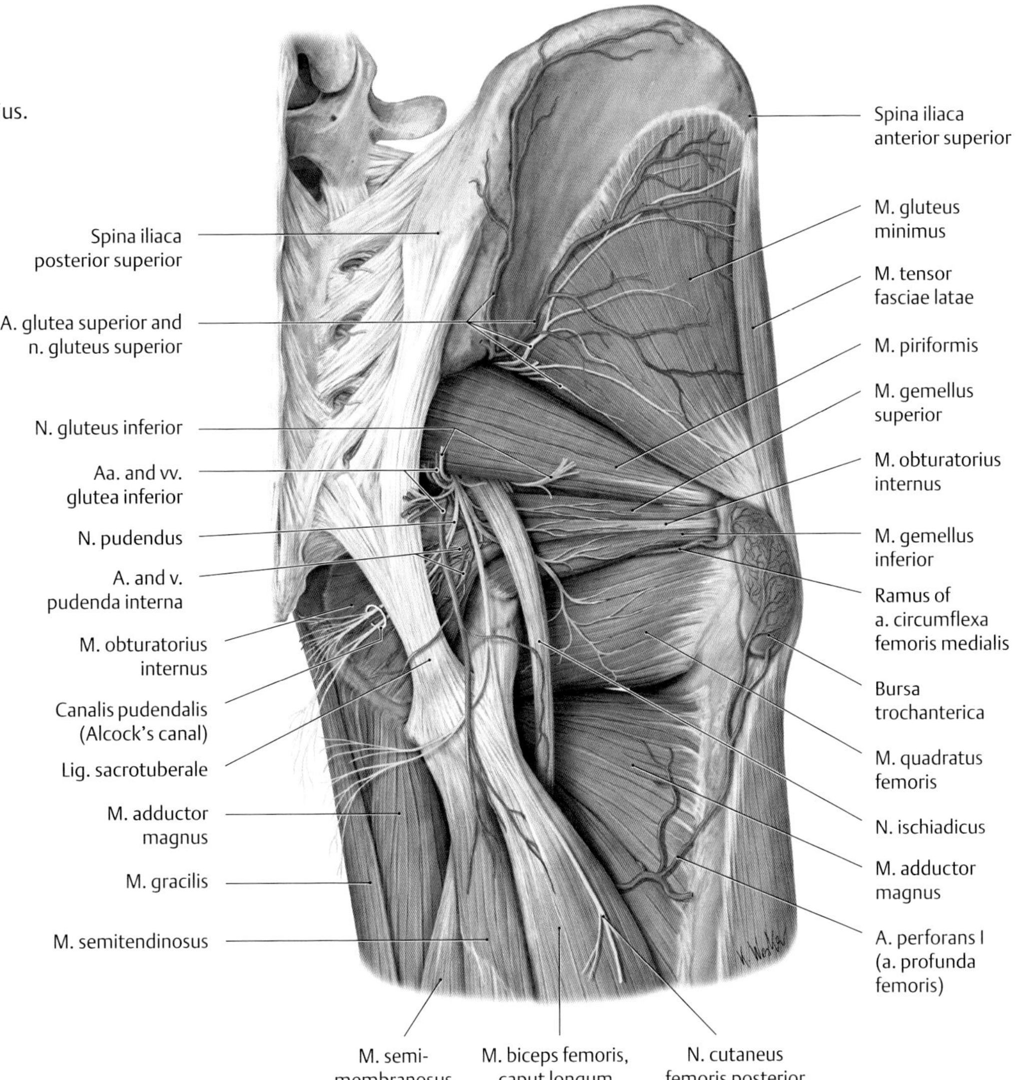

Spina iliaca posterior superior
A. glutea superior and n. gluteus superior
N. gluteus inferior
Aa. and vv. glutea inferior
N. pudendus
A. and v. pudenda interna
M. obturatorius internus
Canalis pudendalis (Alcock's canal)
Lig. sacrotuberale
M. adductor magnus
M. gracilis
M. semitendinosus
M. semimembranosus
M. biceps femoris, caput longum
N. cutaneus femoris posterior
Spina iliaca anterior superior
M. gluteus minimus
M. tensor fasciae latae
M. piriformis
M. gemellus superior
M. obturatorius internus
M. gemellus inferior
Ramus of a. circumflexa femoris medialis
Bursa trochanterica
M. quadratus femoris
N. ischiadicus
M. adductor magnus
A. perforans I (a. profunda femoris)

Topography of the Anterior & Posterior Thigh

Fig. 27.34 Anterior thigh
Right thigh, anterior view.

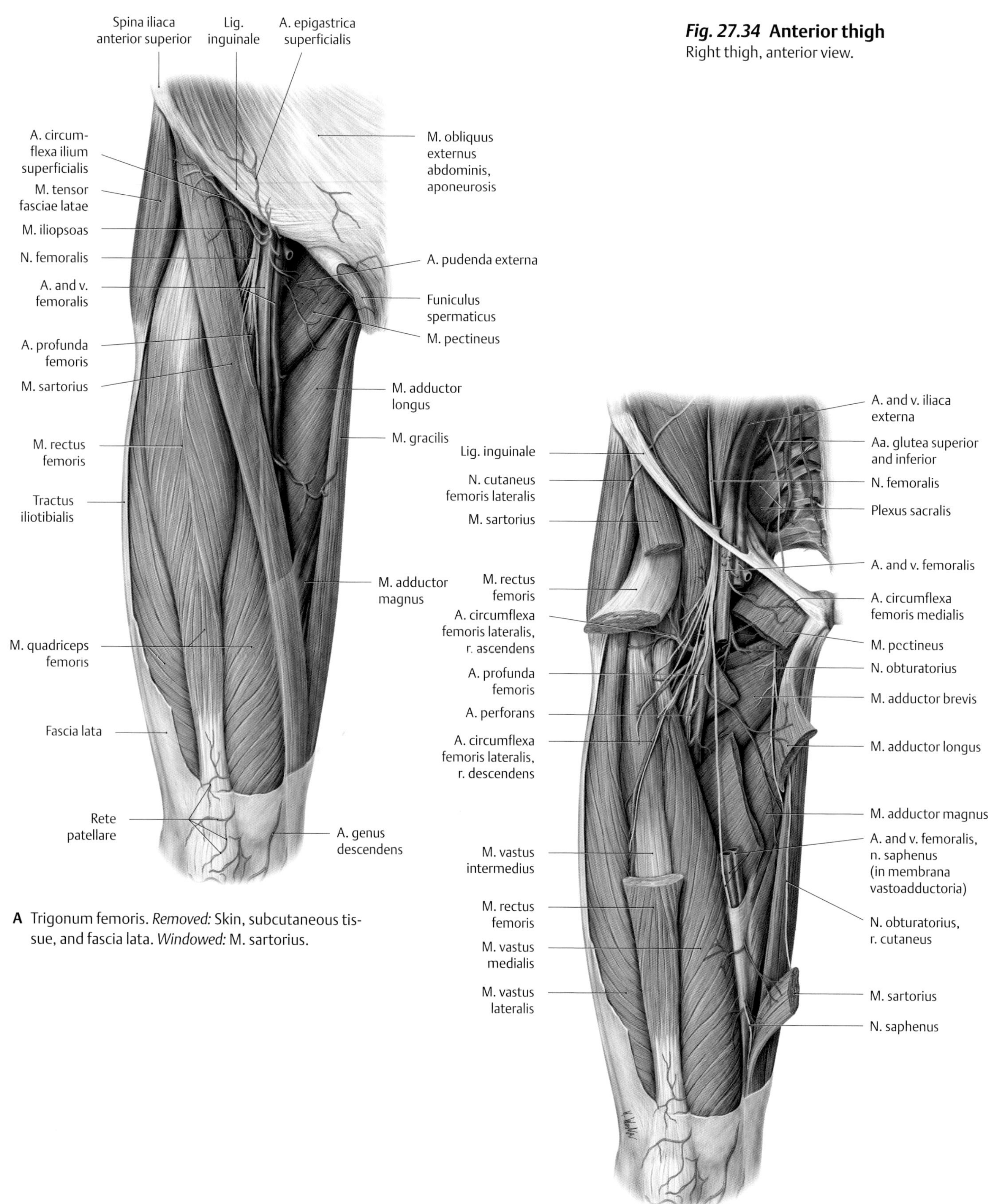
Spina iliaca anterior superior
Lig. inguinale
A. epigastrica superficialis
A. circumflexa ilium superficialis
M. tensor fasciae latae
M. iliopsoas
N. femoralis
A. and v. femoralis
A. profunda femoris
M. sartorius
M. rectus femoris
Tractus iliotibialis
M. quadriceps femoris
Fascia lata
Rete patellare
M. obliquus externus abdominis, aponeurosis
A. pudenda externa
Funiculus spermaticus
M. pectineus
M. adductor longus
M. gracilis
M. adductor magnus
A. genus descendens
Lig. inguinale
N. cutaneus femoris lateralis
M. sartorius
M. rectus femoris
A. circumflexa femoris lateralis, r. ascendens
A. profunda femoris
A. perforans
A. circumflexa femoris lateralis, r. descendens
M. vastus intermedius
M. rectus femoris
M. vastus medialis
M. vastus lateralis
A. and v. iliaca externa
Aa. glutea superior and inferior
N. femoralis
Plexus sacralis
A. and v. femoralis
A. circumflexa femoris medialis
M. pectineus
N. obturatorius
M. adductor brevis
M. adductor longus
M. adductor magnus
A. and v. femoralis, n. saphenus (in membrana vastoadductoria)
N. obturatorius, r. cutaneus
M. sartorius
N. saphenus

A Trigonum femoris. *Removed:* Skin, subcutaneous tissue, and fascia lata. *Windowed:* M. sartorius.

B Neurovasculature of the anterior thigh. *Removed:* Anterior abdominal wall. *Partially removed:* M. sartorius, m. rectus femoris, m. adductor longus, and m. pectineus.

Fig. 27.35 Posterior thigh

Right thigh, posterior view.

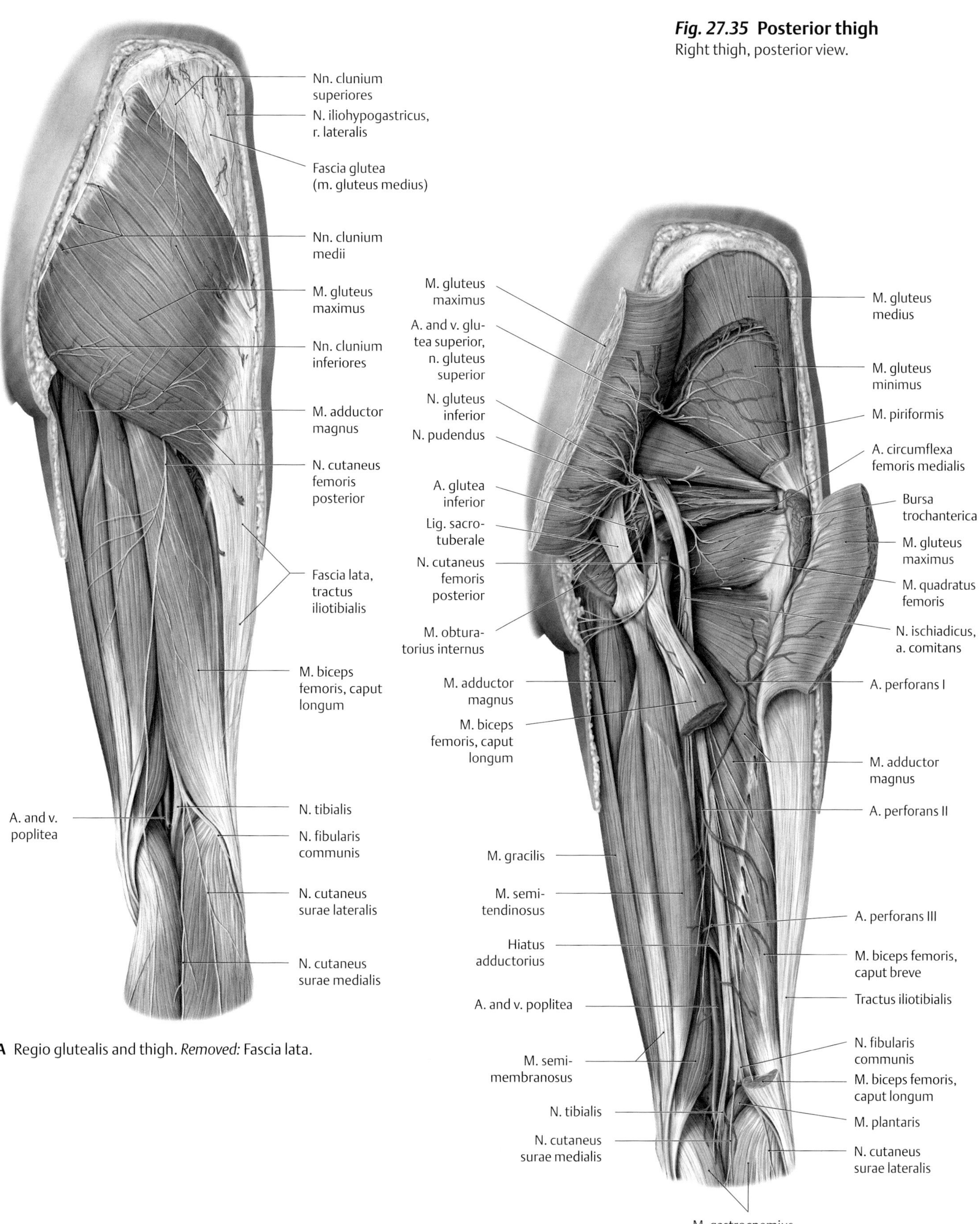
Nn. clunium superiores
N. iliohypogastricus, r. lateralis
Fascia glutea (m. gluteus medius)
Nn. clunium medii
M. gluteus maximus
Nn. clunium inferiores
M. adductor magnus
N. cutaneus femoris posterior
Fascia lata, tractus iliotibialis
M. biceps femoris, caput longum
A. and v. poplitea
N. tibialis
N. fibularis communis
N. cutaneus surae lateralis
N. cutaneus surae medialis
M. gluteus maximus
A. and v. glutea superior, n. gluteus superior
N. gluteus inferior
N. pudendus
A. glutea inferior
Lig. sacrotuberale
N. cutaneus femoris posterior
M. obturatorius internus
M. adductor magnus
M. biceps femoris, caput longum
M. gracilis
M. semitendinosus
Hiatus adductorius
A. and v. poplitea
M. semimembranosus
N. tibialis
N. cutaneus surae medialis
M. gastrocnemius
M. gluteus medius
M. gluteus minimus
M. piriformis
A. circumflexa femoris medialis
Bursa trochanterica
M. gluteus maximus
M. quadratus femoris
N. ischiadicus, a. comitans
A. perforans I
M. adductor magnus
A. perforans II
A. perforans III
M. biceps femoris, caput breve
Tractus iliotibialis
N. fibularis communis
M. biceps femoris, caput longum
M. plantaris
N. cutaneus surae lateralis

A Regio glutealis and thigh. *Removed:* Fascia lata.

B Neurovasculature of the posterior thigh. *Partially removed:* M. gluteus maximus, m. gluteus medius, and m. biceps femoris. *Retracted:* M. semimembranosus.

Topography of the Posterior & Medial Leg

Fig. 27.36 **Posterior compartment**
Right leg, posterior view.

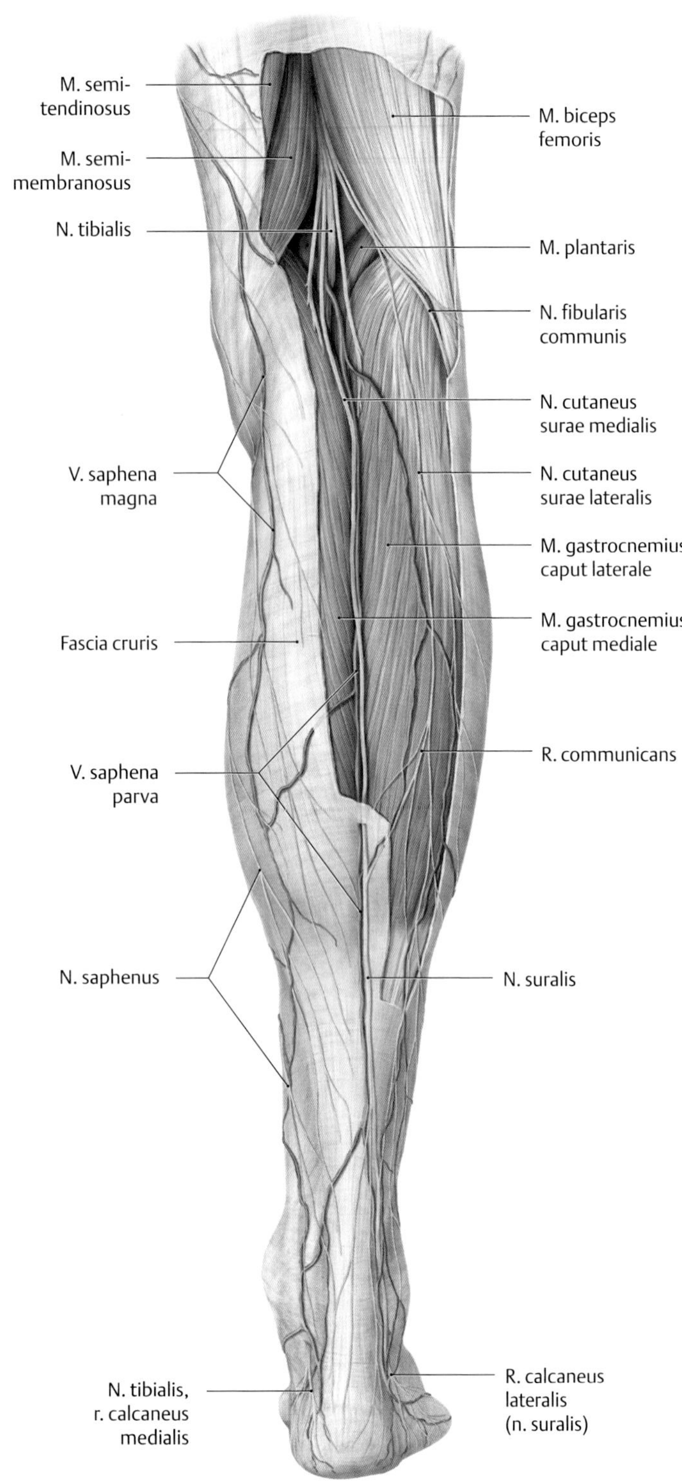
M. semi-
tendinosus
M. semi-
membranosus
N. tibialis
V. saphena
magna
Fascia cruris
V. saphena
parva
N. saphenus
N. tibialis,
r. calcaneus
medialis
M. biceps
femoris
M. plantaris
N. fibularis
communis
N. cutaneus
surae medialis
N. cutaneus
surae lateralis
M. gastrocnemius,
caput laterale
M. gastrocnemius,
caput mediale
R. communicans
N. suralis
R. calcaneus
lateralis
(n. suralis)

A Superficial neurovascular structures.

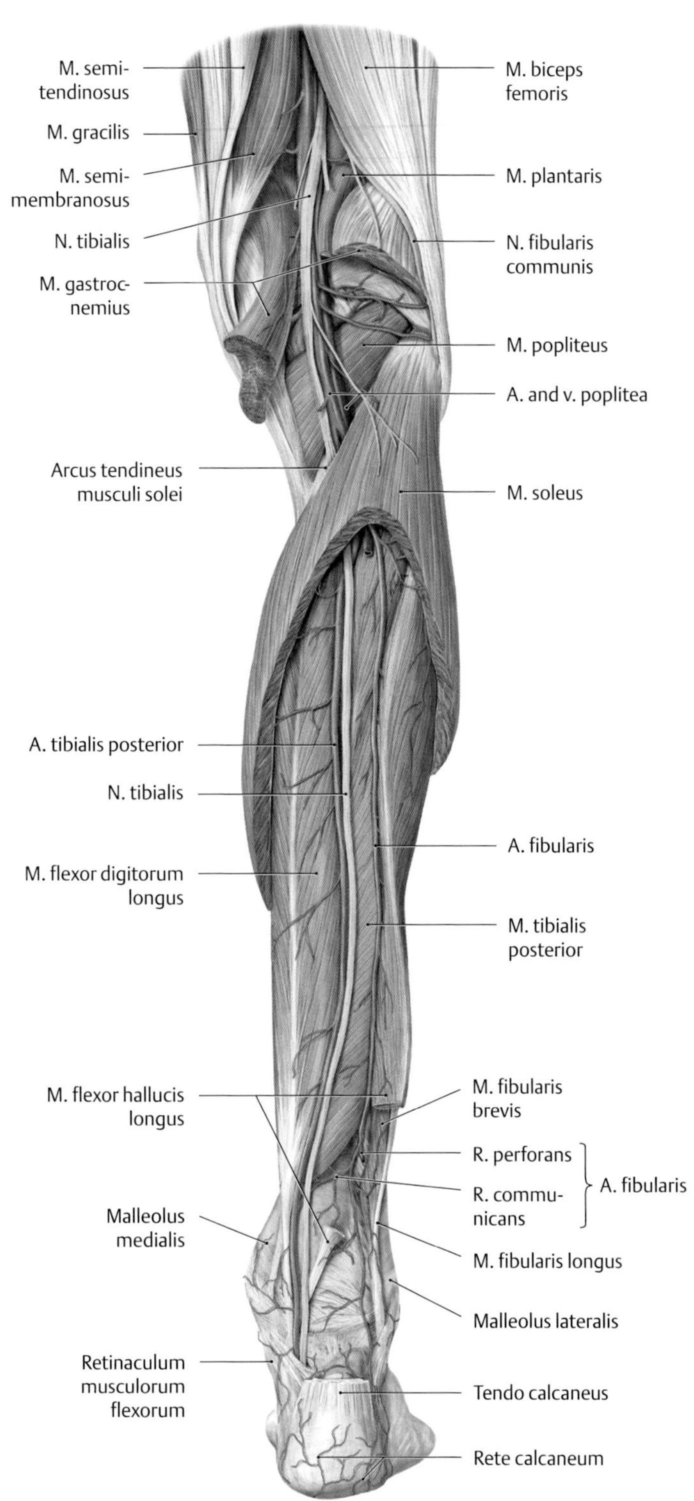
M. semi-
tendinosus
M. gracilis
M. semi-
membranosus
N. tibialis
M. gastroc-
nemius
Arcus tendineus
musculi solei
A. tibialis posterior
N. tibialis
M. flexor digitorum
longus
M. flexor hallucis
longus
Malleolus
medialis
Retinaculum
musculorum
flexorum
M. biceps
femoris
M. plantaris
N. fibularis
communis
M. popliteus
A. and v. poplitea
M. soleus
A. fibularis
M. tibialis
posterior
M. fibularis
brevis
R. perforans
R. commu-
nicans
A. fibularis
M. fibularis longus
Malleolus lateralis
Tendo calcaneus
Rete calcaneum

B Deep neurovascular structures.

Fig. 27.37 Fossa poplitea

Right leg, posterior view.

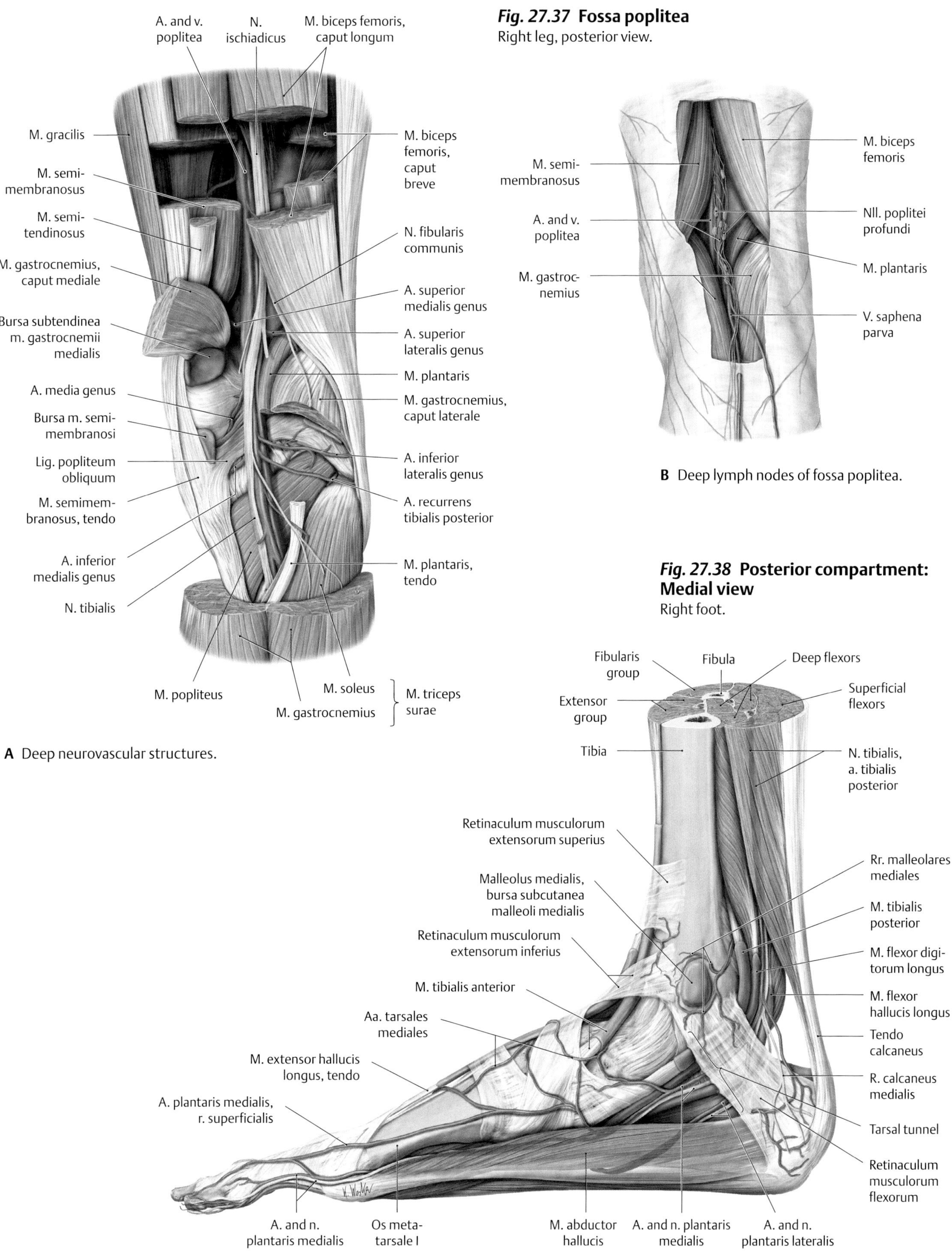
A. and v. poplitea
N. ischiadicus
M. biceps femoris, caput longum
M. gracilis
M. semi-membranosus
M. semi-tendinosus
M. gastrocnemius, caput mediale
Bursa subtendinea m. gastrocnemii medialis
A. media genus
Bursa m. semi-membranosi
Lig. popliteum obliquum
M. semimem-branosus, tendo
A. inferior medialis genus
N. tibialis
M. biceps femoris, caput breve
N. fibularis communis
A. superior medialis genus
A. superior lateralis genus
M. plantaris
M. gastrocnemius, caput laterale
A. inferior lateralis genus
A. recurrens tibialis posterior
M. plantaris, tendo
M. popliteus
M. soleus
M. gastrocnemius
M. triceps surae
M. semi-membranosus
A. and v. poplitea
M. gastroc-nemius
M. biceps femoris
Nll. poplitei profundi
M. plantaris
V. saphena parva
Fibularis group
Fibula
Deep flexors
Superficial flexors
Extensor group
Tibia
N. tibialis, a. tibialis posterior
Retinaculum musculorum extensorum superius
Malleolus medialis, bursa subcutanea malleoli medialis
Retinaculum musculorum extensorum inferius
M. tibialis anterior
Aa. tarsales mediales
M. extensor hallucis longus, tendo
A. plantaris medialis, r. superficialis
Rr. malleolares mediales
M. tibialis posterior
M. flexor digi-torum longus
M. flexor hallucis longus
Tendo calcaneus
R. calcaneus medialis
Tarsal tunnel
Retinaculum musculorum flexorum
A. and n. plantaris medialis
Os meta-tarsale I
M. abductor hallucis
A. and n. plantaris medialis
A. and n. plantaris lateralis

A Deep neurovascular structures.

B Deep lymph nodes of fossa poplitea.

Fig. 27.38 Posterior compartment: Medial view

Right foot.

Topography of the Lateral & Anterior Leg

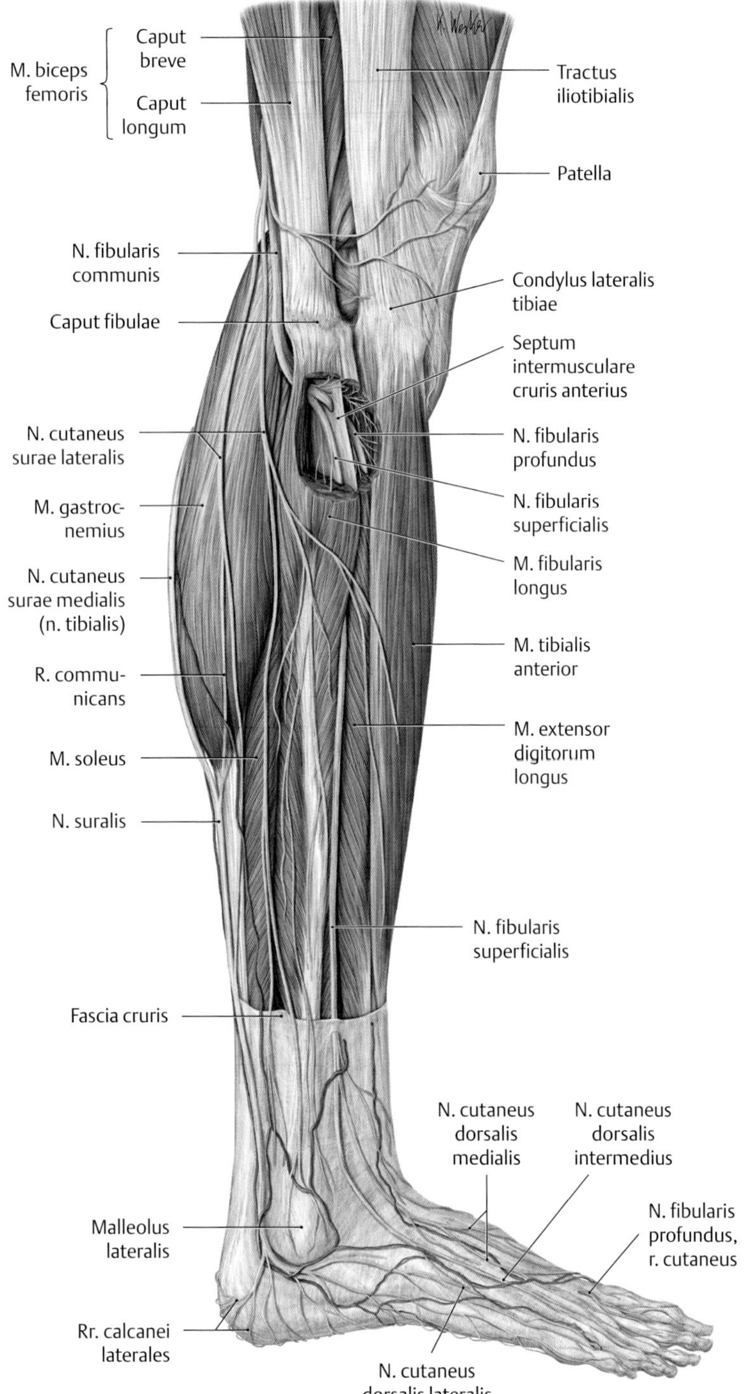
M. biceps femoris
Caput breve
Caput longum
Tractus iliotibialis
Patella
N. fibularis communis
Condylus lateralis tibiae
Caput fibulae
Septum intermusculare cruris anterius
N. cutaneus surae lateralis
N. fibularis profundus
N. fibularis superficialis
M. gastrocnemius
M. fibularis longus
N. cutaneus surae medialis (n. tibialis)
M. tibialis anterior
R. communicans
M. extensor digitorum longus
M. soleus
N. suralis
N. fibularis superficialis
Fascia cruris
N. cutaneus dorsalis medialis
N. cutaneus dorsalis intermedius
N. fibularis profundus, r. cutaneus
Malleolus lateralis
Rr. calcanei laterales
N. cutaneus dorsalis lateralis

Fig. 27.39 **Neurovasculature of the leg: Lateral view**
Right limb. *Removed:* Origins of the m. fibularis longus and m. extensor digitorum longus.

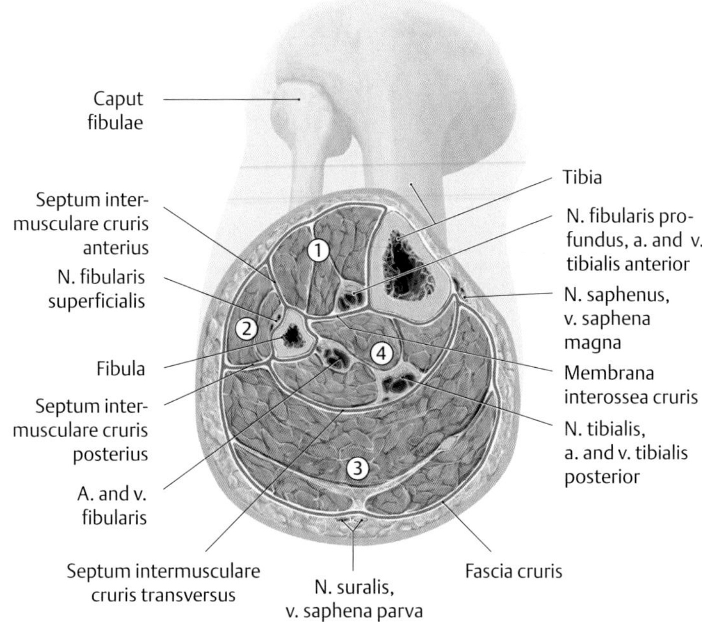
Caput fibulae
Tibia
Septum intermusculare cruris anterius
N. fibularis profundus, a. and v. tibialis anterior
N. fibularis superficialis
N. saphenus, v. saphena magna
Fibula
Membrana interossea cruris
Septum intermusculare cruris posterius
N. tibialis, a. and v. tibialis posterior
A. and v. fibularis
Septum intermusculare cruris transversus
N. suralis, v. saphena parva
Fascia cruris
1
2
3
4

Table 27.10 Compartments of the leg

Compartment		Muscular contents	Neurovascular contents
① Compartimentum cruris anterius		M. tibialis anterior	N. fibularis profundus A. and v. tibialis anterior.
		M. extensor digitorum longus	
		M. extensor hallucis longus	
		M. fibularis tertius	
② Compartimentum cruris laterale		M. fibularis longus	N. fibularis superficialis
		M. fibularis brevis	
Compartimentum crusis posterius	③ Pars superficialis	M. triceps surae (m. gastrocnemius and m. soleus)	–
		M. plantaris	
	④ Pars profunda	M. tibialis posterior	N. tibialis A. and v. tibialis posterior A. and v. fibularis
		M. flexor digitorum longus	
		M. flexor hallucis longus	

Clinical

Compartment syndrome

Muscle edema or hematoma can lead to a rise in tissue pressure in the compartments of the leg. Subsequent compression of neurovascular structures may cause ischemia and irreversible muscle and nerve damage. Patients with *anterior* compartment syndrome, the most common form, suffer excruciating pain and cannot dorsiflex the toes. Emergency incision of the fascia of the leg may be performed to relieve compression.

Fig. 27.40 Neurovasculature of the leg and foot: Anterior view

Right limb with foot in plantar flexion.

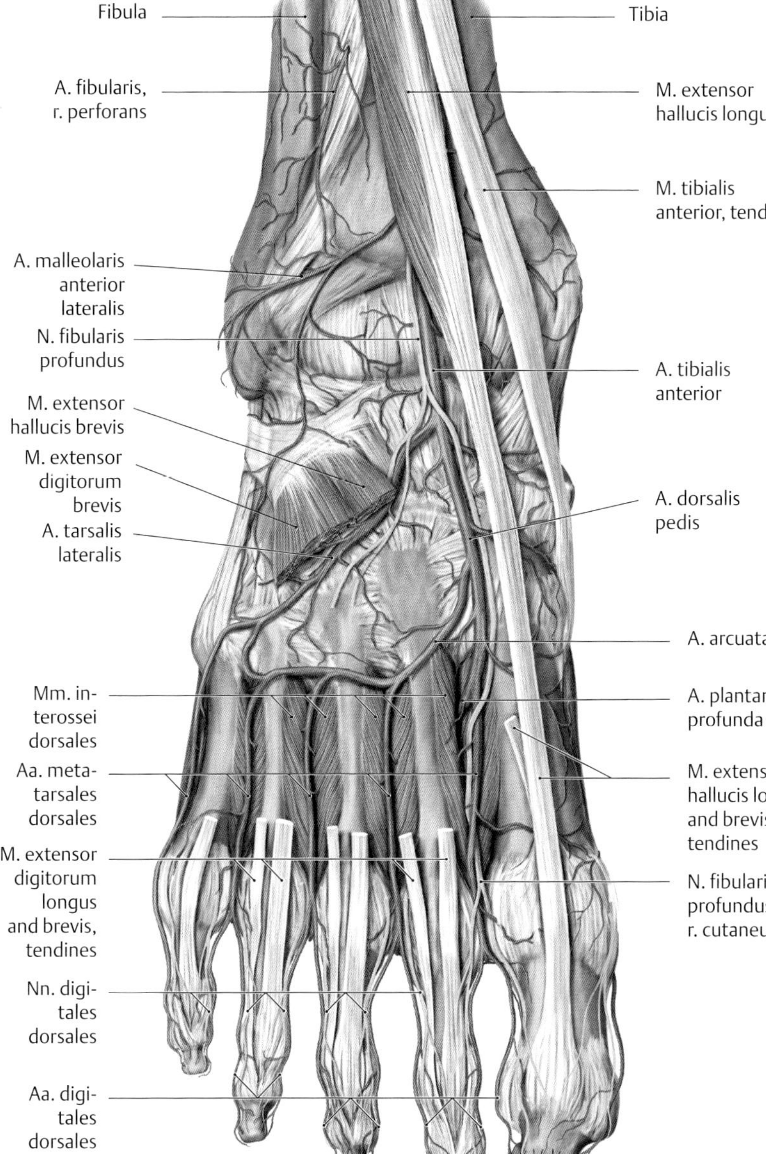
Fibula
A. fibularis, r. perforans
A. malleolaris anterior lateralis
N. fibularis profundus
M. extensor hallucis brevis
M. extensor digitorum brevis
A. tarsalis lateralis
Mm. interossei dorsales
Aa. metatarsales dorsales
M. extensor digitorum longus and brevis, tendines
Nn. digitales dorsales
Aa. digitales dorsales
Tibia
M. extensor hallucis longus
M. tibialis anterior, tendo
A. tibialis anterior
A. dorsalis pedis
A. arcuata
A. plantaris profunda
M. extensor hallucis longus and brevis, tendines
N. fibularis profundus, r. cutaneus

A Neurovasculature of the dorsum.

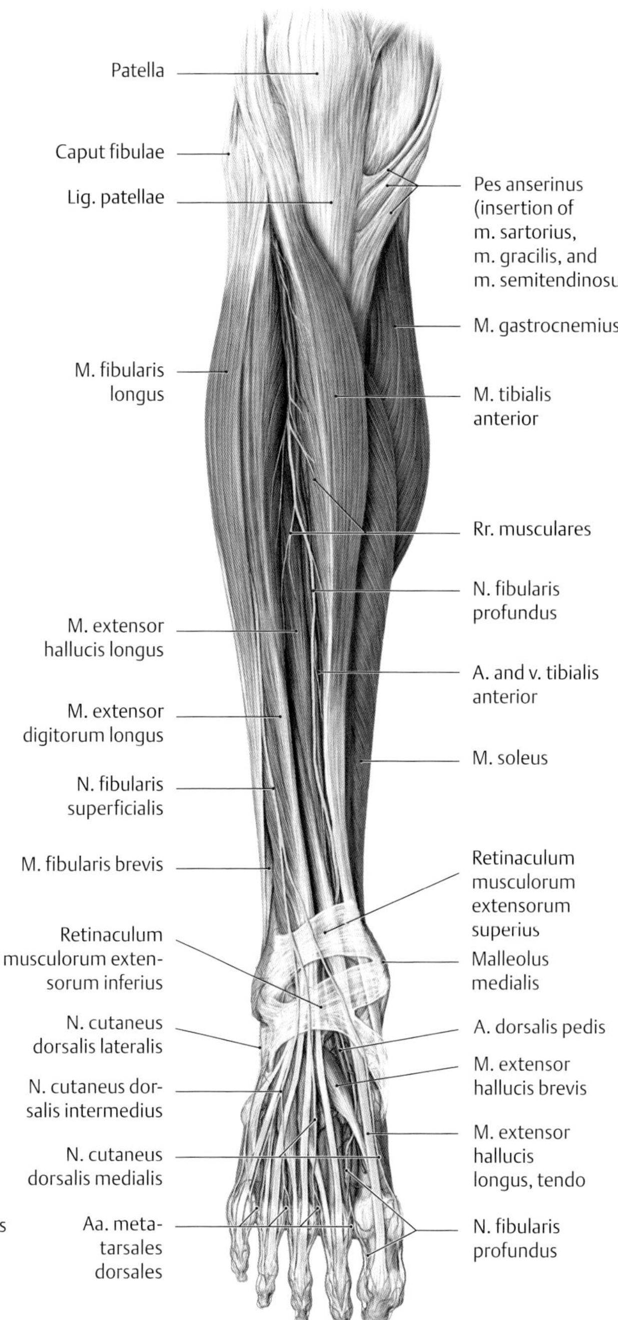
Patella
Caput fibulae
Lig. patellae
M. fibularis longus
M. extensor hallucis longus
M. extensor digitorum longus
N. fibularis superficialis
M. fibularis brevis
Retinaculum musculorum extensorum inferius
N. cutaneus dorsalis lateralis
N. cutaneus dorsalis intermedius
N. cutaneus dorsalis medialis
Aa. metatarsales dorsales
Pes anserinus (insertion of m. sartorius, m. gracilis, and m. semitendinosus)
M. gastrocnemius
M. tibialis anterior
Rr. musculares
N. fibularis profundus
A. and v. tibialis anterior
M. soleus
Retinaculum musculorum extensorum superius
Malleolus medialis
A. dorsalis pedis
M. extensor hallucis brevis
M. extensor hallucis longus, tendo
N. fibularis profundus

B Neurovasculature of the leg. *Removed:* Skin, subcutaneous tissue, and fasciae. *Retracted:* M. tibialis anterior and m. extensor hallucis longus.

Topography of Planta Pedis

Fig. 27.41 Neurovasculature of the foot: Sole
Right foot, plantar view.

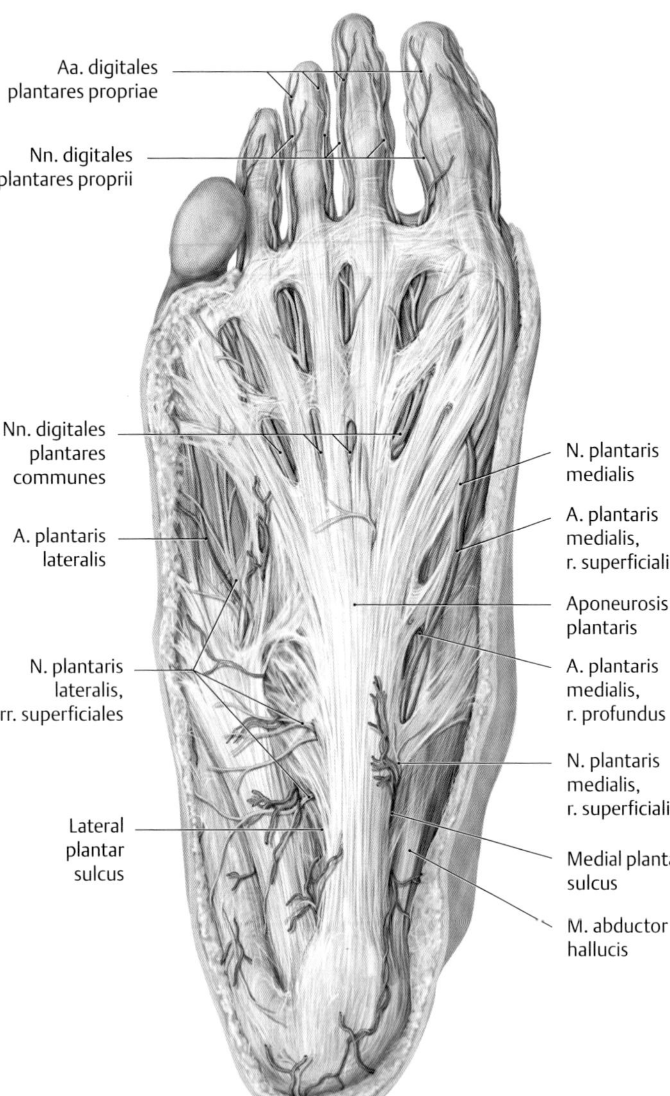
Aa. digitales plantares propriae
Nn. digitales plantares proprii
Nn. digitales plantares communes
A. plantaris lateralis
N. plantaris lateralis, rr. superficiales
Lateral plantar sulcus
N. plantaris medialis
A. plantaris medialis, r. superficialis
Aponeurosis plantaris
A. plantaris medialis, r. profundus
N. plantaris medialis, r. superficialis
Medial plantar sulcus
M. abductor hallucis

A Superficial layer. *Removed:* Skin, subcutaneous tissue, and fascia.

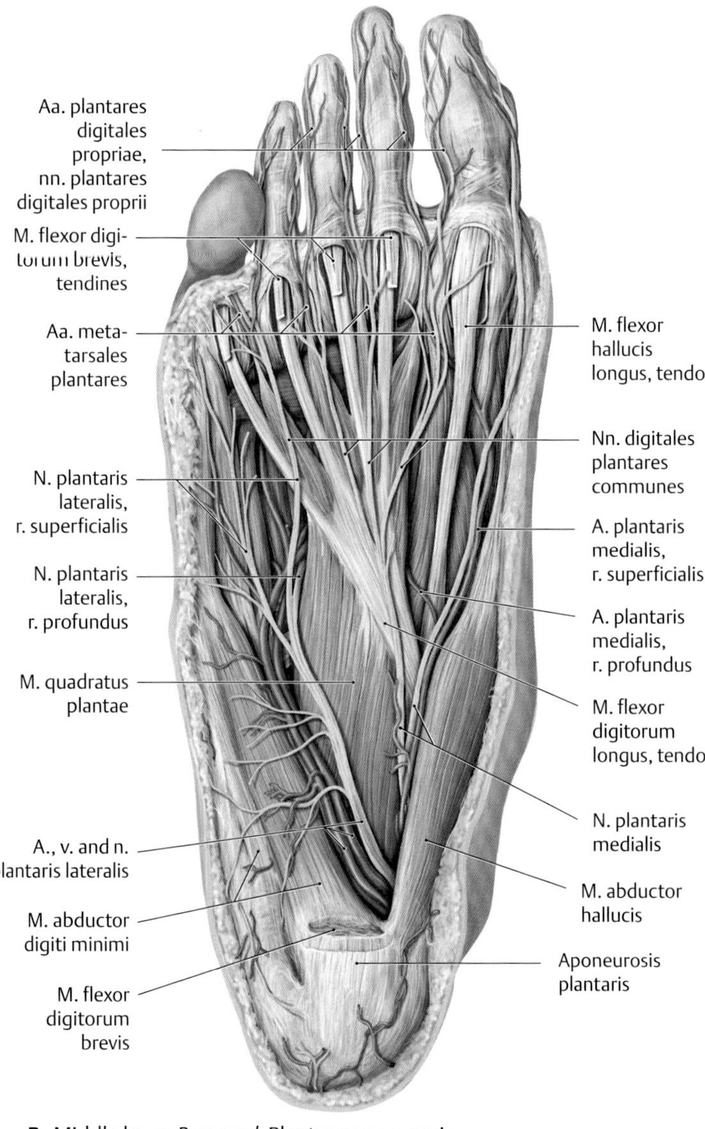
Aa. plantares digitales propriae, nn. plantares digitales proprii
M. flexor digitorum brevis, tendines
Aa. metatarsales plantares
N. plantaris lateralis, r. superficialis
N. plantaris lateralis, r. profundus
M. quadratus plantae
A., v. and n. plantaris lateralis
M. abductor digiti minimi
M. flexor digitorum brevis
M. flexor hallucis longus, tendo
Nn. digitales plantares communes
A. plantaris medialis, r. superficialis
A. plantaris medialis, r. profundus
M. flexor digitorum longus, tendo
N. plantaris medialis
M. abductor hallucis
Aponeurosis plantaris

B Middle layer. *Removed:* Plantar aponeurosis and m. flexor digitorum brevis.

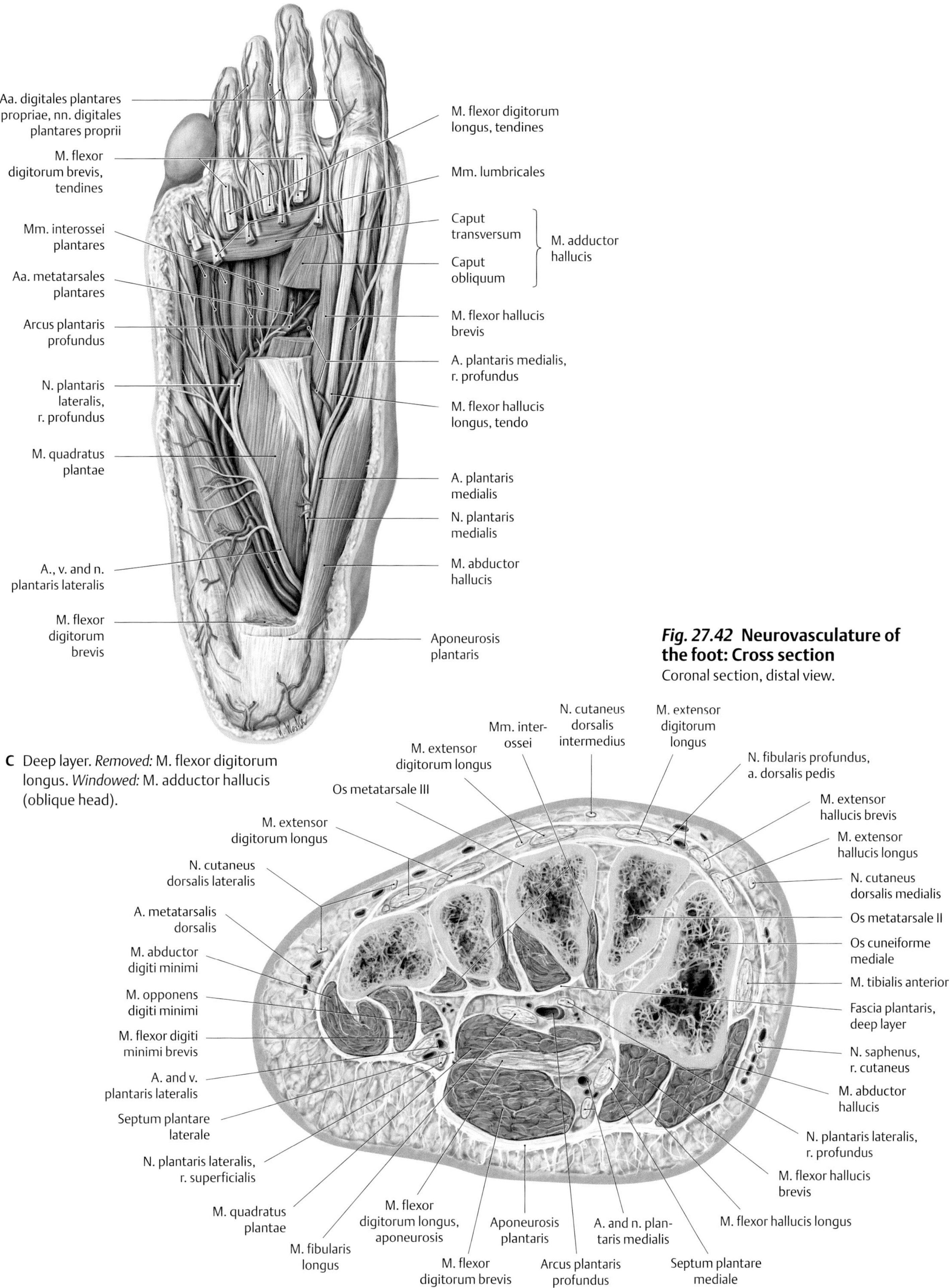
Aa. digitales plantares propriae, nn. digitales plantares proprii
M. flexor digitorum brevis, tendines
Mm. interossei plantares
Aa. metatarsales plantares
Arcus plantaris profundus
N. plantaris lateralis, r. profundus
M. quadratus plantae
A., v. and n. plantaris lateralis
M. flexor digitorum brevis
M. flexor digitorum longus, tendines
Mm. lumbricales
Caput transversum
Caput obliquum
M. adductor hallucis
M. flexor hallucis brevis
A. plantaris medialis, r. profundus
M. flexor hallucis longus, tendo
A. plantaris medialis
N. plantaris medialis
M. abductor hallucis
Aponeurosis plantaris
Mm. interossei
N. cutaneus dorsalis intermedius
M. extensor digitorum longus
M. extensor digitorum longus
N. fibularis profundus, a. dorsalis pedis
Os metatarsale III
M. extensor hallucis brevis
M. extensor digitorum longus
M. extensor hallucis longus
N. cutaneus dorsalis lateralis
N. cutaneus dorsalis medialis
A. metatarsalis dorsalis
Os metatarsale II
M. abductor digiti minimi
Os cuneiforme mediale
M. tibialis anterior
M. opponens digiti minimi
Fascia plantaris, deep layer
M. flexor digiti minimi brevis
N. saphenus, r. cutaneus
A. and v. plantaris lateralis
M. abductor hallucis
Septum plantare laterale
N. plantaris lateralis, r. profundus
N. plantaris lateralis, r. superficialis
M. flexor hallucis brevis
M. quadratus plantae
M. flexor digitorum longus, aponeurosis
Aponeurosis plantaris
A. and n. plantaris medialis
M. flexor hallucis longus
M. fibularis longus
M. flexor digitorum brevis
Arcus plantaris profundus
Septum plantare mediale

C Deep layer. *Removed:* M. flexor digitorum longus. *Windowed:* M. adductor hallucis (oblique head).

Fig. 27.42 **Neurovasculature of the foot: Cross section**
Coronal section, distal view.

Transverse Sections of the Thigh & Leg

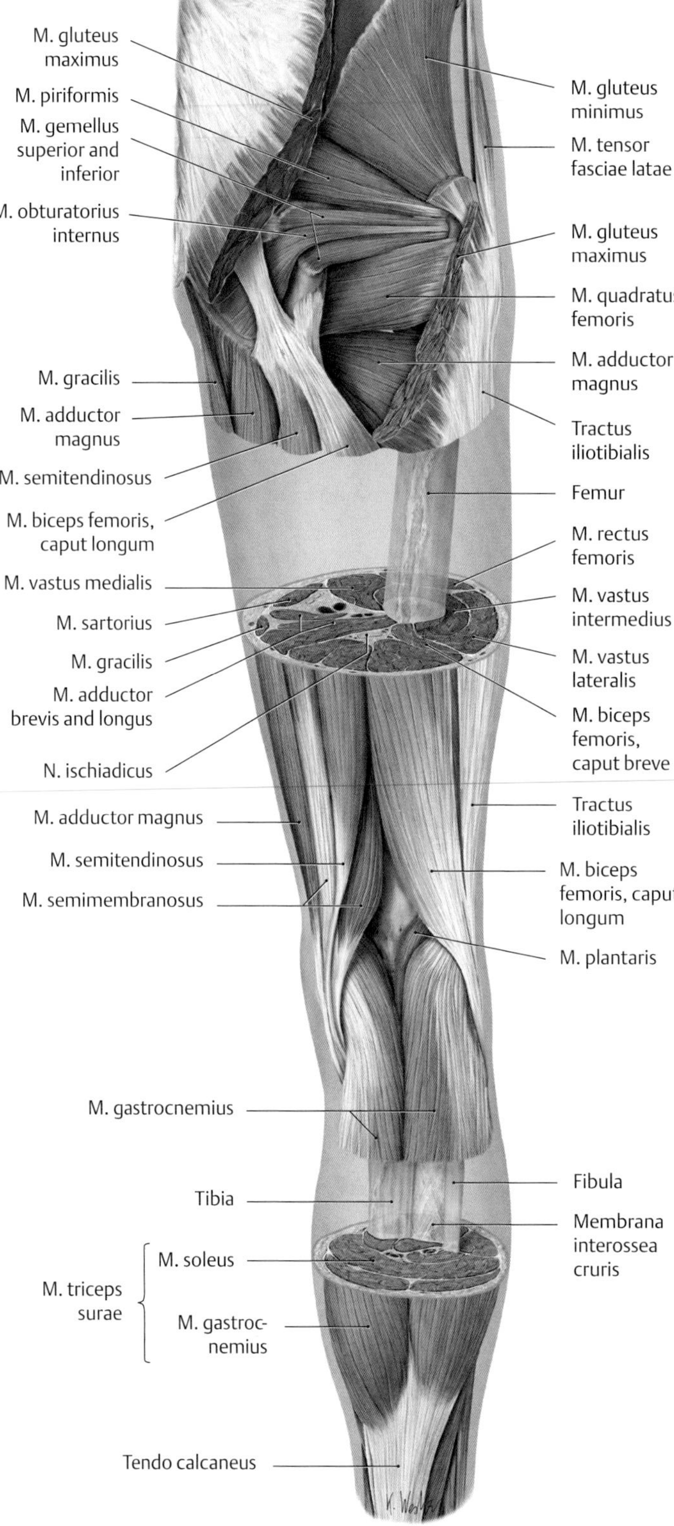

Crista iliaca
M. gluteus medius
M. gluteus maximus
M. piriformis
M. gemellus superior and inferior
M. obturatorius internus
M. gluteus minimus
M. tensor fasciae latae
M. gluteus maximus
M. quadratus femoris
M. adductor magnus
M. gracilis
M. adductor magnus
Tractus iliotibialis
M. semitendinosus
M. biceps femoris, caput longum
Femur
M. rectus femoris
M. vastus medialis
M. sartorius
M. vastus intermedius
M. gracilis
M. vastus lateralis
M. adductor brevis and longus
M. biceps femoris, caput breve
N. ischiadicus
M. adductor magnus
Tractus iliotibialis
M. semitendinosus
M. semimembranosus
M. biceps femoris, caput longum
M. plantaris
M. gastrocnemius
Fibula
Tibia
Membrana interossea cruris
M. triceps surae
M. soleus
M. gastroc-nemius
Tendo calcaneus

Fig. 27.43 **Windowed dissection**
Right limb, posterior view.

***Fig. 27.44* Transverse sections**

Right limb, proximal (superior) view.

M. quadriceps femoris
M. vastus medialis
M. vastus intermedius
M. rectus femoris
M. vastus lateralis
Anterior
Septum intermusculare femoris mediale
M. sartorius
A. and v. femoralis
A. and v. profunda femoris
M. adductor brevis
M. adductor longus
M. gracilis
M. adductor magnus
M. semi-membranosus
M. semitendinosus
Caput longum
Caput breve
M. biceps femoris
Femur
Tractus iliotibialis
N. ischiadicus
Septum intermusculare femoris laterale

A Thigh (plane of section in Fig. 27.43).

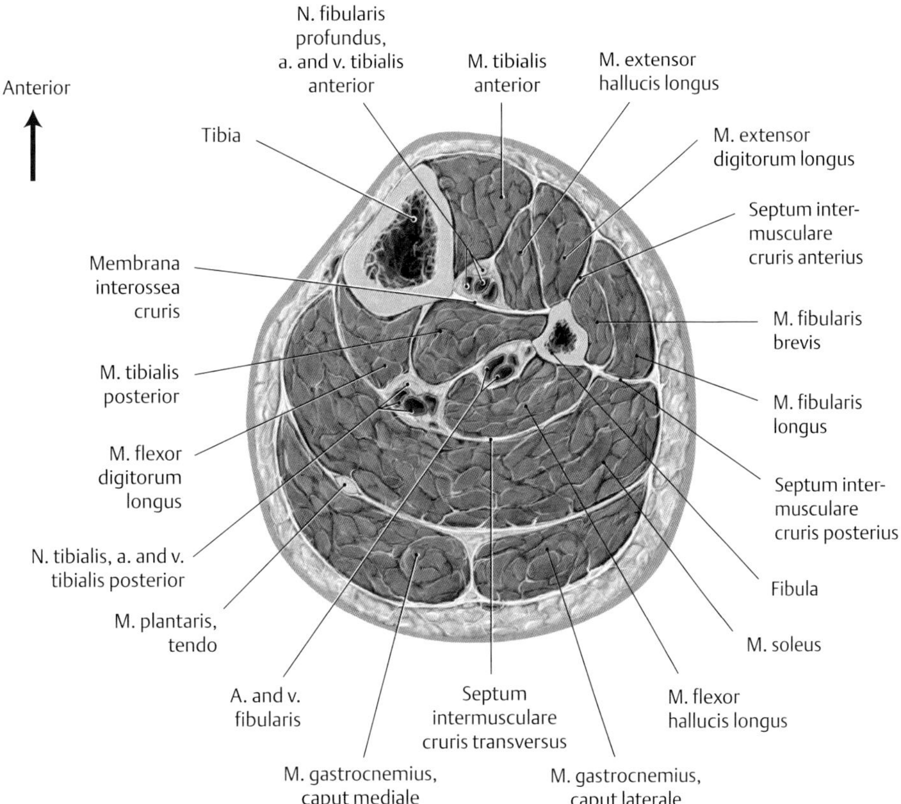
N. fibularis profundus, a. and v. tibialis anterior
M. tibialis anterior
M. extensor hallucis longus
Anterior
Tibia
M. extensor digitorum longus
Septum inter-musculare cruris anterius
Membrana interossea cruris
M. fibularis brevis
M. tibialis posterior
M. fibularis longus
M. flexor digitorum longus
Septum inter-musculare cruris posterius
N. tibialis, a. and v. tibialis posterior
Fibula
M. plantaris, tendo
M. soleus
A. and v. fibularis
Septum intermusculare cruris transversus
M. flexor hallucis longus
M. gastrocnemius, caput mediale
M. gastrocnemius, caput laterale

B Leg (plane of section in Fig. 27.43).

Surface Anatomy

Fig. 28.1 Lower limb: Anterior view

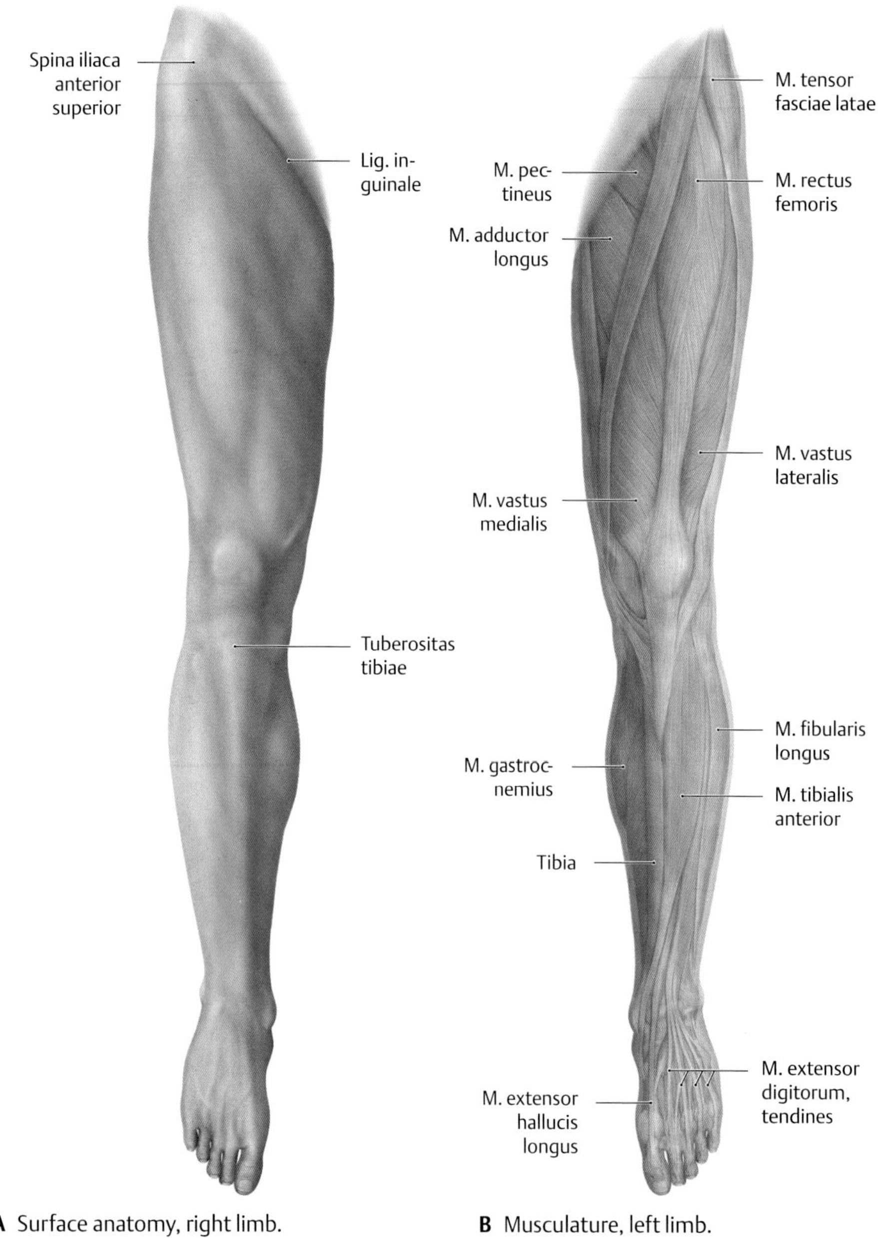
Spina iliaca anterior superior
Lig. inguinale
Tuberositas tibiae
M. pectineus
M. adductor longus
M. vastus medialis
M. gastrocnemius
Tibia
M. extensor hallucis longus
M. tensor fasciae latae
M. rectus femoris
M. vastus lateralis
M. fibularis longus
M. tibialis anterior
M. extensor digitorum, tendines

A Surface anatomy, right limb.

B Musculature, left limb.

Fig. 28.2 Palpable bony prominences

Right limb.

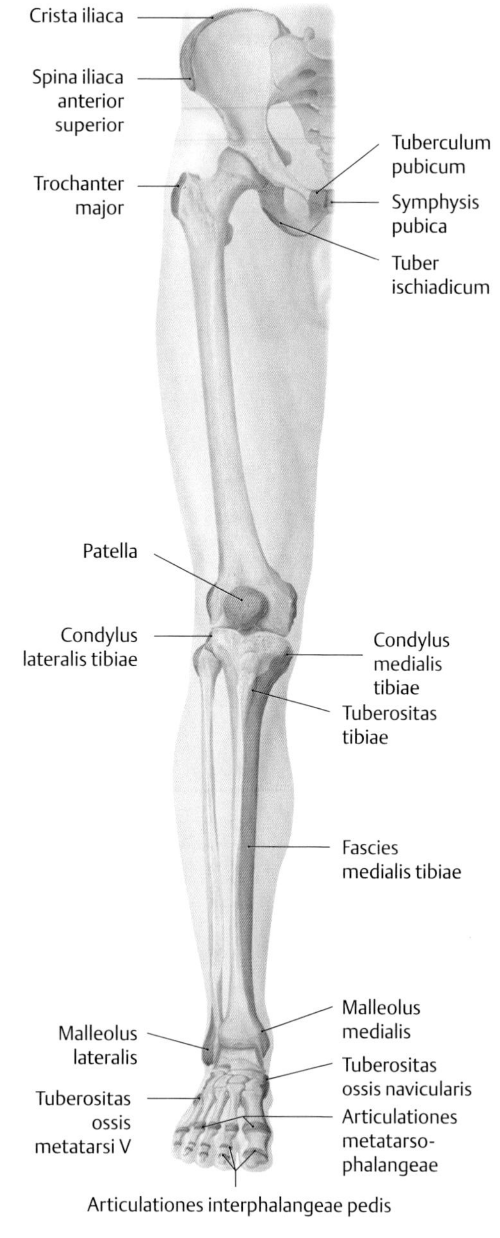
Crista iliaca
Spina iliaca anterior superior
Trochanter major
Tuberculum pubicum
Symphysis pubica
Tuber ischiadicum
Patella
Condylus lateralis tibiae
Condylus medialis tibiae
Tuberositas tibiae
Fascies medialis tibiae
Malleolus lateralis
Malleolus medialis
Tuberositas ossis navicularis
Tuberositas ossis metatarsi V
Articulationes metatarso-phalangeae
Articulationes interphalangeae pedis

A Anterior view.

Q1: The articulatio coxae is not directly palpable. How would you correctly locate caput femoris based on surface anatomy?

Fig. 28.3 **Lower limb: Posterior view**

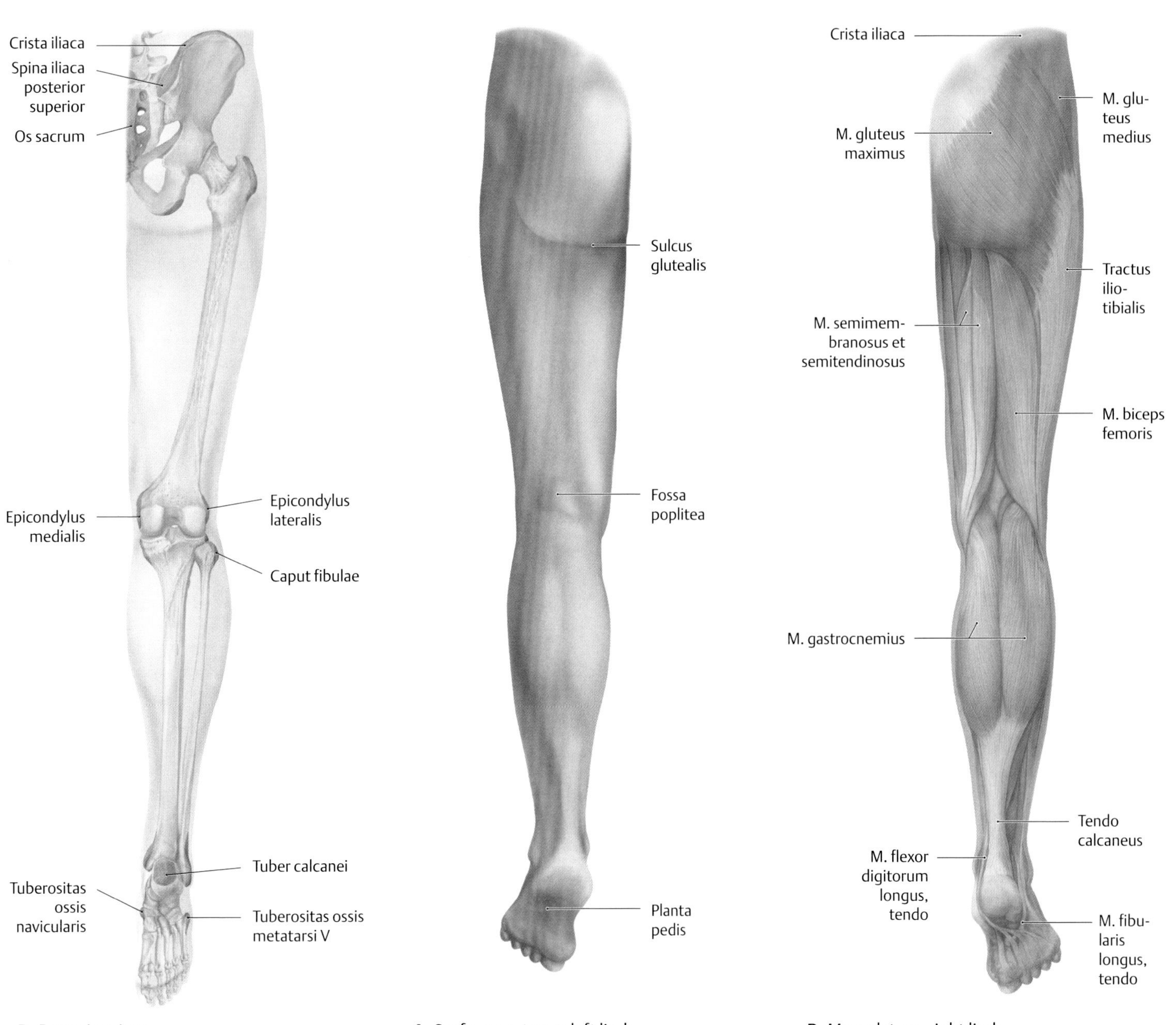
Crista iliaca
Spina iliaca posterior superior
Os sacrum
Epicondylus medialis
Epicondylus lateralis
Caput fibulae
Tuber calcanei
Tuberositas ossis navicularis
Tuberositas ossis metatarsi V
Sulcus glutealis
Fossa poplitea
Planta pedis
Crista iliaca
M. gluteus maximus
M. gluteus medius
Tractus iliotibialis
M. semimembranosus et semitendinosus
M. biceps femoris
M. gastrocnemius
Tendo calcaneus
M. flexor digitorum longus, tendo
M. fibularis longus, tendo

B Posterior view.

A Surface anatomy, left limb.

B Musculature, right limb.

Q2: Which palpable landmarks would you use to locate n. ischiadicus (in regio glutealis), n. fibularis communis (at the knee), and the n. tibialis (at the ankle)?

See answers beginning on p. 626.

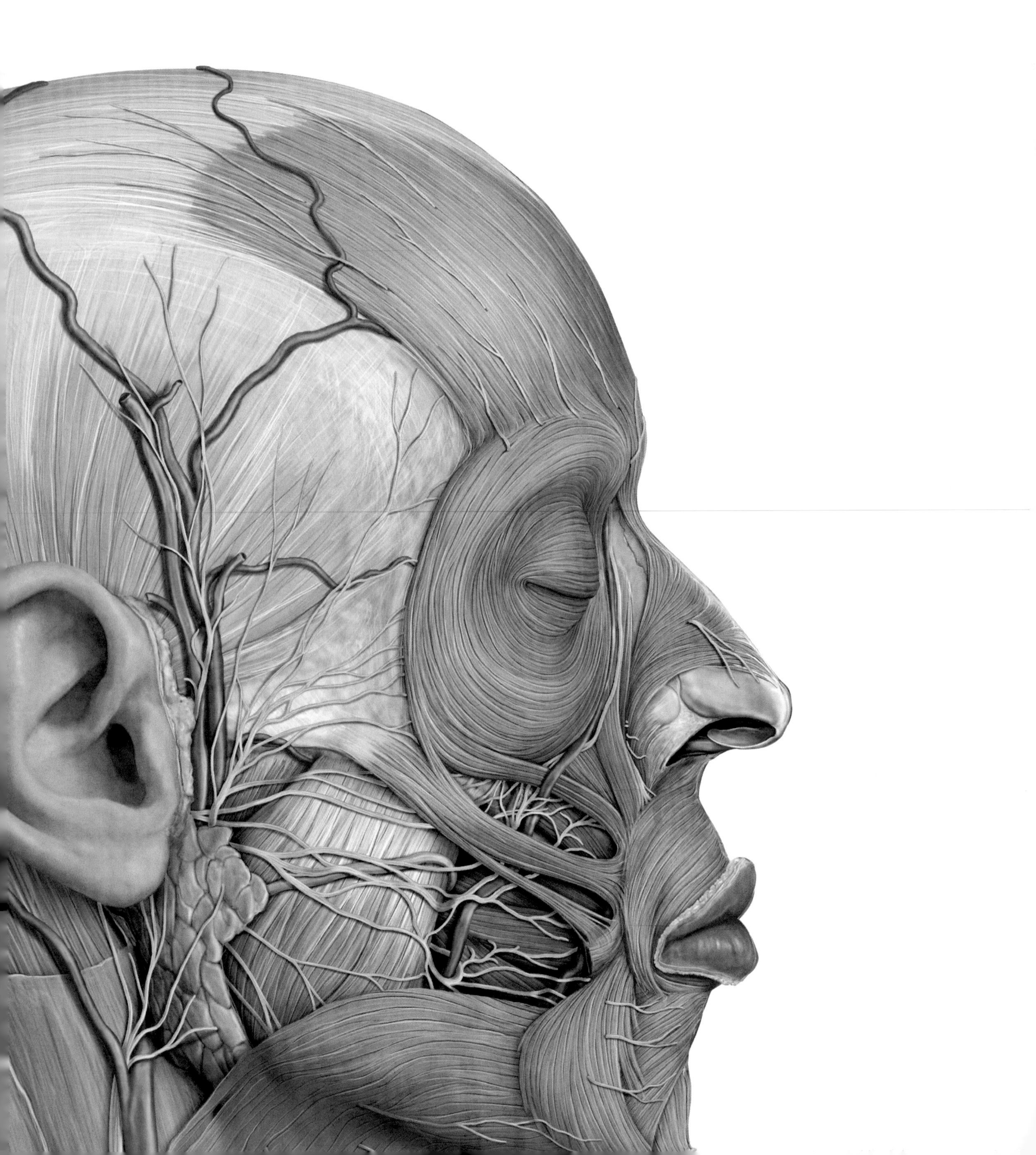

Head & Neck

29 Bones of the Head

Anterior & Lateral Skull 454
Posterior Skull & Calvaria 456
Base of the Skull 458
Os Ethmoidale & Os Sphenoidale 460

30 Muscles of the Skull & Face

Muscles of Facial Expression & of Mastication 462
Muscle Origins & Insertions on the Skull 464
Muscle Facts (I) 466
Muscle Facts (II) 468

31 Cranial Nerves

Cranial Nerves: Overview 470
CN I & II: N. Olfactorius & N. Opticus 472
CN III, IV & VI:
N. Oculomotorius, N. Trochlearis & N. Abducens 474
CN V: N. Trigeminus 476
CN VII: N. Facialis 478
CN VIII: N. Vestibulocochlearis 480
CN IX: N. Glossopharyngeus 482
CN X: N. Vagus 484
CN XI & XII: N. Accessorius & N. Hypoglossus 486

32 Neurovasculature of the Skull & Face

Innervation of the Face 488
Arteries of the Head & Neck 490
A. Carotis Externa:
Anterior, Medial & Posterior Branches 492
A. Carotis Externa: Terminal Branches 494
Veins of the Head & Neck 496
Topography of the Superficial Face 498
Topography of the Parotid Region & Fossa Temporalis 500
Topography of Fossa Infratemporalis 502
Topography of Fossa Pterygopalatina 504

33 Orbit & Eye

Bones of the Orbita 506
Muscles of the Orbita 508
Neurovasculature of the Orbita 510
Topography of the Orbita 512
Orbita & Eyelid 514
Eyeball (Bulbus Oculi) 516
Cornea, Iris & Lens 518

34 Nasal Cavity & Nose

Bones of the Nasal Cavity (Cavitas Nasi) 520
Paranasal Air Sinuses (Sinus Paranasales) 522
Neurovasculature of the Nasal Cavity 524

35 Temporal Bone & Ear

Os Temporale 526
External Ear (Auris Externa) & Auditory Canal 528
Middle Ear (Auris Media):
Tympanic Cavity (Cavitas Tympani) 530
Middle Ear: Ossicular Chain & Membrana Tympanica 532
Arteries of the Middle Ear 534
Inner Ear (Auris Interna) 536

36 Oral Cavity & Pharynx

Bones of the Oral Cavity (Cavitas Oris) 538
Articulatio Temporomandibularis 540
Teeth (Dentes) 542
Muscles of the Oral Cavity 544
Innervation of the Oral Cavity 546
Tongue (Lingua) 548
Topography of the Oral Cavity & Salivary Glands 550
Tonsils & Pharynx 552
Pharyngeal Muscles 554
Neurovasculature of the Pharynx 556

37 Neck

Bones & Ligaments of the Neck 558
Overview & Superficial Muscles of the Neck 560
Suprahyoid & Infrahyoid Muscles of the Neck 562
Deep Muscles of the Neck 564
Arteries & Veins of the Neck 566
Innervation of the Neck 568
Larynx: Cartilage & Structure 570
Larynx: Muscles & Levels 572
Neurovasculature of the Larynx, Thyroid & Parathyroids 574
Topography of the Neck: Regions & Fascia 576
Topography of the Anterior Cervical Region 578
Topography of the Anterior & Lateral Cervical Regions 580
Topography of the Lateral Cervical Region 582
Topography of the Posterior Cervical Region 584
Lymphatics of the Neck 586

38 Surface Anatomy

Surface Anatomy 588

Anterior & Lateral Skull

Fig. 29.1 Lateral skull
Left lateral view.

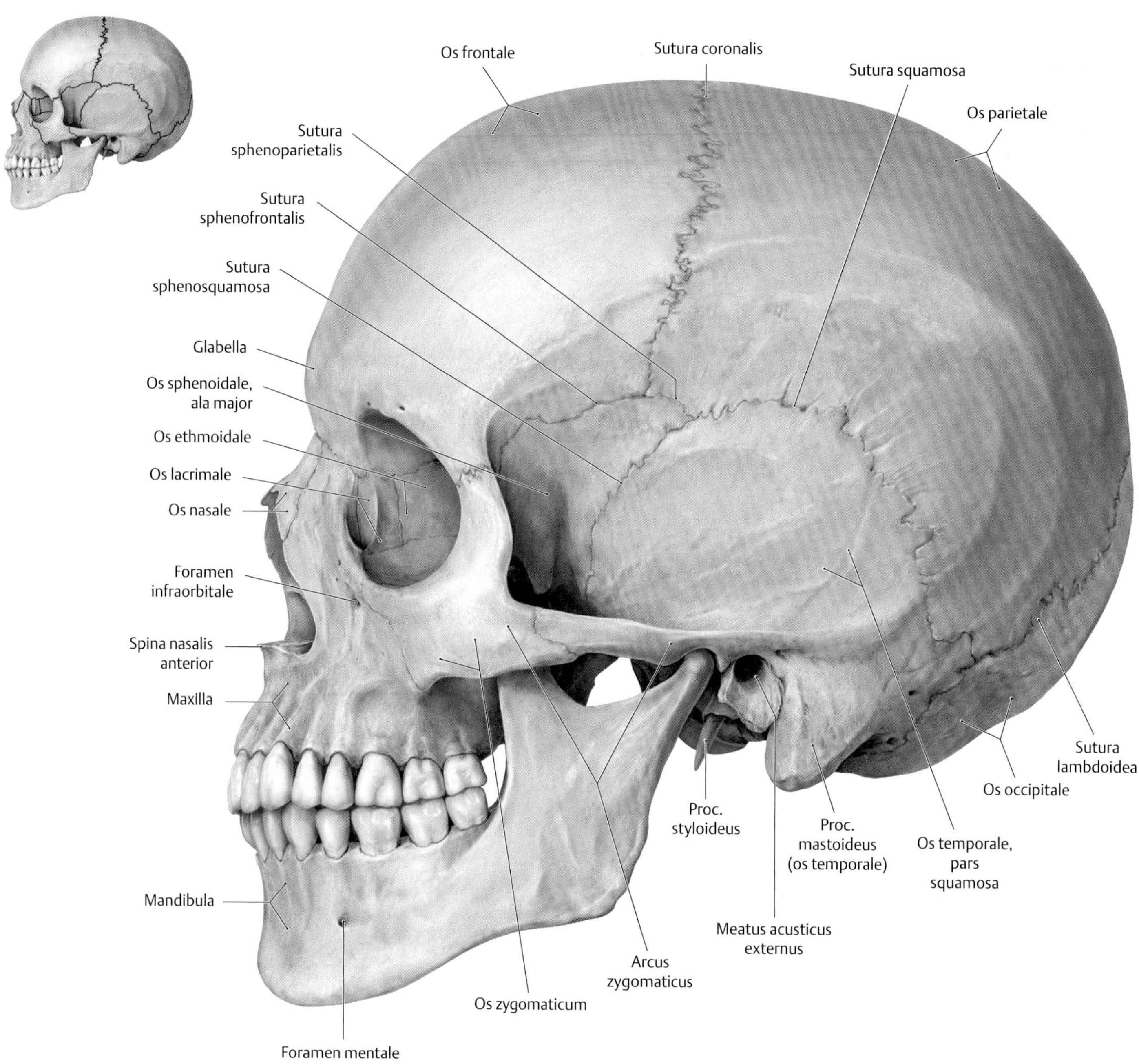
Os frontale
Sutura coronalis
Sutura squamosa
Os parietale
Sutura sphenoparietalis
Sutura sphenofrontalis
Sutura sphenosquamosa
Glabella
Os sphenoidale, ala major
Os ethmoidale
Os lacrimale
Os nasale
Foramen infraorbitale
Spina nasalis anterior
Maxilla
Mandibula
Foramen mentale
Os zygomaticum
Arcus zygomaticus
Meatus acusticus externus
Proc. styloideus
Proc. mastoideus (os temporale)
Os temporale, pars squamosa
Os occipitale
Sutura lambdoidea

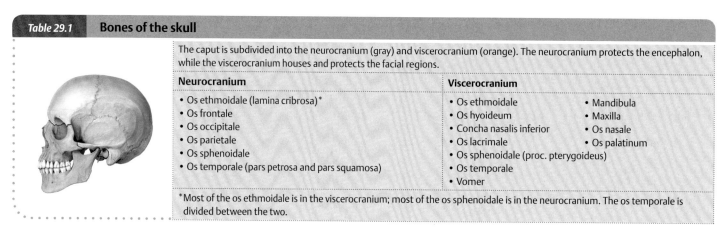

Table 29.1 Bones of the skull

The caput is subdivided into the neurocranium (gray) and viscerocranium (orange). The neurocranium protects the encephalon, while the viscerocranium houses and protects the facial regions.

Neurocranium	Viscerocranium	
• Os ethmoidale (lamina cribrosa)*	• Os ethmoidale	• Mandibula
• Os frontale	• Os hyoideum	• Maxilla
• Os occipitale	• Concha nasalis inferior	• Os nasale
• Os parietale	• Os lacrimale	• Os palatinum
• Os sphenoidale	• Os sphenoidale (proc. pterygoideus)	
• Os temporale (pars petrosa and pars squamosa)	• Os temporale	
	• Vomer	

*Most of the os ethmoidale is in the viscerocranium; most of the os sphenoidale is in the neurocranium. The os temporale is divided between the two.

Fig. 29.2 Anterior skull
Anterior view.

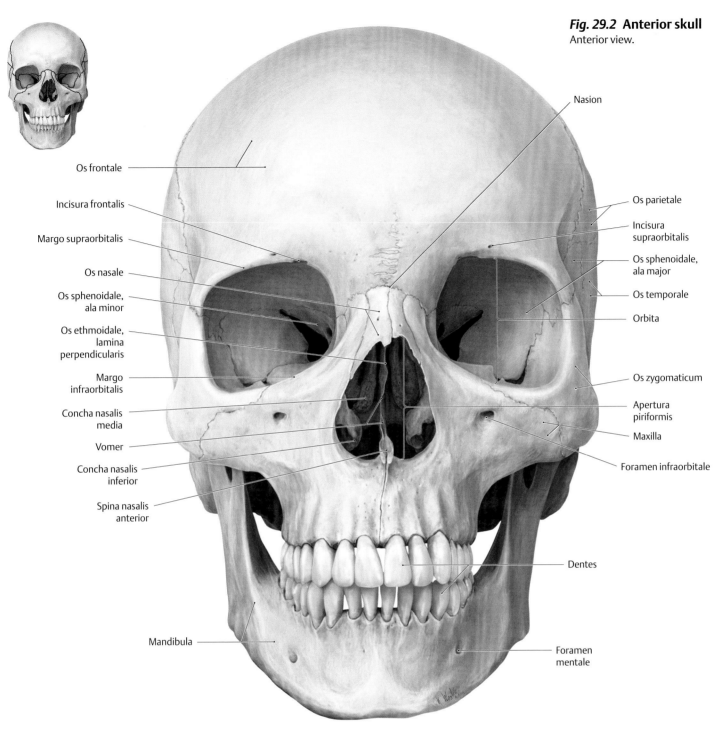

Nasion
Os frontale
Os parietale
Incisura frontalis
Incisura supraorbitalis
Margo supraorbitalis
Os sphenoidale, ala major
Os nasale
Os temporale
Os sphenoidale, ala minor
Orbita
Os ethmoidale, lamina perpendicularis
Margo infraorbitalis
Os zygomaticum
Concha nasalis media
Apertura piriformis
Vomer
Maxilla
Concha nasalis inferior
Foramen infraorbitale
Spina nasalis anterior
Dentes
Mandibula
Foramen mentale

Clinical

Fractures of the face

The framelike construction of the facial skeleton leads to characteristic patterns for fracture lines (classified as Le Fort I, II, and III fractures).

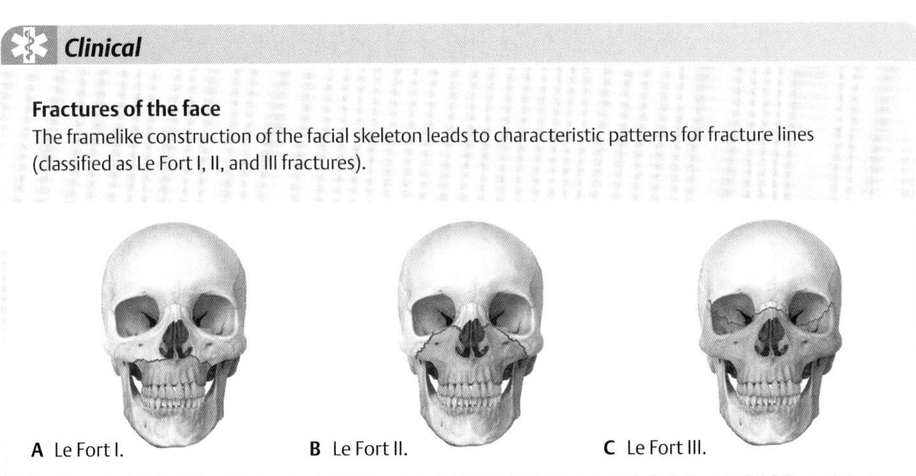

A Le Fort I. **B** Le Fort II. **C** Le Fort III.

Posterior Skull & Calvaria

Fig. 29.3 Posterior skull
Posterior view.

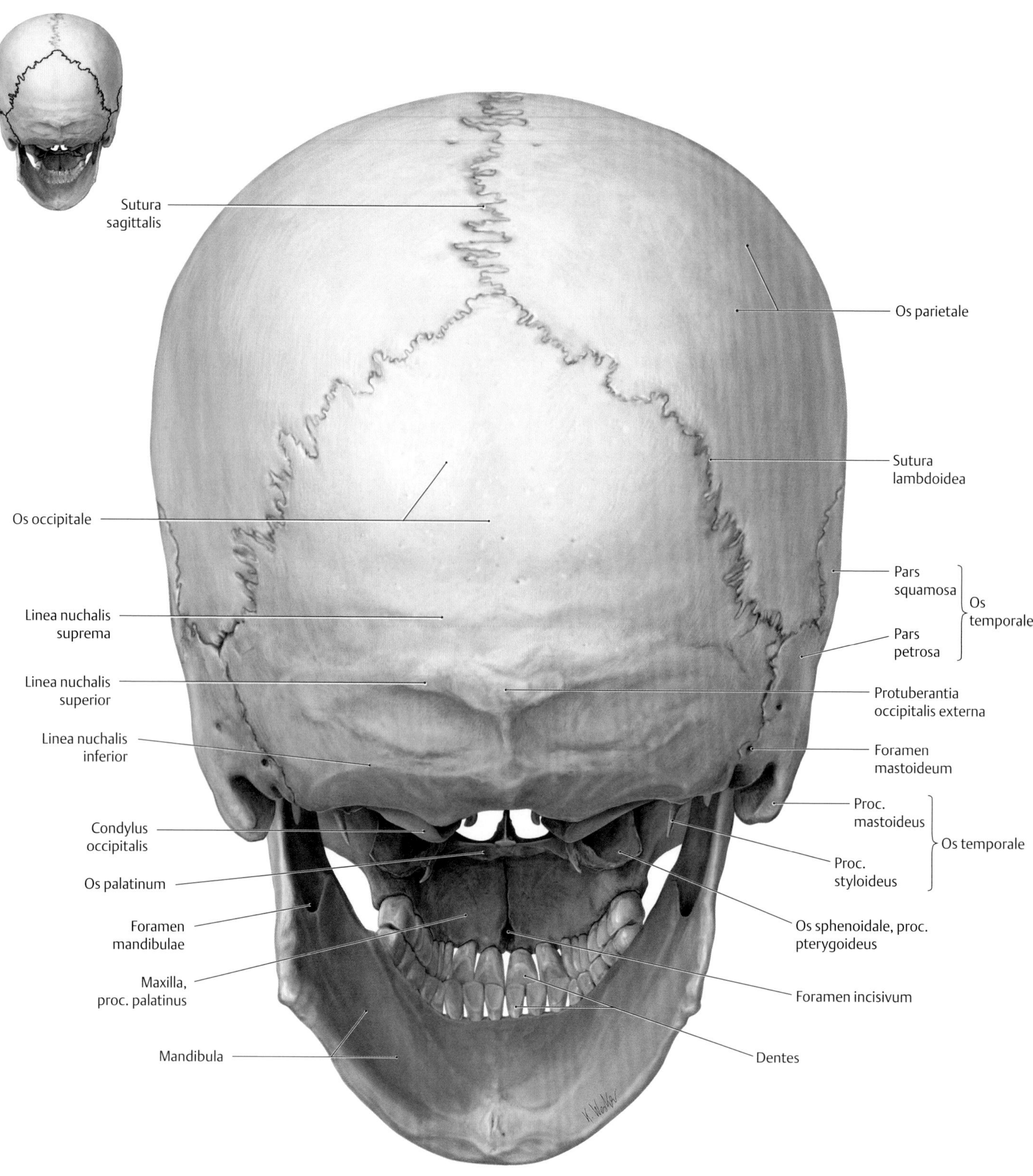
Sutura sagittalis
Os parietale
Sutura lambdoidea
Os occipitale
Pars squamosa
Os temporale
Pars petrosa
Linea nuchalis suprema
Linea nuchalis superior
Protuberantia occipitalis externa
Linea nuchalis inferior
Foramen mastoideum
Proc. mastoideus
Condylus occipitalis
Os temporale
Proc. styloideus
Os palatinum
Os sphenoidale, proc. pterygoideus
Foramen mandibulae
Maxilla, proc. palatinus
Foramen incisivum
Mandibula
Dentes

Fig. 29.4 Calvaria

Fig. 29.5 Structure of the calvaria

Cross section.

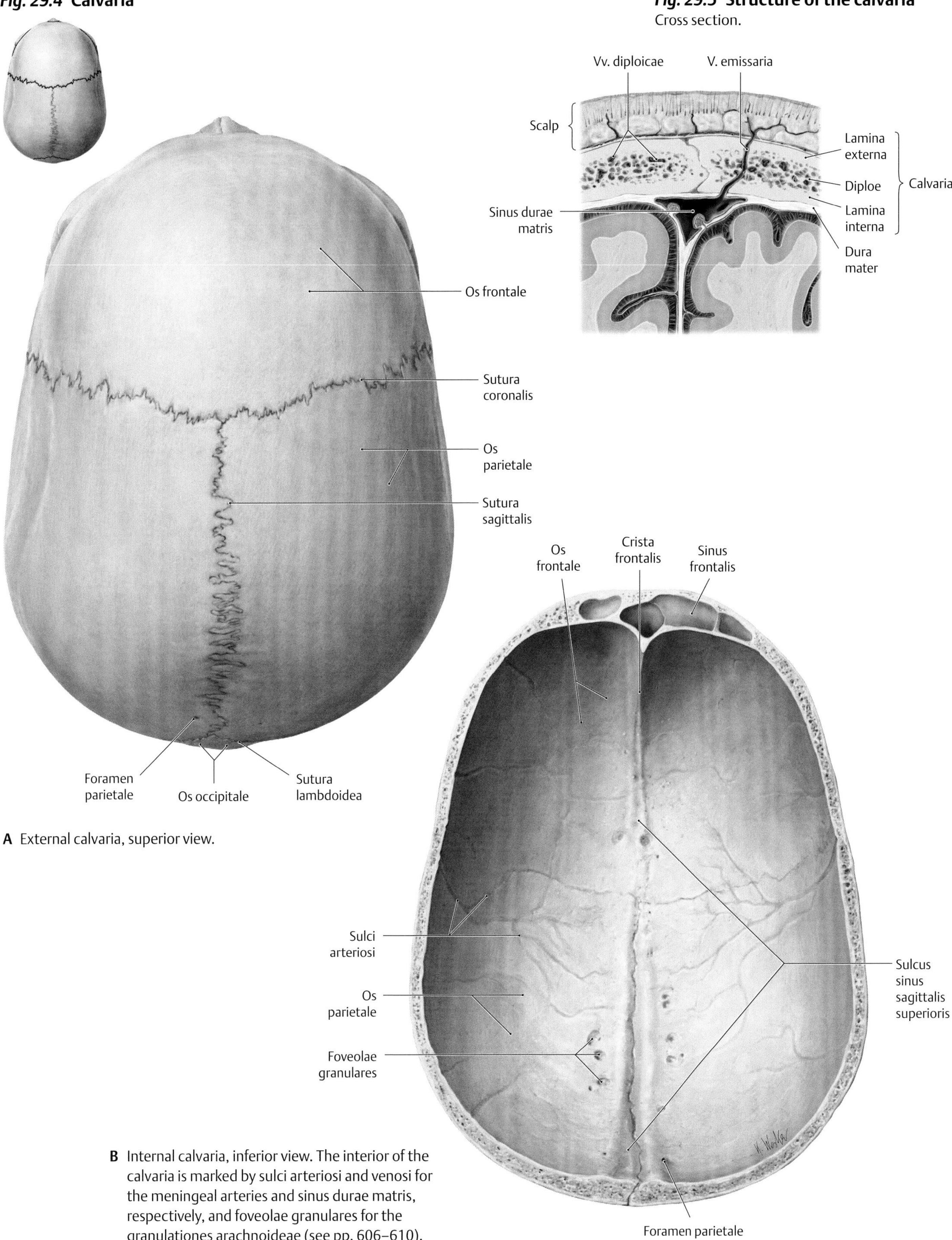

Vv. diploicae
V. emissaria
Scalp
Lamina externa
Diploe
Calvaria
Sinus durae matris
Lamina interna
Dura mater
Os frontale
Sutura coronalis
Os parietale
Sutura sagittalis
Foramen parietale
Os occipitale
Sutura lambdoidea
Os frontale
Crista frontalis
Sinus frontalis
Sulci arteriosi
Os parietale
Foveolae granulares
Sulcus sinus sagittalis superioris
Foramen parietale

A External calvaria, superior view.

B Internal calvaria, inferior view. The interior of the calvaria is marked by sulci arteriosi and venosi for the meningeal arteries and sinus durae matris, respectively, and foveolae granulares for the granulationes arachnoideae (see pp. 606–610).

Base of the Skull

Fig. 29.6 Base of the skull: Exterior
Inferior view. *Revealed:* Foramina and canals for blood vessels (see p. 490) and cranial nerves. *Note:* This view allows visual access into the posterior region of the nasal cavity.

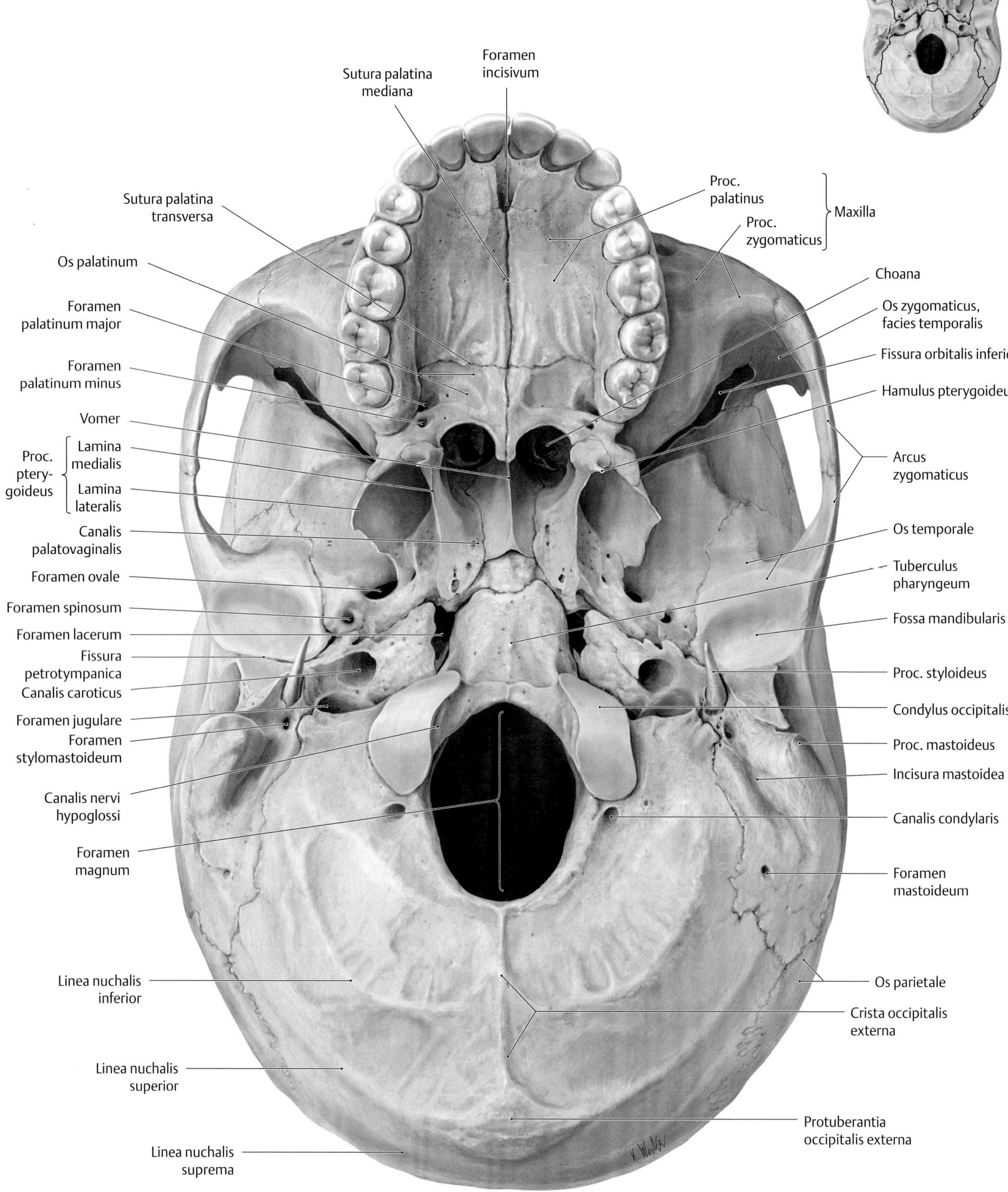
Foramen incisivum
Sutura palatina mediana
Sutura palatina transversa
Proc. palatinus
Proc. zygomaticus
Maxilla
Os palatinum
Choana
Foramen palatinum major
Os zygomaticus, facies temporalis
Fissura orbitalis inferior
Foramen palatinum minus
Hamulus pterygoideus
Vomer
Proc. pterygoideus
Lamina medialis
Lamina lateralis
Arcus zygomaticus
Canalis palatovaginalis
Os temporale
Tuberculus pharyngeum
Foramen ovale
Foramen spinosum
Fossa mandibularis
Foramen lacerum
Fissura petrotympanica
Proc. styloideus
Canalis caroticus
Condylus occipitalis
Foramen jugulare
Foramen stylomastoideum
Proc. mastoideus
Incisura mastoidea
Canalis nervi hypoglossi
Canalis condylaris
Foramen magnum
Foramen mastoideum
Linea nuchalis inferior
Os parietale
Crista occipitalis externa
Linea nuchalis superior
Protuberantia occipitalis externa
Linea nuchalis suprema

Fig. 29.7 Cranial fossae

The interior of the skull base consists of three successive fossae that become progressively deeper in the frontal-to-occipital direction.

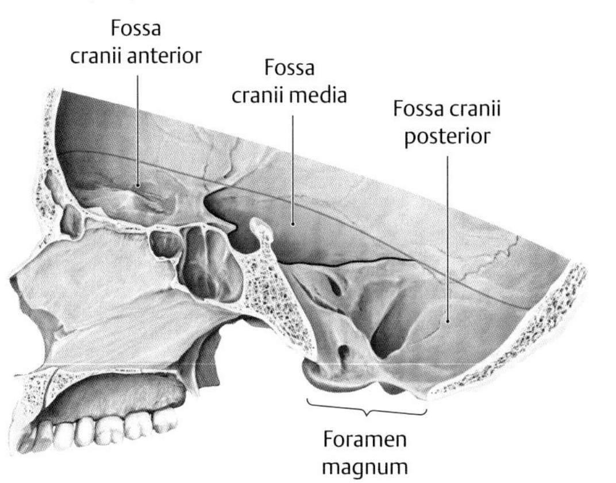
Fossa cranii anterior
Fossa cranii media
Fossa cranii posterior
Foramen magnum

A Midsagittal section, left lateral view.

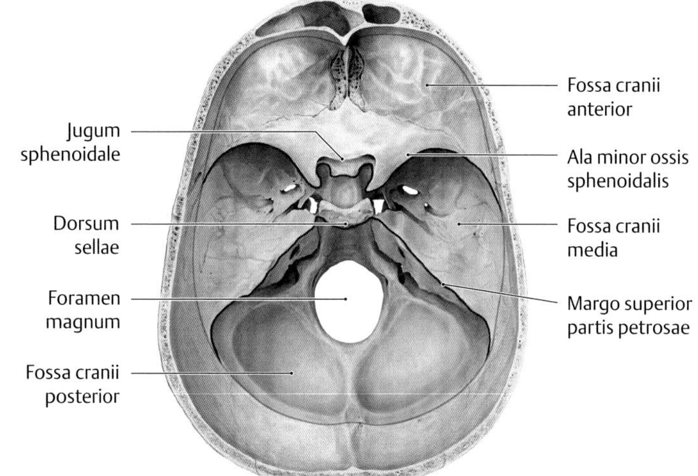
Jugum sphenoidale
Dorsum sellae
Foramen magnum
Fossa cranii posterior
Fossa cranii anterior
Ala minor ossis sphenoidalis
Fossa cranii media
Margo superior partis petrosae

B Superior view of opened skull.

Fig. 29.8 Base of the skull: Interior

Superior view.

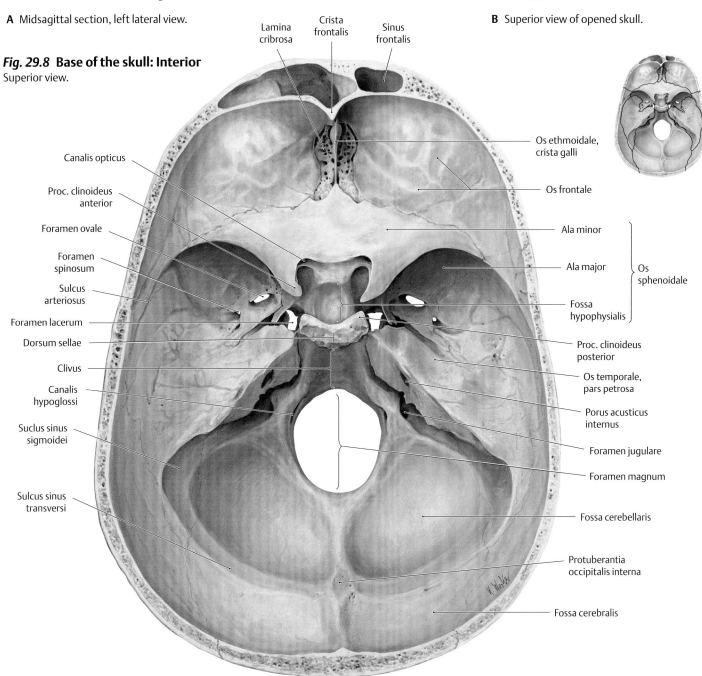

Lamina cribrosa
Crista frontalis
Sinus frontalis
Canalis opticus
Proc. clinoideus anterior
Foramen ovale
Foramen spinosum
Sulcus arteriosus
Foramen lacerum
Dorsum sellae
Clivus
Canalis hypoglossi
Suclus sinus sigmoidei
Sulcus sinus transversi
Os ethmoidale, crista galli
Os frontale
Ala minor
Ala major
Fossa hypophysialis
Os sphenoidale
Proc. clinoideus posterior
Os temporale, pars petrosa
Porus acusticus internus
Foramen jugulare
Foramen magnum
Fossa cerebellaris
Protuberantia occipitalis interna
Fossa cerebralis

Os Ethmoidale & Os Sphenoidale

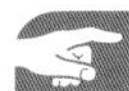

The structurally complex os ethmoidale and os sphenoidale are shown here in isolation. The other bones of the skull are shown in their respective regions: orbita (see pp. 506–507), nasal cavity (see pp. 520–521), oral cavity (see pp. 538–539), and ear (see pp. 526–527).

Fig. 29.9 Os ethmoidale

The os ethmoidale is the central bone of the nose and paranasal air sinuses (see pp. 520–523).

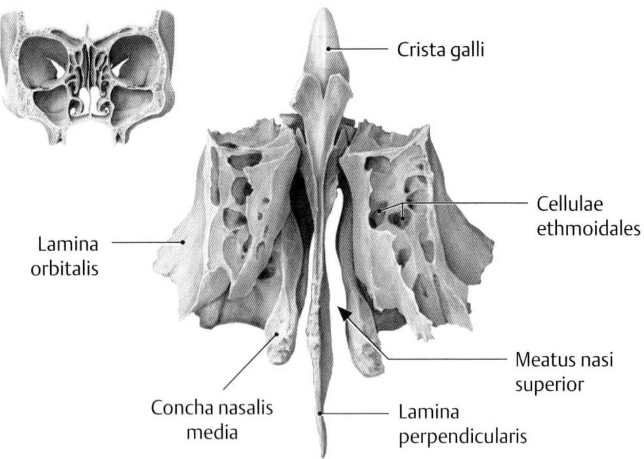
Crista galli
Cellulae ethmoidales
Lamina orbitalis
Meatus nasi superior
Concha nasalis media
Lamina perpendicularis

A Anterior view.

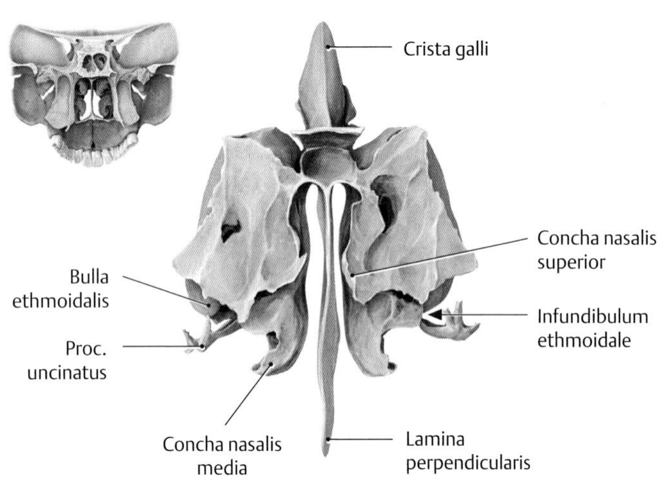
Crista galli
Concha nasalis superior
Bulla ethmoidalis
Infundibulum ethmoidale
Proc. uncinatus
Concha nasalis media
Lamina perpendicularis

C Posterior view.

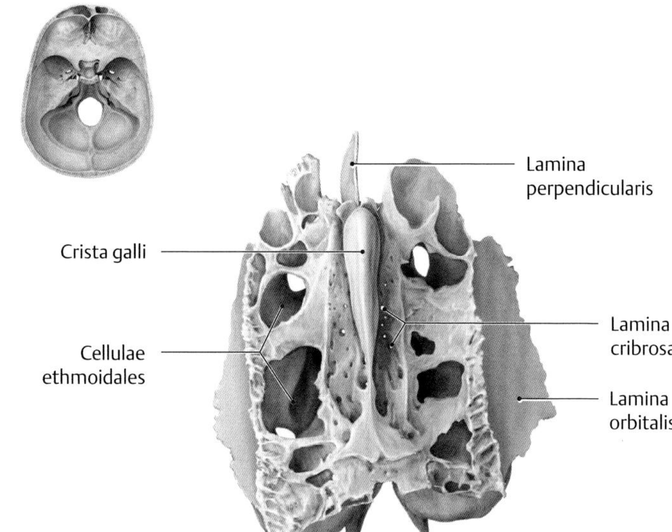
Lamina perpendicularis
Crista galli
Lamina cribrosa
Cellulae ethmoidales
Lamina orbitalis

B Superior view.

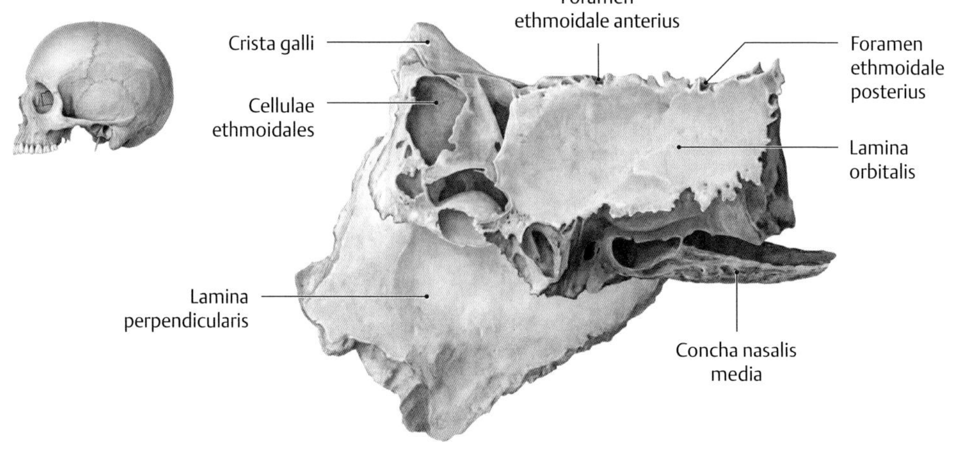
Foramen ethmoidale anterius
Crista galli
Foramen ethmoidale posterius
Cellulae ethmoidales
Lamina orbitalis
Lamina perpendicularis
Concha nasalis media

D Left lateral view.

Fig. 29.10 Os sphenoidale

The os sphenoidale is the most structurally complex bone in the human body.

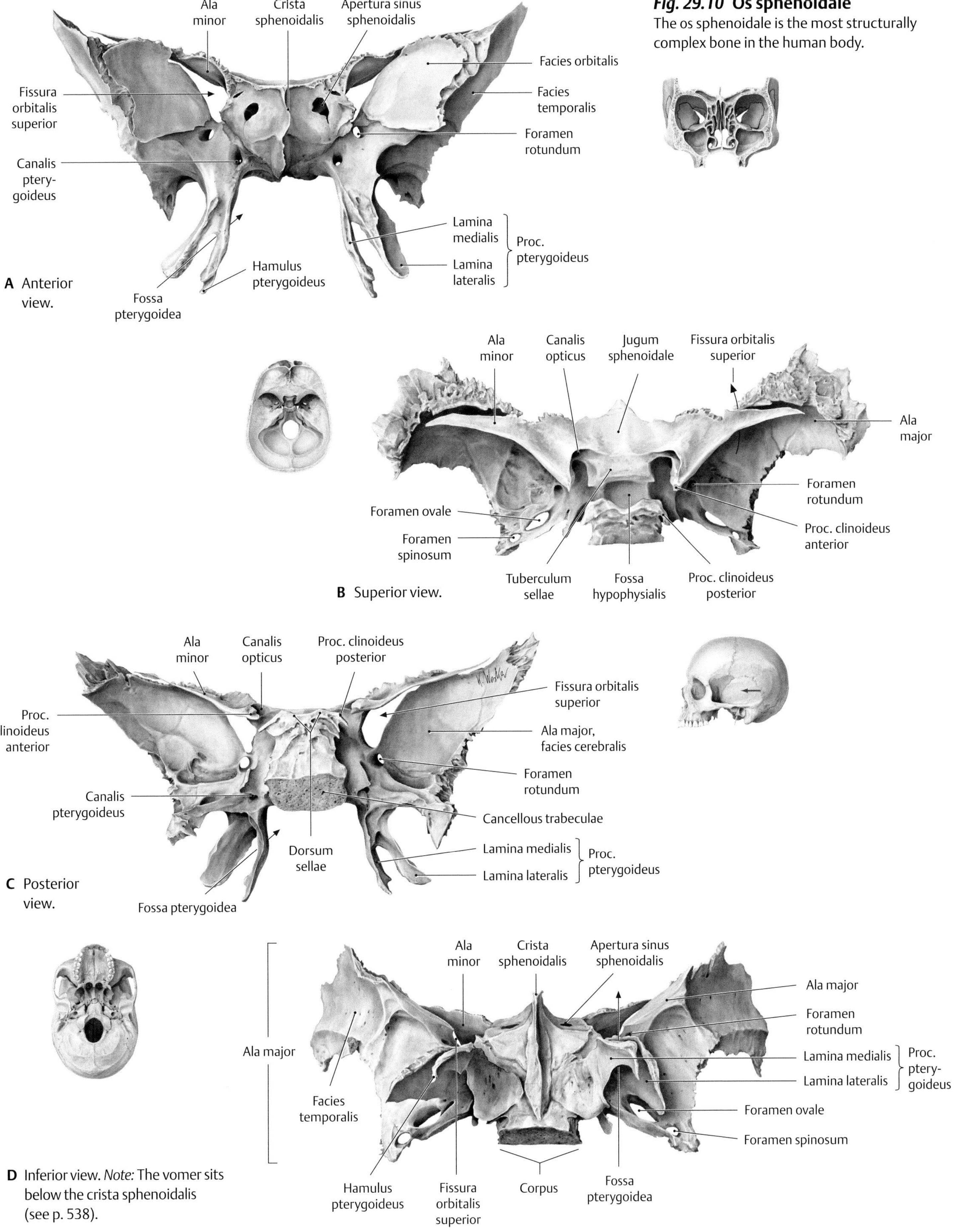
Ala minor
Crista sphenoidalis
Apertura sinus sphenoidalis
Facies orbitalis
Fissura orbitalis superior
Facies temporalis
Foramen rotundum
Canalis pterygoideus
Lamina medialis
Lamina lateralis
Proc. pterygoideus
Hamulus pterygoideus
Fossa pterygoidea
Ala minor
Canalis opticus
Jugum sphenoidale
Fissura orbitalis superior
Ala major
Foramen rotundum
Proc. clinoideus anterior
Foramen ovale
Foramen spinosum
Tuberculum sellae
Fossa hypophysialis
Proc. clinoideus posterior
Ala minor
Canalis opticus
Proc. clinoideus posterior
Fissura orbitalis superior
Proc. clinoideus anterior
Ala major, facies cerebralis
Foramen rotundum
Canalis pterygoideus
Cancellous trabeculae
Dorsum sellae
Lamina medialis
Lamina lateralis
Proc. pterygoideus
Fossa pterygoidea
Ala minor
Crista sphenoidalis
Apertura sinus sphenoidalis
Ala major
Foramen rotundum
Lamina medialis
Lamina lateralis
Proc. pterygoideus
Foramen ovale
Foramen spinosum
Ala major
Facies temporalis
Hamulus pterygoideus
Fissura orbitalis superior
Corpus
Fossa pterygoidea

A Anterior view.

B Superior view.

C Posterior view.

D Inferior view. *Note:* The vomer sits below the crista sphenoidalis (see p. 538).

Muscles of Facial Expression & of Mastication

The muscles of the skull and face are divided into two groups. The muscles of facial expression make up the superficial muscle layer in the face. The muscles of mastication are responsible for the movement of the mandible during mastication (chewing).

Fig. 30.1 Muscles of facial expression (Musculi faciei)

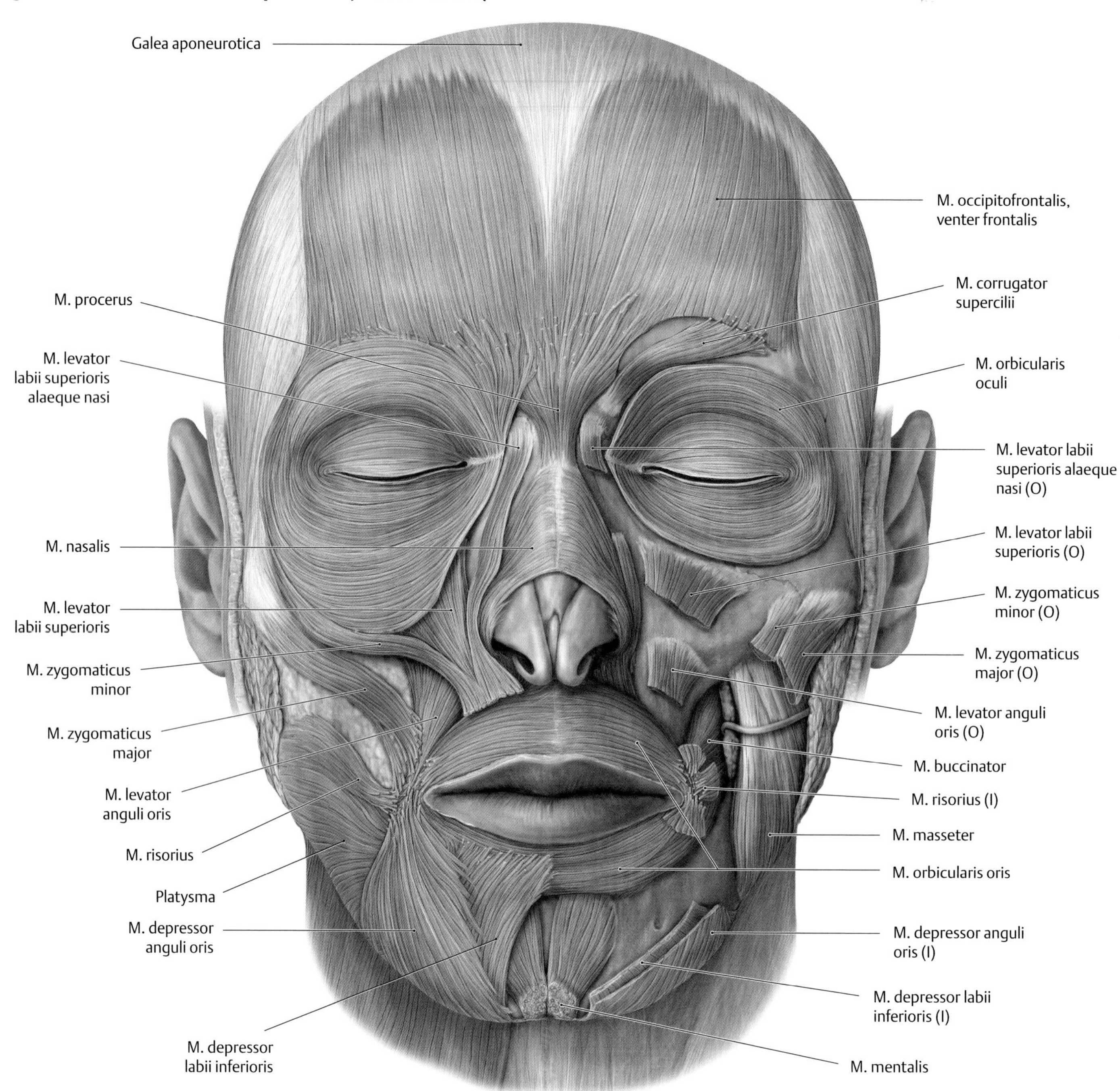
Galea aponeurotica
M. occipitofrontalis, venter frontalis
M. corrugator supercilii
M. procerus
M. orbicularis oculi
M. levator labii superioris alaeque nasi
M. levator labii superioris alaeque nasi (O)
M. nasalis
M. levator labii superioris (O)
M. levator labii superioris
M. zygomaticus minor (O)
M. zygomaticus minor
M. zygomaticus major (O)
M. zygomaticus major
M. levator anguli oris (O)
M. levator anguli oris
M. buccinator
M. risorius (I)
M. risorius
M. masseter
Platysma
M. orbicularis oris
M. depressor anguli oris
M. depressor anguli oris (I)
M. depressor labii inferioris (I)
M. depressor labii inferioris
M. mentalis

A Anterior view. Muscle origins (O) and insertions (I) indicated on left side of face.

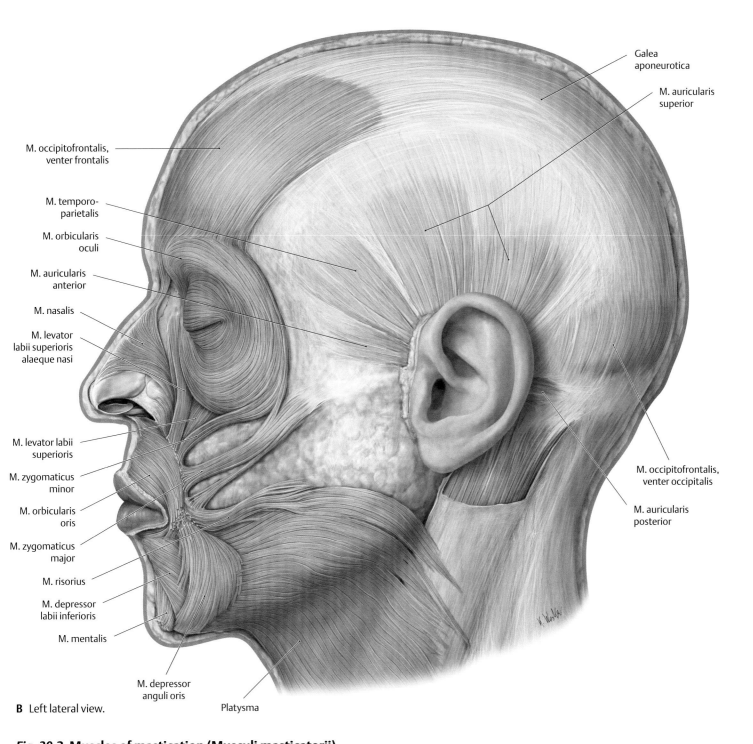

Galea aponeurotica
M. auricularis superior
M. occipitofrontalis, venter frontalis
M. temporoparietalis
M. orbicularis oculi
M. auricularis anterior
M. nasalis
M. levator labii superioris alaeque nasi
M. levator labii superioris
M. zygomaticus minor
M. orbicularis oris
M. zygomaticus major
M. risorius
M. depressor labii inferioris
M. mentalis
M. depressor anguli oris
Platysma
M. occipitofrontalis, venter occipitalis
M. auricularis posterior

B Left lateral view.

Fig. 30.2 Muscles of mastication (Musculi masticatorii)

Left lateral view.

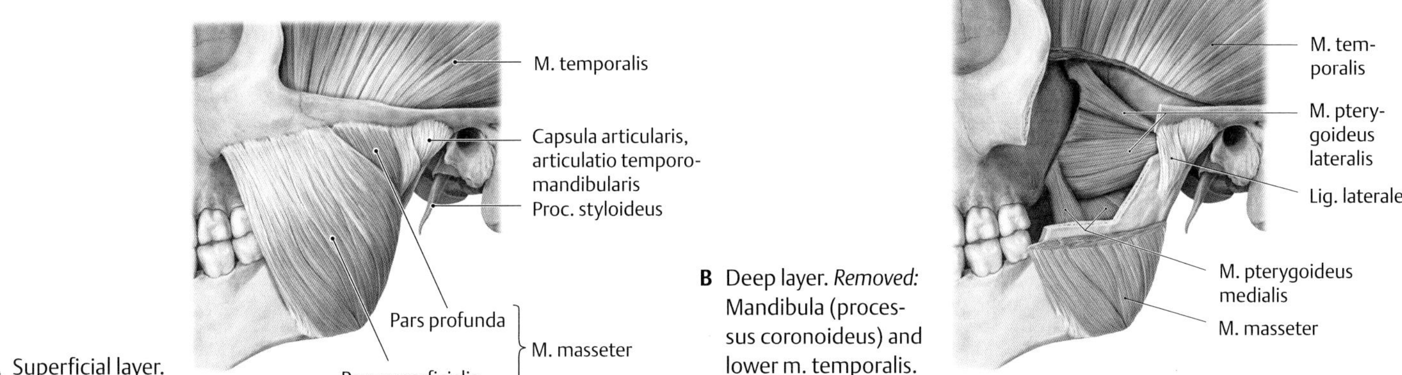
M. temporalis
Capsula articularis, articulatio temporomandibularis
Proc. styloideus
Pars profunda
Pars superficialis
M. masseter
M. temporalis
M. pterygoideus lateralis
Lig. laterale
M. pterygoideus medialis
M. masseter

A Superficial layer.

B Deep layer. *Removed:* Mandibula (processus coronoideus) and lower m. temporalis.

Muscle Origins & Insertions on the Skull

Fig. 30.3 **Lateral skull: Origins and insertions**
Left lateral view. Muscle origins (red), insertions (blue).
Note: There are generally no bony insertions for the muscles of facial expression. These muscles insert into skin and other muscles of facial expression.

Mm. facei: N. facialis (CN VII)

- M. occipitofrontalis, venter occipitalis
- M. corrugator supercilii
- M. orbicularis oculi
  - Pars orbitalis
  - Pars lacrimalis
- M. levator labii superioris alaeque nasi
- M. zygomaticus major
- M. zygomaticus minor
- M. levator anguli oris
- M. nasalis
  - Pars transversa
  - Pars alaris
- M. depressor septi nasi
- M. orbicularis oris
- M. buccinator
- M. mentalis
- M. orbicularis oris
- M. depressor labii inferioris
- M. depressor anguli oris
- Platysma

M. sternocleidomastoideus and m. trapezius: N. accessorius (CN XI)

- M. sternocleidomastoideus
- M. trapezius

Mm. colli and dorsi proprii: Rr. dorsales of nn. spinales cervicales

- M. semispinalis capitis
- M. obliquus capitis superior
- M. rectus capitis posterior major
- M. rectus capitis posterior minor
- M. splenius capitis
- M. longissimus capitis

Mm. masticatorii: N. mandibularis (CN V_3)

- M. masseter
- M. pterygoideus lateralis
- M. temporalis
- M. pterygoideus medialis (see Fig. 30.4)

Fig. 30.4 **Mandibula: Origins and insertions**
Medial view of right hemimandible (inner surface).

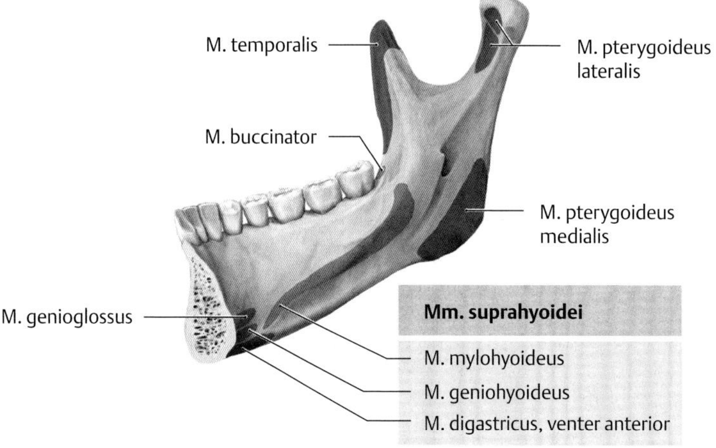
M. temporalis
M. pterygoideus lateralis
M. buccinator
M. pterygoideus medialis
M. genioglossus
Mm. suprahyoidei
M. mylohyoideus
M. geniohyoideus
M. digastricus, venter anterior

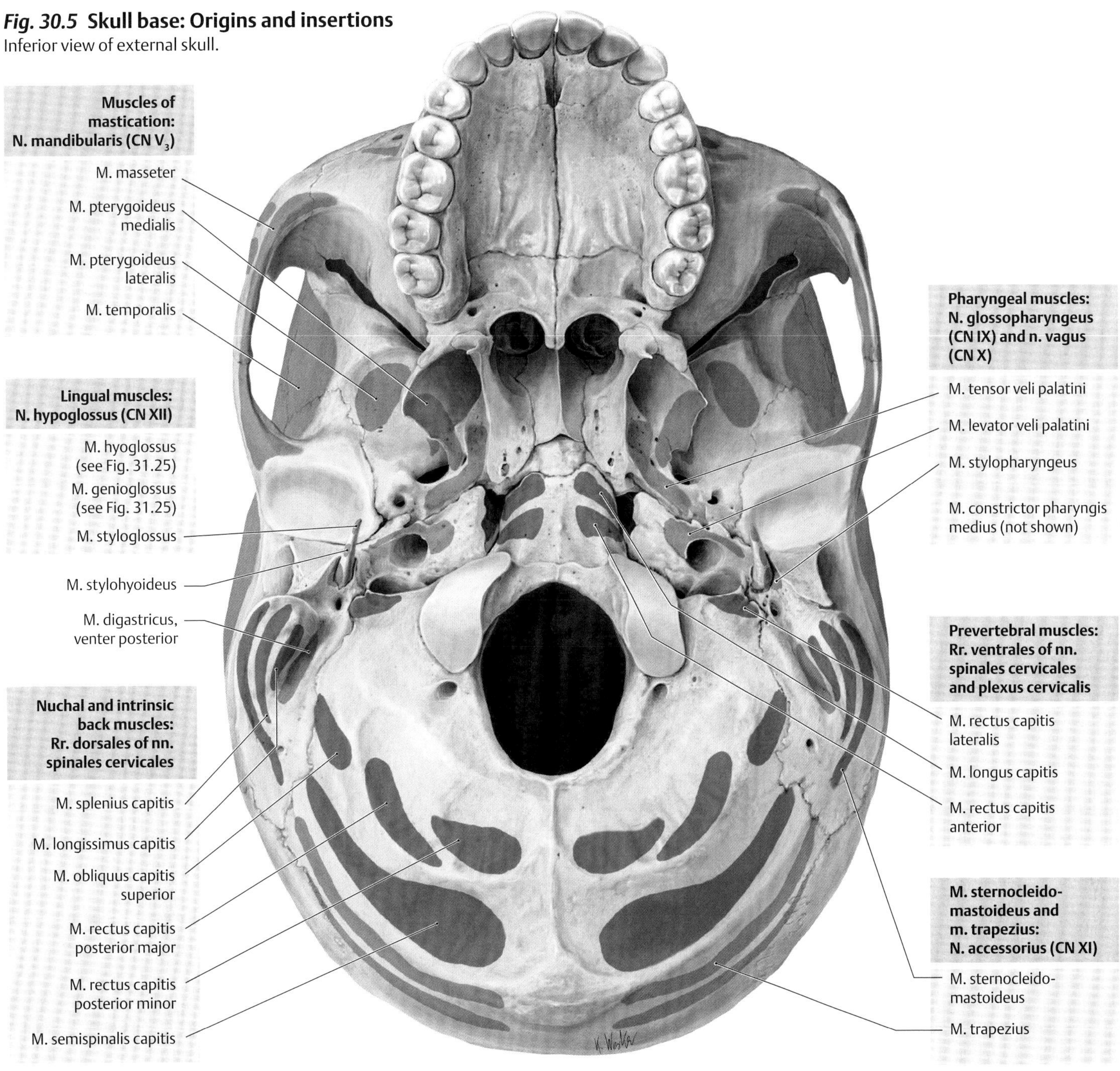

Muscles of mastication: N. mandibularis (CN V_3)
M. masseter
M. pterygoideus medialis
M. pterygoideus lateralis
M. temporalis
Lingual muscles: N. hypoglossus (CN XII)
M. hyoglossus (see Fig. 31.25)
M. genioglossus (see Fig. 31.25)
M. styloglossus
M. stylohyoideus
M. digastricus, venter posterior
Nuchal and intrinsic back muscles: Rr. dorsales of nn. spinales cervicales
M. splenius capitis
M. longissimus capitis
M. obliquus capitis superior
M. rectus capitis posterior major
M. rectus capitis posterior minor
M. semispinalis capitis
Pharyngeal muscles: N. glossopharyngeus (CN IX) and n. vagus (CN X)
M. tensor veli palatini
M. levator veli palatini
M. stylopharyngeus
M. constrictor pharyngis medius (not shown)
Prevertebral muscles: Rr. ventrales of nn. spinales cervicales and plexus cervicalis
M. rectus capitis lateralis
M. longus capitis
M. rectus capitis anterior
M. sternocleido-mastoideus and m. trapezius: N. accessorius (CN XI)
M. sternocleido-mastoideus
M. trapezius

Fig. 30.5 **Skull base: Origins and insertions**
Inferior view of external skull.

Fig. 30.6 **Os hyoideum: Origins and insertions**

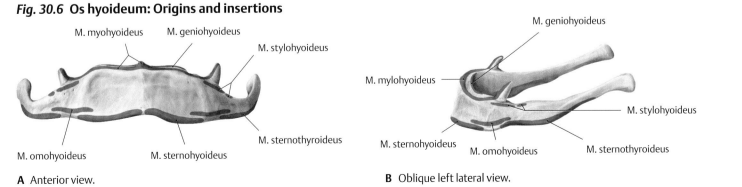

M. myohyoideus
M. geniohyoideus
M. stylohyoideus
M. omohyoideus
M. sternohyoideus
M. sternothyroideus

A Anterior view.

M. geniohyoideus
M. mylohyoideus
M. stylohyoideus
M. sternohyoideus
M. omohyoideus
M. sternothyroideus

B Oblique left lateral view.

Muscle Facts (I)

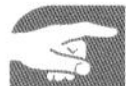

The muscles of facial expression originate on bone and/or fascia, and insert into the subcutaneous tissue of the face. This allows them to produce their effects by pulling on the skin.

Fig. 30.7 **M. occipitofrontalis**
Anterior view.

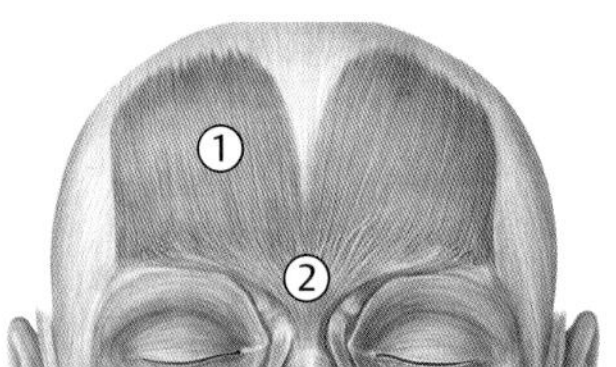
①
②

Fig. 30.8 **Muscles of the palpebral fissure and nose**
Anterior view.

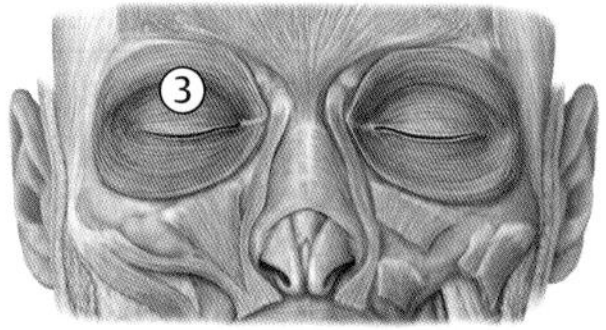
③

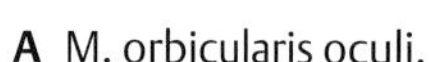

A M. orbicularis oculi.

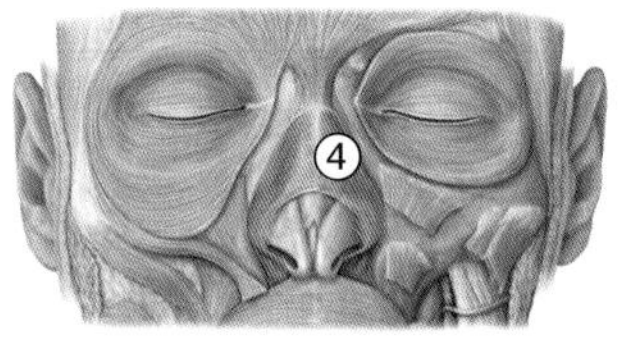
④

B M. nasalis.

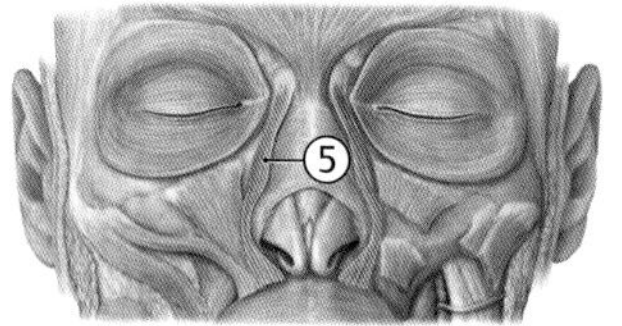
⑤

C M. levator labii superioris alaeque nasi.

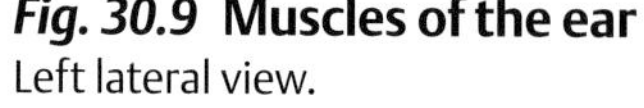

Fig. 30.9 **Muscles of the ear**
Left lateral view.

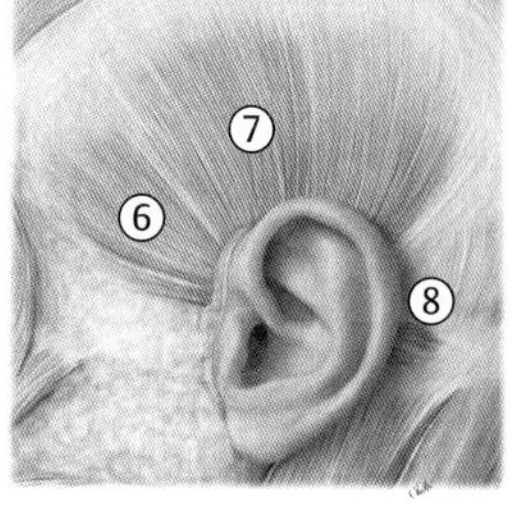
⑦
⑥
⑧

Table 30.1 Muscles of facial expression: Forehead, nose, and ear

Muscle	Origin	Insertion*	Main action(s)**
Calvaria			
① M. occipitofrontalis (venter frontalis)	Galea aponeurotica	Skin and subcutaneous tissue of eyebrows and forehead	Elevates eyebrows, wrinkles skin of forehead
Palpebral fissure and nose			
② M. procerus	Os nasale, cartilago nasi lateralis (upper part)	Skin of lower forehead between eyebrows	Pulls medial angle of eyebrows inferiorly, producing transverse wrinkles over bridge of nose
③ M. orbicularis oculi	Margo orbitalis medialis, lig. palpebrale mediale; os lacrimale	Skin around margo orbitalis, superior and inferior tarsal plates	Acts as orbital sphincter (closes eyelids) • Palpebral portion gently closes • Orbital portion tightly closes (as in winking)
④ M. nasalis	Maxilla (superior region of dens caninus)	Cartilago nasi	Flares nostrils by drawing ala (side) of nose toward nasal septum
⑤ M. levator labii superioris alaeque nasi	Maxilla (proc. frontalis)	Cartilago alaris major and labium superius	Elevates upper lip, opens nostril
Ear			
⑥ M. auricularis anterior	Fascia temporalis (anterior portion)	Spina helicis	Pull ear superiorly and anteriorly
⑦ M. auricularis superior	Galea aponeurotica	Upper portion of auricle	Elevate ear
⑧ M. auricularis posterior	Proc. mastoideus	Concha auriculae	Pull ear superiorly and posteriorly

*There are no bony insertions for the muscles of facial expression.
**All muscles of facial expression are innervated by the n. facialis (CN VII) via rr. temporales, rr. zygomatici, r. buccalis, r. marginalis mandibularis, or r. colli arising from the plexus parotideus (see p. 478).

Fig. 30.10 **Muscles of the mouth**
Left lateral view.

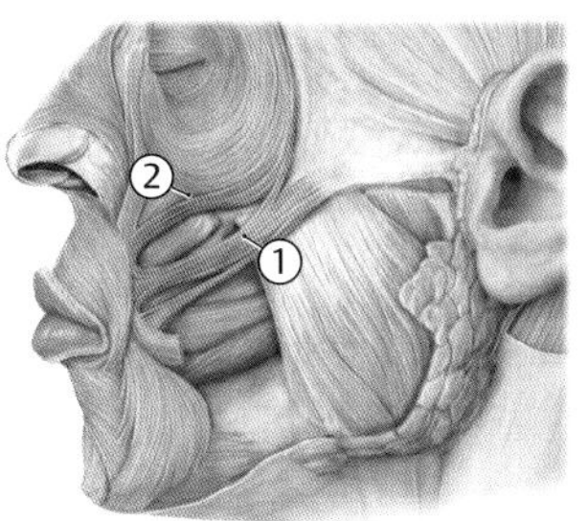

2
1

A Mm. zygomaticus major and minor.

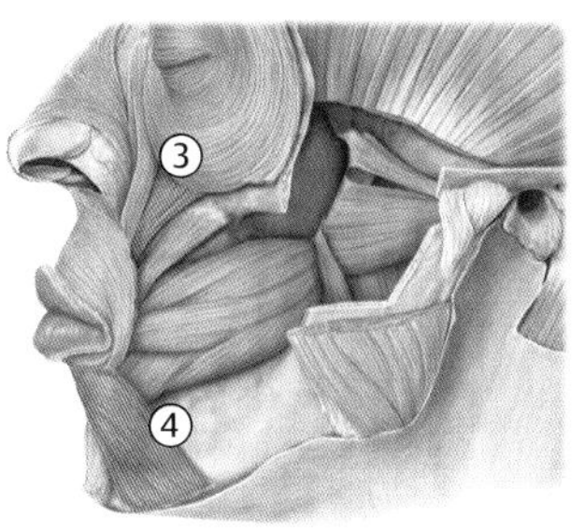

3
4

B M. levator labii superioris and m. depressor labii inferioris.

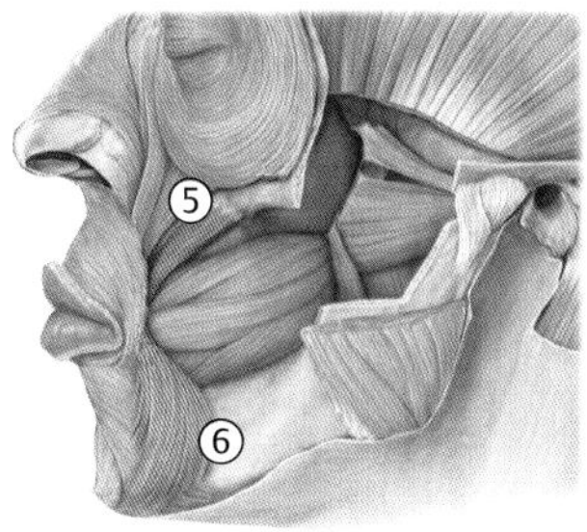

5
6

C Mm. levator and depressor anguli oris.

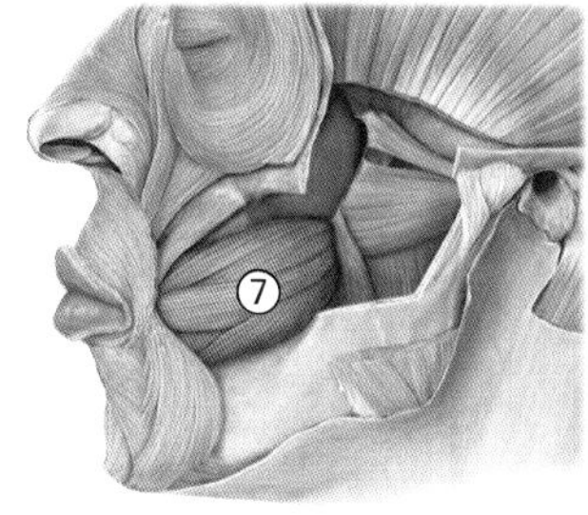

7

D M. buccinator.

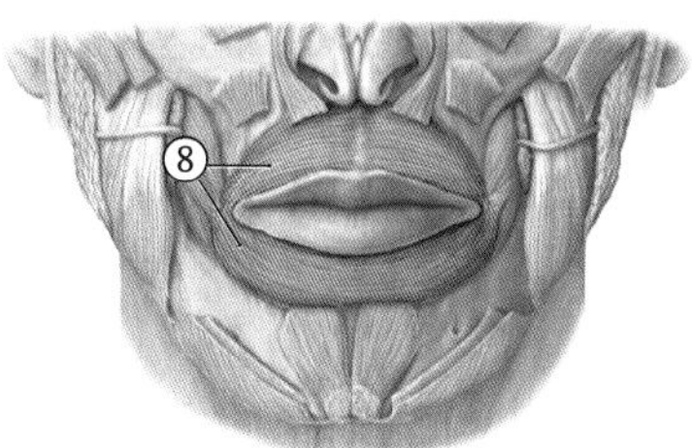

8

E M. orbicularis oris, anterior view.

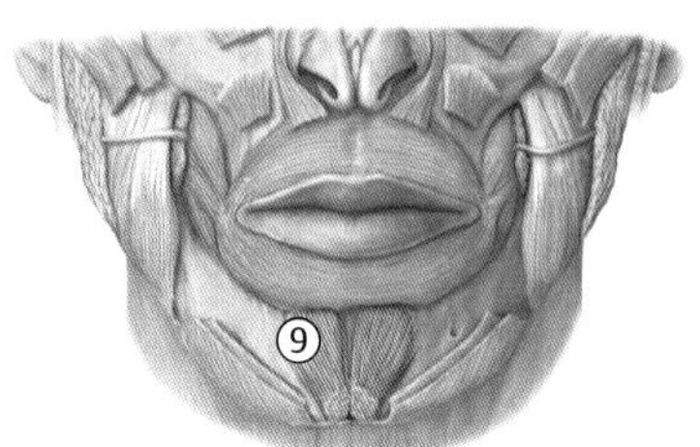

9

F M. mentalis, anterior view.

Table 30.2 **Muscles of facial expression: Mouth and neck**

Muscle	Origin	Insertion*	Main action(s)**
Mouth			
① M. zygomaticus major	Os zygomaticum (facies lateralis, pars posterior)	Skin at angulus oris	Pulls corner of mouth superiorly and laterally
② M. zygomaticus minor		Labium superius medial to angulus oris	Pulls upper lip superiorly
M. levator labii superioris alaeque nasi (see Fig. 30.8C)	Maxilla (proc. frontalis)	Cartilago alaris major and labium superius	Elevates upper lip, opens nostril
③ M. levator labii superioris	Maxilla (proc. frontalis) and regio infraorbitalis	Skin of labium superius, cartilago alaris major	Elevates upper lip, dilates nostril, raises angle of the mouth
④ M. depressor labii inferioris	Mandibula (anterior portion linea obliqua)	Labium inferius at midline; blends with muscle from opposite side	Pulls lower lip inferiorly and laterally
⑤ M. levator anguli oris	Maxilla (below foramen infraorbitale)	Skin at angulus oris	Raises angle of mouth, helps form nasolabial furrow
⑥ M. depressor anguli oris	Mandibula (fossa canina corporis maxillae, dens premolaris I, and dens molaris I)	Skin at angulus oris, Cartilago alaris major; blends with m. orbicularis oris	Pulls angle of mouth inferiorly and laterally
⑦ M. buccinator	Mandibula, procc. alveolares of maxilla and mandibula, raphe pterygomandibularis	Angulus oris, m. orbicularis oris	Presses cheek against molar teeth, working with tongue to keep food between occlusal surfaces and out of oral vestibule; expels air from oral cavity/resists distension when blowing *Unilateral:* Draws mouth to one side
⑧ M. orbicularis oris	Deep surface of skin Superiorly: maxilla (median plane) Inferiorly: mandibula	Mucous membrane of lips	Acts as oral sphincter • Compresses and protrudes lips (e.g., when whistling, sucking, and kissing) • Resists distension (when blowing)
M. risorius (see p. 462)	Fascia parotidea	Skin at angulus oris	Retracts corner of mouth as in grimacing
⑨ M. mentalis	Mandibula (incisive fossa)	Skin of mentum	Elevates and protrudes lower lip
Neck			
Platysma (see p. 463)	Skin over lower neck and upper lateral thorax	Mandibula (inferior border), skin over lower face, angulus oris	Depresses and wrinkles skin of lower face and mouth; tenses skin of neck; aids in forced depression of the mandibula

*There are no bony insertions for the muscles of facial expression.
**All muscles of facial expression are innervated by the n. facialis (CN VII) via rr. temporales, rr. zygomatici, rr. buccales, rr. mandibulares or rr. cervicales arising from plexus parotideus.

Muscle Facts (II)

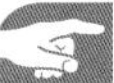

The muscles of mastication are located at various depths in the parotid and infratemporal regions of the face. They attach to mandibula and receive their motor innervation from n. mandibularis of n. trigeminus (CN V_3). The muscles of the oral floor that aid in opening the mouth are found on p. 562.

Table 30.3 Muscles of mastication: Masseter and temporalis

Muscle	Origin	Insertion	Innervation	Action
① M. masseter	Pars superficialis: Arcus zygomaticus (anterior two thirds) Pars profunda: Arcus zygomaticus (posterior one third)	Angulus mandibulae (tuberositas masseterica)	N. mandibularis (CN V_3) via n. massetericus	Elevates (adducts) and protrudes mandibula
② M. temporalis	Linea temporalis	Proc. coronoideus mandibulae (apex and facies medialis)	N. mandibularis (CN V_3) via nn. temporalis profundi.	*Vertical fibers:* Elevate (adduct) mandibula *Horizontal fibers:* Retract (retrude) mandibula *Unilateral:* Lateral movement of mandibula (chewing)

Fig. 30.11 **M. masseter**
Left lateral view.

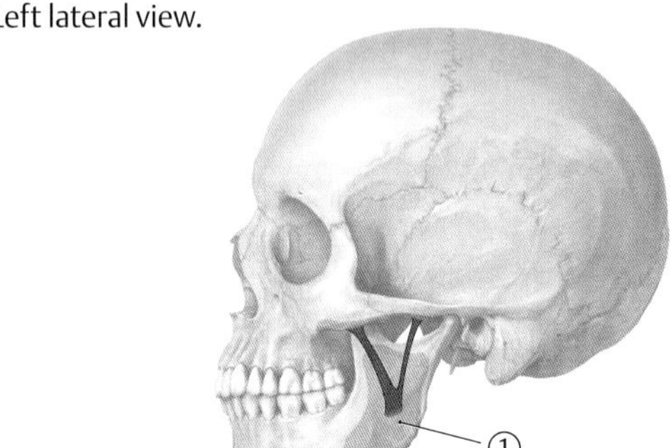
①

A Schematic.

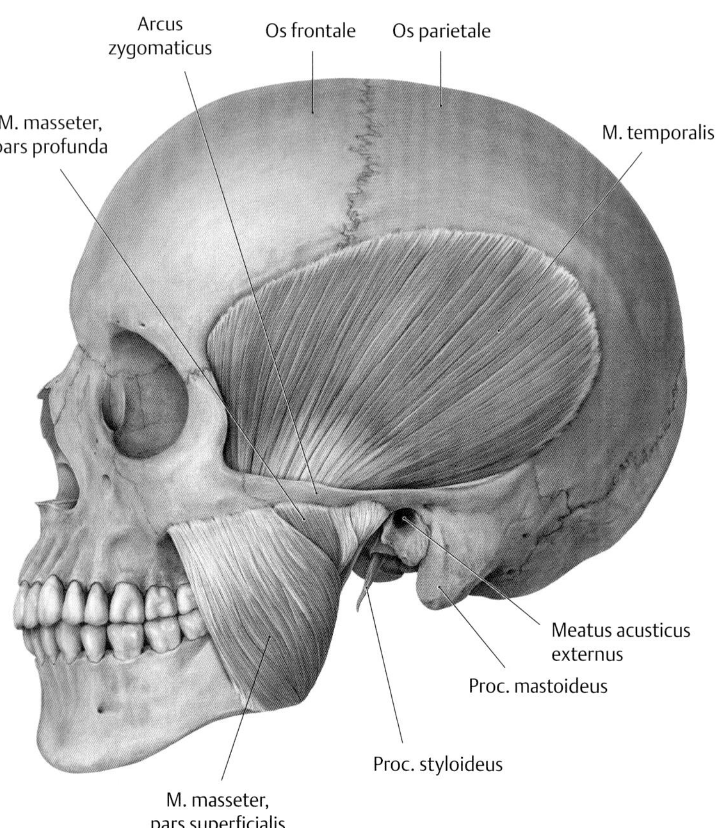
Arcus zygomaticus
Os frontale
Os parietale
M. masseter, pars profunda
M. temporalis
Meatus acusticus externus
Proc. mastoideus
Proc. styloideus
M. masseter, pars superficialis

B M. masseter and m. temporalis.

Fig. 30.12 **M. temporalis**
Left lateral view.

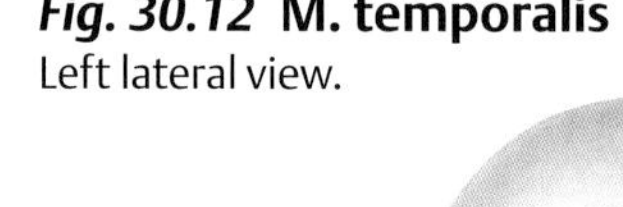

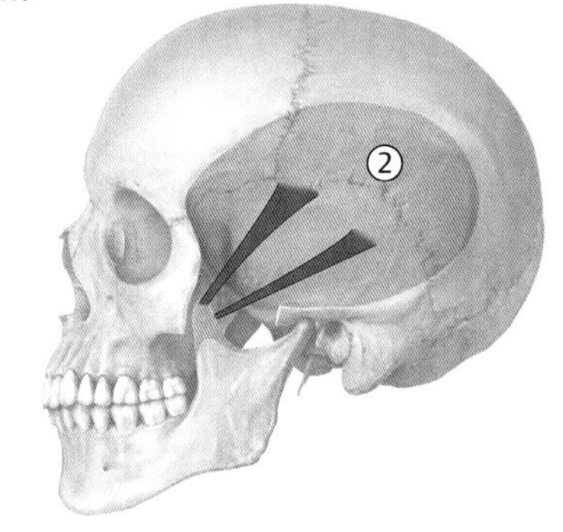
②

A Schematic.

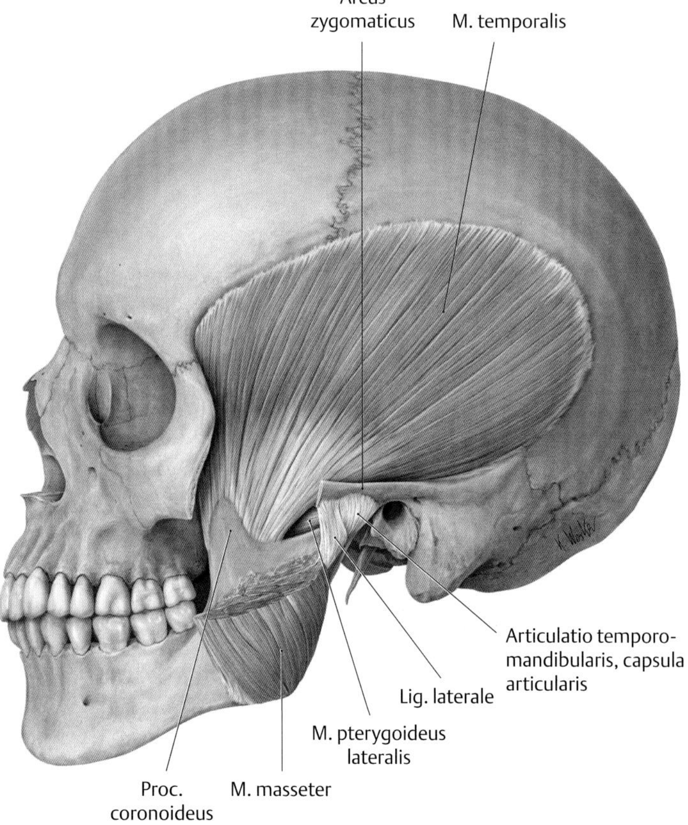
Arcus zygomaticus
M. temporalis
Articulatio temporomandibularis, capsula articularis
Lig. laterale
M. pterygoideus lateralis
Proc. coronoideus
M. masseter

B M. temporalis. *Removed:* M. masseter and arcus zygomaticus.

Table 30.4 Muscles of mastication: Pterygoid muscles

Muscle		Origin	Insertion	Innervation	Action
M. pterygoideus lateralis	③ Pars superior	Crista infratemporalis ossis sphenoidalis	Articulatio temporomandibularis (disus articularis)	N. mandibularis (CN V_3) via n. pterygoideus lateralis	*Bilateral:* Protrudes mandibula (pulls articular disk forward) *Unilateral:* Lateral movements of mandibula (chewing)
	④ Pars inferior	Lamina lateralis of proc. pterygoideus (lateral surface)	Mandibula (proc. condylaris)		
M. pterygoideus medialis	⑤ Pars superficialis	Tuber maxillae	Tuberositas pterygoidea on medial surface of the angulus mandibulae	N. mandibularis (CN V_3) via n. pterygoideus medialis	Elevates (adducts) mandibula
	⑥ Pars profunda	Medial surface of lamina lateralis of proc. pterygoideus and fossa pterygoidea			

Fig. 30.13 **M. pterygoideus lateralis**
Left lateral view.

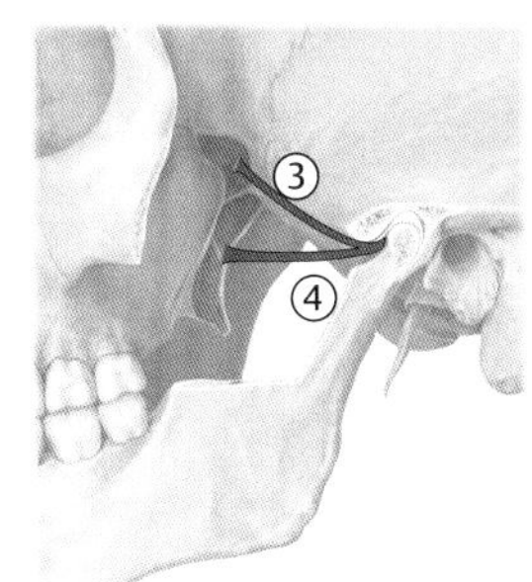
③
④

A Schematic.

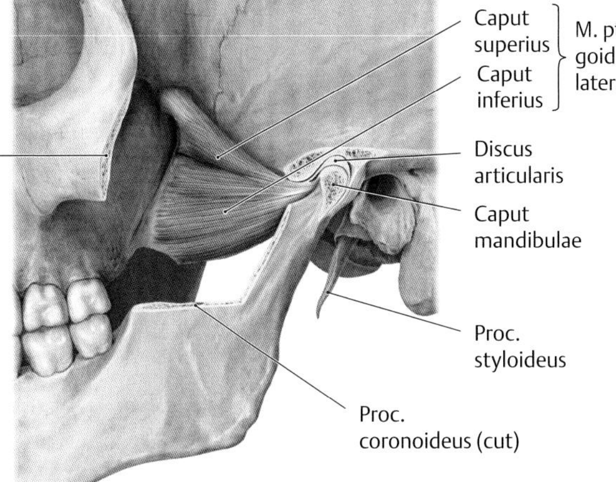
Caput superius
Caput inferius
M. pterygoideus lateralis
Arcus zygomaticus (cut)
Discus articularis
Caput mandibulae
Proc. styloideus
Proc. coronoideus (cut)

B M. pterygoideus lateralis sinister. *Removed:* Processus coronoideus.

Fig. 30.14 **M. pterygoideus medialis**
Left lateral view.

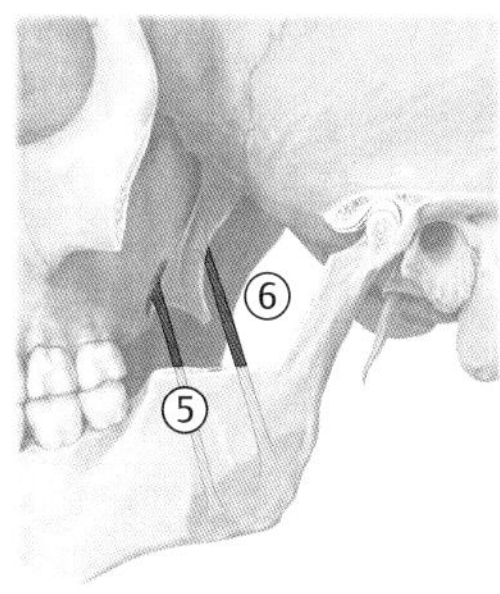
⑥
⑤

A Schematic.

Proc. pterygoideus, lamina lateralis
M. pterygoideus medialis, caput superficialis
M. pterygoideus medialis, caput profundus
Angulus mandibulae

B M. pterygoideus medialis sinister. *Removed:* Processus coronoideus.

Fig. 30.15 **Masticatory muscle sling**
Oblique posterior view.

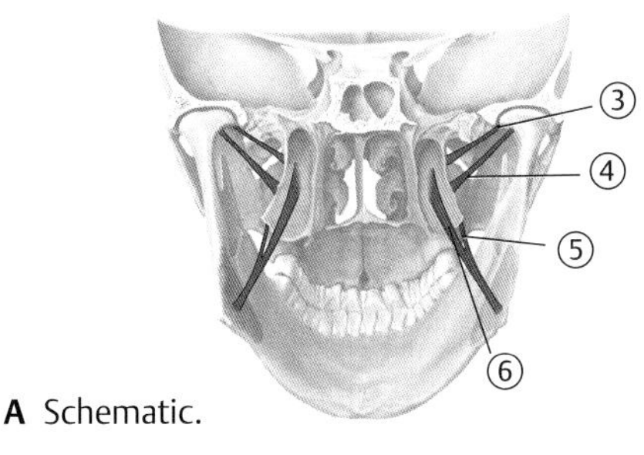
③
④
⑤
⑥

A Schematic.

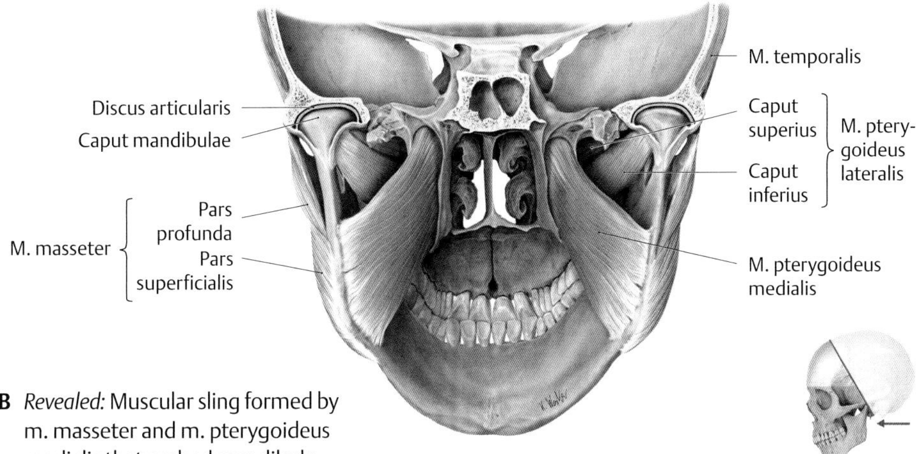
Discus articularis
Caput mandibulae
M. masseter
Pars profunda
Pars superficialis
M. temporalis
Caput superius
Caput inferius
M. pterygoideus lateralis
M. pterygoideus medialis

B *Revealed:* Muscular sling formed by m. masseter and m. pterygoideus medialis that embed mandibula.

Cranial Nerves: Overview

Fig. 31.1 Cranial nerves

Inferior (basal) view. The 12 pairs of cranial nerves (CN) are numbered according to the order of their emergence from the brainstem. *Note:* The sensory and motor fibers of the cranial nerves enter and exit the brainstem at the same sites (in contrast to spinal nerves, whose sensory and motor fibers enter and leave through posterior and anterior roots, respectively).

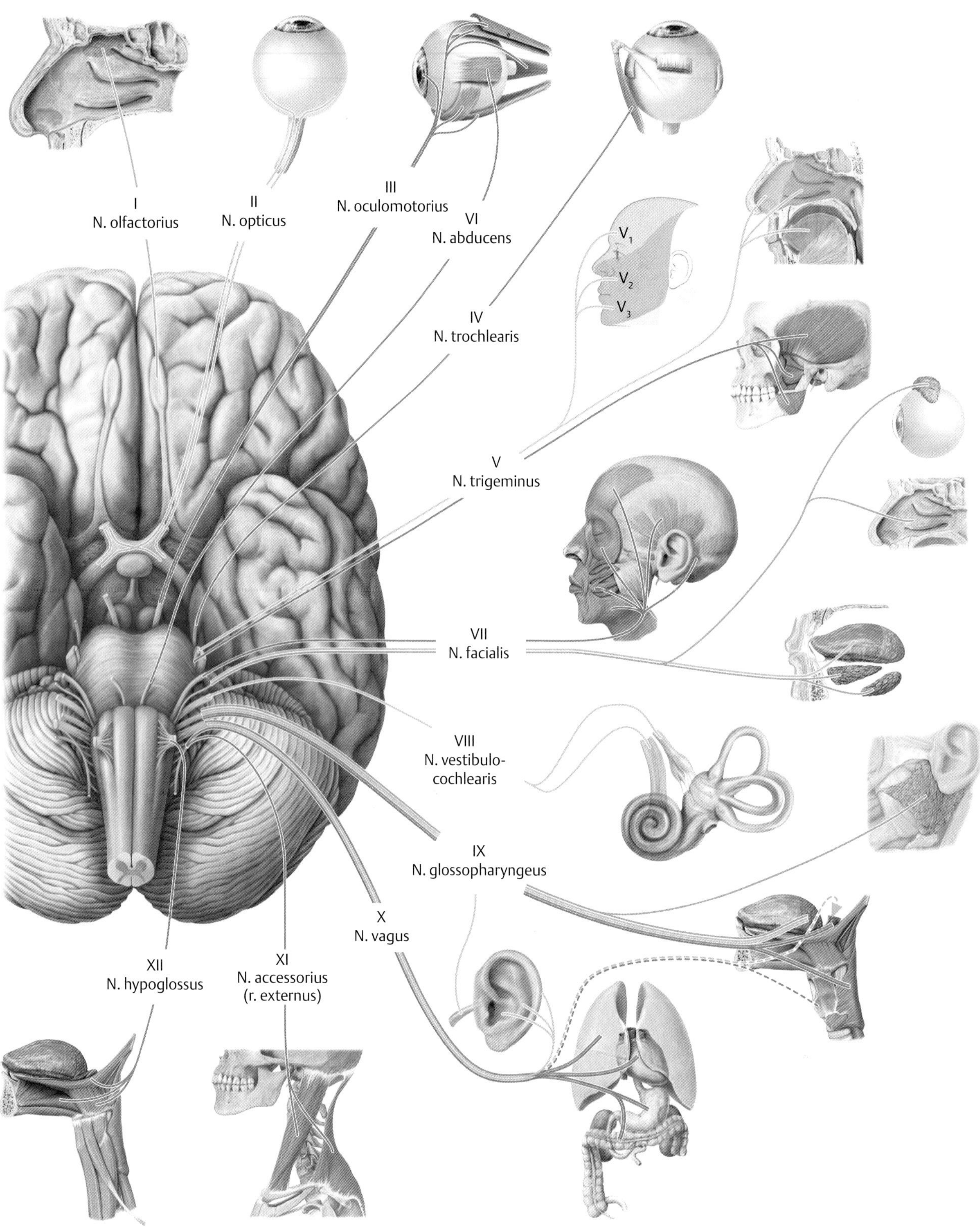
I
N. olfactorius
II
N. opticus
III
N. oculomotorius
VI
N. abducens
V_1
V_2
V_3
IV
N. trochlearis
V
N. trigeminus
VII
N. facialis
VIII
N. vestibulo-
cochlearis
IX
N. glossopharyngeus
X
N. vagus
XI
N. accessorius
(r. externus)
XII
N. hypoglossus

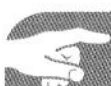

The cranial nerves contain both afferent (sensory) and efferent (motor) axons that belong to either the somatic or the autonomic (visceral) nervous system (see pp. 622–623). The somatic fibers allow interaction with the environment, whereas the visceral fibers regulate the autonomic activity of internal organs. In addition to the general fiber types, the cranial nerves may contain special fiber types associated with particular structures (e.g., auditory apparatus and taste buds). The cranial nerve fibers originate or terminate at specific nuclei, which are similarly classified as either general or special, somatic or visceral, and afferent or efferent.

Table 31.1 Classification of cranial nerve fibers and nuclei

This color coding is used in subsequent chapters to indicate fiber and nuclei classifications.

	Fiber type	Example		Fiber type	Example
	General somatic efferent (somatomotor function)	Innervate skeletal muscles		General somatic afferent (somatic sensation)	Conduct impulses from skin, skeletal muscle spindles
	General visceral efferent (visceromotor function)	Innervate smooth muscle of the viscera, intraocular muscles, heart, glandulae salivariae, etc.		Special somatic afferent	Conduct impulses from retina, auditory and vestibular apparatuses
	Special visceral efferent	Innervate skeletal and cardiac muscle derived from branchial arches		General visceral afferent (visceral sensation)	Conduct impulses from viscera, blood vessels
				Special visceral afferent	Conduct impulses from taste buds, olfactory mucosa

Fig. 31.2 Cranial nerve nuclei

The sensory and motor fibers of cranial nerves III to XII originate and terminate in the brainstem at specific nuclei.

Efferent (motor) nuclei
Afferent (sensory) nuclei
Nuclei of n. oculomotorius (CN III)
Nucleus nervi trochlearis (CN IV)
Nucleus nervi abducentis (CN VI)
Nucleus nervi facialis (CN VII)
Nuclei salivatorii superior and inferior
Nucleus ambiguus
Nucleus dorsalis nervi vagi
Nucleus nervi hypoglossi (CN XII)
Nucleus nervi accessorii (CN XI)
Nuclei of n. trigeminus (CN V)
CN V
CN VII
CN VI
CN VIII
CN IX
CN X
Nucleus spinalis nervi trigemini (CN V)
Nucleus tractus solitarii

A Posterior view with the cerebellum removed.

CN III: Nuclei accessorii nervi oculomotorii (visceral oculomotor nuclei); Nucleus nervi oculomotorii
CN V: Nucleus mesencephalicus nervi trigemini; Nucleus motorius nervi trigemini; Nucleus principalis nervi trigemini
Nucleus salivatorius inferior (CN IX)
Nucleus ambiguus
Nucleus nervi trochlearis (CN IV)
Nucleus nervi abducentis (CN VI)
CN VII: Nucleus nervi facialis; Nucleus salivatorius superior
Nucleus dorsalis nervi vagi (CN X)
Nucleus nervi hypoglossi (CN XII)
Nucleus tractus solitarii
Nucleus spinalis nervi trigemini (CN V)
Nucleus nervi accessorii (CN XI)

B Midsagittal section, left lateral view.

Table 31.2 Cranial nerves

Cranial nerve	Origin	Functional fiber types
CN I: N. olfactorius	Telencephalon*	●
CN II: N. opticus	Diencephalon*	●
CN III: N. oculomotorius	Mesencephalon	● ●
CN IV: N. trochlearis		●
CN V: N. trigeminus	Pons	● ●
CN VI: N. abducens		●
CN VII: N. facialis		● ● ● ●
CN VIII: N. vestibulocochlearis	Medulla oblongata	●
CN IX: N. glossopharyngeus		● ● ● ● ●
CN X: N. vagus		● ● ● ● ●
CN XI: N. accessorius		● ●
CN XII: N. hypoglossus		●

* The n. olfactorius and nn. optici are extensions of the brain rather than true nerves; they are therefore not associated with nuclei in the brainstem.

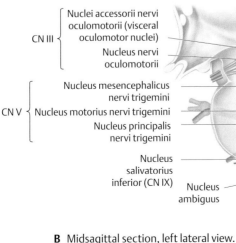

CN I & II: N. Olfactorius & N. Opticus

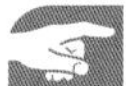

The n. olfactorius and n. opticus are not true peripheral nerves, but extensions (tracts) of the telencephalon and diencephalon, respectively. They are therefore not associated with cranial nerve nuclei in the brainstem.

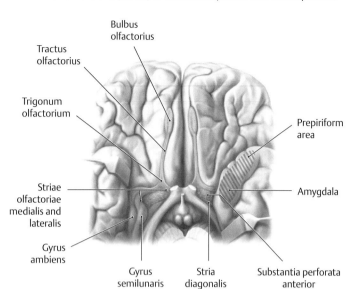

Fig. 31.3 N. olfactorius (CN I)

Fiber bundles in the olfactory mucosa pass from the nasal cavity through lamina cribrosa of os ethmoidale into fossa cranii anterior, where they synapse in bulbus olfactorius. Axons from second-order afferent neurons in bulbus olfactorius pass through tractus olfactorius and striae olfactoria medialis or lateralis, terminating in the cerebral cortex of the prepiriform area, in the amygdala, or in neighboring areas. See p. 617 for the mechanisms of smell.

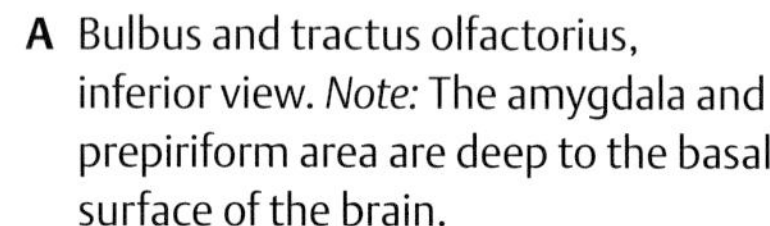

Bulbus olfactorius
Tractus olfactorius
Trigonum olfactorium
Prepiriform area
Striae olfactoriae medialis and lateralis
Amygdala
Gyrus ambiens
Gyrus semilunaris
Stria diagonalis
Substantia perforata anterior

A Bulbus and tractus olfactorius, inferior view. *Note:* The amygdala and prepiriform area are deep to the basal surface of the brain.

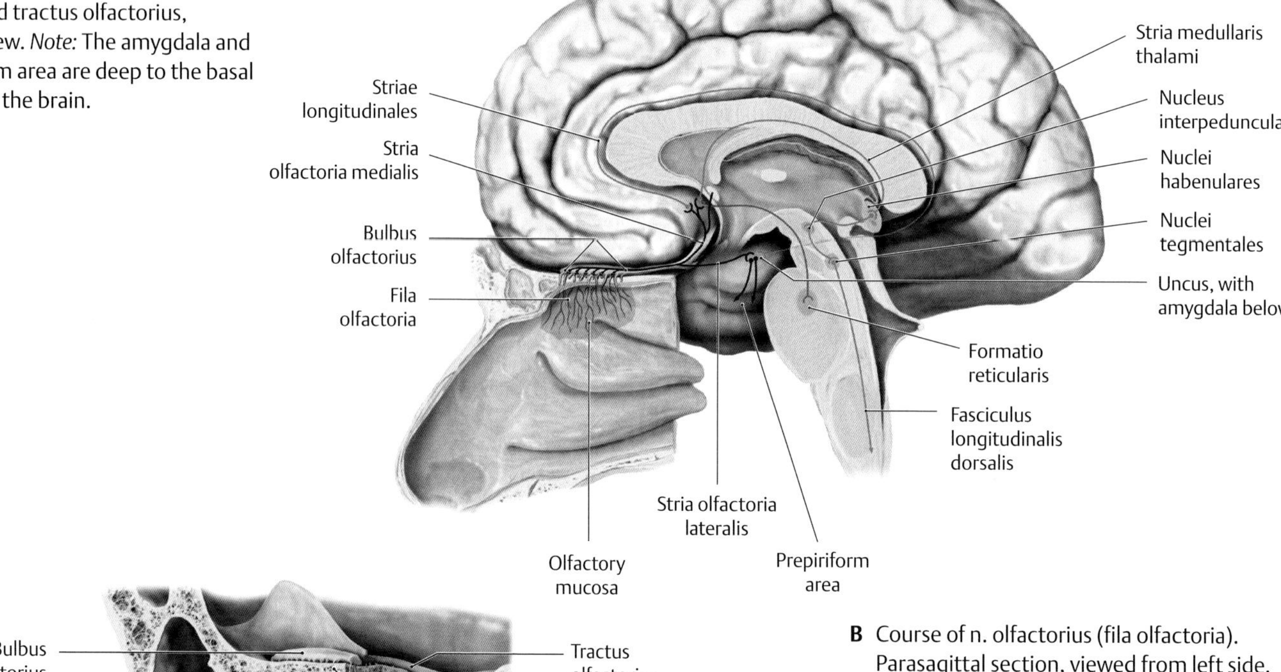

Striae longitudinales
Stria olfactoria medialis
Bulbus olfactorius
Fila olfactoria
Stria medullaris thalami
Nucleus interpeduncularis
Nuclei habenulares
Nuclei tegmentales
Uncus, with amygdala below
Formatio reticularis
Fasciculus longitudinalis dorsalis
Stria olfactoria lateralis
Olfactory mucosa
Prepiriform area

B Course of n. olfactorius (fila olfactoria). Parasagittal section, viewed from left side.

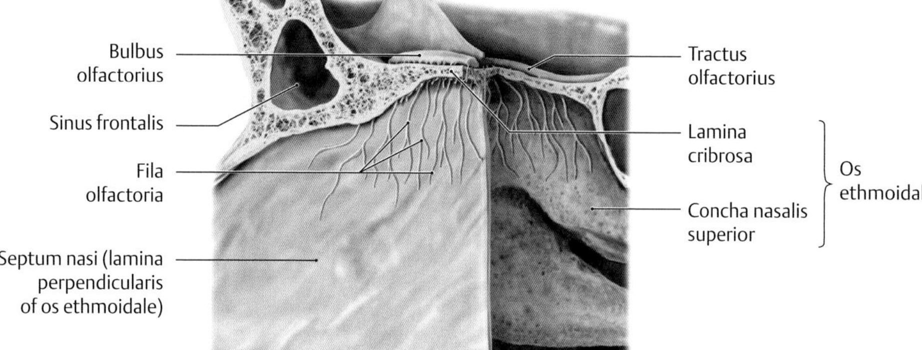

Bulbus olfactorius
Sinus frontalis
Fila olfactoria
Septum nasi (lamina perpendicularis of os ethmoidale)
Tractus olfactorius
Lamina cribrosa
Concha nasalis superior
Os ethmoidale

C Fila olfactoria. Portion of left nasal septum and lateral wall of right nasal cavity, left lateral view.

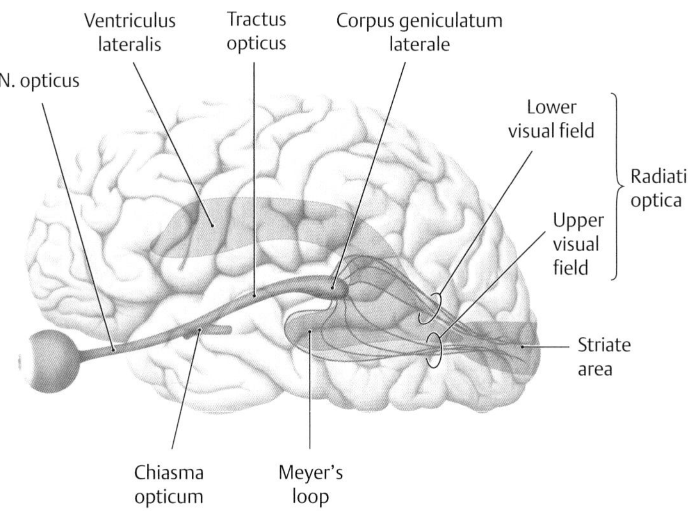
Ventriculus lateralis
Tractus opticus
Corpus geniculatum laterale
N. opticus
Lower visual field
Radiatio optica
Upper visual field
Striate area
Chiasma opticum
Meyer's loop

A N. opticus in the geniculate visual pathway, left lateral view.

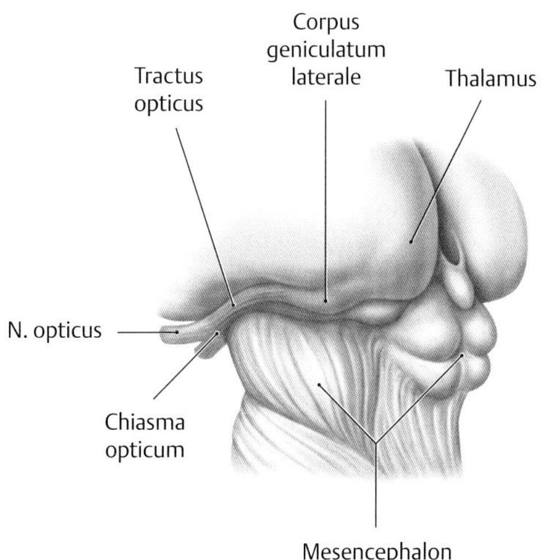
Corpus geniculatum laterale
Tractus opticus
Thalamus
N. opticus
Chiasma opticum
Mesencephalon

B Termination of tractus opticus, left postero-lateral view of the brainstem. The n. opticus contains the axons of retinal ganglion cells, which terminate mainly in the corpus geniculatum laterale of the diencephalon and in the mesencephalon (colliculus superior).

Fig. 31.4 N. opticus (CN II)

The n. opticus passes from the eyeball through canalis opticus into the fossa cranii media. The two optic nerves join below the base of the diencephalon to form the chiasma opticum, before dividing into the left and right tractus opticus. Each of these tracts divides into a lateral and medial root. Many retinal cell ganglion axons cross the midline to the contralateral side of the brain in the optic chiasm. See p. 619 for the mechanisms of sight.

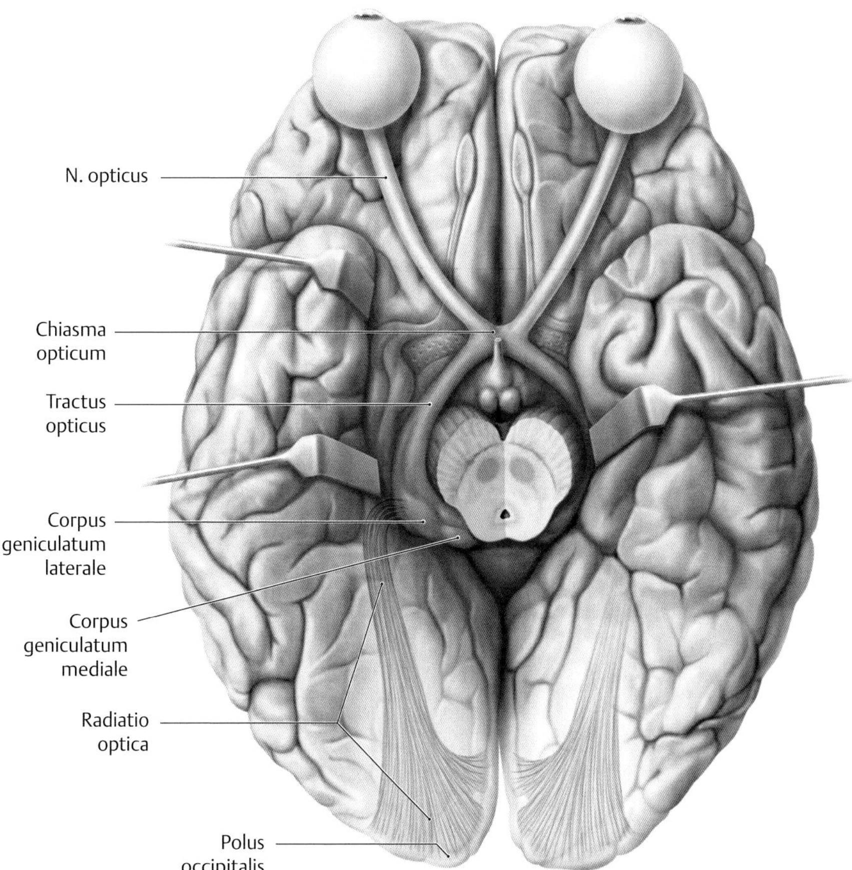
N. opticus
Chiasma opticum
Tractus opticus
Corpus geniculatum laterale
Corpus geniculatum mediale
Radiatio optica
Polus occipitalis

C Course of n. opticus, inferior (basal) view.

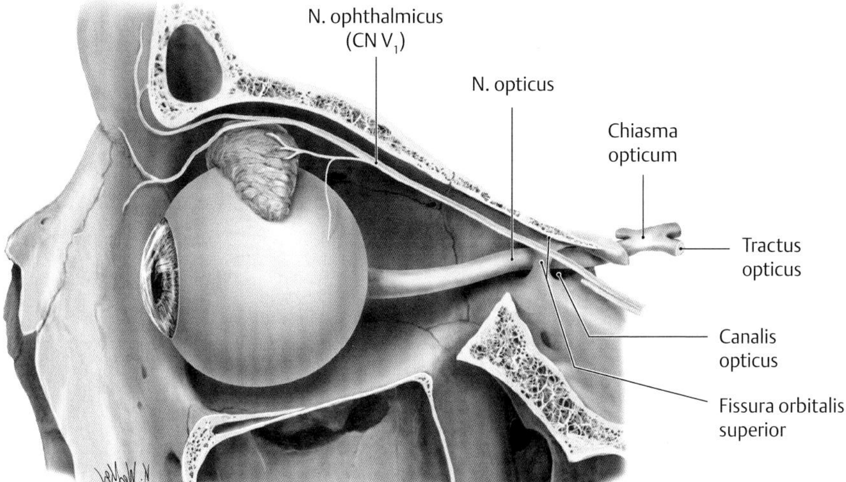
N. ophthalmicus (CN V_1)
N. opticus
Chiasma opticum
Tractus opticus
Canalis opticus
Fissura orbitalis superior

D N. opticus in the left orbita, lateral view. The n. opticus exits the orbita via the canalis opticus. *Note:* The other cranial nerves entering the orbita do so via fissura orbitalis superior.

CN III, IV & VI: N. Oculomotorius, N. Trochlearis & N. Abducens

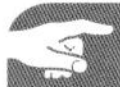

Cranial nerves III, IV, and VI innervate the extraocular muscles (see p. 509). Of the three, only n. oculomotorius (CN III) contains both somatic and visceral efferent fibers; it is also the only cranial nerve of the extraocular muscles to innervate multiple extra- and intraocular muscles.

Fig. 31.5 Nuclei of n. oculomotorius, n. trochlearis, and n. abducens

The n. trochlearis (CN IV) is the only cranial nerve in which all the fibers cross to the opposite side. It is also the only cranial nerve to emerge from the dorsal side of the brainstem and, consequently, has the longest intradural (intracranial) course of any cranial nerve.

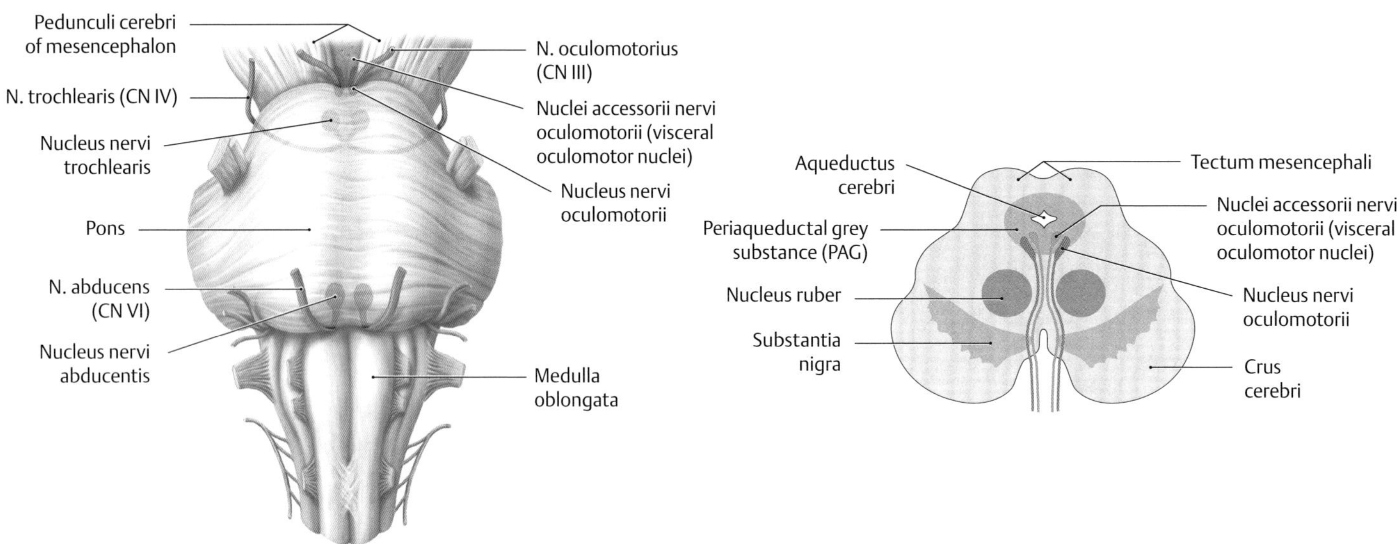
Pedunculi cerebri of mesencephalon
N. trochlearis (CN IV)
Nucleus nervi trochlearis
Pons
N. abducens (CN VI)
Nucleus nervi abducentis
N. oculomotorius (CN III)
Nuclei accessorii nervi oculomotorii (visceral oculomotor nuclei)
Nucleus nervi oculomotorii
Medulla oblongata
Aqueductus cerebri
Periaqueductal grey substance (PAG)
Nucleus ruber
Substantia nigra
Tectum mesencephali
Nuclei accessorii nervi oculomotorii (visceral oculomotor nuclei)
Nucleus nervi oculomotorii
Crus cerebri

A Emergence of the cranial nerves of the extraocular muscles. Anterior view of the brainstem.

B Nuclei of n. oculomotorius. Transverse section, superior view.

Table 31.3 Cranial nerves of the extraocular muscles

Course*	Fibers	Nuclei	Function	Effects of nerve injury
N. oculomotorius (CN III)				
Runs anteriorly from mesencephalon	Somatic efferent	Nucl. nervi oculomotorius	Innervates: • M. levator palpebrae sup. • M. rectus med., sup., and inf. • M. obliquus inf.	Complete oculomotor palsy (paralysis of extra- and intraocular muscles): • Ptosis (drooping of eyelid) • Downward and lateral gaze deviation • Diplopia (double vision) • Mydriasis (pupil dilation) • Accommodation difficulties (ciliary paralysis)
	Visceral efferent	Nuclei accessorii nervi oculomotorii (Edinger-Westphal)	Synapse with neurons of ganglion ciliare. Innervates: • M. spincter pupillae • M. ciliaris	
N. trochlearis (CN IV)				
Emerges from posterior surface of brainstem near midline, courses anteriorly around the pedunculus cerebri	Somatic efferent	Nucl. nervi trochlearis	Innervates: • M. obliquus sup.	• Diplopia • Affected eye is higher and deviated medially (dominance of inferior oblique)
N. abducens (CN VI)				
Follows a long extradural path**	Somatic efferent	Nucleus nervi abducentis	Innervates: • M. rectus lateralis	• Diplopia • Affected eye is deviated superiorly

* All three nerves enter the orbita through the fissura orbitalis superior; CN III and CN VI pass through the anulus tendineus communis of the extraocular muscles.
** The n. abducens follows an extradural course; n. abducens palsy may therefore develop in association with meningitis and subarachnoid hemorrhage.

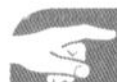

Note: The n. oculomotorius supplies parasympathetic innervation to the intraocular muscles and somatic motor innervation to most of the extraocular muscles (also m. levator palpebrae superioris). Its parasympathetic fibers synapse in ganglion ciliare. Oculomotor nerve palsy may affect exclusively the parasympathetic or somatic fibers, or both concurrently.

Fig. 31.6 Course of the nerves innervating the extraocular muscles
Right orbit.

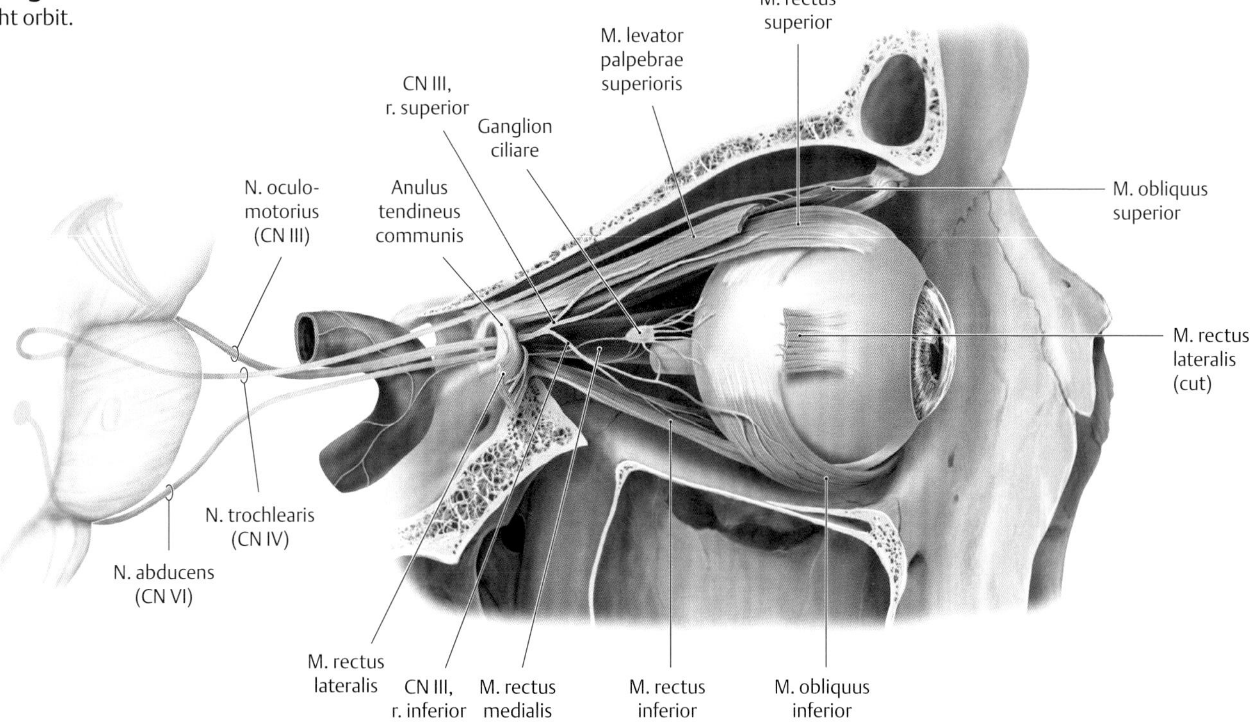
M. rectus superior
M. levator palpebrae superioris
CN III, r. superior
Ganglion ciliare
N. oculo-motorius (CN III)
Anulus tendineus communis
M. obliquus superior
M. rectus lateralis (cut)
N. trochlearis (CN IV)
N. abducens (CN VI)
M. rectus lateralis
CN III, r. inferior
M. rectus medialis
M. rectus inferior
M. obliquus inferior

A Lateral view.

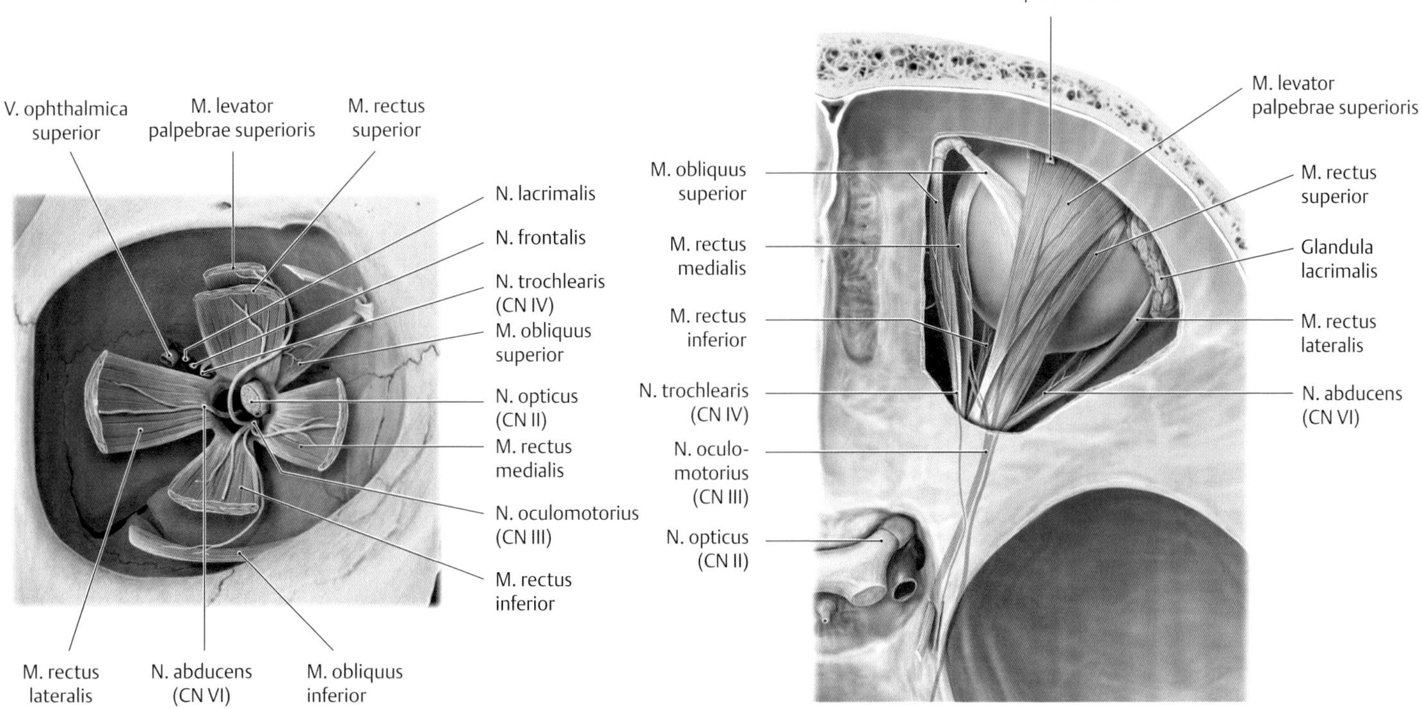
V. ophthalmica superior
M. levator palpebrae superioris
M. rectus superior
N. lacrimalis
N. frontalis
N. trochlearis (CN IV)
M. obliquus superior
N. opticus (CN II)
M. rectus medialis
N. oculomotorius (CN III)
M. rectus inferior
M. rectus lateralis
N. abducens (CN VI)
M. obliquus inferior
N. supraorbitalis
M. levator palpebrae superioris
M. obliquus superior
M. rectus superior
M. rectus medialis
Glandula lacrimalis
M. rectus inferior
M. rectus lateralis
N. trochlearis (CN IV)
N. abducens (CN VI)
N. oculo-motorius (CN III)
N. opticus (CN II)

B Anterior view. CN II exits the orbit via canalis opticus, which lies medial to fissura orbitalis superior (site of emergence of CN III, IV, and VI).

C Superior view of the opened orbit. Note the relationship between canalis opticus and fissura orbitalis superior.

CN V: N. Trigeminus

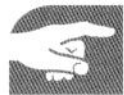

N. trigeminus, the sensory nerve of the head, has three somatic afferent nuclei: the nucleus mesencephalicus, which receives proprioceptive fibers from the muscles of mastication; the nucleus principalis, which chiefly mediates touch; and the nucleus spinalis, which mediates pain and temperature sensation. The nucleus motorius supplies motor innervation to the muscles of mastication.

Fig. 31.7 Nuclei of n. trigeminus

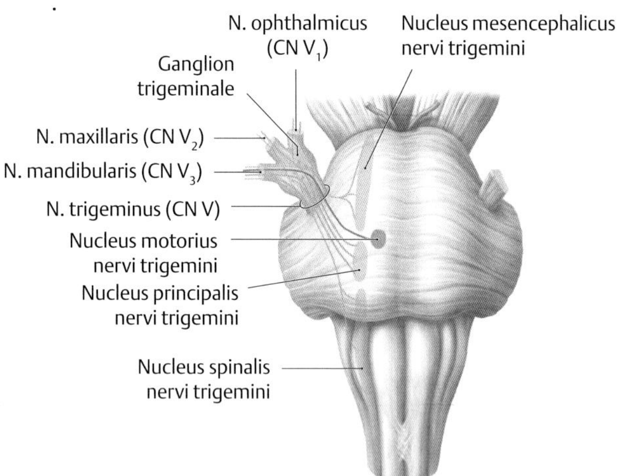
N. ophthalmicus (CN V_1)
Nucleus mesencephalicus nervi trigemini
Ganglion trigeminale
N. maxillaris (CN V_2)
N. mandibularis (CN V_3)
N. trigeminus (CN V)
Nucleus motorius nervi trigemini
Nucleus principalis nervi trigemini
Nucleus spinalis nervi trigemini

A Anterior view of the brainstem.

Ventriculus quartus
Pons
Nucleus mesencephalicus nervi trigemini
Nucleus principalis nervi trigemini
Nucleus motorius nervi trigemini
N. trigeminus (CN V)

B Cross section through pons, superior view.

Fig. 31.8 Divisions of n. trigeminus (CN V)

Right lateral view.

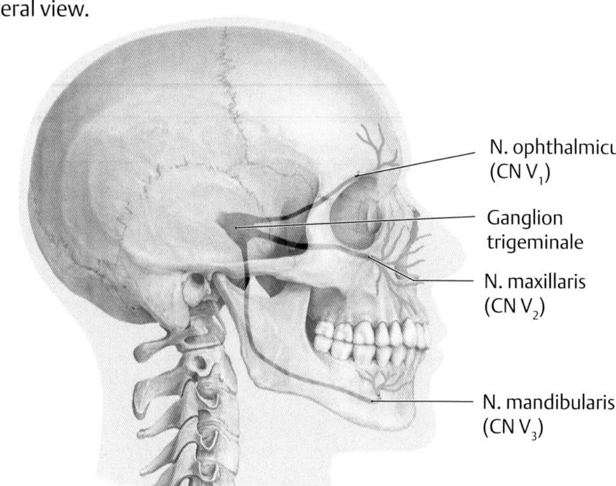
N. ophthalmicus (CN V_1)
Ganglion trigeminale
N. maxillaris (CN V_2)
N. mandibularis (CN V_3)

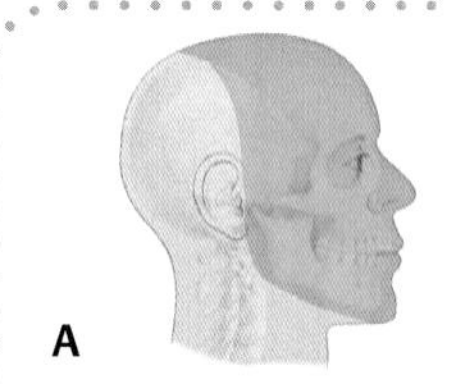
A

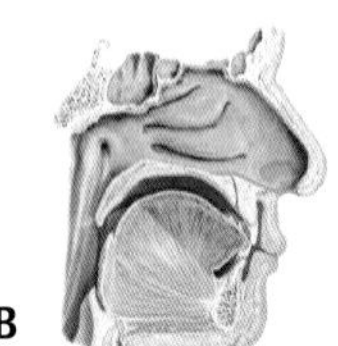
B

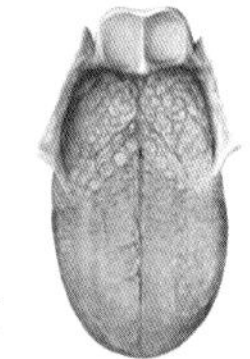
C

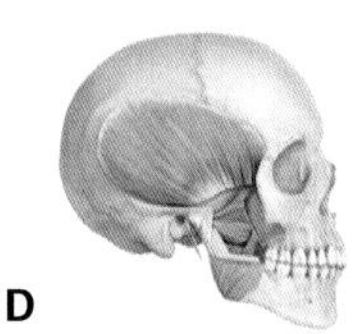
D

Table 31.4 N. trigeminus (CN V)

Course	Fibers	Nuclei	Function	Effects of nerve injury
Exits from Fossa cranii media. **N. ophthalmicus (CN V_1):** Enters orbita through fissura orbitalis superior **N. maxillaris (CN V_2):** Enters fossa pterygopalatina through foramen rotundum **N. mandibularis (CN V_3):** Passes through foramen ovale to inferior surface of basis cranii	Somatic afferent	• Nucl. principalis nervi trigemini (pons) • Nucl. mesencephalicus nervi trigemini • Nucl. spinalis nervi trigemini	Innervates: • Facial skin (**A**) • Nasopharyngeal mucosa (**B**) • Tongue (anterior two thirds) (**C**) Involved in the corneal reflex (reflex closure of eyelid)	• Sensory loss (traumatic nerve lesions) • Herpes zoster ophthalmicus (varicella-zoster virus); herpes zoster of the face
	Special visceral efferent	Nucl. motorius nervi trigemini	Innervates (via CN V_3): • Muscles of mastication (m. temporalis, m. masseter, m. pterygoideus lat. and med. (**D**)) • Oral floor muscles (m. mylohyoideus, m. digastricus (venter anterior)) • M. tensor tympani • M. tensor veli palatini	
	Visceral efferent pathway*	• N. lacrimalis (CN V_1) conveys parasympathetic fibers from CN VII along the n. zygomaticus (CN V_2) to the Glandula lacrimalis • N. lingualis (CN V_3) conveys parasympathetic fibers from CN VII (via the chorda tympani) to glandula submandibularis and glandula sublingualis • N. auriculotemporalis (CN V_3) conveys parasympathetic fibers from CN IX to glandula parotidea		
	Visceral afferent pathway*	Gustatory (taste) fibers from CN VII (via chorda tympani) travel with n. ligualis (CN V_3) to the anterior two thirds of the tongue		

* Fibers of certain cranial nerves adhere to divisions or branches of the n. trigeminus, by which they travel to their destination.

Fig. 31.9 **Course of the trigeminal nerve divisions**
Right lateral view.

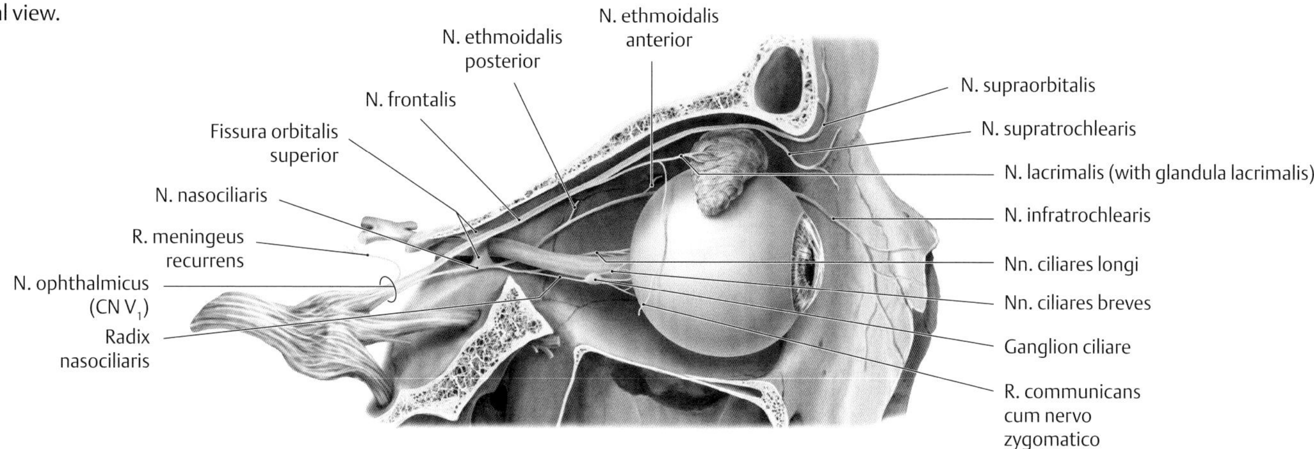
N. ethmoidalis anterior
N. ethmoidalis posterior
N. frontalis
Fissura orbitalis superior
N. nasociliaris
R. meningeus recurrens
N. ophthalmicus (CN V_1)
Radix nasociliaris
N. supraorbitalis
N. supratrochlearis
N. lacrimalis (with glandula lacrimalis)
N. infratrochlearis
Nn. ciliares longi
Nn. ciliares breves
Ganglion ciliare
R. communicans cum nervo zygomatico

A N. ophthalmicus (CN V_1). Partially opened right orbita.

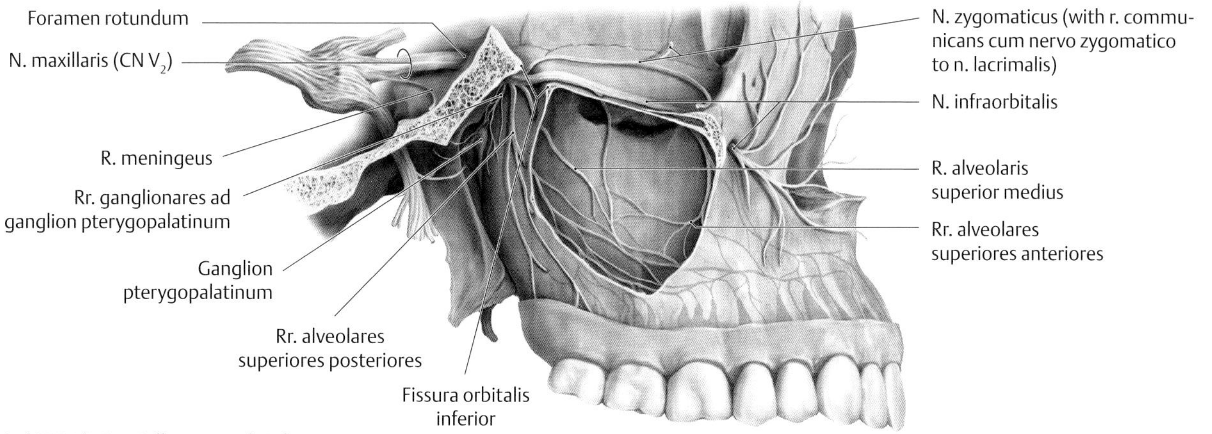
Foramen rotundum
N. maxillaris (CN V_2)
R. meningeus
Rr. ganglionares ad ganglion pterygopalatinum
Ganglion pterygopalatinum
Rr. alveolares superiores posteriores
Fissura orbitalis inferior
N. zygomaticus (with r. communicans cum nervo zygomatico to n. lacrimalis)
N. infraorbitalis
R. alveolaris superior medius
Rr. alveolares superiores anteriores

B N. maxillaris (CN V_2). Partially opened right sinus maxillaris with arcus zygomaticus removed.

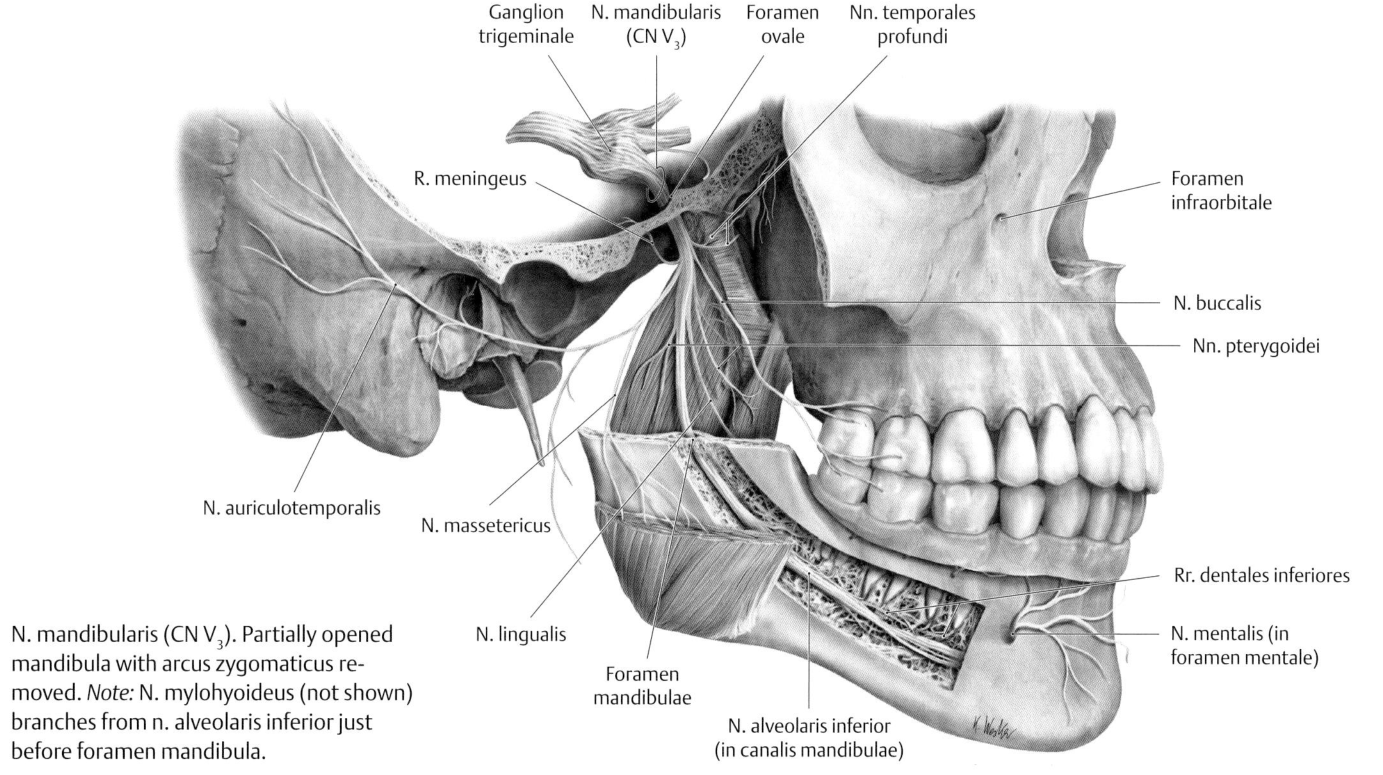
Ganglion trigeminale
N. mandibularis (CN V_3)
Foramen ovale
Nn. temporales profundi
R. meningeus
Foramen infraorbitale
N. buccalis
Nn. pterygoidei
N. auriculotemporalis
N. massetericus
Rr. dentales inferiores
N. lingualis
N. mentalis (in foramen mentale)
Foramen mandibulae
N. alveolaris inferior (in canalis mandibulae)

C N. mandibularis (CN V_3). Partially opened mandibula with arcus zygomaticus removed. *Note:* N. mylohyoideus (not shown) branches from n. alveolaris inferior just before foramen mandibula.

CN VII: N. Facialis

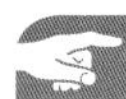

N. facialis mainly conveys special visceral efferent (branchiogenic) fibers from nucleus nervi facialis to the muscles of facial expression. The other visceral efferent (parasympathetic) fibers from nucleus salivatorius superior are grouped with the visceral afferent (gustatory) fibers to form n. intermedius.

Fig. 31.10 Nuclei of n. facialis

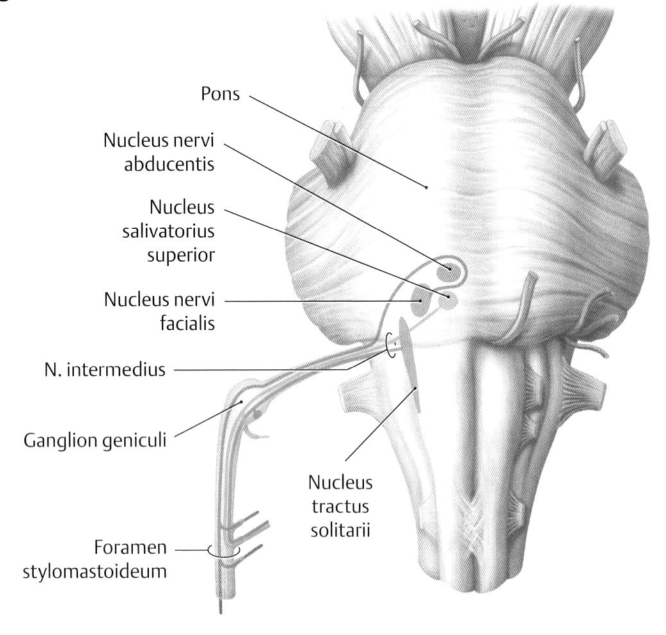
Pons
Nucleus nervi abducentis
Nucleus salivatorius superior
Nucleus nervi facialis
N. intermedius
Ganglion geniculi
Foramen stylomastoideum
Nucleus tractus solitarii

A Anterior view of the brainstem.

Nucleus nervi abducentis
Genu nervi facialis
Nucleus tractus solitarii
Nucleus salivatorius superior
Nucleus nervi facialis

B Cross section through pons, superior view.

Fig. 31.11 Branches of n. facialis

Right lateral view.

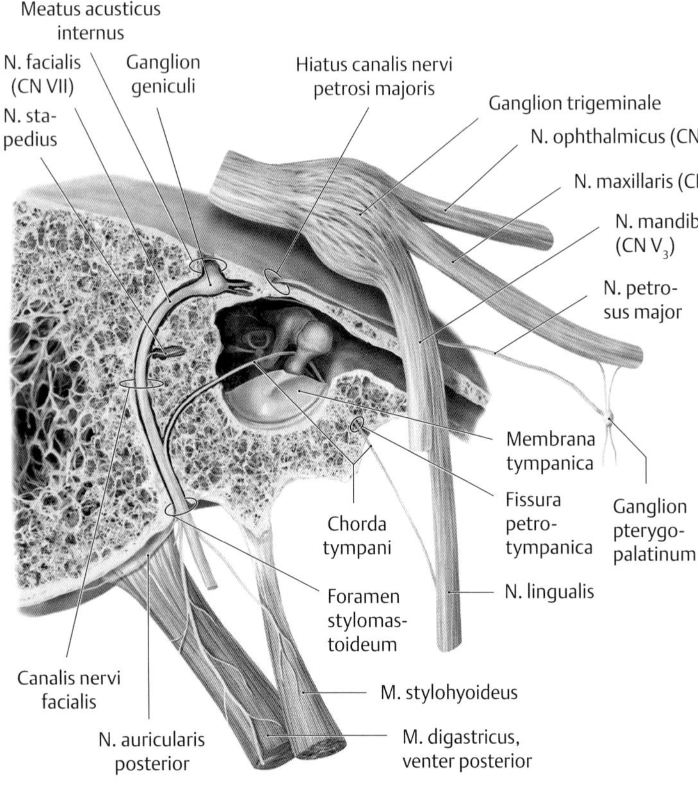
Meatus acusticus internus
N. facialis (CN VII)
Ganglion geniculi
N. stapedius
Hiatus canalis nervi petrosi majoris
Ganglion trigeminale
N. ophthalmicus (CN V_1)
N. maxillaris (CN V_2)
N. mandibularis (CN V_3)
N. petrosus major
Membrana tympanica
Fissura petrotympanica
Ganglion pterygopalatinum
Chorda tympani
Foramen stylomastoideum
N. lingualis
Canalis nervi facialis
M. stylohyoideus
N. auricularis posterior
M. digastricus, venter posterior

A N. facialis in os temporale.

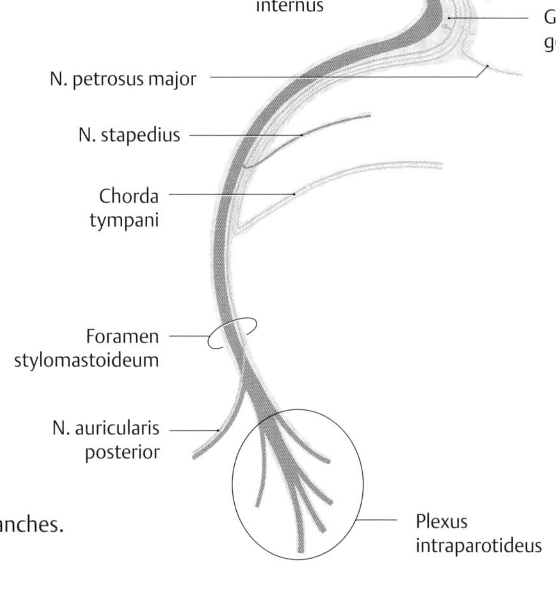
Meatus acusticus internus
Ganglion geniculi
N. petrosus major
N. stapedius
Chorda tympani
Foramen stylomastoideum
N. auricularis posterior
Plexus intraparotideus

B Branches.

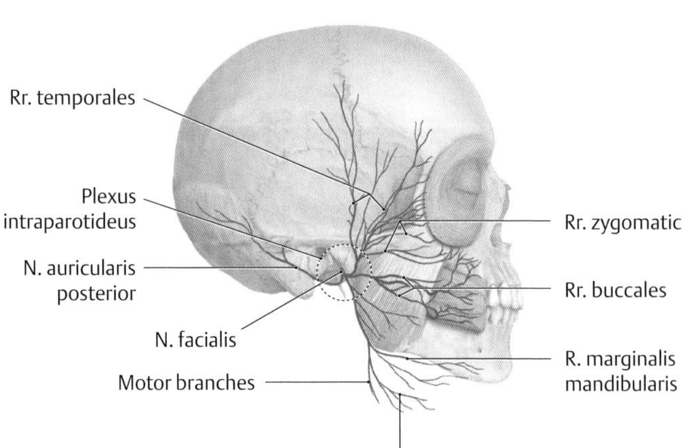
Rr. temporales
Plexus intraparotideus
N. auricularis posterior
N. facialis
Motor branches
Rr. zygomatici
Rr. buccales
R. marginalis mandibularis
R. colli

C Plexus parotideus.

Table 31.5 N. facialis (CN VII)

Course	Fibers	Nuclei	Function	Effects of nerve injury
Emerges in the cerebellopontine angle between the pons and olive; passes through the meatus acusticus internus into the os temporale (pars petrosa), where it divides into: • N. petrosus major • N. stapedius • Chorda tympani Certain visceral efferent fibers pass through the foramen stylomastoideum to the basis cranii, forming the plexus intraparotideus	Special visceral efferent	Nucl. nervi facialis	Innervate: • Muscles of facial expression • M. stylohyoideus • M. diagastricus (venter posterior) • M. stapedius	Peripheral facial nerve injury: paralysis of muscles of facial expression on affected side Associated disturbances of taste, lacrimation, salivation, etc.
	Visceral efferent (parasympathetic)*	Nucl. salivatorius superior	Synapse with neurons in the Ganglion pterygopalatinum or Ganglion submandibulare. Innervate: • Glandula lacrimalis • Glandulae nasales minores • Glandulae palatinae • Glandula submandibularis • Glandula sublingualis • Glandulae salivariae minores of tongue (dorsum)	
	Special visceral afferent*	Nuclei tractus solitarii	Peripheral processes of fibers from Ganglion geniculi form the chorda tympani (gustatory fibers from tongue)	
	Somatic afferent	Sensory fibers from the auricle, skin of the meatus acusticus externus, and outer surface of the membrana tympanica travel via CN VII to the nucl. principalis nervi trigemini		

* Grouped to form n. intermedius, which aggregates with the visceral efferent fibers from the nucl. nervi facialis.

***Fig. 31.12* Course of n. facialis**
Right lateral view. Visceral efferent (parasympathetic) and special visceral afferent (taste) fibers shown in black.

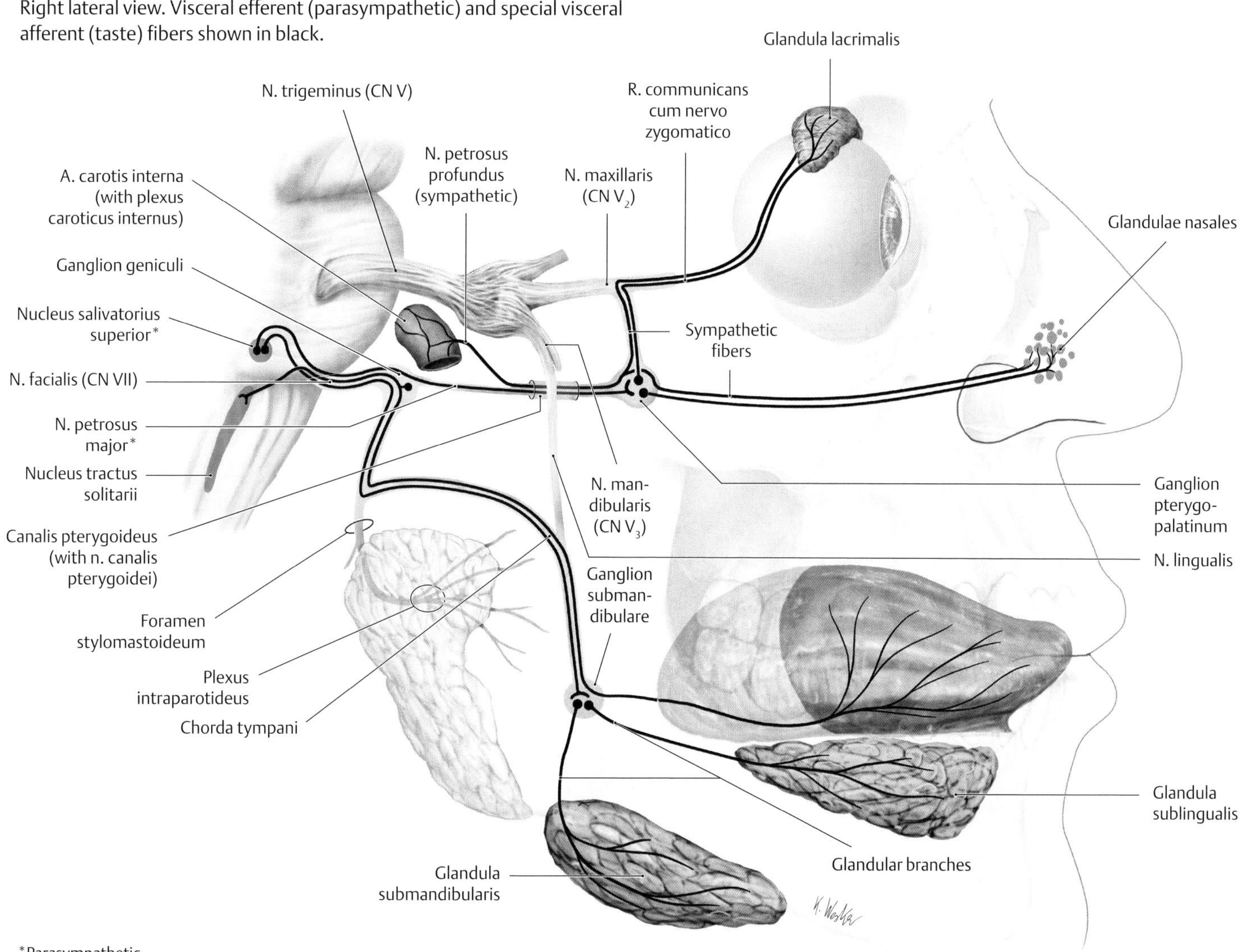
Glandula lacrimalis
N. trigeminus (CN V)
R. communicans cum nervo zygomatico
N. petrosus profundus (sympathetic)
N. maxillaris (CN V_2)
A. carotis interna (with plexus caroticus internus)
Glandulae nasales
Ganglion geniculi
Nucleus salivatorius superior*
Sympathetic fibers
N. facialis (CN VII)
N. petrosus major*
Nucleus tractus solitarii
N. mandibularis (CN V_3)
Ganglion pterygopalatinum
Canalis pterygoideus (with n. canalis pterygoidei)
N. lingualis
Ganglion submandibulare
Foramen stylomastoideum
Plexus intraparotideus
Chorda tympani
Glandula sublingualis
Glandular branches
Glandula submandibularis

*Parasympathetic

CN VIII: N. Vestibulocochlearis

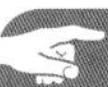

N. vestibulocochlearis is a special somatic afferent nerve that consists of two roots. The n. vestibularis transmits impulses from the vestibular apparatus (balance, see p. 618); the n. cochlearis transmits impulses from the auditory apparatus (hearing, see p. 616).

Fig. 31.13 N. vestibulocochlearis: N. vestibularis

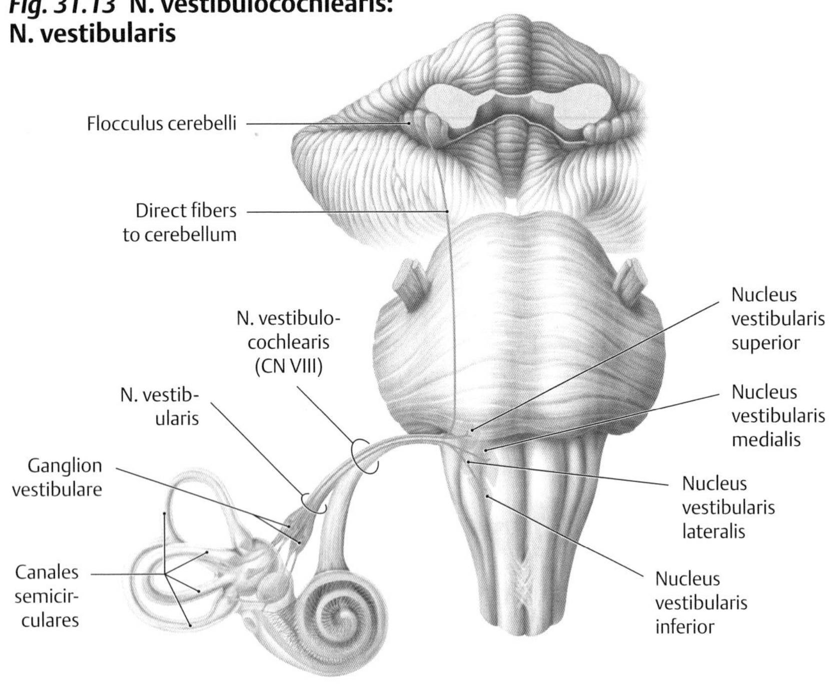

Flocculus cerebelli
Direct fibers to cerebellum
N. vestibulo-cochlearis (CN VIII)
N. vestib-ularis
Ganglion vestibulare
Canales semicir-culares
Nucleus vestibularis superior
Nucleus vestibularis medialis
Nucleus vestibularis lateralis
Nucleus vestibularis inferior

A Anterior view of medulla oblongata and pons with cerebellum.

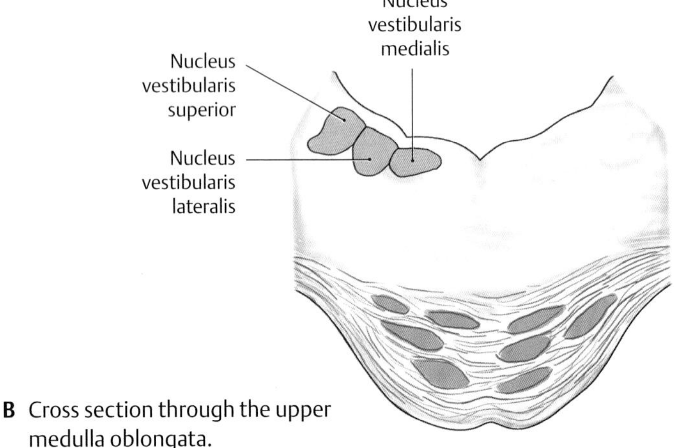

Nucleus vestibularis medialis
Nucleus vestibularis superior
Nucleus vestibularis lateralis

B Cross section through the upper medulla oblongata.

Fig. 31.14 N. vestibulocochlearis: N. cochlearis

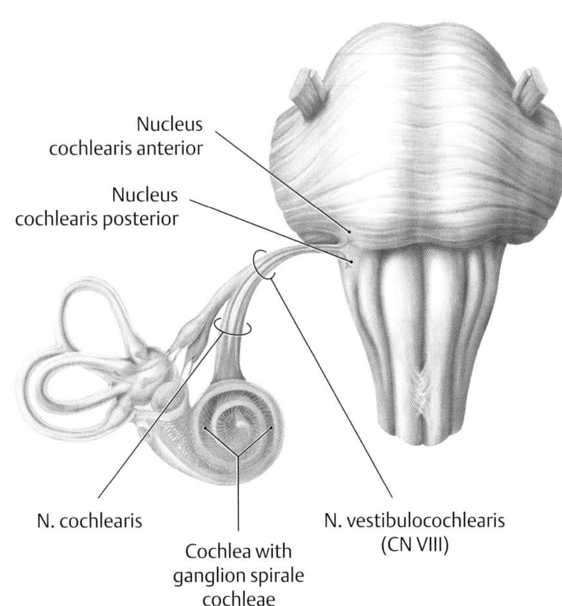

Nucleus cochlearis anterior
Nucleus cochlearis posterior
N. cochlearis
Cochlea with ganglion spirale cochleae
N. vestibulocochlearis (CN VIII)

A Anterior view of medulla oblongata and pons.

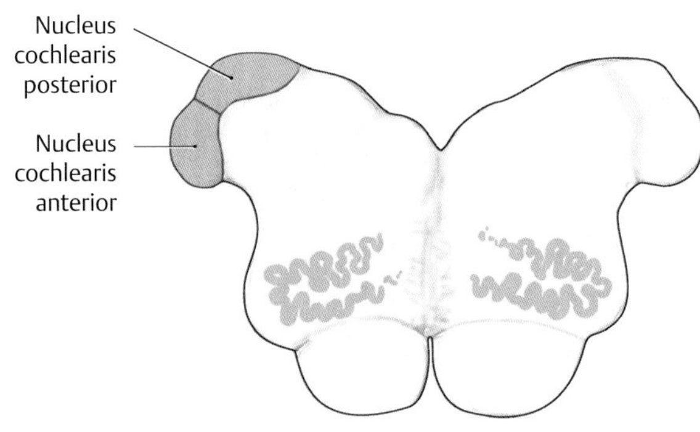

Nucleus cochlearis posterior
Nucleus cochlearis anterior

B Cross section through the upper medulla oblongata.

Table 31.6 **N. vestibulocochlearis (CN VIII)**

Part	Course	Fibers	Nuclei	Function	Effects of nerve injury
Pars vestibularis	Pass from the inner ear through the meatus acusticus internus to the cerebellopontine angle, where they enter the brain	Special somatic afferent	Nucl. vestibularis sup., med., lat., and inf.	Peripheral processes from the canalis semicircularis, sacculus, and utriculus pass to the ganglion vestibulare and then to the four nuclei vestibulares	Dizziness
Pars cochlearis			Nucl. cochlearis posterior and anterior	Peripheral processes beginning at the hair cells of the organ of corti pass to the ganglion spirale and then to the two nuclei cochleares	Hearing loss

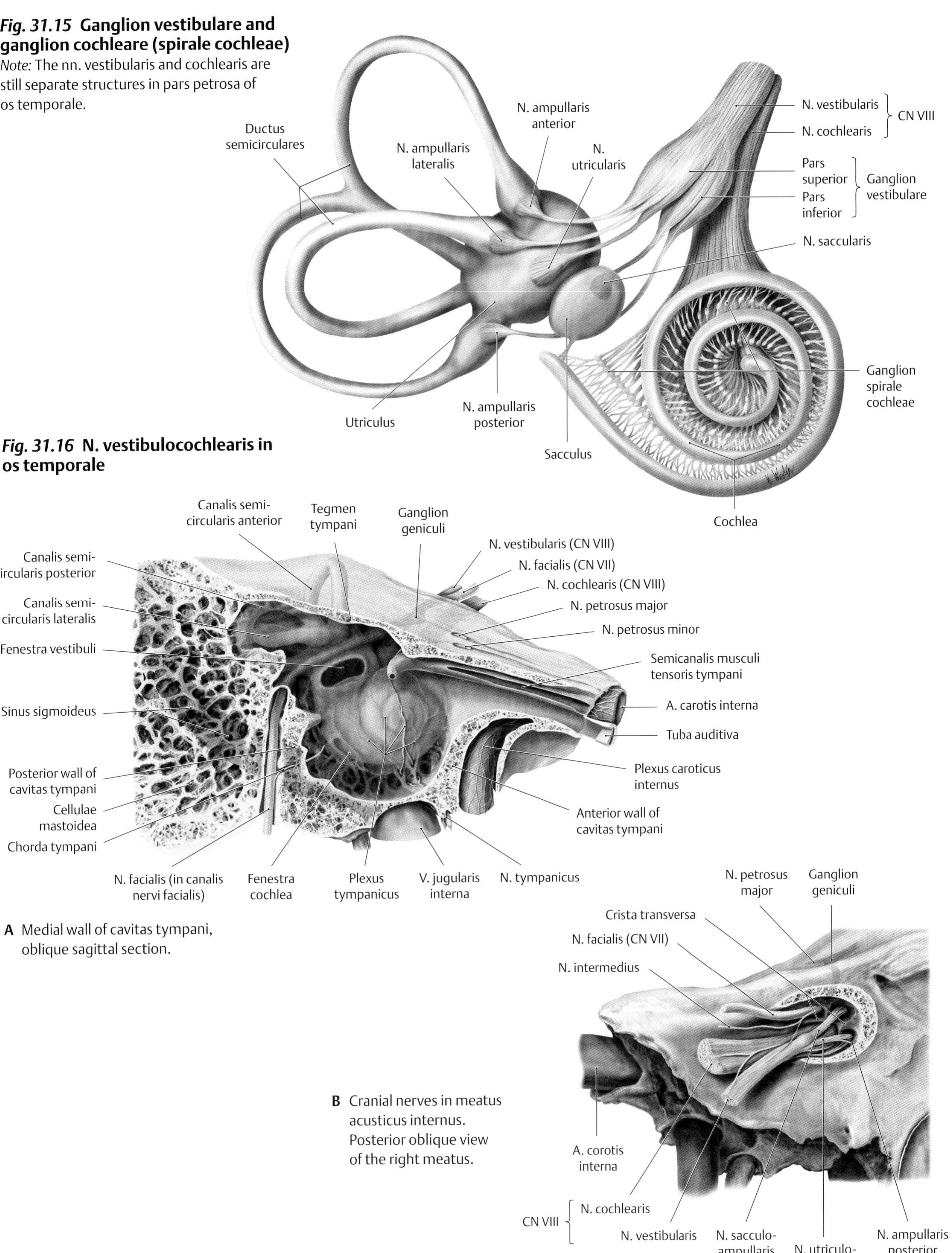
Ductus semicirculares
N. ampullaris lateralis
N. ampullaris anterior
N. utricularis
N. vestibularis
N. cochlearis
CN VIII
Pars superior
Pars inferior
Ganglion vestibulare
N. saccularis
Ganglion spirale cochleae
Utriculus
N. ampullaris posterior
Sacculus
Cochlea
Canalis semi-circularis anterior
Tegmen tympani
Ganglion geniculi
Canalis semi-circularis posterior
Canalis semi-circularis lateralis
Fenestra vestibuli
Sinus sigmoideus
Posterior wall of cavitas tympani
Cellulae mastoidea
Chorda tympani
N. facialis (in canalis nervi facialis)
Fenestra cochlea
Plexus tympanicus
V. jugularis interna
N. tympanicus
N. vestibularis (CN VIII)
N. facialis (CN VII)
N. cochlearis (CN VIII)
N. petrosus major
N. petrosus minor
Semicanalis musculi tensoris tympani
A. carotis interna
Tuba auditiva
Plexus caroticus internus
Anterior wall of cavitas tympani
N. petrosus major
Ganglion geniculi
Crista transversa
N. facialis (CN VII)
N. intermedius
A. corotis interna
CN VIII
N. cochlearis
N. vestibularis
N. sacculo-ampullaris
N. utriculo-ampullaris
N. ampullaris posterior

Fig. 31.15 **Ganglion vestibulare and ganglion cochleare (spirale cochleae)**
Note: The nn. vestibularis and cochlearis are still separate structures in pars petrosa of os temporale.

Fig. 31.16 **N. vestibulocochlearis in os temporale**

A Medial wall of cavitas tympani, oblique sagittal section.

B Cranial nerves in meatus acusticus internus. Posterior oblique view of the right meatus.

CN IX: N. Glossopharyngeus

Fig. 31.17 Nuclei of n. glossopharyngeus

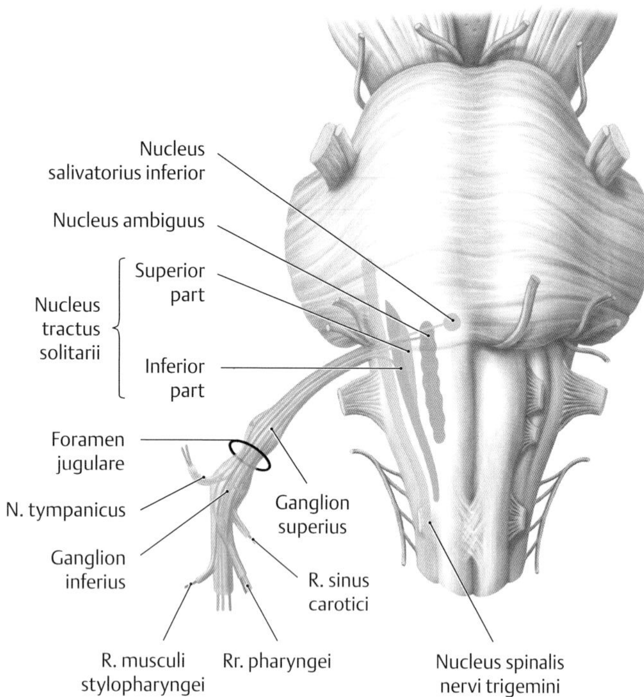
Nucleus salivatorius inferior
Nucleus ambiguus
Nucleus tractus solitarii
Superior part
Inferior part
Foramen jugulare
N. tympanicus
Ganglion inferius
Ganglion superius
R. sinus carotici
R. musculi stylopharyngei
Rr. pharyngei
Nucleus spinalis nervi trigemini

A Anterior view of medulla oblongata.

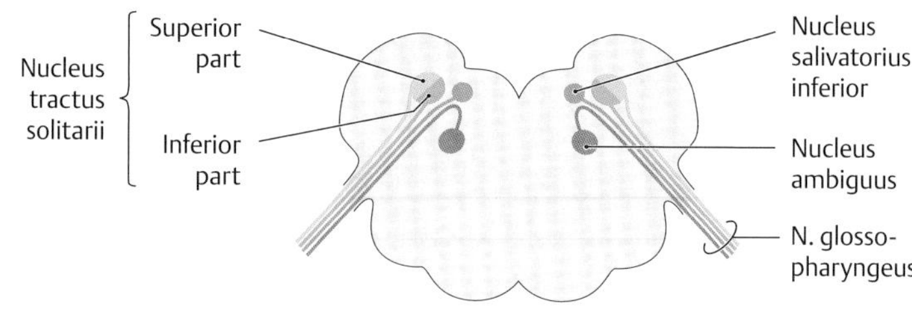
Nucleus tractus solitarii
Superior part
Inferior part
Nucleus salivatorius inferior
Nucleus ambiguus
N. glosso-pharyngeus

B Cross section through medulla oblongata, superior view. *Not shown:* Nuclei of n. trigeminus.

Fig. 31.18 Course of n. glossopharyngeus

Left lateral view. *Note:* Fibers from n. vagus (CN X) combine with fibers from CN IX to form the plexus pharyngeus and supply the sinus caroticus.

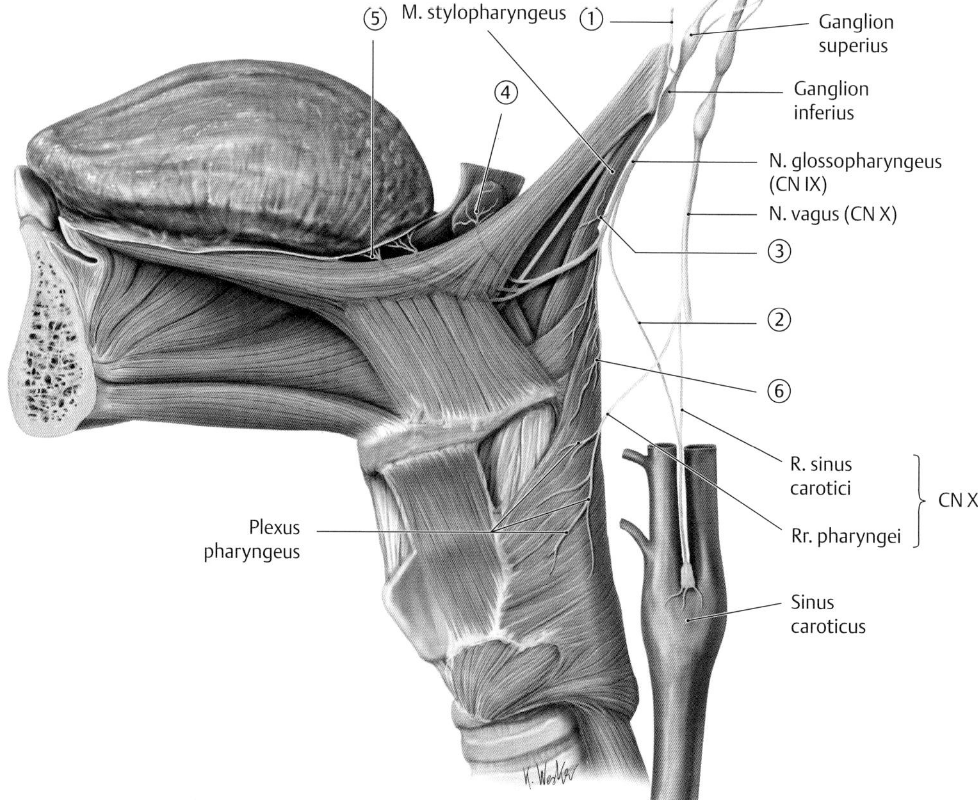
⑤ M. stylopharyngeus ①
④
Ganglion superius
Ganglion inferius
N. glossopharyngeus (CN IX)
N. vagus (CN X)
③
②
⑥
R. sinus carotici
Rr. pharyngei
CN X
Plexus pharyngeus
Sinus caroticus

Table 31.7	Glossopharyngeal nerve branches
①	N. tympanicus
②	R. sinus carotici
③	R. musculi stylopharyngei
④	Rr. tonsillares
⑤	Rr. linguales
⑥	Rr. pharyngeales

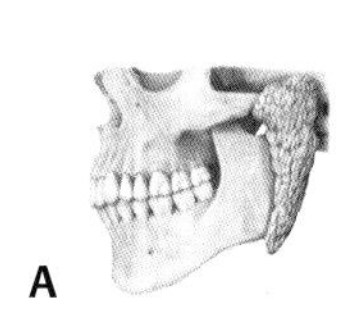
A
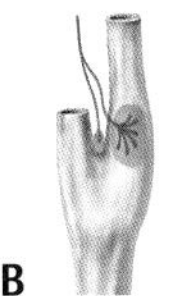
B
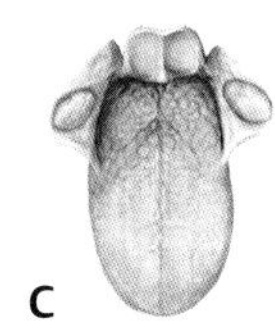
C
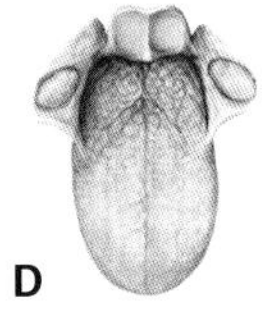
D
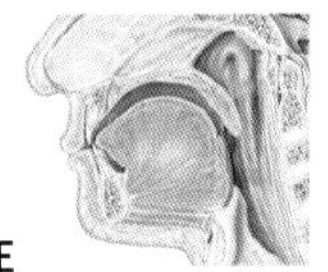
E
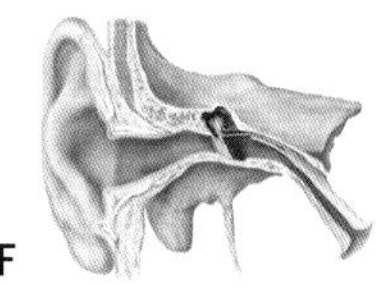
F

Table 31.8 N. glossopharyngeus (CN IX)

Course	Fibers	Nuclei	Function	Effects of nerve injury
Emerges from the medulla oblongata; leaves cavitas cranii through the foramen jugulare	Visceral efferent (parasympathetic)	Nucl. salivatorius inf.	Parasympathetic presynaptic fibers are sent to the ganglion oticum; postsynaptic fibers are distributed to • Glandula parotidea (**A**) • Glandulae buccales • Glandulae labiales	Isolated lesions of CN IX are rare. Lesions are generally accompanied by lesions of CN X and CN XI (cranial part), as all three emerge jointly from the foramen jugulare and are susceptible to injury in basal skull fractures.
	Special visceral efferent (branchiogenic)	Nucl. ambiguus	Innervate: • Constrictor muscles of the pharynx (rr. pharyngeales join with the n. vagus to form the plexus pharyngeus) • M. stylopharyngeus	
	Visceral afferent	Nucl. tractus solitarii (pars inferior)	Receive sensory information from • Chemoreceptors in the Glomus caroticum (**B**) • Pressure receptors in the Sinus caroticus	
	Special visceral afferent	Nucl. tractus solitarii (pars superior)	Receives sensory information from the posterior third of the tongue (via the ganglion inferius) (**C**)	
	Somatic afferent	Nucl. spinalis nervi trigemini	Peripheral processes of the intracranial ganglion superius or the extracranial ganglion inferius arise from • Tongue, soft palate, pharyngeal mucosa, and tonsils (**D,E**) • Mucosa of the internal surface of membrana tympanica, Tuba auditiva (plexus tympanicus) (**F**) • Skin of the external ear and meatus acusticus externus (blends with the n. vagus)	

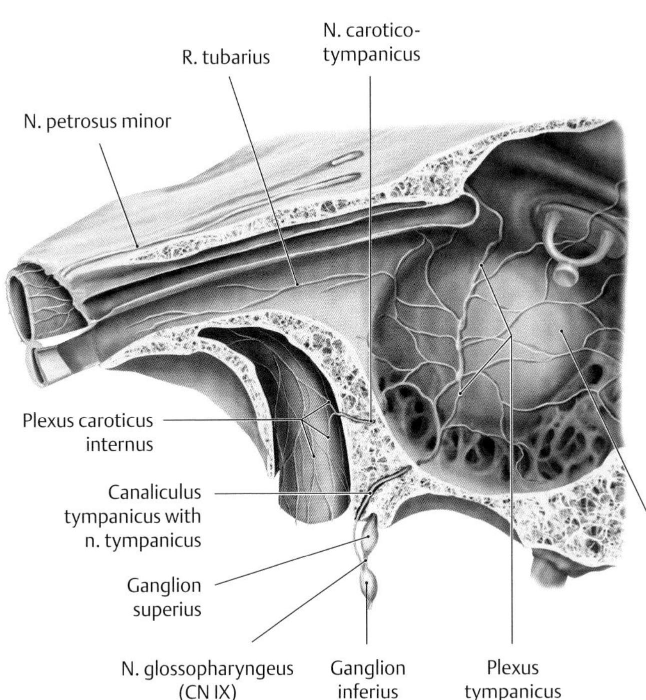
N. petrosus minor
R. tubarius
N. carotico-tympanicus
Plexus caroticus internus
Canaliculus tympanicus with n. tympanicus
Ganglion superius
N. glossopharyngeus (CN IX)
Ganglion inferius
Plexus tympanicus
Promontorium

Fig. 31.19 **N. glossopharyngeus in cavitas tympani**
Left anterolateral view. The n. tympanicus contains visceral efferent (presynaptic parasympathetic) fibers for ganglion oticum, as well as somatic afferent fibers for cavitas tympani and tuba auditiva. It joins with sympathetic fibers from plexus caroticus internus (via nn. caroticotympanici) to form the plexus tympanicus.

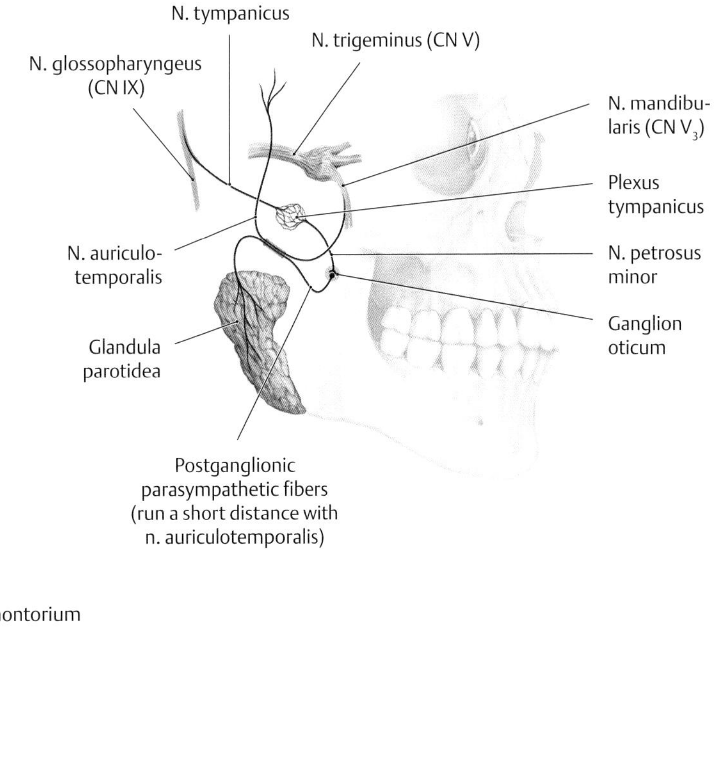
N. tympanicus
N. trigeminus (CN V)
N. glossopharyngeus (CN IX)
N. mandibularis (CN V_3)
Plexus tympanicus
N. auriculotemporalis
N. petrosus minor
Ganglion oticum
Glandula parotidea
Postganglionic parasympathetic fibers (run a short distance with n. auriculotemporalis)

Fig. 31.20 **Visceral efferent (parasympathetic) fibers of CN IX**

CN X: N. Vagus

Fig. 31.21 Nuclei of n. vagus

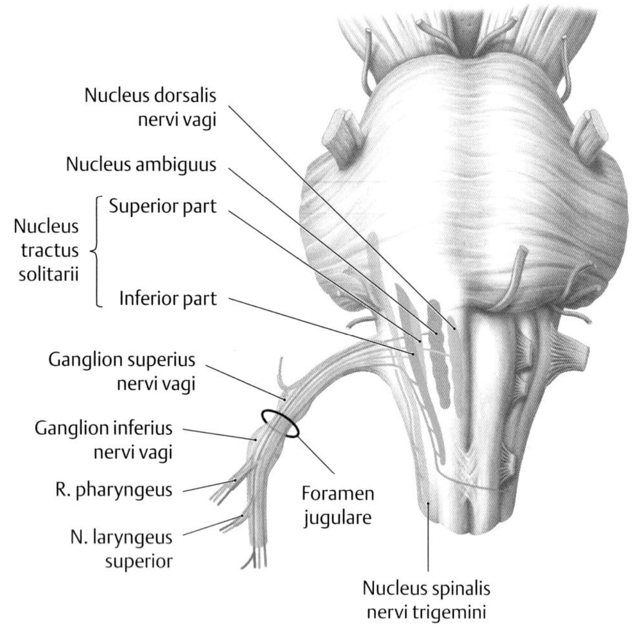
Nucleus dorsalis nervi vagi
Nucleus ambiguus
Nucleus tractus solitarii
Superior part
Inferior part
Ganglion superius nervi vagi
Ganglion inferius nervi vagi
R. pharyngeus
N. laryngeus superior
Foramen jugulare
Nucleus spinalis nervi trigemini

A Anterior view of medulla oblongata.

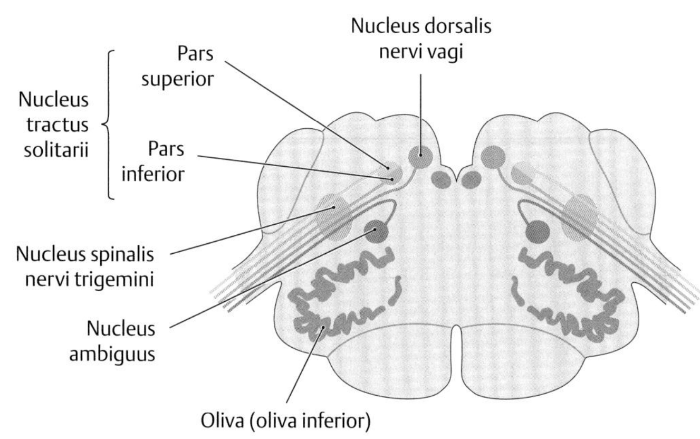
Nucleus tractus solitarii
Pars superior
Pars inferior
Nucleus dorsalis nervi vagi
Nucleus spinalis nervi trigemini
Nucleus ambiguus
Oliva (oliva inferior)

B Cross section through medulla oblongata, superior view.

Table 31.9 N. vagus (CN X)

Course	Fibers	Nuclei	Function	Effects of nerve injury
Emerges from the medulla oblongata; leaves the cavitas cranii through the foramen jugulare. CN X has the most extensive distribution of all the cranial nerves (vagus = "vagabond"), consisting of pars cranialis, cervicalis, thoracica (see p. 91), and abdominalis (see p. 237) parts.	Special visceral efferent (branchiogenic)	Nucl. ambiguus	Innervate: • Pharyngeal muscles (via plexus pharyngeus with CN IX) • Muscles of the soft palate • Laryngeal muscles (n. laryngeus superior supplies the m. cricothyroideus; n. laryngeus inferior supplies all other laryngeal muscles)	The n. laryngeus recurrens supplies visceromotor innervation to the only muscle abducting the vocal cords, the posterior cricoarytenoid. Unilateral destruction of this nerve leads to hoarseness; bilateral destruction leads to respiratory distress (dyspnea).
	Visceral efferent (parasympathetic)	Nucl. dorsalis nervi vagi	Synapse in Ganglia praevertebrales or intramurales. Innervate smooth muscle and glands of • Thoracic viscera (**A**) • Abdominal viscera (**A**)	
	Somatic afferent	Nucl. spinalis nervi trigemini	Ganglion superius (jugulare) receives peripheral fibers from • Dura in fossa cranii posterior (**C**) • Skin of ear (**D**), meatus acusticus externus (**E**)	
	Special visceral afferent	Nucl. tractus solitarii (pars superior)	Ganglion inferius receives peripheral processes from • Taste buds on the epiglottis (**F**)	
	Visceral afferent	Nucl. tractus solitatii (pars inferior)	Ganglion inferius receives peripheral processes from • Mucosa of lower pharynx at its esophageal junction (**G**) • Laryngeal mucosa above (n. laryngeus superior) and below (n. laryngeus inferior) the plica vocalis (**G**) • Pressure receptors in the arcus aortae (**B**) • Chemoreceptors in the corpora paraaortica (**B**) • Thoracic and abdominal viscera (**A**)	

Fig. 31.22 Course of n. vagus

N. vagus gives off four major branches in the neck. The n. laryngeus inferior is the terminal branch of n. laryngeus recurrens. *Note:* The left n. laryngeus recurrens winds around arcus aorta, while the right nerve winds around a. subclavia.

Table 31.10 Vagus nerve branches in the neck

①	Rr. pharyngeales
②	N. laryngeus superior
③R	N. laryngeus recurrens dexter
③L	N. laryngeus recurrens sinister
④	Rr. cardiaci cervicales

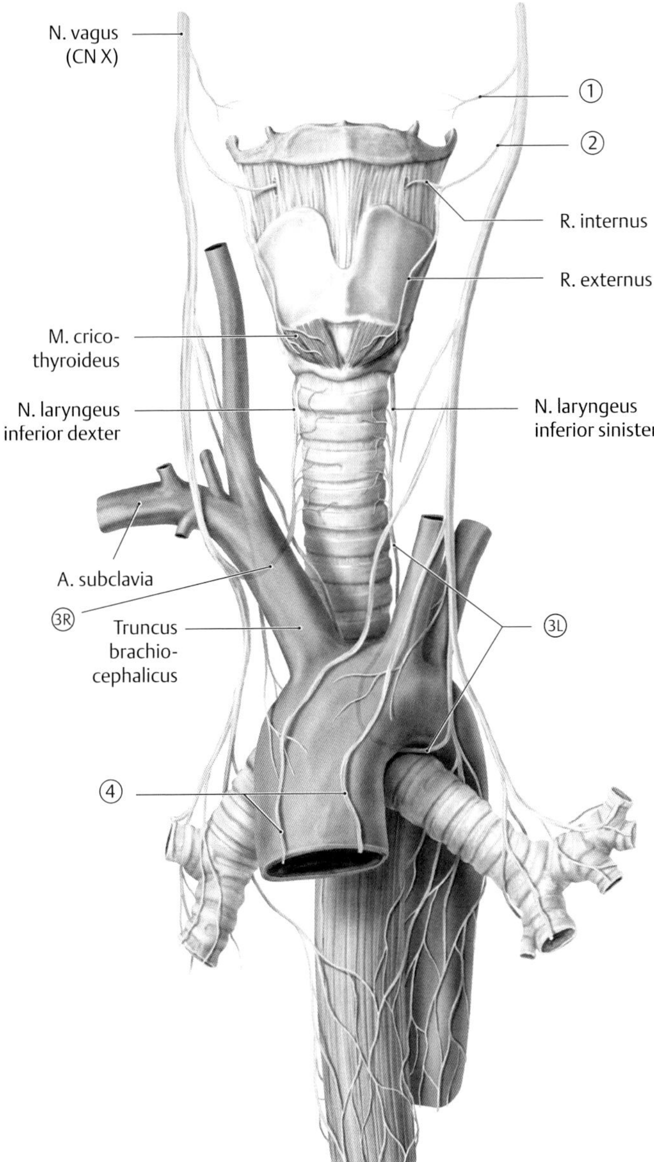
N. vagus (CN X)
①
②
R. internus
R. externus
M. crico-thyroideus
N. laryngeus inferior dexter
N. laryngeus inferior sinister
A. subclavia
③R
Truncus brachio-cephalicus
③L
④

A Branches of n. vagus in the neck. Anterior view.

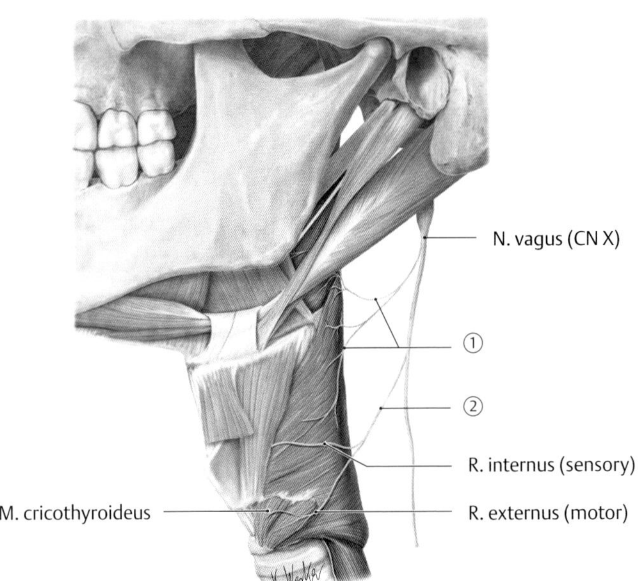
N. vagus (CN X)
①
②
R. internus (sensory)
M. cricothyroideus
R. externus (motor)

B Innervation of the pharyngeal and laryngeal muscles. Left lateral view.

CN XI & XII: N. Accessorius & N. Hypoglossus

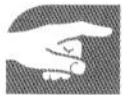

The traditional "cranial root" (radix cranialis) of n. accessorius (CN XI) is now considered a part of n. vagus (CN X) that travels with the spinal root (radix spinalis) for a short distance before splitting. The cranial fibers (r. internus) are distributed via n. vagus while the spinal root fibers continue on as the r. externus of n. accessorius (CN XI).

Fig. 31.23 **N. accessorius**
Posterior view of the brainstem with the cerebellum removed. *Note:* For didactic reasons, the muscles are displayed from the right side.

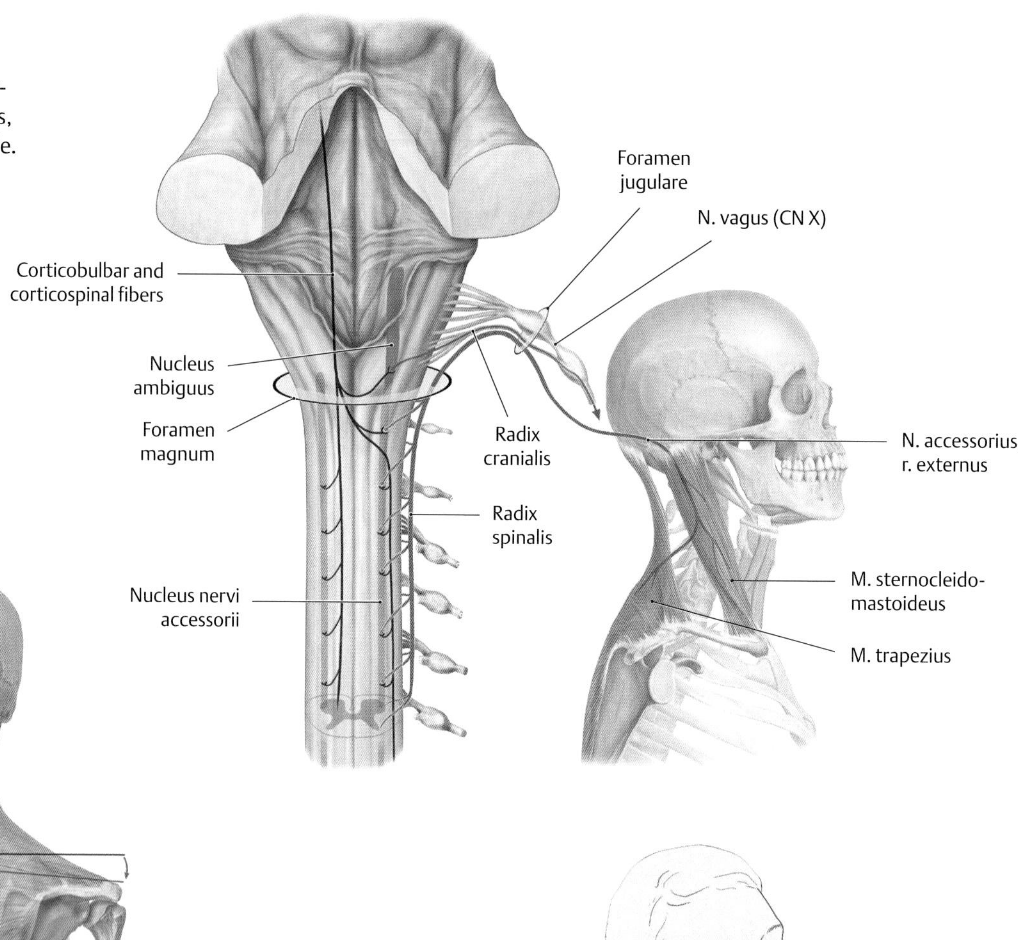

Foramen jugulare
N. vagus (CN X)
Corticobulbar and corticospinal fibers
Nucleus ambiguus
Foramen magnum
Radix cranialis
N. accessorius, r. externus
Radix spinalis
M. sternocleido-mastoideus
Nucleus nervi accessorii
M. trapezius

Fig. 31.24 **Lesions of n. accessorius**
Lesion of the right n. accessorius.

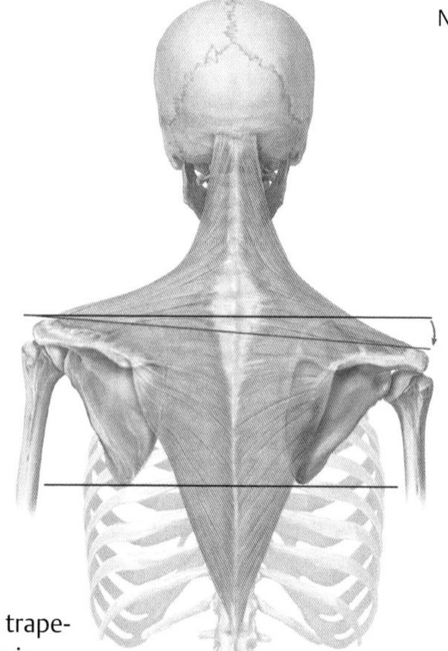

A Paralysis of m. trapezius, posterior view.

B Paralysis of m. sternocleidomastoideus, right anterolateral view.

Table 31.11 **N. accessorius (CN XI)**

Course	Fibers	Nuclei	Function	Effects of nerve injury
The radix spinalis emerges from the spinal cord (at the level of C1–C5/6), passes superiorly, and enters the skull through the foramen magnum, where it joins with the radix cranialis from the medulla oblongata. Both roots leave the skull through the foramen jugulare. Within the foramen jugulare, fibers from the radix cranialis pass to the n. vagus (r. internus). The radix spinalis descends to the regio nuchalis as the r. externus.	Special visceral efferent	Nucl. ambiguus (caudal part)	Join CN X and are distributed with the n. laryngeus recurrens. Innervate: • All laryngeal muscles (except m. cricothyroideus)	*Trapezius paralysis:* drooping of shoulder on affected side and difficulty raising arm above horizontal plane. This paralysis is a concern during neck operations (e.g., lymph node biopsies). An injury of the accessory nerve will not result in complete trapezius paralysis (the muscle is also innervated by segments C3 and C4/5). *Sternocleidomastoid paralysis:* torticollis (wry neck, i.e., difficulty turning head). Unilateral lesions cause flaccid paralysis (the muscle is supplied exclusively by the accessory nerve). Bilateral lesions make it difficult to hold the head upright.
	Somatic efferent	Nucl. nervi accessorii	Form the r. externus of the n. accessorius. Innervate: • M. trapezius • M. sternocleidomastoideus	

Fig. 31.25 N. hypoglossus

Posterior view of the brainstem with the cerebellum removed. *Note:* C1, which innervates m. thyrohyoideus and m. geniohyoideus, runs briefly with n. hypoglossus.

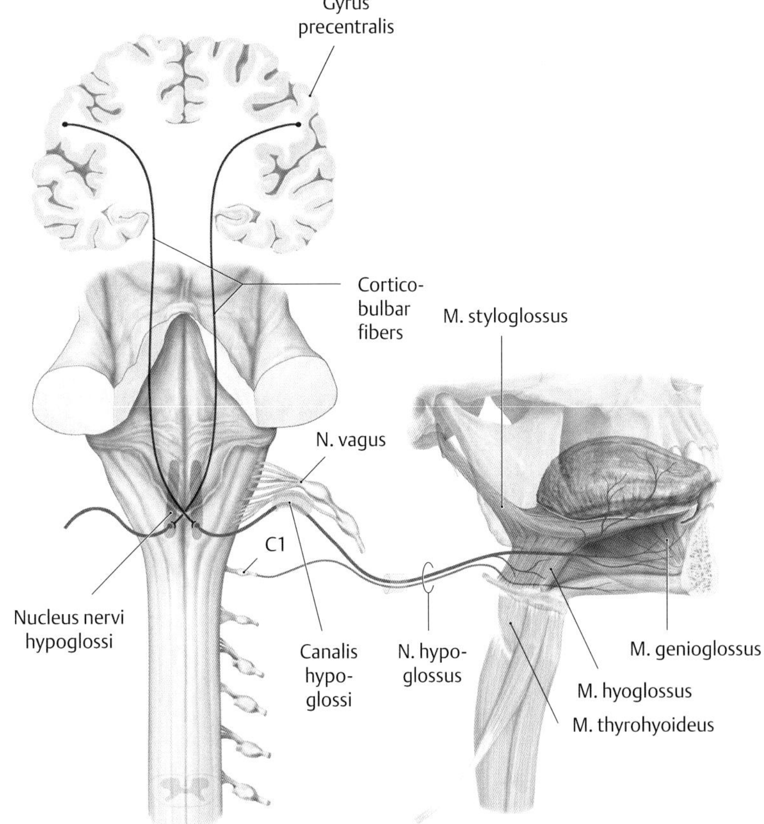
Gyrus precentralis
Cortico-bulbar fibers
M. styloglossus
N. vagus
C1
Nucleus nervi hypoglossi
Canalis hypo-glossi
N. hypo-glossus
M. genioglossus
M. hyoglossus
M. thyrohyoideus

Fig. 31.26 Nuclei of n. hypoglossus

Note: The nucleus nervi hypoglossi is innervated by cortical neurons from the contralateral side.

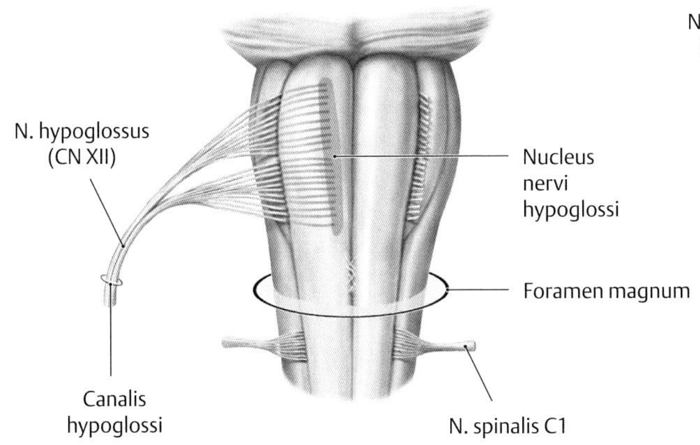
N. hypoglossus (CN XII)
Nucleus nervi hypoglossi
Foramen magnum
Canalis hypoglossi
N. spinalis C1

A Anterior view.

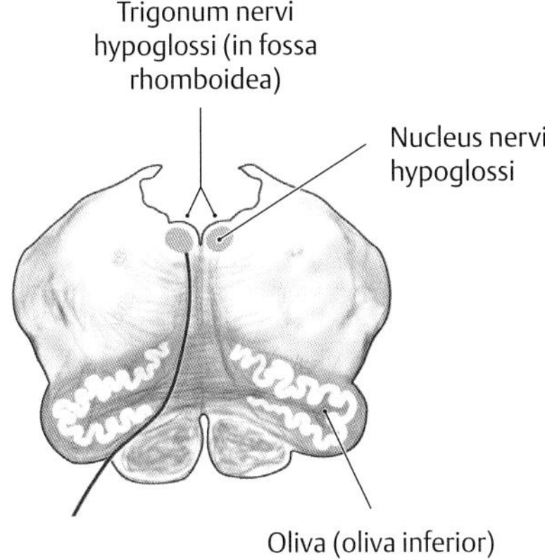
Trigonum nervi hypoglossi (in fossa rhomboidea)
Nucleus nervi hypoglossi
Oliva (oliva inferior)

B Cross section through medulla oblongata.

Fig. 31.27 Lesions of n. hypoglossus

Superior view.

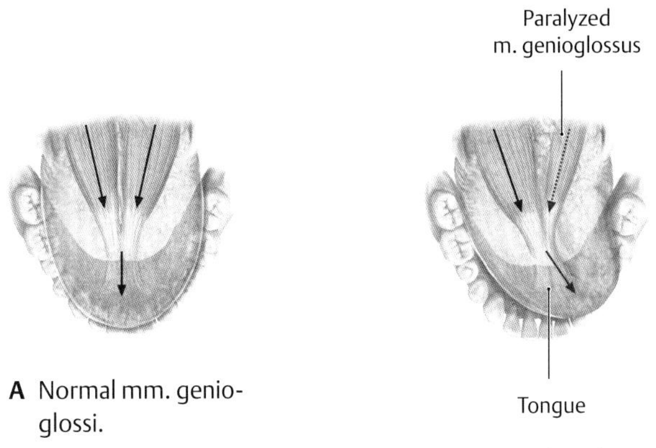
Paralyzed m. genioglossus
Tongue

A Normal mm. genioglossi.

B Unilateral nuclear or peripheral lesion.

Table 31.12 N. hypoglossus (CN XII)

Course	Fibers	Nuclei	Function	Effects of nerve injury
Emerges from the medulla oblongata, leaves the cavitas cranii through the canalis nervi hypoglossi, and descends laterally to the n. vagus. CN XII enters the radix linguae above the os hyoideum.	Somatic efferent	Nucl. nervi hypoglossi	Innervates: • Intrinsic and extrinsic muscles of the tongue (except the m. palatoglossus, supplied by CN X)	Central hypoglossal paralysis (supranuclear): tongue deviates *away* from the side of the lesion Nuclear or peripheral paralysis: tongue deviates *toward* the affected side (due to preponderance of muscle on healthy side) Flaccid paralysis: both nuclei injured; tongue cannot be protruded

Innervation of the Face

Fig. 32.1 Motor innervation of the face

Left lateral view. Five branches of n. facialis (CN VII) provide motor innervation to the muscles of facial expression. N. mandibularis of the trigeminal nerve (CN V_3) supplies motor innervation to the muscles of mastication.

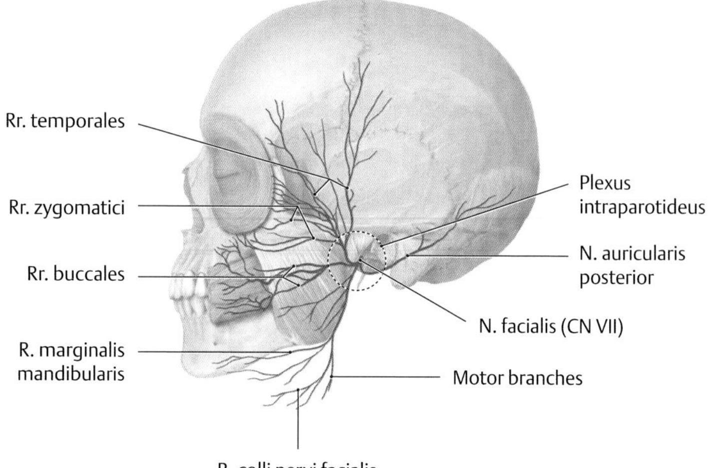

Rr. temporales
Rr. zygomatici
Rr. buccales
R. marginalis mandibularis
Plexus intraparotideus
N. auricularis posterior
N. facialis (CN VII)
Motor branches
R. colli nervi facialis

A Motor innervation of the muscles of facial expression.

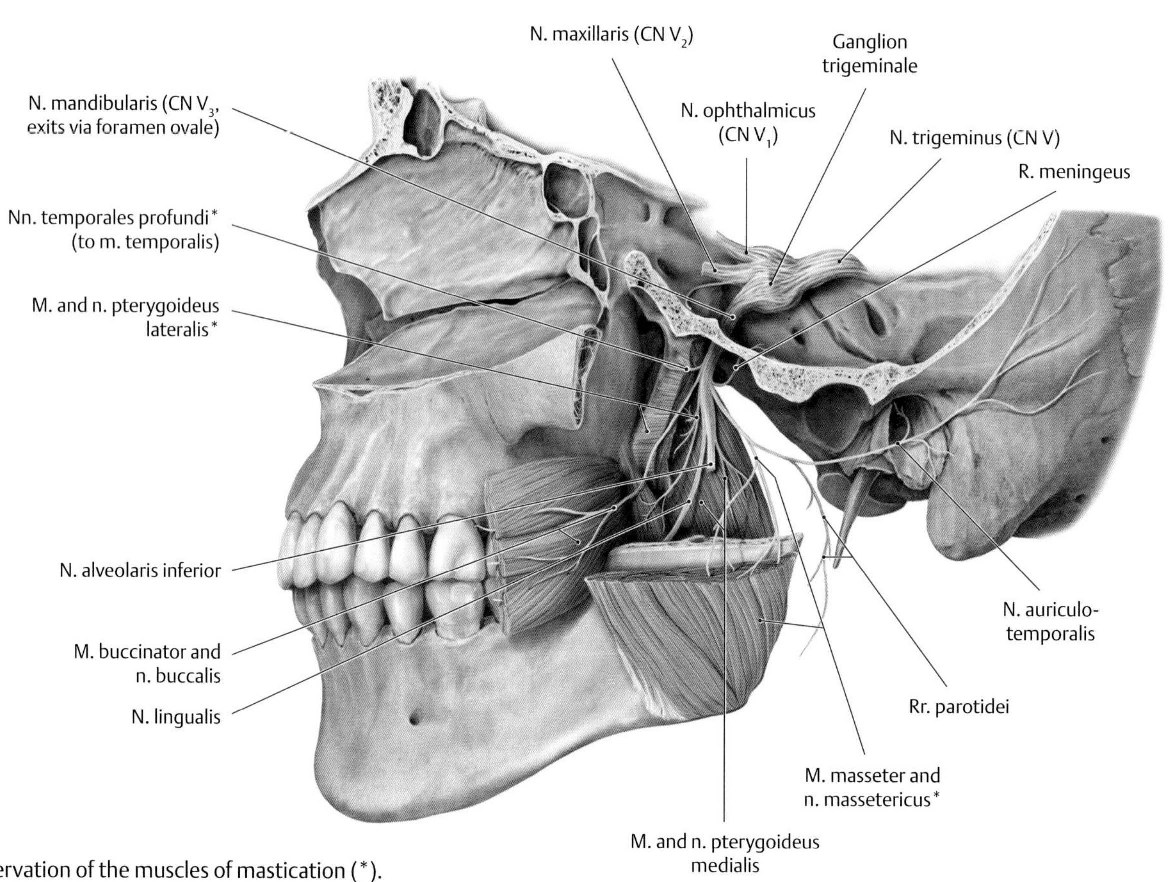

N. maxillaris (CN V_2)
Ganglion trigeminale
N. mandibularis (CN V_3, exits via foramen ovale)
N. ophthalmicus (CN V_1)
N. trigeminus (CN V)
R. meningeus
Nn. temporales profundi* (to m. temporalis)
M. and n. pterygoideus lateralis*
N. alveolaris inferior
M. buccinator and n. buccalis
N. lingualis
N. auriculo-temporalis
Rr. parotidei
M. masseter and n. massetericus*
M. and n. pterygoideus medialis

B Motor innervation of the muscles of mastication (*).

Fig. 32.2 Sensory innervation of the face

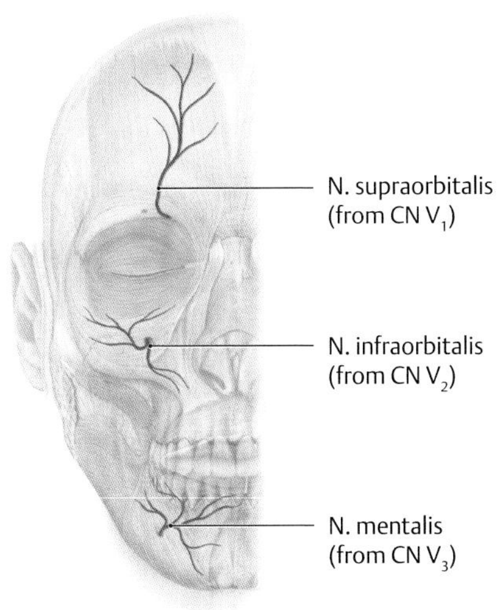

N. supraorbitalis (from CN V_1)
N. infraorbitalis (from CN V_2)
N. mentalis (from CN V_3)

A Sensory branches of n. trigeminus, anterior view. The sensory branches of the three divisions emerge from foramina supraorbitalis, infraorbitalis, and mentalis, respectively.

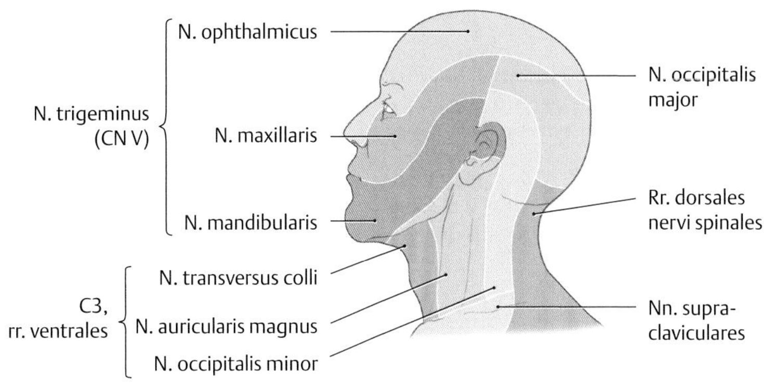

N. trigeminus (CN V)
N. ophthalmicus
N. maxillaris
N. mandibularis
C3, rr. ventrales
N. transversus colli
N. auricularis magnus
N. occipitalis minor
N. occipitalis major
Rr. dorsales nervi spinales
Nn. supra-claviculares

B Sensory innervation of the head and neck, left lateral view. The occiput and nuchal regions are supplied by the rami dorsales (blue) of the spinal nerves (n. occipitalis major is the ramus dorsalis of C2).

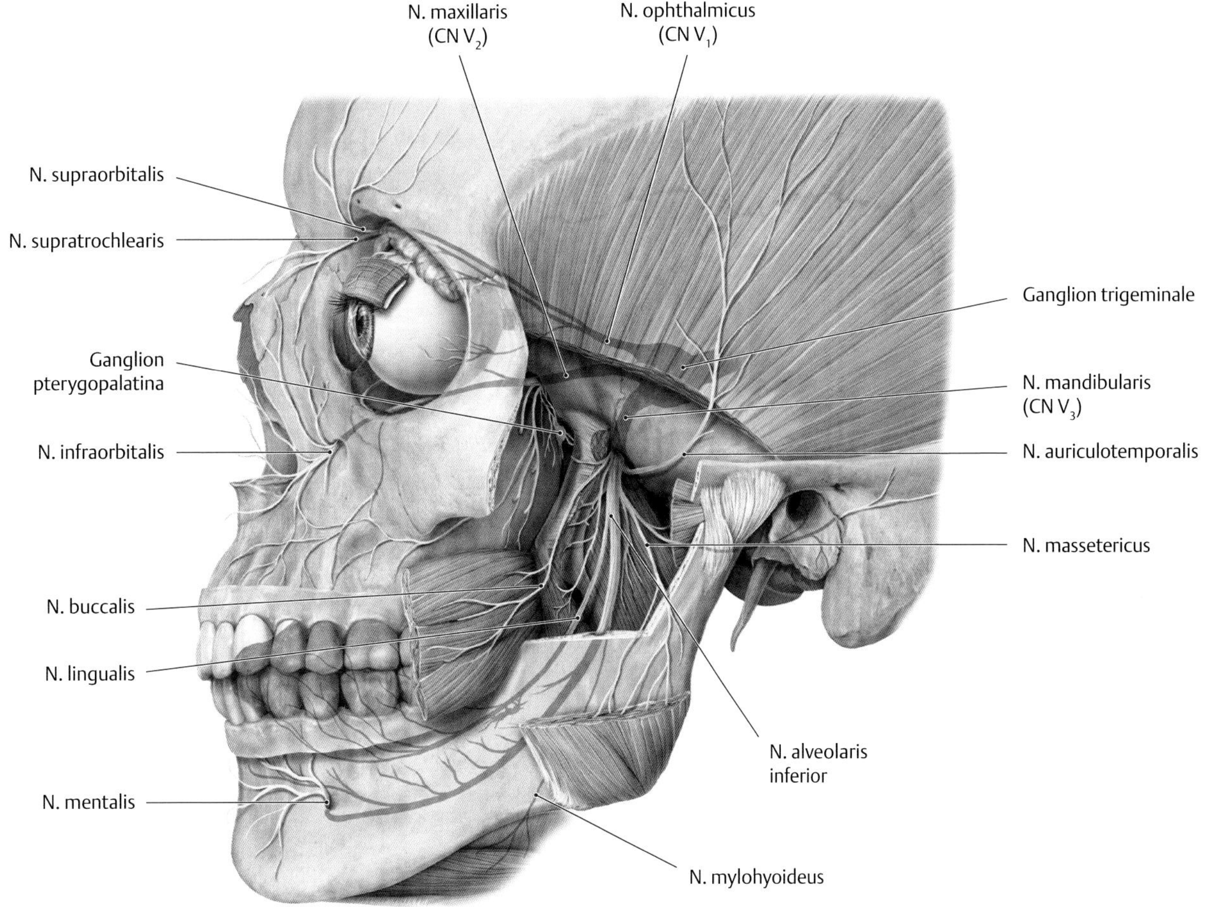

N. maxillaris (CN V_2)
N. ophthalmicus (CN V_1)
N. supraorbitalis
N. supratrochlearis
Ganglion pterygopalatina
N. infraorbitalis
N. buccalis
N. lingualis
N. mentalis
Ganglion trigeminale
N. mandibularis (CN V_3)
N. auriculotemporalis
N. massetericus
N. alveolaris inferior
N. mylohyoideus

C Divisions of n. trigeminus, left lateral view.

Arteries of the Head & Neck

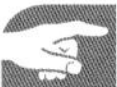

The head and neck are supplied by branches of a. carotis communis. A. carotis communis splits at the bifurcatio carotidis into two branches: a. carotis interna and a. carotis externa. A. carotis interna chiefly supplies the brain (p. 606), although its branches anastomose with a. carotis externa in the orbita and septum nasi. A. carotis externa is the major supplier of structures of the head and neck.

Fig. 32.3 A. carotis interna

Left lateral view. The most important extracerebral branch of a. carotis interna is the a. ophthalmica, which supplies the upper septum nasi (p. 524) and the orbita (p. 512). See pp. 608–609 for arteries of the brain.

A. ophthalmica
A. angularis
A. carotis interna
A. carotis externa
A. facialis
A. carotis communis
A. vertebralis
A. subclavia

A Schematic.

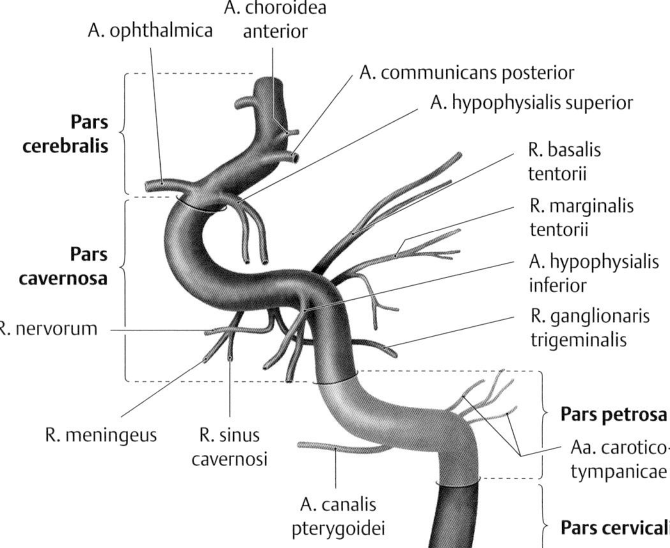
A. ophthalmica
A. choroidea anterior
A. communicans posterior
A. hypophysialis superior
Pars cerebralis
R. basalis tentorii
R. marginalis tentorii
Pars cavernosa
A. hypophysialis inferior
R. nervorum
R. ganglionaris trigeminalis
Pars petrosa
R. meningeus
R. sinus cavernosi
Aa. carotico-tympanicae
A. canalis pterygoidei
Pars cervicalis

B Parts and branches of a. carotis interna.

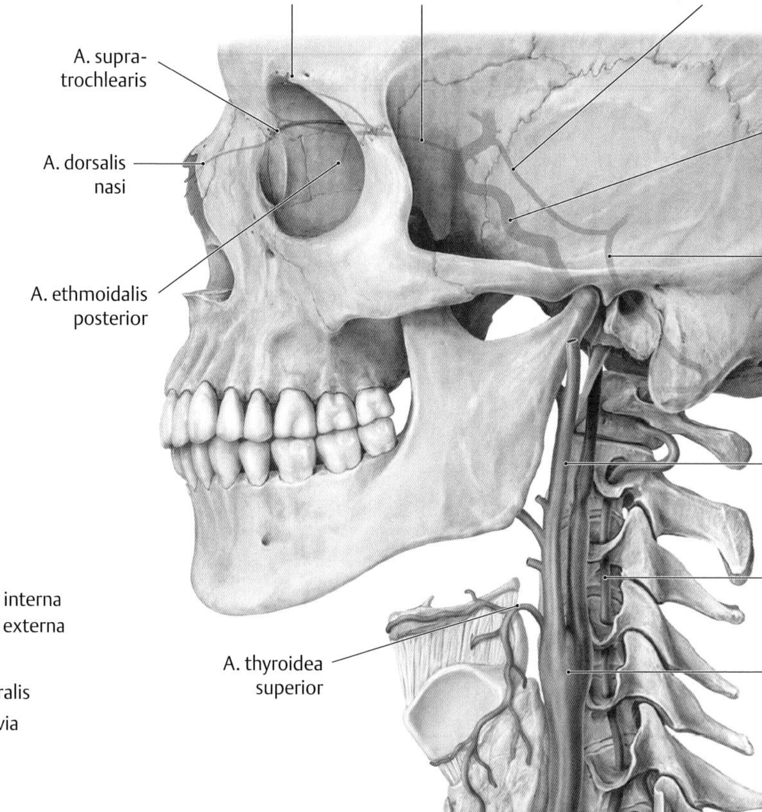
A. supra-orbitalis
A. ophthalmica
A. communicans posterior
A. supra-trochlearis
A. carotis interna
A. dorsalis nasi
A. basilaris
A. ethmoidalis posterior
A. carotis externa
A. vertebralis
A. thyroidea superior
Bifurcatio carotidis
A. vertebralis
A. subclavia

C Course of a. carotis interna.

Clinical

Carotid artery atherosclerosis

The carotid artery is often affected by atherosclerosis, a hardening of arterial walls due to plaque formation. The examiner can determine the status of the arteries using ultrasound. *Note:* The absence of atherosclerosis in the carotid artery does not preclude coronary heart disease or atherosclerotic changes in other locations.

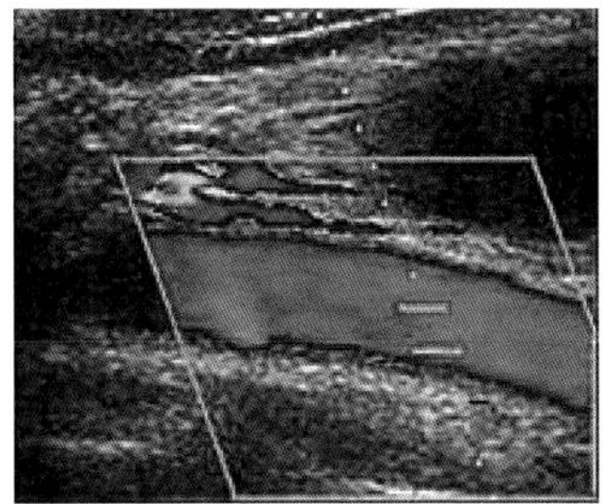

A A. carotis communis with "normal" flow.

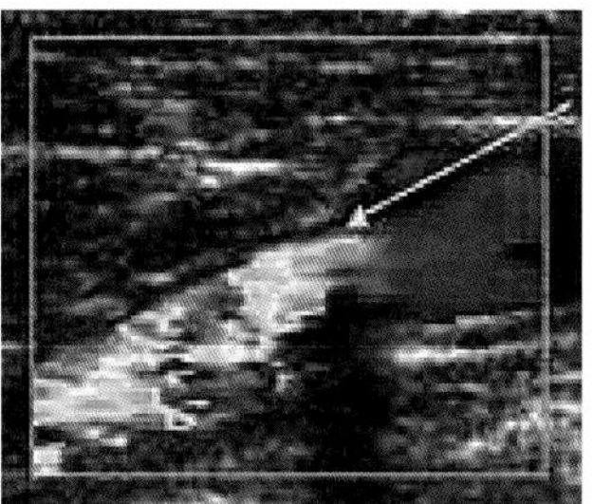

B Calcified plaque in the carotid bulb.

Fig. 32.4 A. carotis externa: Overview

Left lateral view.

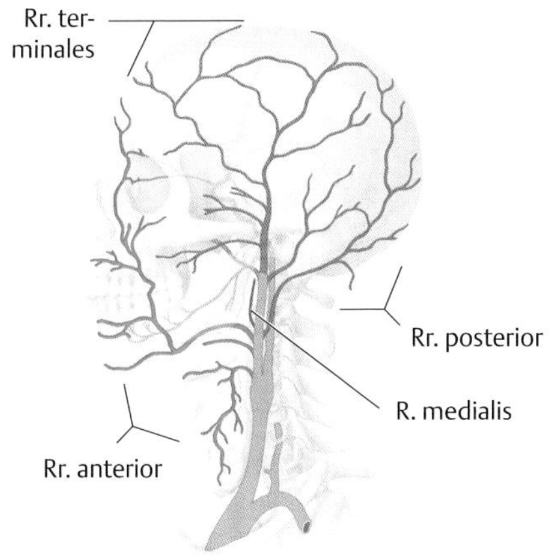
Rr. terminales
Rr. posterior
R. medialis
Rr. anterior

A Schematic of a. carotis externa.

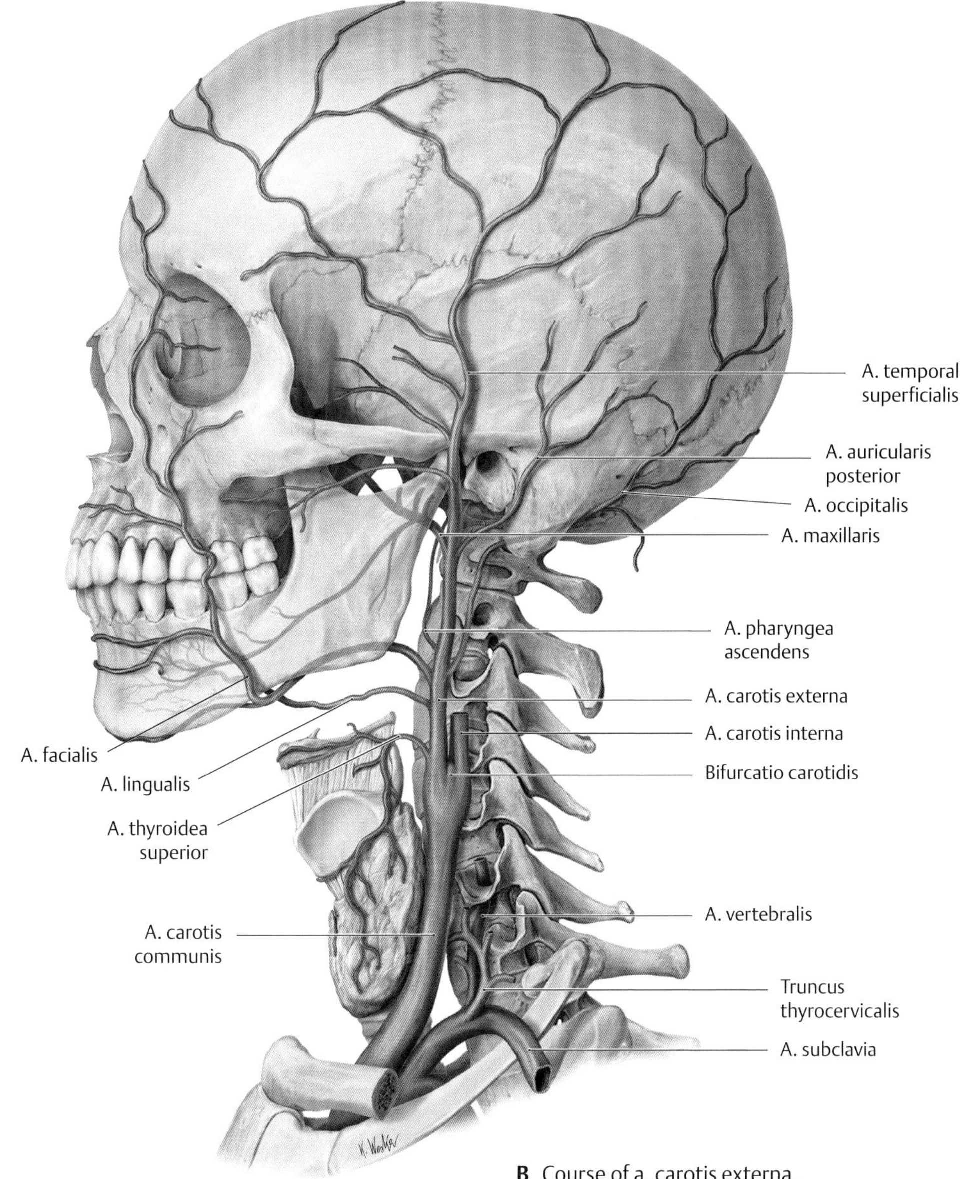
A. temporalis superficialis
A. auricularis posterior
A. occipitalis
A. maxillaris
A. pharyngea ascendens
A. carotis externa
A. carotis interna
Bifurcatio carotidis
A. facialis
A. lingualis
A. thyroidea superior
A. carotis communis
A. vertebralis
Truncus thyrocervicalis
A. subclavia

B Course of a. carotis externa.

Table 32.1	**Rr. of the A. carotis externa**
Group	**Artery**
Anterior (p. 492)	A. thyroidea superior
	A. lingualis
	A. facialis
Medial (p. 492)	A. pharyngea ascendens
Posterior (p. 493)	A. occipitalis
	A. auricularis posterior
Terminal (p. 494)	A. maxillaris
	A. temporalis superficialis

A. Carotis Externa: Anterior, Medial & Posterior Branches

Fig. 32.5 **Anterior and medial branches**
Left lateral view. The arteries of the anterior aspect supply the anterior structures of the head and neck, including the orbita (p. 510), ear (p. 534), larynx (p. 575), pharynx (p. 556), and oral cavity. *Note:* The a. angularis anastomoses with the a. dorsalis nasi of a. carotis interna (via a. ophthalmica).

A. supra-trochlearis
A. dorsalis nasi
A. angularis
A. infraorbitalis
A. labialis superior
A. labialis inferior
A. alveolaris inferior
A. submentalis
A. lingualis
A. thyroidea superior
A. temporalis superficialis
A. maxillaris
A. auricularis posterior
A. pharyngea ascendens
A. occipitalis
A. facialis
A. lingualis
A. carotis interna
A. carotis communis

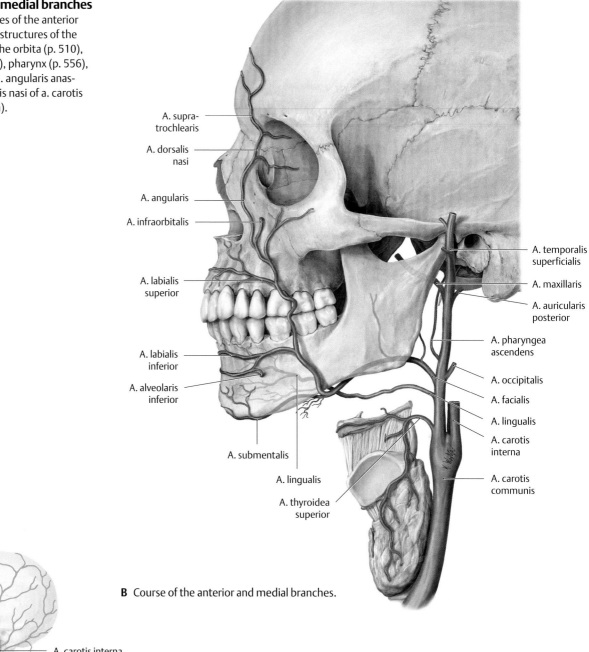

B Course of the anterior and medial branches.

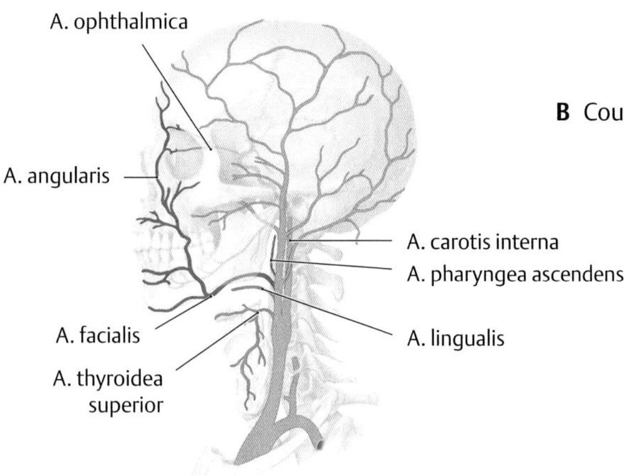
A. ophthalmica
A. angularis
A. carotis interna
A. pharyngea ascendens
A. facialis
A. lingualis
A. thyroidea superior

A Arteries of the anterior and medial branches. The copious blood supply to the face makes facial injuries bleed profusely, but heal quickly. There are extensive anastomoses between branches of a. carotis externa, and between a. carotis externa and branches of a. ophthalmica.

Fig. 32.6 Posterior branches

Left lateral view. The posterior branches of a. carotis externa supply the ear (p. 534), posterior skull (p. 499), and posterior neck muscles (p. 585).

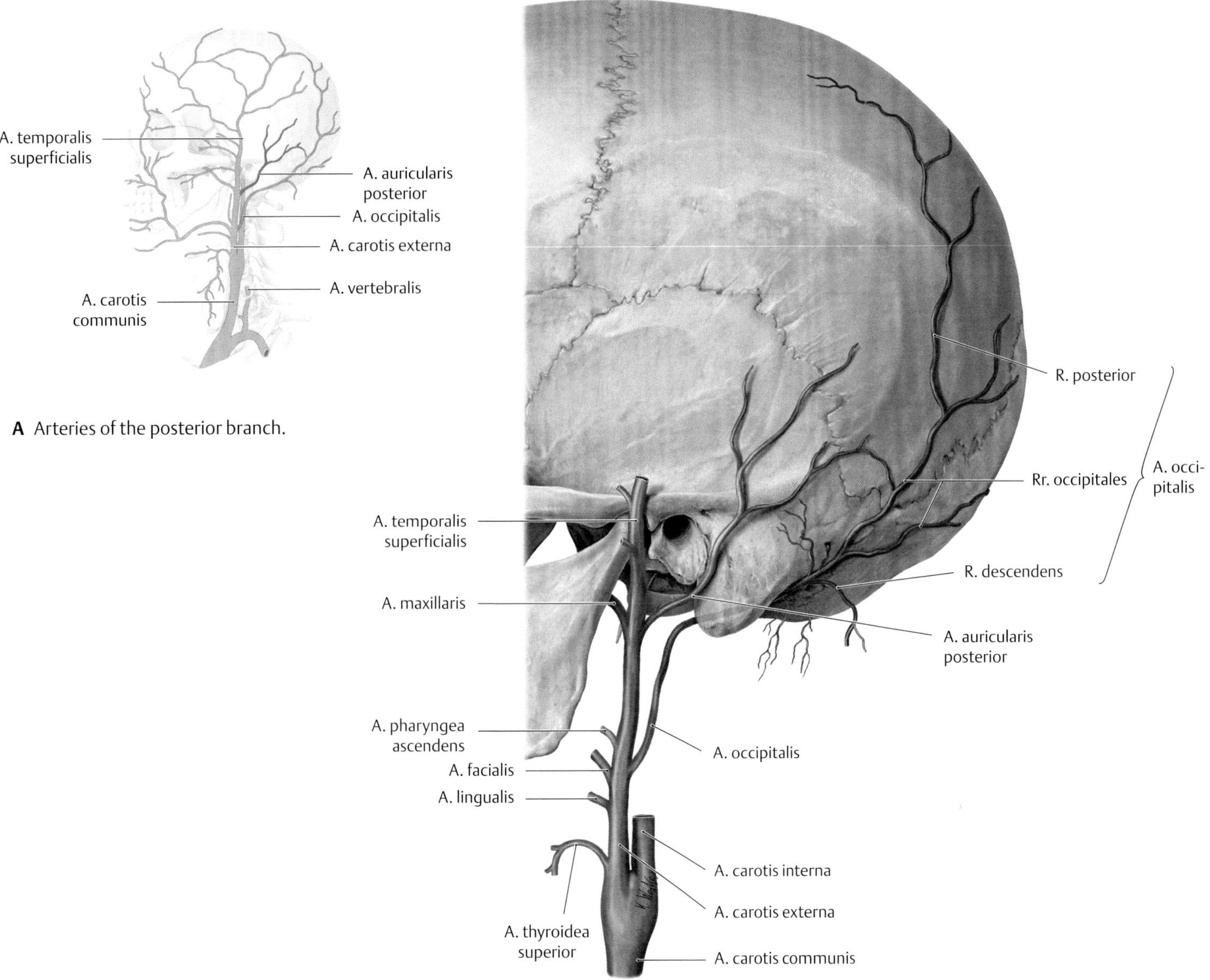

A. temporalis superficialis
A. auricularis posterior
A. occipitalis
A. carotis externa
A. vertebralis
A. carotis communis
R. posterior
Rr. occipitales
A. occipitalis
R. descendens
A. temporalis superficialis
A. maxillaris
A. auricularis posterior
A. pharyngea ascendens
A. facialis
A. lingualis
A. occipitalis
A. carotis interna
A. carotis externa
A. thyroidea superior
A. carotis communis

A Arteries of the posterior branch.

B Course of the posterior branches.

Table 32.2 Rr. anterior, medial, and posterior of the a. carotis externa

Branch	Artery	Divisions and distribution
R. anterior	A. thyroidea superior	R. glandularis anterior (to glandula thyroidea); a. laryngea superior; r. sternocleidomastoideus
	A. lingualis	Rr. dorsales linguae (to base of tongue, epiglottis); a. sublingualis (to glandula sublingualis, tongue, oral floor, oral cavity)
	A. facialis	A. palatina ascendens (to pharyngeal wall, soft palate, Tuba auditiva); rr. tonsillares (to tonsilla palatina); a. submentalis (to oral floor, glandula submandibularis); aa. labiales; a. angularis (radix nasi)
R. medius	A. pharyngea ascendens	Rr. pharyngei; a. tympanica inferior (to mucosa of inner ear); a. meningea posterior
R. posterior	A. occipitalis	Rr. occipitales; r. descendens (to posterior neck muscles)
	A. auricularis posterior	A. stylomastoidea (to n. facialis in canalis nervi facialis); a. tympanica posterior; r. auricularis; r. occipitalis; r. parotideus
For terminal branches, see Table 32.3.		

A. Carotis Externa: Terminal Branches

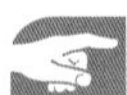

The terminal branches of the external carotid artery consist of two major arteries: a. temporalis superficialis and a. maxillaris. A. temporalis superficialis supplies the lateral skull. A. maxillaris is a major artery for internal structures of the face.

Fig. 32.7 A. temporalis superficialis

Left lateral view. Inflammation of a. temporalis superficialis due to temporal arteritis can cause severe headaches. The course of the frontal branch of the artery can often be seen superficially under the skin of elderly patients.

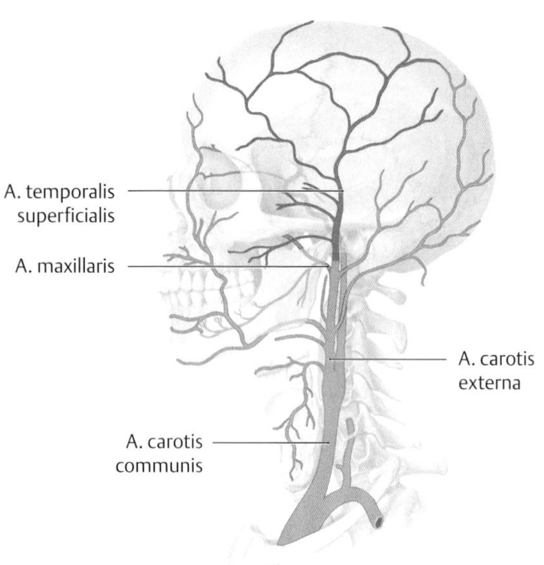
A. temporalis superficialis
A. maxillaris
A. carotis externa
A. carotis communis

A Arteries of the terminal branch.

B Course of a. temporalis superficialis.

Table 32.3 Rr. terminales of the a. carotis externa

Branch	Artery		Divisions and distribution	
Rr. terminales	A. temporalis superficialis		A. transversa faciei (to soft tissues below the arcus zygomaticus); rr. frontales; rr. parietales; a. zygomaticoorbitalis (to paries orbitalis lateralis)	
	A. maxillaris	Pars mandibularis	A. alveolaris inferior (to mandibula, teeth, gingiva); a. meningea media; a. auricularis profunda (to articulatio temporomandibulare, meatus acusticus externus); a. tympanica anterior	
		Pars pterygoidea	A. masseterica; aa. temporales profundae; rr. pterygoidei; a. buccalis	
		Pars pterygopalatina	A. alveolaris superior posterior (to maxillary molars, sinus maxillaris, gingiva); a. infraorbitalis (to alveoli dentales)	
			A. palatina descendens	A. palatina major (to hard palate)
				A. palatina minor (to soft palate, tonsilla palatina, pharyngeal wall)
			A. sphenopalatina	Aa. nasales posteriores laterales (to lateral wall of nasal cavity, conchae)
				Rr. septales posteriores (to septum nasi)

Fig. 32.8 A. maxillaris

Left lateral view. A. maxillaris consists of three parts: mandibular (blue), pterygoid (green), and pterygopalatine (yellow).

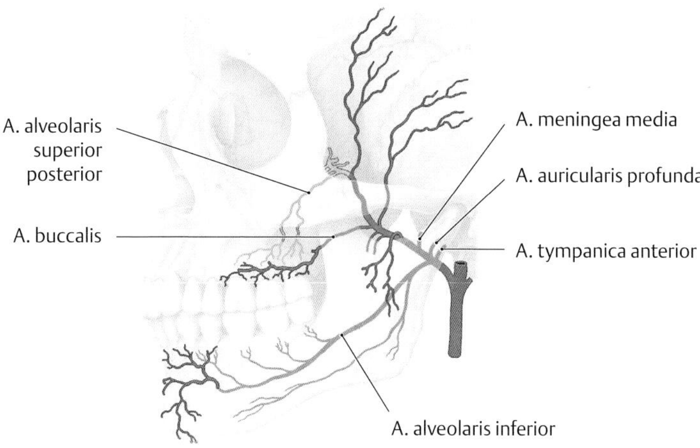

A. alveolaris superior posterior
A. buccalis
A. meningea media
A. auricularis profunda
A. tympanica anterior
A. alveolaris inferior

A Divisions of a. maxillaris.

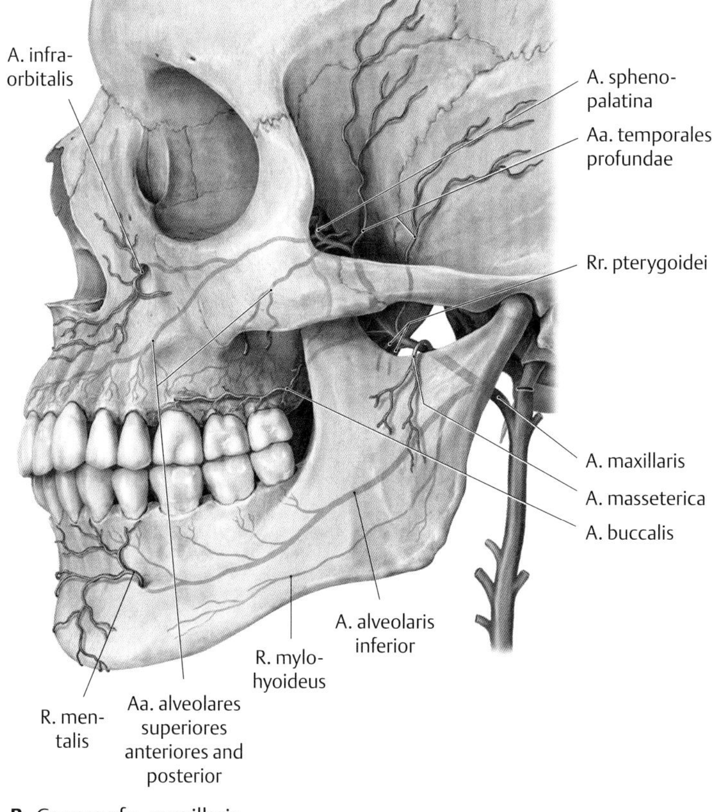

A. infra-orbitalis
A. spheno-palatina
Aa. temporales profundae
Rr. pterygoidei
A. maxillaris
A. masseterica
A. buccalis
A. alveolaris inferior
R. mylo-hyoideus
R. men-talis
Aa. alveolares superiores anteriores and posterior

B Course of a. maxillaris.

Clinical

A. meningea media

The a. meningea media supplies the meninges and overlying calvaria. Rupture of the artery (generally due to head trauma) results in an epidural hematoma.

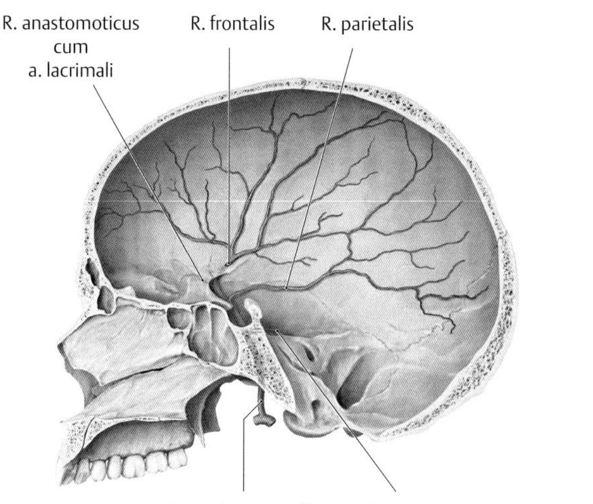

R. anastomoticus cum a. lacrimali
R. frontalis
R. parietalis
A. meningea media
R. petrosus

A Right a. meningea media, medial view of opened skull.

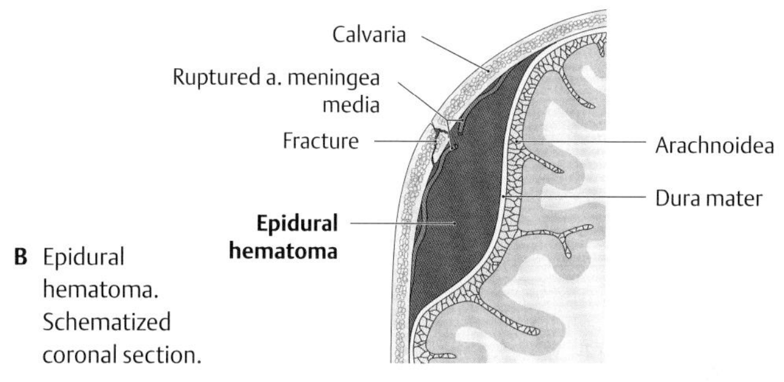

Calvaria
Ruptured a. meningea media
Fracture
Arachnoidea
Dura mater
Epidural hematoma

B Epidural hematoma. Schematized coronal section.

A. sphenopalatina

The a. sphenopalatina supplies the wall of the nasal cavity. Excessive nasopharyngeal bleeding from the branches of a. sphenopalatina may necessitate ligation of a. maxillaris in fossa pterygopalatina.

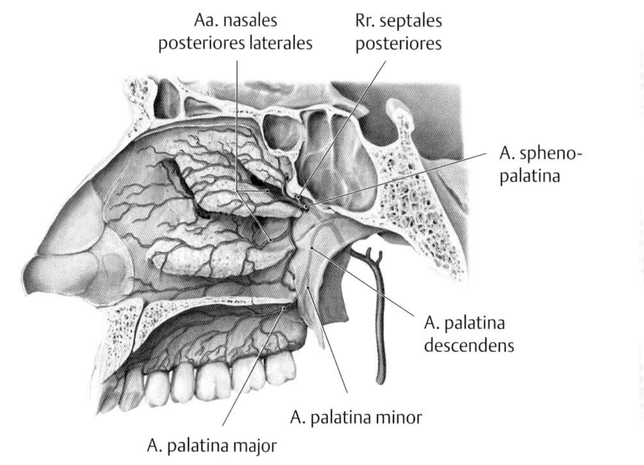

Aa. nasales posteriores laterales
Rr. septales posteriores
A. spheno-palatina
A. palatina descendens
A. palatina minor
A. palatina major

C Lateral wall of nasal cavity, left lateral view.

Veins of the Head & Neck

Fig. 32.9 Veins of the head and neck
Left lateral view. The veins of the head and neck drain into v. brachiocephalica. *Note:* The left and right vv. brachiocephalicae are not symmetrical.

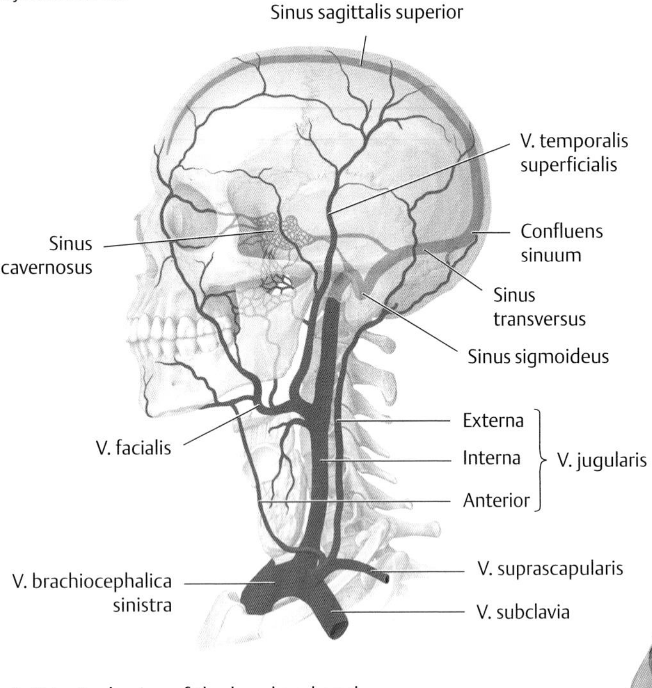
Sinus sagittalis superior
V. temporalis superficialis
Sinus cavernosus
Confluens sinuum
Sinus transversus
Sinus sigmoideus
V. facialis
Externa
Interna
Anterior
V. jugularis
V. brachiocephalica sinistra
V. suprascapularis
V. subclavia

A Principal veins of the head and neck.

Table 32.4	**Principal superficial veins**	
Vein	**Region drained**	**Location**
V. jugularis interna	Interior of skull (including brain)	Within vagina carotica
V. jugularis externa	Superficial head	Within fascia cervicalis superficialis
V. jugularis anterior	Neck, portions of head	

Vv. opthalmicae superior and inferior
Plexus pterygoideus
V. angularis
V. facialis
V. submentalis
V. jugularis anterior
V. brachiocephalica sinistra
V. temporalis superficialis
V. maxillaris
V. occipitalis
V. auricularis posterior
V. retromandibularis
V. thyroidea superior
V. jugularis interna
V. jugularis externa
V. supra-scapularis
V. subclavia

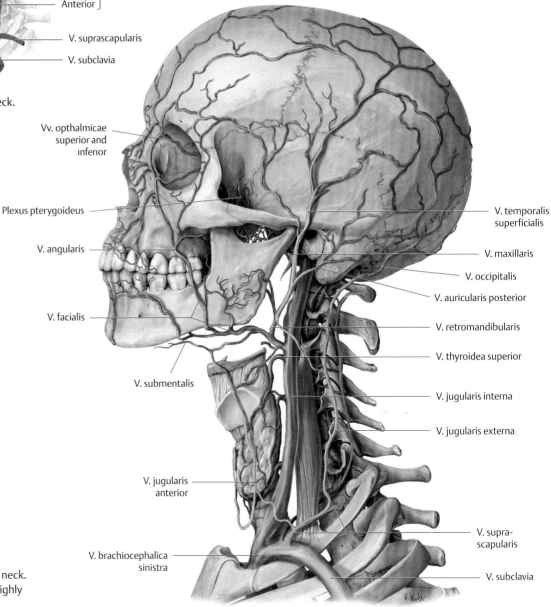

B Superficial veins of the head and neck. *Note:* The course of the veins is highly variable.

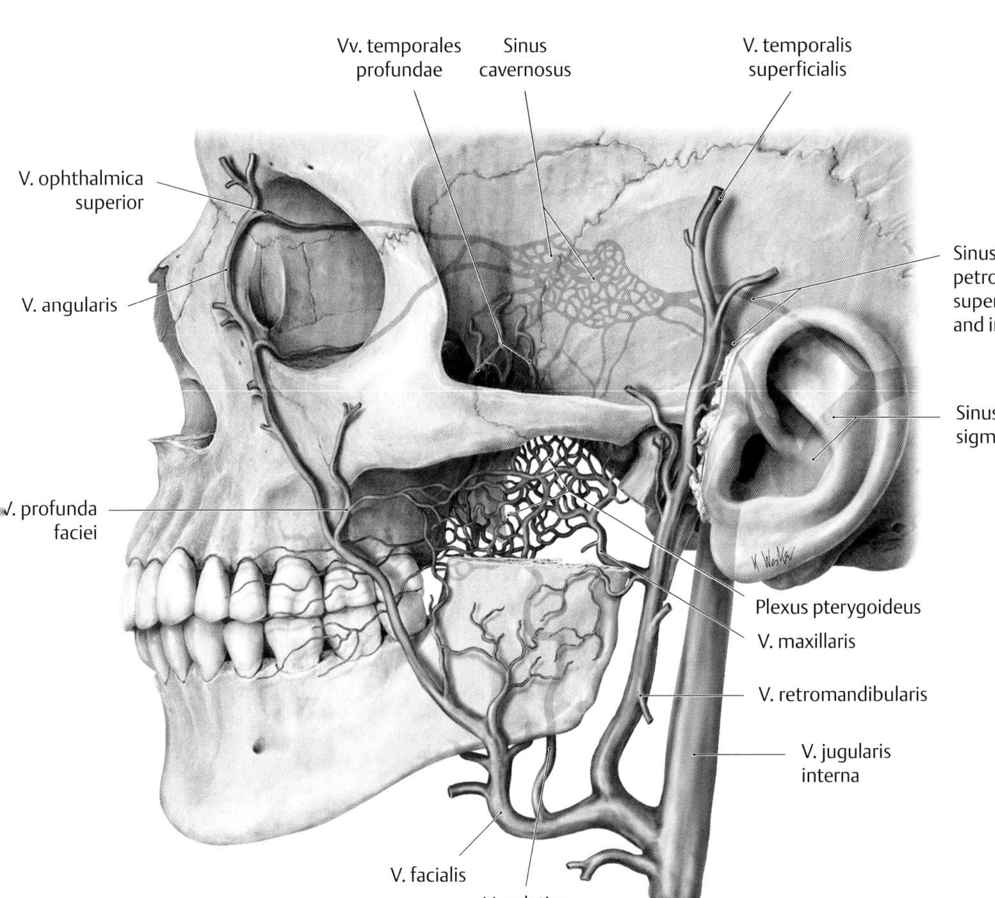
Vv. temporales profundae
Sinus cavernosus
V. temporalis superficialis
V. ophthalmica superior
V. angularis
Sinus petrosi superior and inferior
Sinus sigmoideus
V. profunda faciei
Plexus pterygoideus
V. maxillaris
V. retromandibularis
V. jugularis interna
V. facialis
V. palatina externa

Fig. 32.10 **Deep veins of the head**
Left lateral view. *Removed:* Upper ramus, processus condylaris and processus coronoideus of mandibula. The plexus pterygoideus is a venous network situated between ramus mandibulae and the muscles of mastication. Sinus cavernosus connects branches of v. facialis to sinus sigmoideus.

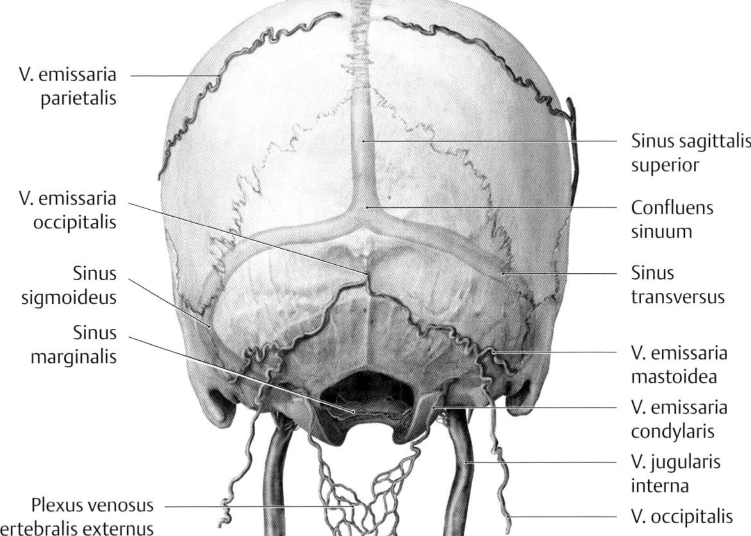
V. emissaria parietalis
Sinus sagittalis superior
V. emissaria occipitalis
Confluens sinuum
Sinus sigmoideus
Sinus transversus
Sinus marginalis
V. emissaria mastoidea
V. emissaria condylaris
V. jugularis interna
Plexus venosus vertebralis externus
V. occipitalis

Fig. 32.11 **Veins of the occiput**
Posterior view. The superficial veins of the occiput communicate with sinus durae matris via vv. emissariae that drain to vv. diploicae (calvaria, p. 457). *Note:* The plexus venosus vertebralis externus traverses the entire length of the spine (p. 611).

Table 32.5 Venous anastomoses

The extensive venous anastomoses in this region provide routes for the spread of infections.

Extracranial vein	Connecting vein	Venous sinus
V. angularis	V. ophthalmica superior and inferior	Sinus cavernosus*
Vv. of palatine tonsil	Plexus pterygoideus; v. ophthalmica inferior	
V. temporalis superficialis	Vv. emissariae parietales	Sinus sagittalis superior
V. occipitalis	V. emissaria occipitalis	Sinus transversus, confluens sinuum
V. auricularis posterior	V. emissaria mastoidea	Sinus sigmoideus
Plexus venosus vertebralis externus	V. emissaria condylaris	

*Deep spread of bacterial infection from the facial region may result in sinus cavernosus thrombosis.

Topography of the Superficial Face

Fig. 32.12 **Superficial neurovasculature of the face**
Anterior view. *Removed:* Skin and fatty subcutaneous tissue; muscles of facial expression (left side).

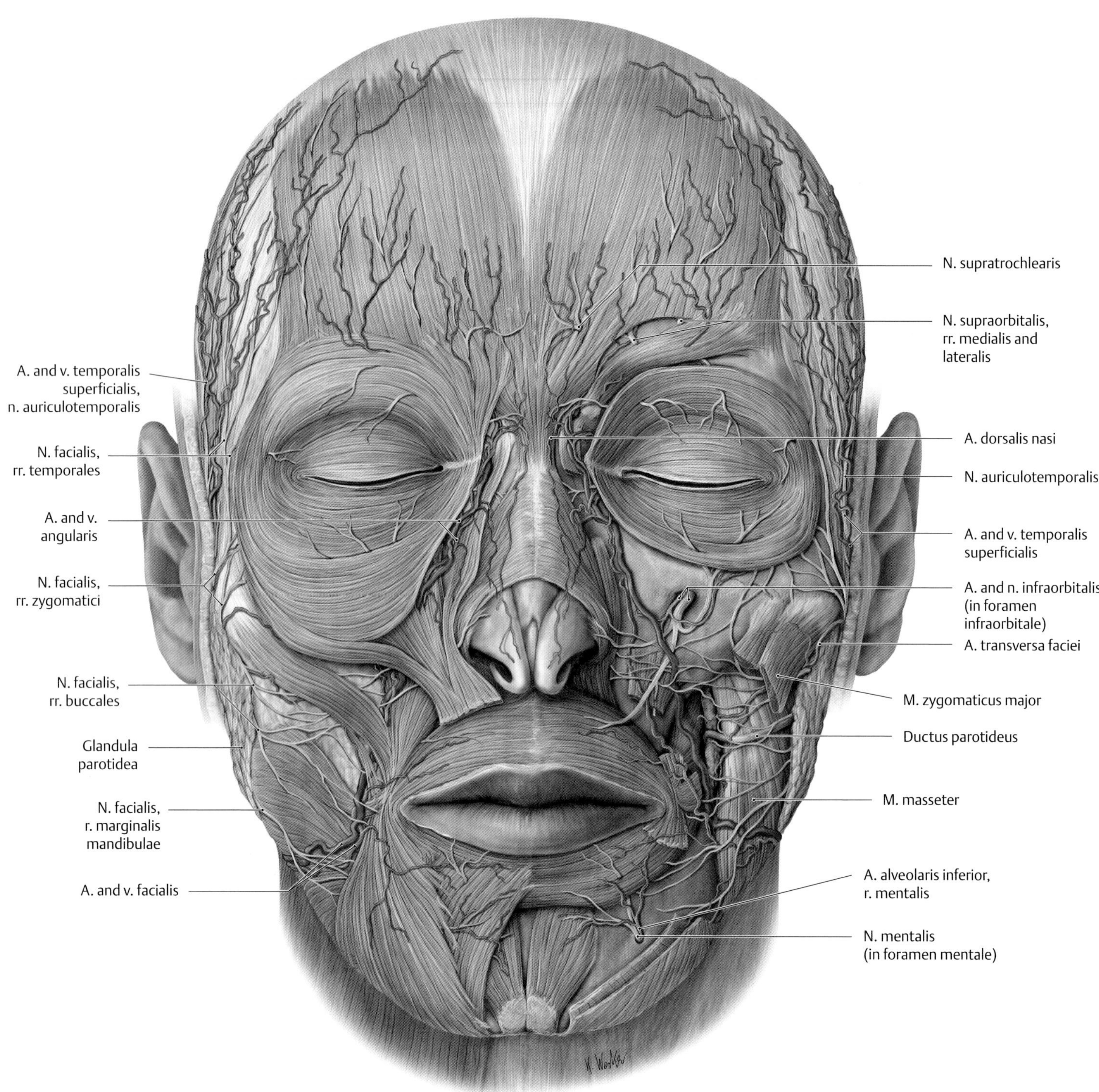
N. supratrochlearis
N. supraorbitalis, rr. medialis and lateralis
A. and v. temporalis superficialis, n. auriculotemporalis
A. dorsalis nasi
N. facialis, rr. temporales
N. auriculotemporalis
A. and v. angularis
A. and v. temporalis superficialis
N. facialis, rr. zygomatici
A. and n. infraorbitalis (in foramen infraorbitale)
A. transversa faciei
N. facialis, rr. buccales
M. zygomaticus major
Glandula parotidea
Ductus parotideus
N. facialis, r. marginalis mandibulae
M. masseter
A. and v. facialis
A. alveolaris inferior, r. mentalis
N. mentalis (in foramen mentale)

Fig. 32.13 **Superficial neurovasculature of the head**
Left lateral view.

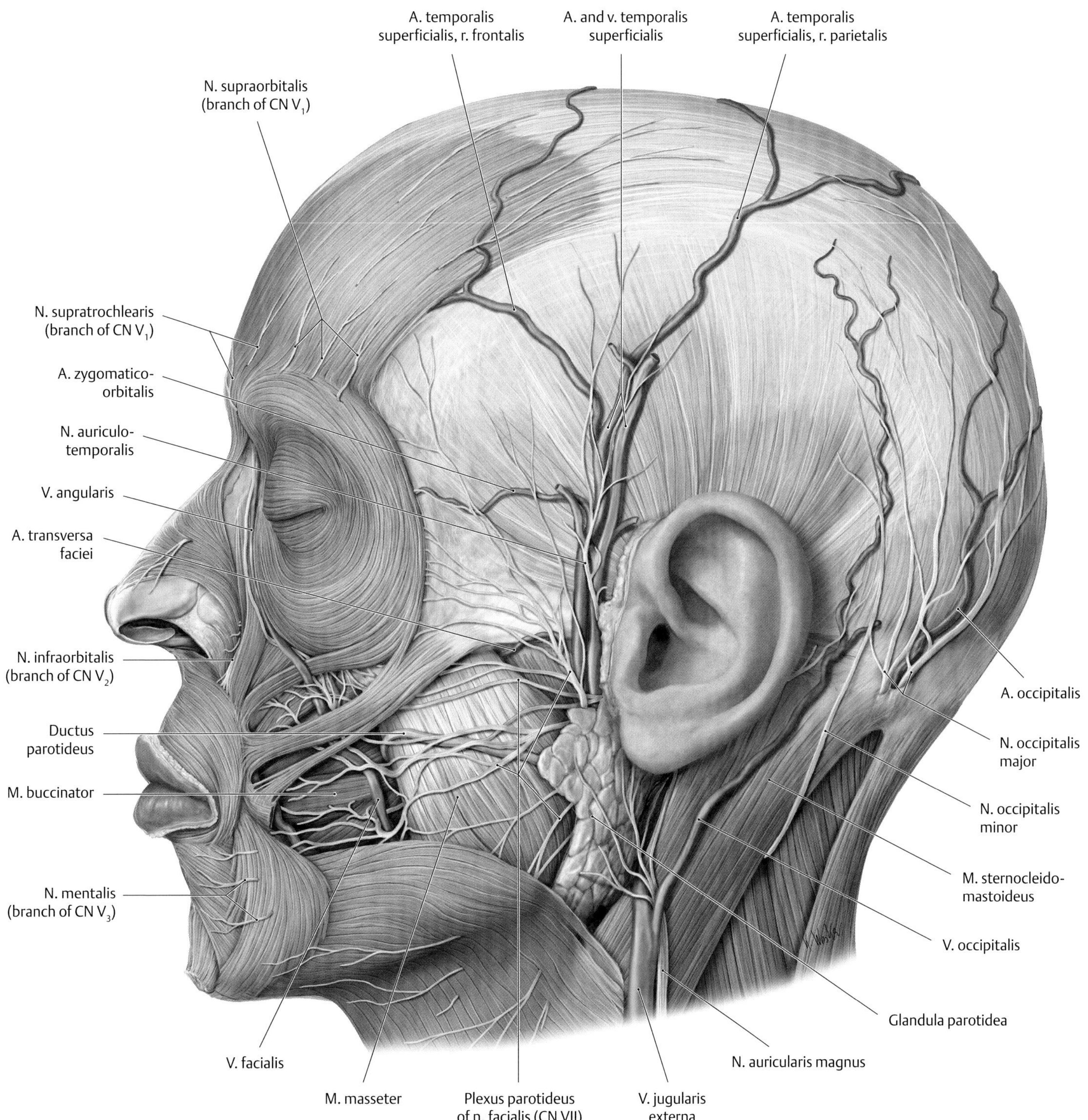
A. temporalis superficialis, r. frontalis
A. and v. temporalis superficialis
A. temporalis superficialis, r. parietalis
N. supraorbitalis (branch of CN V_1)
N. supratrochlearis (branch of CN V_1)
A. zygomatico-orbitalis
N. auriculo-temporalis
V. angularis
A. transversa faciei
N. infraorbitalis (branch of CN V_2)
Ductus parotideus
M. buccinator
N. mentalis (branch of CN V_3)
V. facialis
M. masseter
Plexus parotideus of n. facialis (CN VII)
V. jugularis externa
N. auricularis magnus
Glandula parotidea
V. occipitalis
M. sternocleido-mastoideus
N. occipitalis minor
N. occipitalis major
A. occipitalis

Topography of the Parotid Region & Fossa Temporalis

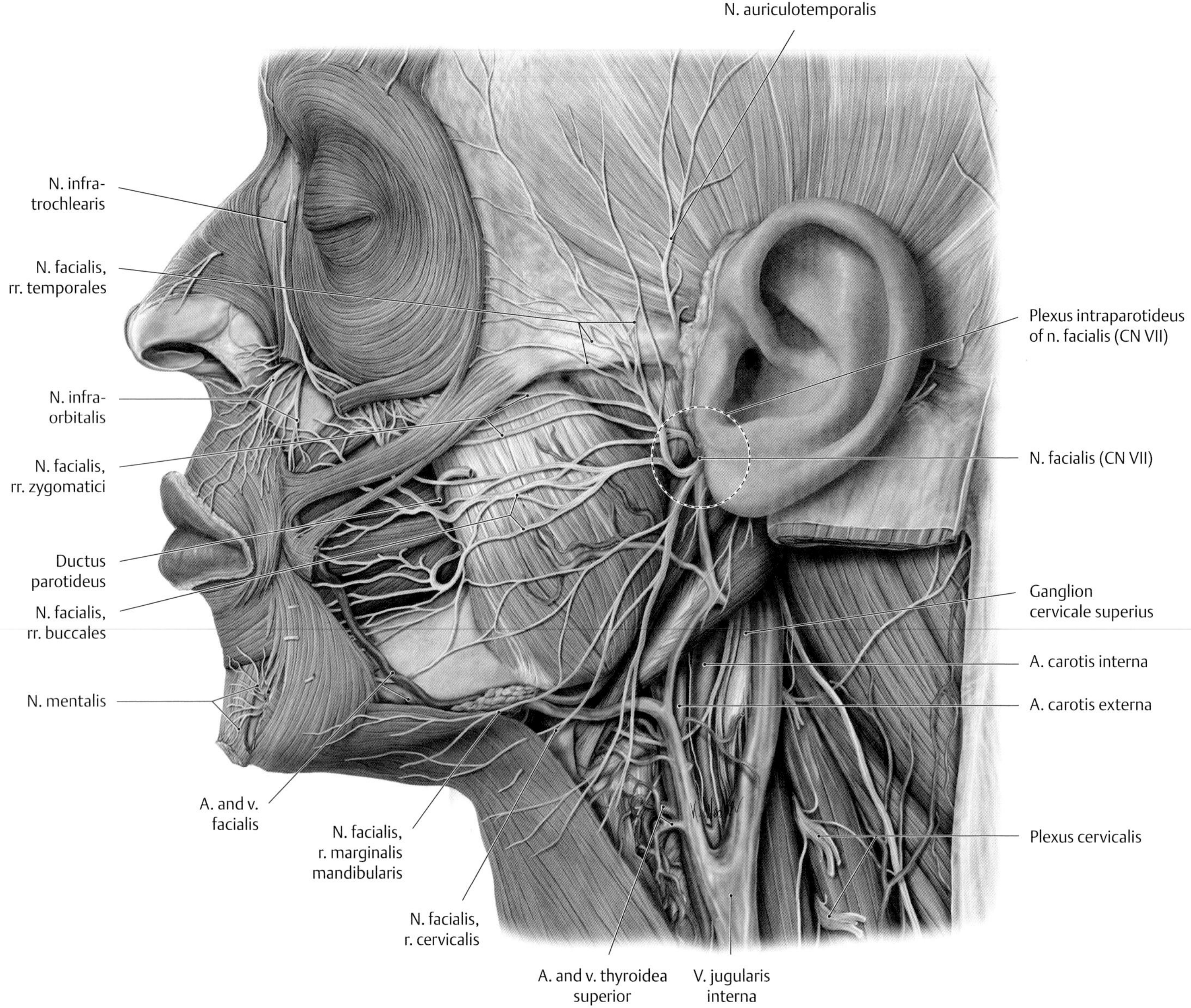
N. auriculotemporalis
N. infra-
trochlearis
N. facialis,
rr. temporales
Plexus intraparotideus
of n. facialis (CN VII)
N. infra-
orbitalis
N. facialis (CN VII)
N. facialis,
rr. zygomatici
Ductus
parotideus
Ganglion
cervicale superius
N. facialis,
rr. buccales
A. carotis interna
N. mentalis
A. carotis externa
A. and v.
facialis
N. facialis,
r. marginalis
mandibularis
Plexus cervicalis
N. facialis,
r. cervicalis
A. and v. thyroidea
superior
V. jugularis
interna

Fig. 32.14 **Parotid region**
Left lateral view. *Removed:* Glandula parotidea, m. sternocleidomastoideus, and veins of the head. *Revealed:* Parotid bed and trigonum caroticum.

Fig. 32.15 Fossa temporalis

Left lateral view. *Removed:* M. sternocleidomastoid and m. masseter. *Revealed:* Fossa temporalis and articulatio temporomandibularis (p. 540).

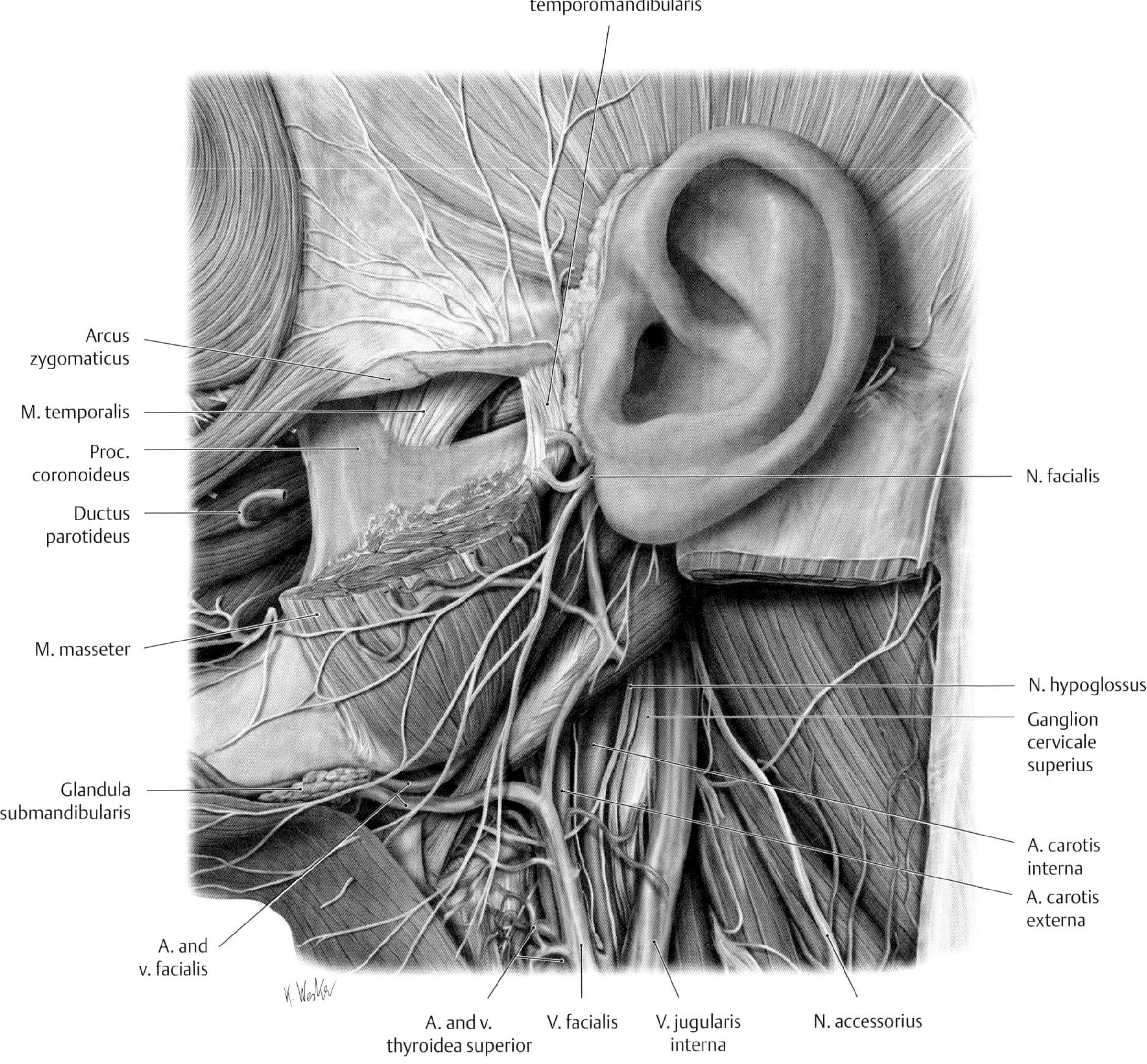

Joint capsule, articulatio temporomandibularis
Arcus zygomaticus
M. temporalis
Proc. coronoideus
Ductus parotideus
M. masseter
Glandula submandibularis
A. and v. facialis
A. and v. thyroidea superior
V. facialis
V. jugularis interna
N. accessorius
N. facialis
N. hypoglossus
Ganglion cervicale superius
A. carotis interna
A. carotis externa

Topography of Fossa Infratemporalis

Fig. 32.16 **Fossa infratemporalis: Superficial layer**
Left lateral view. *Removed:* Ramus mandibulae. *Note:* The n. mylohyoideus (see p. 547) branches from n. alveolaris inferior just before foramen mandibulae.

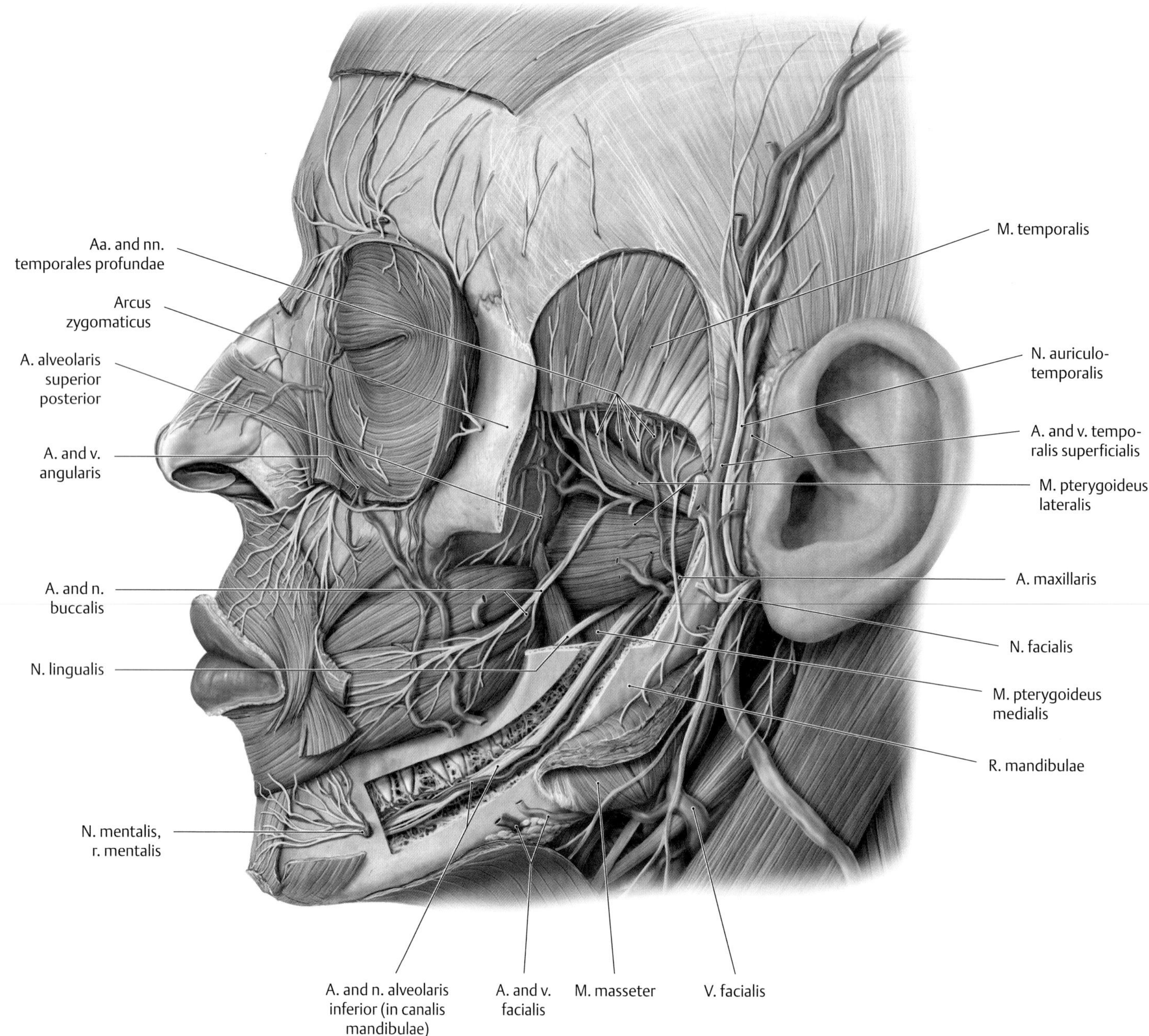
Aa. and nn. temporales profundae
Arcus zygomaticus
A. alveolaris superior posterior
A. and v. angularis
A. and n. buccalis
N. lingualis
N. mentalis, r. mentalis
M. temporalis
N. auriculo-temporalis
A. and v. temporalis superficialis
M. pterygoideus lateralis
A. maxillaris
N. facialis
M. pterygoideus medialis
R. mandibulae
A. and n. alveolaris inferior (in canalis mandibulae)
A. and v. facialis
M. masseter
V. facialis

Fig. 32.17 **Deep layer**

Left lateral view. *Removed:* M. pterygoideus lateralis (both heads). *Revealed:* Deep fossa infratemporalis and n. mandibularis as it enters canalis mandibulae via foramen ovale in the roof of the fossa.

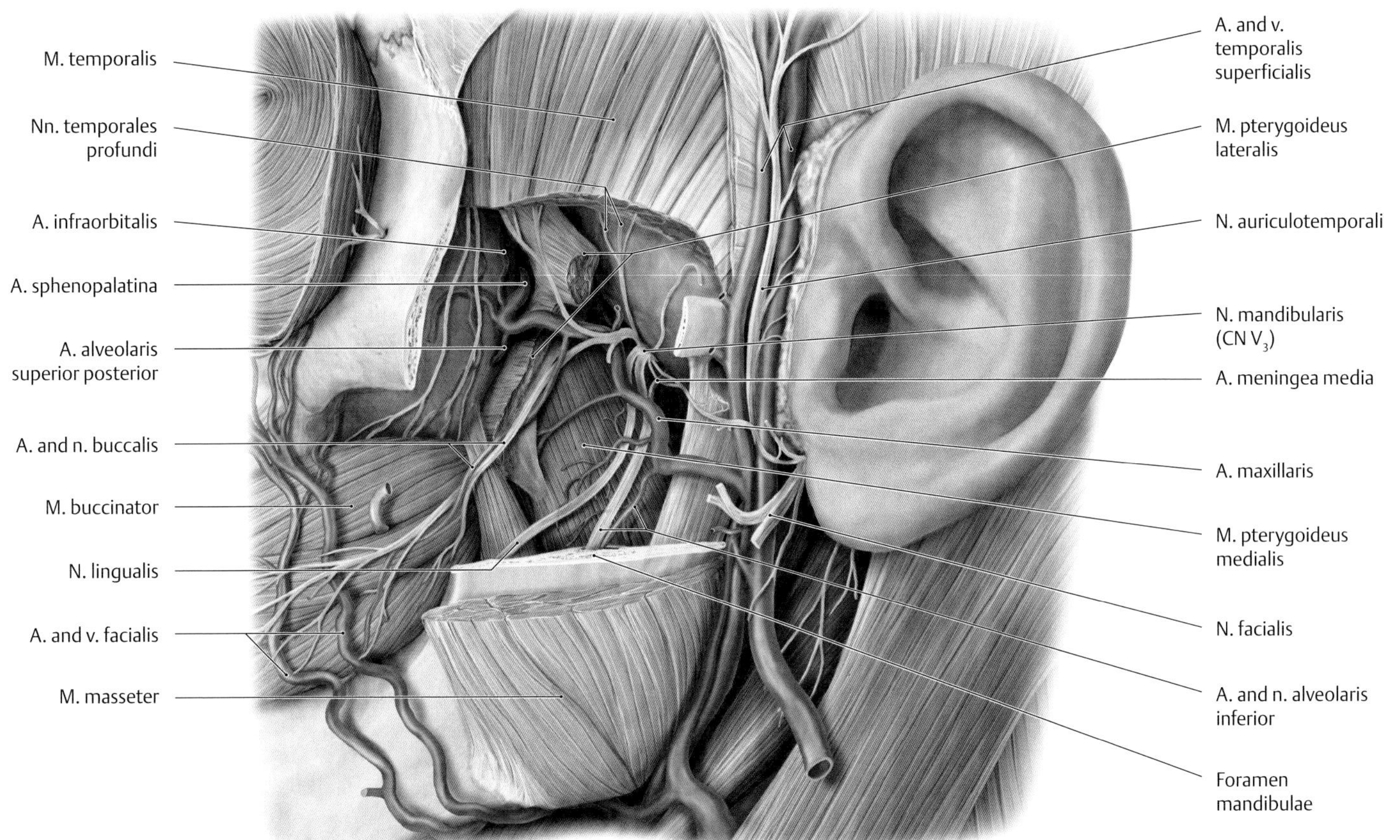
M. temporalis
Nn. temporales profundi
A. infraorbitalis
A. sphenopalatina
A. alveolaris superior posterior
A. and n. buccalis
M. buccinator
N. lingualis
A. and v. facialis
M. masseter
A. and v. temporalis superficialis
M. pterygoideus lateralis
N. auriculotemporalis
N. mandibularis (CN V_3)
A. meningea media
A. maxillaris
M. pterygoideus medialis
N. facialis
A. and n. alveolaris inferior
Foramen mandibulae

Fig. 32.18 **N. mandibularis (CN V_3) in fossa infratemporalis**

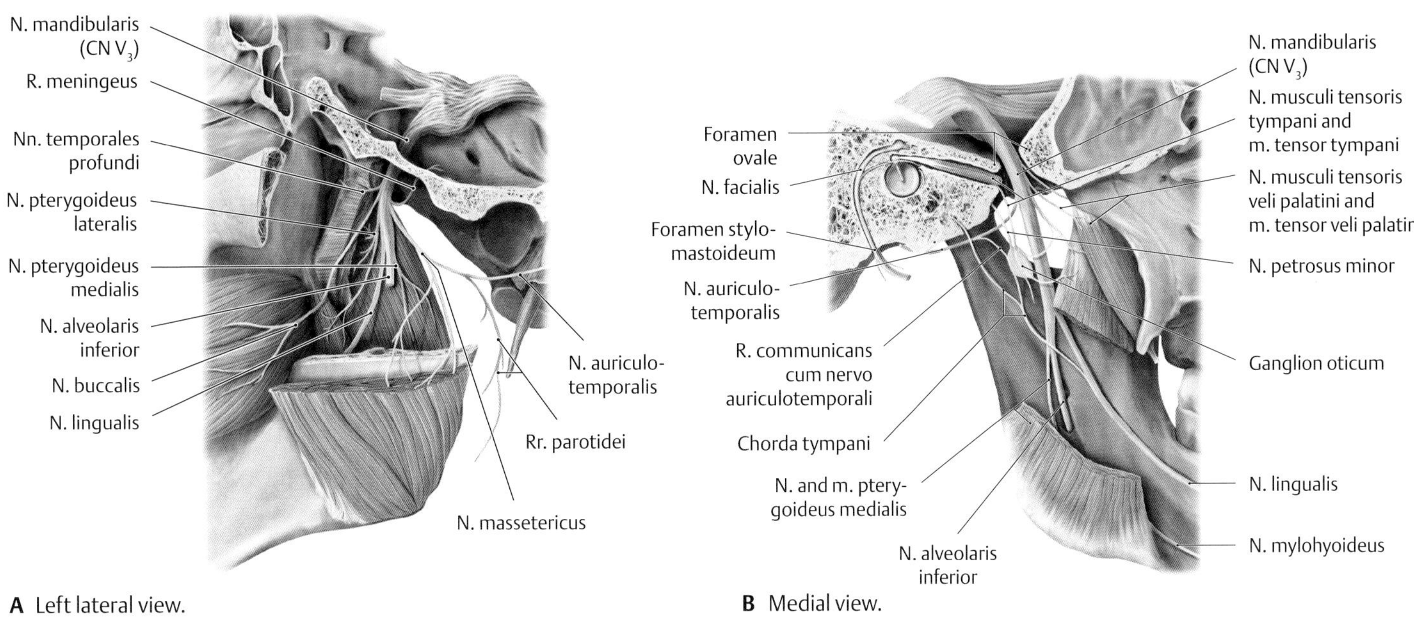
N. mandibularis (CN V_3)
R. meningeus
Nn. temporales profundi
N. pterygoideus lateralis
N. pterygoideus medialis
N. alveolaris inferior
N. buccalis
N. lingualis
N. auriculo-temporalis
Rr. parotidei
N. massetericus
Foramen ovale
N. facialis
Foramen stylo-mastoideum
N. auriculo-temporalis
R. communicans cum nervo auriculotemporali
Chorda tympani
N. and m. ptery-goideus medialis
N. alveolaris inferior
N. mandibularis (CN V_3)
N. musculi tensoris tympani and m. tensor tympani
N. musculi tensoris veli palatini and m. tensor veli palatini
N. petrosus minor
Ganglion oticum
N. lingualis
N. mylohyoideus

A Left lateral view.

B Medial view.

Topography of Fossa Pterygopalatina

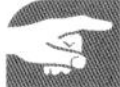

The fossa pterygopalatina is a small pyramidal space just inferior to the apex of the orbita. It is continuous with fossa infratemporalis, with no clear line of demarcation between them. Fossa pterygopalatina is a crossroads for neurovascular structures traveling between fossa cranii media, orbita, nasal cavity, and oral cavity.

Table 32.6 Borders of the Fossa pterygopalatina

Direction	Boundaries	Direction	Boundaries
Superior	Os sphenoidale (ala major), junction with Fissura orbitalis inferior	Posterior	Proc. pterygoideus (lamina lateralis)
Anterior	Tuber maxillae	Lateral	Communicates with the fossa infratemporalis via the fissura pterygomaxillaris
Medial	Os palatinum (lamina perpendicularis)	Inferior	None; opens into the spatium retropharyngeum

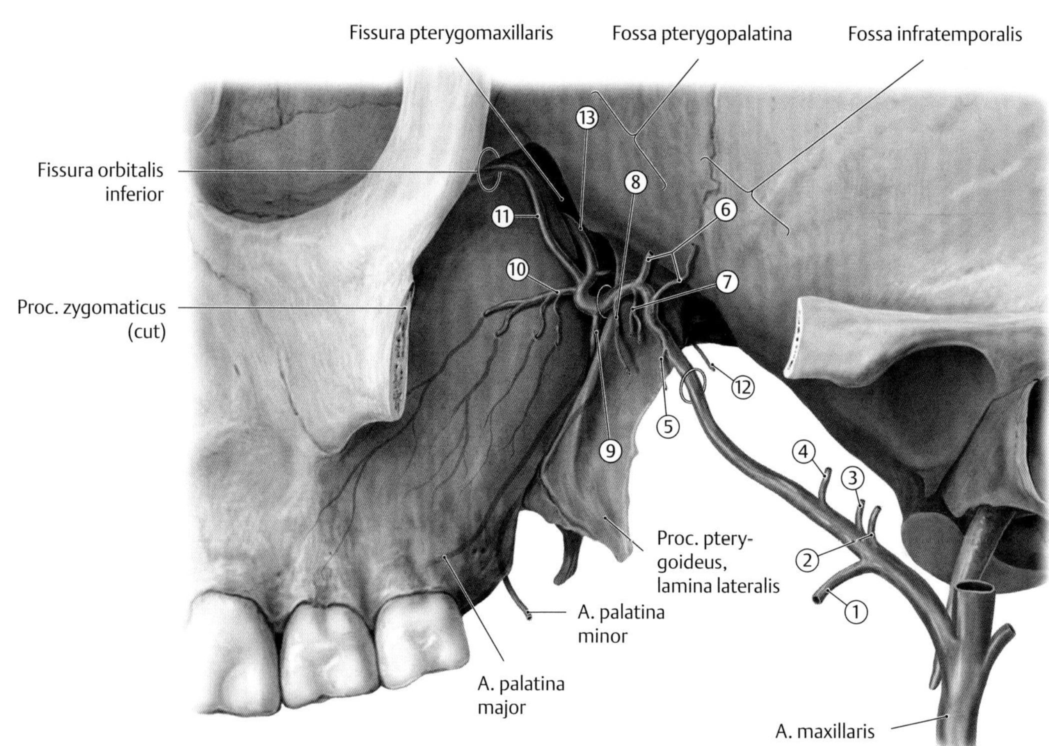

Fissura pterygomaxillaris
Fossa pterygopalatina
Fossa infratemporalis
Fissura orbitalis inferior
Proc. zygomaticus (cut)
Proc. pterygoideus, lamina lateralis
A. palatina minor
A. palatina major
A. maxillaris
①
②
③
④
⑤
⑥
⑦
⑧
⑨
⑩
⑪
⑫
⑬

Fig. 32.19 **Arteries in fossa pterygopalatina**
Left lateral view into area. A. maxillaris passes over m. pterygoideus lateralis in fossa infratemporalis (see Fig. 32.16) and enters fossa pterygopalatina through fissura pterygomaxillaris.

Table 32.7 Rr. of the a. maxillaris

Part	Artery		Distribution
Pars mandibularis	① A. alveolaris inferior		Mandibula, teeth, gingiva
	② A. tympanica anterior		Cavitas tympanica
	③ A. auricularis profunda		Articulatio temporomandibulare, meatus acusticus externus
	④ A. meningea media		Calvaria, dura, fossa cranii ant. and med.
Pars pterygoidea	⑤ A. masseterica		M. masseter
	⑥ Aa. temporales profundae		M. temporalis
	⑦ Rr. pterygoidei		M. pterygoideus
	⑧ A. buccalis		Buccal mucosa
Pars pterygopalatina	⑨ A. palatina descendens	A. palatina major	Hard palate
		A. palatina minor	Soft palate, tonsilla palatina, pharyngeal wall
	⑩ A. alveolaris superior posterior		Maxillary molars, sinus maxillaris, Gingiva
	⑪ A. infraorbitalis		Alveoli dentales of maxilla
	⑫ A. canalis pterygoidei		
	⑬ A. sphenopalatina	Aa. nasales posteriores laterales	Paries lateralis of cavitas nasalis, choanae
		Rr. septales posteriores	Septum nasi

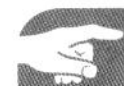

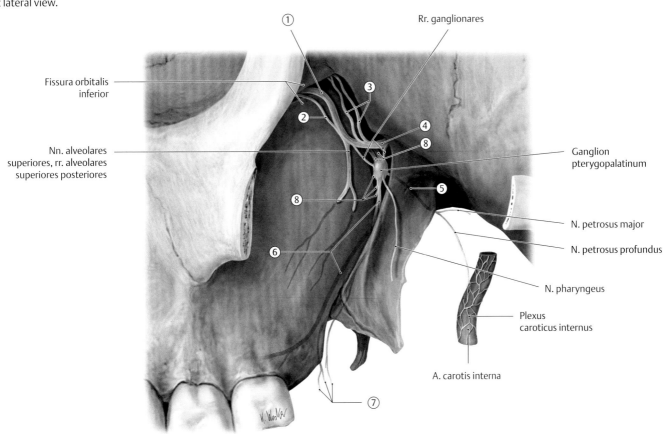

N. maxillaris of n. trigeminus (CN V_2, see p. 477) passes from fossa cranii media through the foramen rotundum into fossa pterygopalatina. The parasympathetic ganglion pterygopalatinum receives presynaptic fibers from the n. petrosus major (the parasympathetic root of n. intermedius of n. facialis). The preganglionic fibers of ganglion pterygopalatinum synapse with ganglion cells that innervate the lacrimal, small palatal, and small nasal glands. The sympathetic fibers of n. petrosus profundus (sympathetic root) and sensory fibers of n. maxillaris (sensory root) pass through ganglion pterygopalatinum without synapsing.

Fig. 32.20 **Nerves in the pterygopalatine fossa**
Left lateral view.

①
Rr. ganglionares
Fissura orbitalis inferior
③
②
④
⑧
Nn. alveolares superiores, rr. alveolares superiores posteriores
Ganglion pterygopalatinum
⑤
⑧
N. petrosus major
N. petrosus profundus
⑥
N. pharyngeus
Plexus caroticus internus
A. carotis interna
⑦

Table 32.8 Passage of neurovascular structures into fossa pterygopalatina

Origin of structures	Passageway	Transmitted nerves	Transmitted vessels
Orbita	Fissura orbitalis inferior	① N. infraorbitalis	A. infraorbitalis (and accompanying vv.)
		② N. zygomaticus	V. ophthalmica inferior
		③ Rr. orbitales (from CN V_2)	
Fossa cranii media	Foramen rotundum	④ N. maxillaris (CN V_2)	
Basis cranii	Canalis pterygoideus	⑤ N. canalis pterygoidei (n. petrosus major and n. petrosus minor)	A. canalis pterygoidei (with accompanying vv.)
Palatum	Foramen palatinum majus	⑥ N. palatinus major	A. palatina descendens
			A. palatina major
	Foramen palatinum minus	⑦ N. palatinus minor	Aa. patatinae minores (r. terminalis of a. palatina descendens)
Cavitas nasalis	Foramen sphenopalatinum	⑧ Medial and lateral rr. nasales posteriores superiores and inferiores (from n. nasopalatinus, CN V_2)	A. sphenopalatina (with accompanying vv.)

Bones of the Orbita

Fig. 33.1 Bones of the orbita

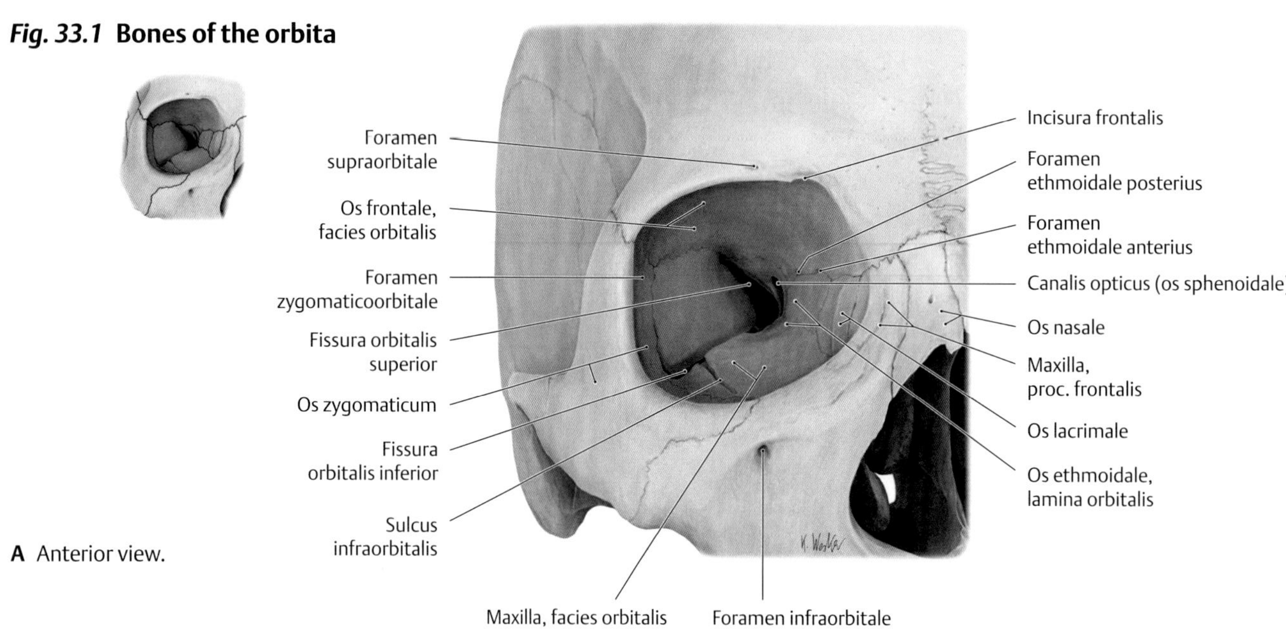
Foramen supraorbitale
Os frontale, facies orbitalis
Foramen zygomaticoorbitale
Fissura orbitalis superior
Os zygomaticum
Fissura orbitalis inferior
Sulcus infraorbitalis
Maxilla, facies orbitalis
Foramen infraorbitale
Incisura frontalis
Foramen ethmoidale posterius
Foramen ethmoidale anterius
Canalis opticus (os sphenoidale)
Os nasale
Maxilla, proc. frontalis
Os lacrimale
Os ethmoidale, lamina orbitalis

A Anterior view.

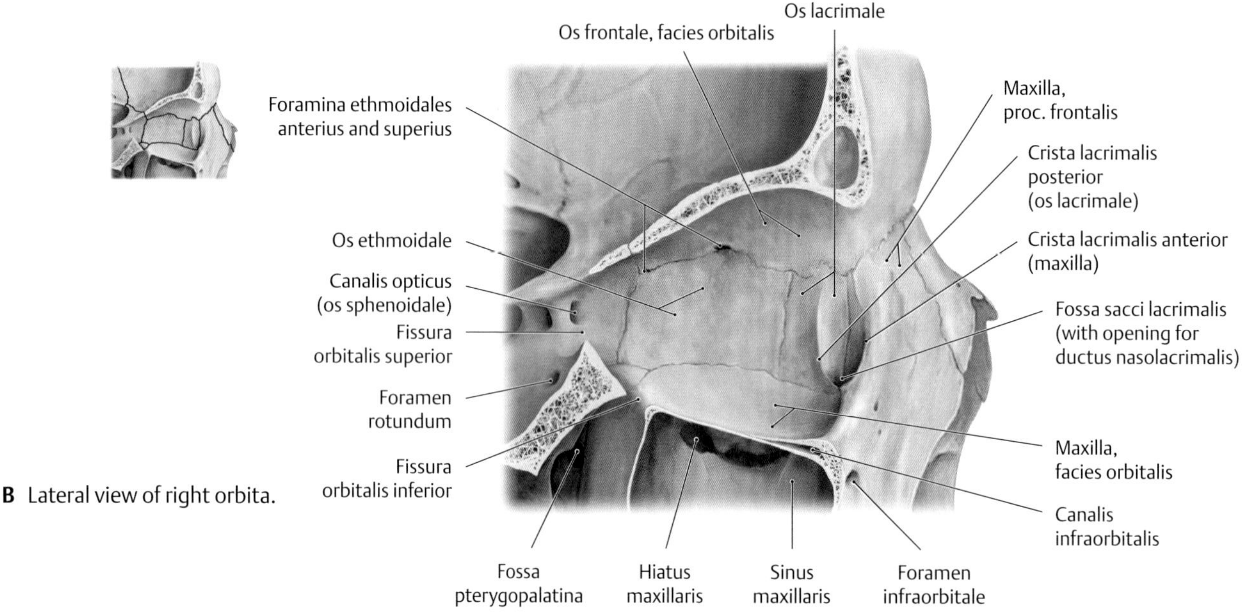
Os lacrimale
Os frontale, facies orbitalis
Foramina ethmoidales anterius and superius
Os ethmoidale
Canalis opticus (os sphenoidale)
Fissura orbitalis superior
Foramen rotundum
Fissura orbitalis inferior
Fossa pterygopalatina
Hiatus maxillaris
Sinus maxillaris
Foramen infraorbitale
Maxilla, proc. frontalis
Crista lacrimalis posterior (os lacrimale)
Crista lacrimalis anterior (maxilla)
Fossa sacci lacrimalis (with opening for ductus nasolacrimalis)
Maxilla, facies orbitalis
Canalis infraorbitalis

B Lateral view of right orbita.

Table 33.1 Openings in the orbita for neurovascular structures

Opening*	Nerves		Vessels
Canalis opticus	N. opticus (CN II)		A. ophthalmica
Fissura orbitalis superior	N. oculomotorius (CN III) N. trochlearis (CN IV) N. abducens (CN VI)	N. trigeminus, ophthalmic division (CN V_1) • N. lacrimalis • N. frontalis • N. nasociliaris	V. ophthalmica superior
Fissura orbitalis inferior	N. infraorbitalis (CN V_2) N. zygomaticus (CN V_2)		A. and v. infraorbitalis, v. ophthalmica inferior
Canalis infraorbitalis	N. infraorbitalis (CN V_2), a., and v.		
Foramen supraorbitale	N. supraorbitalis (r. lateralis)		A. supraorbitalis
Incisura frontalis	N. supraorbitalis (r. medialis)		A. supratrochlearis
Foramen ethmoidale anterior	N., a., and v. ethmoidalis anterior		
Foramen ethmoidale posterior	N., a., and v. ethmoidalis posterior		

* The canalis nasolacrimalis transmits the duchtus nasolacrimalis.

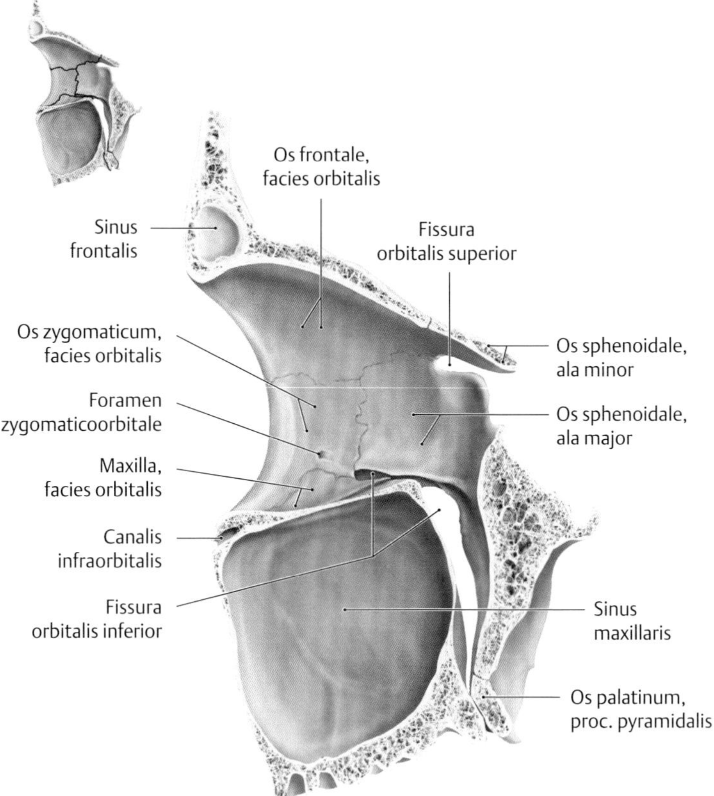

Os frontale, facies orbitalis
Sinus frontalis
Fissura orbitalis superior
Os zygomaticum, facies orbitalis
Os sphenoidale, ala minor
Foramen zygomaticoorbitale
Os sphenoidale, ala major
Maxilla, facies orbitalis
Canalis infraorbitalis
Fissura orbitalis inferior
Sinus maxillaris
Os palatinum, proc. pyramidalis

C Medial view of right orbita.

Table 33.2	**Structures surrounding the orbita**
Direction	**Bordering structure**
Superior	Sinus frontalis
	Fossa cranii anterior
Medial	Sinus ethmoidalis
Inferior	Sinus maxillaris
Certain deeper structures also have a clinically important relationship to the orbita:	
Sinus sphenoidalis	Glandula pituitaria
Fossa cranii media	Sinus cavernosus
Chiasma opticum	Fossa pterygopalatina

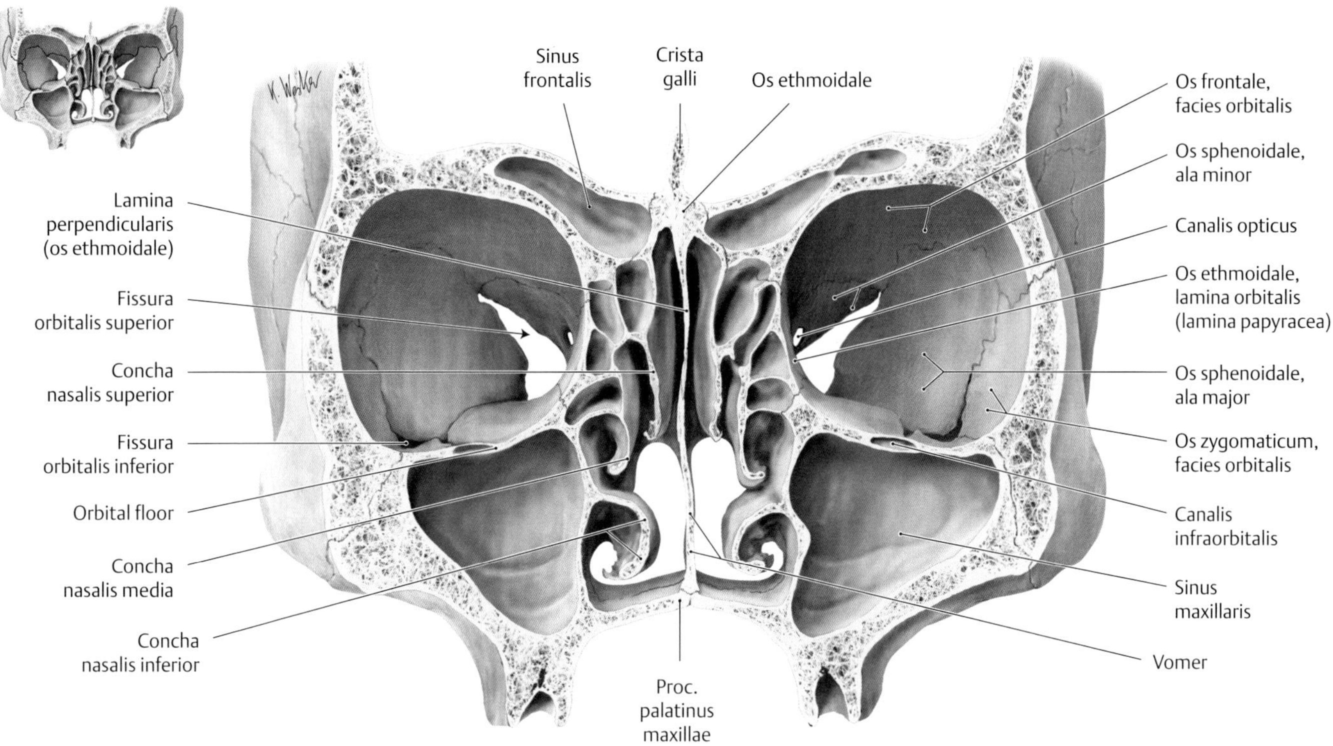

Sinus frontalis
Crista galli
Os ethmoidale
Os frontale, facies orbitalis
Os sphenoidale, ala minor
Lamina perpendicularis (os ethmoidale)
Canalis opticus
Os ethmoidale, lamina orbitalis (lamina papyracea)
Fissura orbitalis superior
Concha nasalis superior
Os sphenoidale, ala major
Fissura orbitalis inferior
Os zygomaticum, facies orbitalis
Orbital floor
Canalis infraorbitalis
Concha nasalis media
Sinus maxillaris
Concha nasalis inferior
Vomer
Proc. palatinus maxillae

D Coronal section, anterior view.

Muscles of the Orbita

Fig. 33.2 Extraocular muscles

Right eye, superior view (except **A**). The eyeball is moved by six extrinsic muscles: four rectus (mm. rectus superior, inferior, medialis, and lateralis) and two oblique (mm. obliquus superior and inferior).

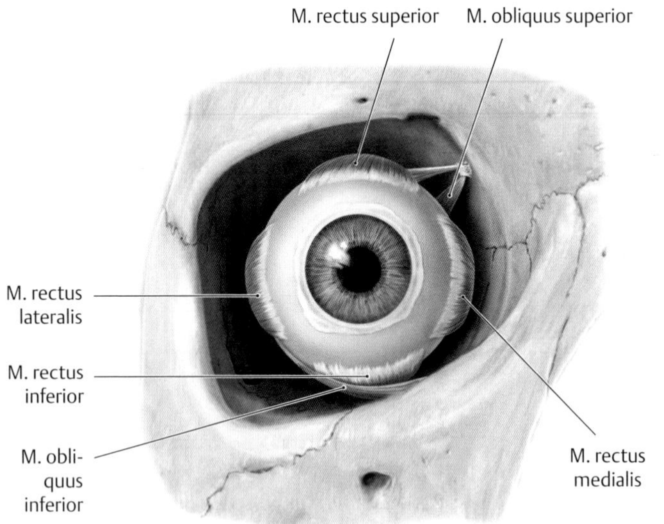

M. rectus superior
M. obliquus superior
M. rectus lateralis
M. rectus inferior
M. obli-quus inferior
M. rectus medialis

A Anterior view.

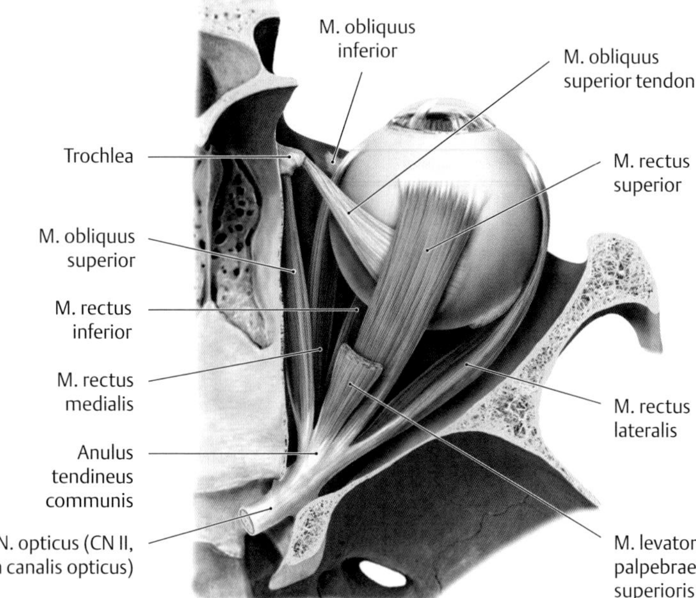

M. obliquus inferior
M. obliquus superior tendon
Trochlea
M. rectus superior
M. obliquus superior
M. rectus inferior
M. rectus medialis
M. rectus lateralis
Anulus tendineus communis
N. opticus (CN II, in canalis opticus)
M. levator palpebrae superioris

B Superior view of opened orbita.

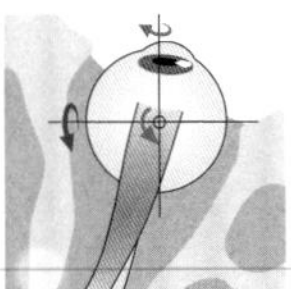

C M. rectus superior.

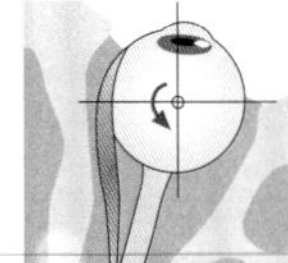

D M. rectus medialis.

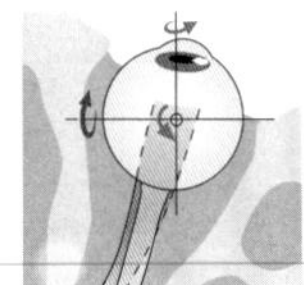

E M. rectus inferior.

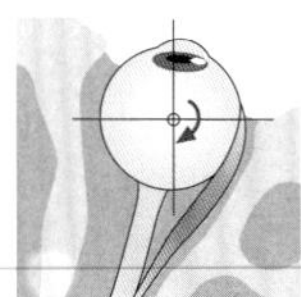

F M. rectus lateralis.

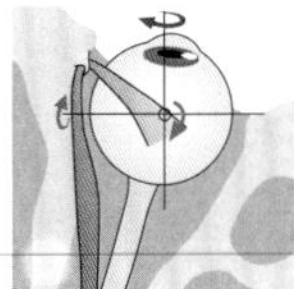

G M. obliquus superior.

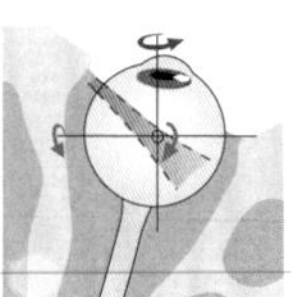

H M. obliquus inferior.

Table 33.3 Extraocular muscles

Muscle	Origin	Insertion	Primary action (red)	Secondary action (blue)	Innervation
M. rectus superior	Anulus tendineus communis	Sclera of the eye	Elevation	Adduction and medial rotation	N. oculomotorius (CN III), r. superior
M. rectus medialis			Adduction	–	N. oculomotorius (CN III), r. inferior
M. rectus inferior			Depression	Adduction and lateral rotation	
M. rectus lateralis			Abduction	–	N. abducens (CN VI)
M. obliquus superior	Os sphenoidale*		Depression and abduction	Medial rotation	N. trochlearis (CN IV)
M. obliquus inferior	Margo orbitalis medialis		Elevation and abduction	Lateral rotation	N. oculomotorius (CN III), r. inferior

* The tendon of insertion of the m. obliquus superior passes through a tendinous loop (trochlea) attached to the margo orbitalis superomedialis.

Fig. 33.3 Cardinal directions of gaze

There are six cardinal directions of gaze, all of which are tested during clinical evaluation of ocular motility. *Note:* Each gaze requires activation of two different muscles (not a muscle pair) and therefore two cranial nerves.

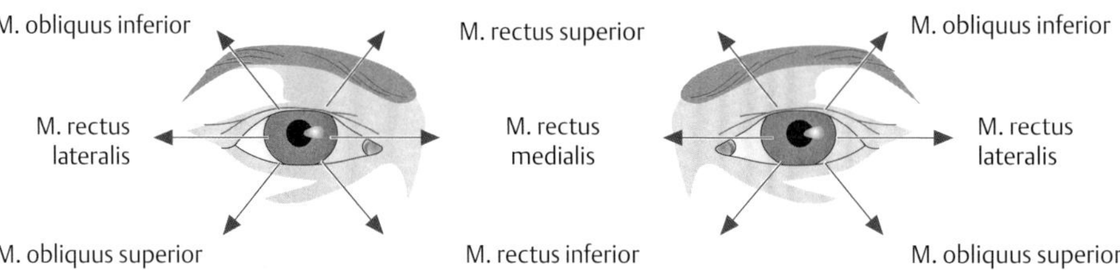

M. obliquus inferior
M. rectus superior
M. obliquus inferior
M. rectus lateralis
M. rectus medialis
M. rectus lateralis
M. obliquus superior
M. rectus inferior
M. obliquus superior

Fig. 33.4 **Innervation of the extraocular muscles**
Right eye, lateral view with the temporal wall of the orbita removed.

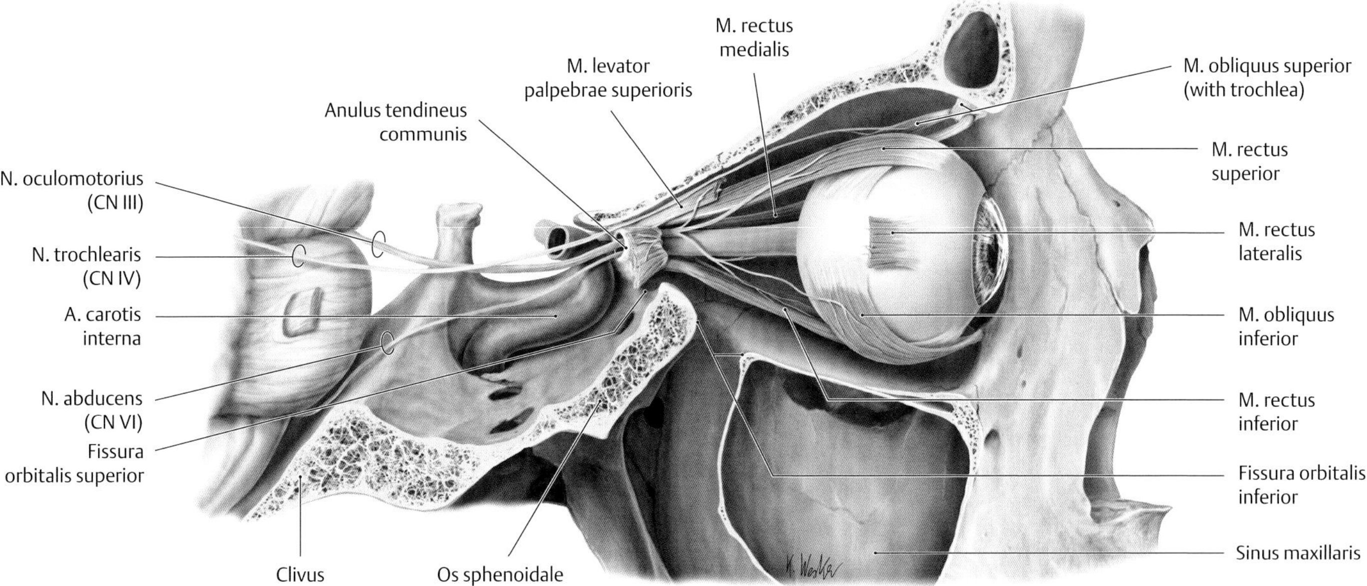
M. rectus medialis
M. levator palpebrae superioris
Anulus tendineus communis
N. oculomotorius (CN III)
N. trochlearis (CN IV)
A. carotis interna
N. abducens (CN VI)
Fissura orbitalis superior
Clivus
Os sphenoidale
M. obliquus superior (with trochlea)
M. rectus superior
M. rectus lateralis
M. obliquus inferior
M. rectus inferior
Fissura orbitalis inferior
Sinus maxillaris

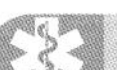

Clinical

N. oculomotorius palsies

N. oculomotorius palsies may result from a lesion involving an eye muscle or its associated cranial nerve (at the nucleus or along the course of the nerve). If one extraocular muscle is weak or paralyzed, deviation of the eye will be noted. Impairment of the coordinated actions of the extraocular muscles may cause the visual axis of one eye to deviate from its normal position. The patient will therefore perceive a double image (diplopia).

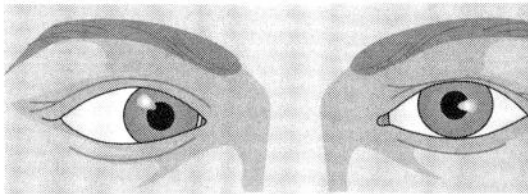

A N. abducens palsy. *Disabled:* M. rectus lateralis.

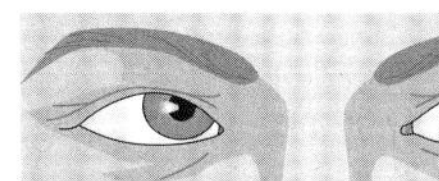
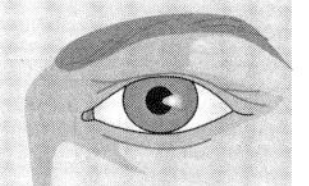

B N. trochlearis palsy. *Disabled:* M. obliquus superior.

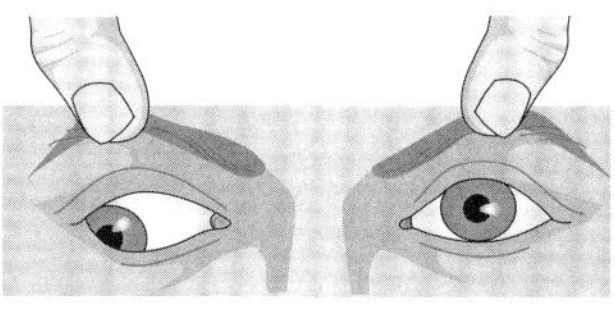

C Complete n. oculomotorius palsy. *Disabled:* Mm. rectus superior and inferior and m. obliquus inferior.

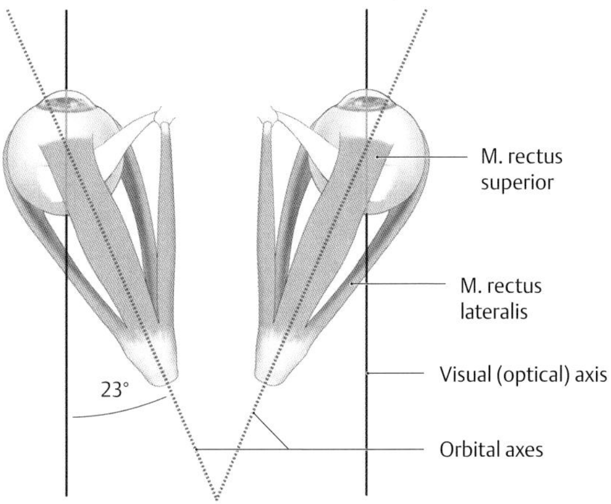
M. rectus superior
M. rectus lateralis
Visual (optical) axis
Orbital axes
23°

D Normal visual and orbital axes.

Neurovasculature of the Orbita

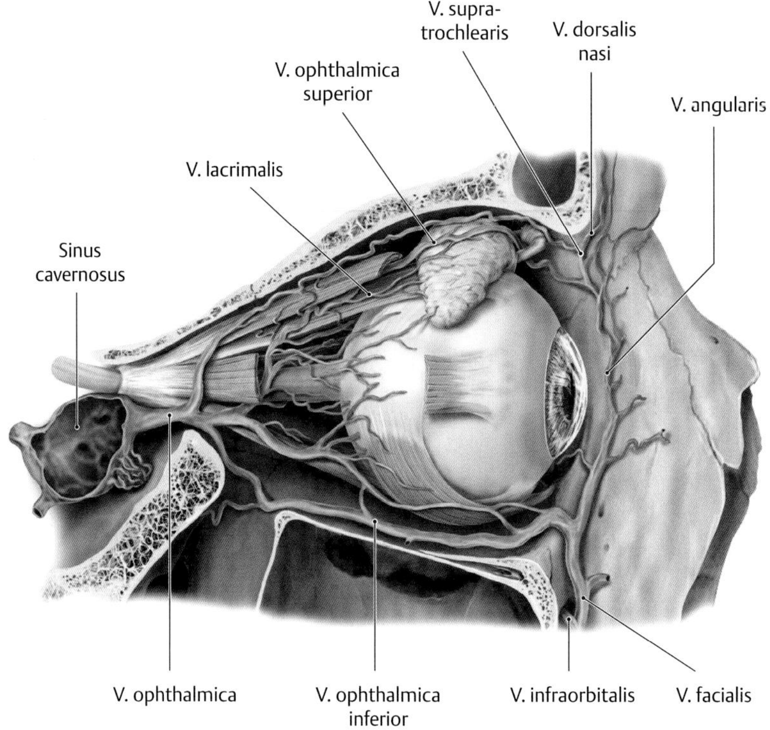
V. supra-
trochlearis
V. dorsalis
nasi
V. ophthalmica
superior
V. angularis
V. lacrimalis
Sinus
cavernosus
V. ophthalmica
V. ophthalmica
inferior
V. infraorbitalis
V. facialis

Fig. 33.5 **Veins of the orbita**
Lateral view of the right orbita. *Removed:* Lateral orbital wall. *Opened:* Sinus maxillaris.

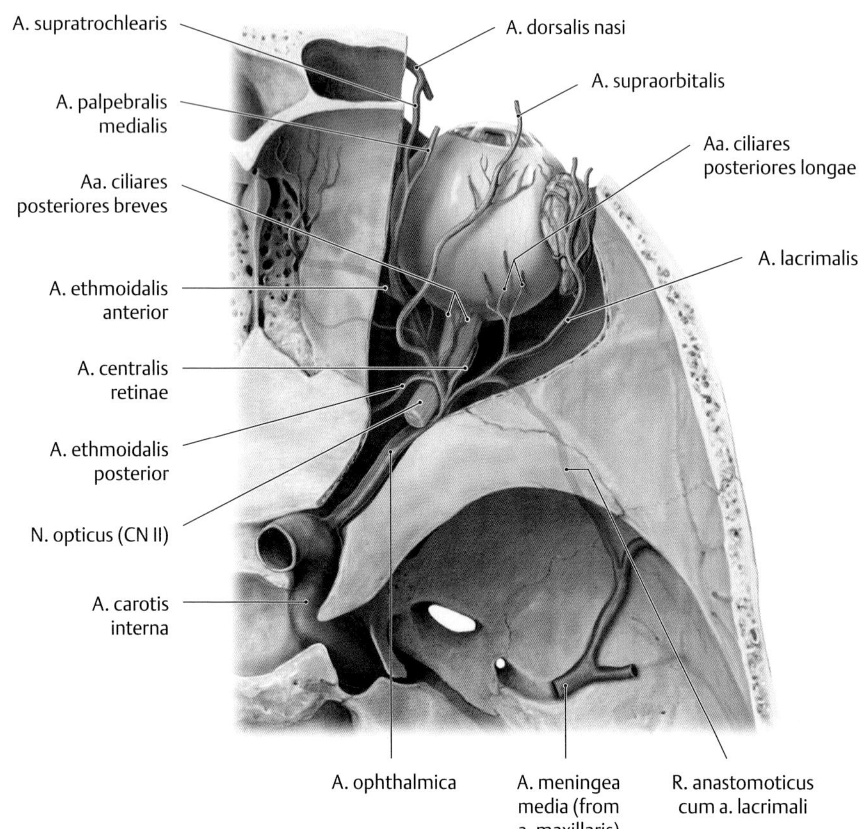
A. supratrochlearis
A. dorsalis nasi
A. supraorbitalis
A. palpebralis
medialis
Aa. ciliares
posteriores longae
Aa. ciliares
posteriores breves
A. lacrimalis
A. ethmoidalis
anterior
A. centralis
retinae
A. ethmoidalis
posterior
N. opticus (CN II)
A. carotis
interna
A. ophthalmica
A. meningea
media (from
a. maxillaris)
R. anastomoticus
cum a. lacrimali

Fig. 33.6 **Arteries of the orbita**
Superior view of the right orbita. *Opened:* Canalis opticus and orbital roof.

Fig. 33.7 Innervation of the orbita

Lateral view of the right orbita. *Removed:* Temporal bony wall.

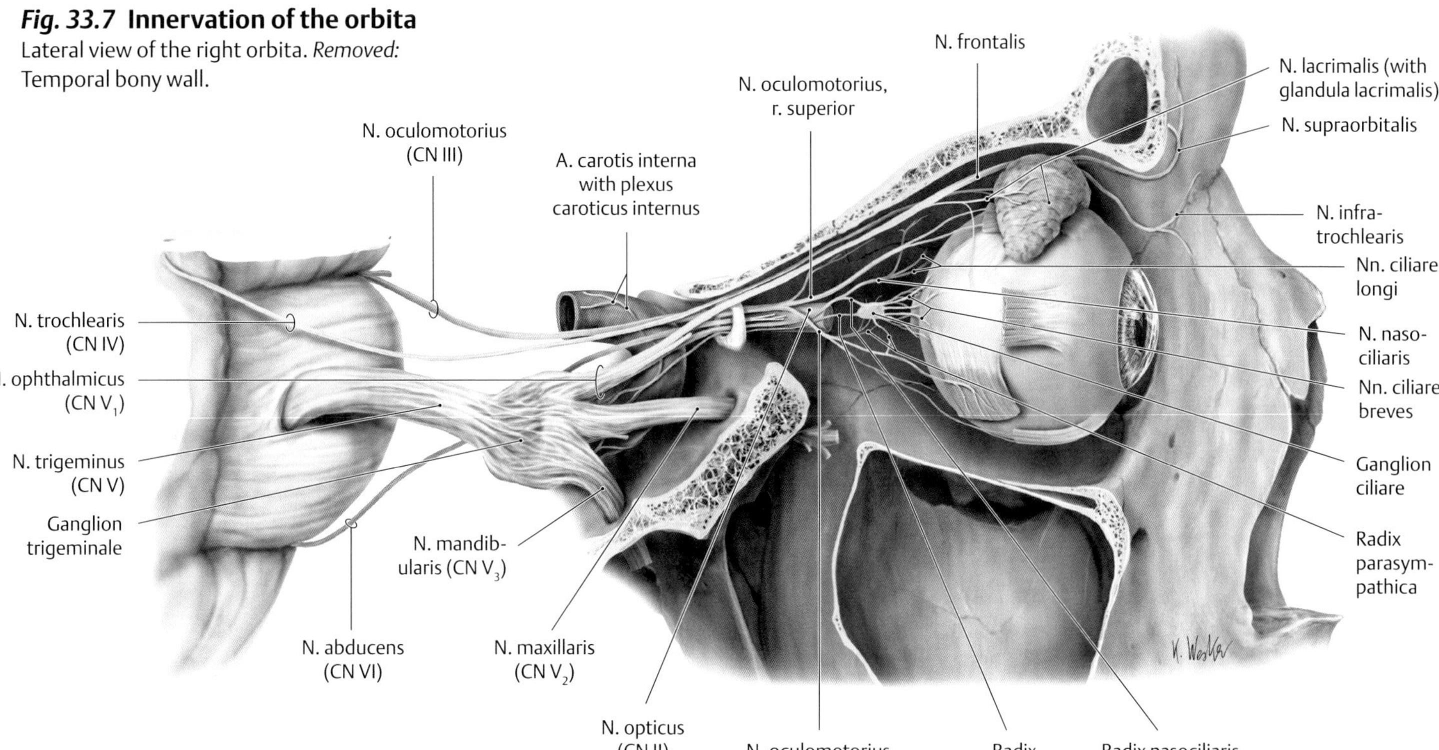
N. frontalis
N. oculomotorius, r. superior
N. lacrimalis (with glandula lacrimalis)
N. supraorbitalis
N. oculomotorius (CN III)
A. carotis interna with plexus caroticus internus
N. infra-trochlearis
Nn. ciliares longi
N. trochlearis (CN IV)
N. naso-ciliaris
N. ophthalmicus (CN V_1)
Nn. ciliares breves
N. trigeminus (CN V)
Ganglion ciliare
Ganglion trigeminale
N. mandib-ularis (CN V_3)
Radix parasym-pathica
N. abducens (CN VI)
N. maxillaris (CN V_2)
N. opticus (CN II)
N. oculomotorius, r. inferior
Radix sympathica
Radix nasociliaris (sensoria)

Fig. 33.8 Cranial nerves in the orbit

Superior view of fossae cranii anterior and posterior. *Removed:* Sinus cavernosus (lateral and superior walls), orbital roof, and periorbita (portions). The trigeminal ganglion has been retracted laterally.

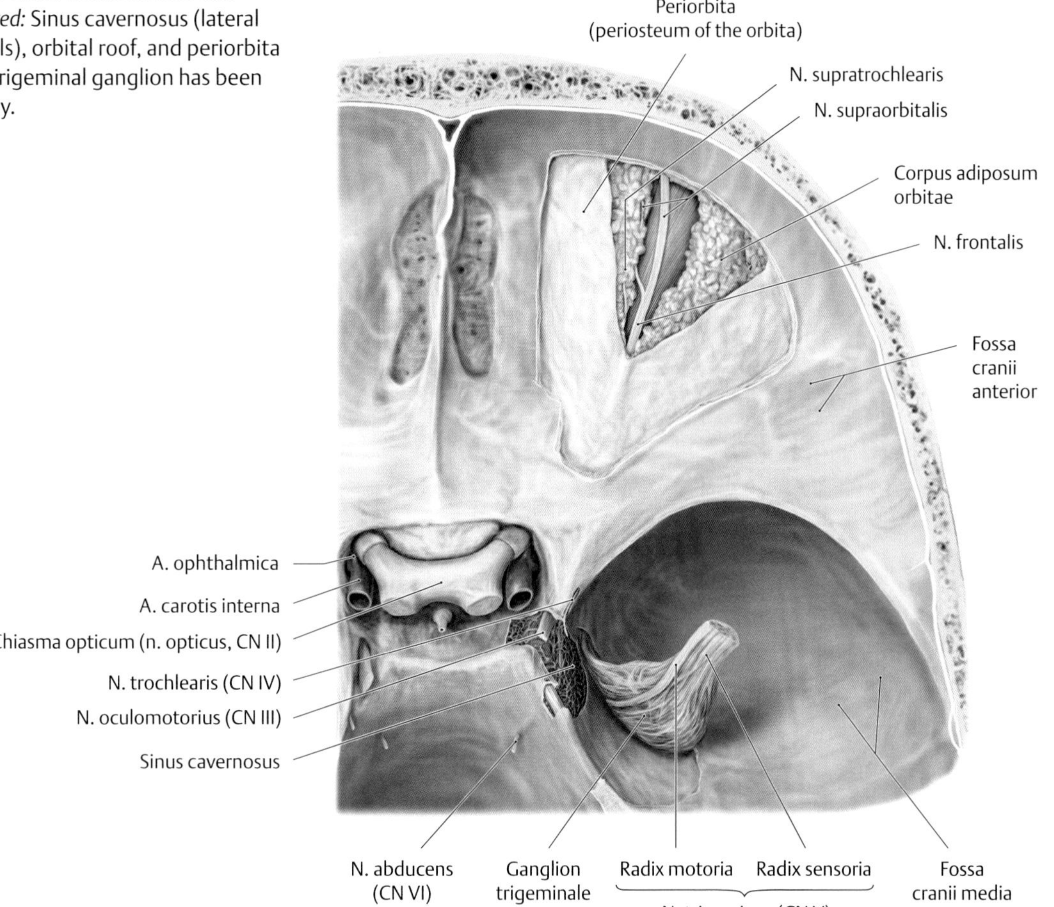
Periorbita (periosteum of the orbita)
N. supratrochlearis
N. supraorbitalis
Corpus adiposum orbitae
N. frontalis
Fossa cranii anterior
A. ophthalmica
A. carotis interna
Chiasma opticum (n. opticus, CN II)
N. trochlearis (CN IV)
N. oculomotorius (CN III)
Sinus cavernosus
N. abducens (CN VI)
Ganglion trigeminale
Radix motoria
Radix sensoria
N. trigeminus (CN V)
Fossa cranii media

Topography of the Orbita

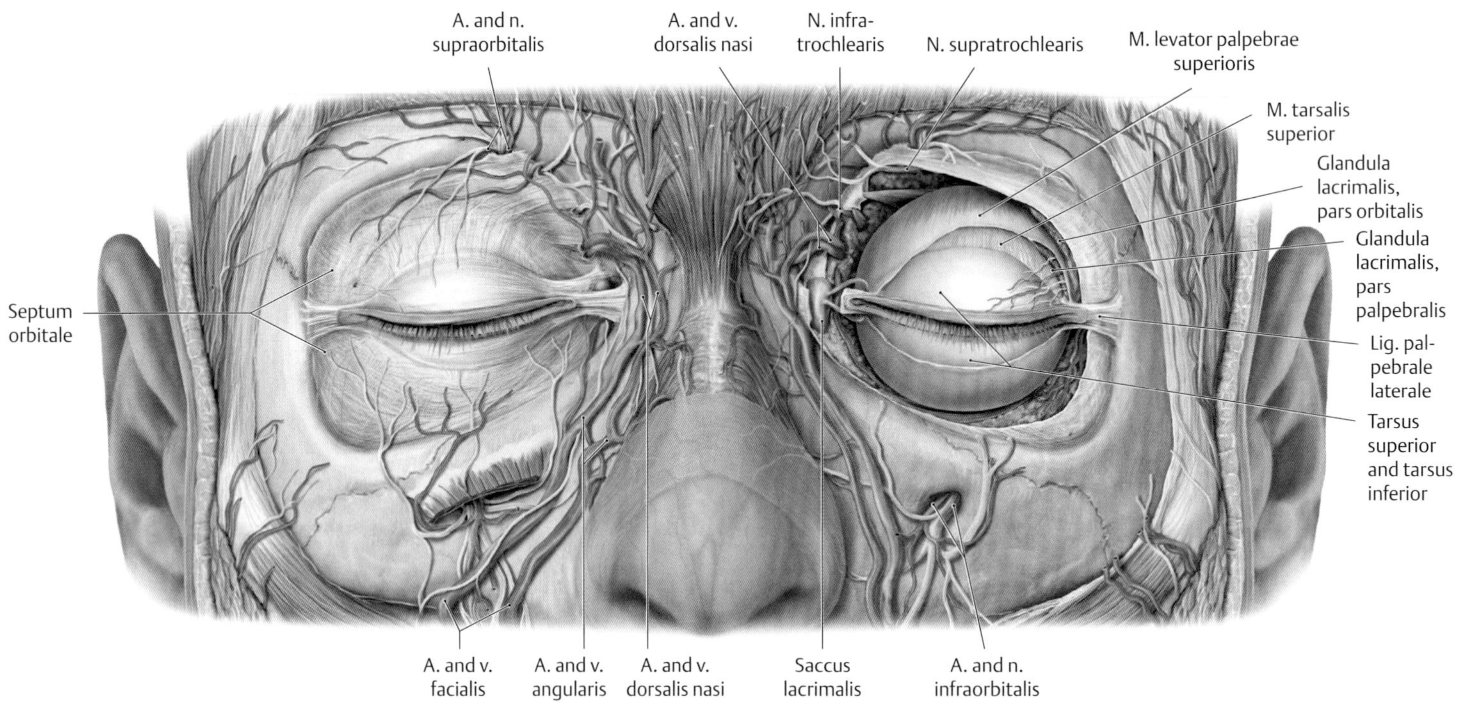
A. and n. supraorbitalis
A. and v. dorsalis nasi
N. infra-trochlearis
N. supratrochlearis
M. levator palpebrae superioris
M. tarsalis superior
Glandula lacrimalis, pars orbitalis
Glandula lacrimalis, pars palpebralis
Lig. pal-pebrale laterale
Tarsus superior and tarsus inferior
Septum orbitale
A. and v. facialis
A. and v. angularis
A. and v. dorsalis nasi
Saccus lacrimalis
A. and n. infraorbitalis

Fig. 33.9 **Neurovascular structures of the orbita**
Anterior view. *Right side:* M. orbicularis oculi removed. *Left side:* Septum orbitale partially removed.

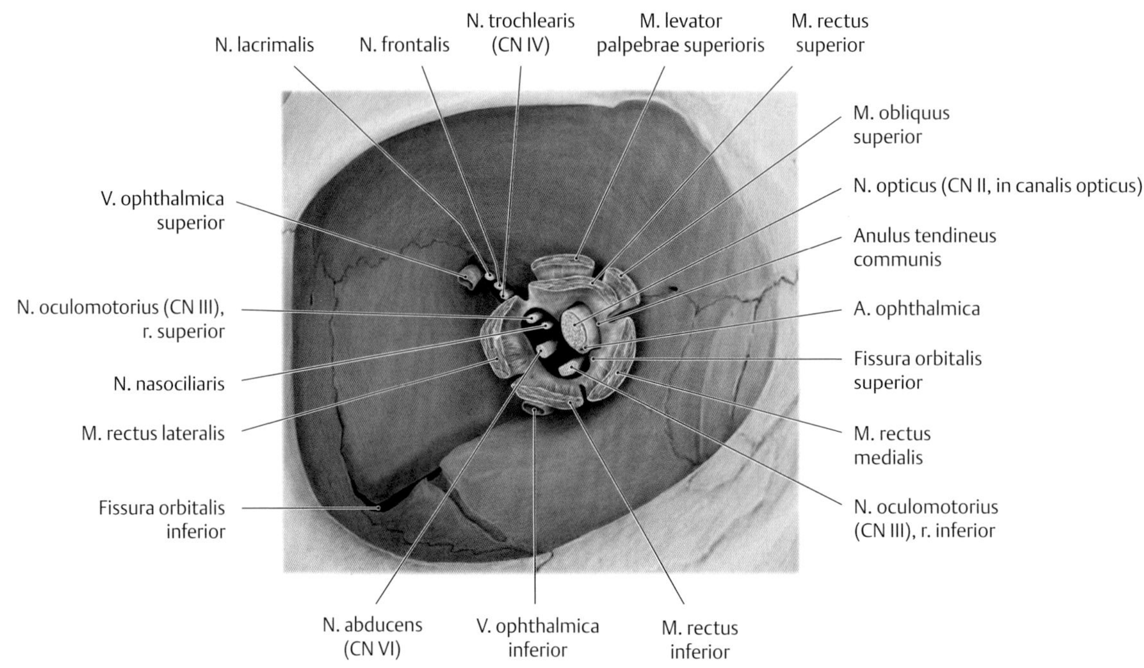
N. lacrimalis
N. frontalis
N. trochlearis (CN IV)
M. levator palpebrae superioris
M. rectus superior
M. obliquus superior
N. opticus (CN II, in canalis opticus)
Anulus tendineus communis
A. ophthalmica
Fissura orbitalis superior
M. rectus medialis
N. oculomotorius (CN III), r. inferior
V. ophthalmica superior
N. oculomotorius (CN III), r. superior
N. nasociliaris
M. rectus lateralis
Fissura orbitalis inferior
N. abducens (CN VI)
V. ophthalmica inferior
M. rectus inferior

Fig. 33.10 **Passage of neurovascular structures through the orbita**
Anterior view. *Removed:* Orbital contents. *Note:* N. opticus and a. ophthalmica travel in canalis opticus. The remaining structures pass through fissura orbitalis superior.

Fig. 33.11 **Neurovascular contents of the orbita**
Superior view. *Removed:* Bony roof of orbita, peritorbita, and corpus adiposum orbitae.

V. ophthalmica superior
Aa. and nn. supraorbitales
N. infratrochlearis
Lamina cribrosa
A. and n. ethmoidalis anterior
A. and n. supratrochlearis
A. and n. ethmoidalis posterior
A. supraorbitalis
N. nasociliaris
N. trochlearis (CN IV)
M. levator palpebrae superioris
A. and n. lacrimalis, glandula lacrimalis
M. rectus superior
N. abducens (CN VI)
V. ophthalmica inferior
N. frontalis

A Upper level.

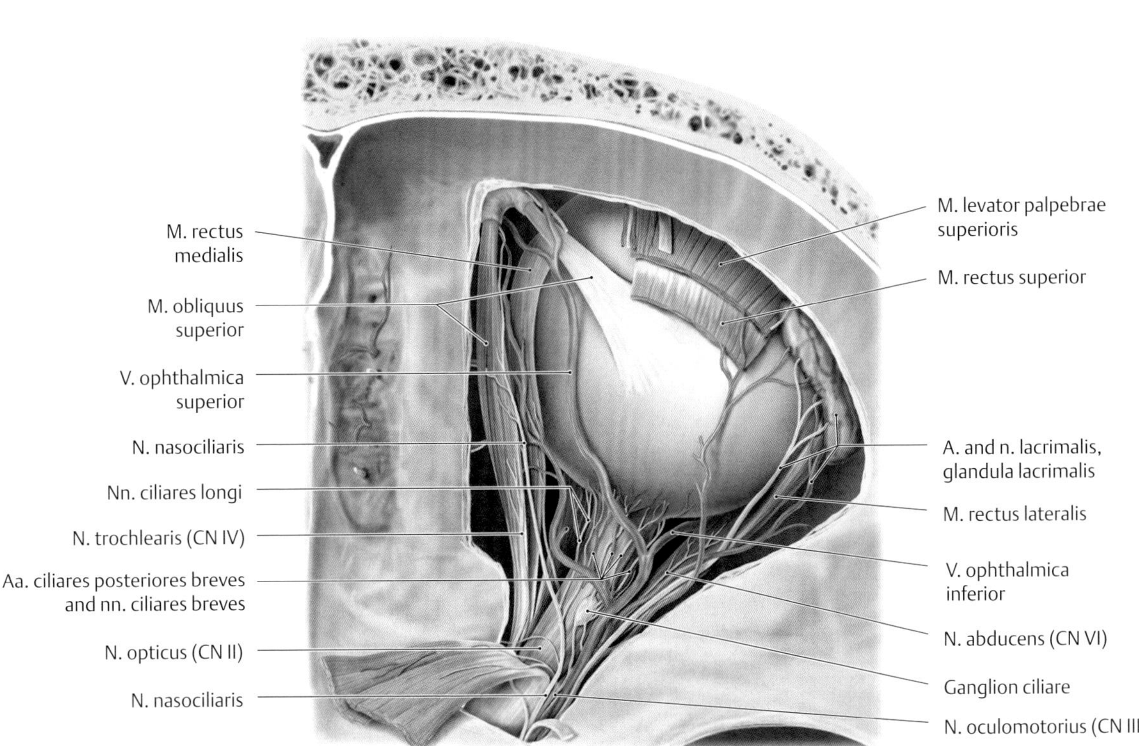
M. rectus medialis
M. obliquus superior
V. ophthalmica superior
N. nasociliaris
Nn. ciliares longi
N. trochlearis (CN IV)
Aa. ciliares posteriores breves and nn. ciliares breves
N. opticus (CN II)
N. nasociliaris
M. levator palpebrae superioris
M. rectus superior
A. and n. lacrimalis, glandula lacrimalis
M. rectus lateralis
V. ophthalmica inferior
N. abducens (CN VI)
Ganglion ciliare
N. oculomotorius (CN III)

B Middle level. *Reflected:* M. levator palpebrae superioris and m. rectus superior. *Revealed:* N. opticus.

Orbita & Eyelid

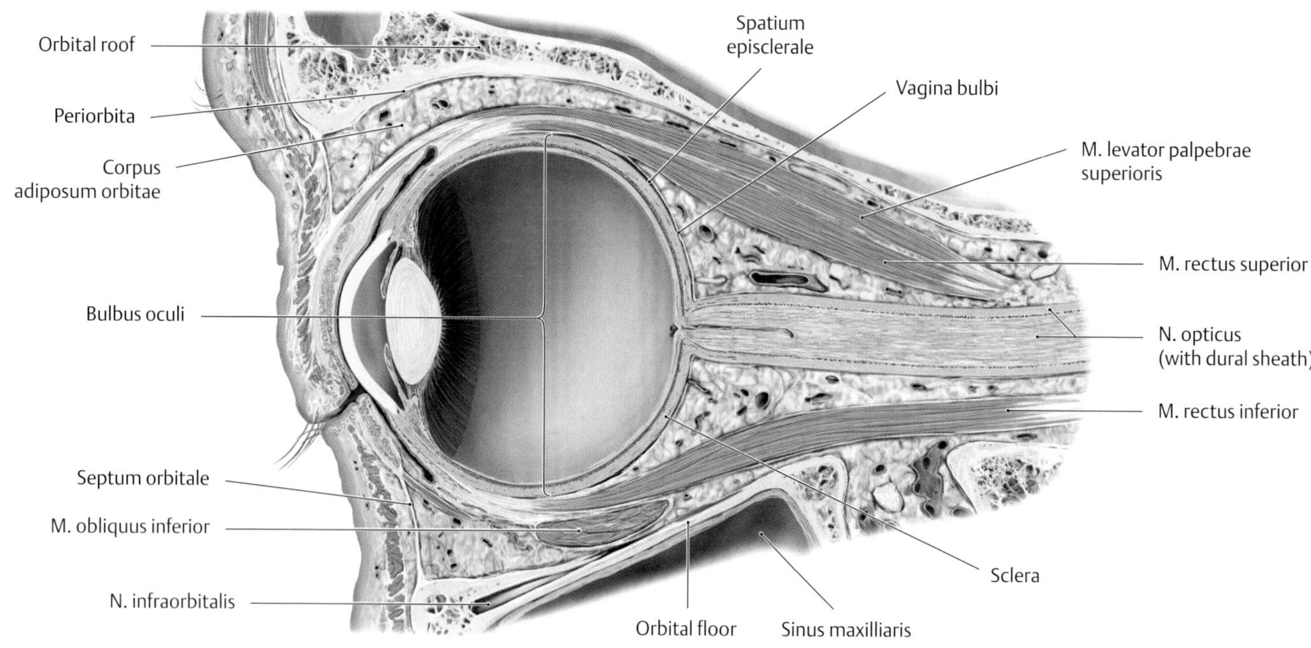
Orbital roof
Periorbita
Corpus adiposum orbitae
Bulbus oculi
Septum orbitale
M. obliquus inferior
N. infraorbitalis
Spatium episclerale
Vagina bulbi
M. levator palpebrae superioris
M. rectus superior
N. opticus (with dural sheath)
M. rectus inferior
Sclera
Orbital floor
Sinus maxilliaris

Fig. 33.12 **Topography of the orbita**
Sagittal section through the right orbita, medial view.

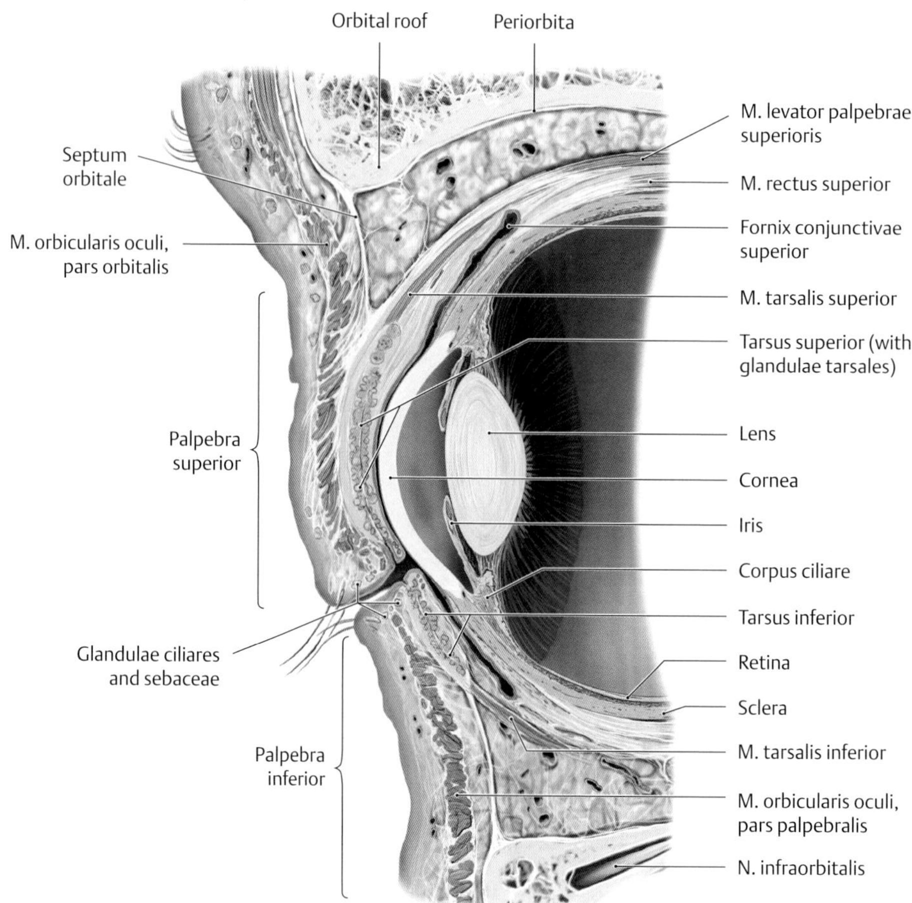
Orbital roof
Periorbita
Septum orbitale
M. orbicularis oculi, pars orbitalis
Palpebra superior
Glandulae ciliares and sebaceae
Palpebra inferior
M. levator palpebrae superioris
M. rectus superior
Fornix conjunctivae superior
M. tarsalis superior
Tarsus superior (with glandulae tarsales)
Lens
Cornea
Iris
Corpus ciliare
Tarsus inferior
Retina
Sclera
M. tarsalis inferior
M. orbicularis oculi, pars palpebralis
N. infraorbitalis

Fig. 33.13 **Eyelids and tunica conjuctiva**
Sagittal section through the anterior orbital cavity.

Fig. 33.14 **Lacrimal apparatus**
Right eye, anterior view. *Removed:* Orbital septum (partial). *Divided:* M. levator palpebrae superioris (tendon of insertion).

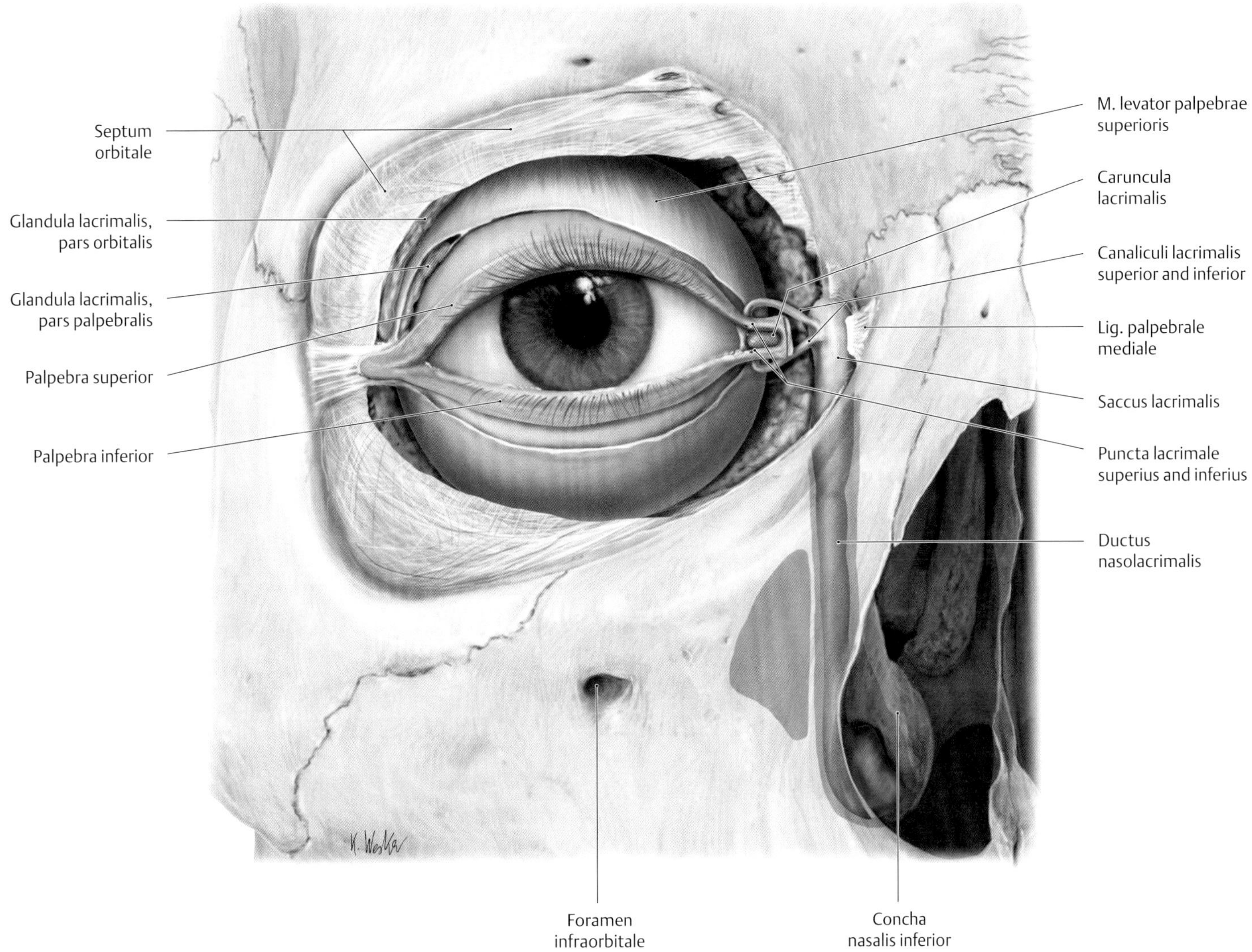

Septum orbitale
Glandula lacrimalis, pars orbitalis
Glandula lacrimalis, pars palpebralis
Palpebra superior
Palpebra inferior
M. levator palpebrae superioris
Caruncula lacrimalis
Canaliculi lacrimalis superior and inferior
Lig. palpebrale mediale
Saccus lacrimalis
Puncta lacrimale superius and inferius
Ductus nasolacrimalis
Foramen infraorbitale
Concha nasalis inferior

Clinical

Lacrimal drainage

Perimenopausal women are frequently subject to chronically dry eyes (*keratoconjunctivitis sicca*), due to insufficient tear production by the glandula lacrimalis. Acute inflammation of the glandula lacrimalis (due to bacteria) is less common and characterized by intense inflammation and extreme tenderness to palpation. The upper eyelid shows a characteristic S-curve.

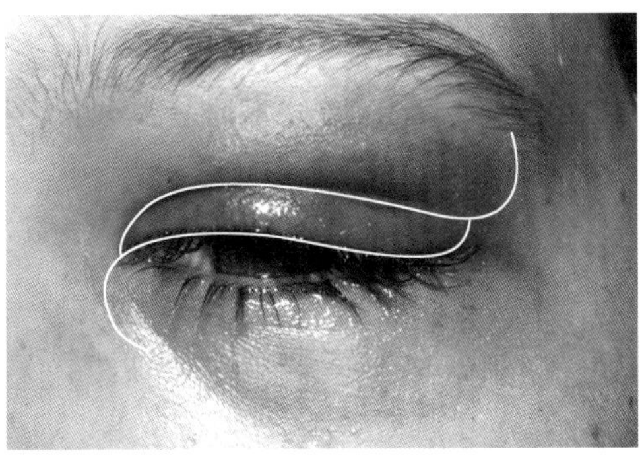

Eyeball (Bulbus Oculi)

Fig. 33.15 **Structure of the eyeball (bulbus oculi)**
Transverse section through right eyeball, superior view.
Note: The orbital axis (running along n. opticus through the discus nervi optici) deviates from the optical axis (running down the center of the eye to the fovea centralis) by 23 degrees.

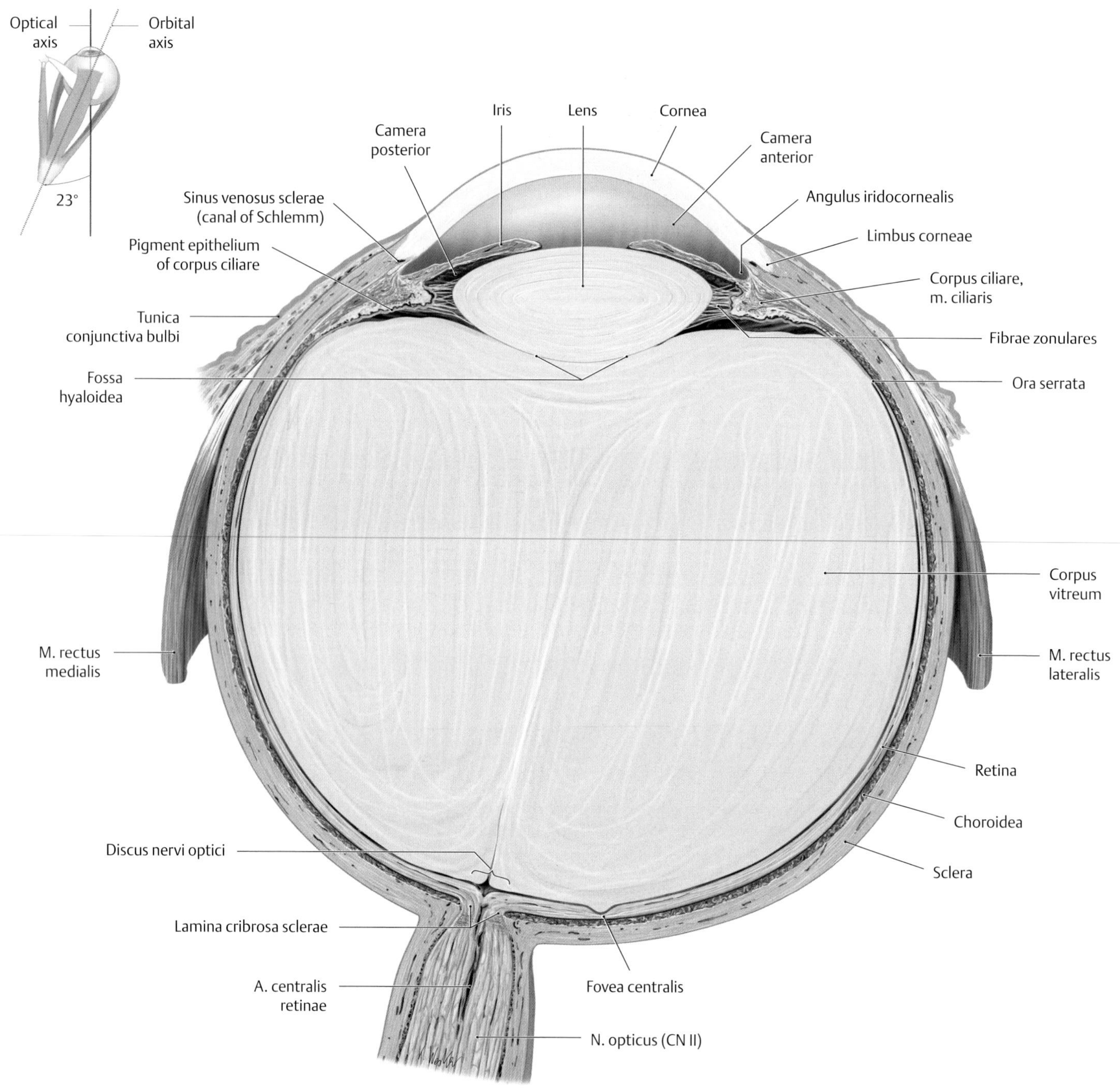

Optical axis
Orbital axis
23°
Iris
Lens
Cornea
Camera posterior
Camera anterior
Sinus venosus sclerae (canal of Schlemm)
Angulus iridocornealis
Limbus corneae
Pigment epithelium of corpus ciliare
Corpus ciliare, m. ciliaris
Tunica conjunctiva bulbi
Fibrae zonulares
Fossa hyaloidea
Ora serrata
Corpus vitreum
M. rectus medialis
M. rectus lateralis
Retina
Choroidea
Sclera
Discus nervi optici
Lamina cribrosa sclerae
A. centralis retinae
Fovea centralis
N. opticus (CN II)

Fig. 33.16 **Blood vessels of the eyeball**
Transverse section at the level of n. opticus, superior view. The arteries of the eye arise from a. ophthalmica, a terminal branch of a. carotis interna. Blood is drained by four to eight vv. vorticosae that open into vv. ophthalmicae superior and inferior.

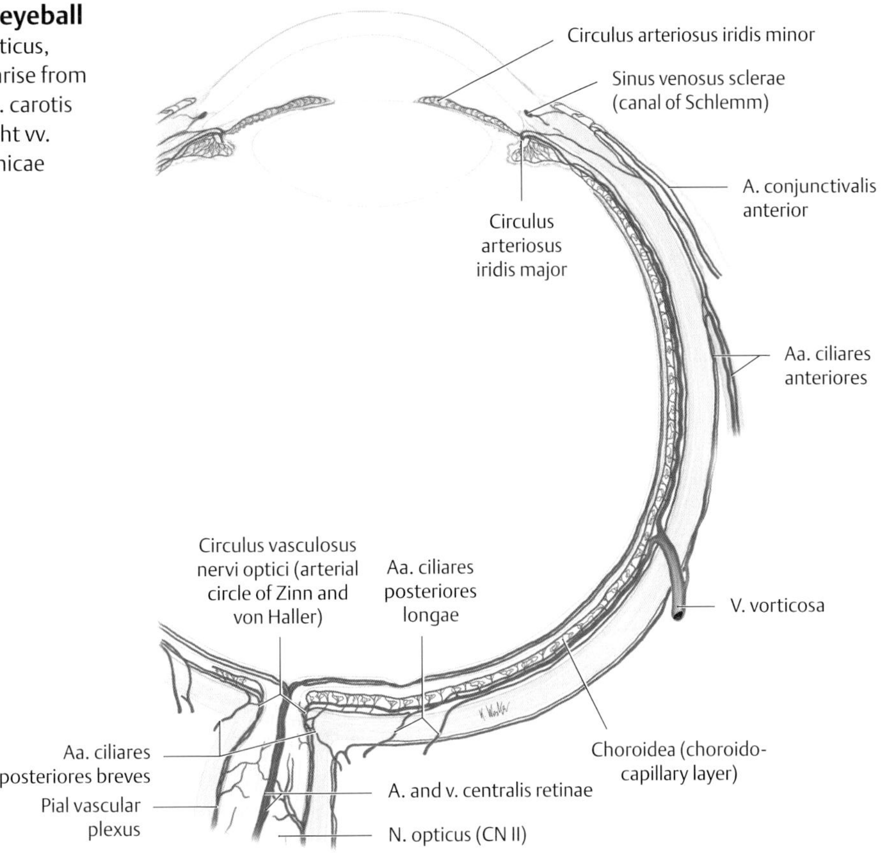
Circulus arteriosus iridis minor
Sinus venosus sclerae (canal of Schlemm)
A. conjunctivalis anterior
Circulus arteriosus iridis major
Aa. ciliares anteriores
Circulus vasculosus nervi optici (arterial circle of Zinn and von Haller)
Aa. ciliares posteriores longae
V. vorticosa
Aa. ciliares posteriores breves
Pial vascular plexus
A. and v. centralis retinae
N. opticus (CN II)
Choroidea (choroido-capillary layer)

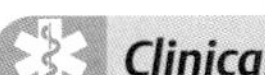

Clinical

Fundus oculi

The fundus oculi is the only place in the body where capillaries can be examined directly. Examination of fundus oculi permits observation of vascular changes that may be caused by high blood pressure or diabetes. Examination of the discus nervi optici is important in determining intracranial pressure and diagnosing multiple sclerosis.

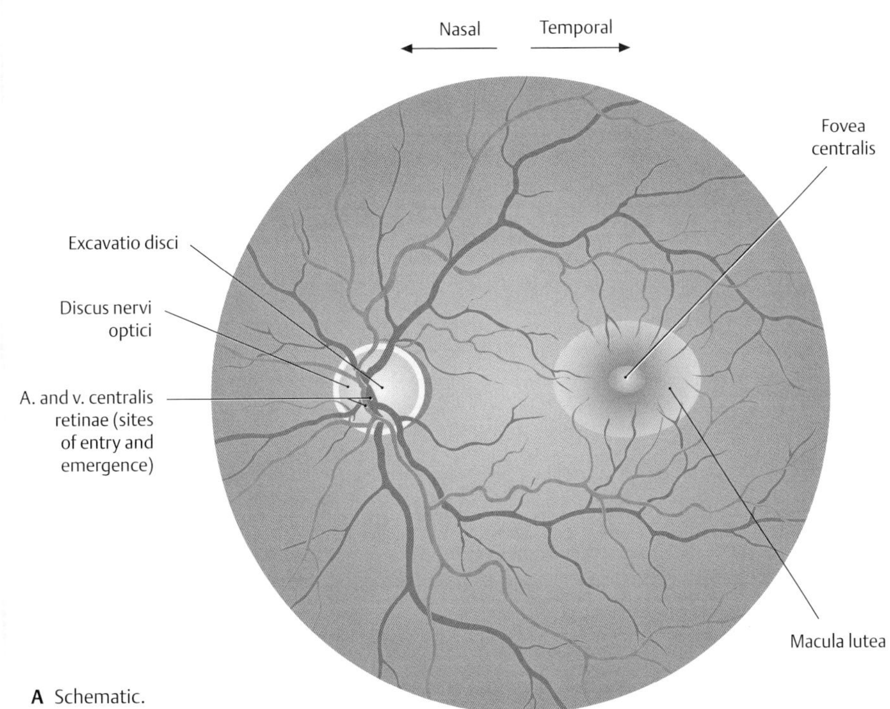
Nasal
Temporal
Fovea centralis
Excavatio disci
Discus nervi optici
A. and v. centralis retinae (sites of entry and emergence)
Macula lutea

A Schematic.

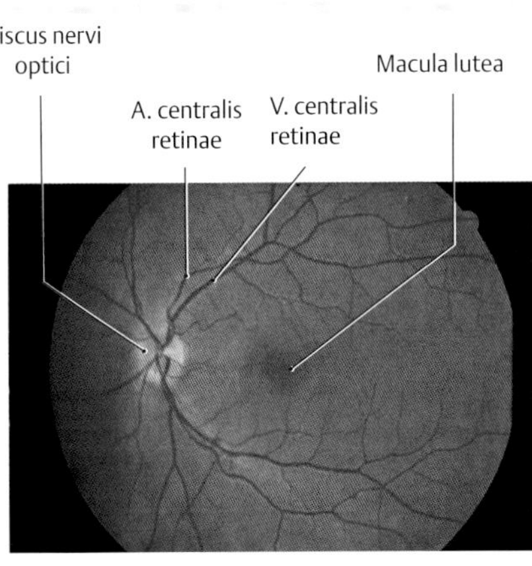
Discus nervi optici
Macula lutea
A. centralis retinae
V. centralis retinae

B Normal optic fundus in the ophthalmoscopic examination.

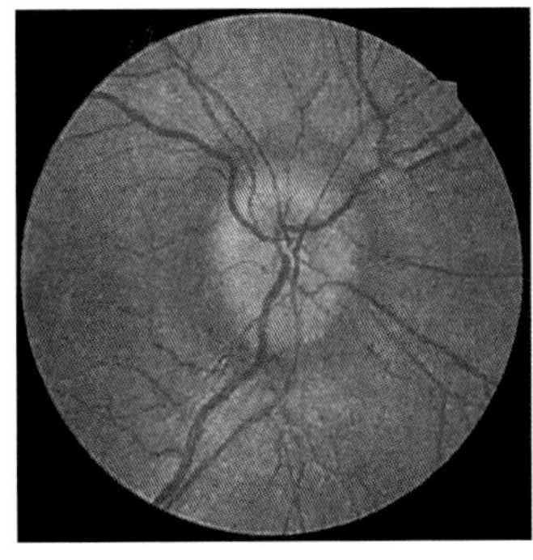

C High intracranial pressure; the edges of the optic disk appear less sharp.

Cornea, Iris & Lens

Fig. 33.17 **Cornea, iris, and lens**
Transverse section through the anterior segment of the eye. Anterosuperior view.

Fig. 33.18 **Iris**
Transverse section through the anterior segment of the eye. Anterosuperior view.

Clinical

Glaucoma

Aqueous humor produced in the camera posterior passes through the pupil into the camera anterior. It seeps through the spaces of the reticulum trabeculare into the sinus venosus sclerae (canal of Schlemm) before passing into the vv. episclerales. Obstruction of aqueous humor drainage causes an increase in intraocular pressure (glaucoma), which constricts n. opticus in the lamina cribrosa sclerae. This constriction eventually leads to blindness. The most common glaucoma (approximately 90% of cases) is chronic (open-angle) glaucoma. The more rare acute glaucoma is characterized by red eye, strong headache and/or eye pain, nausea, dilated episcleral veins, and edema of the cornea.

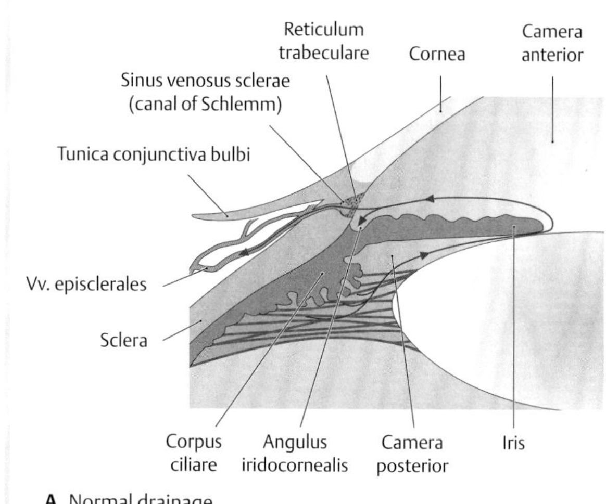

Reticulum trabeculare
Cornea
Camera anterior
Sinus venosus sclerae (canal of Schlemm)
Tunica conjunctiva bulbi
Vv. episclerales
Sclera
Corpus ciliare
Angulus iridocornealis
Camera posterior
Iris

A Normal drainage.

B Chronic (open-angle) glaucoma. Drainage through the trabecular meshwork is impaired.

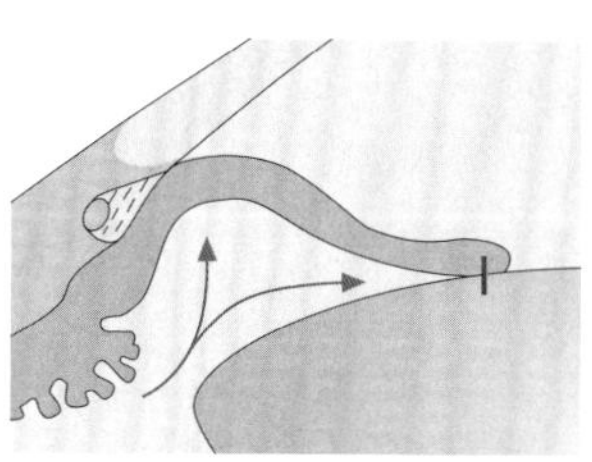

C Acute (angle-closure) glaucoma. The chamber angle is obstructed by iris tissue. Aqueous fluid cannot drain into the anterior chamber, which pushes portions of the iris upward, blocking the chamber angle.

Fig. 33.19 **Pupilla**
Pupilla size is regulated by two intraocular muscles of the iris: m. sphincter pupillae, which narrows the pupil (parasympathetic innervation), and m. dilator pupillae, which enlarges it (sympathetic innervation).

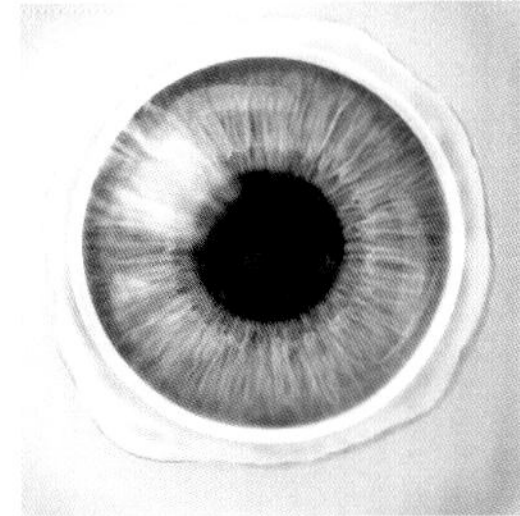

A Normal pupil size.

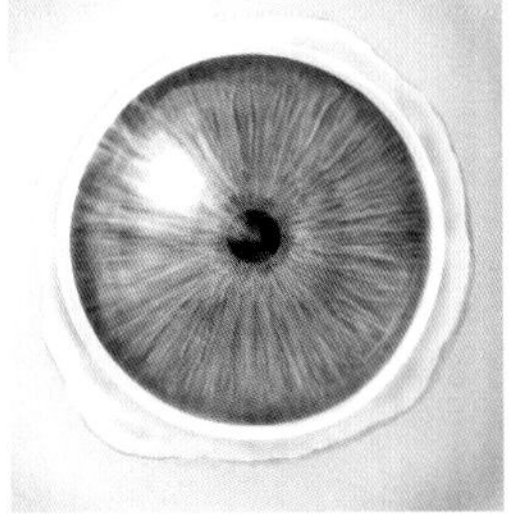

B Maximum constriction (miosis).

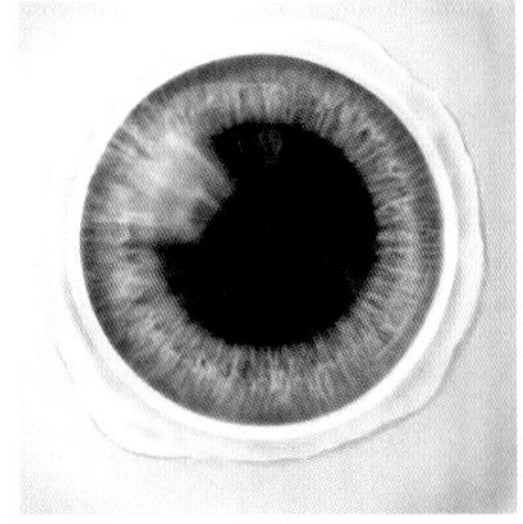

C Maximum dilation (mydriasis).

Fig. 33.20 **Lens and corpus ciliare**
Posterior view. The curvature of the lens is regulated by the muscle fibers (m. ciliaris) of the annular corpus ciliare.

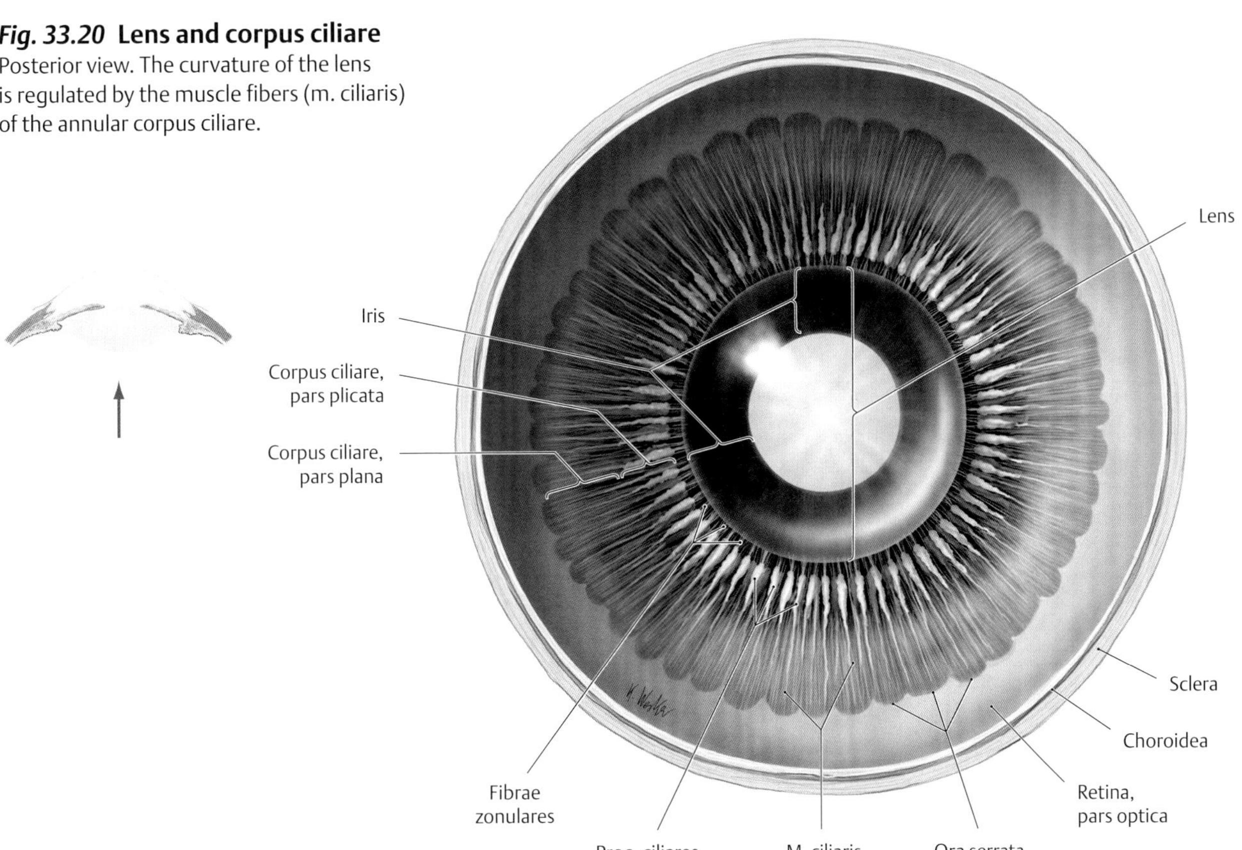

Lens
Iris
Corpus ciliare, pars plicata
Corpus ciliare, pars plana
Sclera
Choroidea
Retina, pars optica
Fibrae zonulares
Proc. ciliares
M. ciliaris
Ora serrata

Fig. 33.21 **Light refraction by the lens**
Transverse section, superior view. In the normal (emmetropic) eye, light rays are refracted by the lens (and cornea) to a focal point on the retinal surface (fovea centralis). Tensing of the fibrae zonulares, with relaxation of the m. ciliaris, flattens the lens in response to parallel rays arriving from a distant source (far vision). Contraction of m. ciliaris, with relaxation of fibrae zonulares, causes the lens to assume a more rounded shape (near vision).

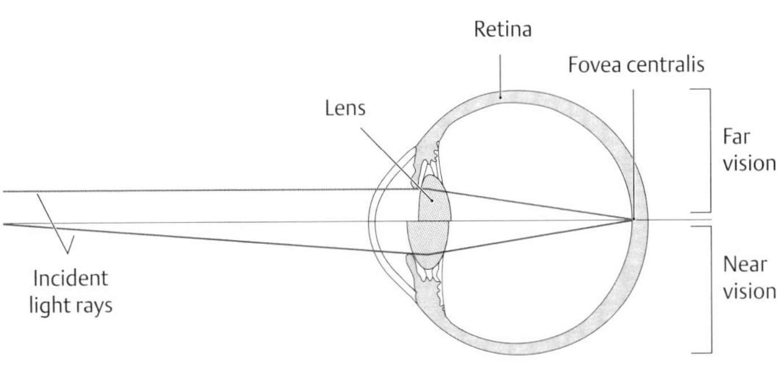

Retina
Fovea centralis
Lens
Far vision
Near vision
Incident light rays

A Normal dynamics of the lens.

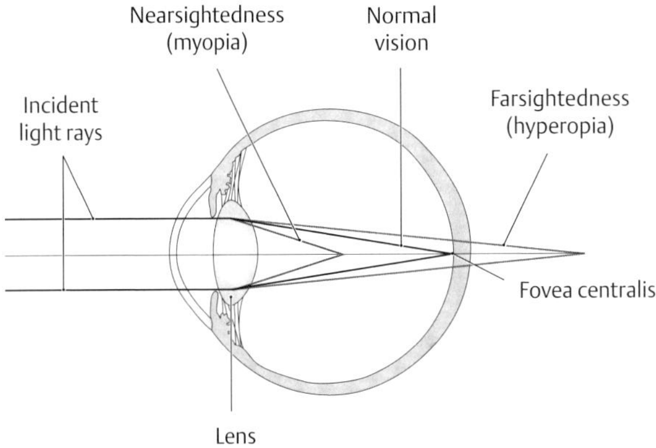

Nearsightedness (myopia)
Normal vision
Incident light rays
Farsightedness (hyperopia)
Fovea centralis
Lens

B Abnormal lens dynamics.

Bones of the Nasal Cavity (Cavitas Nasi)

Fig. 34.1 Skeleton of the nose

The skeleton of the nose is composed of an upper bony portion and a lower cartilaginous portion. The proximal portions of the nostrils (alae) are composed of connective tissue with small embedded pieces of cartilage.

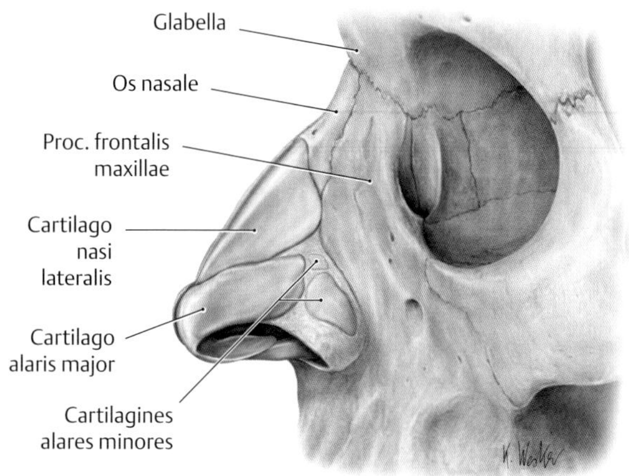
Glabella
Os nasale
Proc. frontalis maxillae
Cartilago nasi lateralis
Cartilago alaris major
Cartilagines alares minores

A Left lateral view.

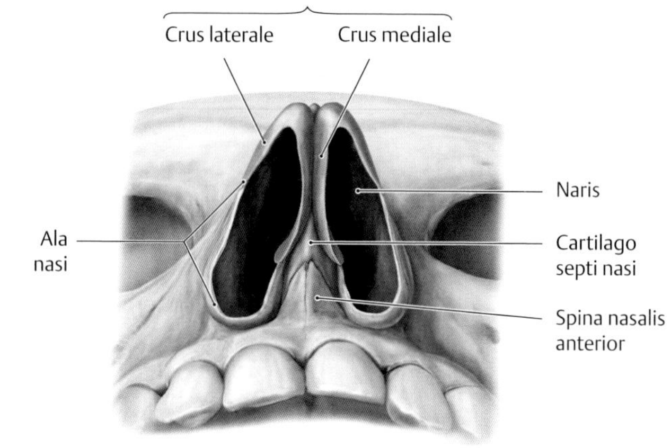
Cartilago alaris major
Crus laterale
Crus mediale
Naris
Ala nasi
Cartilago septi nasi
Spina nasalis anterior

B Inferior view.

Fig. 34.2 Bones of the nasal cavity (cavitas nasi)

The left and right nasal cavities are flanked by lateral walls and separated by septum nasi. Air enters the nasal cavity through the anterior nasal aperture and travels through three passages: the meatus nasi superior, medius, and inferior (arrows). These passages are separated by the superior, media, and inferior conchae nasi. Air leaves the nose through the choanae, entering the nasopharynx.

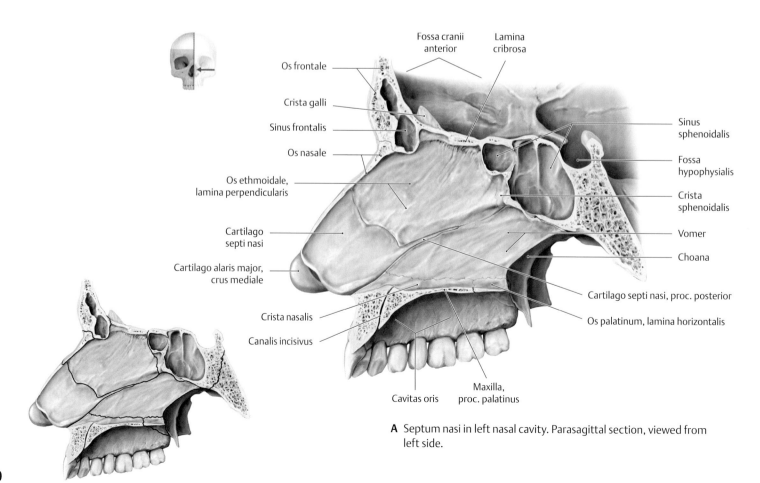

Fossa cranii anterior
Lamina cribrosa
Os frontale
Crista galli
Sinus frontalis
Os nasale
Os ethmoidale, lamina perpendicularis
Cartilago septi nasi
Cartilago alaris major, crus mediale
Crista nasalis
Canalis incisivus
Cavitas oris
Maxilla, proc. palatinus
Sinus sphenoidalis
Fossa hypophysialis
Crista sphenoidalis
Vomer
Choana
Cartilago septi nasi, proc. posterior
Os palatinum, lamina horizontalis

A Septum nasi in left nasal cavity. Parasagittal section, viewed from left side.

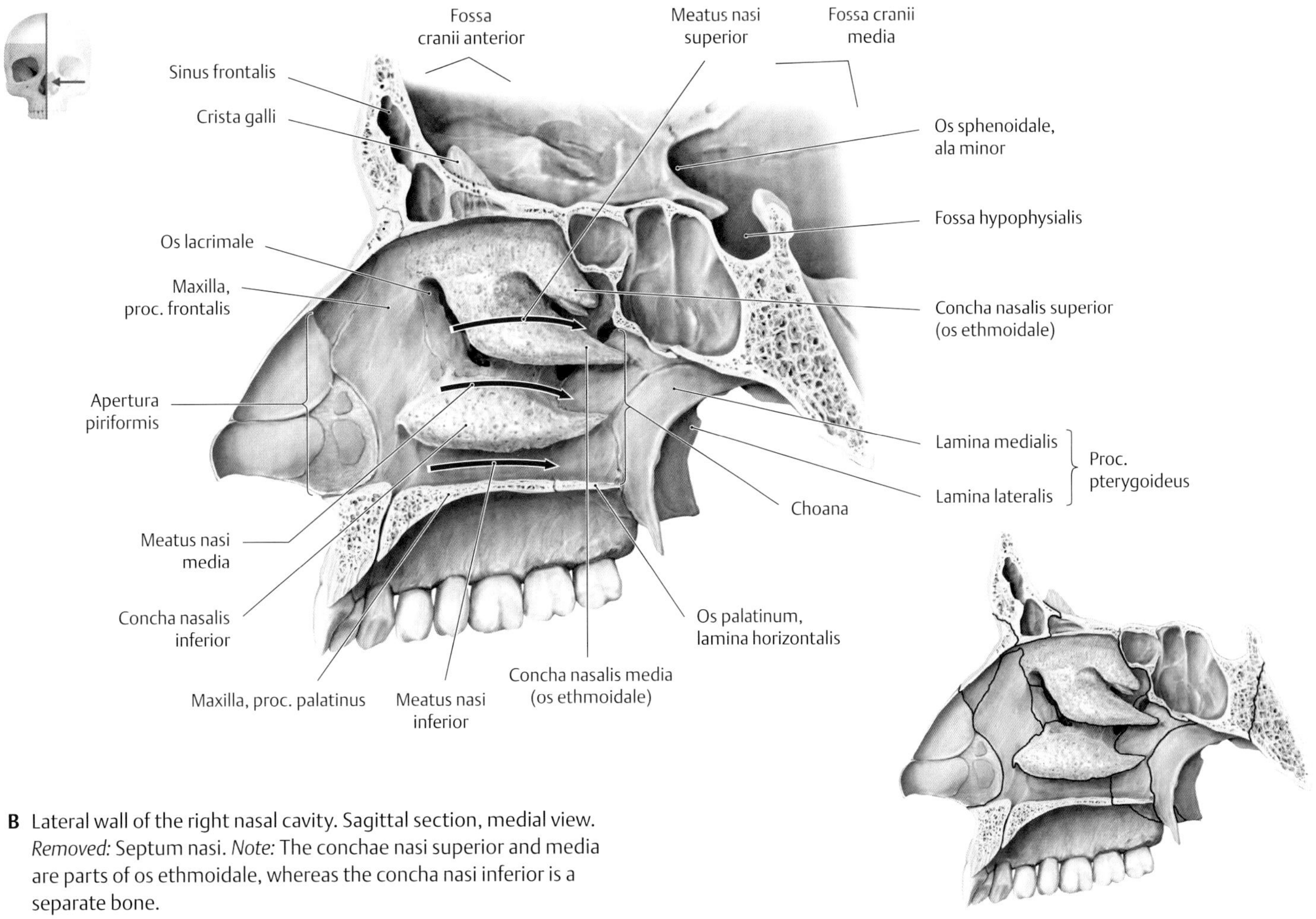

Fossa cranii anterior
Meatus nasi superior
Fossa cranii media
Sinus frontalis
Crista galli
Os sphenoidale, ala minor
Fossa hypophysialis
Os lacrimale
Maxilla, proc. frontalis
Concha nasalis superior (os ethmoidale)
Apertura piriformis
Lamina medialis
Lamina lateralis
Proc. pterygoideus
Choana
Meatus nasi media
Concha nasalis inferior
Os palatinum, lamina horizontalis
Maxilla, proc. palatinus
Meatus nasi inferior
Concha nasalis media (os ethmoidale)

B Lateral wall of the right nasal cavity. Sagittal section, medial view. *Removed:* Septum nasi. *Note:* The conchae nasi superior and media are parts of os ethmoidale, whereas the concha nasi inferior is a separate bone.

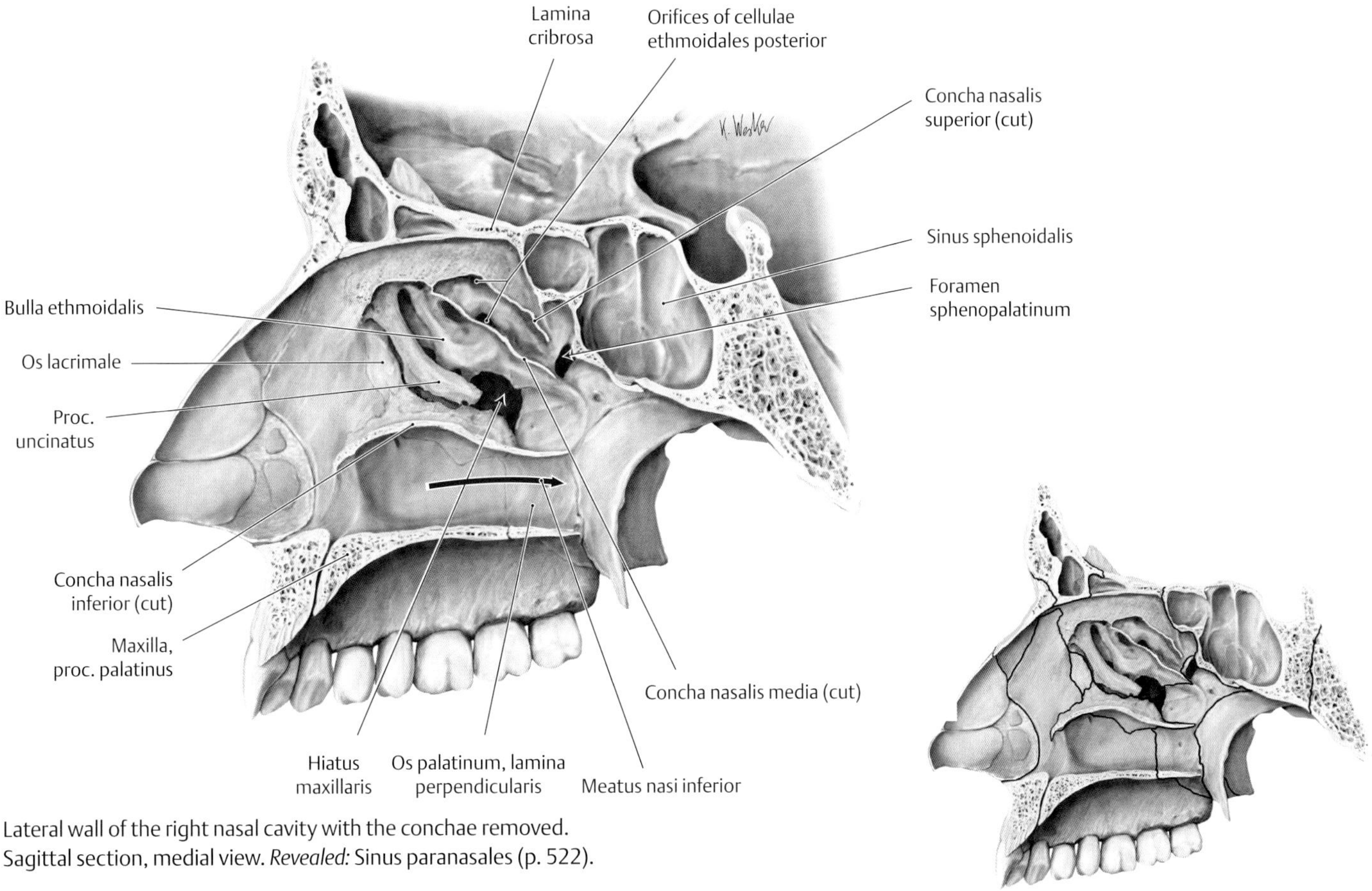

Lamina cribrosa
Orifices of cellulae ethmoidales posterior
Concha nasalis superior (cut)
Sinus sphenoidalis
Foramen sphenopalatinum
Bulla ethmoidalis
Os lacrimale
Proc. uncinatus
Concha nasalis inferior (cut)
Maxilla, proc. palatinus
Concha nasalis media (cut)
Hiatus maxillaris
Os palatinum, lamina perpendicularis
Meatus nasi inferior

C Lateral wall of the right nasal cavity with the conchae removed. Sagittal section, medial view. *Revealed:* Sinus paranasales (p. 522).

Paranasal Air Sinuses (Sinus Paranasales)

Fig. 34.3 Location of the paranasal sinuses

The paranasal sinuses [sinus frontalis, sinus (cellulae) ethmoidalis, sinus maxillaris, and sinus sphenoidalis] are air-filled cavities that reduce the weight of the skull.

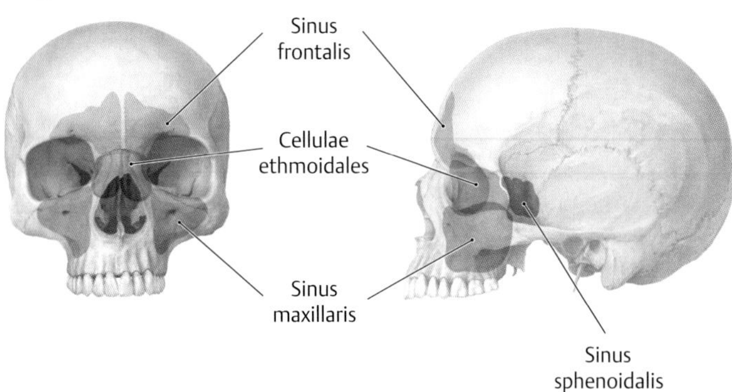
Sinus frontalis
Cellulae ethmoidales
Sinus maxillaris
Sinus sphenoidalis

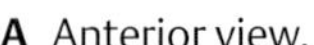

A Anterior view.

B Left lateral view.

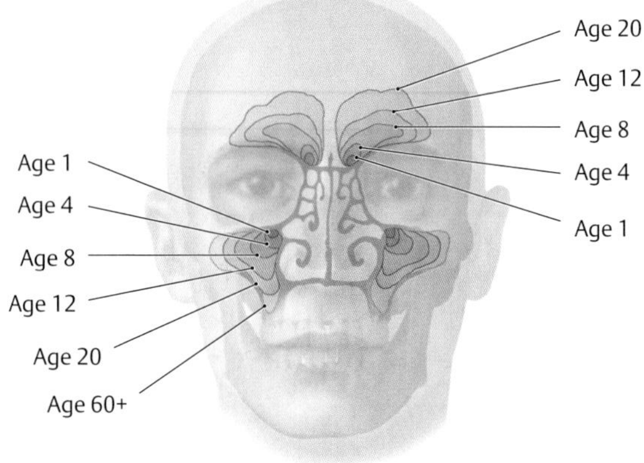
Age 20
Age 12
Age 8
Age 4
Age 1
Age 1
Age 4
Age 8
Age 12
Age 20
Age 60+

C Pneumatization of the sinuses. Sinus frontalis and maxillaris develop gradually over the course of cranial growth.

Table 34.1 Opening of nasal structures into the nose

Nasal passage	Sinuses/duct
Recessus sphenoethmoidalis	Sinus sphenoidalis (blue)
Meatus nasi superior	Sinus ethmoidalis posterior (green)
Meatus nasi medius	Sinus ethmoidalis anterior and medius (green)
	Sinus frontalis (yellow)
	Sinus maxillaris (orange)
Meatus nasi inferior	Ductus nasolacrimalis (red)

Fig. 34.4 Paranasal sinuses

Mucosal secretions from the sinuses and ductus nasolacrimalis open into the nose.

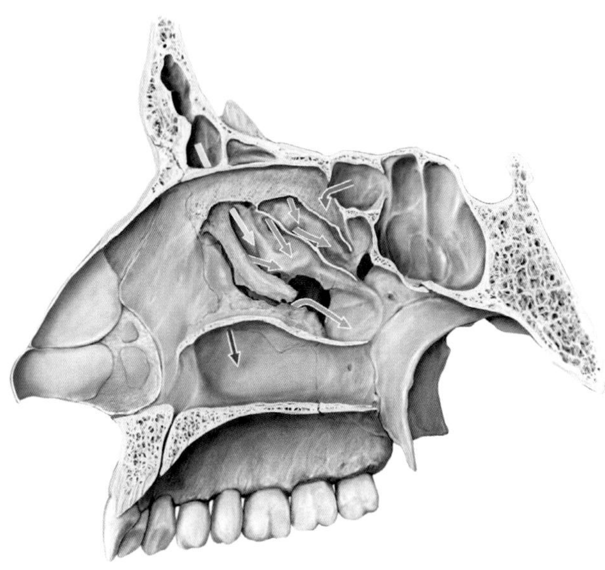

A Openings of the paranasal sinuses and ductus nasolacrimalis. Sagittal section, medial view of the right nasal cavity.

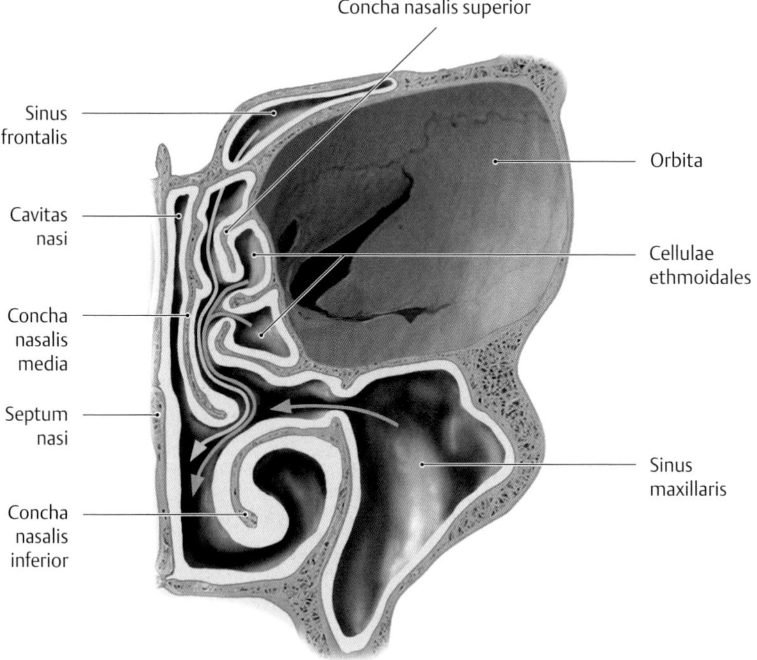
Concha nasalis superior
Sinus frontalis
Orbita
Cavitas nasi
Cellulae ethmoidales
Concha nasalis media
Septum nasi
Sinus maxillaris
Concha nasalis inferior

B Paranasal sinuses and osteomeatal unit in the left nasal cavity. Coronal section, anterior view.

Fig. 34.5 Bony structure of the paranasal sinuses

Coronal section, anterior view.

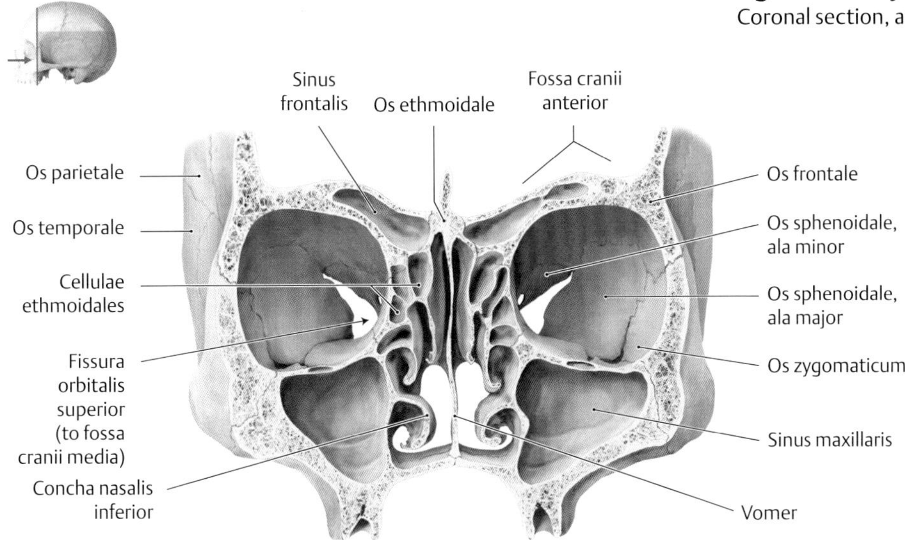
Sinus frontalis
Os ethmoidale
Fossa cranii anterior
Os parietale
Os temporale
Cellulae ethmoidales
Fissura orbitalis superior (to fossa cranii media)
Concha nasalis inferior
Os frontale
Os sphenoidale, ala minor
Os sphenoidale, ala major
Os zygomaticum
Sinus maxillaris
Vomer

A Bones of the paranasal sinuses.

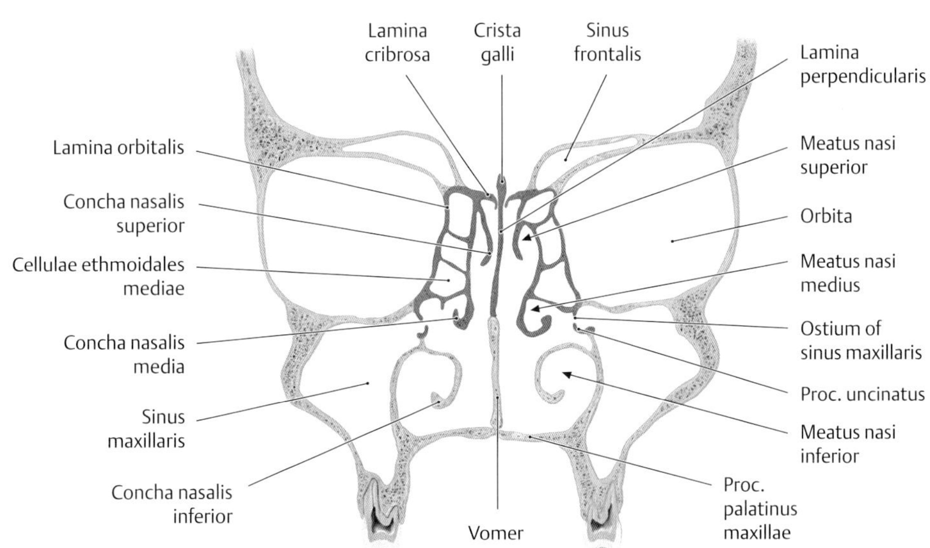
Lamina cribrosa
Crista galli
Sinus frontalis
Lamina perpendicularis
Lamina orbitalis
Concha nasalis superior
Cellulae ethmoidales mediae
Concha nasalis media
Sinus maxillaris
Concha nasalis inferior
Vomer
Meatus nasi superior
Orbita
Meatus nasi medius
Ostium of sinus maxillaris
Proc. uncinatus
Meatus nasi inferior
Proc. palatinus maxillae

B Os ethmoidale (red) in the paranasal sinuses.

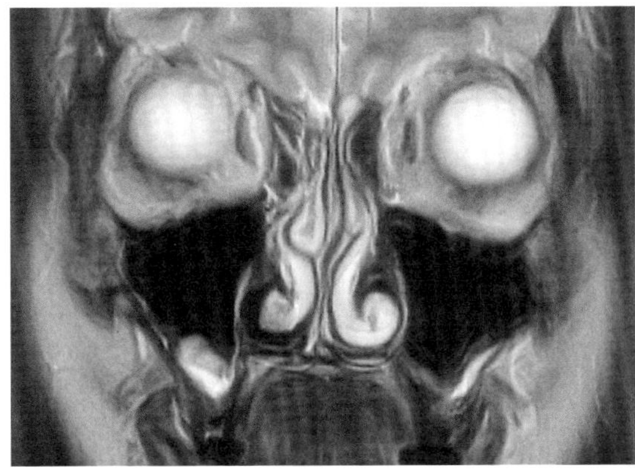

C MRI through the paranasal sinuses.

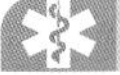

Clinical

Deviated septum

The normal position of septum nasi creates two roughly symmetrical nasal cavities. Extreme lateral deviation of the septum may result in obstruction of the nasal passages. This may be corrected by removing portions of the cartilage (septoplasty).

Sinusitis

When the mucosa in cellulae ethmoidales becomes swollen due to inflammation (*sinusitis*), it blocks the flow of secretions from sinus frontalis and maxillaris in the osteomeatal unit (see Fig. 34.4). This may cause microorganisms to become trapped, causing secondary inflammations. In patients with chronic sinusitis, the narrow sites can be surgically widened to establish more effective drainage routes.

Neurovasculature of the Nasal Cavity

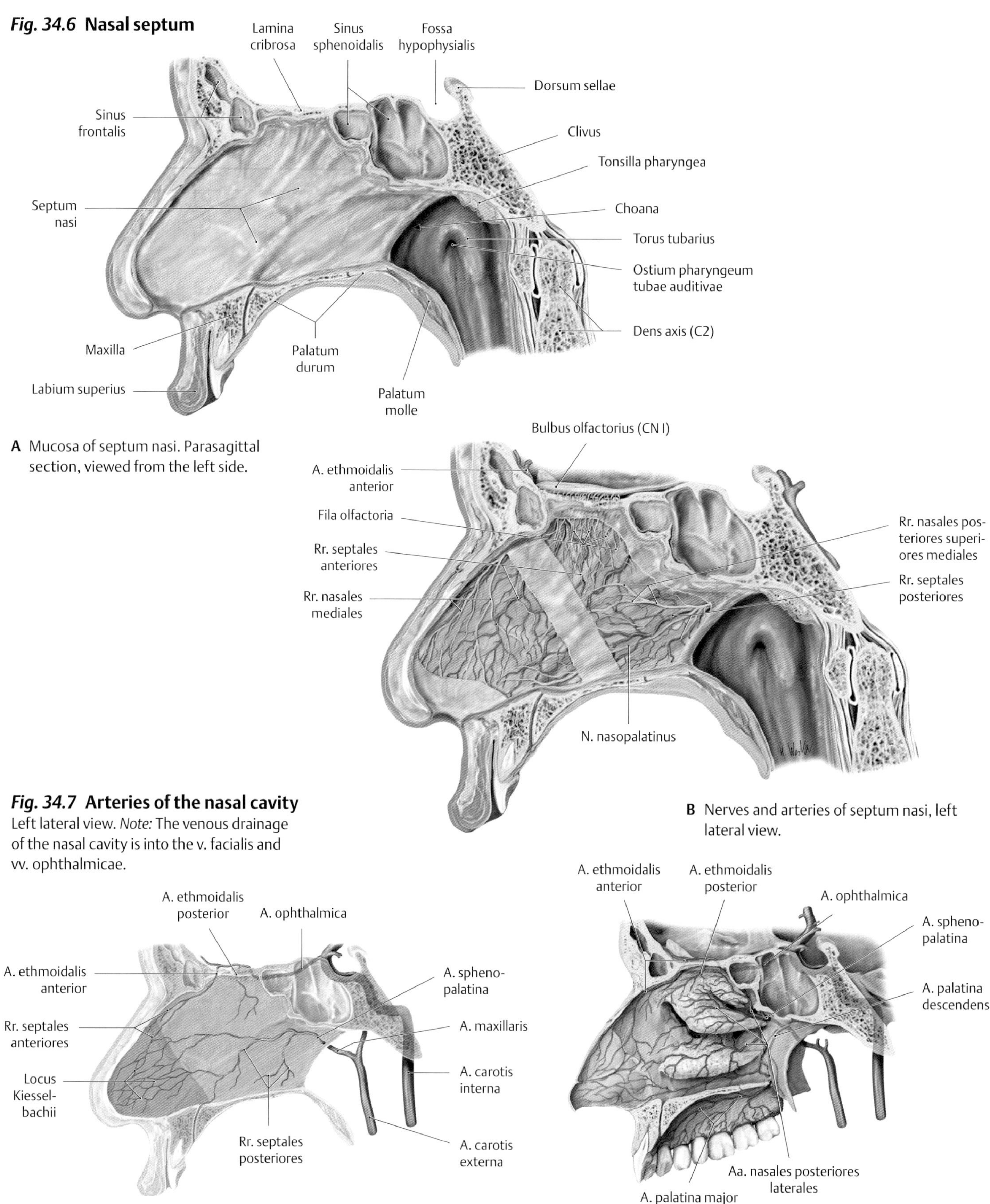
Lamina cribrosa
Sinus sphenoidalis
Fossa hypophysialis
Dorsum sellae
Sinus frontalis
Clivus
Tonsilla pharyngea
Septum nasi
Choana
Torus tubarius
Ostium pharyngeum tubae auditivae
Dens axis (C2)
Maxilla
Palatum durum
Labium superius
Palatum molle
Bulbus olfactorius (CN I)
A. ethmoidalis anterior
Fila olfactoria
Rr. septales anteriores
Rr. nasales mediales
Rr. nasales posteriores superiores mediales
Rr. septales posteriores
N. nasopalatinus
A. ethmoidalis anterior
A. ethmoidalis posterior
A. ophthalmica
A. ethmoidalis posterior
A. ophthalmica
A. spheno-palatina
A. ethmoidalis anterior
A. spheno-palatina
A. palatina descendens
Rr. septales anteriores
A. maxillaris
Locus Kiesselbachii
A. carotis interna
Rr. septales posteriores
A. carotis externa
Aa. nasales posteriores laterales
A. palatina major

Fig. 34.6 **Nasal septum**

A Mucosa of septum nasi. Parasagittal section, viewed from the left side.

B Nerves and arteries of septum nasi, left lateral view.

Fig. 34.7 **Arteries of the nasal cavity**
Left lateral view. *Note:* The venous drainage of the nasal cavity is into the v. facialis and vv. ophthalmicae.

A Arteries of septum nasi.

B Arteries of the right lateral nasal wall.

Fig. 34.8 Lateral nasal wall

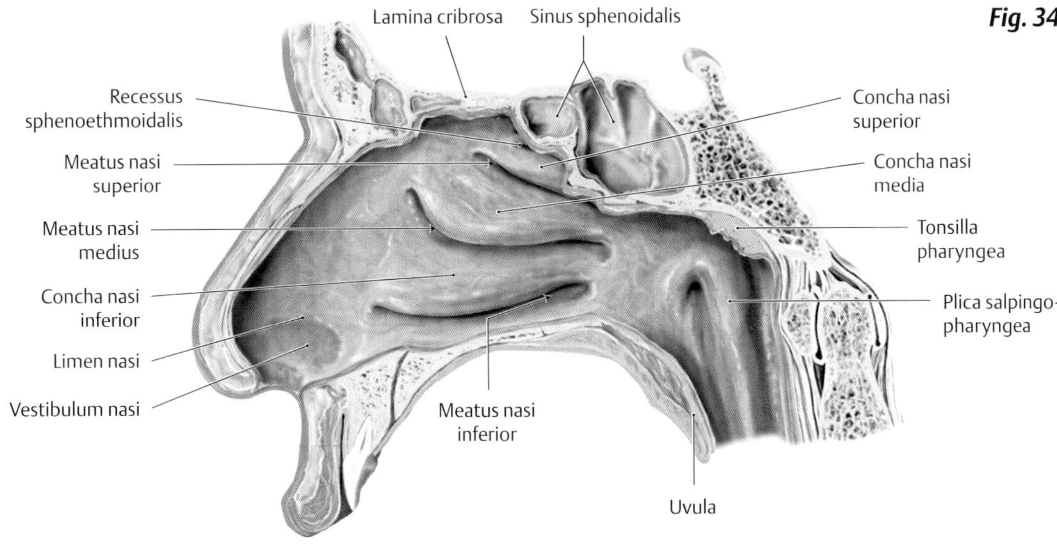
Lamina cribrosa
Sinus sphenoidalis
Recessus sphenoethmoidalis
Meatus nasi superior
Meatus nasi medius
Concha nasi inferior
Limen nasi
Vestibulum nasi
Meatus nasi inferior
Uvula
Concha nasi superior
Concha nasi media
Tonsilla pharyngea
Plica salpingo-pharyngea

A Mucosa of the lateral nasal wall. Sagittal section, viewed from the left side.

Bulbus olfactorius (CN I)
Fila olfactoria, a. ethmoidalis posterior
A. ethmoidalis anterior
Rr. nasales posteriores inferiores, aa. nasales posteriores laterales
Ganglion pterygo-palatinum
A. palatina descendens, n. palatinus major and nn. palatini minores
A. palatina major and n. palatinus major

B Nerves and arteries of the lateral nasal wall, left lateral view.

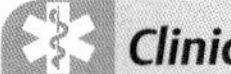

Clinical

Nosebleeds

Vascular supply to the nasal cavity arises from both aa. carotis interna and externa. The anterior part of septum nasi contains a very vascularized region referred to as Locus Kiesselbachii. This area is the most common site of significant nosebleeds.

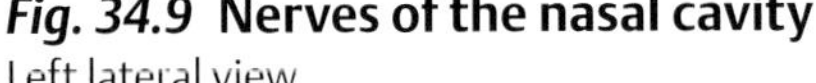

Fig. 34.9 Nerves of the nasal cavity

Left lateral view.

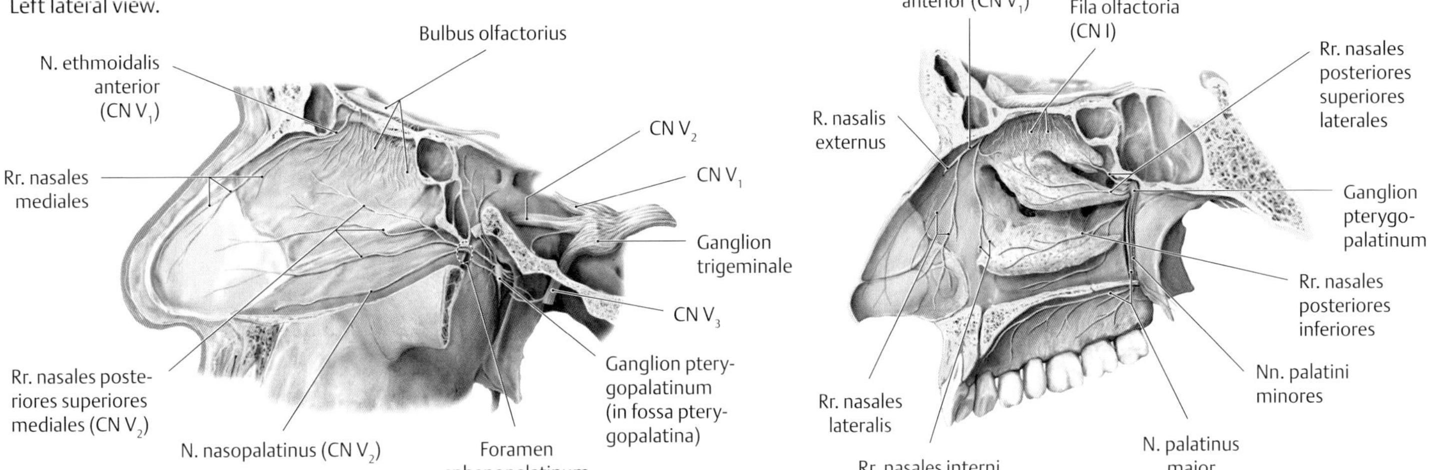
Bulbus olfactorius
N. ethmoidalis anterior (CN V_1)
Rr. nasales mediales
CN V_2
CN V_1
Ganglion trigeminale
CN V_3
Ganglion pterygopalatinum (in fossa pterygopalatina)
Rr. nasales posteriores superiores mediales (CN V_2)
N. nasopalatinus (CN V_2)
Foramen sphenopalatinum
N. ethmoidalis anterior (CN V_1)
Fila olfactoria (CN I)
R. nasalis externus
Rr. nasales posteriores superiores laterales
Ganglion pterygo-palatinum
Rr. nasales posteriores inferiores
Nn. palatini minores
N. palatinus major
Rr. nasales lateralis
Rr. nasales interni

A Nerves of septum nasi.

B Nerves of the lateral nasal wall.

Os Temporale

***Fig. 35.1* Os temporale**
Left bone. The os temporale consists of three major parts: pars squamousa, pars petrosa, and pars tympanica (see Fig. 35.2).

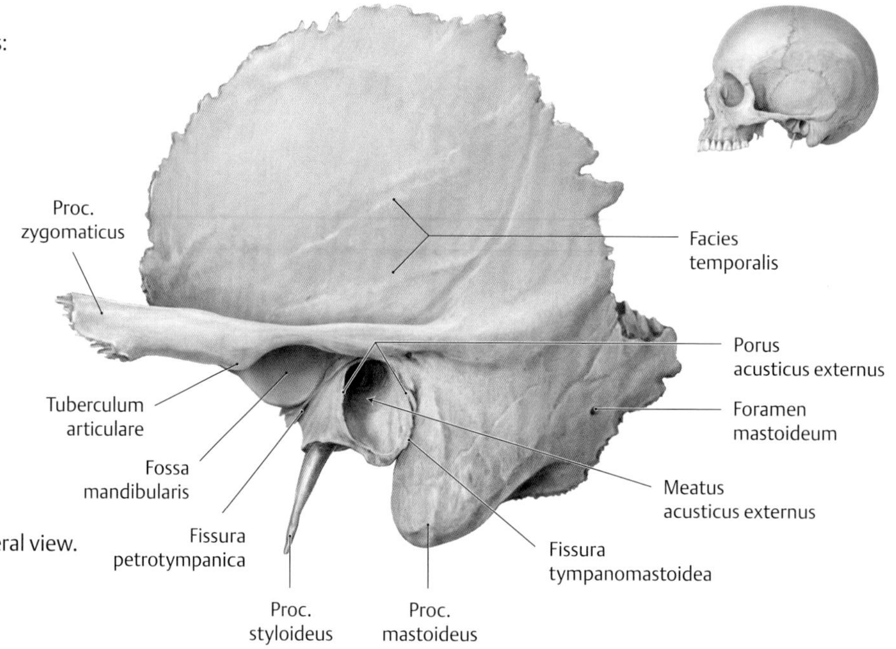

Proc. zygomaticus
Facies temporalis
Porus acusticus externus
Foramen mastoideum
Meatus acusticus externus
Tuberculum articulare
Fossa mandibularis
Fissura petrotympanica
Fissura tympanomastoidea
Proc. styloideus
Proc. mastoideus

A Left lateral view.

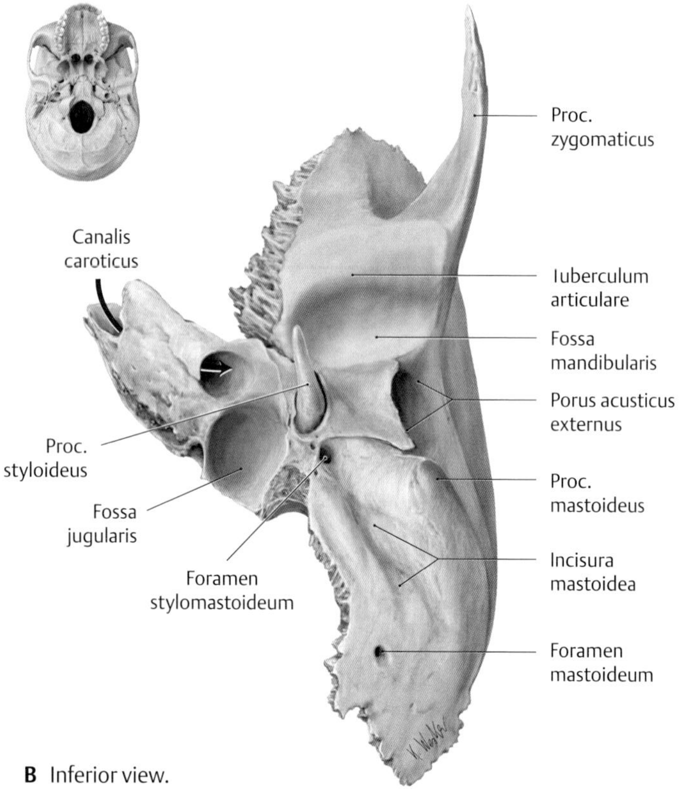

Proc. zygomaticus
Canalis caroticus
Iuberculum articulare
Fossa mandibularis
Porus acusticus externus
Proc. styloideus
Proc. mastoideus
Fossa jugularis
Incisura mastoidea
Foramen stylomastoideum
Foramen mastoideum

B Inferior view.

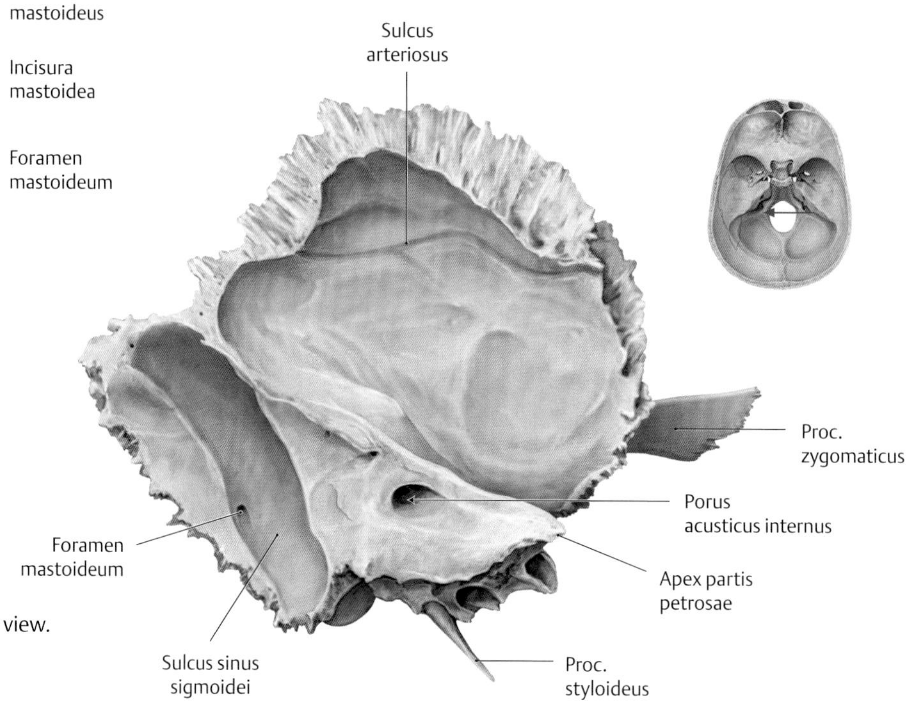

Sulcus arteriosus
Proc. zygomaticus
Porus acusticus internus
Foramen mastoideum
Apex partis petrosae
Sulcus sinus sigmoidei
Proc. styloideus

C Medial view.

Fig. 35.2 **Parts of os temporale**

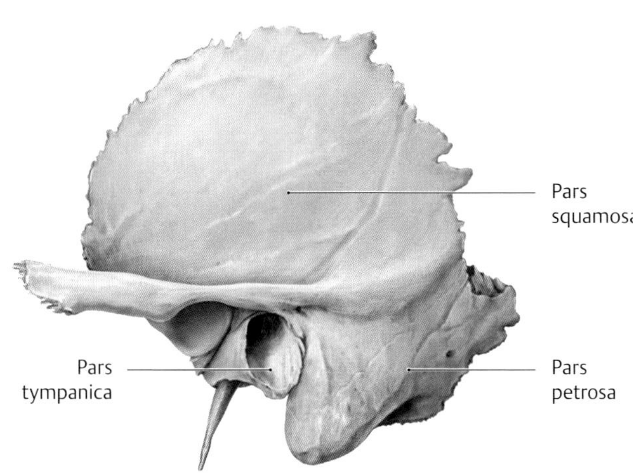
Pars squamosa
Pars tympanica
Pars petrosa

A Left lateral view.

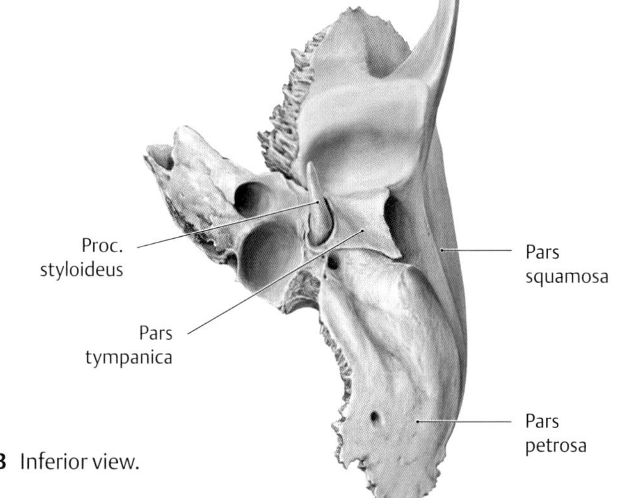
Proc. styloideus
Pars tympanica
Pars squamosa
Pars petrosa

B Inferior view.

Clinical

Structures in os temporale

The processus mastoideus contains mastoid air cells (cellulae mastoideae) that communicate with the middle ear; the middle ear in turn communicates with the nasopharynx via the tuba auditiva. Bacteria may use this pathway to move from the nasopharynx into the middle ear. In severe cases, bacteria may pass from the mastoid air cells into the cranial cavity, causing meningitis.

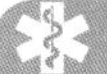

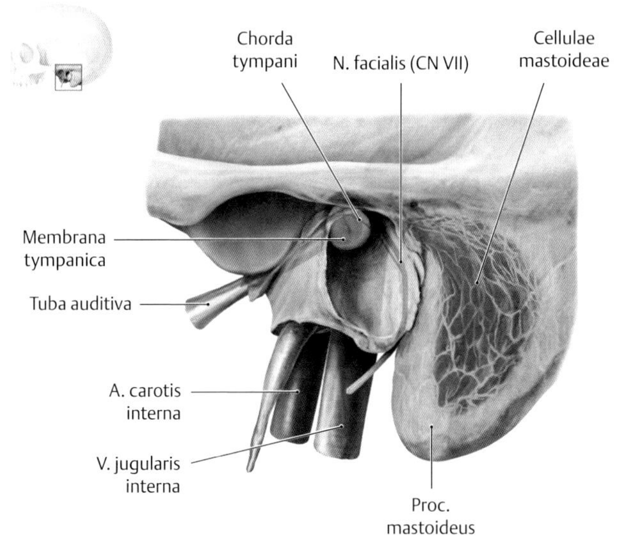
Chorda tympani
N. facialis (CN VII)
Cellulae mastoideae
Membrana tympanica
Tuba auditiva
A. carotis interna
V. jugularis interna
Proc. mastoideus

A

Irrigation of the auditory canal with warm (44°C) or cool (30°C) water can induce a thermal current in the endolympha of the canalis semicircularis, causing the patient to manifest vestibular nystagmus (jerky eye movements, vestibulo-ocular reflex). This caloric testing is important in the diagnosis of unexplained vertigo. The patient must be oriented so that the canalis semicircularis of interest lies in the vertical plane.

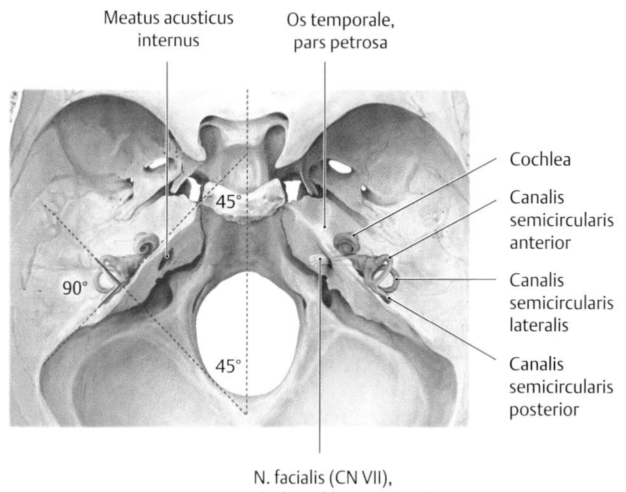
Meatus acusticus internus
Os temporale, pars petrosa
Cochlea
Canalis semicircularis anterior
Canalis semicircularis lateralis
Canalis semicircularis posterior
45°
90°
45°
N. facialis (CN VII), n. vestibulocochlearis (CN VIII)

B

The pars petrosa of os temporale contains the middle and inner ear as well as the membrana tympanica. The bony canales semicirculares are oriented at an approximately 45-degree angle from the coronal, transverse, and sagittal planes.

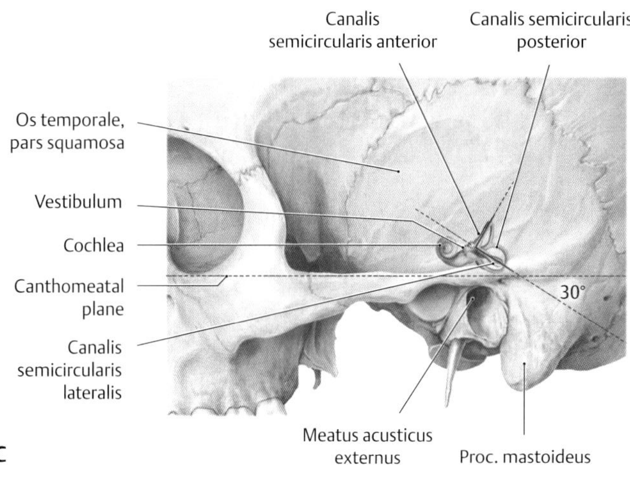
Canalis semicircularis anterior
Canalis semicircularis posterior
Os temporale, pars squamosa
Vestibulum
Cochlea
Canthomeatal plane
30°
Canalis semicircularis lateralis
Meatus acusticus externus
Proc. mastoideus

C

External Ear (Auris Externa) & Auditory Canal

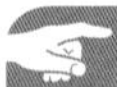

The auditory apparatus is divided into three main parts: external, middle, and inner ear. The external and middle ear are part of the sound conduction apparatus, and the inner ear is the actual organ of hearing (see p. 619). The inner ear also contains the vestibular apparatus, the organ of balance (see p. 618).

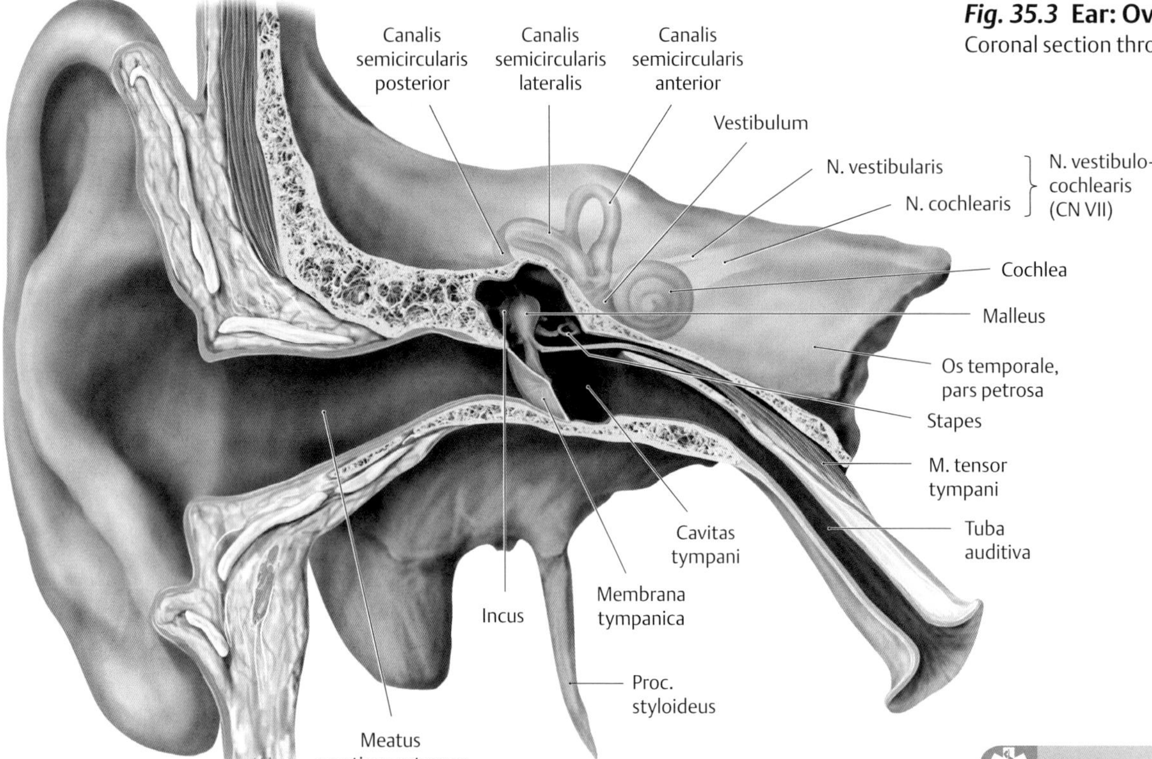
Canalis semicircularis posterior
Canalis semicircularis lateralis
Canalis semicircularis anterior
Vestibulum
N. vestibularis
N. cochlearis
N. vestibulo-cochlearis (CN VII)
Cochlea
Malleus
Os temporale, pars petrosa
Stapes
M. tensor tympani
Tuba auditiva
Cavitas tympani
Membrana tympanica
Incus
Proc. styloideus
Meatus acusticus externus

Fig. 35.3 **Ear: Overview**
Coronal section through right ear, anterior view.

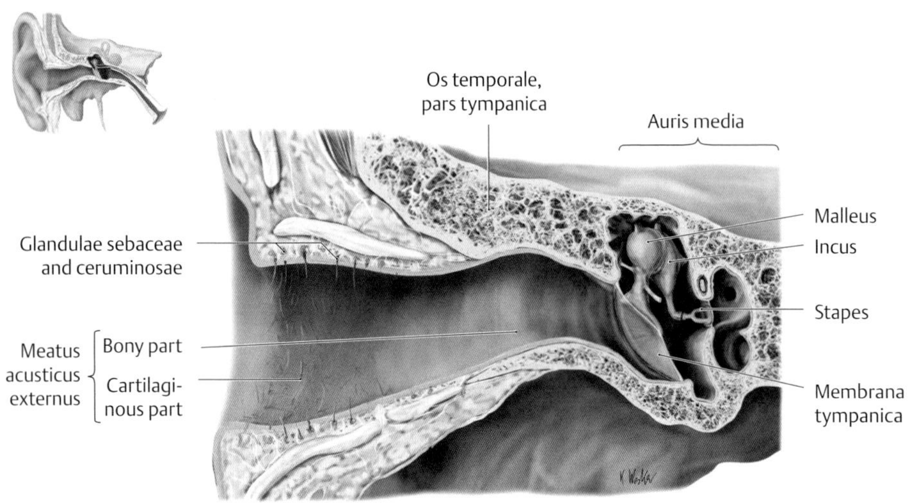
Os temporale, pars tympanica
Auris media
Malleus
Incus
Stapes
Membrana tympanica
Glandulae sebaceae and ceruminosae
Meatus acusticus externus
Bony part
Cartilagi-nous part

Fig. 35.4 **Meatus acusticus externus**
Coronal section through right ear, anterior view. The membrana tympanica separates the meatus acusticus externus from the cavitas tympani (middle ear). The outer third of the meatus acusticus externus is cartilaginous, and the inner two thirds are osseous (pars tympanica of os temporale).

Clinical

Curvature of the meatus acusticus externus
The meatus acusticus externus is most curved in its cartilaginous portion. When an otoscope is being inserted, the auricula should be pulled backward and upward so the speculum can be introduced into a straightened canal.

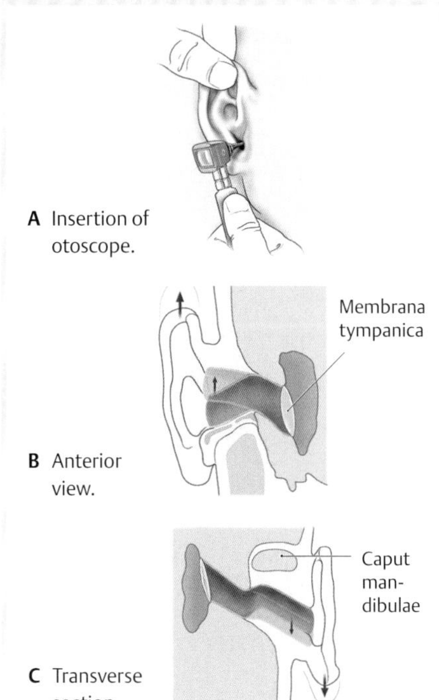
Membrana tympanica
Caput man-dibulae

A Insertion of otoscope.

B Anterior view.

C Transverse section.

Fig. 35.5 Structure of the auricula

The auricula of the ear encloses a cartilaginous framework that forms a funnel-shaped receptor for acoustic vibrations. The muscles of the auricula are considered muscles of facial expression, although they are vestigial in humans.

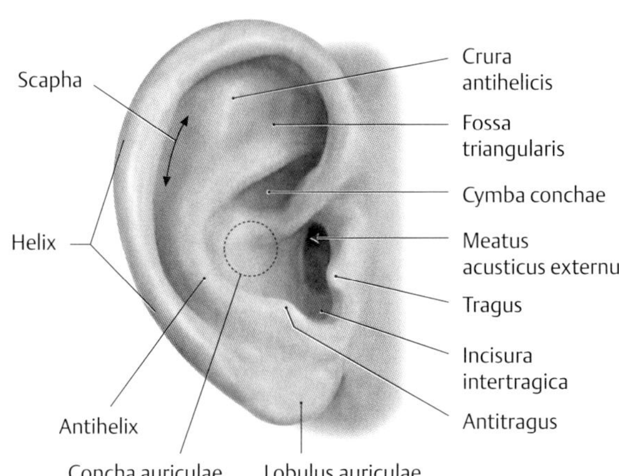
Scapha
Helix
Antihelix
Concha auriculae
Lobulus auriculae
Crura antihelicis
Fossa triangularis
Cymba conchae
Meatus acusticus externus
Tragus
Incisura intertragica
Antitragus

A Right auricula, right lateral view.

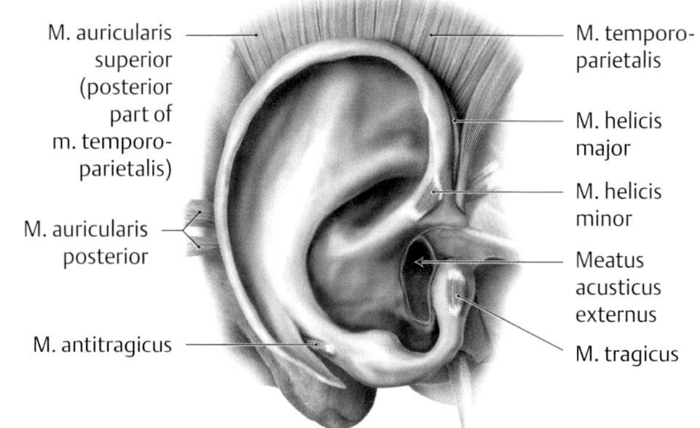
M. auricularis superior (posterior part of m. temporo-parietalis)
M. auricularis posterior
M. antitragicus
M. temporo-parietalis
M. helicis major
M. helicis minor
Meatus acusticus externus
M. tragicus

B Cartilage and muscles of the auricula, right lateral view.

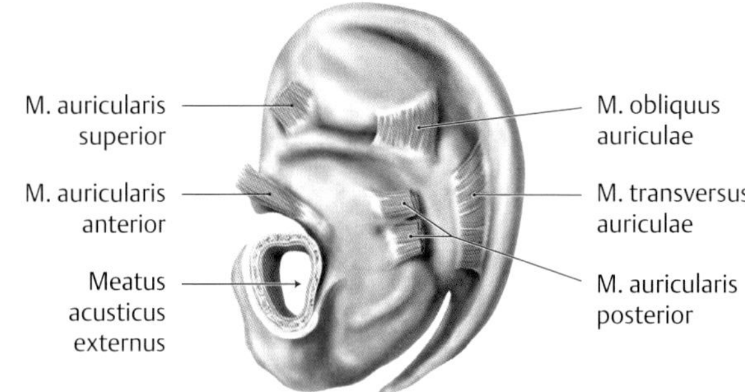
M. auricularis superior
M. auricularis anterior
Meatus acusticus externus
M. obliquus auriculae
M. transversus auriculae
M. auricularis posterior

C Cartilage and muscles of the auricula, medial view of posterior surface.

Fig. 35.6 Arteries of the auricula

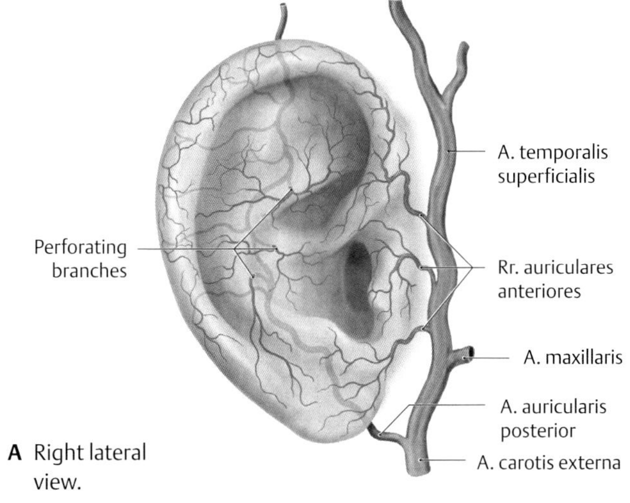
Perforating branches
A. temporalis superficialis
Rr. auriculares anteriores
A. maxillaris
A. auricularis posterior
A. carotis externa

A Right lateral view.

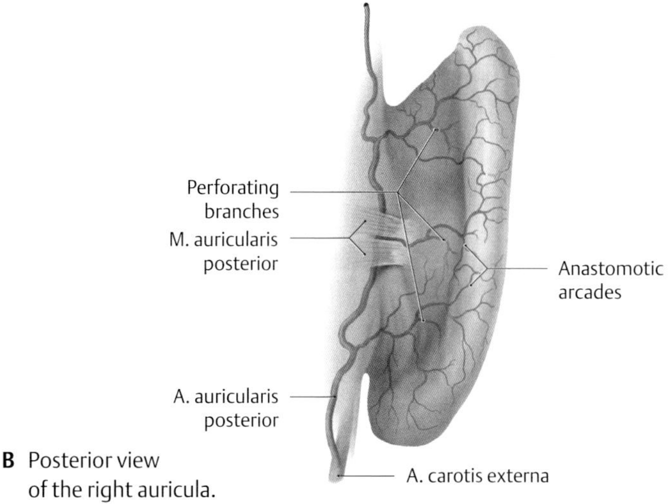
Perforating branches
M. auricularis posterior
A. auricularis posterior
Anastomotic arcades
A. carotis externa

B Posterior view of the right auricula.

Fig. 35.7 Innervation of the auricula

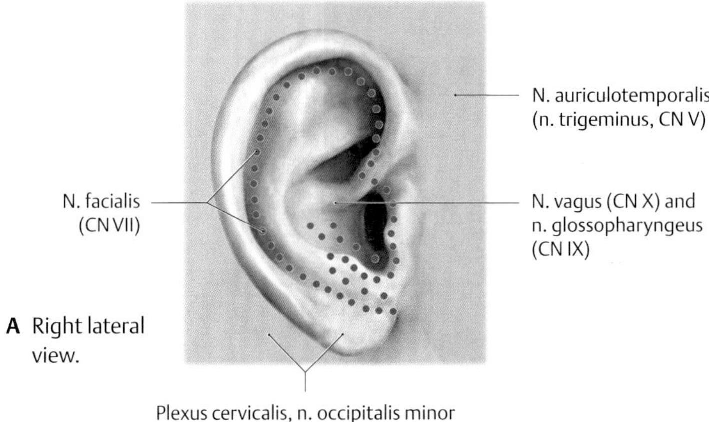
N. facialis (CN VII)
N. auriculotemporalis (n. trigeminus, CN V)
N. vagus (CN X) and n. glossopharyngeus (CN IX)
Plexus cervicalis, n. occipitalis minor and n. auricularis magnus

A Right lateral view.

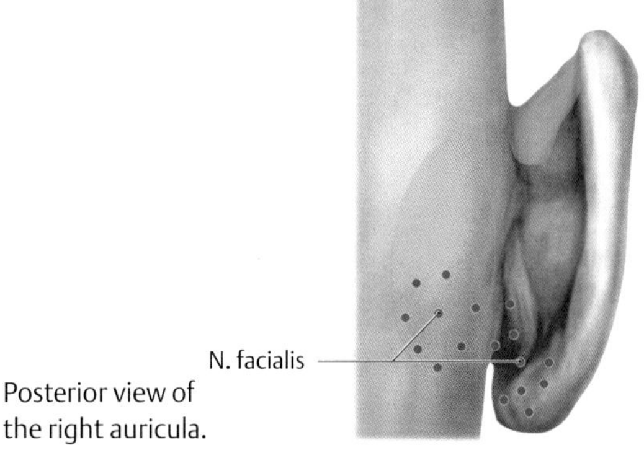
N. facialis

B Posterior view of the right auricula.

Middle Ear (Auris Media): Tympanic Cavity (Cavitas Tympani)

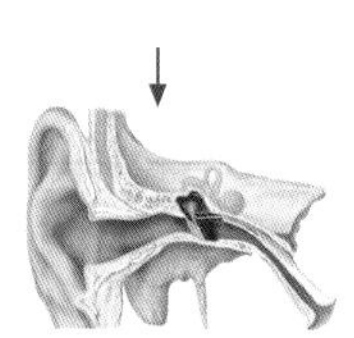

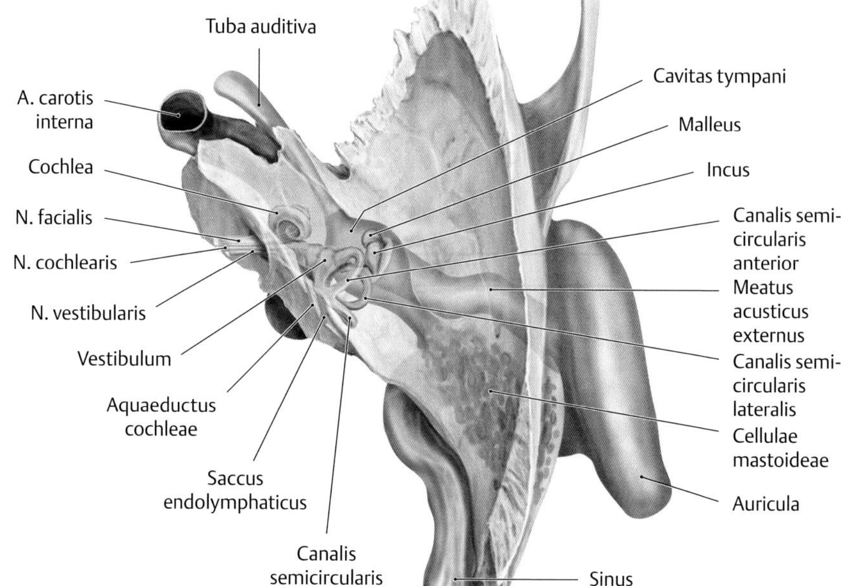

Tuba auditiva
A. carotis interna
Cochlea
N. facialis
N. cochlearis
N. vestibularis
Vestibulum
Aquaeductus cochleae
Saccus endolymphaticus
Canalis semicircularis posterior
Cavitas tympani
Malleus
Incus
Canalis semi-circularis anterior
Meatus acusticus externus
Canalis semi-circularis lateralis
Cellulae mastoideae
Auricula
Sinus sigmoideus

Fig. 35.8 **Middle ear**
Right pars petrosa, superior view. The tympanic cavity of the middle ear communicates anteriorly with the pharynx via the tuba auditiva and posteriorly with the cellulae mastoideae.

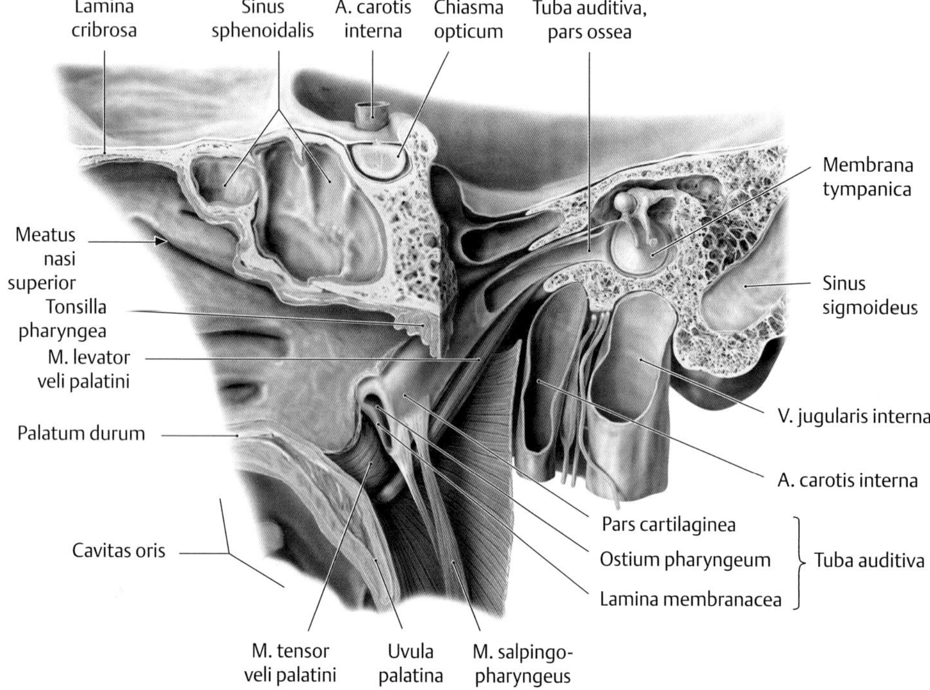

Lamina cribrosa
Sinus sphenoidalis
A. carotis interna
Chiasma opticum
Tuba auditiva, pars ossea
Meatus nasi superior
Tonsilla pharyngea
M. levator veli palatini
Palatum durum
Cavitas oris
M. tensor veli palatini
Uvula palatina
M. salpingo-pharyngeus
Membrana tympanica
Sinus sigmoideus
V. jugularis interna
A. carotis interna
Pars cartilaginea
Ostium pharyngeum
Lamina membranacea
Tuba auditiva

Fig. 35.9 **Tympanic cavity and tuba auditiva**
Medial view of opened tympanic cavity.

Table 35.1 **Boundaries of the Cavitas tympani**

During chronic suppurative otitis media (inflammation of the middle ear), pathogenic bacteria may spread to adjacent regions.

Direction	Wall	Anatomical boundary	Neighboring structures	Infection
Anterior	Carotid	Opening to tuba auditiva	Canalis caroticus	
Lateral	Paries caroticus	Membrana tympanica	Meatus acusticus externus	
Superior	Paries tegmentalis	Tegmen tympani	Fossa cranii media	Meningitis, cerebral abscess (especially of temporal lobe)
Medial	Paries labyrinthicus	Prominentia canalis semicircularis lateralis	Inner ear	
			CSF space (via petrous apex)	Abducent paralysis, trigeminal nerve irritation, visual disturbances (Gradenigo's syndrome)
Inferior	Paries jugularis	Os temporale, pars tympanica	Bulbus superior v. jugularae	
			Sinus sigmoideus	Sinus thrombosis
Posterior	Paries mastoidea	Antrum mastoideum	Cellulae mastoideae	Mastoiditis
			Canalis n. facialis	Facial paralysis

CSF = cerebrospinal fluid.

Fig. 35.10 Tympanic cavity (cavitas tympani)

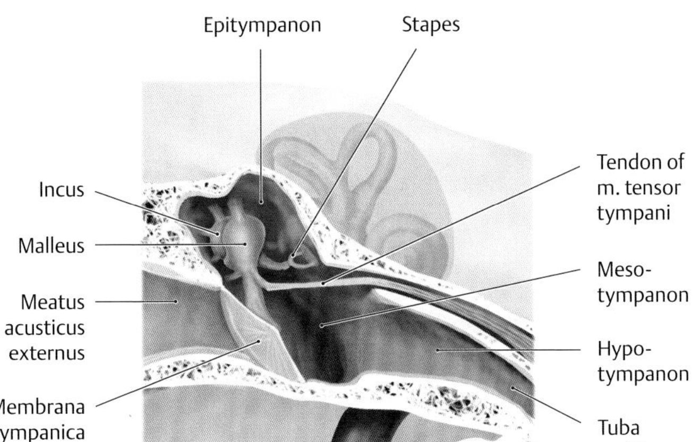
Epitympanon
Stapes
Incus
Malleus
Meatus acusticus externus
Membrana tympanica
Tendon of m. tensor tympani
Meso-tympanon
Hypo-tympanon
Tuba auditiva

A Levels of the tympanic cavity. Anterior view. The tympanic cavity is divided into three levels: epi-, meso-, and hypotympanum.

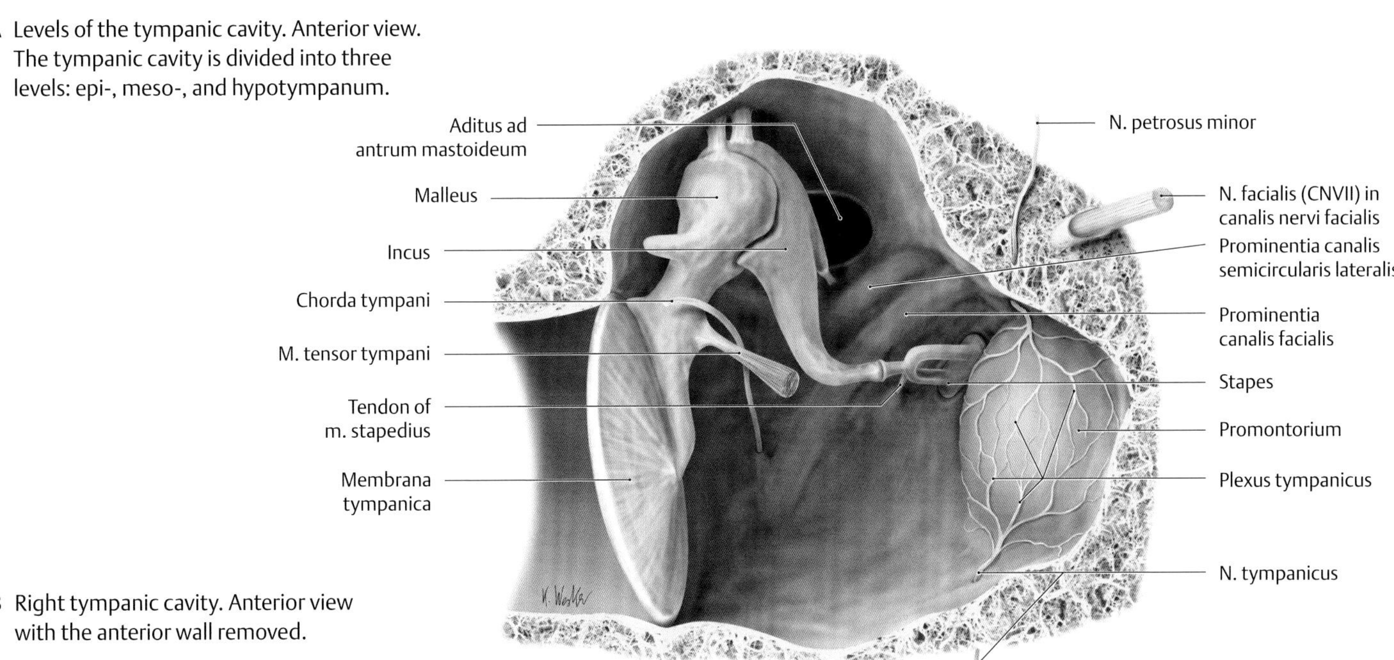
Aditus ad antrum mastoideum
Malleus
Incus
Chorda tympani
M. tensor tympani
Tendon of m. stapedius
Membrana tympanica
N. petrosus minor
N. facialis (CNVII) in canalis nervi facialis
Prominentia canalis semicircularis lateralis
Prominentia canalis facialis
Stapes
Promontorium
Plexus tympanicus
N. tympanicus

B Right tympanic cavity. Anterior view with the anterior wall removed.

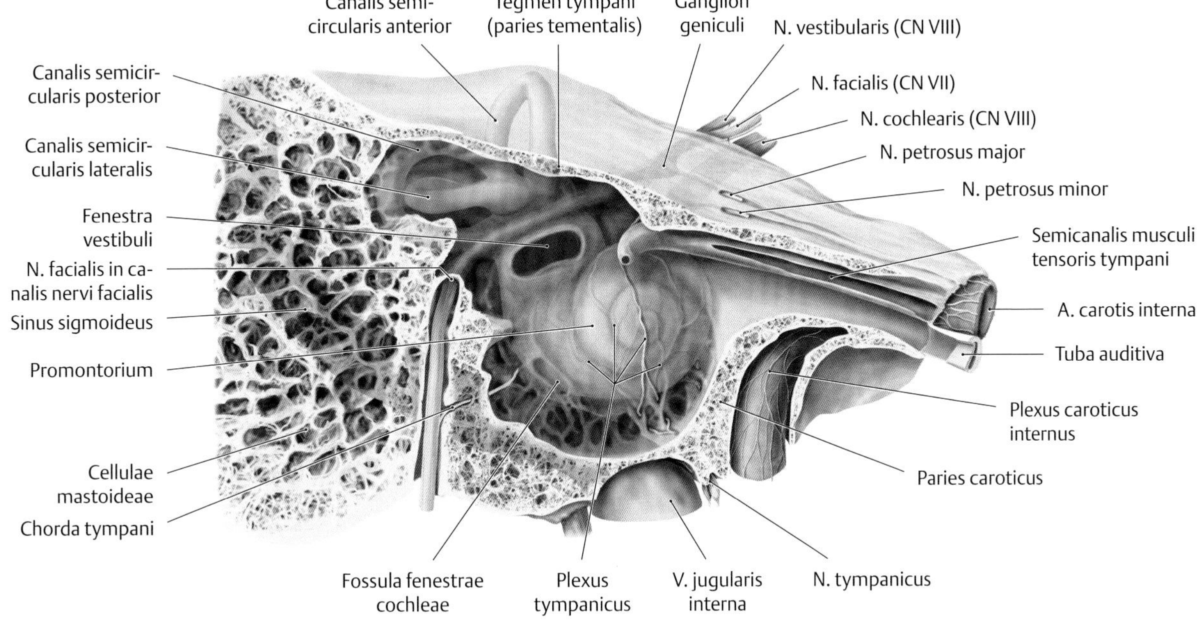
Canalis semicircularis anterior
Tegmen tympani (paries tementalis)
Ganglion geniculi
N. vestibularis (CN VIII)
N. facialis (CN VII)
N. cochlearis (CN VIII)
N. petrosus major
N. petrosus minor
Semicanalis musculi tensoris tympani
A. carotis interna
Tuba auditiva
Plexus caroticus internus
Paries caroticus
Canalis semicircularis posterior
Canalis semicircularis lateralis
Fenestra vestibuli
N. facialis in canalis nervi facialis
Sinus sigmoideus
Promontorium
Cellulae mastoideae
Chorda tympani
Fossula fenestrae cochleae
Plexus tympanicus
V. jugularis interna
N. tympanicus

C Anatomical relationships of the tympanic cavity. Oblique sagittal section showing the medial wall.

Middle Ear: Ossicular Chain & Membrana Tympanica

Fig. 35.11 Auditory ossicles (ossicula auditus)

Left ear. The ossicular chain consists of three small bones that establish an articular connection between membrana tympanica and the oval window (fenestra vestibuli).

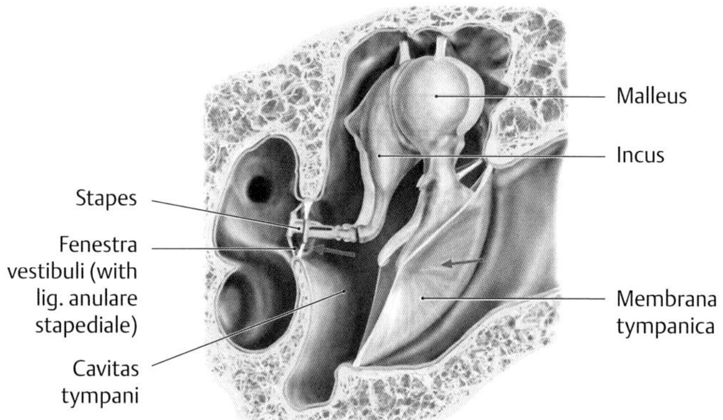
Malleus
Incus
Stapes
Fenestra vestibuli (with lig. anulare stapediale)
Membrana tympanica
Cavitas tympani

A Auditory ossicles in the middle ear. Anterior view of the left ear.

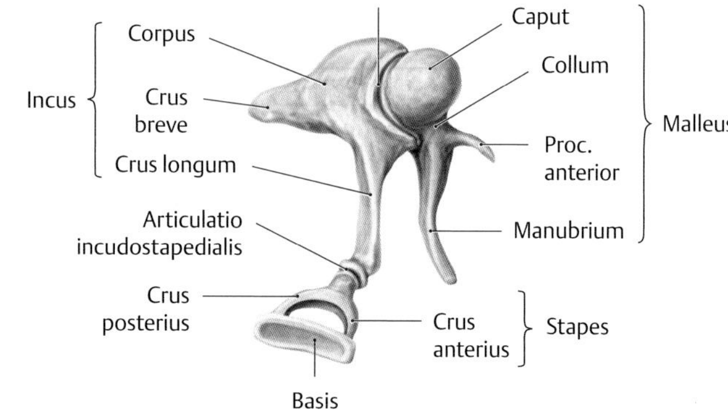
Articulatio incudomallearis
Incus
Corpus
Crus breve
Crus longum
Caput
Collum
Malleus
Proc. anterior
Manubrium
Articulatio incudostapedialis
Crus posterius
Crus anterius
Stapes
Basis

B Bones of the ossicular chain. Medial view of the left ossicular chain.

Fig. 35.12 Malleus ("hammer")

Left ear.

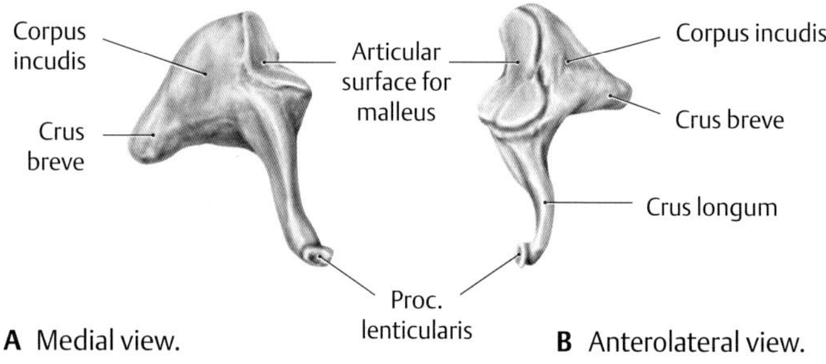
Collum mallei
Articular surface for incus
Proc. lateralis
Manubrium mallei
Caput mallei
Collum mallei
Proc. lateralis
Proc. anterior

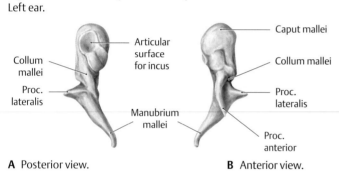

A Posterior view. **B** Anterior view.

Fig. 35.13 Incus ("anvil")

Left ear.

Corpus incudis
Crus breve
Articular surface for malleus
Proc. lenticularis
Corpus incudis
Crus breve
Crus longum

A Medial view. **B** Anterolateral view.

Fig. 35.14 Stapes ("stirrup")

Left ear.

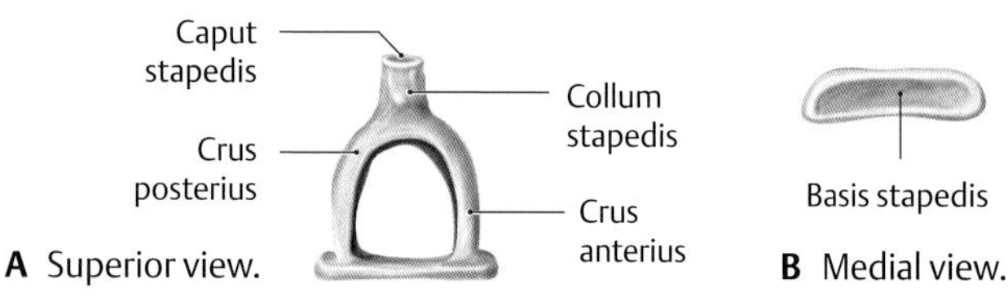
Caput stapedis
Crus posterius
Collum stapedis
Crus anterius
Basis stapedis

A Superior view. **B** Medial view.

Fig. 35.15 Membrana tympanica

Right membrana tympanica. Membrana tympanica is divided into four quadrants: anterosuperior (I), anteroinferior (II), posteroinferior (III), and posterosuperior (IV).

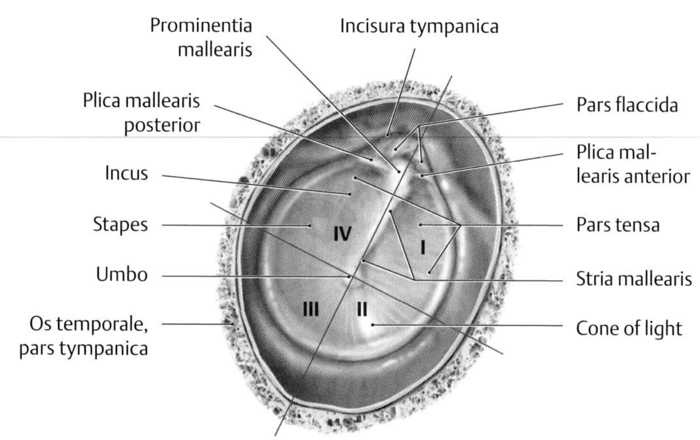
Prominentia mallearis
Incisura tympanica
Plica mallearis posterior
Pars flaccida
Plica mallearis anterior
Incus
Stapes
Pars tensa
Umbo
Stria mallearis
Os temporale, pars tympanica
Cone of light
IV
I
III
II

A Lateral view of the right membrana tympanica.

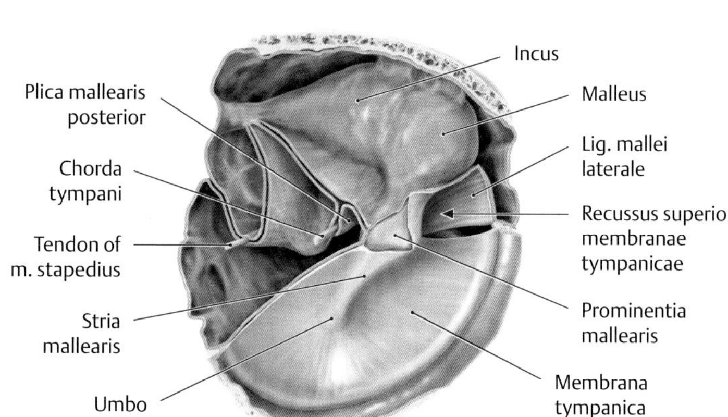
Incus
Malleus
Plica mallearis posterior
Lig. mallei laterale
Chorda tympani
Recussus superior membranae tympanicae
Tendon of m. stapedius
Prominentia mallearis
Stria mallearis
Membrana tympanica
Umbo

B Mucosal lining of the tympanic cavity. Posterolateral view with membrana tympanica partially removed.

Fig. 35.16 Ossicular chain in the tympanic cavity
Lateral view of the right ear. *Revealed:* Ligaments of the ossicular chain and muscles of the middle ear (m. stapedius and m. tensor tympani).

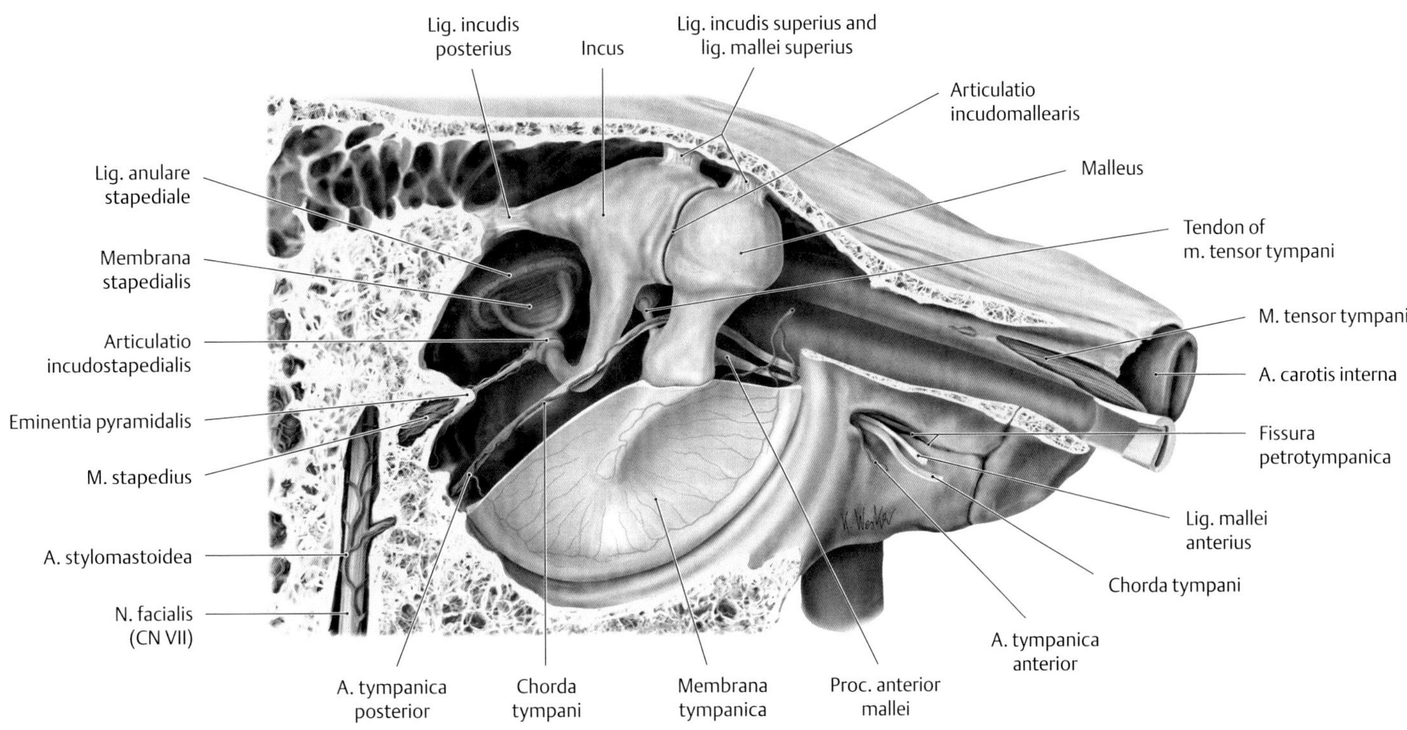
Lig. incudis posterius
Incus
Lig. incudis superius and lig. mallei superius
Articulatio incudomallearis
Malleus
Tendon of m. tensor tympani
M. tensor tympani
A. carotis interna
Fissura petrotympanica
Lig. mallei anterius
Chorda tympani
A. tympanica anterior
Proc. anterior mallei
Membrana tympanica
Chorda tympani
A. tympanica posterior
N. facialis (CN VII)
A. stylomastoidea
M. stapedius
Eminentia pyramidalis
Articulatio incudostapedialis
Membrana stapedialis
Lig. anulare stapediale

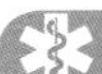

Clinical

Ossicular chain in hearing

Sound waves funneled into the meatus acusticus externus set the membrana tympanica into vibration. The ossicular chain transmits the vibrations to the oval window, which communicates them to the fluid column of the inner ear. Sound waves in fluid meet with higher impedance; they must therefore be amplified in the middle ear. The difference in surface area between membrana tympanica and the oval window increases the sound pressure 17-fold. A total amplification factor of 22 is achieved through the lever action of the ossicular chain. If the ossicular chain fails to transform the sound pressure between membrana tympanica and the basis stapedis, the patient will experience conductive hearing loss of magnitude 20 dB. See p. 619 for hearing.

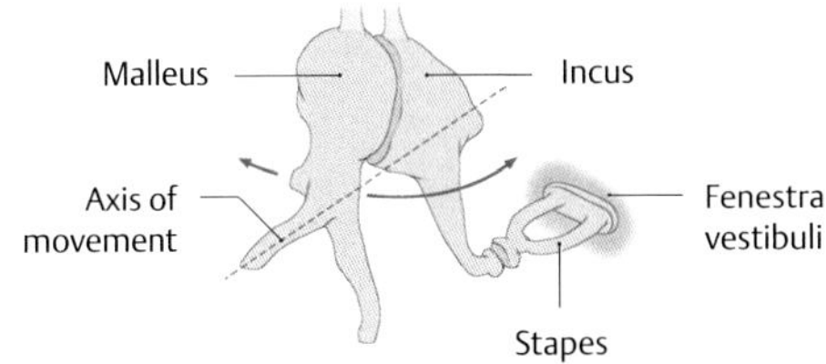
Malleus
Incus
Axis of movement
Fenestra vestibuli
Stapes

A Vibration of membrana tympanica causes a rocking movement in the ossicular chain. The mechanical advantage of the lever action of the ossicular chain amplifies the sound waves by a factor of 1.3.

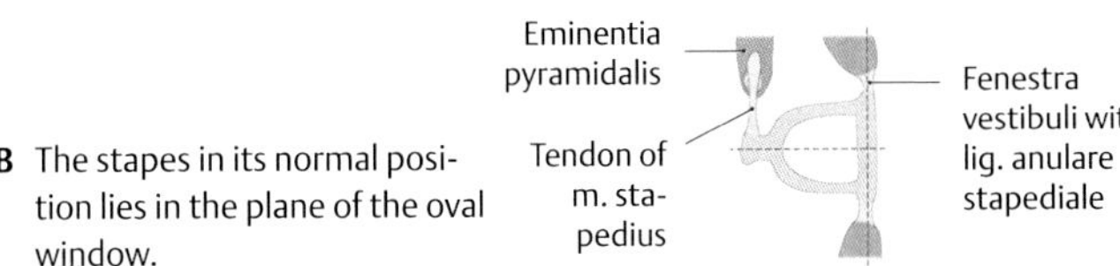
Eminentia pyramidalis
Tendon of m. stapedius
Fenestra vestibuli with lig. anulare stapediale

B The stapes in its normal position lies in the plane of the oval window.

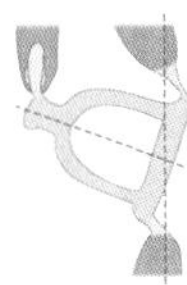

C Rocking of the ossicular chain causes the stapes to tilt. The movement of the basis stapedis against the membrane of the oval window (membrana stapedialis) induces corresponding waves in the fluid column of the inner ear.

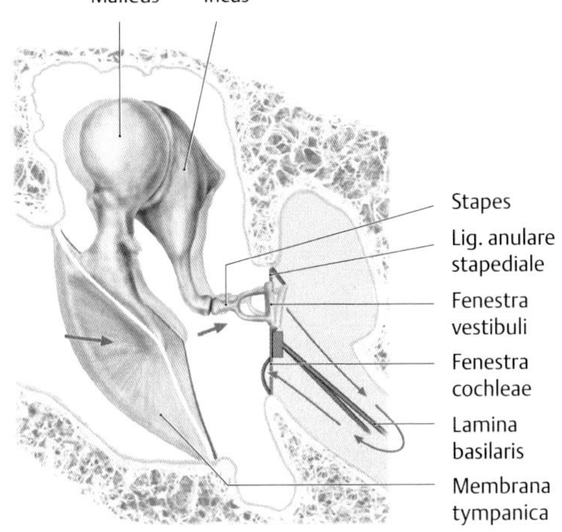
Malleus
Incus
Stapes
Lig. anulare stapediale
Fenestra vestibuli
Fenestra cochleae
Lamina basilaris
Membrana tympanica

D Propagation of sound waves by the ossicular chain.

Arteries of the Middle Ear

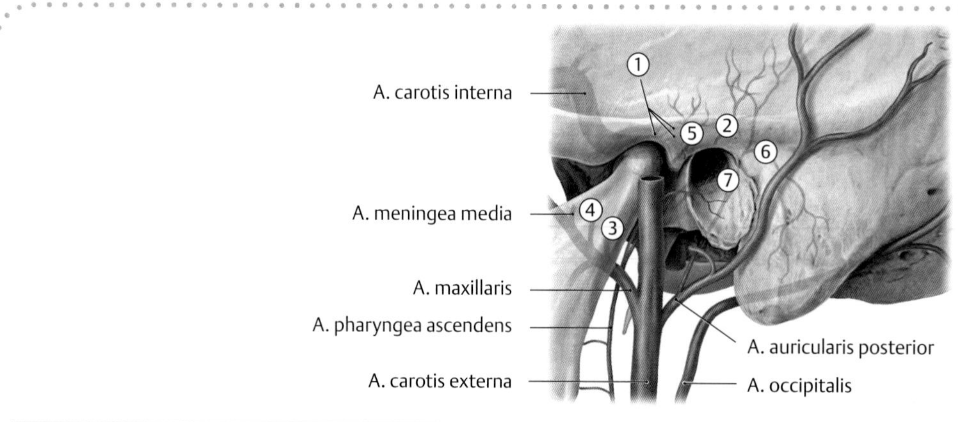

A. carotis interna
A. meningea media
A. maxillaris
A. pharyngea ascendens
A. carotis externa
A. auricularis posterior
A. occipitalis
①
②
③
④
⑤
⑥
⑦

Table 35.2 Principal arteries of the middle ear

Origin	Artery			Distribution
A. carotis interna	① Aa. caroticotympanicae			Cavitas tympani (paries caroticus), tuba auditiva
A. carotis externa	A. pharyngea ascendens (r. medius)	② A. tympanica inferior		Cavitas tympani (paries jugularis), promotorium
	A. maxillaris (r. terminalis)	③ A. auricularis profunda		Cavitas tympani (paries jugularis), membrana tympanica
		④ A. tympanica anterior		Membrana tympanica, antrum mastoideum, malleus, incus
		A. meningea media	⑤ A. tympanica superior	Cavitas tympani (paries tegmentalis), m. tensor tympani, stapes
	A. auricularis posterior (r. posterior)	A. stylomastoidea	⑥ A. stylomastoidea	Cavitas tympani (paries mastoideus), cellulae mastoideae, m. stapedius, stapes
			⑦ A. tympanica posterior	Chorda tympani, membrana tympanica, malleus

Fig. 35.17 **Arteries of the middle ear: Ossicular chain and membrana tympanica**

Medial view of the right membrana tympanica. With inflammation, the arteries of membrana tympanica may become so dilated that their course can be observed (as shown here).

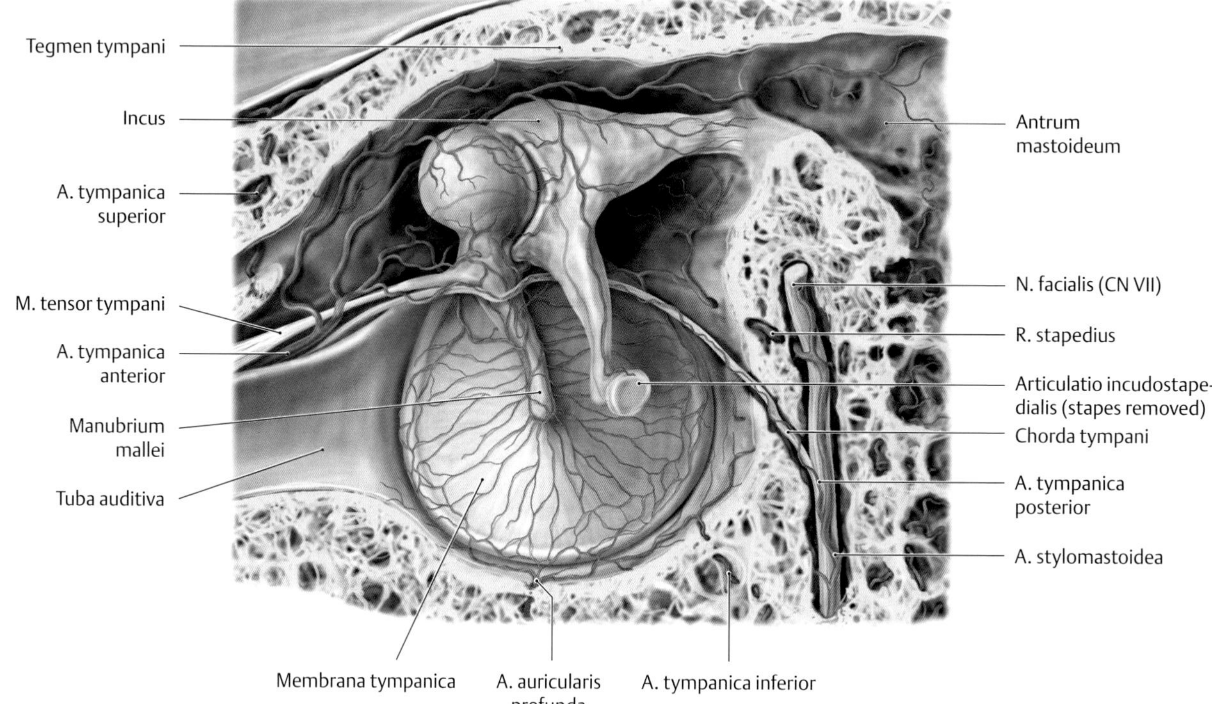

Tegmen tympani
Incus
A. tympanica superior
M. tensor tympani
A. tympanica anterior
Manubrium mallei
Tuba auditiva
Antrum mastoideum
N. facialis (CN VII)
R. stapedius
Articulatio incudostapedialis (stapes removed)
Chorda tympani
A. tympanica posterior
A. stylomastoidea
Membrana tympanica
A. auricularis profunda
A. tympanica inferior

Fig. 35.18 **Arteries of the middle ear: Tympanic cavity**
Right petrous bone, anterior view. *Removed:* Malleus, incus, portions of chorda tympani, and a. tympanica anterior.

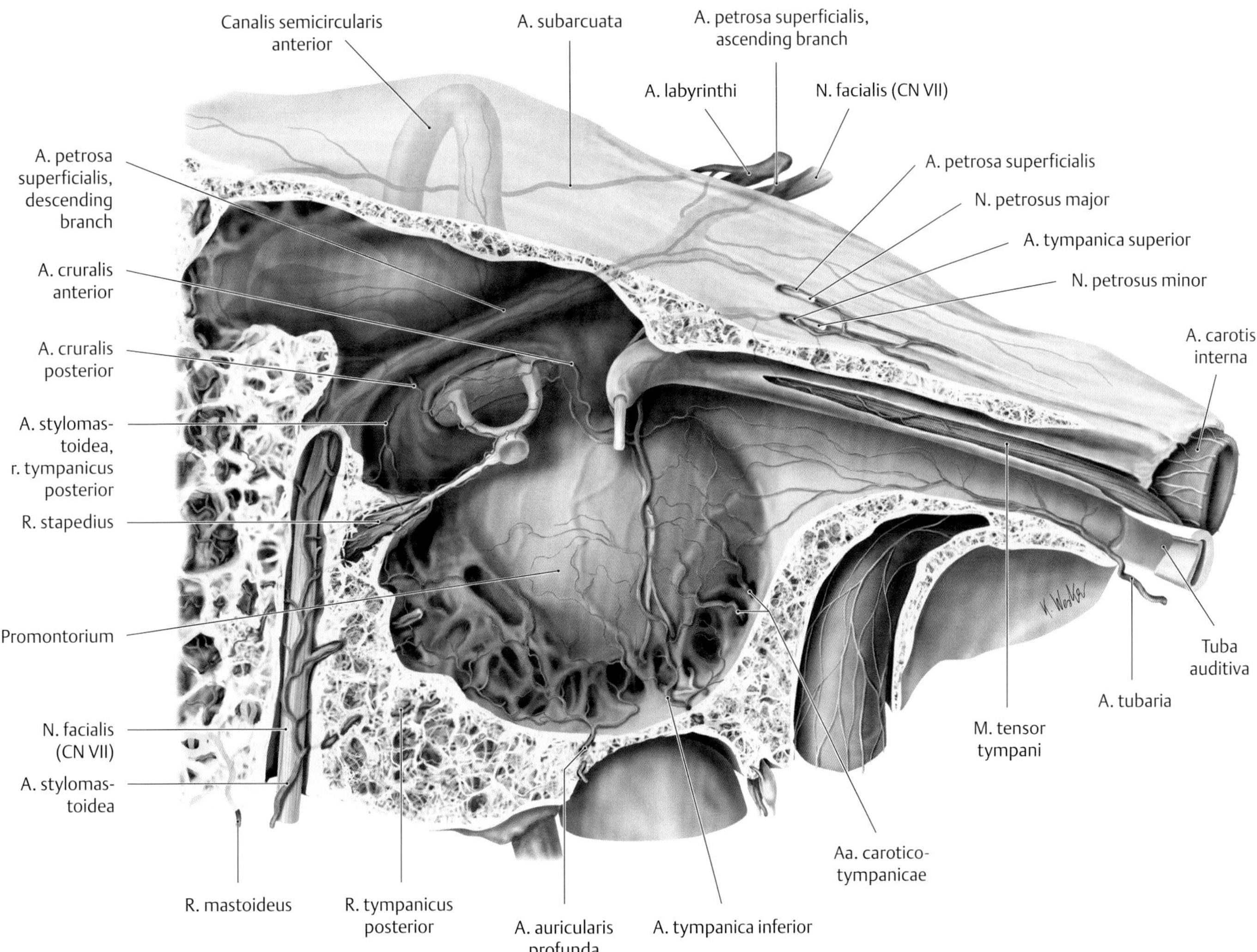
Canalis semicircularis anterior
A. subarcuata
A. petrosa superficialis, ascending branch
A. labyrinthi
N. facialis (CN VII)
A. petrosa superficialis
N. petrosus major
A. tympanica superior
N. petrosus minor
A. carotis interna
A. petrosa superficialis, descending branch
A. cruralis anterior
A. cruralis posterior
A. stylomastoidea, r. tympanicus posterior
R. stapedius
Promontorium
N. facialis (CN VII)
A. stylomastoidea
R. mastoideus
R. tympanicus posterior
A. auricularis profunda
A. tympanica inferior
Aa. caroticotympanicae
M. tensor tympani
A. tubaria
Tuba auditiva

Inner Ear (Auris Interna)

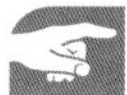

The inner ear consists of the vestibular apparatus (for balance) and the auditory apparatus (for hearing). Both are formed by a membranous labyrinth filled with endolympha floating within a bony labyrinth filled with perilympha and embedded in pars petrosa of os temporale.

Fig. 35.19 Vestibular apparatus

Right lateral view.

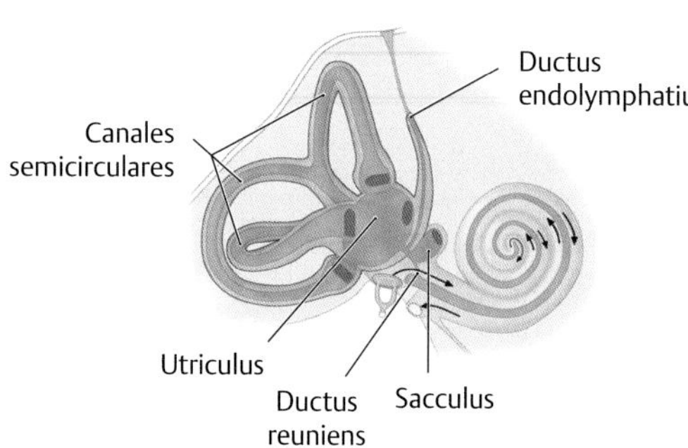
Ductus endolymphatius
Canales semicirculares
Utriculus
Ductus reuniens
Sacculus

A Schematic. Cristae ampullares and maculae of utriculus and sacculus shown in red.

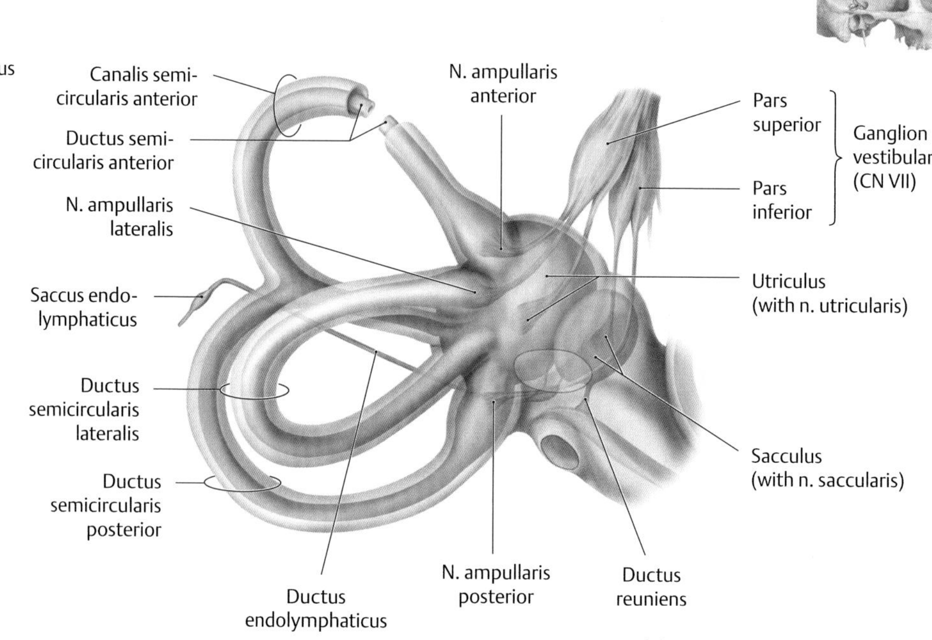
Canalis semicircularis anterior
Ductus semicircularis anterior
N. ampullaris lateralis
Saccus endolymphaticus
Ductus semicircularis lateralis
Ductus semicircularis posterior
Ductus endolymphaticus
N. ampullaris anterior
N. ampullaris posterior
Ductus reuniens
Pars superior
Pars inferior
Ganglion vestibulare (CN VII)
Utriculus (with n. utricularis)
Sacculus (with n. saccularis)

B Structure of the vestibular apparatus.

Fig. 35.20 Auditory apparatus

The cochlear labyrinth and its bony shell form the cochlea, which contains the sensory epithelium of the auditory apparatus (organ of Corti).

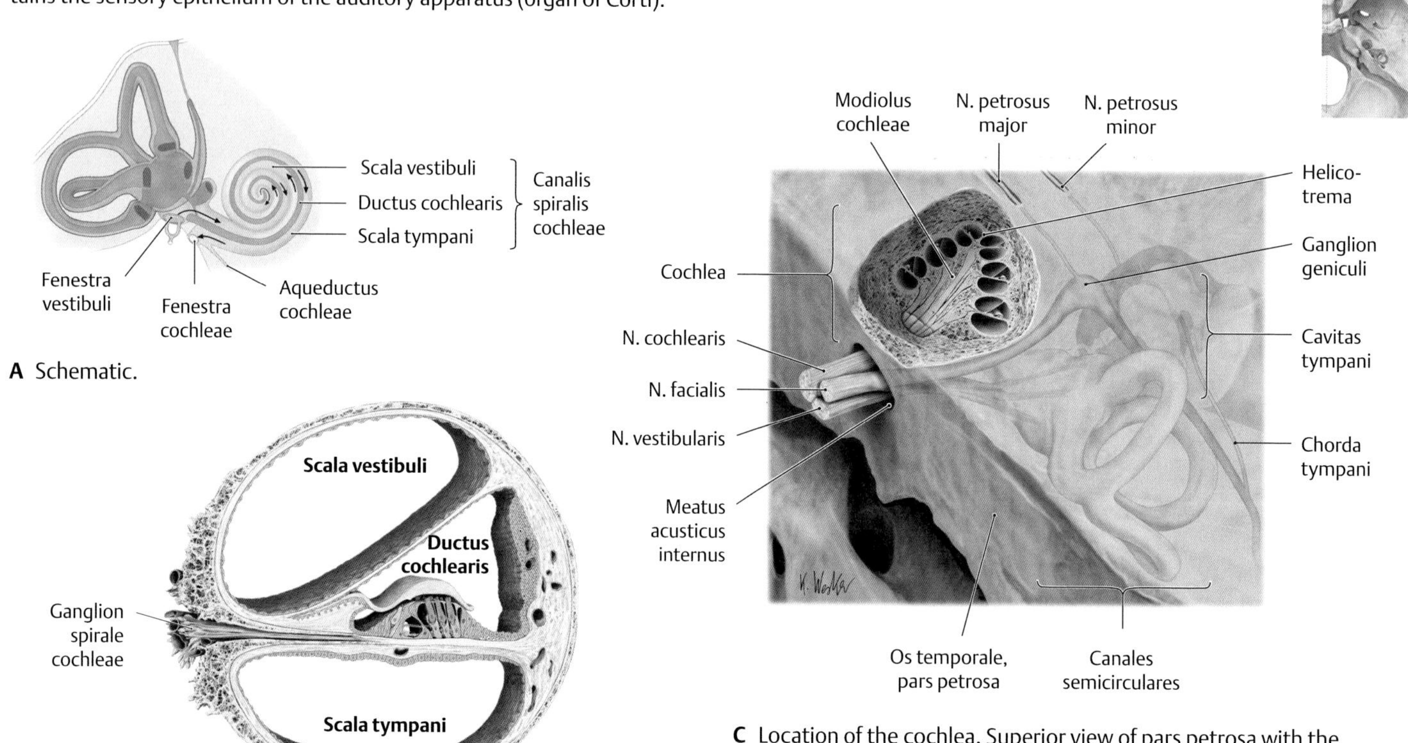
Scala vestibuli
Ductus cochlearis
Scala tympani
Canalis spiralis cochleae
Fenestra vestibuli
Fenestra cochleae
Aqueductus cochleae
Scala vestibuli
Ductus cochlearis
Ganglion spirale cochleae
Scala tympani
Modiolus cochleae
N. petrosus major
N. petrosus minor
Helicotrema
Ganglion geniculi
Cavitas tympani
Chorda tympani
Cochlea
N. cochlearis
N. facialis
N. vestibularis
Meatus acusticus internus
Os temporale, pars petrosa
Canales semicirculares

A Schematic.

B Compartments of the canalis spiralis cochleae, cross section.

C Location of the cochlea. Superior view of pars petrosa with the cochlea sectioned transversely. The bony canal of the cochlea (canalis spiralis cochlea) makes 2.5 turns around its bony axis (modiolus cochleae).

Fig. 35.21 Innervation of the membranous labyrinth

Right ear, anterior view. N. vestibulocochlearis (CN VIII; see p. 480) transmits afferent impulses from the inner ear to the brainstem through the meatus acousticus internus. N. vestibulocochlearis is divided into the n. vestibularis and n. cochlearis. *Note:* The sensory organs in the semicircular canals respond to angular acceleration, and the macular organs (sacculus and utriculus) respond to horizontal and vertical linear acceleration.

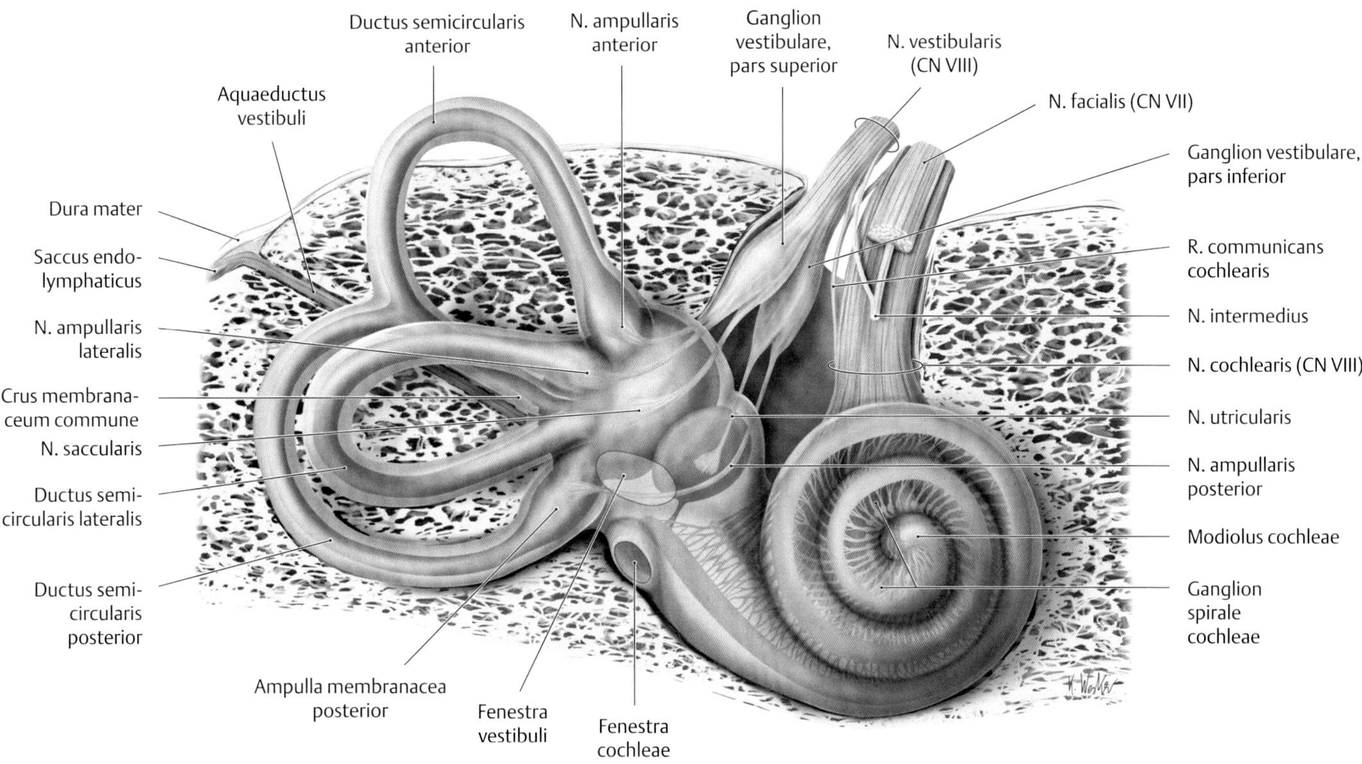
Ductus semicircularis anterior
N. ampullaris anterior
Ganglion vestibulare, pars superior
N. vestibularis (CN VIII)
N. facialis (CN VII)
Ganglion vestibulare, pars inferior
R. communicans cochlearis
N. intermedius
N. cochlearis (CN VIII)
N. utricularis
N. ampullaris posterior
Modiolus cochleae
Ganglion spirale cochleae
Aquaeductus vestibuli
Dura mater
Saccus endo-lymphaticus
N. ampullaris lateralis
Crus membranaceum commune
N. saccularis
Ductus semicircularis lateralis
Ductus semicircularis posterior
Ampulla membranacea posterior
Fenestra vestibuli
Fenestra cochleae

Fig. 35.22 Blood vessels of the inner ear

Right anterior view. The labyrinth receives its blood supply from the a. labyrinthi, a branch of the a. inferior anterior cerebelli (see p. 608).

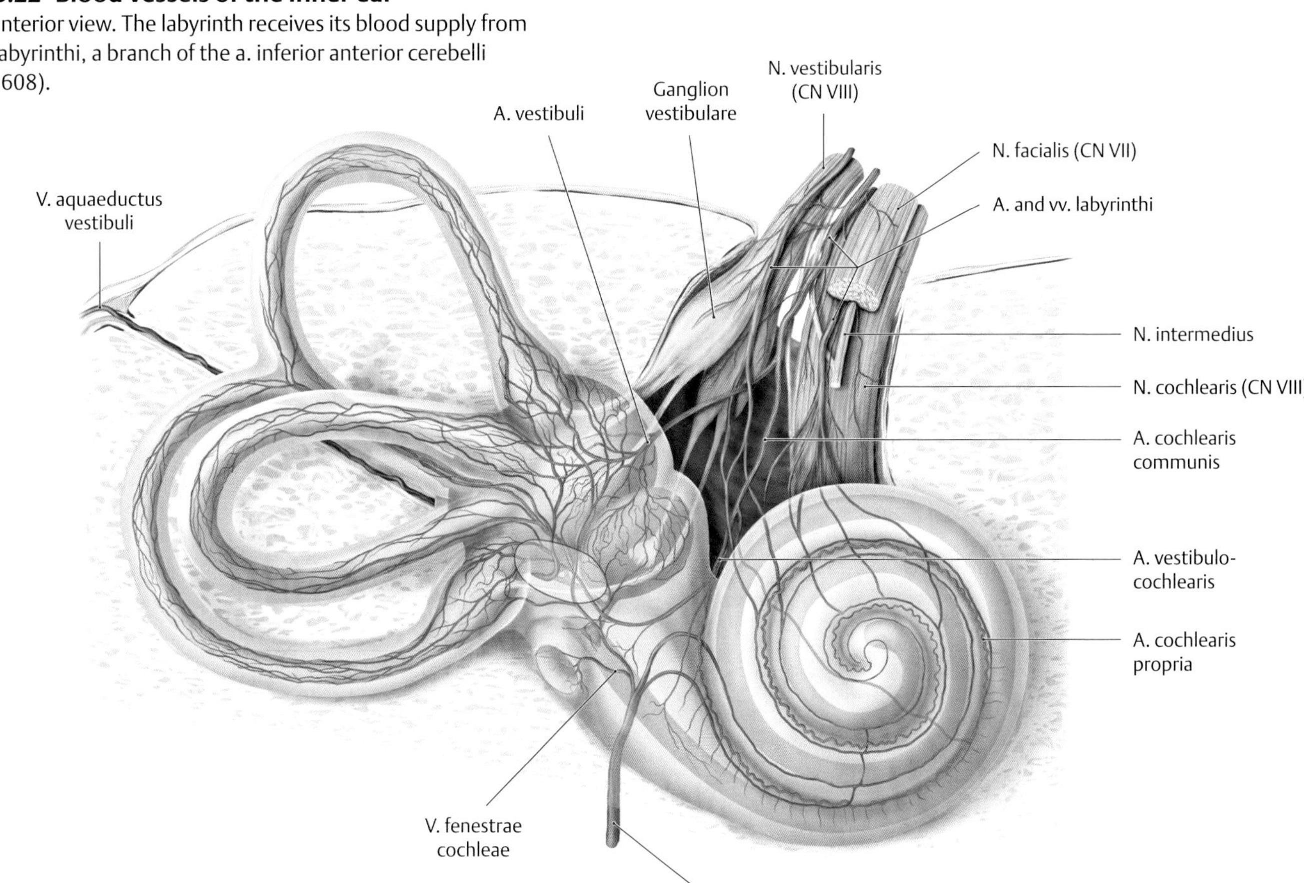
A. vestibuli
Ganglion vestibulare
N. vestibularis (CN VIII)
N. facialis (CN VII)
A. and vv. labyrinthi
N. intermedius
N. cochlearis (CN VIII)
A. cochlearis communis
A. vestibulo-cochlearis
A. cochlearis propria
V. aquaeductus vestibuli
V. fenestrae cochleae
V. aquaeductus cochleae

Bones of the Oral Cavity (Cavitas Oris)

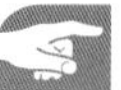

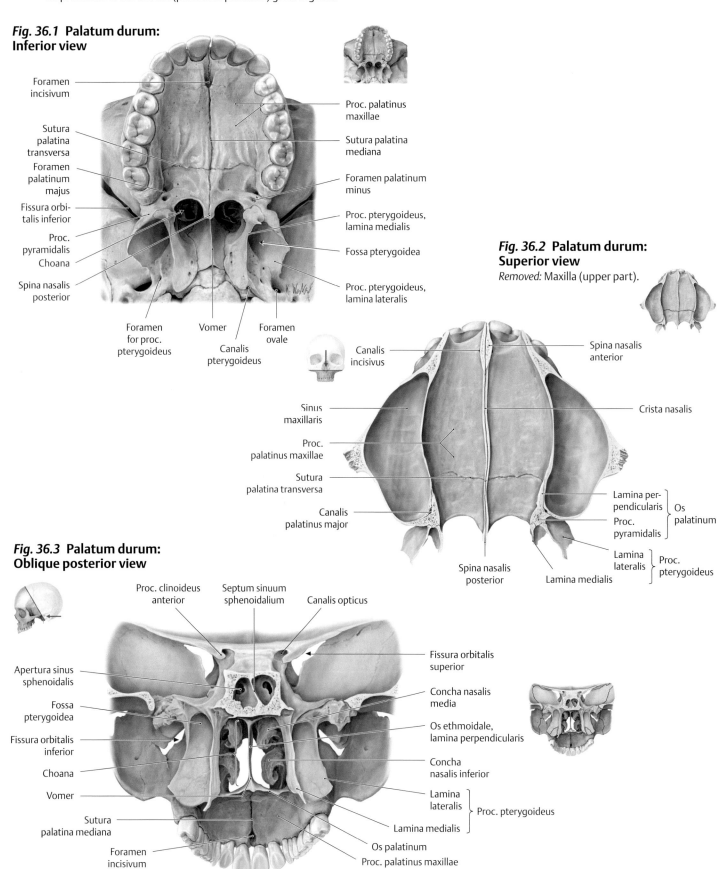

The floor of the nasal cavity (the maxilla and palatine bone) forms the roof of the oral cavity, the palatum durum. The two horizontal processes of the maxilla (processus palatinus) grow together during development, eventually fusing at the sutura palatina mediana. Failure to fuse results in a cleft palate.

Fig. 36.1 **Palatum durum: Inferior view**

Foramen incisivum
Sutura palatina transversa
Foramen palatinum majus
Fissura orbitalis inferior
Proc. pyramidalis
Choana
Spina nasalis posterior
Foramen for proc. pterygoideus
Vomer
Canalis pterygoideus
Foramen ovale
Proc. palatinus maxillae
Sutura palatina mediana
Foramen palatinum minus
Proc. pterygoideus, lamina medialis
Fossa pterygoidea
Proc. pterygoideus, lamina lateralis

Fig. 36.2 **Palatum durum: Superior view**
Removed: Maxilla (upper part).

Canalis incisivus
Sinus maxillaris
Proc. palatinus maxillae
Sutura palatina transversa
Canalis palatinus major
Spina nasalis posterior
Lamina medialis
Spina nasalis anterior
Crista nasalis
Lamina perpendicularis, Proc. pyramidalis — Os palatinum
Lamina lateralis — Proc. pterygoideus

Fig. 36.3 **Palatum durum: Oblique posterior view**

Proc. clinoideus anterior
Septum sinuum sphenoidalium
Canalis opticus
Apertura sinus sphenoidalis
Fossa pterygoidea
Fissura orbitalis inferior
Choana
Vomer
Sutura palatina mediana
Foramen incisivum
Fissura orbitalis superior
Concha nasalis media
Os ethmoidale, lamina perpendicularis
Concha nasalis inferior
Lamina lateralis, Lamina medialis — Proc. pterygoideus
Os palatinum
Proc. palatinus maxillae

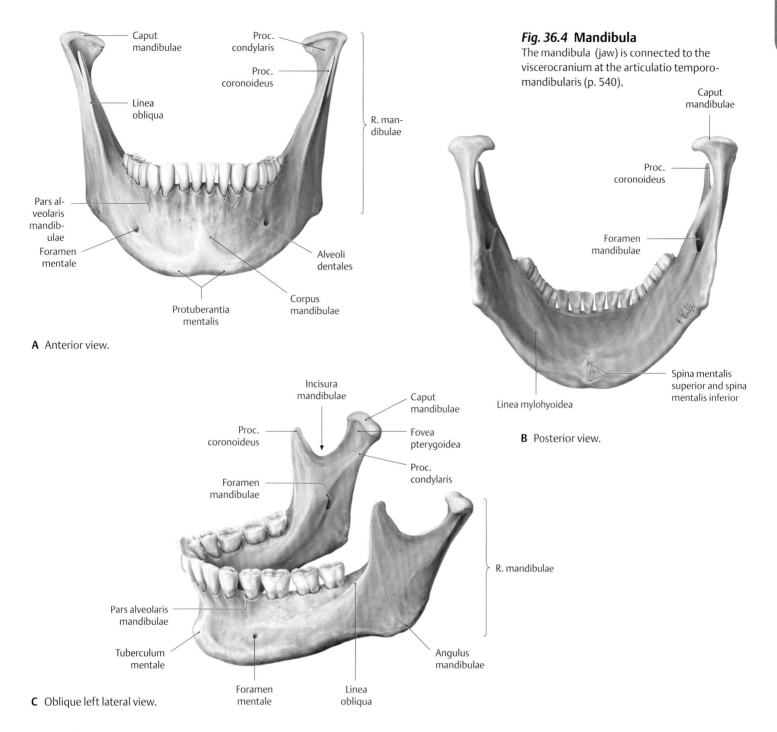

Fig. 36.4 **Mandibula**

The mandibula (jaw) is connected to the viscerocranium at the articulatio temporomandibularis (p. 540).

Caput mandibulae
Proc. condylaris
Proc. coronoideus
Linea obliqua
R. mandibulae
Pars alveolaris mandibulae
Foramen mentale
Alveoli dentales
Corpus mandibulae
Protuberantia mentalis

A Anterior view.

Caput mandibulae
Proc. coronoideus
Foramen mandibulae
Linea mylohyoidea
Spina mentalis superior and spina mentalis inferior

B Posterior view.

Incisura mandibulae
Proc. coronoideus
Caput mandibulae
Fovea pterygoidea
Proc. condylaris
Foramen mandibulae
R. mandibulae
Pars alveolaris mandibulae
Tuberculum mentale
Angulus mandibulae
Foramen mentale
Linea obliqua

C Oblique left lateral view.

Fig. 36.5 **Os hyoideum**

The os hyoideum is suspended in the neck by muscles between the floor of the mouth and the larynx. Although not listed among the cranial bones, os hyoideum gives attachment to the muscles of the oral floor. The cornu majus and corpus of os hyoideum are palpable in the neck.

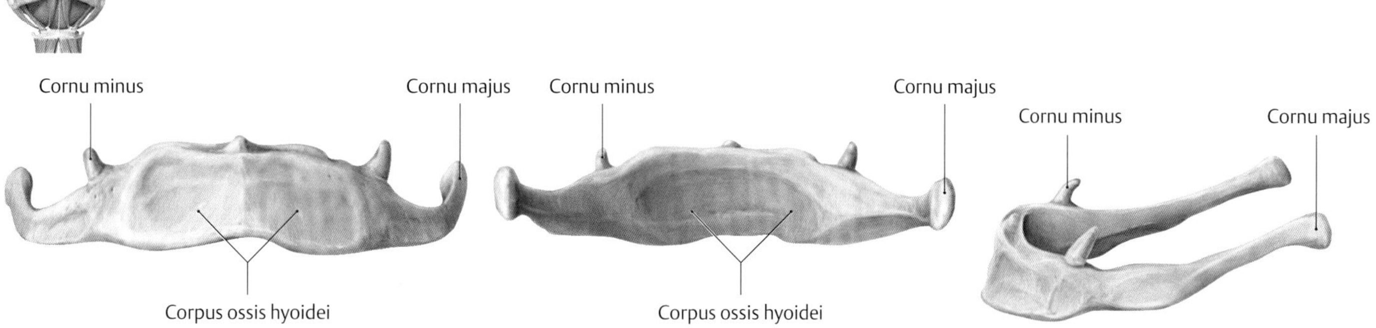
Cornu minus
Cornu majus
Corpus ossis hyoidei
Cornu minus
Cornu majus
Corpus ossis hyoidei
Cornu minus
Cornu majus

A Anterior view.

B Posterior view.

C Oblique left lateral view.

Articulatio Temporomandibularis

Fig. 36.6 Articulatio temporomandibularis

The caput mandibulae articulates with the fossa mandibularis in the articulatio temporomandibularis.

Tuberculum articulare
Fossa mandibularis
Discus articularis
Caput mandibulae

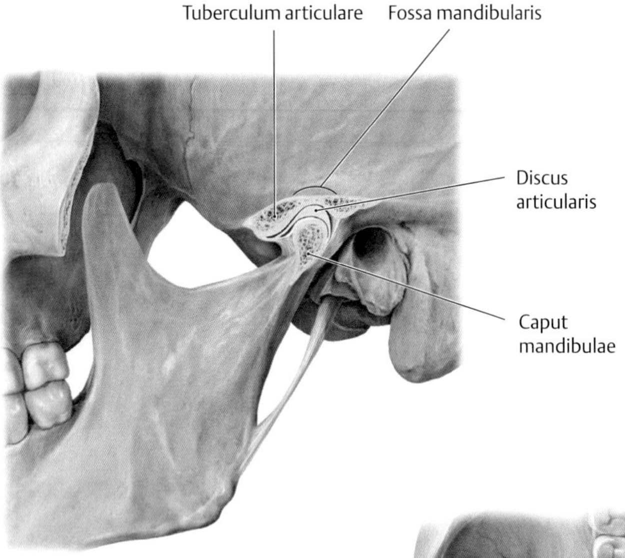

A Sagittally sectioned articulatio temporomandibularis, left lateral view.

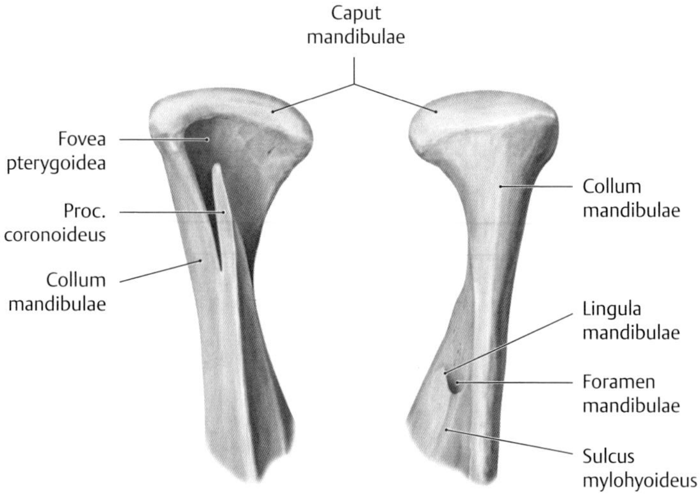

Caput mandibulae
Fovea pterygoidea
Proc. coronoideus
Collum mandibulae
Collum mandibulae
Lingula mandibulae
Foramen mandibulae
Sulcus mylohyoideus

B Caput mandibulae, anterior view.

C Caput mandibulae, posterior view.

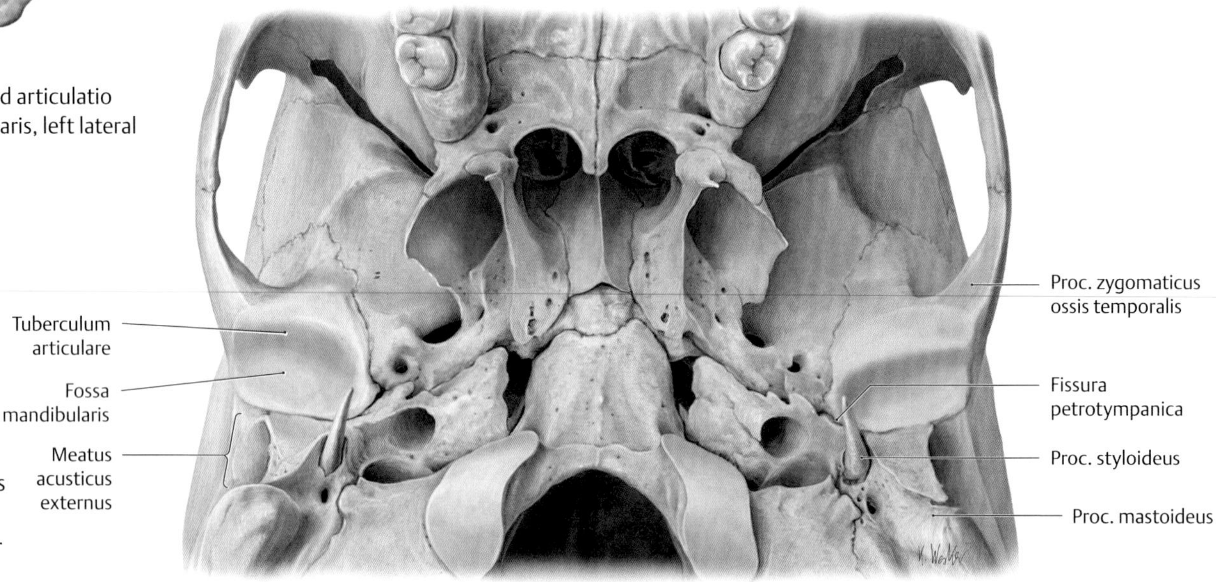

Tuberculum articulare
Fossa mandibularis
Meatus acusticus externus
Proc. zygomaticus ossis temporalis
Fissura petrotympanica
Proc. styloideus
Proc. mastoideus

D Fossa mandibularis of the articulatio temporomandibularis, inferior view.

Fig. 36.7 Ligaments of articulatio temporomandibularis

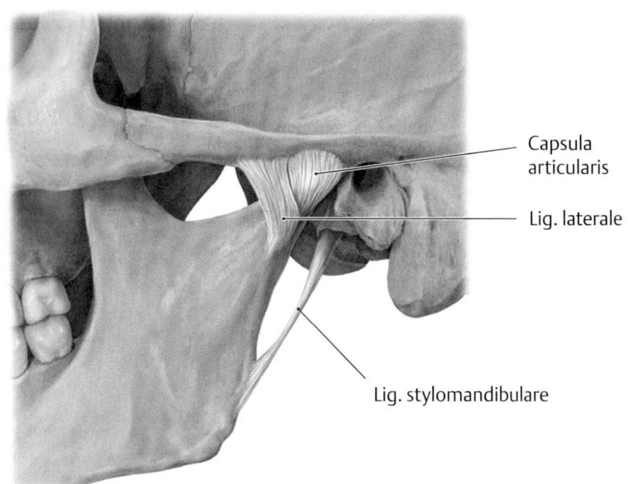
Capsula articularis
Lig. laterale
Lig. stylomandibulare

A Lateral view of the left articulatio temporomandibularis.

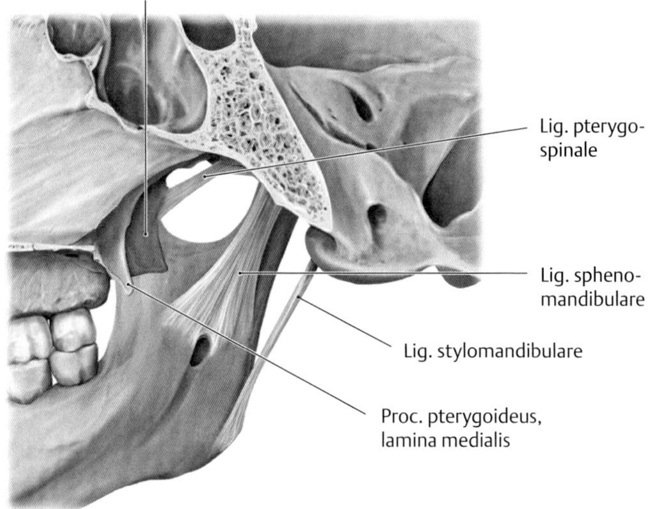
Proc. pterygoideus, lamina lateralis
Lig. pterygo-spinale
Lig. spheno-mandibulare
Lig. stylomandibulare
Proc. pterygoideus, lamina medialis

B Medial view of the right articulatio temporomandibularis.

Fig. 36.8 Movement of articulatio temporomandibularis

Left lateral view. Up to 15 degrees of abduction, caput mandibulae remains in the fossa mandibularis. Past 15 degrees, caput mandibulae glides forward onto the tuberculum articulare.

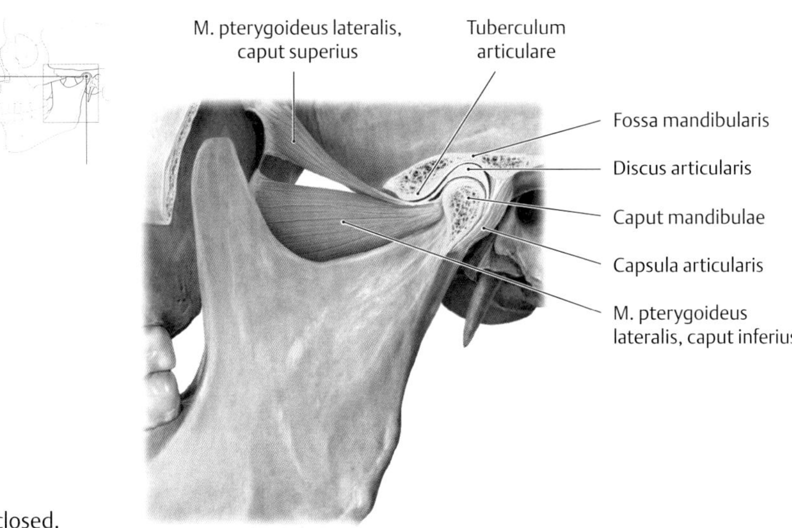
M. pterygoideus lateralis, caput superius
Tuberculum articulare
Fossa mandibularis
Discus articularis
Caput mandibulae
Capsula articularis
M. pterygoideus lateralis, caput inferius

A Mouth closed.

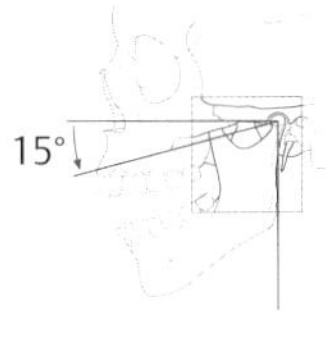
15°

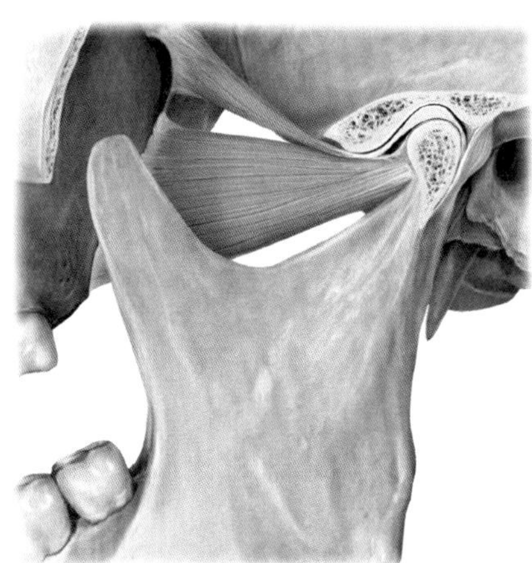

B Mouth opened to 15 degrees.

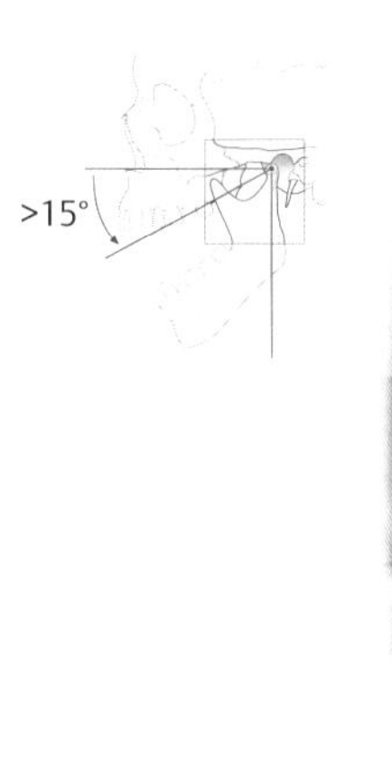
>15°
Tuberculum articulare
Fossa mandibularis
Discus articularis
Capsula articularis

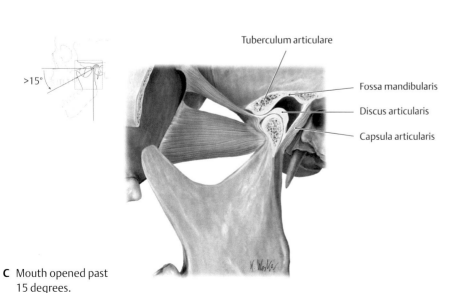

C Mouth opened past 15 degrees.

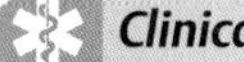

Clinical

Dislocation of articulatio temporomandibularis

Dislocation may occur if caput mandibulae slides past the tuberculum articulare. The mandibula then becomes locked in a protruded position, a condition reduced by pressing on the mandibular row of teeth.

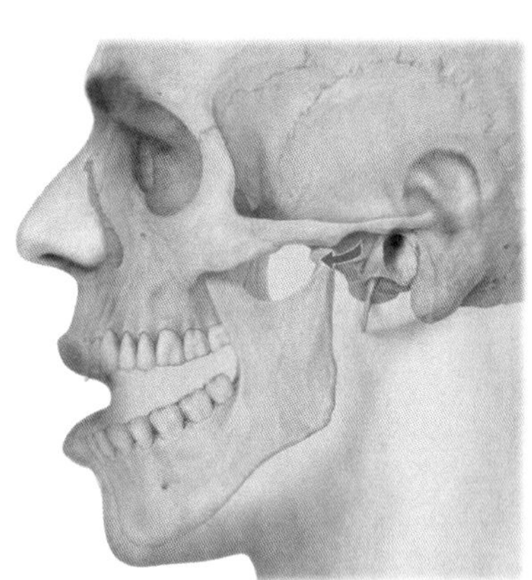

Fig. 36.9 Innervation of the joint capsule of articulatio temporomandibularis

Superior view.

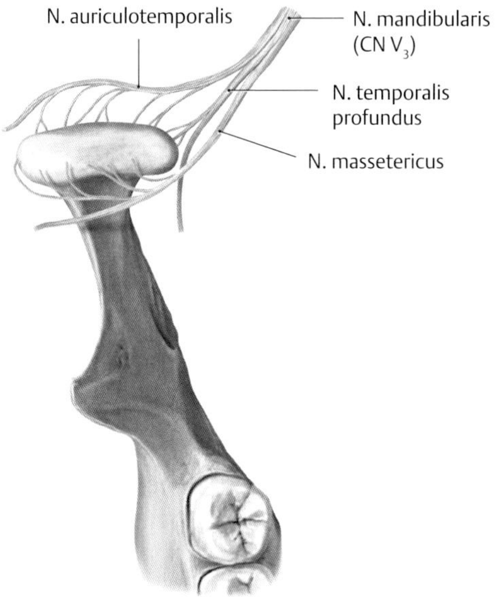
N. auriculotemporalis
N. mandibularis (CN V3)
N. temporalis profundus
N. massetericus

Teeth (Dentes)

Fig. 36.10 Structure of a tooth

Each tooth consists of hard tissue (enamel, dentin, cementum) and soft tissue (dental pulp) arranged into a crown, neck (cervix), and root.

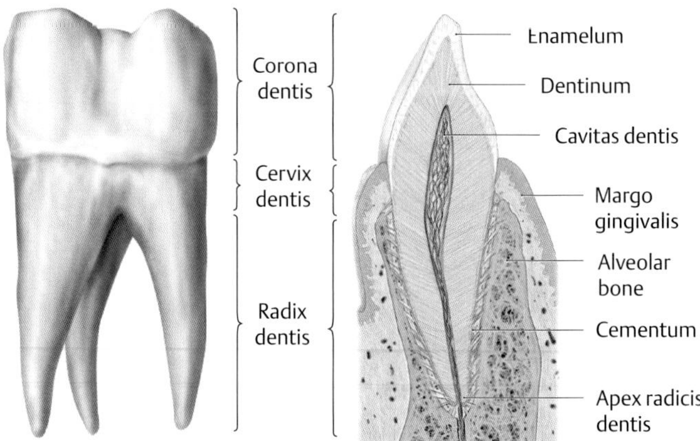

Corona dentis
Cervix dentis
Radix dentis
Enamelum
Dentinum
Cavitas dentis
Margo gingivalis
Alveolar bone
Cementum
Apex radicis dentis

A Principal parts of a tooth (molar).

B Histology of a tooth (mandibular dens incisivus).

Fig. 36.11 Permanent teeth

Each half of the maxilla and mandibula contains a set of three anterior teeth (two dentes incisivi, one dens caninus) and five posterior (postcanine) teeth (two dentes premolares, three dentes molares).

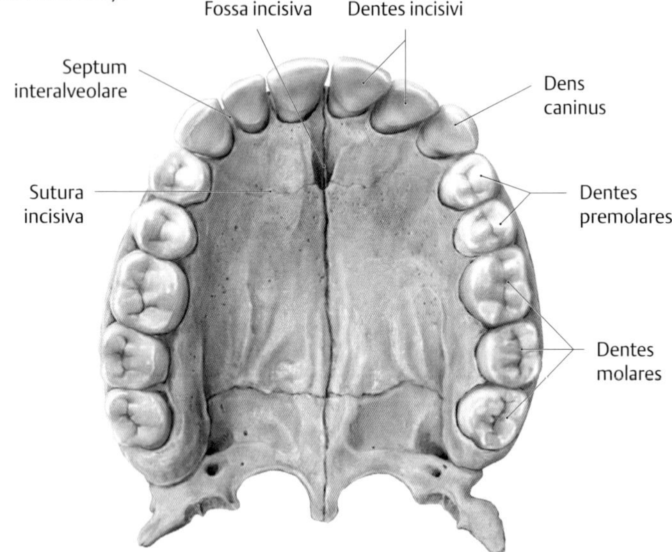

Fossa incisiva
Dentes incisivi
Septum interalveolare
Dens caninus
Sutura incisiva
Dentes premolares
Dentes molares

A Maxillary teeth. Inferior view of maxilla.

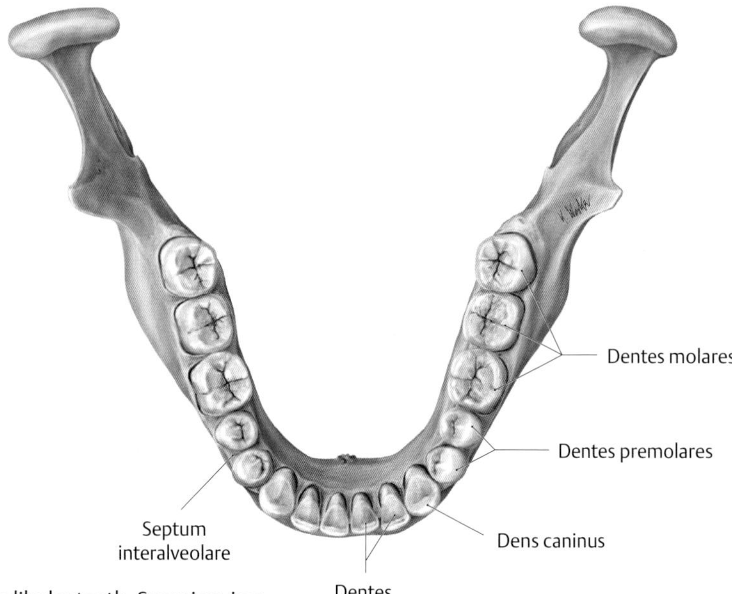

Dentes molares
Dentes premolares
Dens caninus
Septum interalveolare
Dentes incisivi

B Mandibular teeth. Superior view of mandibula.

Fig. 36.12 Tooth surfaces

The top of the tooth is known as the occlusal surface.

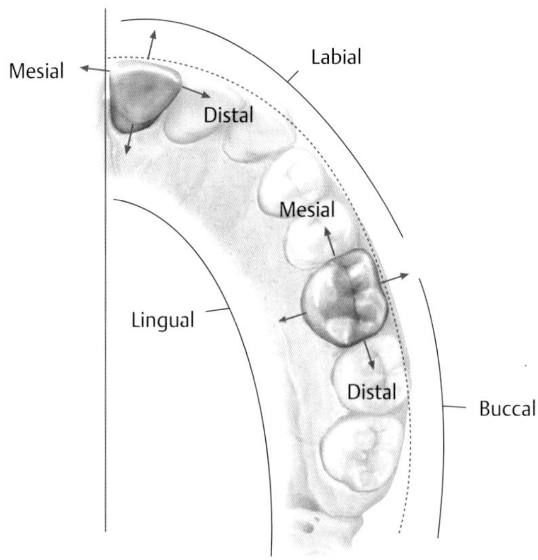

Mesial
Labial
Distal
Mesial
Lingual
Distal
Buccal

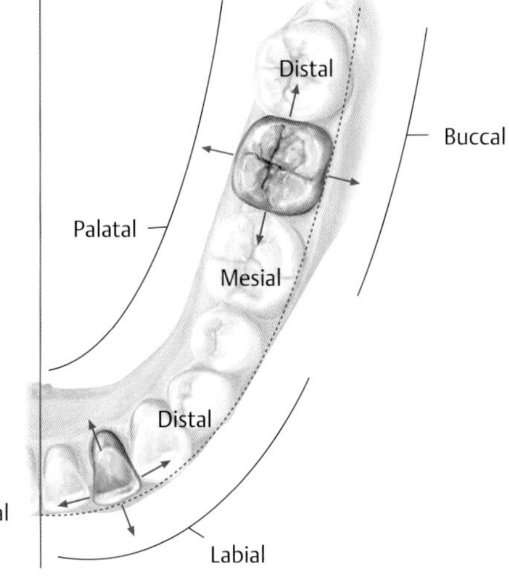

Distal
Buccal
Palatal
Mesial
Distal
Mesial
Labial

Fig. 36.13 Coding of the teeth
In the United States, the 32 permanent teeth are numbered sequentially (not assigned to quadrants). *Note:* The 20 deciduous (baby) teeth are coded A to J (upper arch), and K to T in a similar clockwise fashion. The third upper right molar is 1; the second upper right premolar is A.

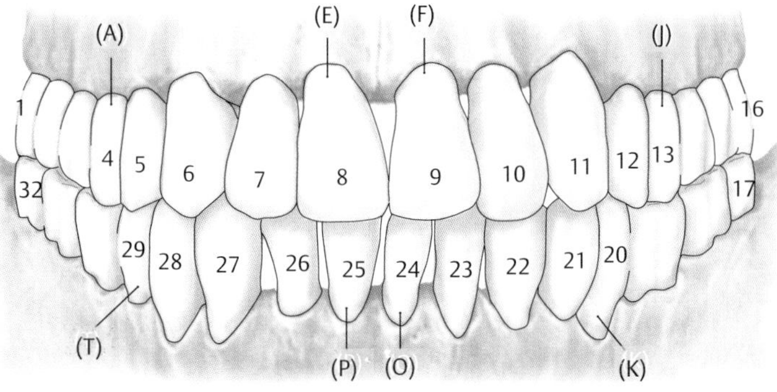
(A)
(E)
(F)
(J)
1
4
5
6
7
8
9
10
11
12
13
16
32
17
29
28
27
26
25
24
23
22
21
20
(T)
(P)
(O)
(K)

Fig. 36.14 Dental panoramic tomogram
The dental panoramic tomogram (DPT) is a survey radiograph that allows preliminary assessment of the temporomandibular joints, maxillary sinuses, maxillomandibular bone, and dental status (carious lesions, location of wisdom teeth, etc.). *DPT courtesy of Dr. U. J. Rother, Director of the Department of Diagnostic Radiology, Center for Dentistry and Oromaxillofacial Surgery, Eppendorf University Medical Center, Hamburg, Germany.*

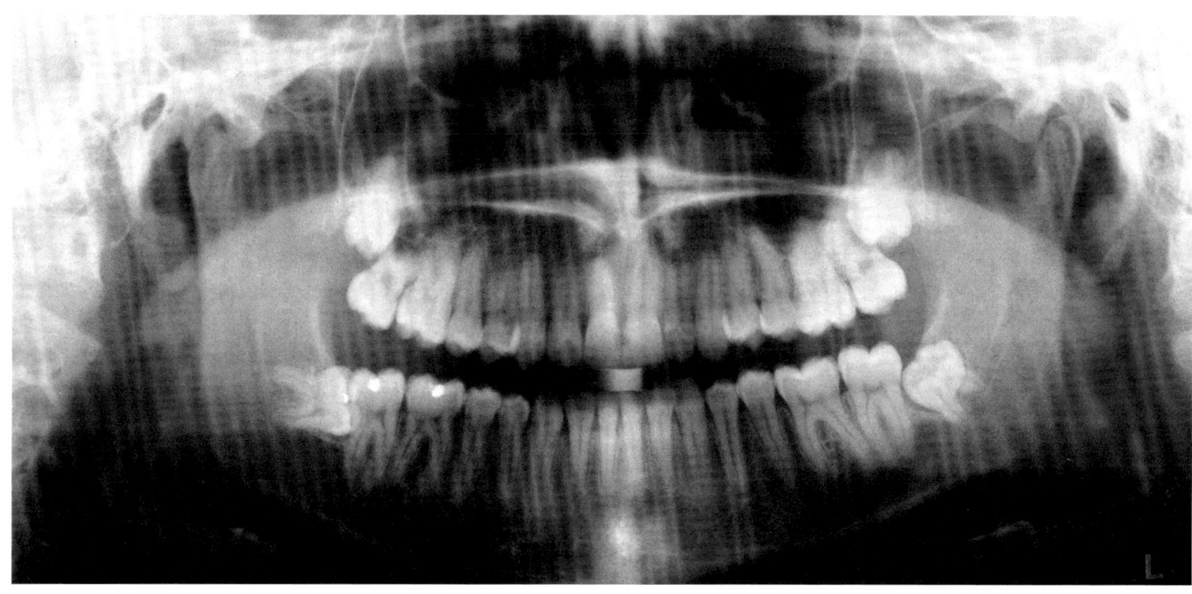

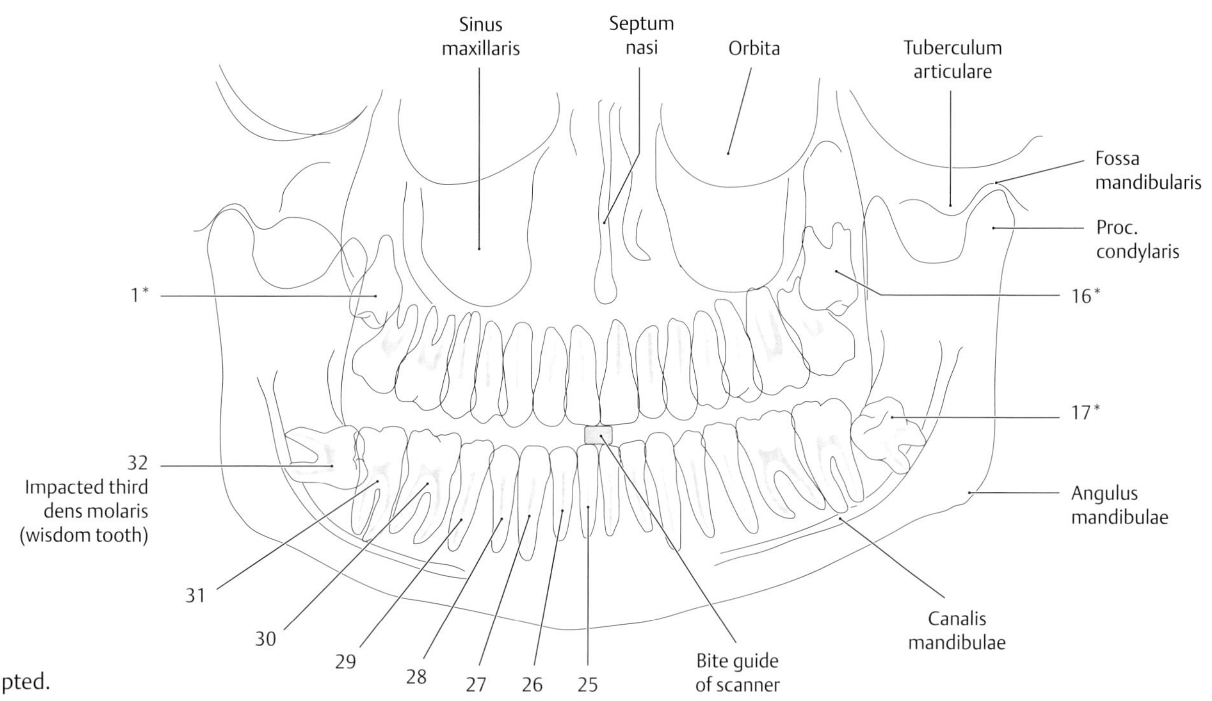
Sinus maxillaris
Septum nasi
Orbita
Tuberculum articulare
Fossa mandibularis
Proc. condylaris
1*
16*
17*
32
Impacted third dens molaris (wisdom tooth)
Angulus mandibulae
31
30
29
28
27
26
25
Bite guide of scanner
Canalis mandibulae

*Not fully erupted.

Muscles of the Oral Cavity

Fig. 36.15 **Muscles of the oral floor**
See pp. 562–563 for the infrahyoid muscles.

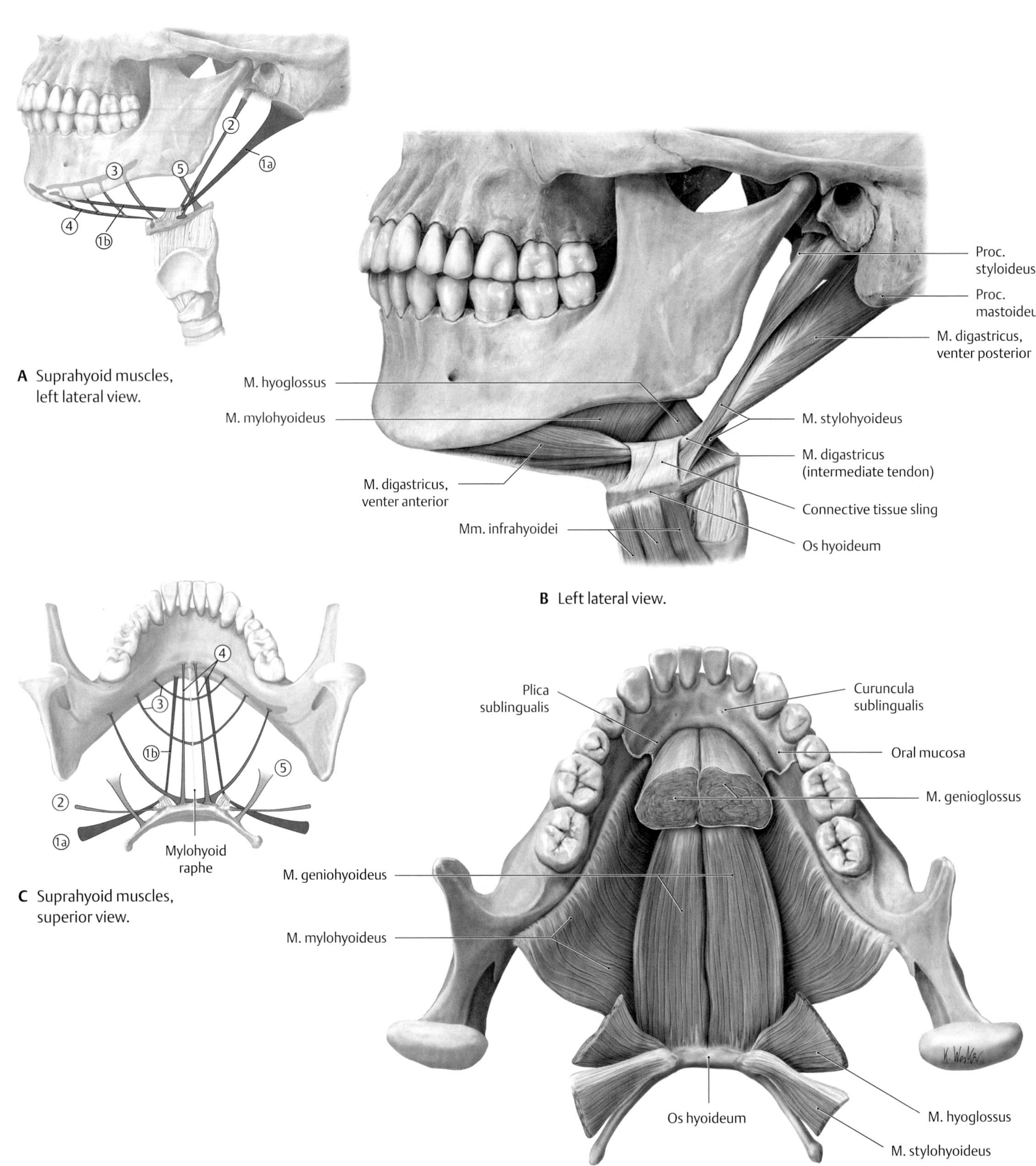

②
①a
③
⑤
④
①b
Proc. styloideus
Proc. mastoideus
M. digastricus, venter posterior
M. hyoglossus
M. mylohyoideus
M. stylohyoideus
M. digastricus (intermediate tendon)
M. digastricus, venter anterior
Connective tissue sling
Mm. infrahyoidei
Os hyoideum
Mylohyoid raphe
Plica sublingualis
Curuncula sublingualis
Oral mucosa
M. genioglossus
M. geniohyoideus
M. mylohyoideus
Os hyoideum
M. hyoglossus
M. stylohyoideus

A Suprahyoid muscles, left lateral view.

B Left lateral view.

C Suprahyoid muscles, superior view.

D Superior view of mandibula and os hyoideum.

Table 36.1 Suprahyoid muscles

Muscle		Origin	Insertion		Innervation	Action
① M. diagastricus	(1a) Venter anterior	Mandibula (fossa digastrica)	Os hyoideum (corpus)	Via an intermediate tendon with a fibrous loop	N. mylohyoideus (from CN V_3)	Elevates hyoid bone (during swallowing), assists in opening mandibula
	(1b) Venter posterior	Os temporale (incisura mastoidea, medial to proc. mastoideus)			N. facialis (CN VII)	
② M. stylohyoideus		Os temporale (proc. styloideus)		Via a split tendon		
③ M. mylohyoideus		Mandibula (linea mylohyoidea)		Via median tendon of insertion (raphe mylohyoidea)	N. mylohyoideus (from CN V_3)	Tightens and elevates oral floor, draws hyoid bone forward (during swallowing), assists in opening mandible and moving it side to side (mastication)
④ M. geniohyoideus		Mandibula (spina mentalis inferior)		Os hyoideum (corpus)	R. ventralis of C1 via n. hypoglossus (CN XII)	Draws hyoid bone forward (during swallowing), assists in opening mandible
⑤ M. hyoglossus		Os hyoideum (superior border of cornu majus)	Sides of tongue		N. hypoglossus (CN XII)	Depresses the tongue

Fig. 36.16 Muscles of palatum molle
Inferior view. The palatum molle forms the posterior boundary of the oral cavity, separating it from the oropharynx.

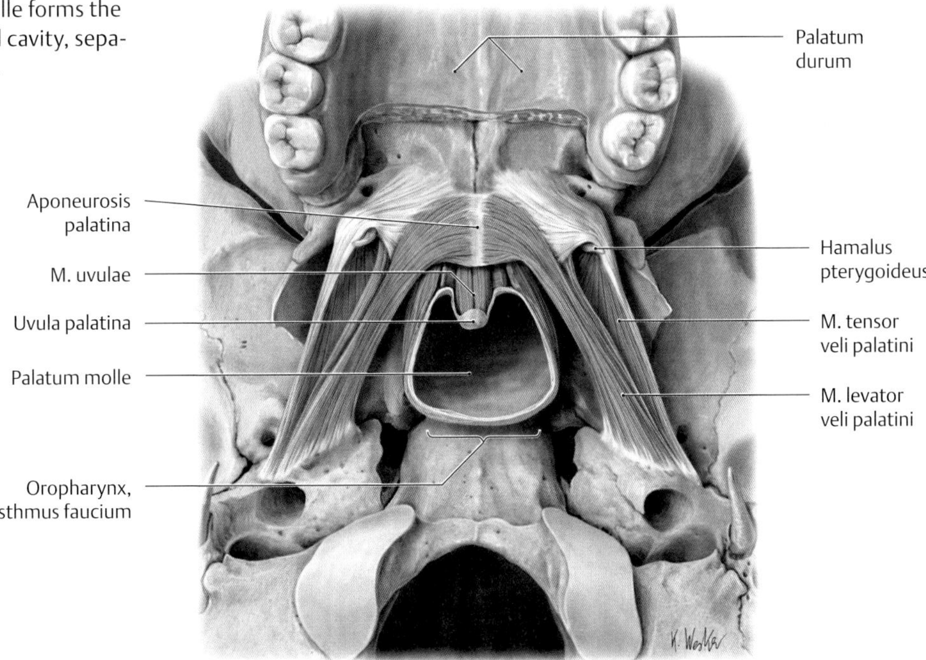

Palatum durum
Aponeurosis palatina
M. uvulae
Uvula palatina
Palatum molle
Oropharynx, isthmus faucium
Hamalus pterygoideus
M. tensor veli palatini
M. levator veli palatini

Table 36.2 Muscles of the Palatum molle

Muscle	Origin	Insertion	Innervation	Action
M. tensor veli palatini	Lamina medialis of proc. pterygoideus (fossa scaphoidea); spina ossis sphenoidalis; cartilage of tuba auditiva	Aponeurosis palatina	N. pterygoideus medialis (CN V_3 via ganglion oticum)	Tightens soft palate; opens inlet to pharyngotympanic tube (during swallowing, yawning)
M. levator veli palatini	Cartilage of tuba auditiva; os temporale (pars petrosa)		N. accessorius (CN XI, pars cranialis) via plexus pharyngeus (n. vagus, CN X)	Raises soft palate to horizontal position
M. uvulae	Uvula (mucosa)	Aponeurosis palatina; spina nasalis posterior		Shortens and raises uvula
M. palatoglossus*	Tongue (side)	Aponeurosis palatina		Elevates tongue (posterior portion); pulls soft palate onto tongue
M. palatopharyngeus*				Tightens soft palate; during swallowing pulls pharyngeal walls superiorly, anteriorly, and medially

*See pp. 548, 555.

Innervation of the Oral Cavity

Fig. 36.17 N. trigeminus in the oral cavity
Right lateral view.

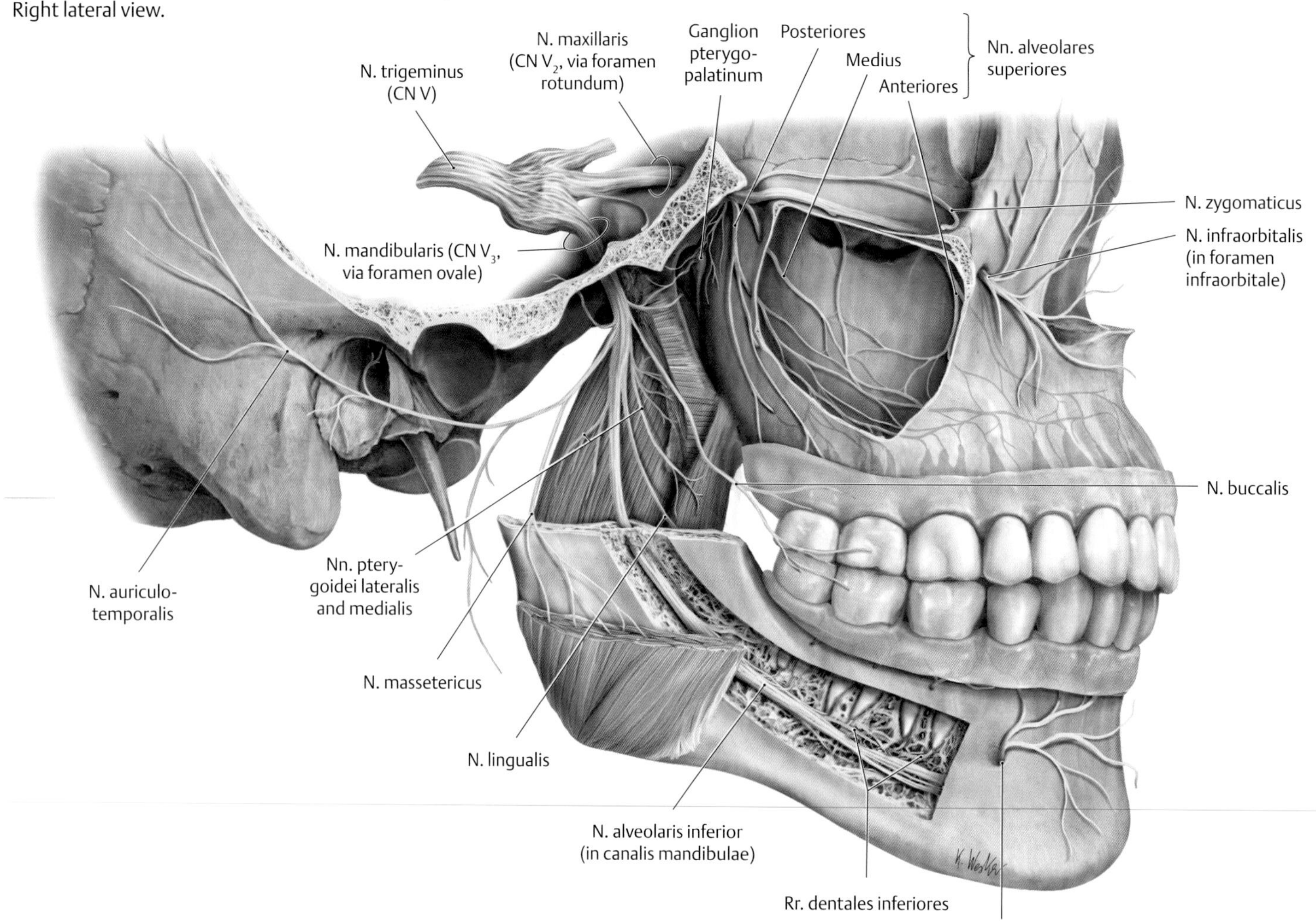
N. trigeminus (CN V)
N. maxillaris (CN V_2, via foramen rotundum)
Ganglion pterygo-palatinum
Posteriores
Medius
Anteriores
Nn. alveolares superiores
N. zygomaticus
N. infraorbitalis (in foramen infraorbitale)
N. mandibularis (CN V_3, via foramen ovale)
N. buccalis
N. auriculo-temporalis
Nn. pterygoidei lateralis and medialis
N. massetericus
N. lingualis
N. alveolaris inferior (in canalis mandibulae)
Rr. dentales inferiores
N. mentalis (in foramen mentale)

Fig. 36.18 Neurovasculature of palatum durum
Inferior view. The palatum durum receives sensory innervation primarily from terminal branches of n. maxillaris (CN V_2). The arteries of the hard palate arise from a. maxillaris.

N. infra-orbitalis: Rr. labiales superiores; Rr. alveolares superiores anteriores and R. alveolaris superior medius; Rr. alveoares superiores posteriores
N. buccalis
N. nasopalatinus
N. palatinus major
Nn. palatini minores

A Sensory innervation. *Note:* N. buccalis is a branch of n. mandibularis (CN V_3).

Rr. septales posteriores (a. nasopalatina)
N. nasopalatinus
Foramen incisivum
Sutura palatina mediana
A. palatina major and n. palatinus major
Foramen palatinum majus
Foramen palatinum minus
Aa. palatinae minores and nn. palatini minores
Vomer
Proc. pterygoideus

B Nerves and arteries.

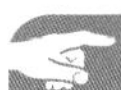

The muscles of the oral floor have a complex nerve supply with contributions from n. mandibularis (CN V_3), n. facialis (CN VII), and C1 spinal nerve via n. hypoglossus (CN XII).

Fig. 36.19 Innervation of the oral floor muscles

Ganglion trigeminale
N. mandibularis (CN V_3)
N. alveolaris inferior
Chorda tympani (CN VII)
N. lingualis
N. mylohyoideus
Ganglion submandibulare
M. mylohyoideus
M. digastricus, venter anterior

A N. mylohyoideus (CN V_3). Left lateral view with the left half of mandibula removed.

Ganglion geniculi
Plexus tympanicus
Ganglion trigeminale
N. facialis (CN VII)
Cellulae mastoideae
N. mandibularis (CN V_3)
Chorda tympani
Foramen stylomastoideum
N. lingualis
N. glossopharyngeus (CN IX)
Proc. mastoideus
R. stylohyoideus (with m. stylohyoideus)
R. digastricus (with venter posterior of m. digastricus)

B N. facialis (CN VII). Sagittal section through the right pars petrosa at the level of processus mastoideus, medial view.

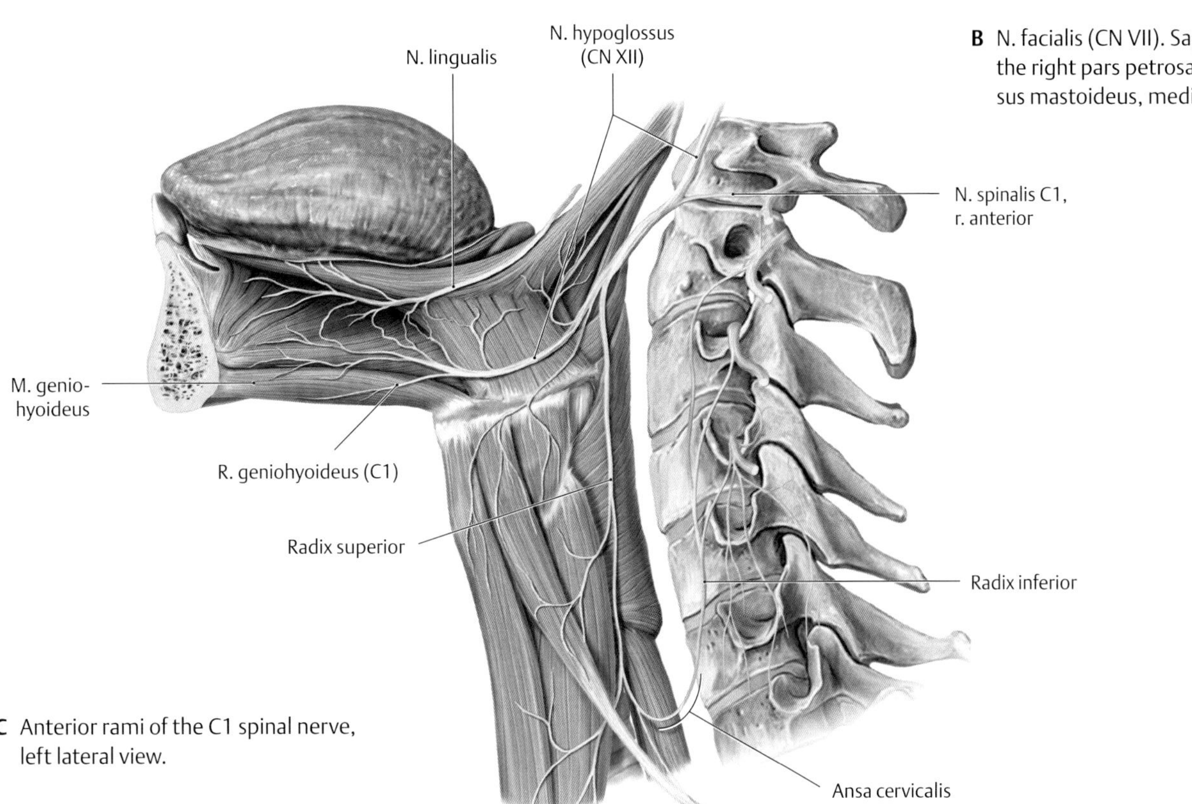
N. lingualis
N. hypoglossus (CN XII)
N. spinalis C1, r. anterior
M. genio-hyoideus
R. geniohyoideus (C1)
Radix superior
Radix inferior
Ansa cervicalis

C Anterior rami of the C1 spinal nerve, left lateral view.

Tongue (Lingua)

The dorsum of the tongue is covered by a highly specialized mucosa that supports its sensory functions (taste and fine tactile discrimination; see p. 616). The tongue is endowed with a very powerful muscular body to support its motor properties during mastication, swallowing, and speaking.

Fig. 36.20 Structure of the tongue

The V-shaped sulcus terminalis divides the tongue into an anterior (oral, pars presulcalis) and a posterior (pharyngeal, pars postsulcalis) part.

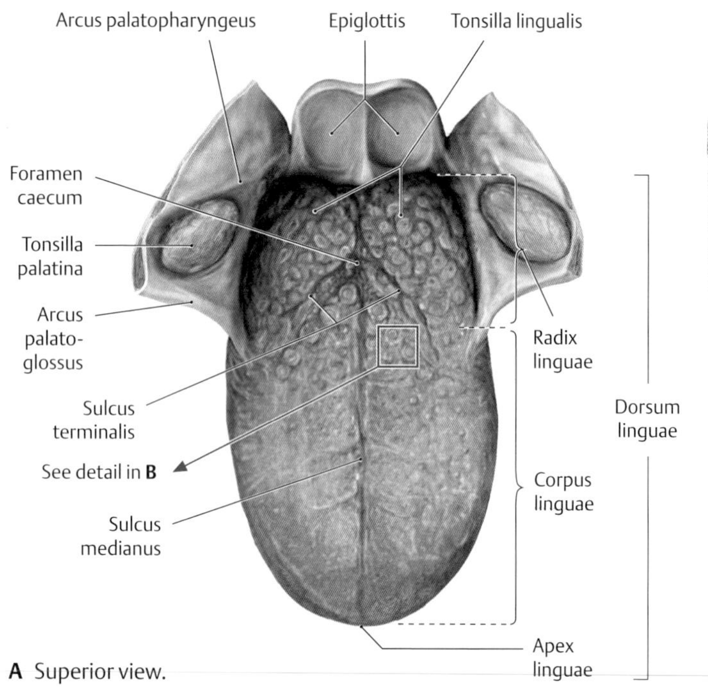
Arcus palatopharyngeus
Epiglottis
Tonsilla lingualis
Foramen caecum
Tonsilla palatina
Arcus palato-glossus
Sulcus terminalis
See detail in B
Sulcus medianus
Radix linguae
Corpus linguae
Dorsum linguae
Apex linguae

A Superior view.

Papillae filiformes
Papilla vallata
Papilla fungiformis
Tunica mucosa linguae
Aponeurosis linguae
Mm. linguae

B Papillae linguales, sectional block diagram. The connective tissue between the mucosal surface and musculature contains many small seromucous glands (not shown).

Fig. 36.21 Muscles of the tongue

The extrinsic lingual muscles (m. genioglossus, m. hyoglossus, m. palatoglossus, and m. styloglossus) have bony attachments and move the tongue as a whole. The intrinsic lingual muscles (mm. longitudinales superior and inferior, m. transversus linguae, and m. verticalis linguae) have no bony attachments and alter the shape of the tongue.

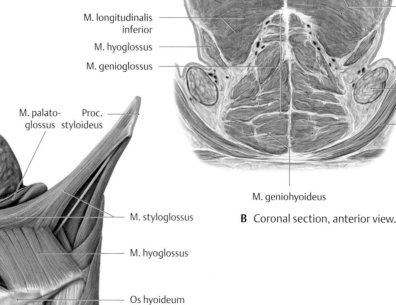

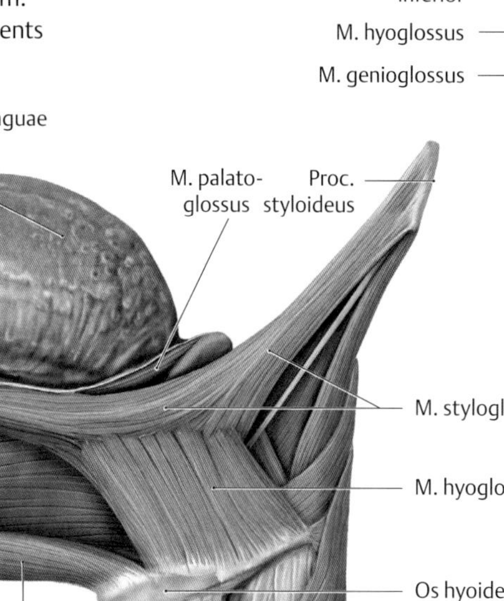
Dorsum linguae
Apex linguae
M. palato-glossus
Proc. styloideus
Mandibula
M. styloglossus
M. hyoglossus
Os hyoideum
M. genio-glossus
M. genio-hyoideus

A Left lateral view.

Aponeurosis linguae
Tunica mucosa linguae
M. longitudinalis superior
Septum linguae
M. longitudinalis inferior
M. hyoglossus
M. genioglossus
M. verticalis linguae
M. trans-versus linguae
Glandula sublingualis
M. mylo-hyoideus
M. geniohyoideus

B Coronal section, anterior view.

Fig. 36.22 Somatosensory and taste innervation of the tongue

Anterior view.

Taste

Somatic sensation

N. vagus (CN X)

N. vagus (CN X)

N. glossopharyngeus (CN IX)

N. glossopharyngeus (CN IX)

N. lingualis (from n. mandibularis, CN V_3)

N. facialis (CN VII, via chorda tympani)

Fig. 36.23 Neurovasculature of the tongue

The lingual muscles receive somatomotor innervation from n. hypoglossus (CN XII), with the exception of m. palatoglossus (supplied by n. vagus, CN X).

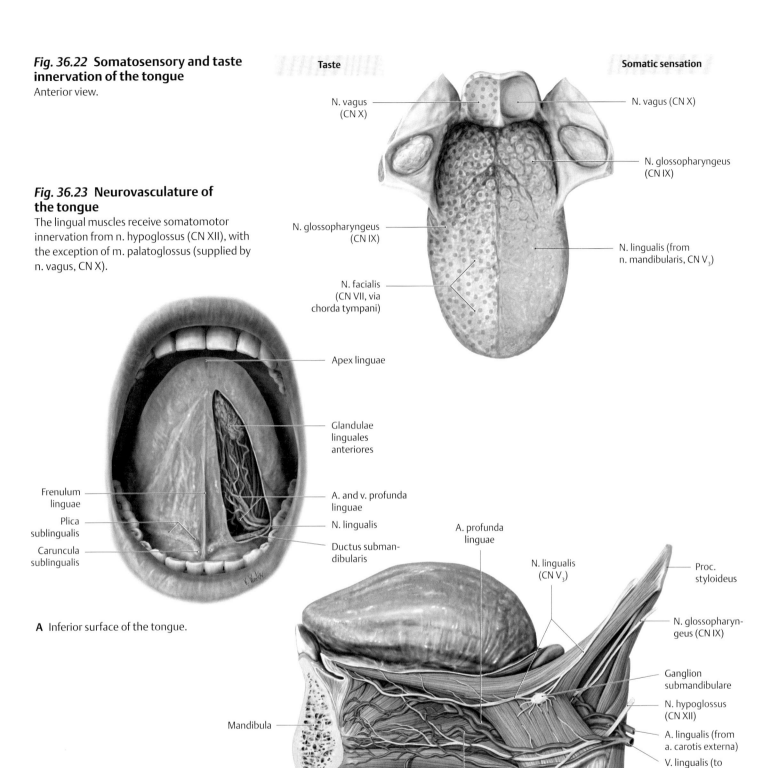

Apex linguae

Glandulae linguales anteriores

Frenulum linguae

A. and v. profunda linguae

Plica sublingualis

N. lingualis

Caruncula sublingualis

Ductus submandibularis

A Inferior surface of the tongue.

A. profunda linguae

N. lingualis (CN V_3)

Proc. styloideus

N. glossopharyngeus (CN IX)

Ganglion submandibulare

N. hypoglossus (CN XII)

Mandibula

A. lingualis (from a. carotis externa)

V. lingualis (to v. jugularis interna)

Os hyoideum

A. and v. submentalis

A. sublingualis

B Left lateral view.

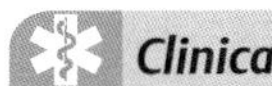

Clinical

Unilateral n. hypoglossus palsy

Damage to n. hypoglossus causes paralysis of m. genioglossus on the affected side. The healthy (innervated) m. genioglossus on the unaffected side will therefore dominate. Upon protrusion, the tongue will deviate *toward* the paralyzed side.

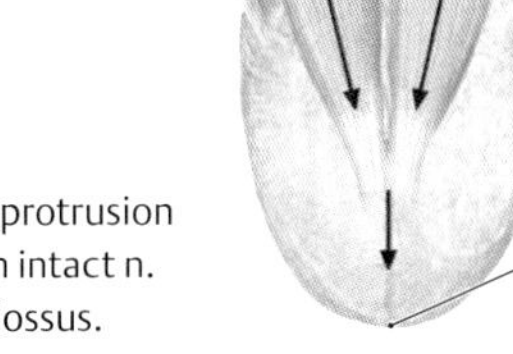
Apex
linguae

A Active protrusion with an intact n. hypoglossus.

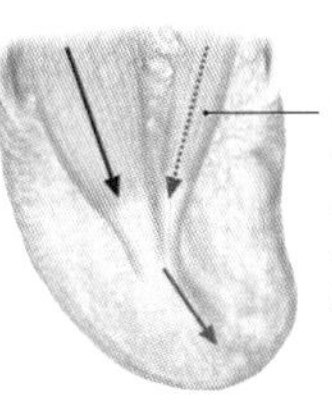
Paralyzed
m. genio-
glossus on
affected
side

B Active protrusion with a unilateral lesion of n. hypoglossus.

Topography of the Oral Cavity & Salivary Glands

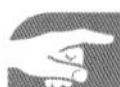

The oral cavity is located below the nasal cavity and anterior to the pharynx. It is bounded by the hard and soft palates, the tongue and muscles of the oral floor, and the uvula.

Fig. 36.24 Oral cavity

Midsagittal section, left lateral view.

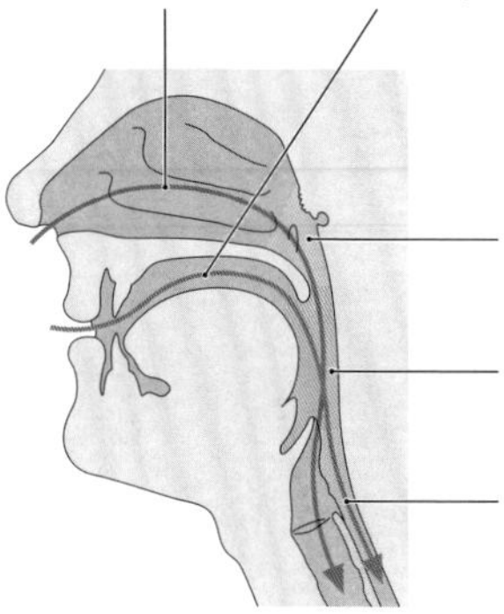

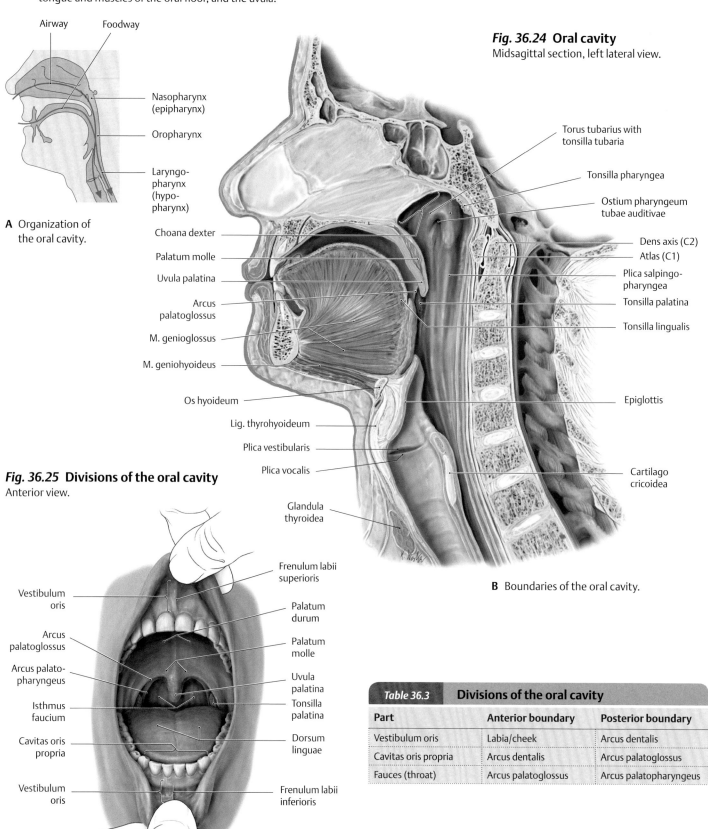

Airway
Foodway
Nasopharynx (epipharynx)
Oropharynx
Laryngo-pharynx (hypo-pharynx)

A Organization of the oral cavity.

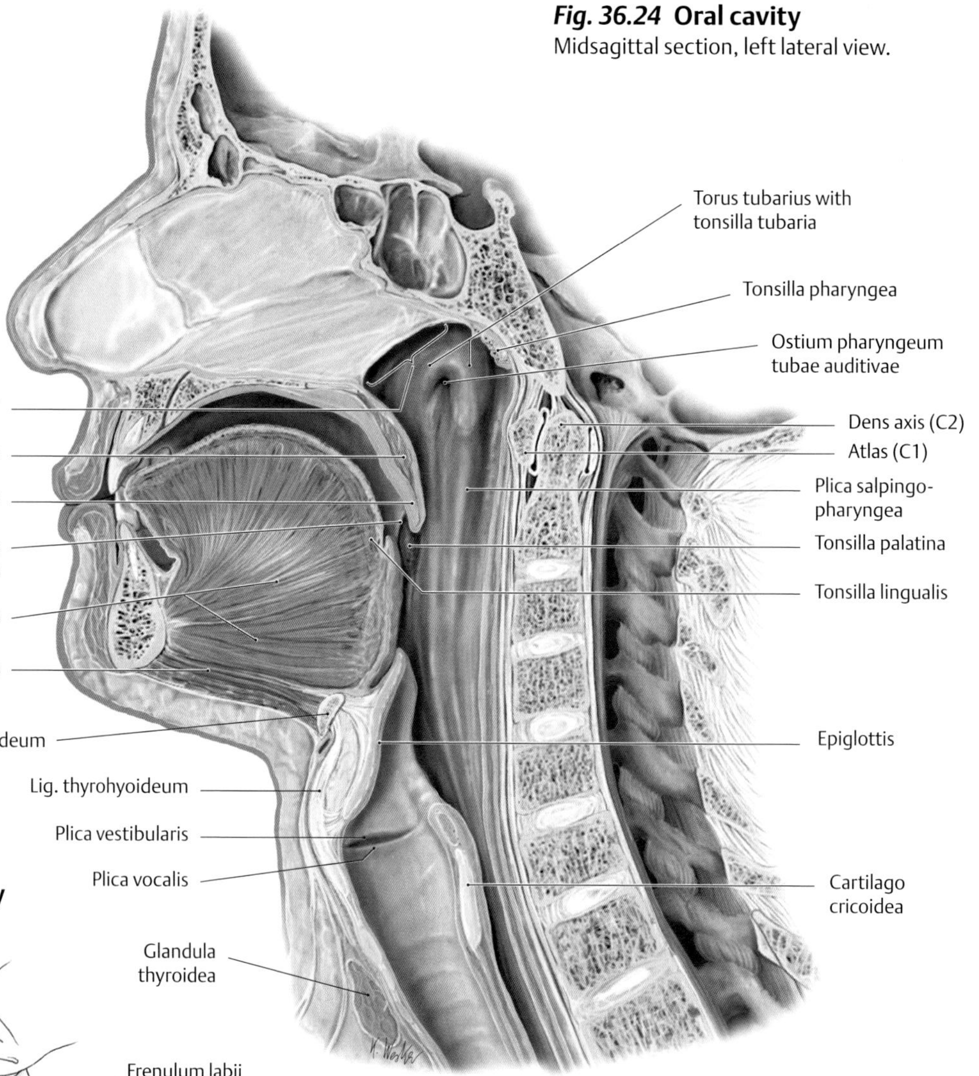

Choana dexter
Palatum molle
Uvula palatina
Arcus palatoglossus
M. genioglossus
M. geniohyoideus
Os hyoideum
Lig. thyrohyoideum
Plica vestibularis
Plica vocalis
Glandula thyroidea
Torus tubarius with tonsilla tubaria
Tonsilla pharyngea
Ostium pharyngeum tubae auditivae
Dens axis (C2)
Atlas (C1)
Plica salpingo-pharyngea
Tonsilla palatina
Tonsilla lingualis
Epiglottis
Cartilago cricoidea

B Boundaries of the oral cavity.

Fig. 36.25 Divisions of the oral cavity

Anterior view.

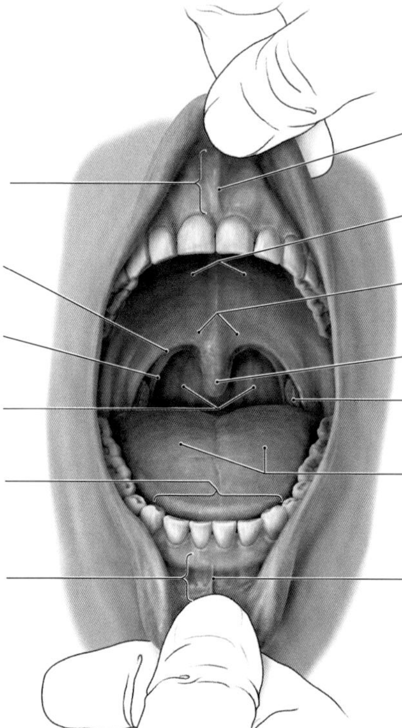

Vestibulum oris
Arcus palatoglossus
Arcus palato-pharyngeus
Isthmus faucium
Cavitas oris propria
Vestibulum oris
Frenulum labii superioris
Palatum durum
Palatum molle
Uvula palatina
Tonsilla palatina
Dorsum linguae
Frenulum labii inferioris

Table 36.3 Divisions of the oral cavity

Part	Anterior boundary	Posterior boundary
Vestibulum oris	Labia/cheek	Arcus dentalis
Cavitas oris propria	Arcus dentalis	Arcus palatoglossus
Fauces (throat)	Arcus palatoglossus	Arcus palatopharyngeus

The three large, paired salivary glands are the glandulae parotidea, submandibularis, and sublingualis. The glandula parotidea is a purely serous (watery) salivary gland. The glandula sublingualis is predominantly mucous; the glandula submandibularis is a mixed seromucous gland.

Fig. 36.26 Salivary glands

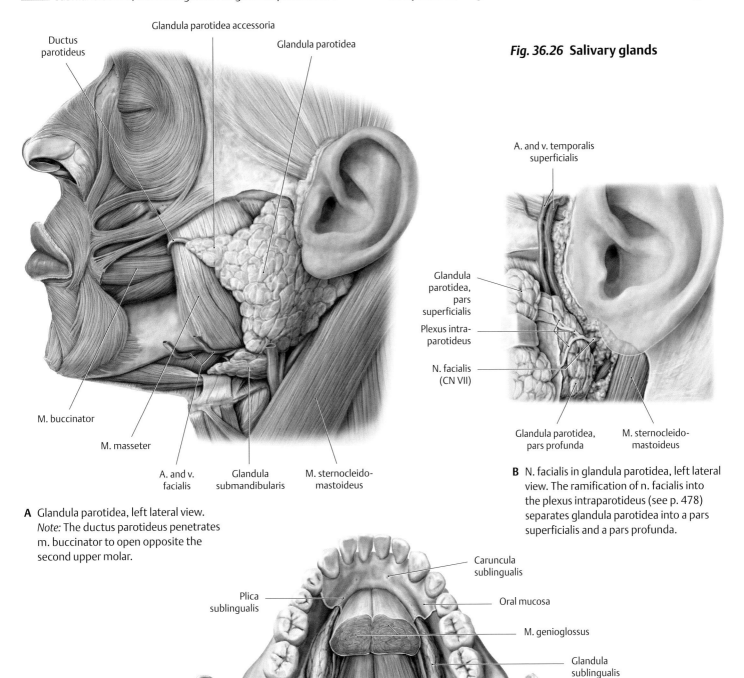

Glandula parotidea accessoria
Ductus parotideus
Glandula parotidea
M. buccinator
M. masseter
A. and v. facialis
Glandula submandibularis
M. sternocleido-mastoideus

A Glandula parotidea, left lateral view.
Note: The ductus parotideus penetrates m. buccinator to open opposite the second upper molar.

A. and v. temporalis superficialis
Glandula parotidea, pars superficialis
Plexus intra-parotideus
N. facialis (CN VII)
Glandula parotidea, pars profunda
M. sternocleido-mastoideus

B N. facialis in glandula parotidea, left lateral view. The ramification of n. facialis into the plexus intraparotideus (see p. 478) separates glandula parotidea into a pars superficialis and a pars profunda.

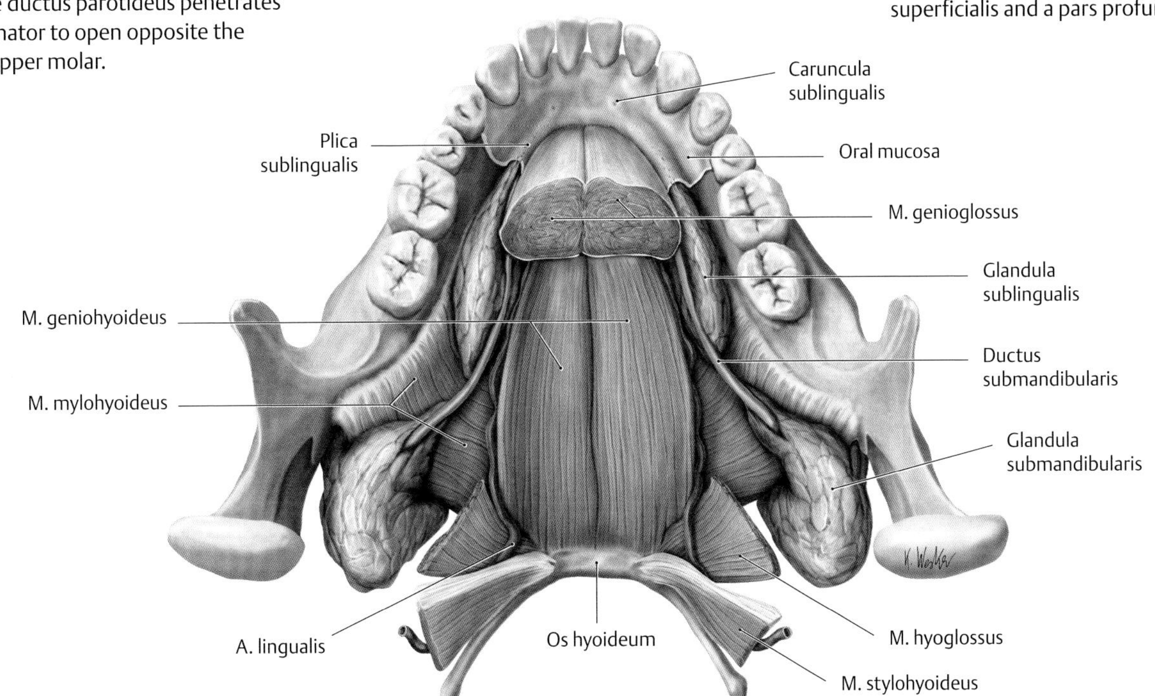
Caruncula sublingualis
Plica sublingualis
Oral mucosa
M. genioglossus
Glandula sublingualis
M. geniohyoideus
Ductus submandibularis
M. mylohyoideus
Glandula submandibularis
A. lingualis
Os hyoideum
M. hyoglossus
M. stylohyoideus

C Glandulae submandibularis and sublingualis, superior view with tongue removed.

Tonsils & Pharynx

Fig. 36.27 Tonsils

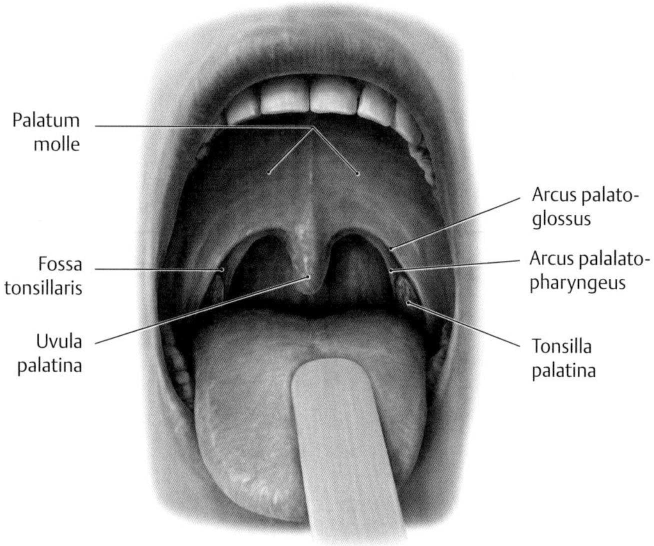

Palatum molle
Fossa tonsillaris
Uvula palatina
Arcus palato-glossus
Arcus palalato-pharyngeus
Tonsilla palatina

A Tonsilla palatina, anterior view.

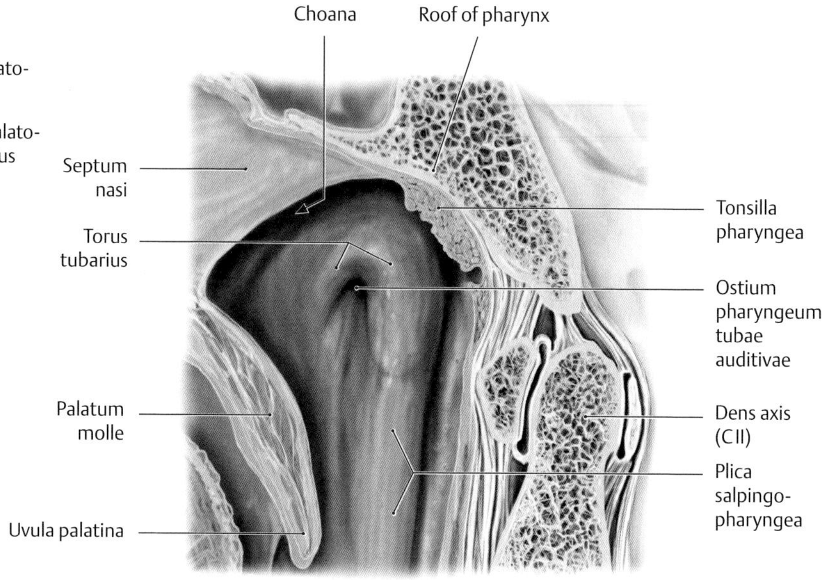

Choana
Roof of pharynx
Septum nasi
Torus tubarius
Palatum molle
Uvula palatina
Tonsilla pharyngea
Ostium pharyngeum tubae auditivae
Dens axis (C II)
Plica salpingo-pharyngea

B Tonsilla pharyngea. Sagittal section through the roof of the pharynx.

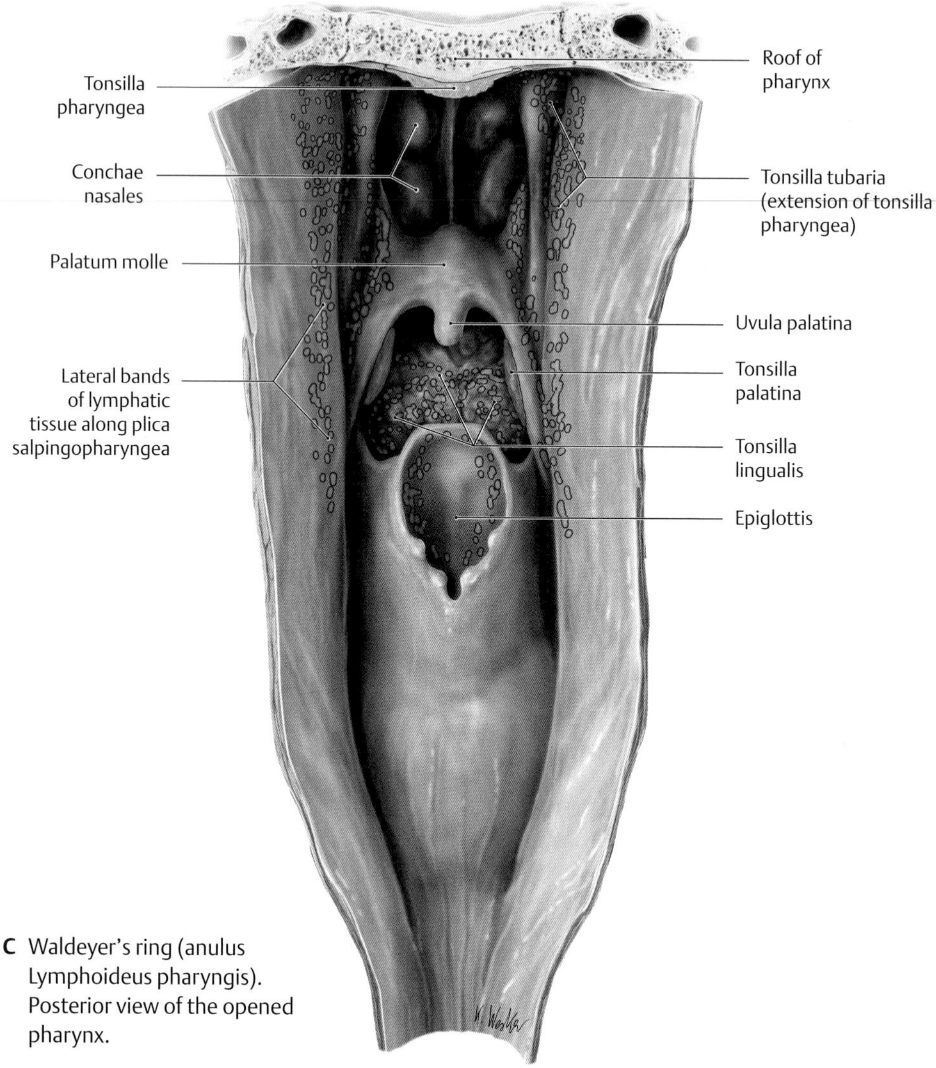

Tonsilla pharyngea
Conchae nasales
Palatum molle
Lateral bands of lymphatic tissue along plica salpingopharyngea
Roof of pharynx
Tonsilla tubaria (extension of tonsilla pharyngea)
Uvula palatina
Tonsilla palatina
Tonsilla lingualis
Epiglottis

C Waldeyer's ring (anulus Lymphoideus pharyngis). Posterior view of the opened pharynx.

Table 36.4 **Structures in Waldeyer's ring**

Tonsil	#
Tonsilla pharyngea	1
Tonsillae tubariae	2
Tonsillae palatinae	2
Tonsilla lingualis	1
Lateral bands	2

Clinical

Tonsil infections

Abnormal enlargement of the tonsillae palatinae due to severe viral or bacterial infection can result in obstruction of the oropharynx, causing difficulty swallowing.

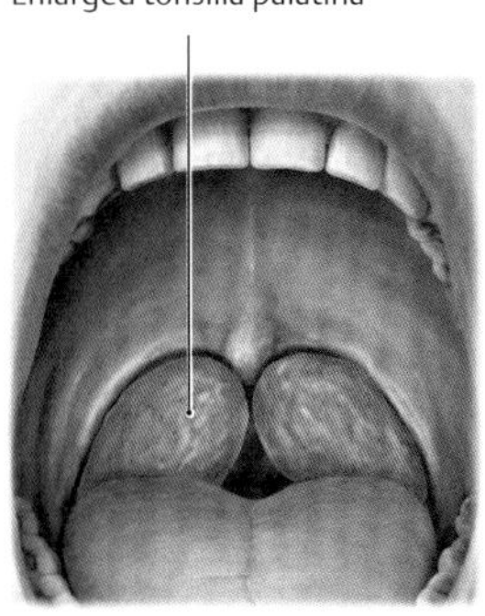
Enlarged tonsilla palatina

A

Particularly well developed in young children, tonsilla pharyngea begins to regress at 6 to 7 years of age. Abnormal enlargement is common, with the tonsil bulging into the nasopharynx and obstructing air passages, forcing the child to "mouth breathe."

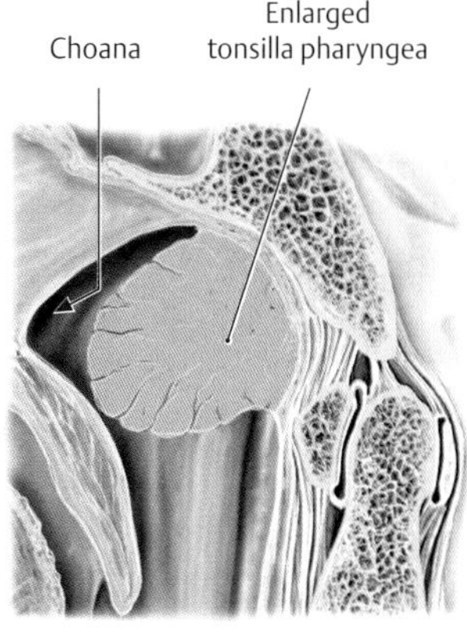
Choana
Enlarged tonsilla pharyngea

B

Fig. 36.28 **Pharyngeal mucosa**
Posterior view of the opened pharynx. The anterior portion of the muscular tube contains three openings: choanae (to the nasal cavity), isthmus faucium (to the oral cavity), and aditus Laryngis (to the laryngeal inlet).

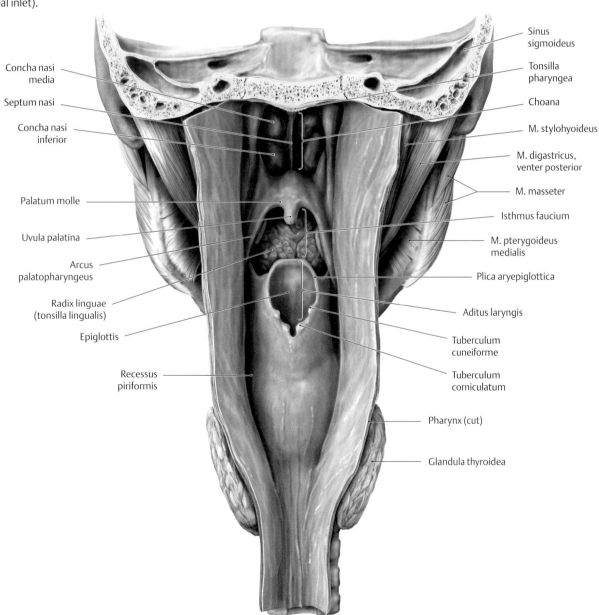

Concha nasi media
Septum nasi
Concha nasi inferior
Palatum molle
Uvula palatina
Arcus palatopharyngeus
Radix linguae (tonsilla lingualis)
Epiglottis
Recessus piriformis
Sinus sigmoideus
Tonsilla pharyngea
Choana
M. stylohyoideus
M. digastricus, venter posterior
M. masseter
Isthmus faucium
M. pterygoideus medialis
Plica aryepiglottica
Aditus laryngis
Tuberculum cuneiforme
Tuberculum corniculatum
Pharynx (cut)
Glandula thyroidea

Pharyngeal Muscles

Fig. 36.29 **Pharyngeal muscles: Left lateral view**

The pharyngeal musculature consists of the pharyngeal constrictors and the relatively weak pharyngeal elevators.

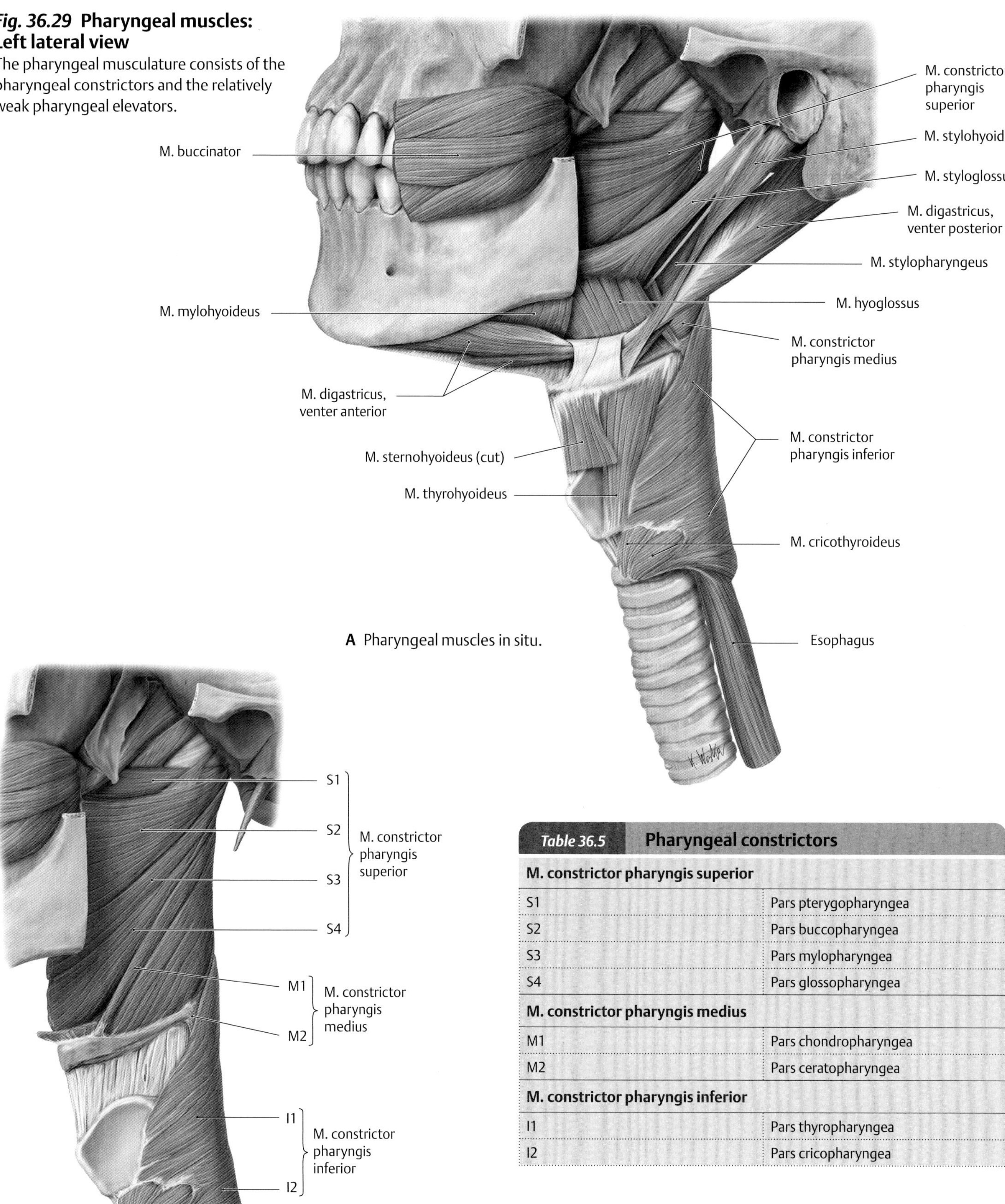
M. buccinator
M. mylohyoideus
M. digastricus, venter anterior
M. sternohyoideus (cut)
M. thyrohyoideus
M. constrictor pharyngis superior
M. stylohyoideus
M. styloglossus
M. digastricus, venter posterior
M. stylopharyngeus
M. hyoglossus
M. constrictor pharyngis medius
M. constrictor pharyngis inferior
M. cricothyroideus
Esophagus
S1
S2
S3
S4
M. constrictor pharyngis superior
M1
M2
M. constrictor pharyngis medius
I1
I2
M. constrictor pharyngis inferior

A Pharyngeal muscles in situ.

B Subdivisions of the pharyngeal constrictors.

Table 36.5	**Pharyngeal constrictors**
M. constrictor pharyngis superior	
S1	Pars pterygopharyngea
S2	Pars buccopharyngea
S3	Pars mylopharyngea
S4	Pars glossopharyngea
M. constrictor pharyngis medius	
M1	Pars chondropharyngea
M2	Pars ceratopharyngea
M. constrictor pharyngis inferior	
I1	Pars thyropharyngea
I2	Pars cricopharyngea

Fig. 36.30 **Pharyngeal muscles: Posterior view**

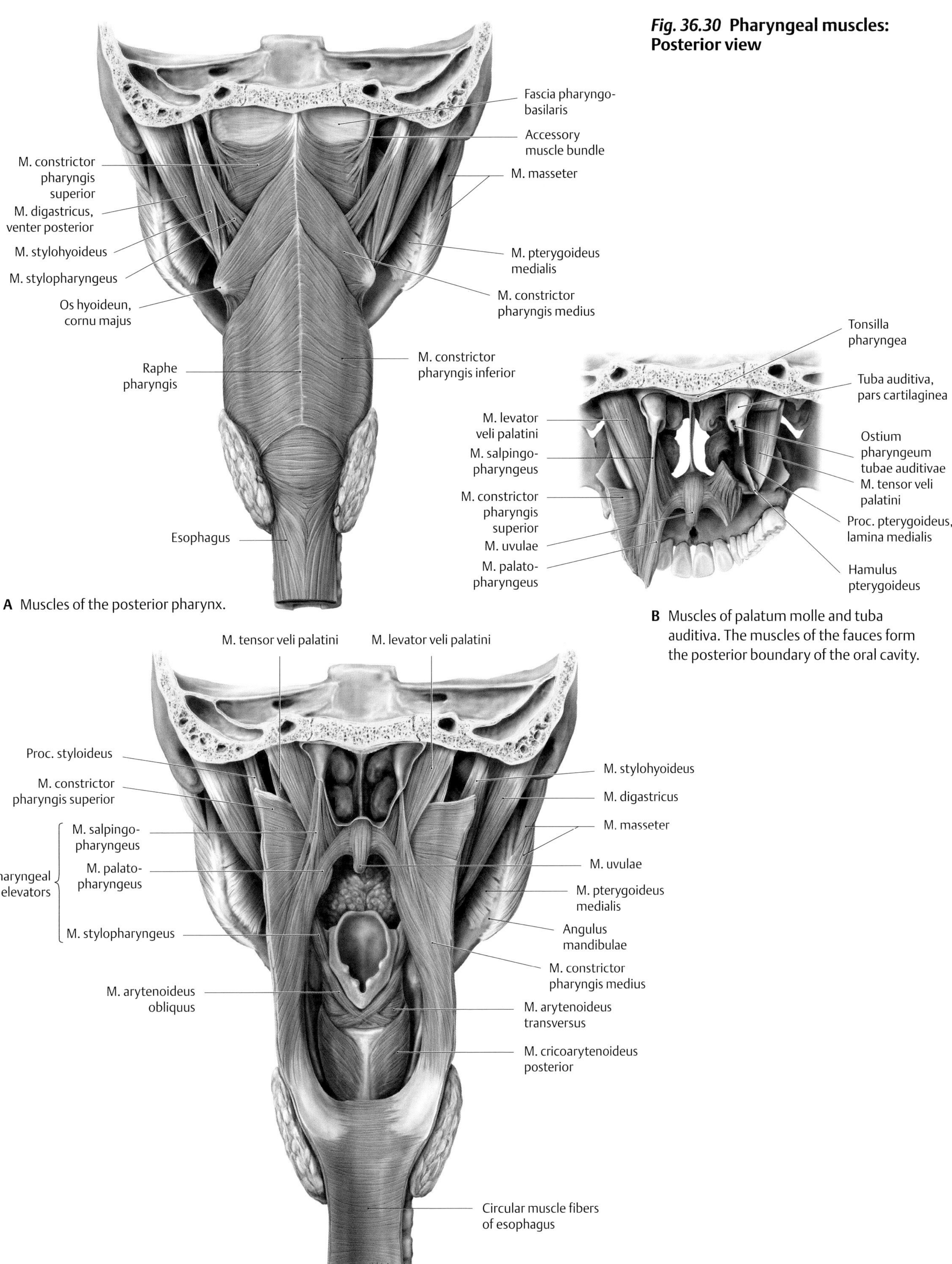
Fascia pharyngo-basilaris
Accessory muscle bundle
M. masseter
M. constrictor pharyngis superior
M. digastricus, venter posterior
M. stylohyoideus
M. stylopharyngeus
M. pterygoideus medialis
M. constrictor pharyngis medius
Os hyoideun, cornu majus
M. constrictor pharyngis inferior
Raphe pharyngis
Esophagus
Tonsilla pharyngea
Tuba auditiva, pars cartilaginea
M. levator veli palatini
Ostium pharyngeum tubae auditivae
M. salpingo-pharyngeus
M. tensor veli palatini
M. constrictor pharyngis superior
Proc. pterygoideus, lamina medialis
M. uvulae
M. palato-pharyngeus
Hamulus pterygoideus
M. tensor veli palatini
M. levator veli palatini
Proc. styloideus
M. stylohyoideus
M. constrictor pharyngis superior
M. digastricus
M. masseter
M. salpingo-pharyngeus
Pharyngeal elevators
M. palato-pharyngeus
M. uvulae
M. pterygoideus medialis
M. stylopharyngeus
Angulus mandibulae
M. constrictor pharyngis medius
M. arytenoideus obliquus
M. arytenoideus transversus
M. cricoarytenoideus posterior
Circular muscle fibers of esophagus

A Muscles of the posterior pharynx.

B Muscles of palatum molle and tuba auditiva. The muscles of the fauces form the posterior boundary of the oral cavity.

C Muscles in the opened pharynx.

Neurovasculature of the Pharynx

Fig. 36.31 **Neurovasculature in the parapharyngeal space**
Posterior view. *Removed:* Columna vertebralis and posterior structures.

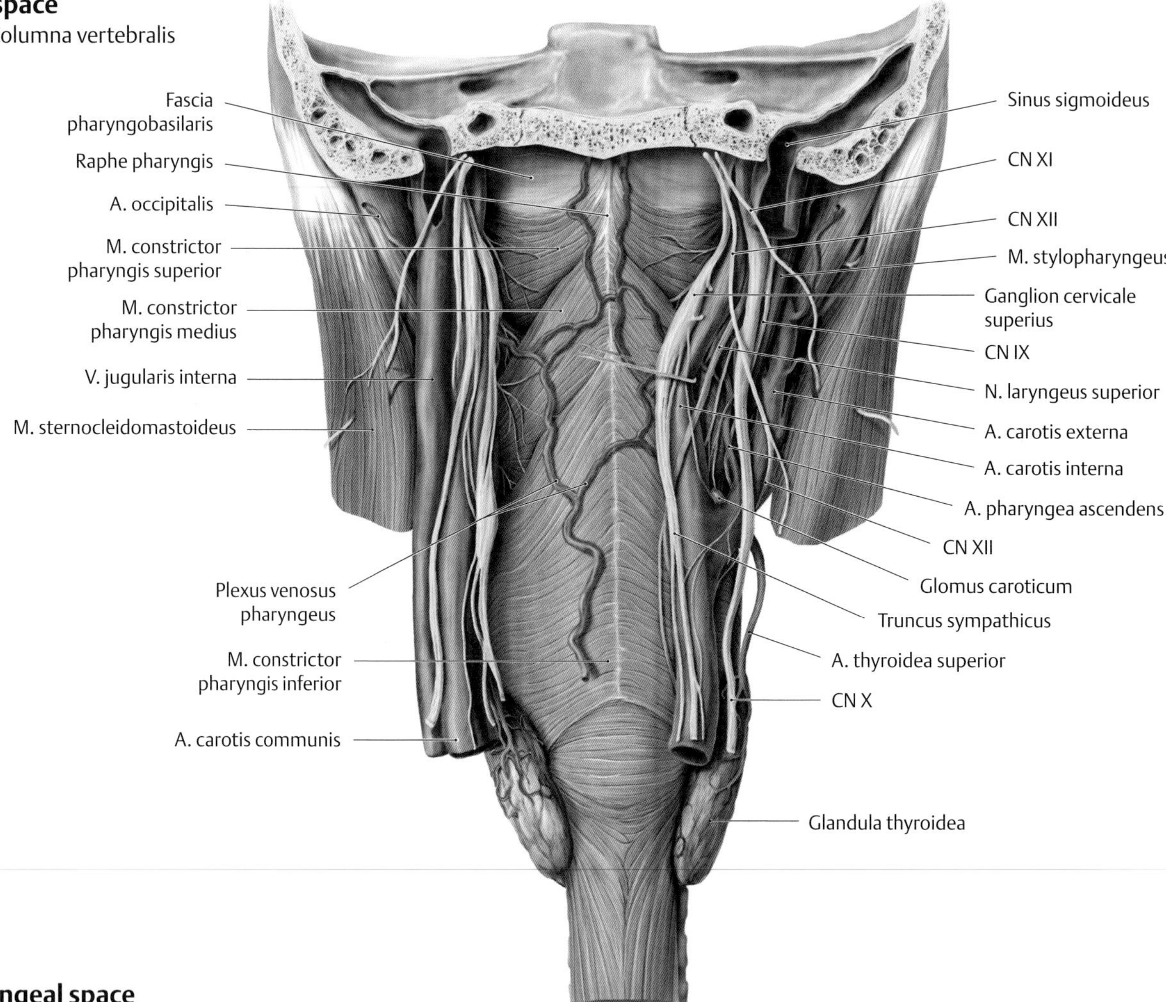
Fascia pharyngobasilaris
Raphe pharyngis
A. occipitalis
M. constrictor pharyngis superior
M. constrictor pharyngis medius
V. jugularis interna
M. sternocleidomastoideus
Plexus venosus pharyngeus
M. constrictor pharyngis inferior
A. carotis communis
Sinus sigmoideus
CN XI
CN XII
M. stylopharyngeus
Ganglion cervicale superius
CN IX
N. laryngeus superior
A. carotis externa
A. carotis interna
A. pharyngea ascendens
CN XII
Glomus caroticum
Truncus sympathicus
A. thyroidea superior
CN X
Glandula thyroidea

Fig. 36.32 **Parapharyngeal space**
Transverse section, superior view.

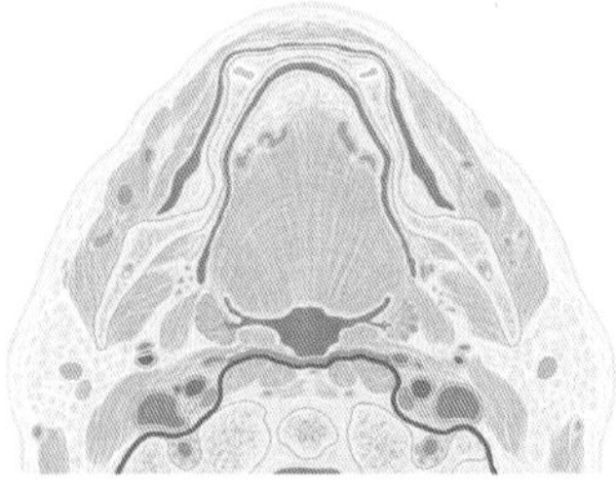

A Parapharyngeal space. The parapharyngeal space consists of a retropharyngeal (green) and a lateropharyngeal space. The lateropharyngeal space is further subdivided into an anterior (yellow) and a posterior (orange) part. Note the deep layer of fascia cervicalis (prevertebral lamina, red).

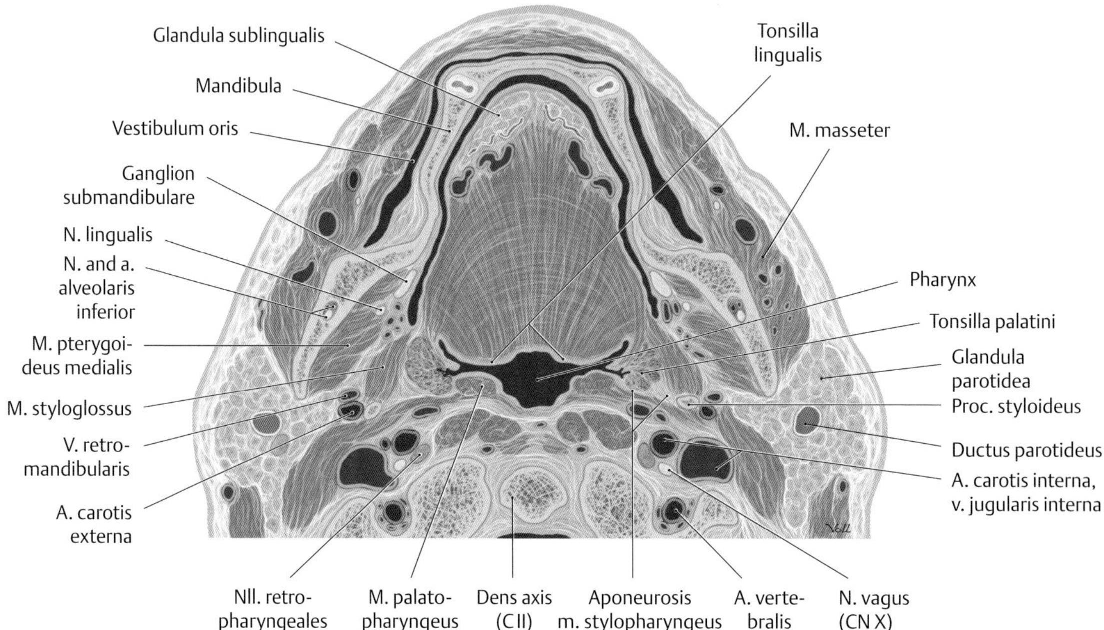
Glandula sublingualis
Mandibula
Vestibulum oris
Ganglion submandibulare
N. lingualis
N. and a. alveolaris inferior
M. pterygoideus medialis
M. styloglossus
V. retromandibularis
A. carotis externa
Tonsilla lingualis
M. masseter
Pharynx
Tonsilla palatini
Glandula parotidea
Proc. styloideus
Ductus parotideus
A. carotis interna, v. jugularis interna
Nll. retropharyngeales
M. palatopharyngeus
Dens axis (C II)
Aponeurosis m. stylopharyngeus
A. vertebralis
N. vagus (CN X)

B Superior view of the transverse section at the level of fossa tonsillaris.

Fig. 36.33 **Neurovasculature of the opened pharynx**
Posterior view.

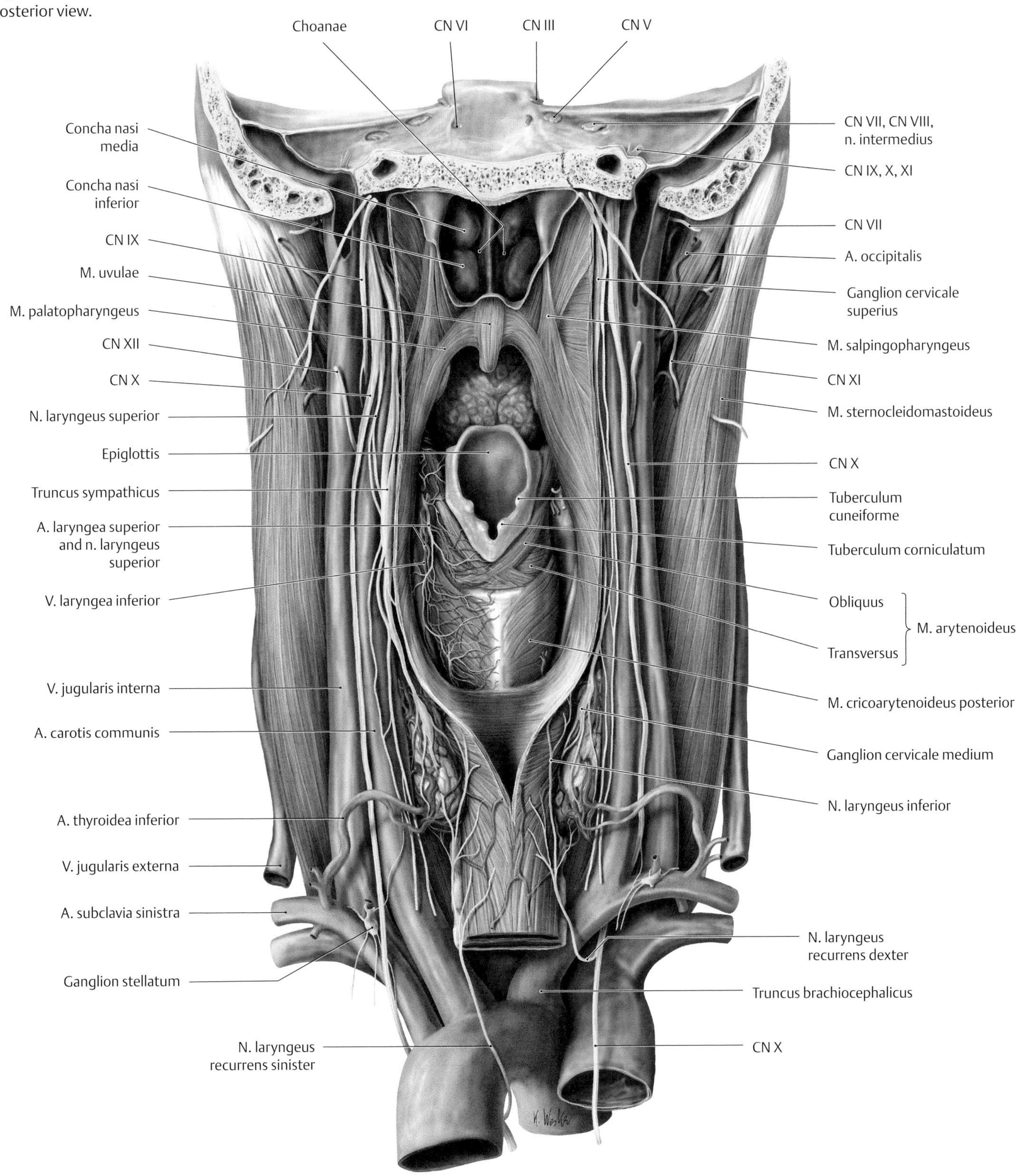

Choanae
CN VI
CN III
CN V
Concha nasi media
Concha nasi inferior
CN IX
M. uvulae
M. palatopharyngeus
CN XII
CN X
N. laryngeus superior
Epiglottis
Truncus sympathicus
A. laryngea superior and n. laryngeus superior
V. laryngea inferior
V. jugularis interna
A. carotis communis
A. thyroidea inferior
V. jugularis externa
A. subclavia sinistra
Ganglion stellatum
N. laryngeus recurrens sinister
CN VII, CN VIII, n. intermedius
CN IX, X, XI
CN VII
A. occipitalis
Ganglion cervicale superius
M. salpingopharyngeus
CN XI
M. sternocleidomastoideus
CN X
Tuberculum cuneiforme
Tuberculum corniculatum
Obliquus
Transversus
M. arytenoideus
M. cricoarytenoideus posterior
Ganglion cervicale medium
N. laryngeus inferior
N. laryngeus recurrens dexter
Truncus brachiocephalicus
CN X

CN III = N. oculomotorius, CN V = N. trigeminus, CN VI = N. abducens,
CN VII = N. facialis, CN VIII = N. vestibulocochlearis, CN IX = N. glossopharyngeus,
CN X = N. vagus, CN XI = N. accessorius, CN XII = N. hypoglossus
See Chapter 31 for the cranial nerves.

Bones & Ligaments of the Neck

Fig. 37.1 Boundaries of the neck

Left lateral view.

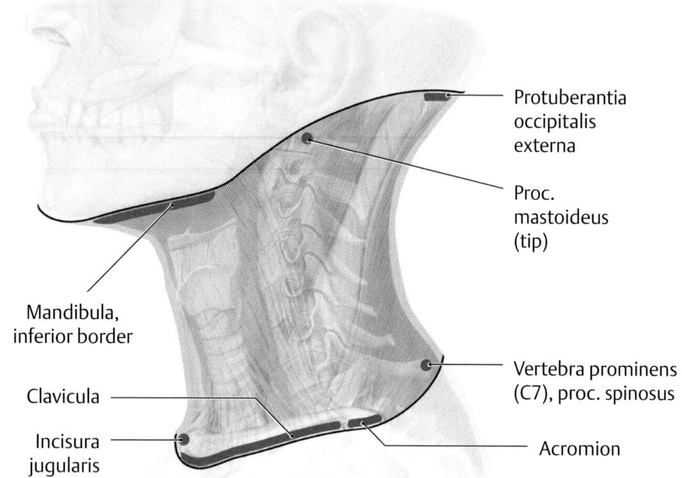
Protuberantia occipitalis externa
Proc. mastoideus (tip)
Mandibula, inferior border
Vertebra prominens (C7), proc. spinosus
Clavicula
Incisura jugularis
Acromion

Table 37.1	Bones and joints of the neck	
Columna vertebralis cervicalis		p. 6
Os hyoideum		p. 539
Articulationes craniovertebrales	Articulatio atlantooccipitalis	p. 16
	Articulatio atlantoaxialis	
Uncovertebral joints		p. 15
Articulationes zygapophysialis (intervertebral facet)		p. 14
Larynx		p. 571

Fig. 37.2 Bony structures of the neck

Left lateral view.

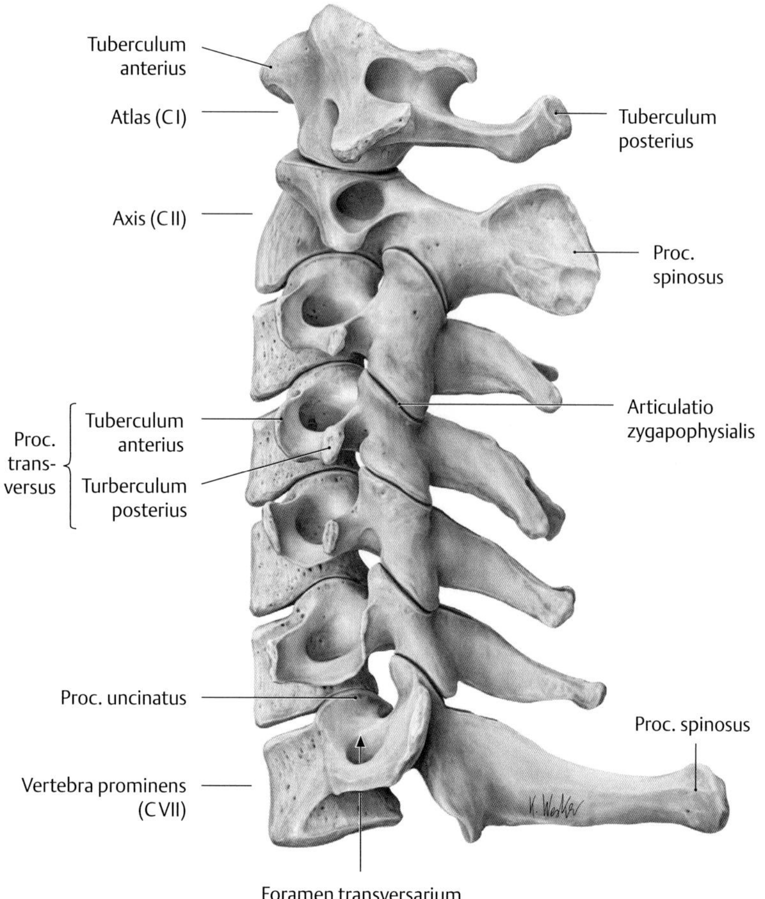
Tuberculum anterius
Atlas (C I)
Tuberculum posterius
Axis (C II)
Proc. spinosus
Proc. transversus
Tuberculum anterius
Turberculum posterius
Articulatio zygapophysialis
Proc. uncinatus
Proc. spinosus
Vertebra prominens (C VII)
Foramen transversarium

A Cervical spine. The seven vertebrae of the cervical spine are specialized for bearing the weight of the head.

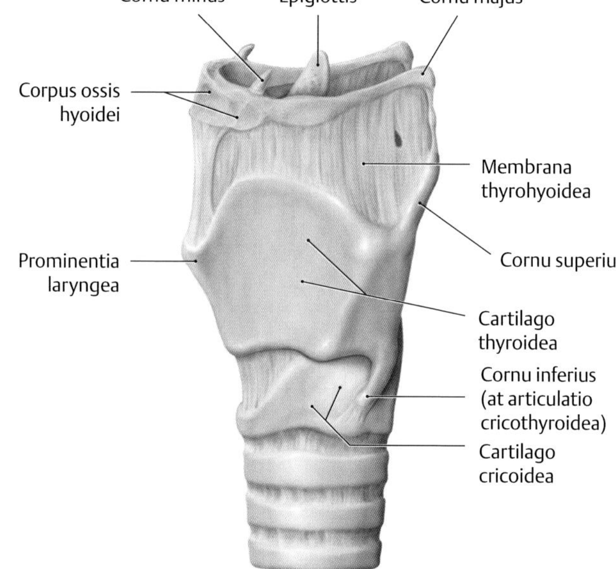
Cornu minus
Epiglottis
Cornu majus
Corpus ossis hyoidei
Membrana thyrohyoidea
Cornu superius
Prominentia laryngea
Cartilago thyroidea
Cornu inferius (at articulatio cricothyroidea)
Cartilago cricoidea

B Os hyoideum and larynx. The os hyoideum provides a site for bony attachment for the supra- and infrahyoid muscles. *Note:* The larynx is suspended from the os hyoideum, primarily by the membrana thyrohyoidea.

Fig. 37.3 **Ligaments of the cervical spine**
Midsagittal section, viewed from the left side. For the ligaments of the craniovertebral joints, see p. 16.

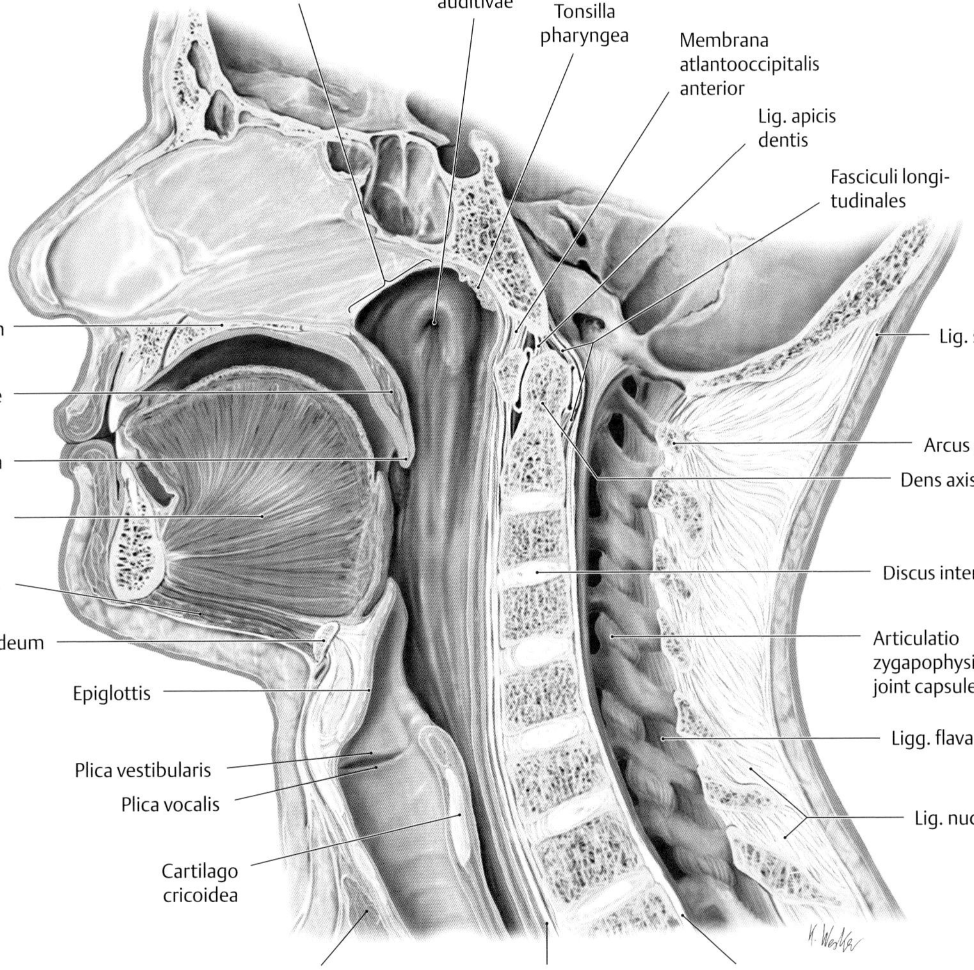

Choana dexter
Ostium pharyngeum tubae auditivae
Tonsilla pharyngea
Membrana atlantooccipitalis anterior
Lig. apicis dentis
Fasciculi longitudinales
Palatum durum
Palatum molle
Uvula palatina
Corpus linguae
M. mylohyoideus
Os hyoideum
Epiglottis
Plica vestibularis
Plica vocalis
Cartilago cricoidea
Glandula thyroidea
Lig. longitudinale anterius
Lig. longitudinale posterius
Lig. supraspinale
Arcus posterior atlantis (C I)
Dens axis (C II)
Discus intervertebralis
Articulatio zygapophysialis, joint capsule
Ligg. flava
Lig. nuchae

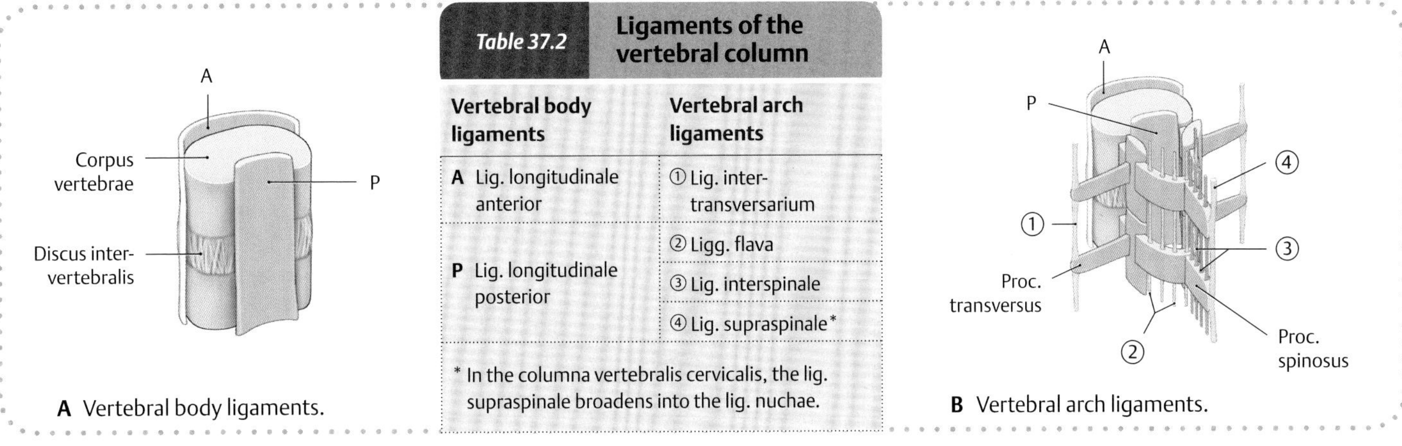
A
Corpus vertebrae
P
Discus intervertebralis
A
P
④
①
③
Proc. transversus
②
Proc. spinosus

A Vertebral body ligaments.

Table 37.2	Ligaments of the vertebral column
Vertebral body ligaments	**Vertebral arch ligaments**
A Lig. longitudinale anterior	① Lig. intertransversarium
P Lig. longitudinale posterior	② Ligg. flava
	③ Lig. interspinale
	④ Lig. supraspinale*

* In the columna vertebralis cervicalis, the lig. supraspinale broadens into the lig. nuchae.

B Vertebral arch ligaments.

Overview & Superficial Muscles of the Neck

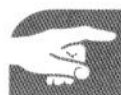

From a topographical standpoint, there are six major muscle groups in the neck. Functionally, however, the platysma belongs to the muscles of facial expression, m. trapezius belongs to the muscles of the shoulder girdle, and the nuchal muscles belong to the intrinsic back muscles. The mm. suboccipitales (short nuchal and craniovertebral joint muscles) are included in this chapter with the deep muscles of the neck.

Table 37.3 Classification of neck muscles

I	**Superficial neck muscles**			**III**	**Suprahyoid muscles**	
	Platysma, m. sternocleidomastoideus, m. trapezius		Fig. 37.4		M. digastricus, m. geniohyoideus, m. mylohyoideus, m. stylohyoideus	Fig. 37.7A
II	**Nuchal muscles (intrinsic back muscles)**			**IV**	**Infrahyoid muscles**	
	⑥ M. semispinalis capitis	⑦ M. semispinalis cervicis	See p. 32		M. sternohyoideus, m. sternothyroideus, m. thyrohyoideus, m. omohyoideus	Fig. 37.7B
	⑧ M. splenius capitis	⑨ M. splenius cervicis		**V**	**Prevertebral muscles**	
	⑩ M. longissimus capitis	⑪ M. longissimus cervicis	See p. 30		M. longus capitis, m. longus coli, m. rectus capitis anterior and lateralis	Fig. 37.9A
	⑫ M. iliocostalis cervicis			**VI**	**Lateral (deep) neck muscles**	
	Mm. suboccipitales (short nuchal and craniovertebral joint muscles)		Fig. 37.9C		M. scalenus anterior, medius, and posterior	Fig. 37.9B

Fig. 37.4 **Superficial neck muscles**
See Table 37.4 for details.

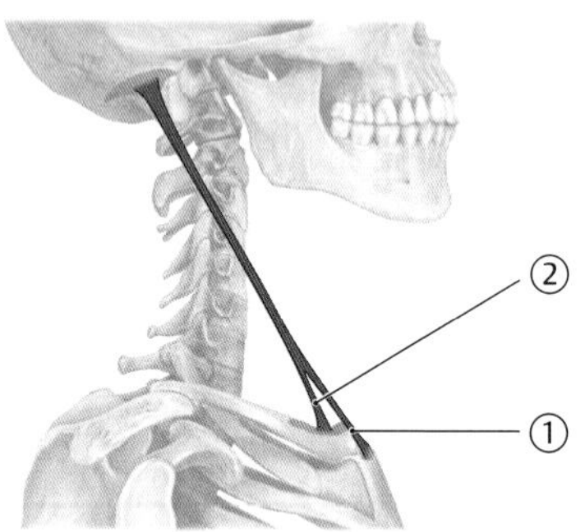

②
①

A M. sternocleidomastoideus.

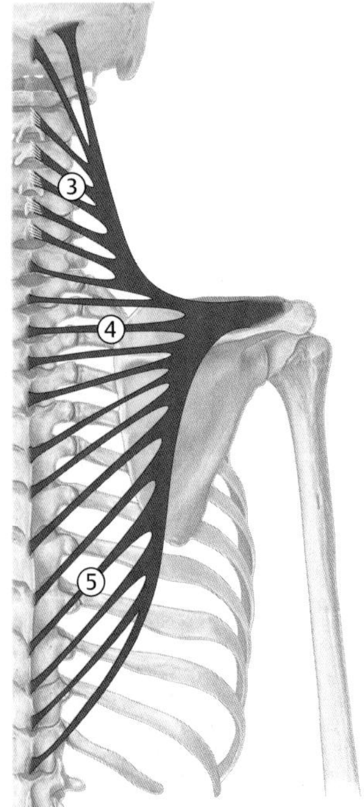

③
④
⑤

B M. trapezius.

Fig. 37.5 **Nuchal muscles**

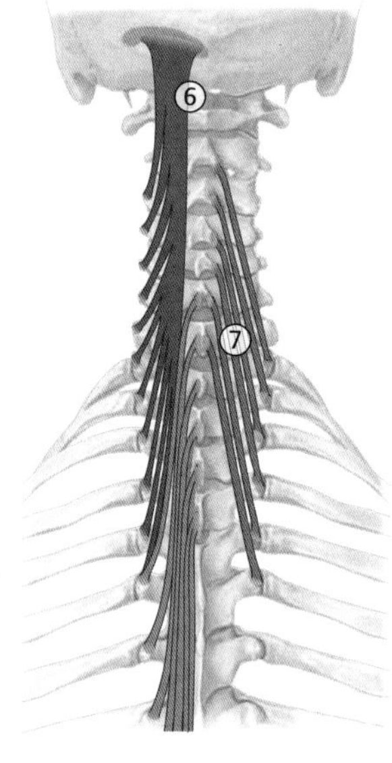

⑥
⑦

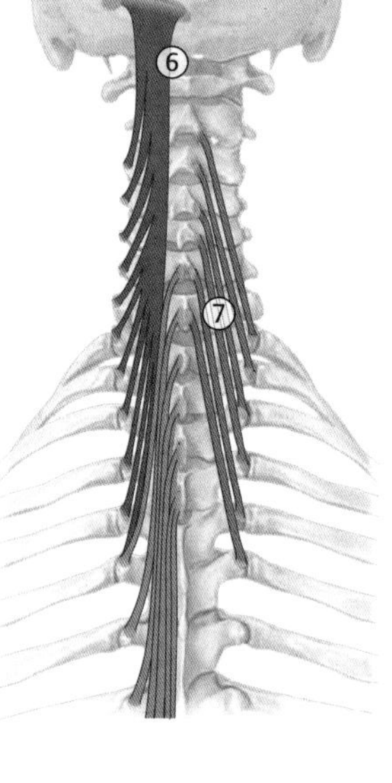

A Mm. semispinalis capitas and cervicis.

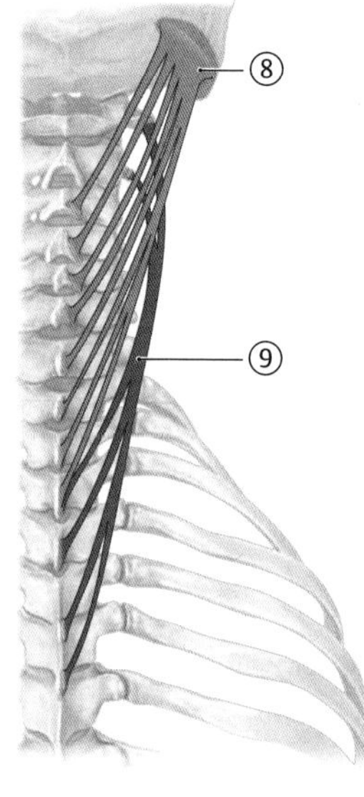

⑧
⑨

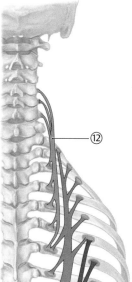

B M. splenius capitis and cervicis.

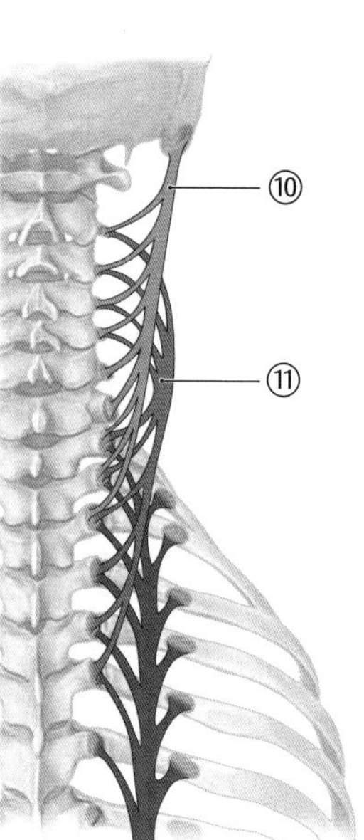

⑩
⑪

C M. longissimus capitas and cervicis.

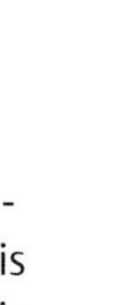

⑫

D M. iliocostalis cervicis.

Fig. 37.6 **Superficial musculature of the neck**

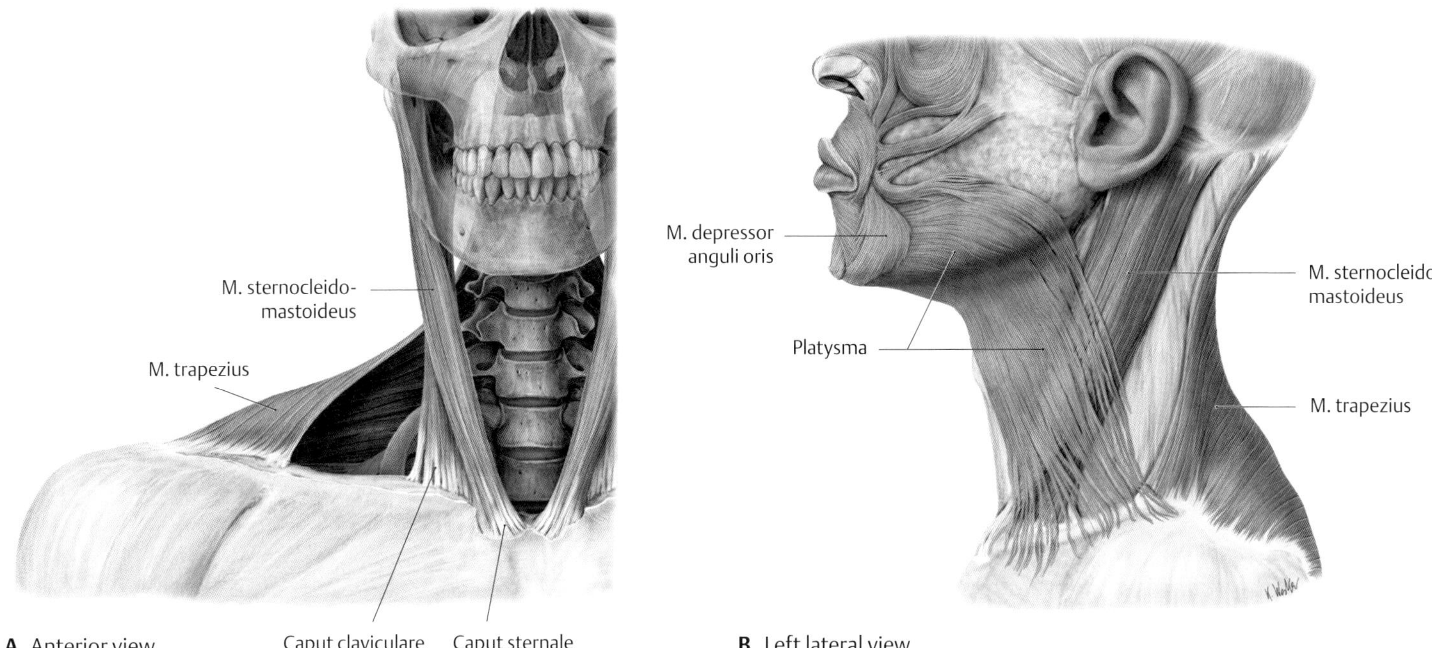
M. sternocleido-
mastoideus
M. trapezius
Caput claviculare
Caput sternale
M. depressor
anguli oris
Platysma
M. sternocleido-
mastoideus
M. trapezius

A Anterior view.

B Left lateral view.

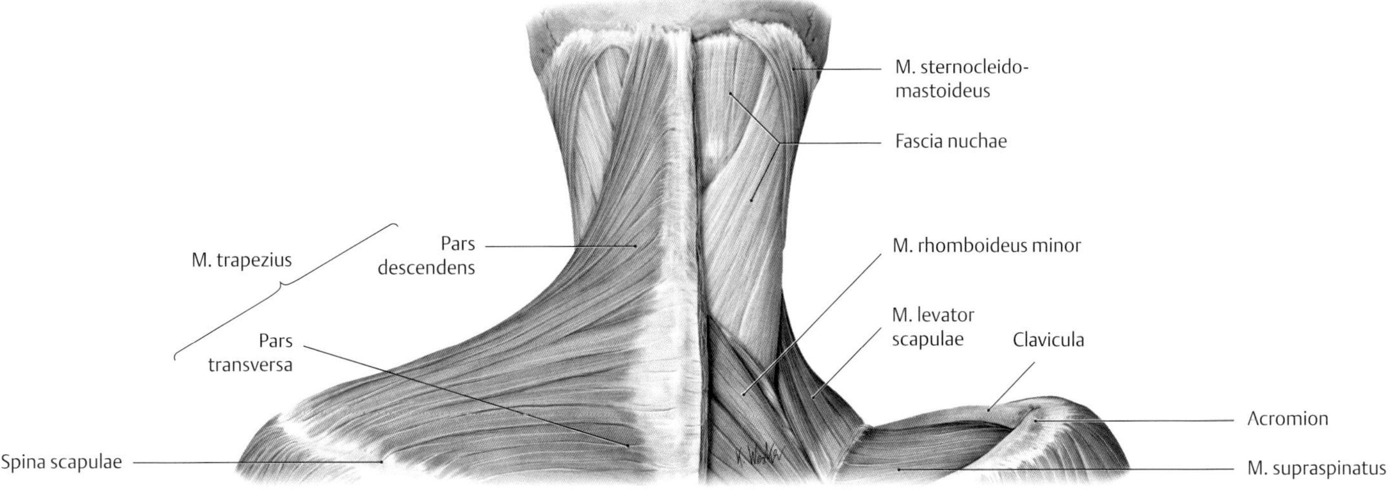
M. sternocleido-
mastoideus
Fascia nuchae
M. trapezius
Pars
descendens
Pars
transversa
M. rhomboideus minor
M. levator
scapulae
Clavicula
Acromion
Spina scapulae
M. supraspinatus

C Posterior view. *Removed:* M. trapezius (right side).

Table 37.4 Superficial neck muscles

Muscle		Origin	Insertion	Innervation	Action
Platysma		Skin over lower neck and upper lateral thorax	Mandibula (inferior border), skin over lower face and angulus oris	R. cervicalis of n. facialis (CN VII)	Depresses and wrinkles skin of lower face and mouth, tenses skin of neck, aids forced depression of mandibula
M. sternocleido-mastoideus	① Caput sternale	Manubrium sterni	Os temporale (proc. mastoideus), os occipitale (linea nuchalis superior)	*Motor:* N. accessorius (CN IX) *Pain and proprioception:* Plexus cervicalis (C2, C3)	*Unilateral:* Tilts head to same side, rotates head to opposite side *Bilateral:* Extends head, aids in respiration when head is fixed
	② Caput claviculare	Clavicula (medial one third)			
M. trapezius	③ Pars descendens	Os occipitale, procc. spinosi of C I–C VII	Clavicula (lateral one third)		Draws scapula obliquely upward, rotates glenoid cavity inferiorly

* The pars transversa ④ and pars ascendens ⑤ are described on p. 276.

Suprahyoid & Infrahyoid Muscles of the Neck

Table 37.5 Suprahyoid muscles

The suprahyoid muscles are also considered accessory muscles of mastication.

Muscle		Origin	Insertion		Innervation	Action
M. diagas-tricus	(1a) Venter anterior	Mandibula (Fossa digastrica)	Os hyoideum (corpus)	Via an intermediate tendon with a fibrous loop	N. mylohyoideus (from CN V_3)	Elevates hyoid bone (during swallowing), assists in opening mandibula
	(1b) Venter posterior	Os temporale (incisura mastoidea, medial to proc. mastoideus)			N. facialis (CN VII)	
② M. stylohyoideus		Os temporale (proc. styloideus)		Via a split tendon		
③ M. mylohyoideus		Mandibula (linea mylohyoidea)		Via median tendon of insertion (raphe mylohyoidea)	N. mylohyoideus (from CN V_3)	Tightens and elevates oral floor, draws hyoid bone forward (during swallowing), assists in opening mandibula and moving it side to side (mastication)
④ M. geniohyoideus		Mandibula (spina mentalis inferior)		Directly	R. ventralis of C1 via (via CN XII)	Draws hyoid bone forward (swallowing), assists in opening mandibula

Fig. 37.7 **Supra- and infrahyoid muscles**

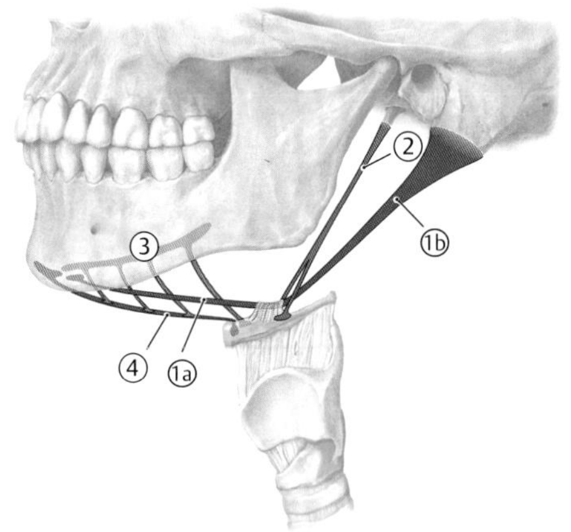

2
1b
3
4
1a

A Suprahyoid muscles, left lateral view.

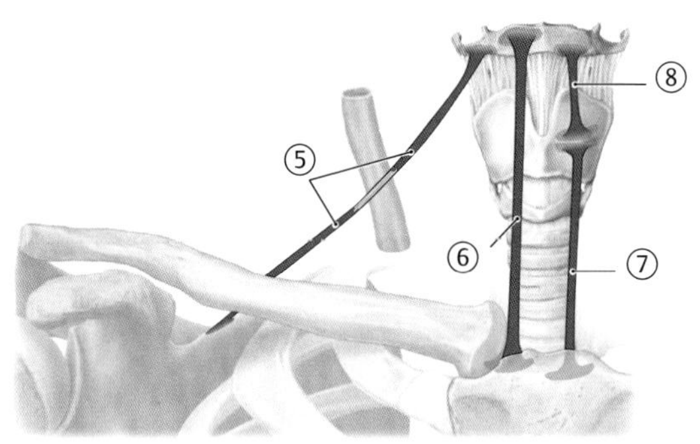

8
5
6
7

B Infrahyoid muscles, anterior view.

Table 37.6 Infrahyoid muscles

Muscle	Origin	Insertion	Innervation	Action
⑤ M. omohyoideus	Scapula (margo superior)	Os hyoideum (corpus)	Ansa cervicalis of plexus cervicalis (C1–C3)	Depresses (fixes) hyoid, draws larynx and hyoid down for phonation and terminal phases of swallowing*
⑥ M. sternohyoideus	Manubrium sterni and articulatio sternoclaviculare (posterior surface)			
⑦ M. sternothyroideus	Manubrium sterni (posterior surface)	Cartilago thyroidea (linea obliqua)	Ansa cervicalis (C2–C3)	
⑧ M. thyrohyoideus	Cartilago thyroidea (linea obliqua)	Os hyoideum (corpus)	C1 via n. hypoglossus (CN XII)	Depresses and fixes hyoid, raises the larynx during swallowing

* The m. omohyoideus also tenses the fascia cervicalis (with an intermediate tendon).

Fig. 37.8 **Supra- and infrahyoid muscles**

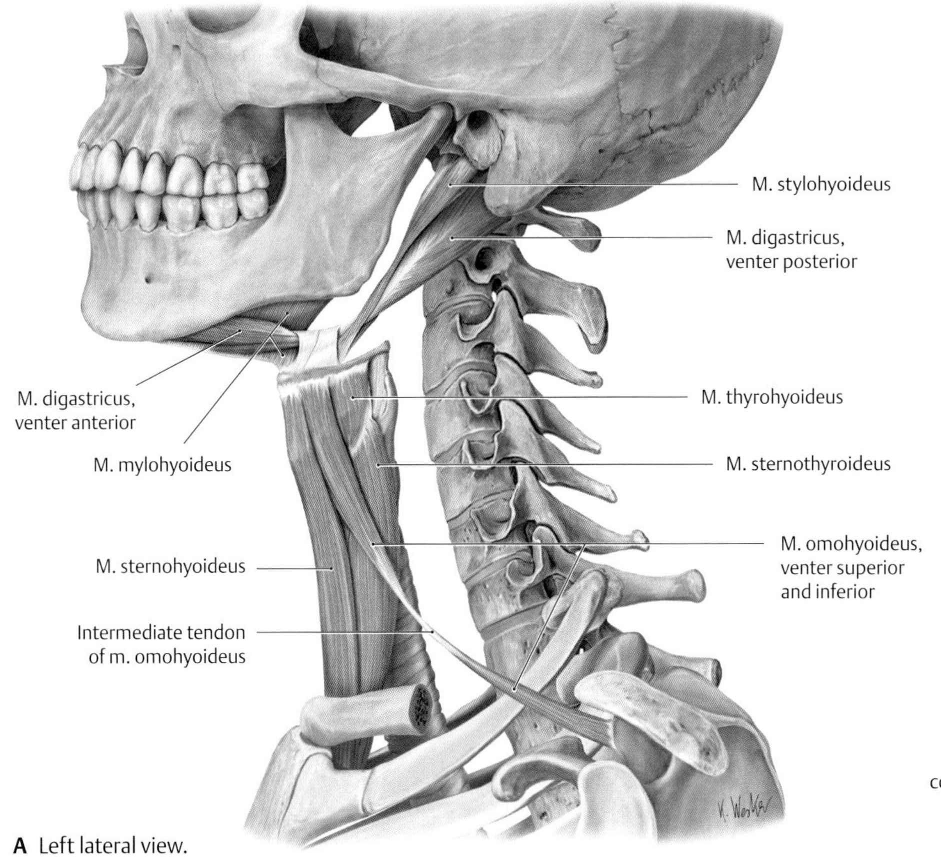

M. stylohyoideus
M. digastricus, venter posterior
M. digastricus, venter anterior
M. thyrohyoideus
M. mylohyoideus
M. sternothyroideus
M. omohyoideus, venter superior and inferior
M. sternohyoideus
Intermediate tendon of m. omohyoideus

A Left lateral view.

Proc. coronoideus
M. geniohyoideus
Linea mylohyoidea
Caput mandibulae
R. mandibulae
M. mylohyoideus
Corpus ossis hyoidei

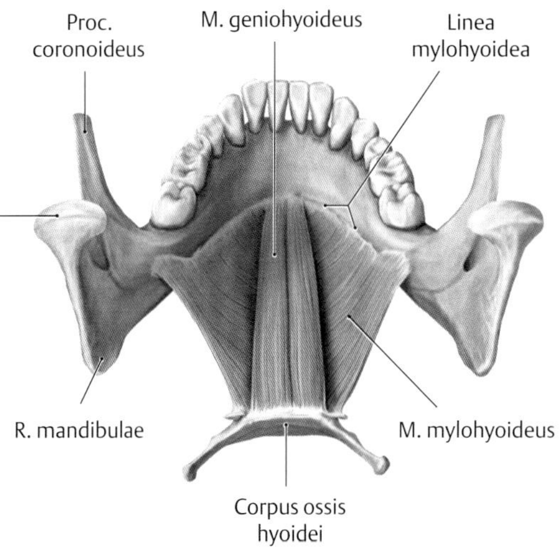

B M. mylohyoideus and m. geniohyoideus (oral floor), posterosuperior view.

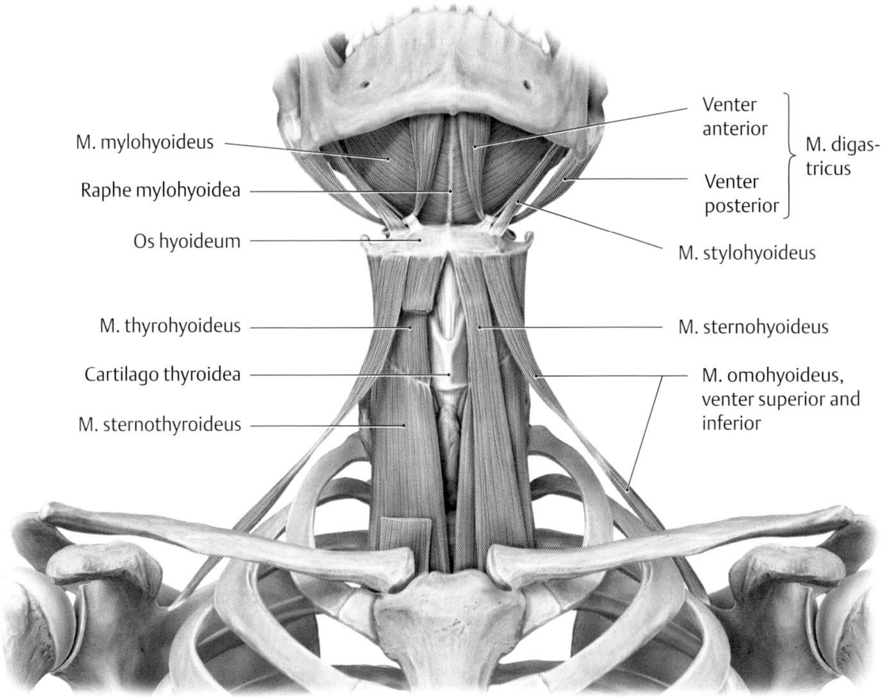

M. mylohyoideus
Venter anterior
Venter posterior
M. digastricus
Raphe mylohyoidea
Os hyoideum
M. stylohyoideus
M. thyrohyoideus
M. sternohyoideus
Cartilago thyroidea
M. omohyoideus, venter superior and inferior
M. sternothyroideus

C Anterior view. M. sternohyoideus has been cut (right).

Deep Muscles of the Neck

Fig. 37.9 **Deep muscles of the neck**

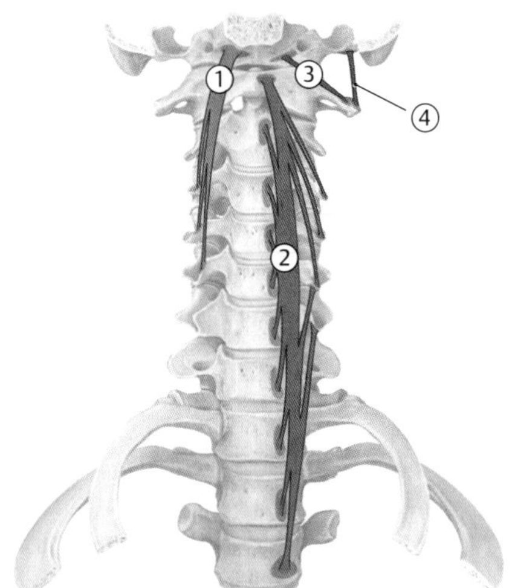
1
2
3
4
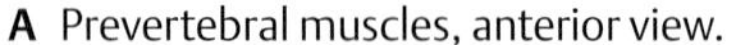

A Prevertebral muscles, anterior view.

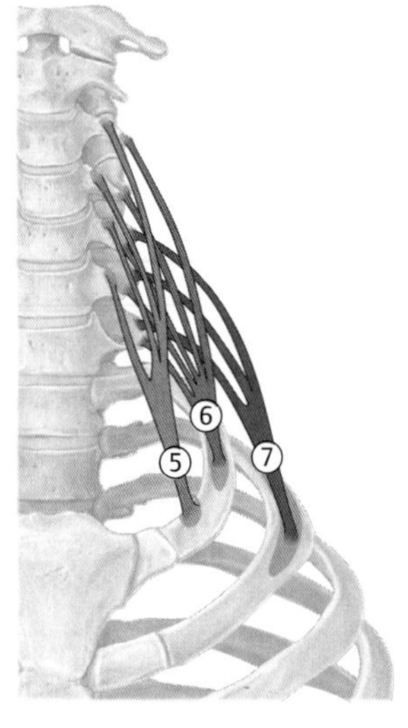
5
6
7

B Mm. scaleni, anterior view.

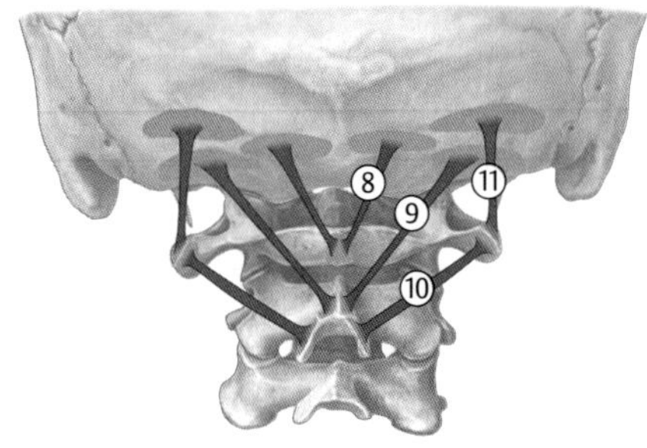
8
9
10
11

C Mm. suboccipitales, posterior view.

Table 37.7 **Deep muscles of the neck**

Muscle		Origin	Insertion	Innervation	Action
Prevertebral muscles					
① M. longus capitis		CIII–CVI (tuberculum anterius of proc. transversus)	Os occipitale (pars basilaris)	Direct branches from plexus cervicalis (C1–C3)	Flexion of head at atlanto-occipital joints
② M. longus colli	Pars verticalis (intermedia)	CV–TIII (tuberculum anterius of corpus vertebrae)	CI–CIV (anterior surfaces)	Direct branches from plexus cervicalis (C2–C6)	*Unilateral:* Tilts and rotates cervical spine to opposite side *Bilateral:* Forward flexion of cervical spine
	Pars obliqua superior	CIII–CV (tuberculum anterius of proc. transversus)	Atlas (tuberculum anterius)		
	Pars obliqua inferior	TI–TIII (anterior surfaces of corpus vertebrae)	CV–CVI (tuberculum anterius of proc. transversus)		
③ M. rectus capitis anterior		CI (massa lateralis atlantis)	Os occipitale (basilar part)	R. ventralis of C1 and C2	*Unilateral:* Lateral flexion at the atlanto-occipital joint *Bilateral:* Flexion at the atlanto-occipital joint
④ M. rectus capitis lateralis		CI (proc. transversus)	Os occipitale (pars basilaris, lateral to proc. condylaris)		
MM. scaleni					
⑤ M. scalenus anterior		CIII–CVI (tuberculum anterius of proc. transversus)	Costa I (tuberculum musculi scaleni)	Direct branches from plexus cervicalis and plexus brachialis (C3–C8)	*With ribs mobile:* Elevates upper ribs (during forced inspiration) *With ribs fixed:* Bends cervical spine to same side (unilateral), flexes neck (bilateral)
⑥ M. scalenus medius		CI–CII (proc. transversus), CIII–CVII (tuberculum posterius of proc. transversus)	Costa I (posterior to sulcus arteriae subclaviae)		
⑦ M. scalenus posterior		CV–CVII (tuberculum posterius of proc. transversus)	Costa II (outer surface)		
Mm. suboccipitales (short nuchal and craniovertebral joint muscles)					
⑧ M. rectus capitis posterior minor		CI (tuberculum posterius)	Os occipitale (inner third of linea)	R. dorsalis of C1 (n. suboccipitalis)	*Unilateral:* Rotates head to same side *Bilateral:* Extends head
⑨ M. rectus capitis posterior major		CII (proc. spinosus)	Os occipitale (middle third of linea nuchalis inferior)		
⑩ M. obliquus capitis inferior			CI (proc. transversus)		
⑪ M. obliquus capitis superior		CI (proc. transversus)	Os occipitale (above insertion of m. rectus capitis posterior major)		*Unilateral:* Tilts head to same side, rotates it to opposite side *Bilateral:* Extends head

Fig. 37.10 Deep muscles of the neck

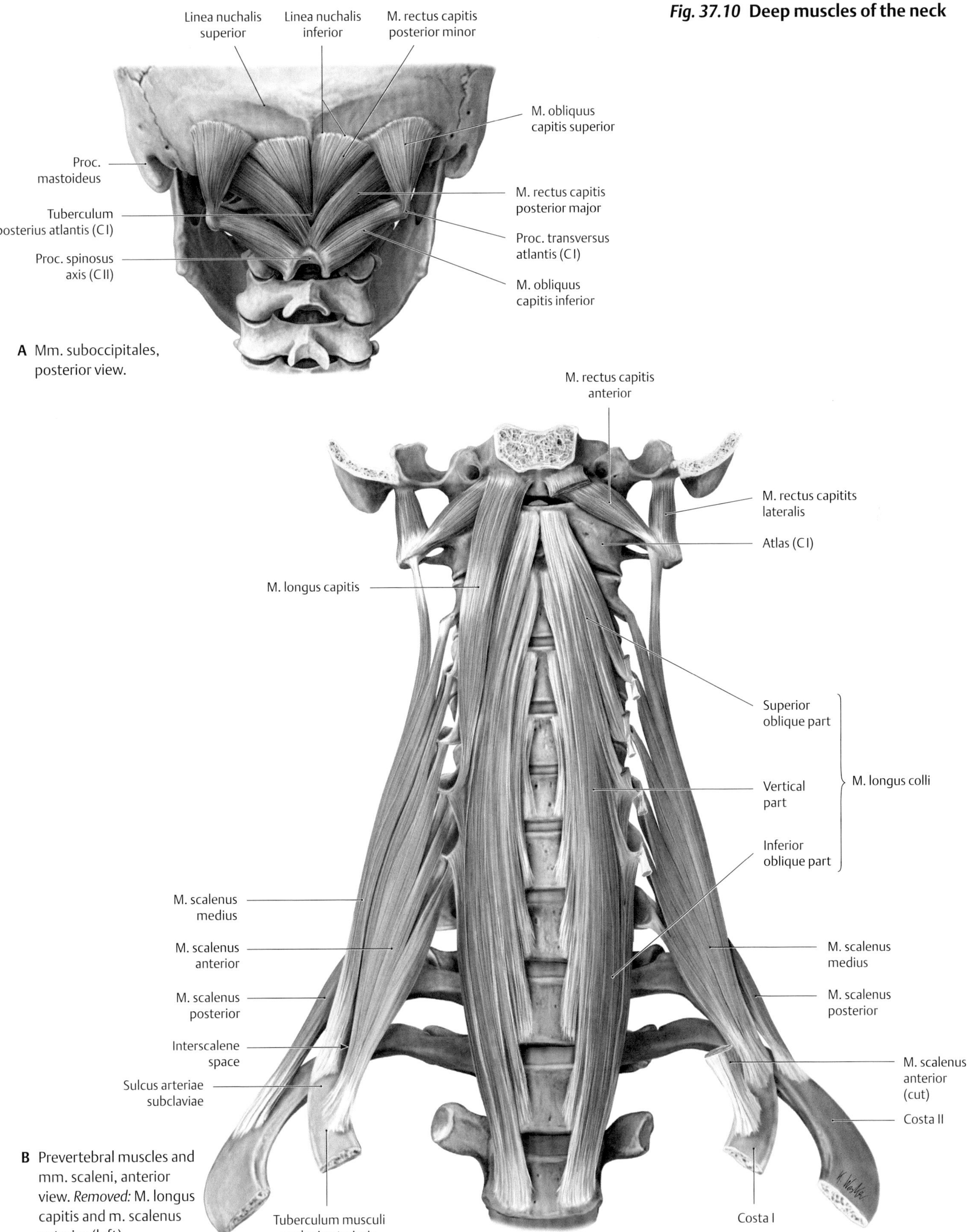
Linea nuchalis superior
Linea nuchalis inferior
M. rectus capitis posterior minor
M. obliquus capitis superior
Proc. mastoideus
M. rectus capitis posterior major
Tuberculum posterius atlantis (C I)
Proc. transversus atlantis (C I)
Proc. spinosus axis (C II)
M. obliquus capitis inferior
M. rectus capitis anterior
M. rectus capitits lateralis
Atlas (C I)
M. longus capitis
Superior oblique part
Vertical part
Inferior oblique part
M. longus colli
M. scalenus medius
M. scalenus anterior
M. scalenus posterior
Interscalene space
Sulcus arteriae subclaviae
M. scalenus medius
M. scalenus posterior
M. scalenus anterior (cut)
Costa II
Tuberculum musculi scaleni anterioris
Costa I

A Mm. suboccipitales, posterior view.

B Prevertebral muscles and mm. scaleni, anterior view. *Removed:* M. longus capitis and m. scalenus anterior (left).

Arteries & Veins of the Neck

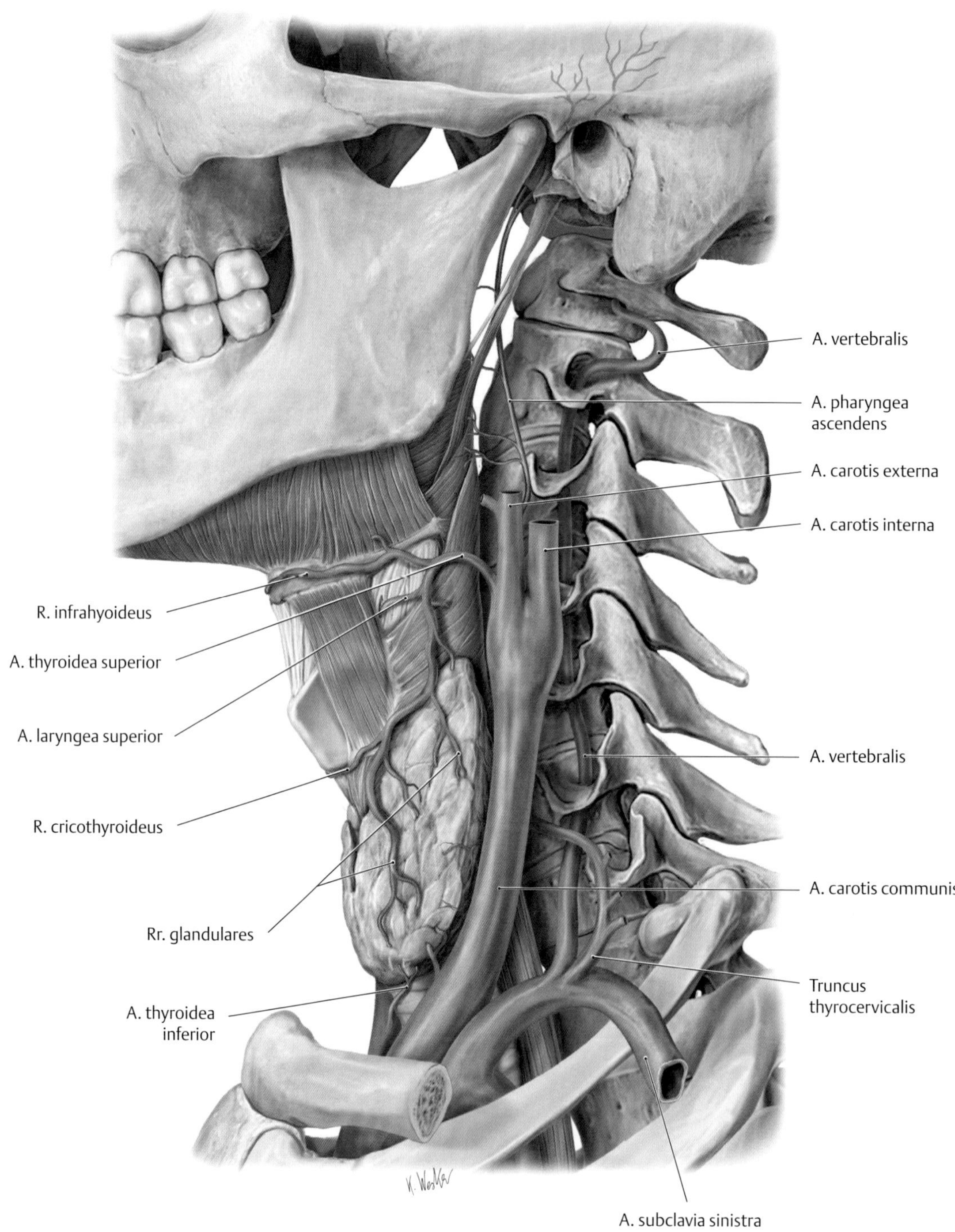
A. vertebralis
A. pharyngea ascendens
A. carotis externa
A. carotis interna
R. infrahyoideus
A. thyroidea superior
A. laryngea superior
A. vertebralis
R. cricothyroideus
A. carotis communis
Rr. glandulares
Truncus thyrocervicalis
A. thyroidea inferior
A. subclavia sinistra

Fig. 37.11 **Arteries of the neck**
Left lateral view. The structures of the neck are primarily supplied by a. carotis externa (anterior branches) and a. subclavia (a. vertebralis, truncus thyrocervicalis, and truncus costocervicalis).

Fig. 37.12 **Veins of the neck**
Left lateral view. The principal veins of the neck are the vv. jugulares interna, externa, and anterior.

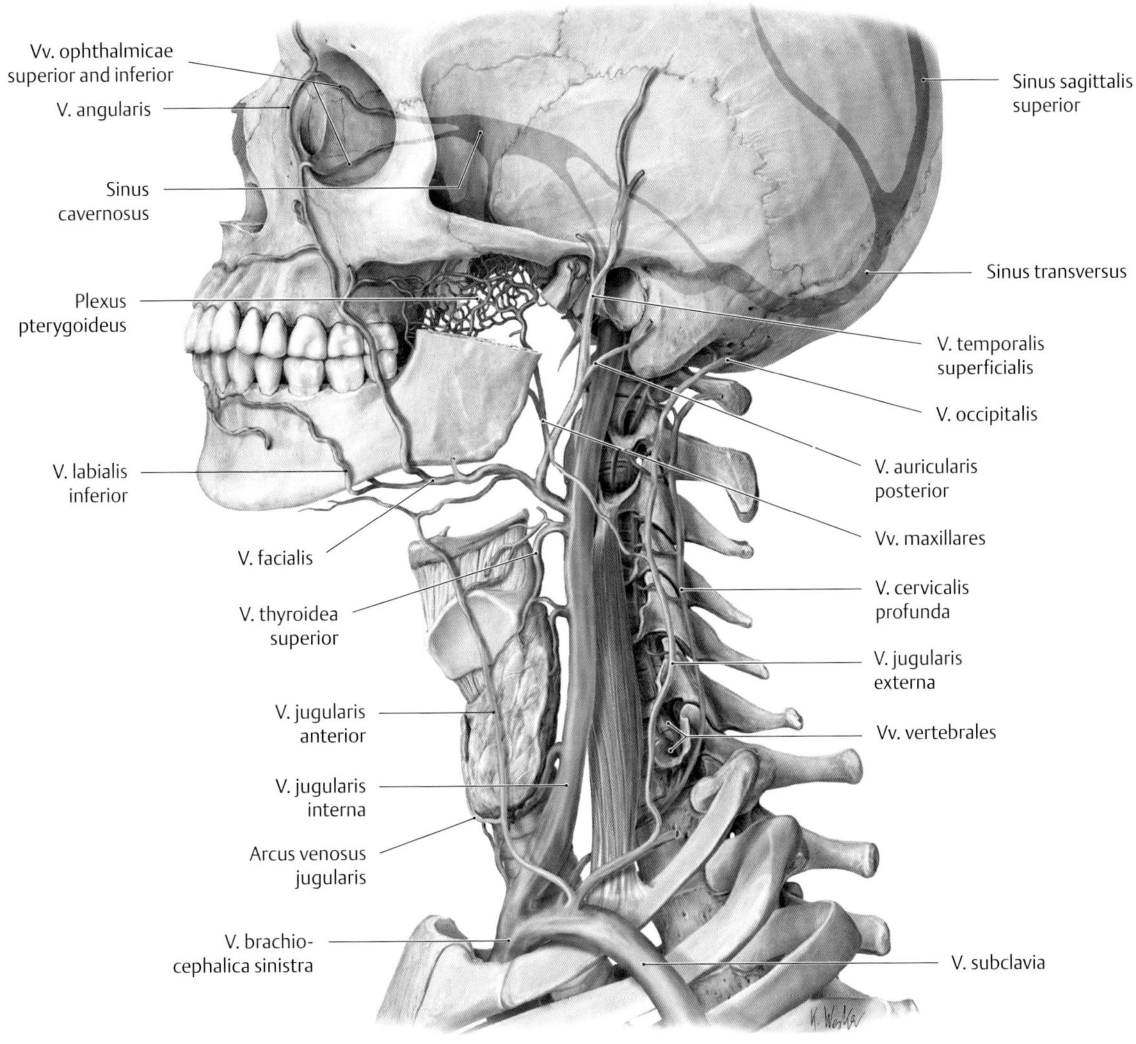
Vv. ophthalmicae superior and inferior
V. angularis
Sinus cavernosus
Plexus pterygoideus
V. labialis inferior
V. facialis
V. thyroidea superior
V. jugularis anterior
V. jugularis interna
Arcus venosus jugularis
V. brachio-cephalica sinistra
Sinus sagittalis superior
Sinus transversus
V. temporalis superficialis
V. occipitalis
V. auricularis posterior
Vv. maxillares
V. cervicalis profunda
V. jugularis externa
Vv. vertebrales
V. subclavia

Clinical

Impeded blood flow and veins of the neck
When clinical factors (e.g., chronic lung disease, mediastinal tumors, or infections) impede the flow of blood to the right heart, blood dams up in the v. cava superior, and consequently, the vv. jugulares. This causes conspicuous swelling in the vv. jugulares (and sometimes more minor veins).

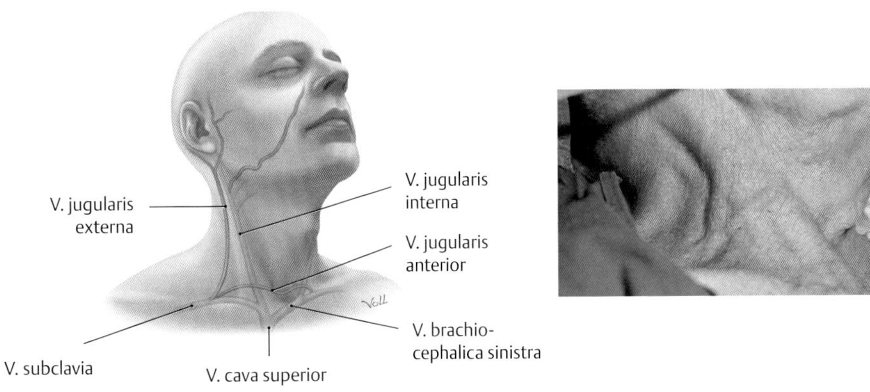
V. jugularis externa
V. jugularis interna
V. jugularis anterior
V. brachio-cephalica sinistra
V. subclavia
V. cava superior

Innervation of the Neck

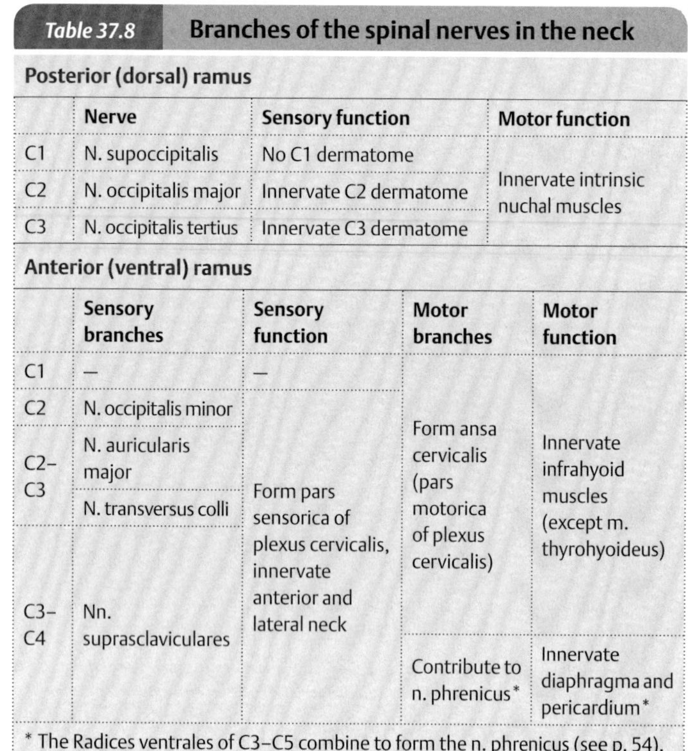

Table 37.8 Branches of the spinal nerves in the neck

Posterior (dorsal) ramus

	Nerve	Sensory function	Motor function
C1	N. supocciptalis	No C1 dermatome	Innervate intrinsic nuchal muscles
C2	N. occipitalis major	Innervate C2 dermatome	
C3	N. occipitalis tertius	Innervate C3 dermatome	

Anterior (ventral) ramus

	Sensory branches	Sensory function	Motor branches	Motor function
C1	–	–	Form ansa cervicalis (pars motorica of plexus cervicalis)	Innervate infrahyoid muscles (except m. thyrohyoideus)
C2	N. occipitalis minor	Form pars sensorica of plexus cervicalis, innervate anterior and lateral neck		
C2–C3	N. auricularis major			
	N. transversus colli			
C3–C4	Nn. suprasclaviculares			
			Contribute to n. phrenicus*	Innervate diaphragma and pericardium*

* The Radices ventrales of C3–C5 combine to form the n. phrenicus (see p. 54).

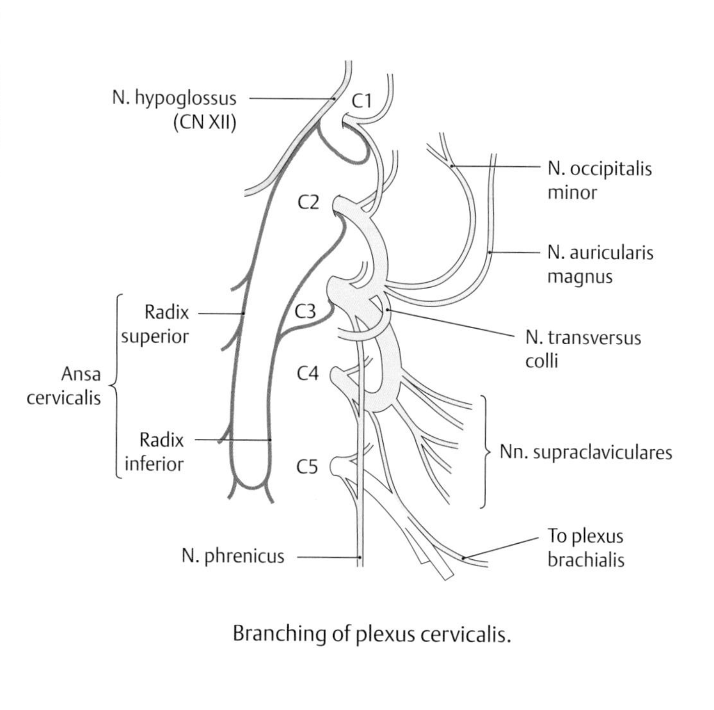
N. hypoglossus (CN XII)
C1
C2
C3
C4
C5
N. occipitalis minor
N. auricularis magnus
N. transversus colli
Nn. supraclaviculares
To plexus brachialis
N. phrenicus
Ansa cervicalis
Radix superior
Radix inferior

Branching of plexus cervicalis.

Fig. 37.13 **Innervation of the nuchal region**
Posterior view.

N. ophthalmicus (CN V_1)
C2
C3
C4

A Dermatomes.

N. ophthalmicus (CN V_1)
N. occipitalis major
N. occipitalis minor
Nn. spinales, rr. dorsales
N. auricularis magnus
Nn. supraclaviculares

B Cutaneous nerve territories.

N. occipitalis minor
N. suboccipitalis (in suboccipital triangle)
N. auricularis magnus
N. occipitalis major
N. occipitalis tertius
Nn. supraclaviculares
N. spinalis C5, r. dorsalis

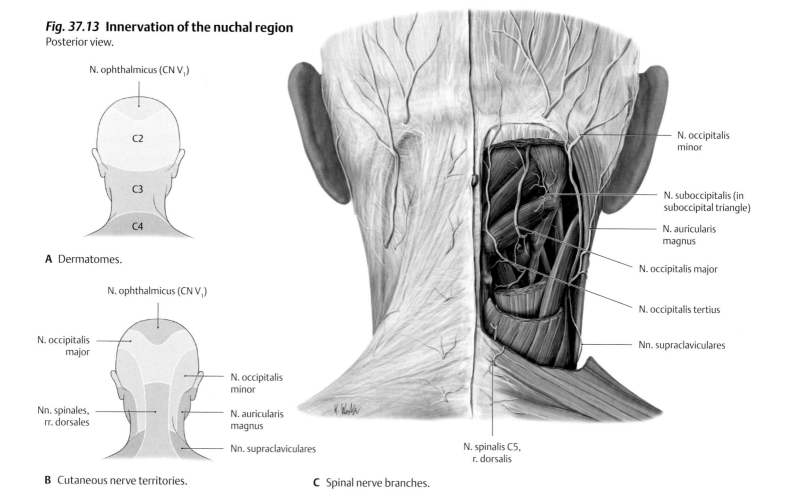

C Spinal nerve branches.

Fig. 37.14 **Sensory innervation of the anterolateral neck**
Left lateral view.

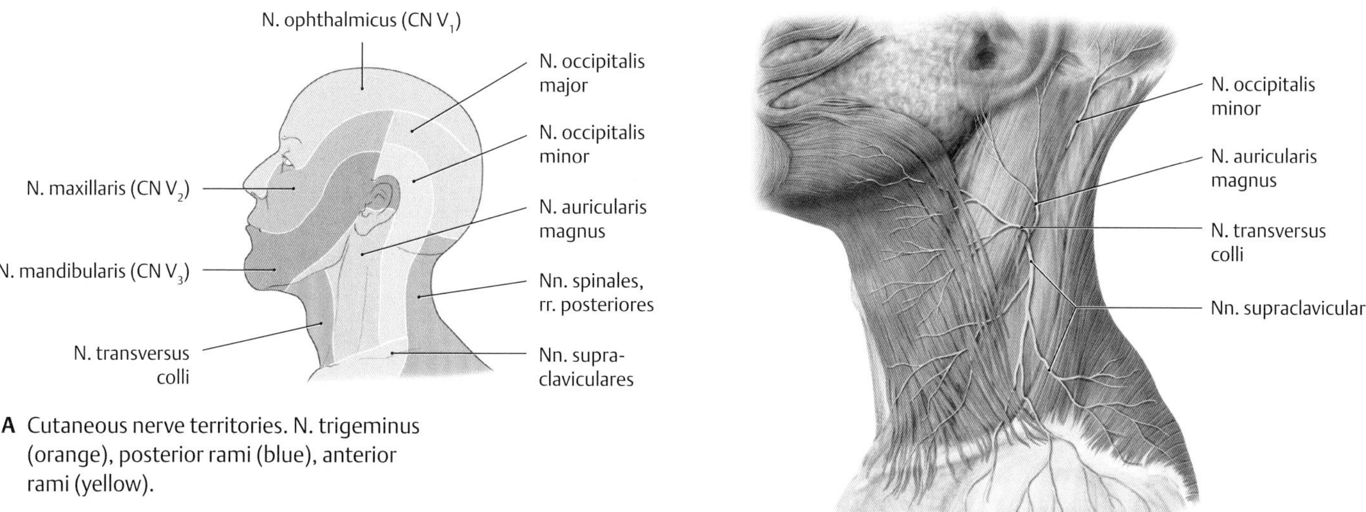
N. ophthalmicus (CN V_1)
N. occipitalis major
N. occipitalis minor
N. maxillaris (CN V_2)
N. auricularis magnus
N. mandibularis (CN V_3)
Nn. spinales, rr. posteriores
N. transversus colli
Nn. supraclaviculares
N. occipitalis minor
N. auricularis magnus
N. transversus colli
Nn. supraclavicularis

A Cutaneous nerve territories. N. trigeminus (orange), posterior rami (blue), anterior rami (yellow).

B Sensory branches of plexus cervicalis.

Fig. 37.15 **Motor innervation of the anterolateral neck**
Left lateral view.

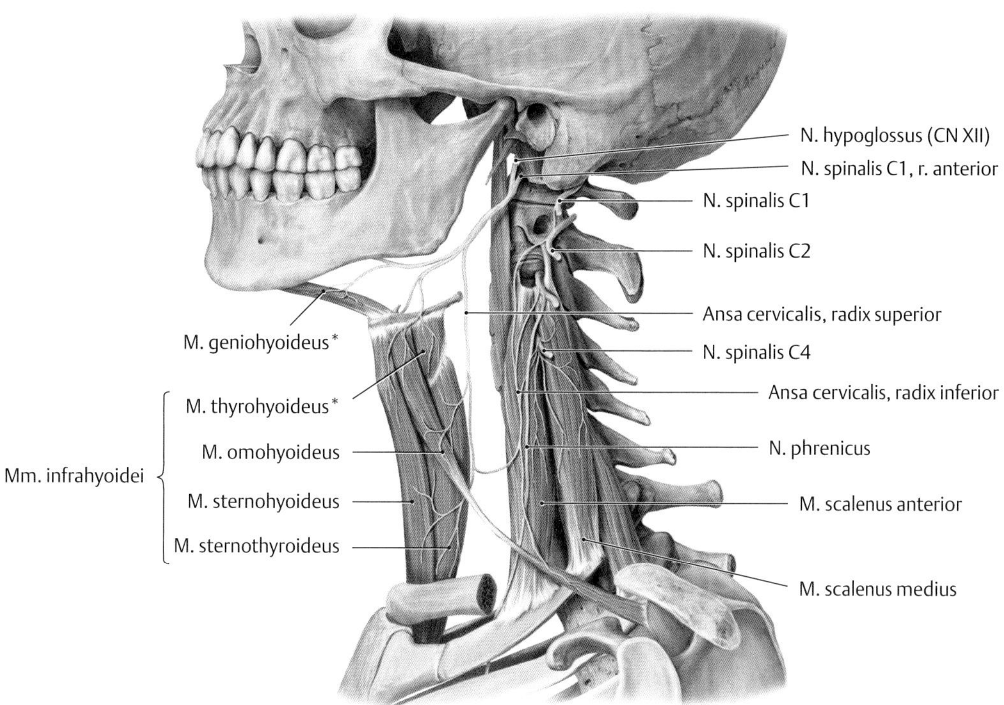
N. hypoglossus (CN XII)
N. spinalis C1, r. anterior
N. spinalis C1
N. spinalis C2
Ansa cervicalis, radix superior
M. geniohyoideus*
N. spinalis C4
M. thyrohyoideus*
Ansa cervicalis, radix inferior
M. omohyoideus
N. phrenicus
Mm. infrahyoidei
M. sternohyoideus
M. scalenus anterior
M. sternothyroideus
M. scalenus medius

* Innervated by the ramus anterior of C1 (distributed by n. hypoglossus).

Larynx: Cartilage & Structure

***Fig. 37.16* Laryngeal cartilages**
Left lateral view. The larynx consists of five laryngeal cartilages: cartilago epiglottica, cartilago thyroidea, cartilago cricoidea, and the paired cartilago arytenoidea and cartilago corniculata. They are connected to each other, trachea, and os hyoideum.

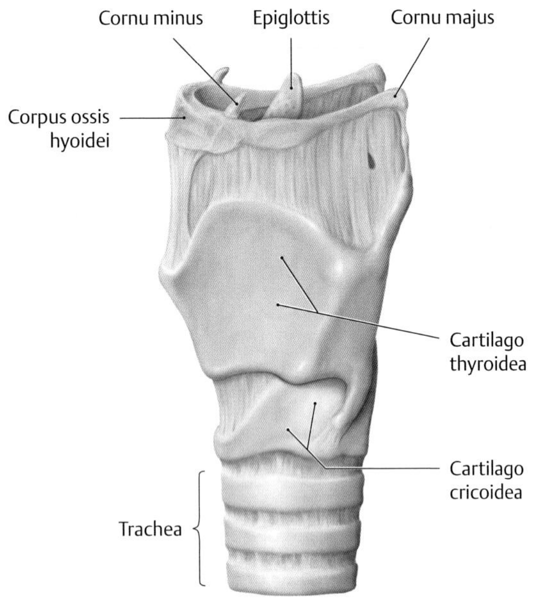
Cornu minus
Epiglottis
Cornu majus
Corpus ossis hyoidei
Cartilago thyroidea
Cartilago cricoidea
Trachea

***Fig. 37.17* Cartilago epiglottica**
The elastic cartilago epiglottica comprises the internal skeleton of the epiglottis, providing resilience to return it to its initial position after swallowing.

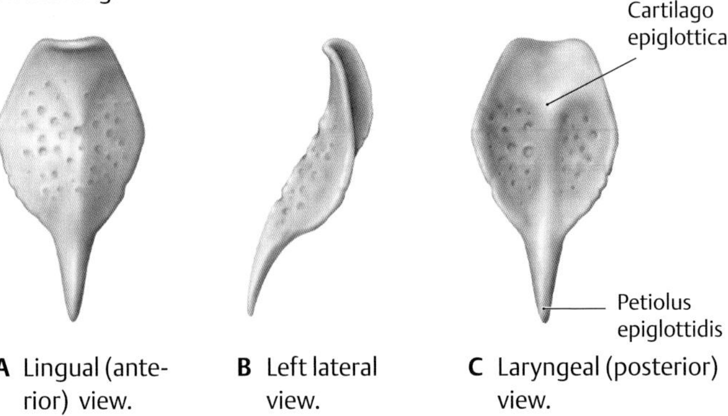
Cartilago epiglottica
Petiolus epiglottidis

A Lingual (anterior) view. **B** Left lateral view. **C** Laryngeal (posterior) view.

***Fig. 37.18* Cartilago thyroidea**
Left oblique view.

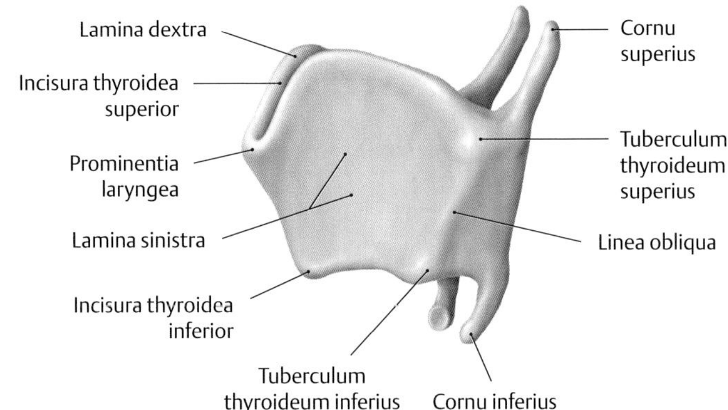
Lamina dextra
Incisura thyroidea superior
Prominentia laryngea
Lamina sinistra
Incisura thyroidea inferior
Tuberculum thyroideum inferius
Cornu inferius
Cornu superius
Tuberculum thyroideum superius
Linea obliqua

***Fig. 37.19* Cartilago cricoidea**

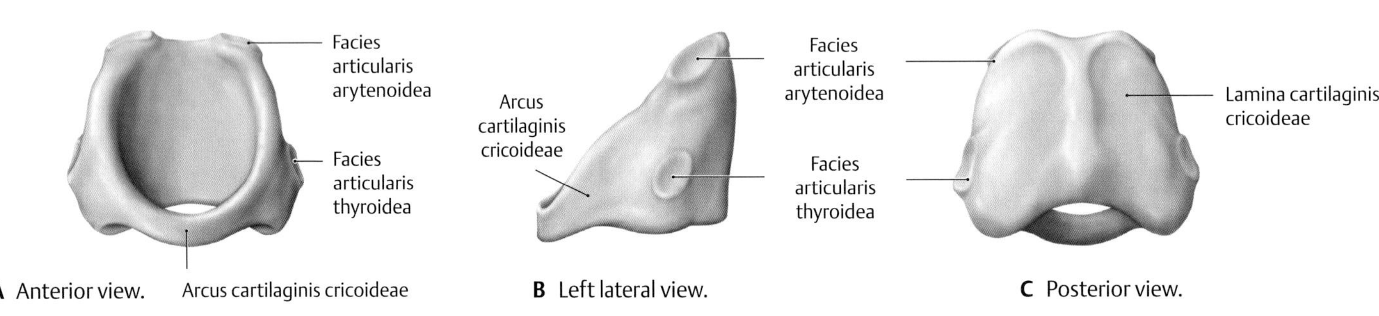
Facies articularis arytenoidea
Facies articularis thyroidea
Arcus cartilaginis cricoideae
Arcus cartilaginis cricoideae
Facies articularis arytenoidea
Facies articularis thyroidea
Lamina cartilaginis cricoideae

A Anterior view. **B** Left lateral view. **C** Posterior view.

***Fig. 37.20* Cartilagines arytenoidea and corniculata**
Right cartilages.

Cartilago corniculata
Apex cartilaginis arytenoideae
Colliculus
Facies anterolateralis
Cartilago arytenoidea
Proc. vocalis
Proc. muscularis
Facies medialis
Cartilago corniculata
Facies posterior
Proc. vocalis
Facies articularis
Proc. muscularis

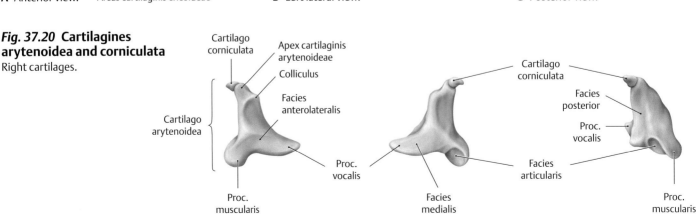

A Right lateral view. **B** Medial view. **C** Posterior view.

Fig. 37.21 **Structure of the larynx**

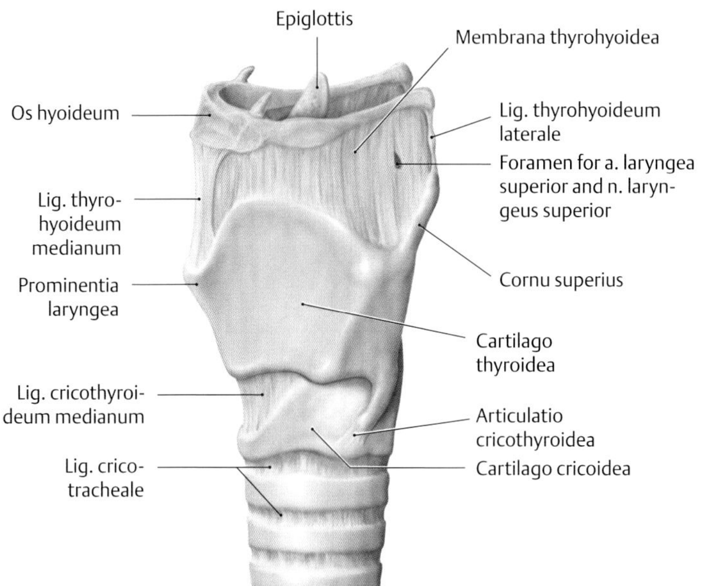
Epiglottis
Membrana thyrohyoidea
Os hyoideum
Lig. thyrohyoideum laterale
Foramen for a. laryngea superior and n. laryngeus superior
Lig. thyro-hyoideum medianum
Cornu superius
Prominentia laryngea
Cartilago thyroidea
Lig. cricothyroideum medianum
Articulatio cricothyroidea
Lig. crico-tracheale
Cartilago cricoidea

A Left anterior oblique view.

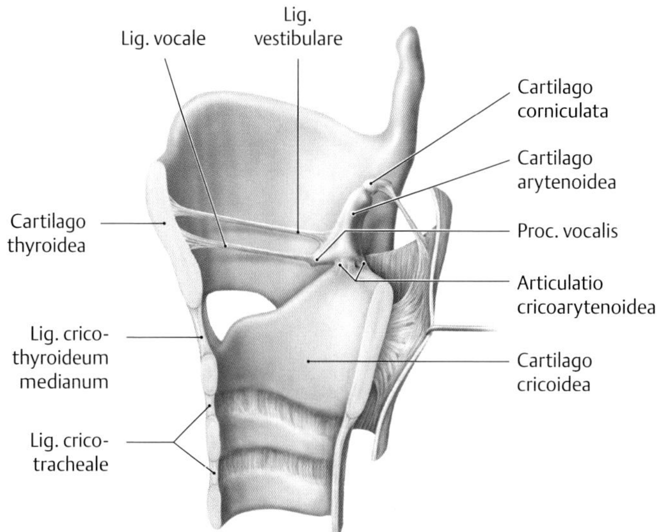
Lig. vocale
Lig. vestibulare
Cartilago corniculata
Cartilago arytenoidea
Cartilago thyroidea
Proc. vocalis
Articulatio cricoarytenoidea
Lig. crico-thyroideum medianum
Cartilago cricoidea
Lig. crico-tracheale

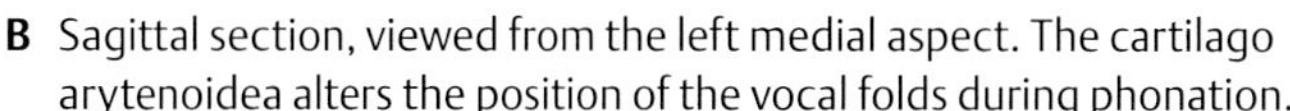
B Sagittal section, viewed from the left medial aspect. The cartilago arytenoidea alters the position of the vocal folds during phonation.

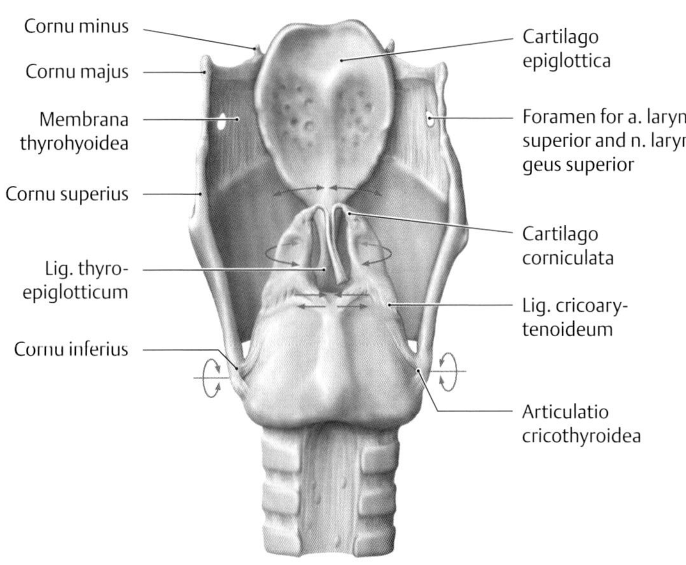
Cornu minus
Cornu majus
Cartilago epiglottica
Membrana thyrohyoidea
Foramen for a. laryngea superior and n. laryngeus superior
Cornu superius
Cartilago corniculata
Lig. thyro-epiglotticum
Lig. cricoary-tenoideum
Cornu inferius
Articulatio cricothyroidea

C Posterior view. Arrows indicate the directions of movement in the various joints.

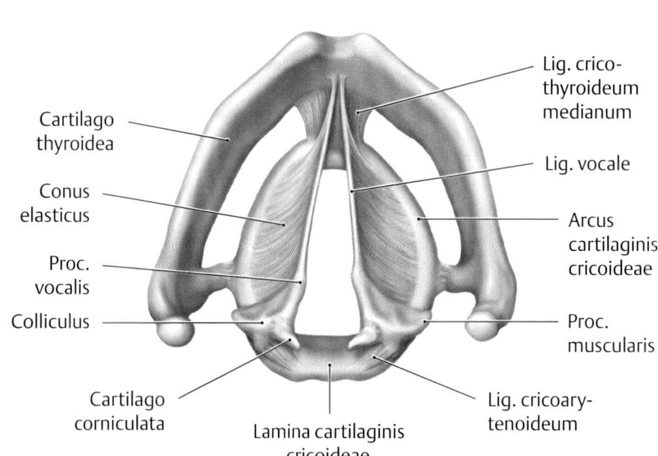
Lig. crico-thyroideum medianum
Cartilago thyroidea
Lig. vocale
Conus elasticus
Arcus cartilaginis cricoideae
Proc. vocalis
Colliculus
Proc. muscularis
Cartilago corniculata
Lamina cartilaginis cricoideae
Lig. cricoary-tenoideum

D Superior view.

Larynx: Muscles & Levels

Fig. 37.22 Laryngeal muscles

The laryngeal muscles move the laryngeal cartilages relative to one another, affecting the tension and/or position of the vocal folds. Muscles that move the larynx as a whole (infra- and suprahyoid muscles) are described on p. 562.

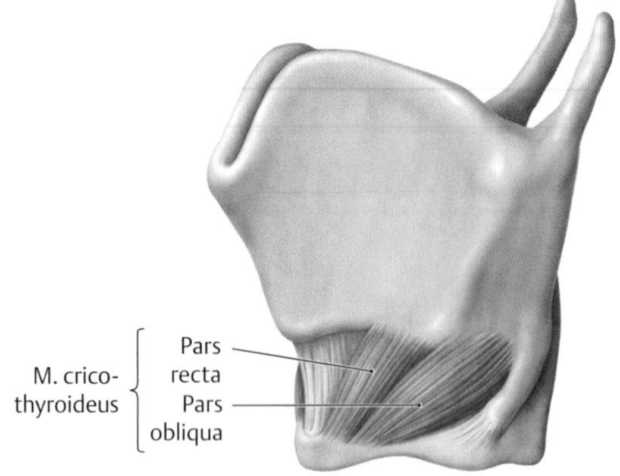
M. crico-
thyroideus
Pars
recta
Pars
obliqua

A Extrinsic laryngeal muscles, left lateral oblique view.

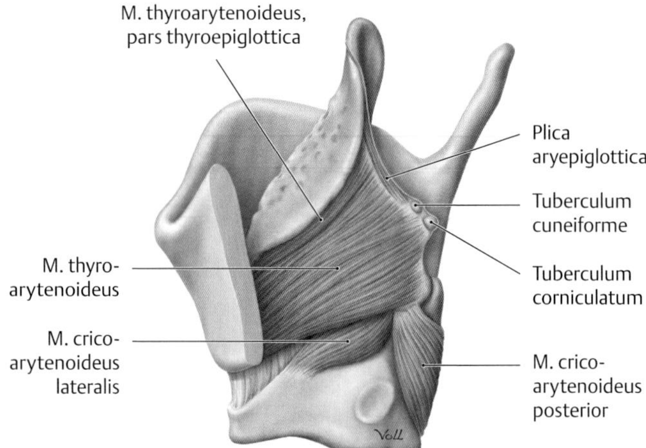
M. thyroarytenoideus,
pars thyroepiglottica
Plica
aryepiglottica
Tuberculum
cuneiforme
Tuberculum
corniculatum
M. thyro-
arytenoideus
M. crico-
arytenoideus
lateralis
M. crico-
arytenoideus
posterior

B Intrinsic laryngeal muscles, left lateral view. *Removed:* Cartilago thyroidea (left half). *Revealed:* Epiglottis and m. thyroarytenoideus.

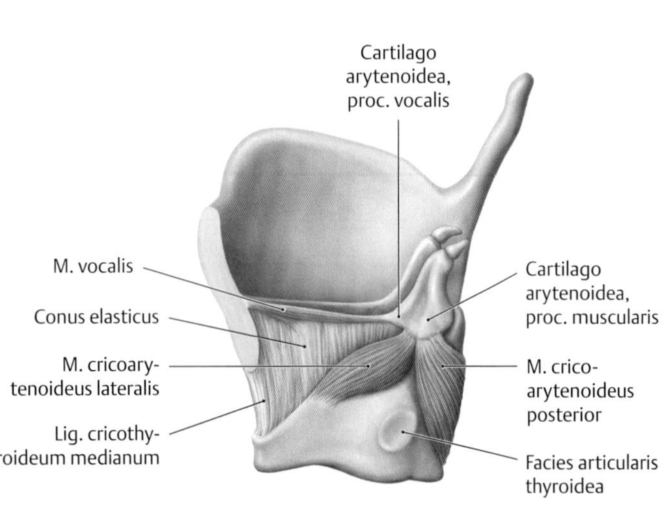
Cartilago
arytenoidea,
proc. vocalis
M. vocalis
Conus elasticus
M. cricoary-
tenoideus lateralis
Lig. cricothy-
roideum medianum
Cartilago
arytenoidea,
proc. muscularis
M. crico-
arytenoideus
posterior
Facies articularis
thyroidea

C Left lateral view with the epiglottis removed.

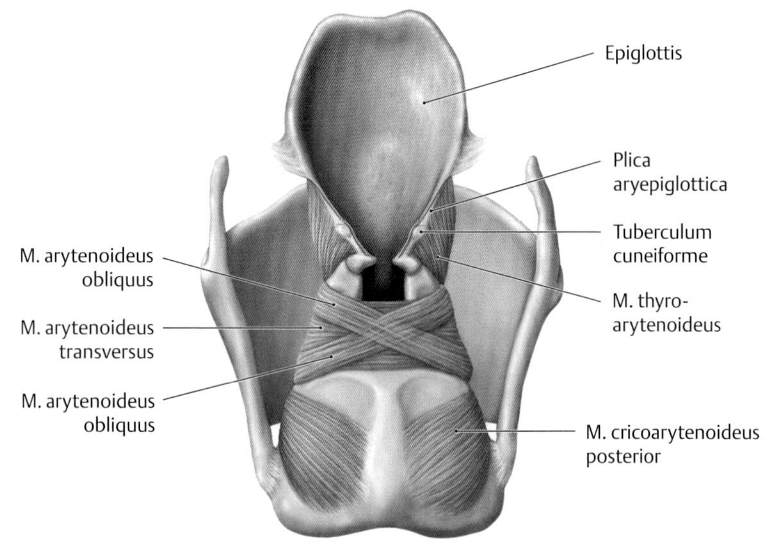
Epiglottis
Plica
aryepiglottica
Tuberculum
cuneiforme
M. thyro-
arytenoideus
M. arytenoideus
obliquus
M. arytenoideus
transversus
M. arytenoideus
obliquus
M. cricoarytenoideus
posterior

D Posterior view.

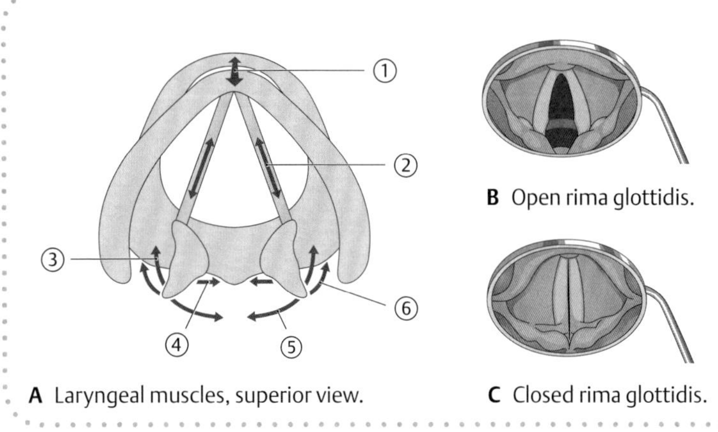
①
②
③
④
⑤
⑥

A Laryngeal muscles, superior view.

B Open rima glottidis.

C Closed rima glottidis.

Table 37.9 Actions of the laryngeal muscles

Muscle	Action	Effect on rima glottidis
① M. cricothyroideus*	Tightens the plicae vocales	None
② M. vocalis		
③ M. thyroarytaenoideus	Adducts the plicae vocales	Closes
④ M. arytaenoideus transversus		
⑤ M. cricoarytaenoideus posterior	Abducts the plicae vocales	Opens
⑥ M. cricoarytaenoideus lateralis	Adducts the plicae vocales	Closes

* The m. cricothyroideus is the only extrinsic laryngeal muscle.

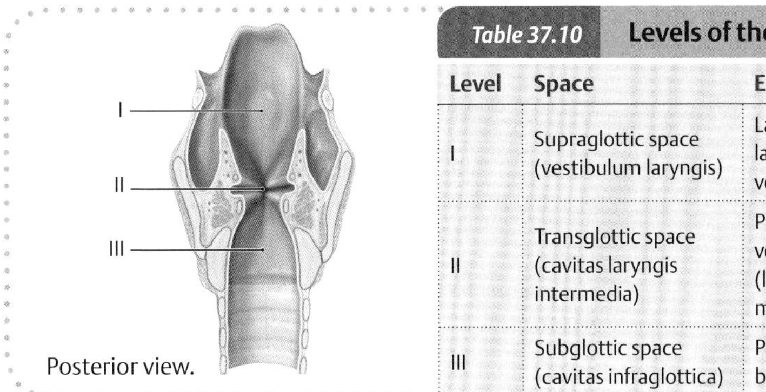
I
II
III
Posterior view.

Table 37.10 Levels of the larynx

Level	Space	Extent
I	Supraglottic space (vestibulum laryngis)	Laryngeal inlet (aditus laryngis) to plicae vestibulares
II	Transglottic space (cavitas laryngis intermedia)	Plicae vestibulares across ventriculus laryngis (lateral evagination of mucosa) to plicae vocales
III	Subglottic space (cavitas infraglottica)	Plicae vocales to inferior border of cartilago cricoidea

Fig. 37.23 Cavitas laryngis

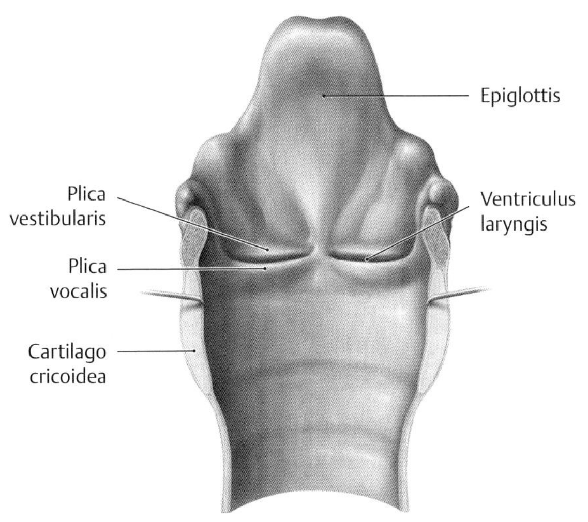
Epiglottis
Plica vestibularis
Ventriculus laryngis
Plica vocalis
Cartilago cricoidea

A Posterior view with the larynx splayed open.

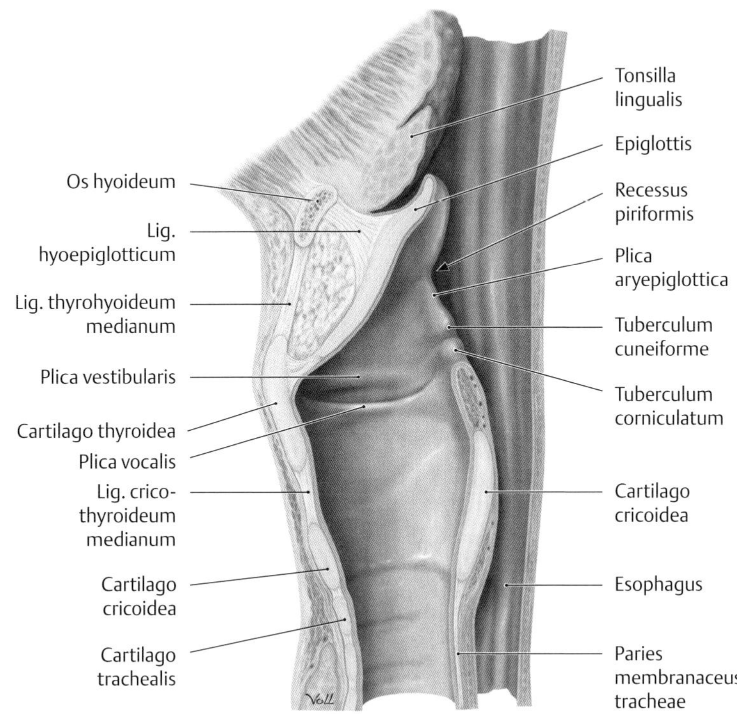
Tonsilla lingualis
Epiglottis
Os hyoideum
Recessus piriformis
Lig. hyoepiglotticum
Plica aryepiglottica
Lig. thyrohyoideum medianum
Tuberculum cuneiforme
Plica vestibularis
Tuberculum corniculatum
Cartilago thyroidea
Plica vocalis
Lig. crico-thyroideum medianum
Cartilago cricoidea
Cartilago cricoidea
Esophagus
Cartilago trachealis
Paries membranaceus tracheae
Voll

B Midsagittal section viewed from the left side.

Fig. 37.24 Plicae vestibularis and vocalis

Coronal section, superior view.

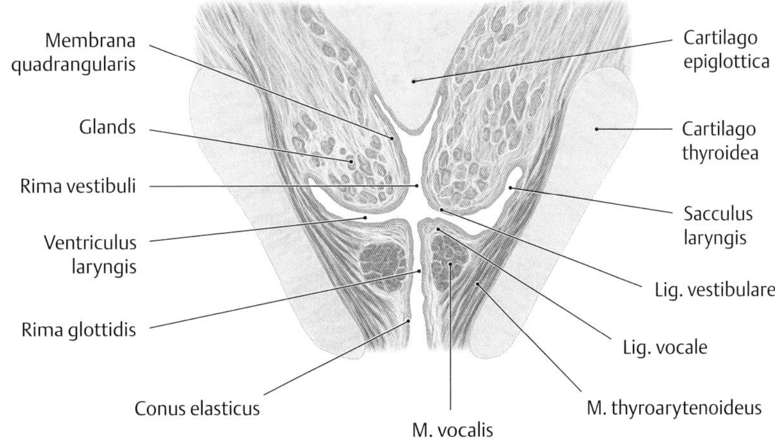
Membrana quadrangularis
Cartilago epiglottica
Glands
Cartilago thyroidea
Rima vestibuli
Sacculus laryngis
Ventriculus laryngis
Lig. vestibulare
Rima glottidis
Lig. vocale
Conus elasticus
M. thyroarytenoideus
M. vocalis

Neurovasculature of the Larynx, Thyroid & Parathyroids

Fig. 37.25 **Glandulae thyroidea and parathyroidea**

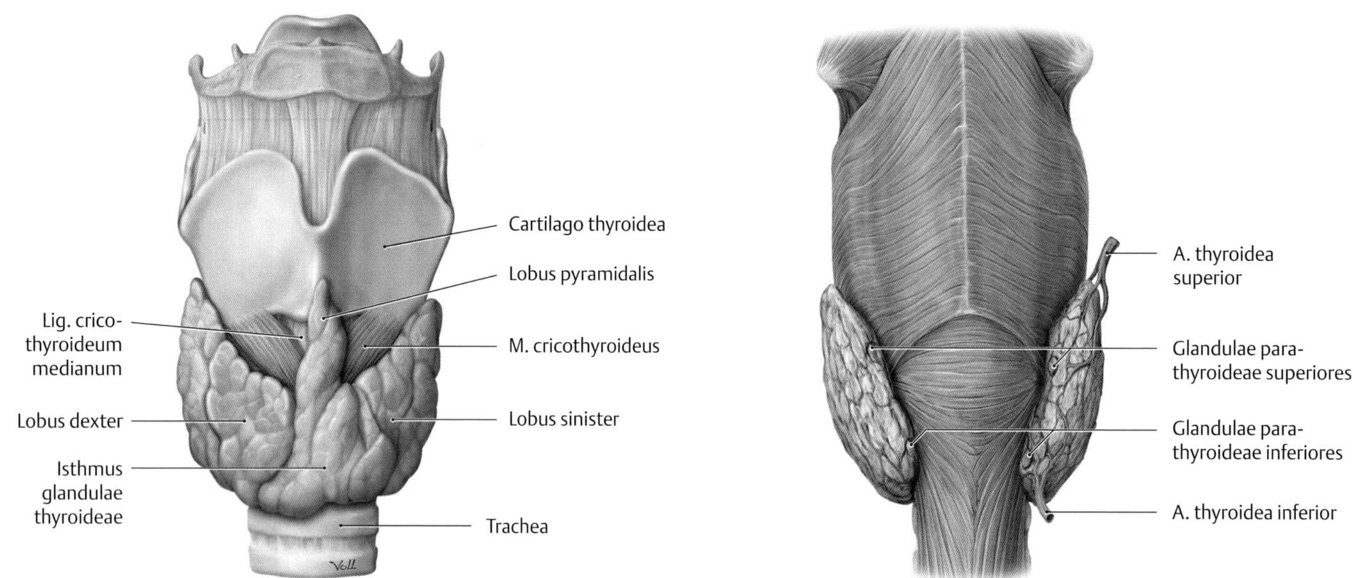
Cartilago thyroidea
Lobus pyramidalis
Lig. crico-thyroideum medianum
M. cricothyroideus
Lobus dexter
Lobus sinister
Isthmus glandulae thyroideae
Trachea
A. thyroidea superior
Glandulae para-thyroideae superiores
Glandulae para-thyroideae inferiores
A. thyroidea inferior

A Glandula thyroidea, anterior view.

B Glandulae thyroidea and parathyroidea, posterior view.

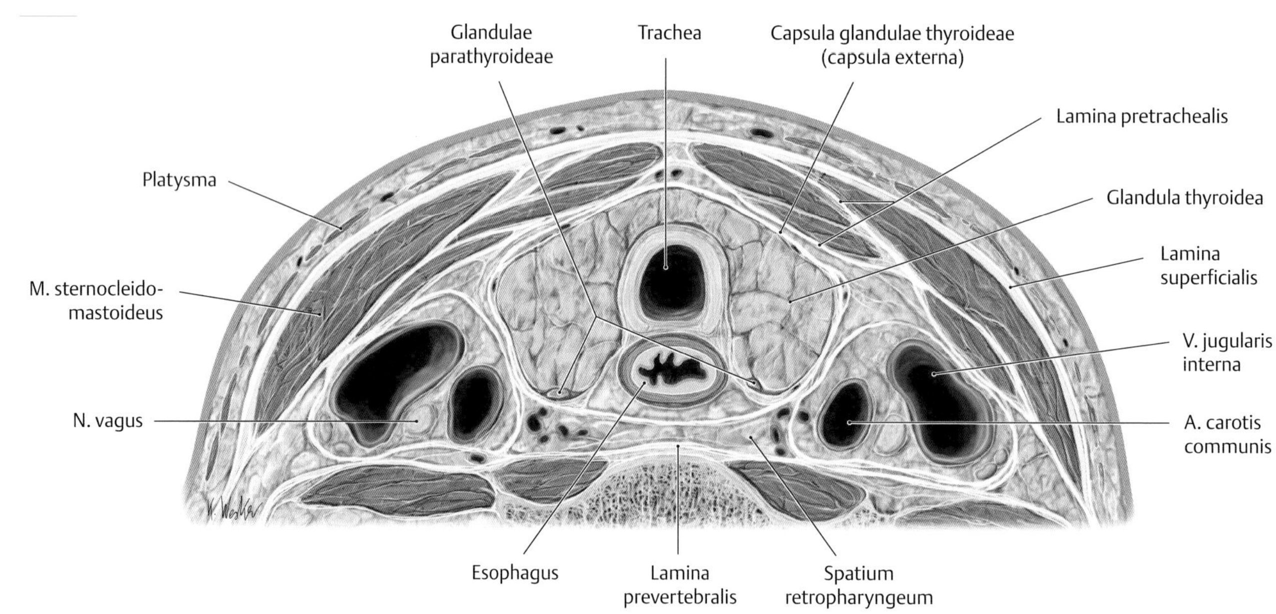
Glandulae parathyroideae
Trachea
Capsula glandulae thyroideae (capsula externa)
Lamina pretrachealis
Platysma
Glandula thyroidea
Lamina superficialis
M. sternocleido-mastoideus
V. jugularis interna
N. vagus
A. carotis communis
Esophagus
Lamina prevertebralis
Spatium retropharyngeum

C Topographical relations of glandulae thyroidea and parathyroidea. See p. 577 for the layers of fascia cervicalis.

Fig. 37.26 Arteries and nerves

Anterior view.

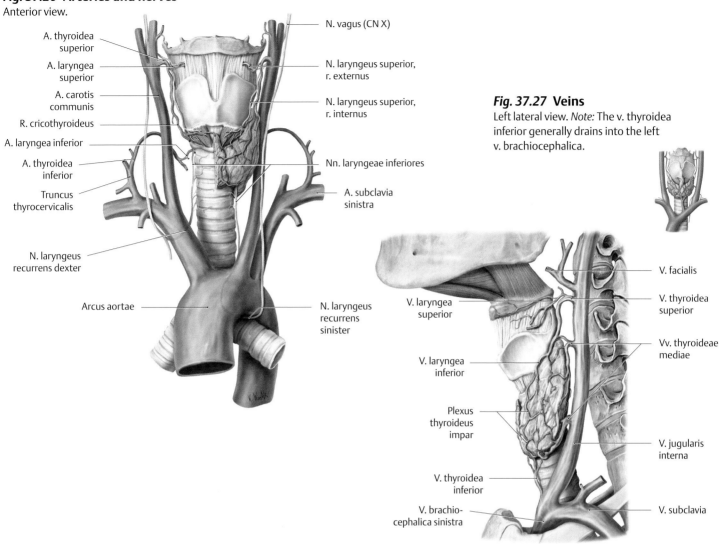

A. thyroidea superior
A. laryngea superior
A. carotis communis
R. cricothyroideus
A. laryngea inferior
A. thyroidea inferior
Truncus thyrocervicalis
N. laryngeus recurrens dexter
Arcus aortae
N. vagus (CN X)
N. laryngeus superior, r. externus
N. laryngeus superior, r. internus
Nn. laryngeae inferiores
A. subclavia sinistra
N. laryngeus recurrens sinister

Fig. 37.27 Veins

Left lateral view. *Note:* The v. thyroidea inferior generally drains into the left v. brachiocephalica.

V. laryngea superior
V. laryngea inferior
Plexus thyroideus impar
V. thyroidea inferior
V. brachio-cephalica sinistra
V. facialis
V. thyroidea superior
Vv. thyroideae mediae
V. jugularis interna
V. subclavia

Fig. 37.28 Neurovasculature

Left lateral view.

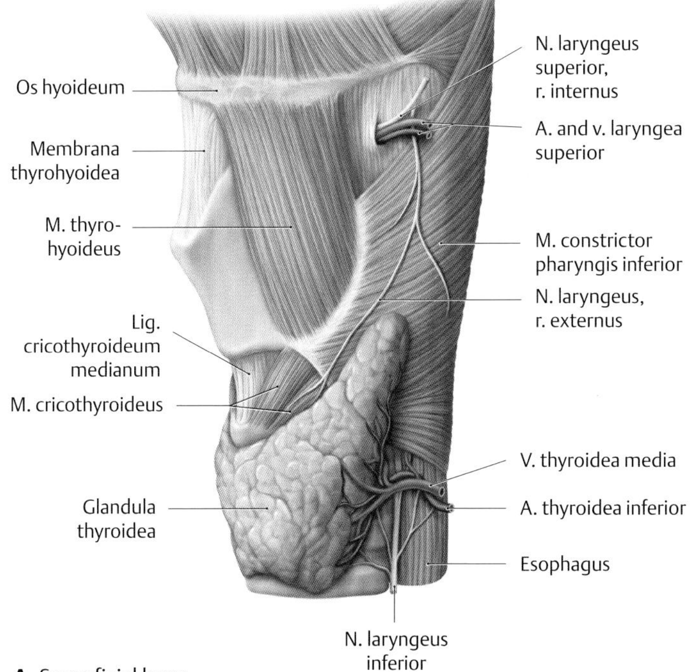

Os hyoideum
Membrana thyrohyoidea
M. thyro-hyoideus
Lig. cricothyroideum medianum
M. cricothyroideus
Glandula thyroidea
N. laryngeus superior, r. internus
A. and v. laryngea superior
M. constrictor pharyngis inferior
N. laryngeus, r. externus
V. thyroidea media
A. thyroidea inferior
Esophagus
N. laryngeus inferior

A Superficial layer.

Epiglottis
Os hyoideum
Lig. thyrohyoideum medianum
M. thyro-arytenoideus
M. cricoaryte-noideus lateralis
Lig. cricothyroideum medianum
M. cricothyroideus
Rr. tracheales
N. laryngeus superior, r. internus
A. and v. laryngea superior
R. communicans cum nervo laryngeo recurrente (Galen's anastomosis)
M. cricoarytenoi-deus posterior
Esophagus
V. thyroidea media
A. thyroidea inferior
N. laryngeus inferior

B Deep layer. *Removed:* M. cricothyroideus and left lamina of cartilago thyroidea. *Retracted:* Pharyngeal mucosa.

Topography of the Neck: Regions & Fascia

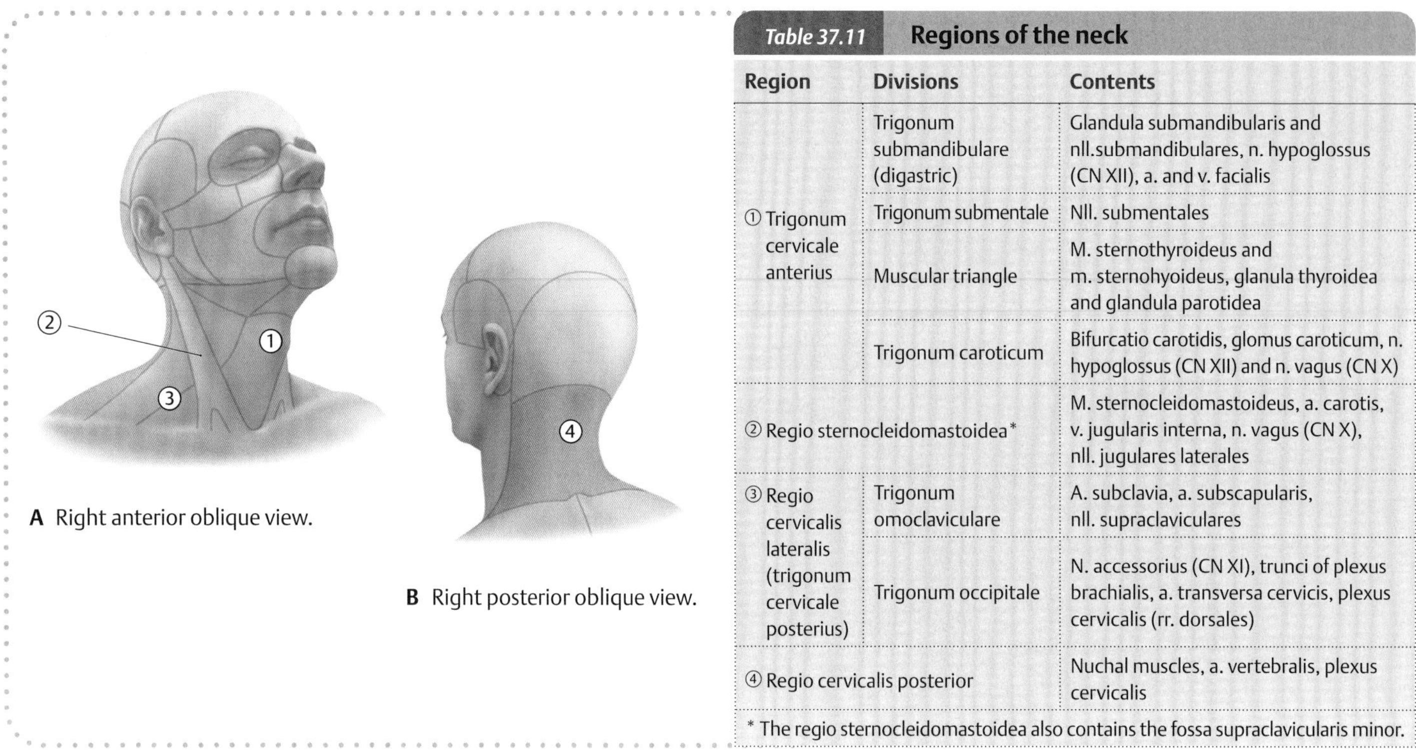
②
①
③
④

A Right anterior oblique view.

B Right posterior oblique view.

Table 37.11 Regions of the neck

Region	Divisions	Contents
① Trigonum cervicale anterius	Trigonum submandibulare (digastric)	Glandula submandibularis and nll.submandibulares, n. hypoglossus (CN XII), a. and v. facialis
	Trigonum submentale	Nll. submentales
	Muscular triangle	M. sternothyroideus and m. sternohyoideus, glanula thyroidea and glandula parotidea
	Trigonum caroticum	Bifurcatio carotidis, glomus caroticum, n. hypoglossus (CN XII) and n. vagus (CN X)
② Regio sternocleidomastoidea*		M. sternocleidomastoideus, a. carotis, v. jugularis interna, n. vagus (CN X), nll. jugulares laterales
③ Regio cervicalis lateralis (trigonum cervicale posterius)	Trigonum omoclaviculare	A. subclavia, a. subscapularis, nll. supraclaviculares
	Trigonum occipitale	N. accessorius (CN XI), trunci of plexus brachialis, a. transversa cervicis, plexus cervicalis (rr. dorsales)
④ Regio cervicalis posterior		Nuchal muscles, a. vertebralis, plexus cervicalis

* The regio sternocleidomastoidea also contains the fossa supraclavicularis minor.

***Fig. 37.29* Cervical regions**

Trigonum submandibulare
M. digastricus
Trigonum submentale
Os hyoideum
M. sternocleido-mastoideus
Trigonum caroticum
Trigonum omoclaviculare
Fossa supra-clavicularis minor
Trigonum musculare
M. trapezius

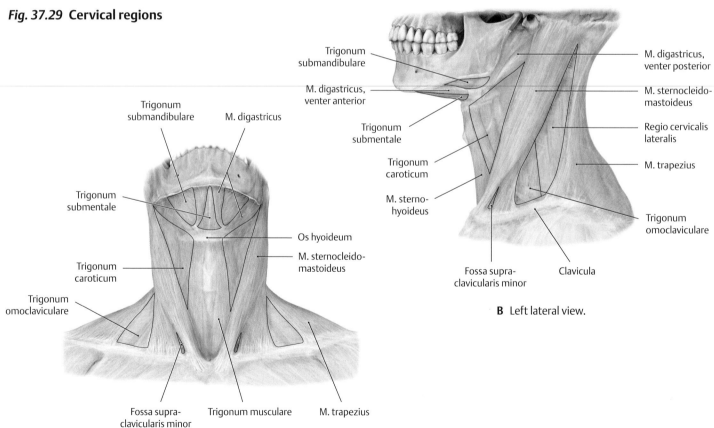

A Anterior view.

Trigonum submandibulare
M. digastricus, venter anterior
Trigonum submentale
Trigonum caroticum
M. sterno-hyoideus
M. digastricus, venter posterior
M. sternocleido-mastoideus
Regio cervicalis lateralis
M. trapezius
Trigonum omoclaviculare
Fossa supra-clavicularis minor
Clavicula

B Left lateral view.

Table 37.12 Fascia cervicalis profunda

The fascia cervicalis profunda is divided into four laminae that enclose the structures of the neck.

Layer	Lamina	Type of fascia	Description
① Fascia investiens	Lamina superficialis	Muscular	Envelopes entire neck; splits to enclose m. sternocleidomastoideus and m. trapezius
Pretracheal layer	② Lamina pretrachealis		Encloses infrahyoid muscles
	③ Lamina visceralis	Visceral	Surrounds glandula thyroidea, larynx, trachea, pharynx, and esophagus
④ Prevertebral layer	Lamina prevertebralis	Muscular	Surrounds columna vertebralis cervicalis and associated muscles
⑤ Vagina carotica		Neurovascular	Encloses common a. carotis, v. jugularis interna, and n. vagus

A Transverse section at level of C V vertebra.

B Midsagittal section, left lateral view.

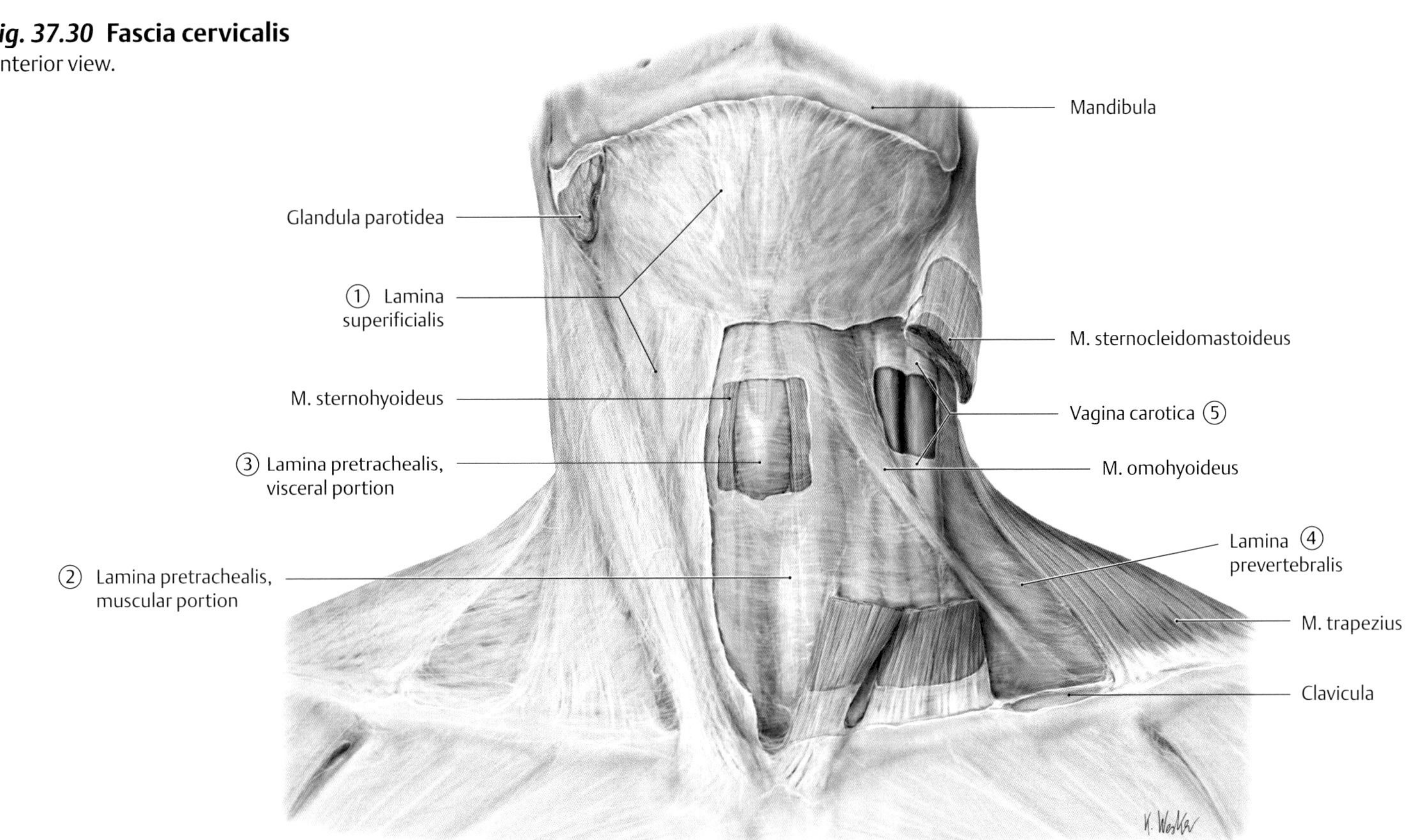

Mandibula
Glandula parotidea
① Lamina superificialis
M. sternocleidomastoideus
M. sternohyoideus
Vagina carotica ⑤
③ Lamina pretrachealis, visceral portion
M. omohyoideus
Lamina ④ prevertebralis
② Lamina pretrachealis, muscular portion
M. trapezius
Clavicula

Fig. 37.30 **Fascia cervicalis**
Anterior view.

Topography of the Anterior Cervical Region

Fig. 37.31 **Regio cervicalis anterior**
Anterior view.

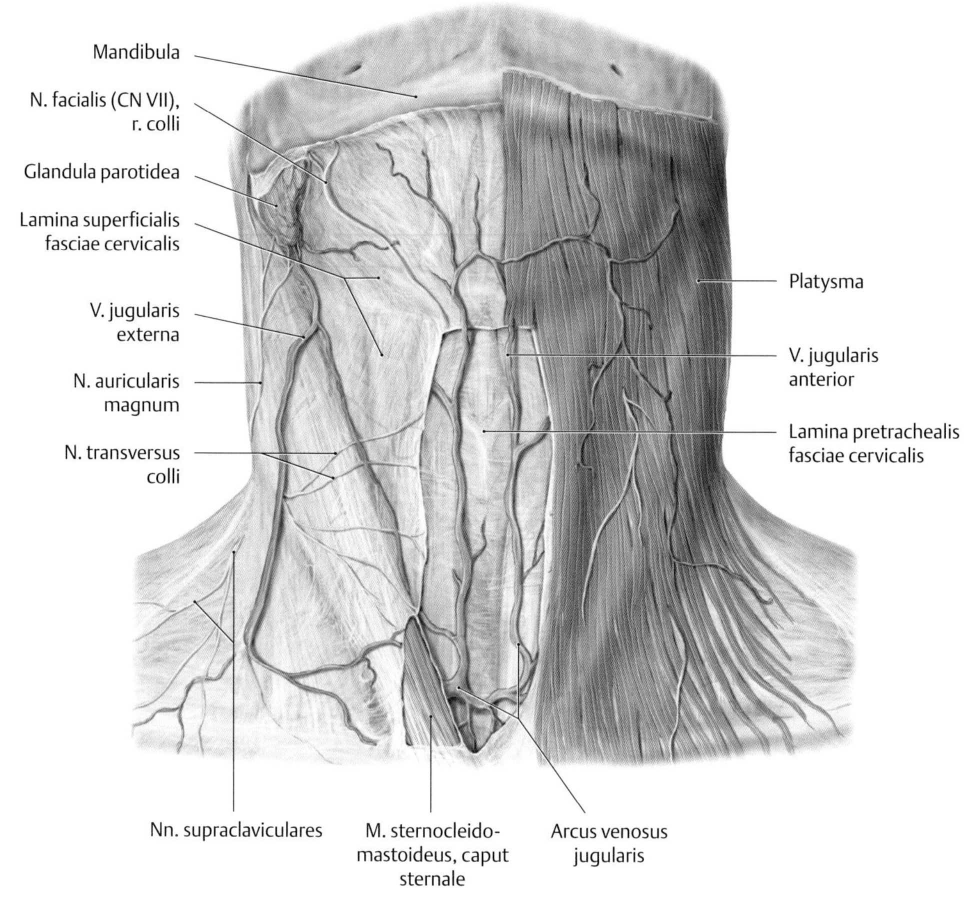
Mandibula
N. facialis (CN VII), r. colli
Glandula parotidea
Lamina superficialis fasciae cervicalis
V. jugularis externa
N. auricularis magnum
N. transversus colli
Nn. supraclaviculares
M. sternocleido-mastoideus, caput sternale
Arcus venosus jugularis
Platysma
V. jugularis anterior
Lamina pretrachealis fasciae cervicalis

A Superficial layer. *Removed:* Subcutaneous platysma (right side) and lamina superficialis of fascia cervicalis (center).

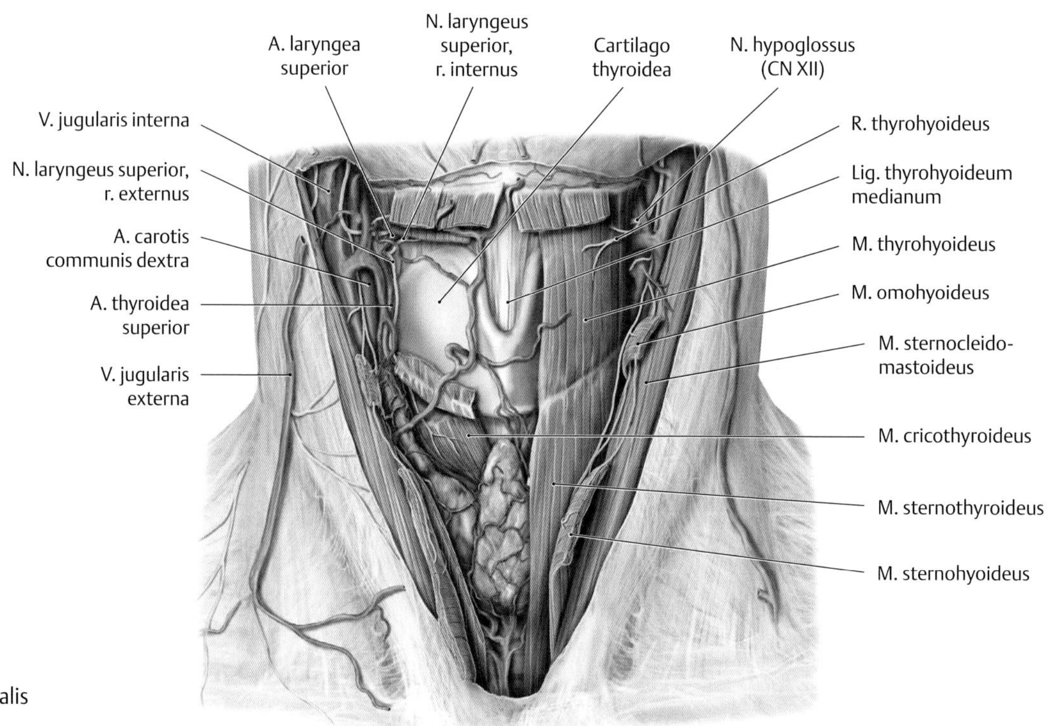
A. laryngea superior
N. laryngeus superior, r. internus
Cartilago thyroidea
N. hypoglossus (CN XII)
V. jugularis interna
N. laryngeus superior, r. externus
A. carotis communis dextra
A. thyroidea superior
V. jugularis externa
R. thyrohyoideus
Lig. thyrohyoideum medianum
M. thyrohyoideus
M. omohyoideus
M. sternocleido-mastoideus
M. cricothyroideus
M. sternothyroideus
M. sternohyoideus

B Deep layer. *Removed:* Lamina pretrachealis (middle layer of fascia cervicalis).

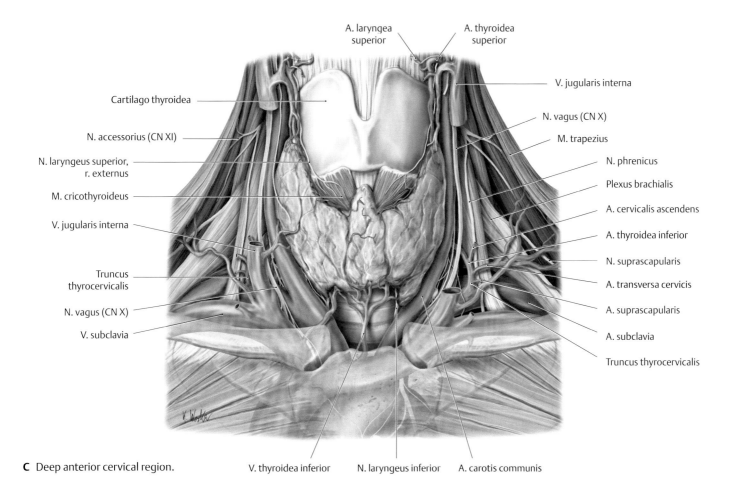

A. laryngea superior
A. thyroidea superior
V. jugularis interna
Cartilago thyroidea
N. vagus (CN X)
N. accessorius (CN XI)
M. trapezius
N. laryngeus superior, r. externus
N. phrenicus
M. cricothyroideus
Plexus brachialis
A. cervicalis ascendens
V. jugularis interna
A. thyroidea inferior
N. suprascapularis
Truncus thyrocervicalis
A. transversa cervicis
N. vagus (CN X)
A. suprascapularis
V. subclavia
A. subclavia
Truncus thyrocervicalis
V. thyroidea inferior
N. laryngeus inferior
A. carotis communis

C Deep anterior cervical region.

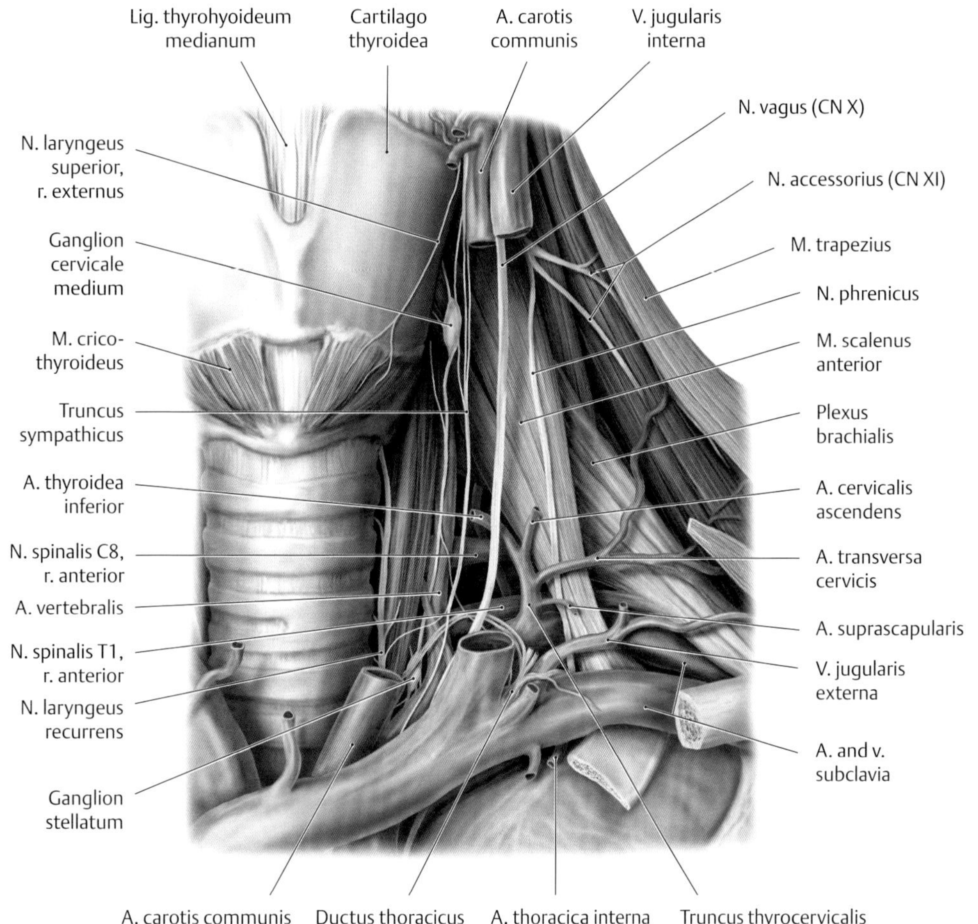

Lig. thyrohyoideum medianum
Cartilago thyroidea
A. carotis communis
V. jugularis interna
N. vagus (CN X)
N. laryngeus superior, r. externus
N. accessorius (CN XI)
M. trapezius
Ganglion cervicale medium
N. phrenicus
M. crico-thyroideus
M. scalenus anterior
Truncus sympathicus
Plexus brachialis
A. thyroidea inferior
A. cervicalis ascendens
N. spinalis C8, r. anterior
A. transversa cervicis
A. vertebralis
A. suprascapularis
N. spinalis T1, r. anterior
V. jugularis externa
N. laryngeus recurrens
A. and v. subclavia
Ganglion stellatum
A. carotis communis
Ductus thoracicus
A. thoracica interna
Truncus thyrocervicalis

D Root of the neck.

Topography of the Anterior & Lateral Cervical Regions

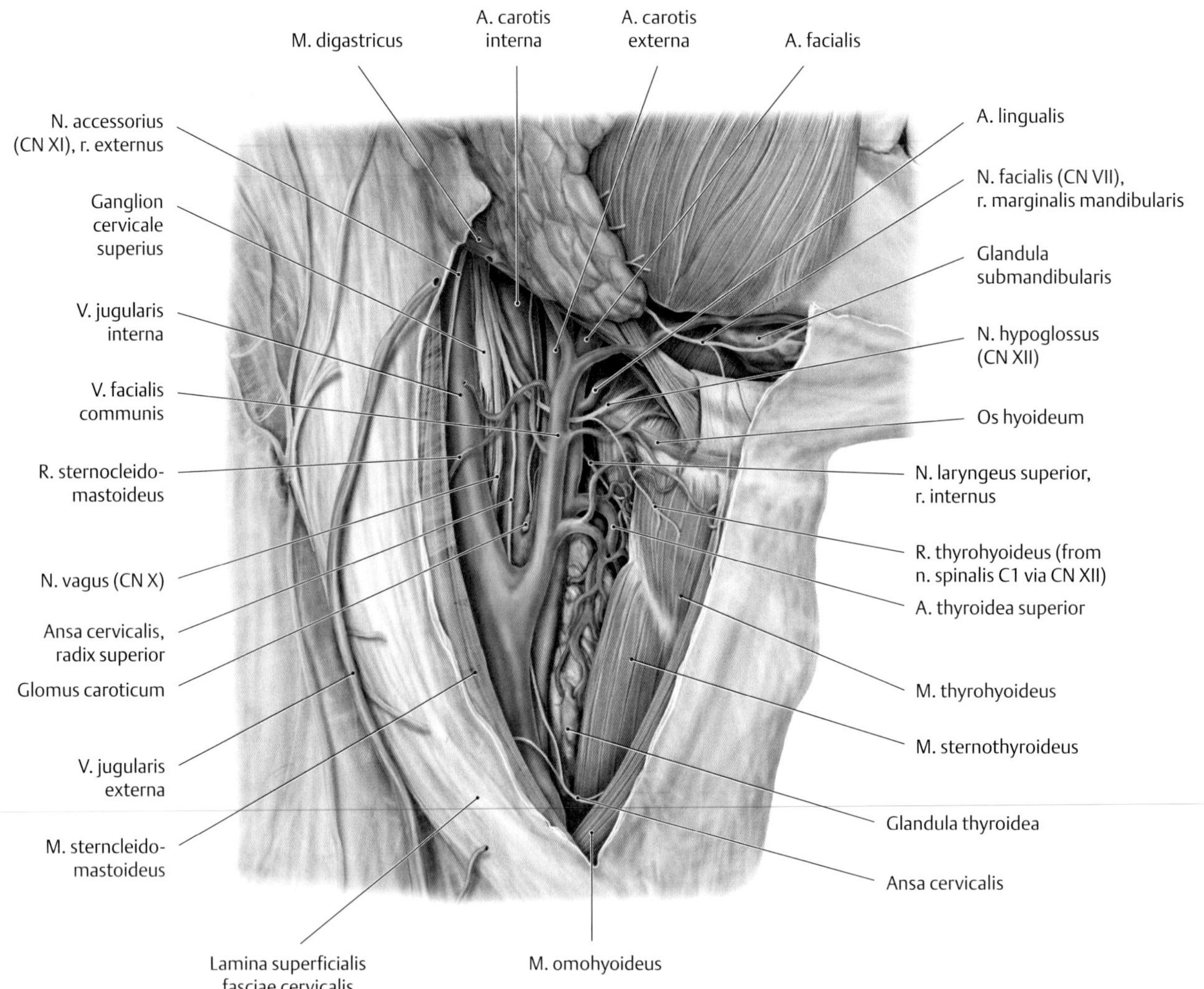
M. digastricus
A. carotis interna
A. carotis externa
A. facialis
A. lingualis
N. accessorius (CN XI), r. externus
N. facialis (CN VII), r. marginalis mandibularis
Ganglion cervicale superius
Glandula submandibularis
V. jugularis interna
N. hypoglossus (CN XII)
V. facialis communis
Os hyoideum
R. sternocleido-mastoideus
N. laryngeus superior, r. internus
R. thyrohyoideus (from n. spinalis C1 via CN XII)
N. vagus (CN X)
A. thyroidea superior
Ansa cervicalis, radix superior
Glomus caroticum
M. thyrohyoideus
M. sternothyroideus
V. jugularis externa
Glandula thyroidea
M. sterncleido-mastoideus
Ansa cervicalis
Lamina superficialis fasciae cervicalis
M. omohyoideus

Fig. 37.32 **Trigonum caroticum**
Right lateral view.

Fig. 37.33 Regio cervicalis lateralis
Right lateral view with m. sternocleidomastoideus windowed.

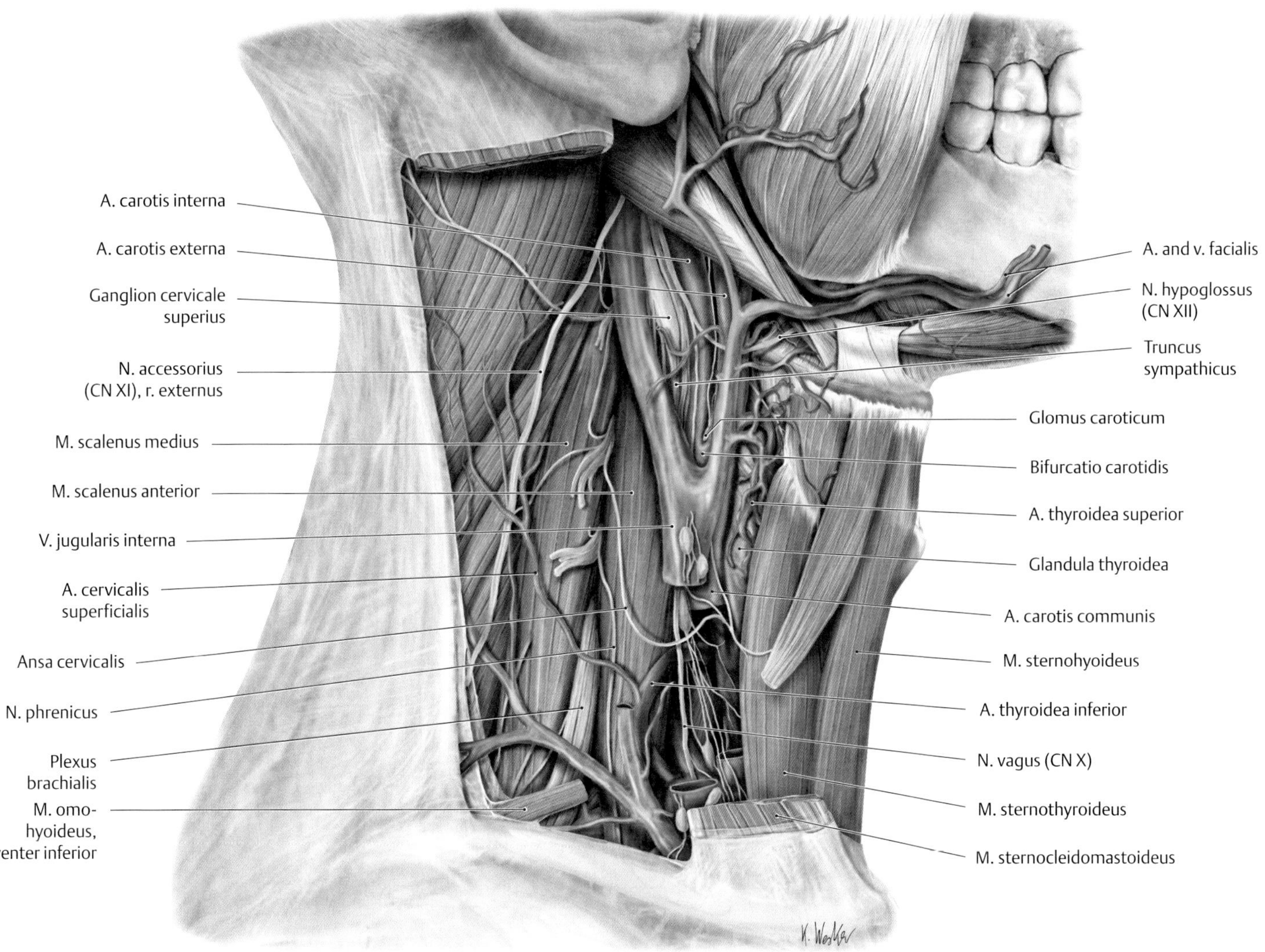
A. carotis interna
A. carotis externa
Ganglion cervicale superius
N. accessorius (CN XI), r. externus
M. scalenus medius
M. scalenus anterior
V. jugularis interna
A. cervicalis superficialis
Ansa cervicalis
N. phrenicus
Plexus brachialis
M. omohyoideus, venter inferior
A. and v. facialis
N. hypoglossus (CN XII)
Truncus sympathicus
Glomus caroticum
Bifurcatio carotidis
A. thyroidea superior
Glandula thyroidea
A. carotis communis
M. sternohyoideus
A. thyroidea inferior
N. vagus (CN X)
M. sternothyroideus
M. sternocleidomastoideus

Topography of the Lateral Cervical Region

Fig. 37.34 **Regio cervicalis lateralis**
Right lateral view. The contents of regio cervicalis lateralis are found in Fig. 37.33.

Glandula parotidea
N. facialis (CN VII), r. colli
M. masseter
N. occipitalis minor
N. auricularis magnus
Punctum nervosum (Erb's point)
Nn. supraclaviculares laterales
M. trapezius, anterior border
V. jugularis externa
M. sternocleido-mastoideus, posterior border
R. communicans cum nervo transverso colli
Lamina superficialis fasciae cervicalis
N. transversus colli
Clavicula
Nn. supraclaviculares intermedii
Nn. supraclaviculare mediales

A Subcutaneous layer.

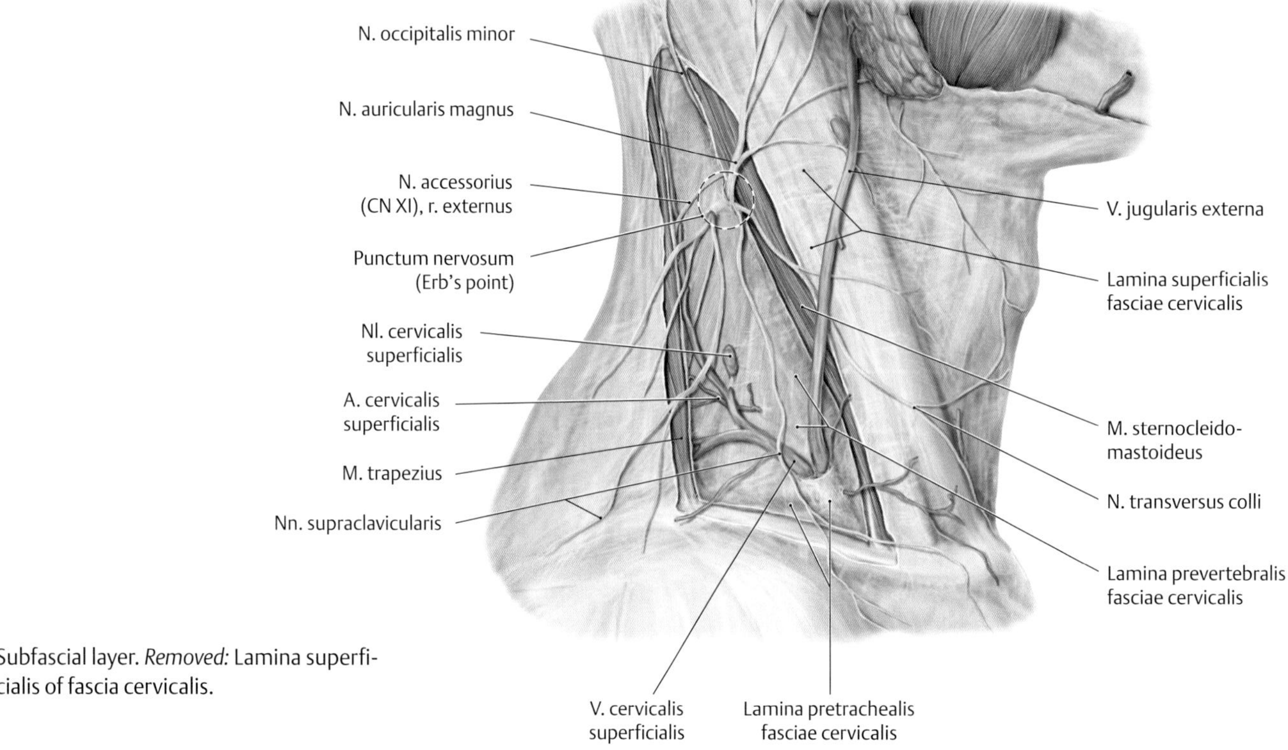
N. occipitalis minor
N. auricularis magnus
N. accessorius (CN XI), r. externus
Punctum nervosum (Erb's point)
Nl. cervicalis superficialis
A. cervicalis superficialis
M. trapezius
Nn. supraclavicularis
V. jugularis externa
Lamina superficialis fasciae cervicalis
M. sternocleido-mastoideus
N. transversus colli
Lamina prevertebralis fasciae cervicalis
V. cervicalis superficialis
Lamina pretrachealis fasciae cervicalis

B Subfascial layer. *Removed:* Lamina superficialis of fascia cervicalis.

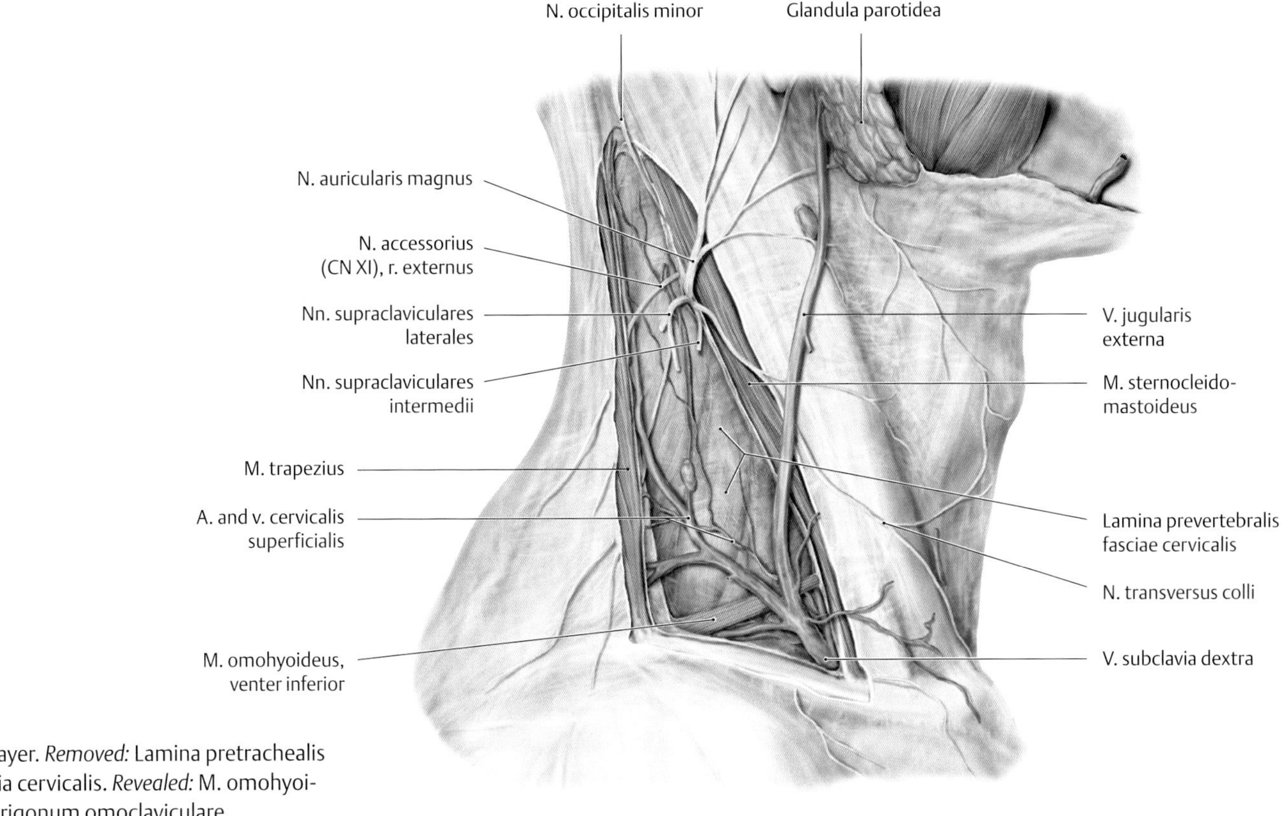
N. occipitalis minor
Glandula parotidea
N. auricularis magnus
N. accessorius (CN XI), r. externus
Nn. supraclaviculares laterales
Nn. supraclaviculares intermedii
M. trapezius
A. and v. cervicalis superficialis
M. omohyoideus, venter inferior
V. jugularis externa
M. sternocleido-mastoideus
Lamina prevertebralis fasciae cervicalis
N. transversus colli
V. subclavia dextra

C Deep layer. *Removed:* Lamina pretrachealis of fascia cervicalis. *Revealed:* M. omohyoideus, trigonum omoclaviculare.

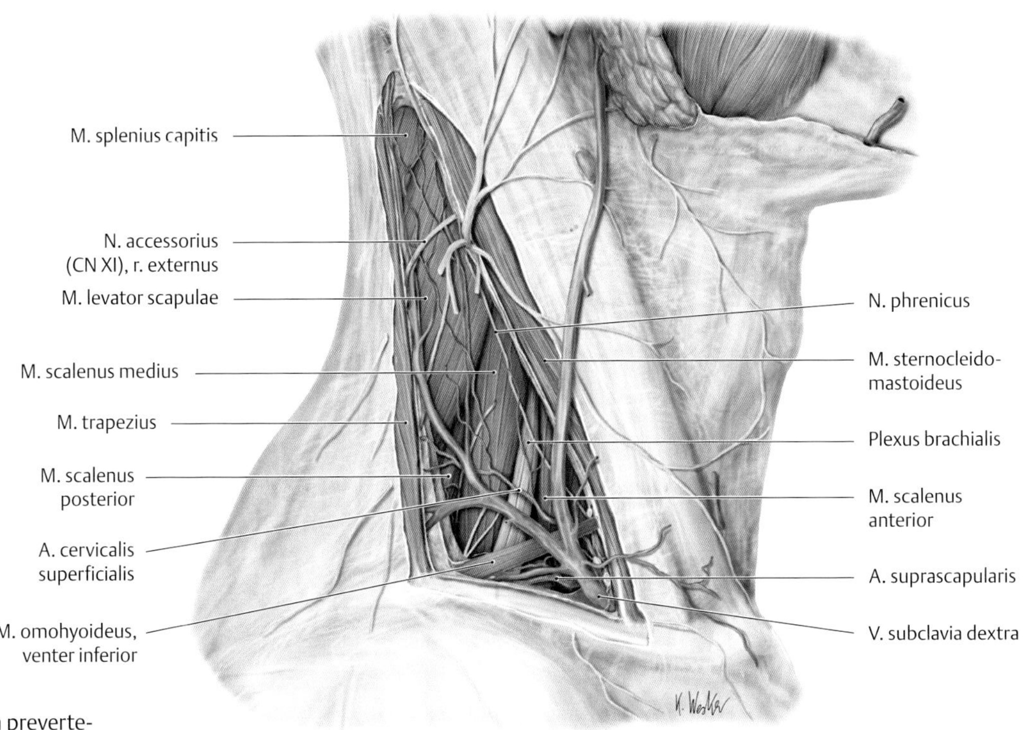
M. splenius capitis
N. accessorius (CN XI), r. externus
M. levator scapulae
M. scalenus medius
M. trapezius
M. scalenus posterior
A. cervicalis superficialis
M. omohyoideus, venter inferior
N. phrenicus
M. sternocleido-mastoideus
Plexus brachialis
M. scalenus anterior
A. suprascapularis
V. subclavia dextra

D Deepest layer. *Removed:* Lamina prevertebralis of fascia cervicalis. *Revealed:* Muscular floor of regio cervicalis lateralis, plexus brachialis and n. phrenicus.

Topography of the Posterior Cervical Region

Fig. 37.35 **Regiones occipitalis and cervicalis posterior**
Posterior view. Subcutaneous layer (left), subfascial layer (right). The occiput is technically a region of the head, but it is included here due to the continuity of the vessels and nerves from the neck.

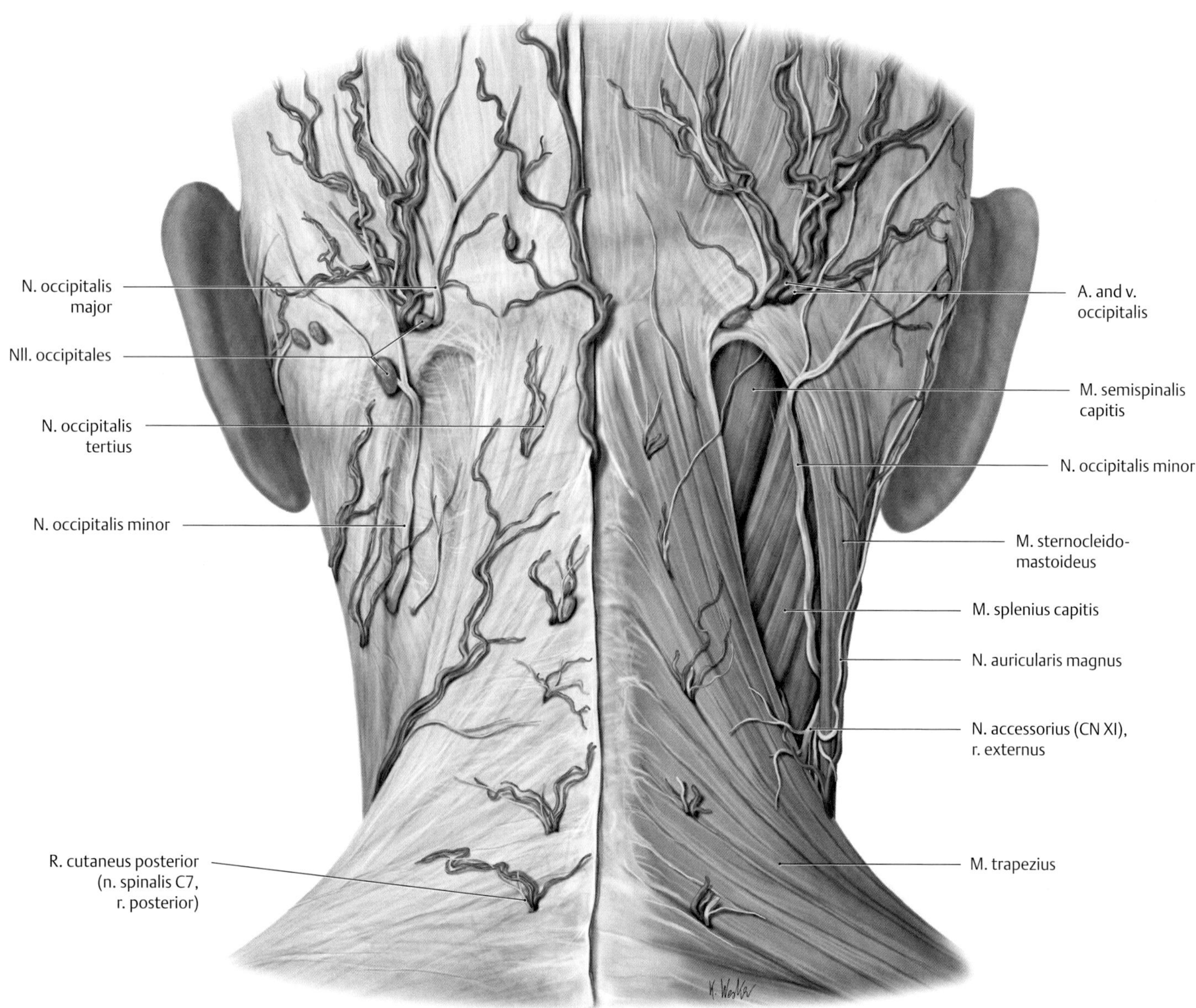
N. occipitalis major
Nll. occipitales
N. occipitalis tertius
N. occipitalis minor
R. cutaneus posterior (n. spinalis C7, r. posterior)
A. and v. occipitalis
M. semispinalis capitis
N. occipitalis minor
M. sternocleido-mastoideus
M. splenius capitis
N. auricularis magnus
N. accessorius (CN XI), r. externus
M. trapezius

Fig. 37.36 **Suboccipital triangle**
Right side, posterior view. The suboccipital triangle is bounded by the suboccipital muscles (m. rectus capitis posterior major and mm. obliquus capitis superior and inferior) and contains a. vertebralis. The left and right aa. vertebrales pass through the membrana atlantooccipitalis posterior and combine to form a. basilaris.

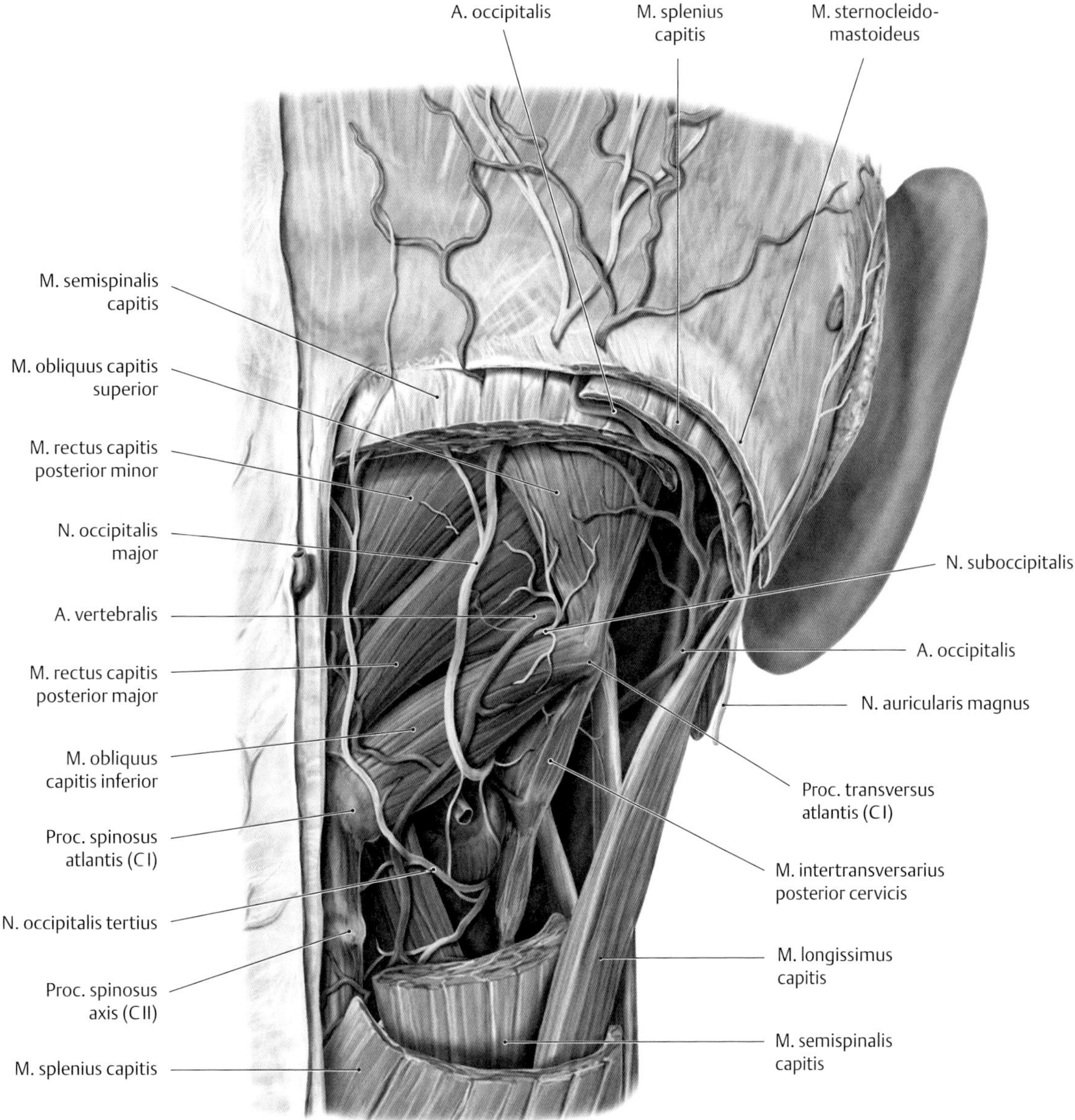
A. occipitalis
M. splenius capitis
M. sternocleido-mastoideus
M. semispinalis capitis
M. obliquus capitis superior
M. rectus capitis posterior minor
N. occipitalis major
A. vertebralis
M. rectus capitis posterior major
M. obliquus capitis inferior
Proc. spinosus atlantis (C I)
N. occipitalis tertius
Proc. spinosus axis (C II)
M. splenius capitis
N. suboccipitalis
A. occipitalis
N. auricularis magnus
Proc. transversus atlantis (C I)
M. intertransversarius posterior cervicis
M. longissimus capitis
M. semispinalis capitis

Lymphatics of the Neck

Fig. 37.37 Lymphatic drainage regions
Right lateral view.

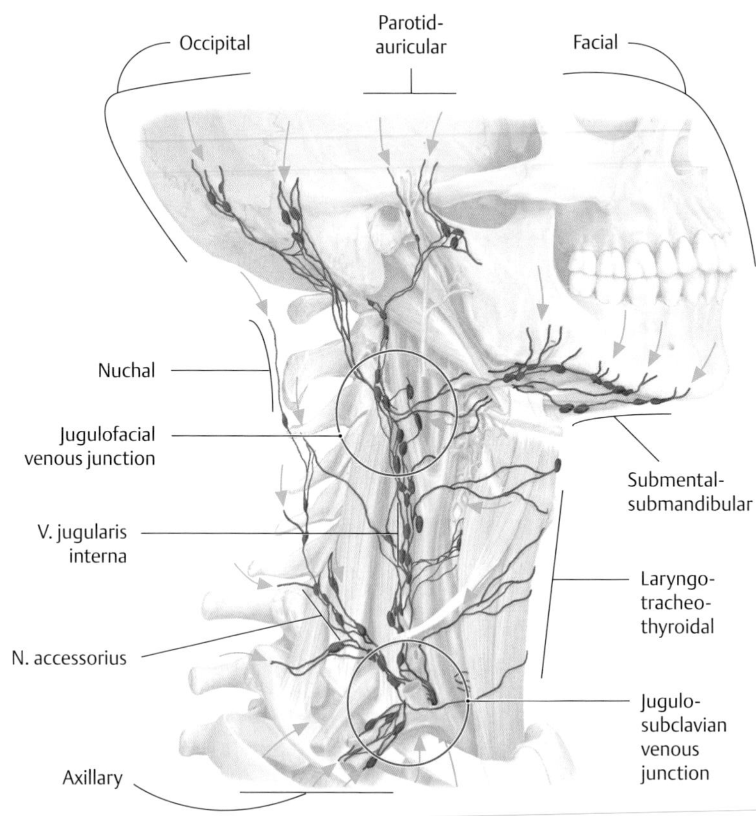
Occipital
Parotid-auricular
Facial
Nuchal
Jugulofacial venous junction
V. jugularis interna
N. accessorius
Axillary
Submental-submandibular
Laryngo-tracheo-thyroidal
Jugulo-subclavian venous junction

Clinical

Tumor metastasis
Lymph from the entire body is channeled to the left and right jugulosubclavian junctions (red circles). Gastric carcinoma may metastasize to the left nll. supraclaviculares, producing an enlarged *sentinel node* (see pp. 73, 231). Systemic lymphomas may also spread to the cervical lymph nodes by this pathway.

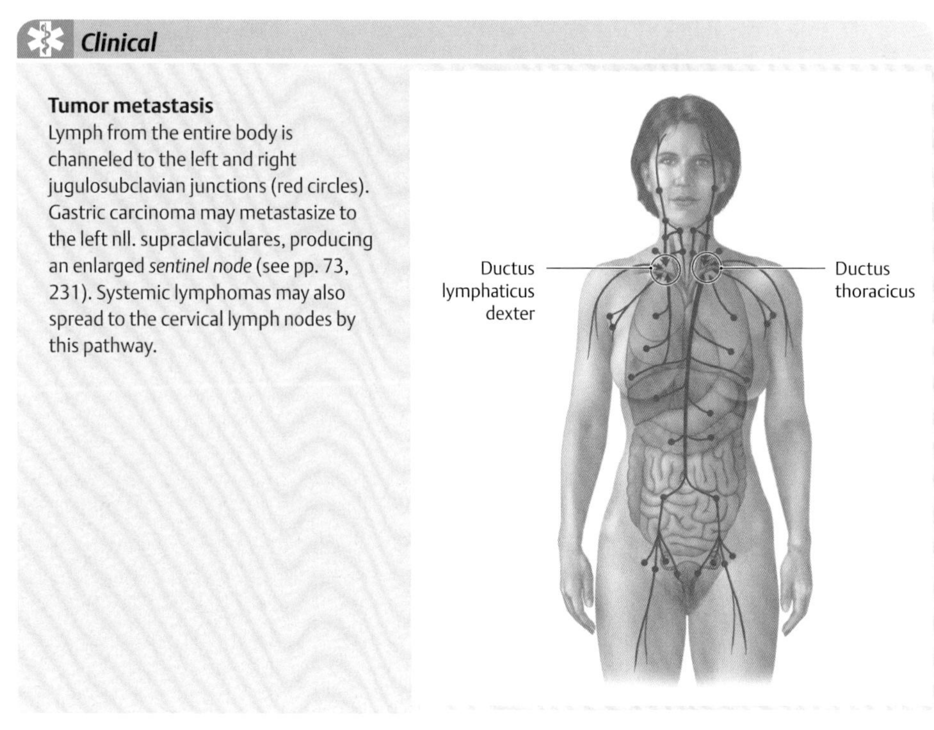
Ductus lymphaticus dexter
Ductus thoracicus

Fig. 37.38 Superficial cervical lymph nodes
Right lateral view.

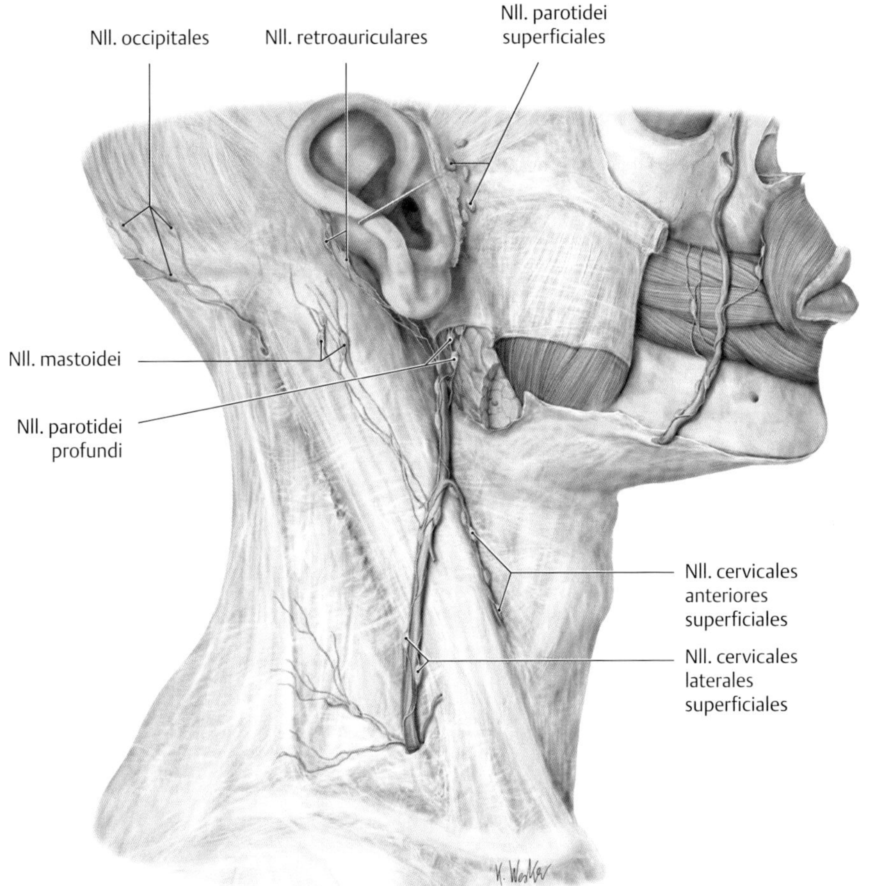

Nll. occipitales
Nll. retroauriculares
Nll. parotidei superficiales
Nll. mastoidei
Nll. parotidei profundi
Nll. cervicales anteriores superficiales
Nll. cervicales laterales superficiales

Table 37.13 Superficial cervical lymph nodes

Lymph nodes (l.n.)	Drainage region
Nll. retroauriculares	Regio occipitalis
Nll. occipitales	
Nll. mastoidei	
Nll. paratoidei superficiales	Regio parotideo-auricularis
Nll. paratoidei profundi	
Nll. anteriores superficiales	Regio sternocleido-mastoidea
Nll. laterales superficiales	

Fig. 37.39 Deep cervical lymph nodes
Right lateral view.

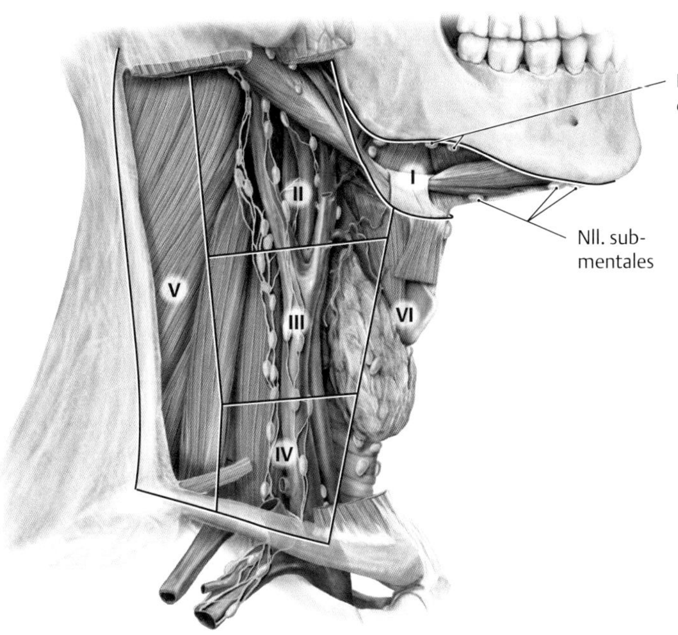

Nll. submandibulares
I
II
Nll. submentales
V
III
VI
IV

Table 37.14 Deep cervical lymph nodes

Level	Lymph nodes (l.n.)		Drainage region
I	Nll. submentales		Face
	Nll. submandibulares		
II	Nll. jugulares laterales	Upper lateral group	Regio nuchalis, laryngo-tracheo-thyroidal region
III		Middle lateral group	
IV		Lower lateral group	
V	Nll. trigoni cervicalis posterioris		Regio nuchalis
VI	Nll. cervicales anteriores		Laryngo-tracheo-thyroidal region

Surface Anatomy

Fig. 38.1 Surface anatomy of the skull and nuchal region

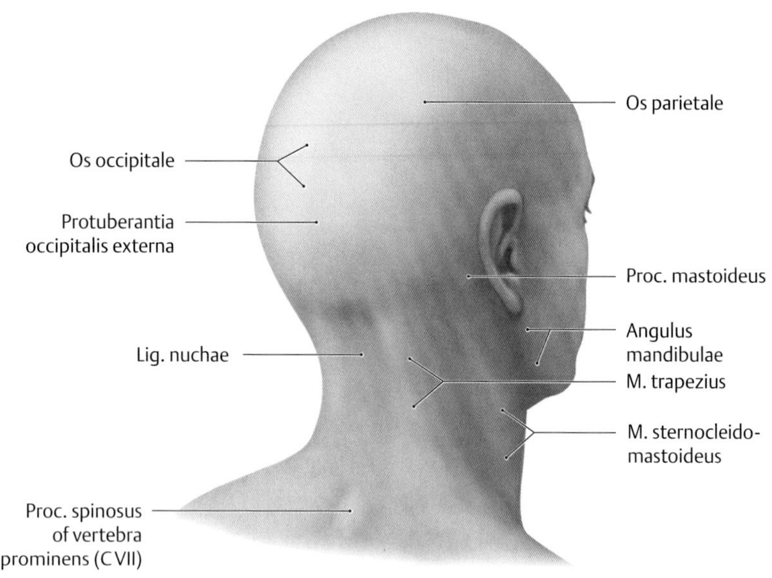
Os parietale
Os occipitale
Protuberantia occipitalis externa
Proc. mastoideus
Angulus mandibulae
Lig. nuchae
M. trapezius
M. sternocleido-mastoideus
Proc. spinosus of vertebra prominens (C VII)

A Surface anatomy. Right posterolateral view.

Q1: Injecting a bolus of anesthetic two thirds of the way up the posterior border of m. sternocleidomastoideus would accomplish what task?

Q2: What palpable bony landmark would you use to auscultate the venous blood in the confluence of the sinuses?

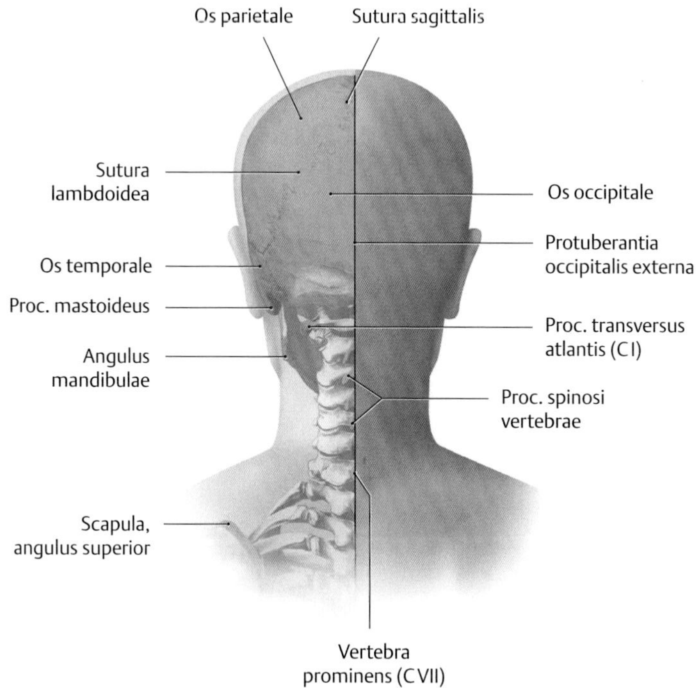
Os parietale
Sutura sagittalis
Sutura lambdoidea
Os occipitale
Protuberantia occipitalis externa
Os temporale
Proc. mastoideus
Proc. transversus atlantis (C I)
Angulus mandibulae
Proc. spinosi vertebrae
Scapula, angulus superior
Vertebra prominens (C VII)

B Palpable bony prominences. Posterior view.

Fig. 38.2 Surface anatomy of the face and neck

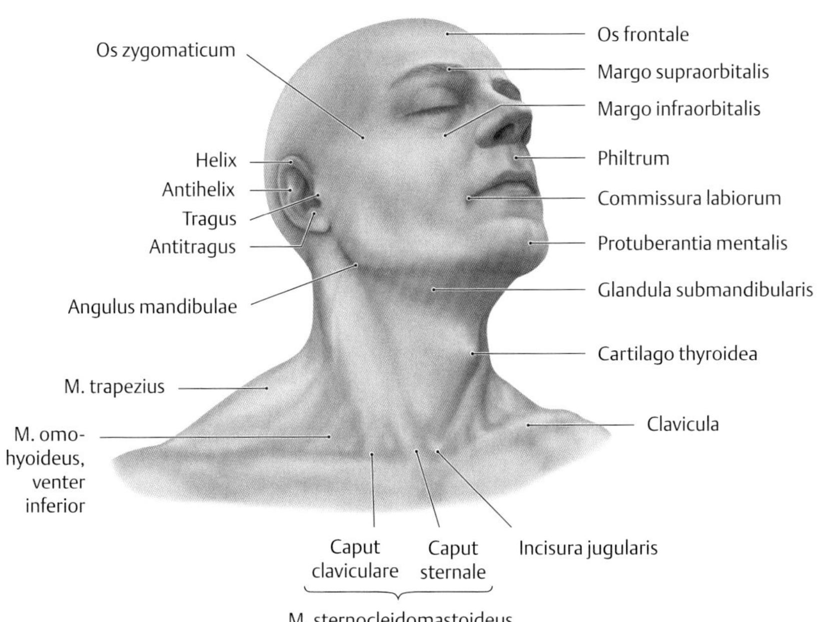
Os zygomaticum
Helix
Antihelix
Tragus
Antitragus
Angulus mandibulae
M. trapezius
M. omo-hyoideus, venter inferior
Os frontale
Margo supraorbitalis
Margo infraorbitalis
Philtrum
Commissura labiorum
Protuberantia mentalis
Glandula submandibularis
Cartilago thyroidea
Clavicula
Incisura jugularis
Caput claviculare
Caput sternale
M. sternocleidomastoideus

A Surface anatomy. Right anterolateral view.

Q3: What are the boundaries of regio cervicalis lateralis (trigonum cervicale posterius)? Name two structures within this region that supply motor innervation to the muscles of the upper limb.

Q4: What are the boundaries of trigonum caroticum? Name one non-vascular component of the vertical neurovascular bundle within vagina carotica located in the trigonum caroticum.

Q5: What is the anatomical structure referred to as the "Adam's apple"?

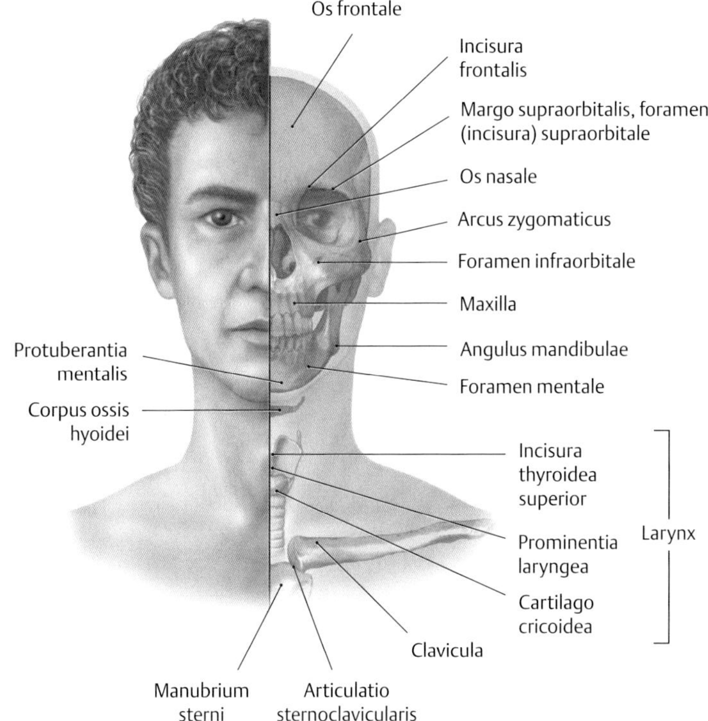
Os frontale
Incisura frontalis
Margo supraorbitalis, foramen (incisura) supraorbitale
Os nasale
Arcus zygomaticus
Foramen infraorbitale
Maxilla
Angulus mandibulae
Foramen mentale
Protuberantia mentalis
Corpus ossis hyoidei
Incisura thyroidea superior
Prominentia laryngea
Cartilago cricoidea
Larynx
Clavicula
Manubrium sterni
Articulatio sternoclavicularis

B Palpable bony prominences. Anterior view.

See answers beginning on p. 626.

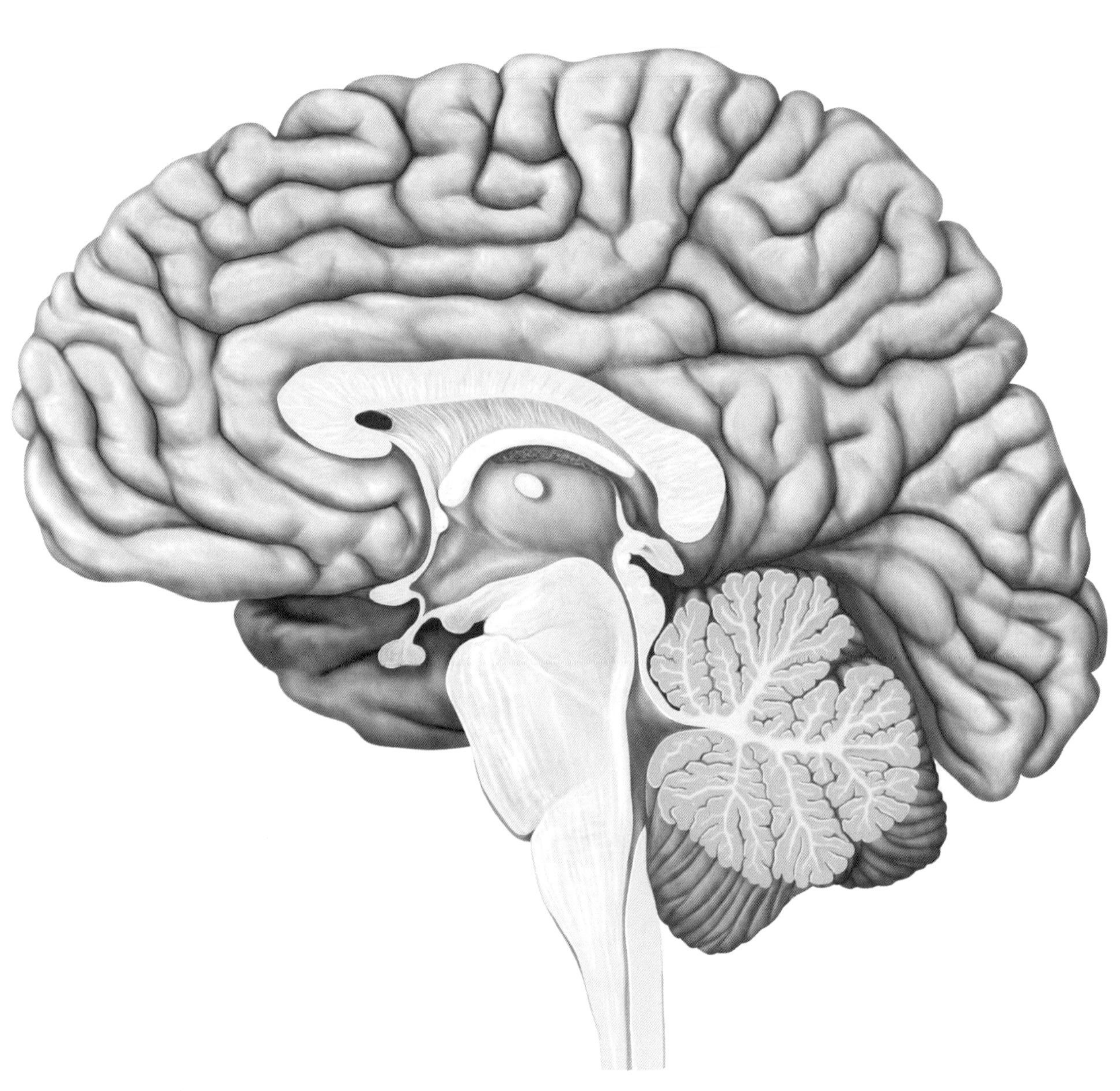

Neuroanatomy

39 Brain & Spinal Cord

Nervous System: Overview ... 592
Telencephalon ... 594
Telencephalon & Diencephalon ... 596
Diencephalon, Brainstem & Cerebellum ... 598
Medulla Spinalis ... 600
Meninges ... 602
Ventricles & CSF Spaces ... 604

40 Blood Vessels of the Brain & Spinal Cord

Sinus Durae Matris & Veins of the Brain ... 606
Arteries of the Brain ... 608
Arteries & Veins of Medulla Spinalis ... 610

41 Functional Systems

Circuitry ... 612
Sensory & Motor Pathways ... 614
Sensory Systems (I) ... 616
Sensory Systems (II) ... 618
Sensory Systems (III) ... 620

42 Autonomic Nervous System

Autonomic Nervous System ... 622

Nervous System: Overview

Fig. 39.1 Central and peripheral nervous systems

The nervous system is divided into the central (CNS) and peripheral (PNS) nervous systems. The CNS consists of the brain and spinal cord, which comprise a functional unit. The PNS consists of the nerves emerging from the brain and spinal cord (cranial and spinal nerves, respectively).

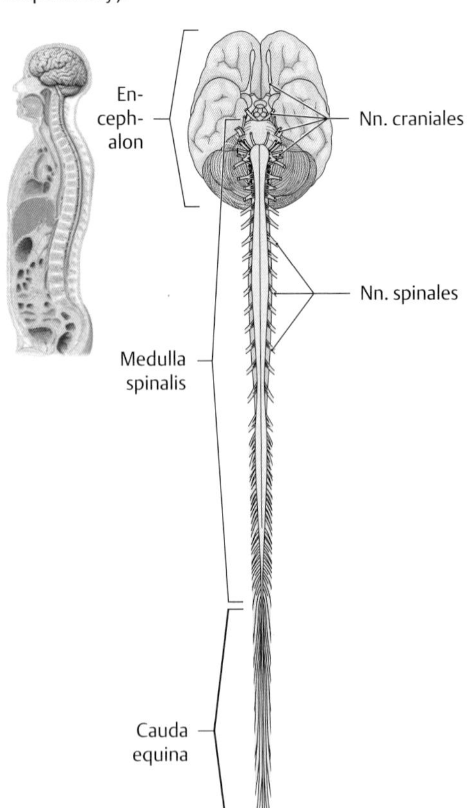
En-
ceph-
alon
Nn. craniales
Nn. spinales
Medulla
spinalis
Cauda
equina

Fig. 39.2 Neurons (nerve cells)

The nervous system is composed of neurons (nerve cells) and supporting neuroglial cells, which vastly outnumber them (10 to 1). Each neuron contains a cell body (soma) with one axon (projecting segment) and one or more dendrites (receptor segments). The release of neurotransmitters at synapses creates an excitatory or inhibitory postsynaptic potential at the target neuron. If this exceeds the depolarization threshold of the neuron, the axon “fires,” initiating the release of a transmitter from its presynaptic knob (bouton).

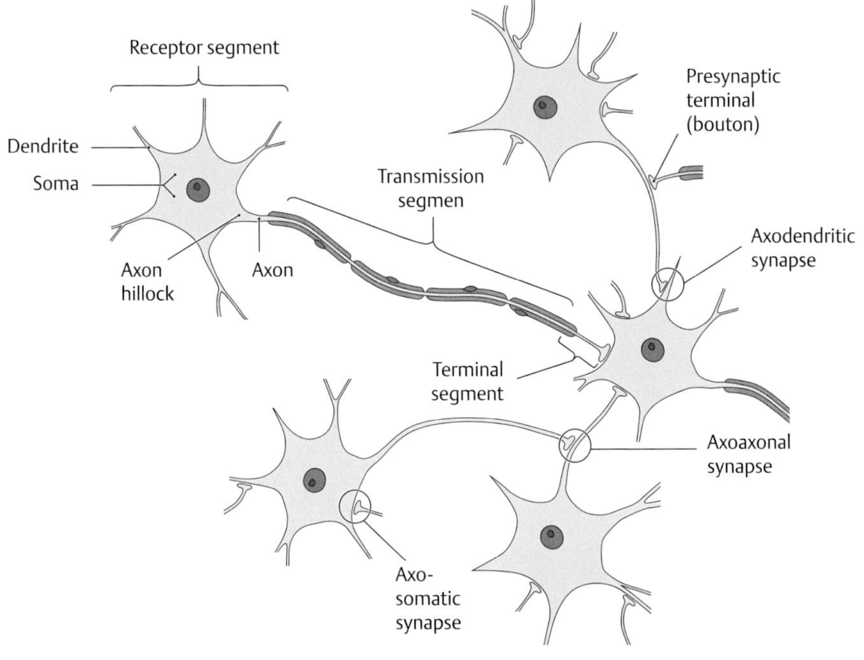
Receptor segment
Dendrite
Soma
Axon
hillock
Axon
Transmission
segmen
Presynaptic
terminal
(bouton)
Axodendritic
synapse
Terminal
segment
Axoaxonal
synapse
Axo-
somatic
synapse

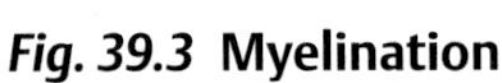

Fig. 39.3 Myelination

Certain glial cells with lipid-rich membranes may myelinate axons (nerve fibers). Myelination electrically insulates axons, thereby increasing impulse conduction speed. In the CNS, one oligodendrocyte myelinates multiple axons; in the PNS, one Schwann cell myelinates one axon.

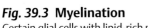

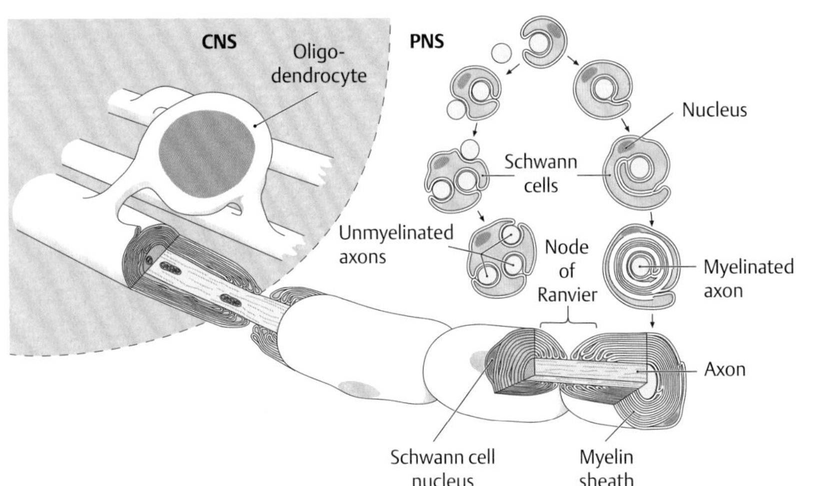
CNS
Oligo-
dendrocyte
PNS
Nucleus
Schwann
cells
Unmyelinated
axons
Node
of
Ranvier
Myelinated
axon
Axon
Schwann cell
nucleus
Myelin
sheath

Fig. 39.4 Substantia alba and grisea in CNS

Nerve cell bodies appear gray in gross inspection, whereas nerve cell processes (axons) and their insulating myelin sheaths appear white.

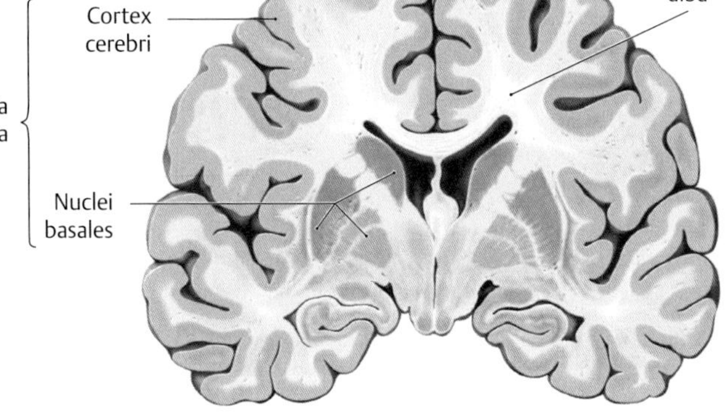
Substantia
alba
Cortex
cerebri
Substantia
grisea
Nuclei
basales

A Coronal section through the brain.

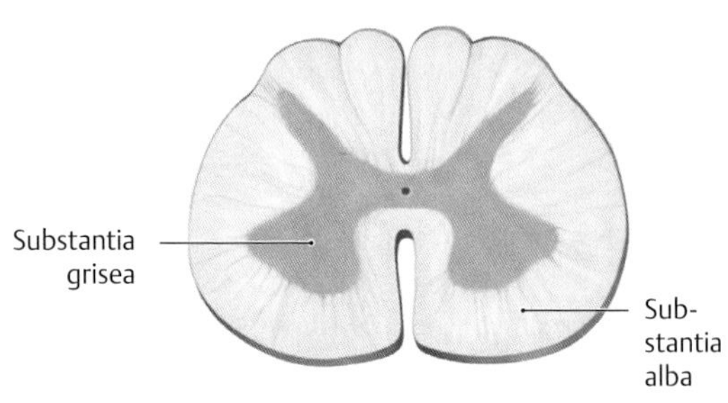
Substantia
grisea
Sub-
stantia
alba

B Transverse section through the spinal cord.

Table 39.1 Development of the brain

	Primary vesicle	Region			Structure
Neural tube	Pros-encephalon (forebrain)	Telencephalon (cerebrum)			Cortex cerebri, substantia alba and nuclei basales
		Diencephalon			Epithalamus (glandula pinealis), thalamus, subthalamus, and hypothalamus
	Mesencephalon (midbrain)*				Tectum mesencephali, tegmentum, and pedunculi cerebri
	Rhombencephalon (hindbrain)	Metencephalon	Cerebellum		Cortex cerebelli, nuclei cerebelli, and pedunculi cerebri
			Pons*		Nuclei and fiber tracts
		Myelencephalon	Medulla oblongata*		

* The mesencephalon, pons, and medulla oblongata are collectively known as the brainstem.

Fig. 39.5 **Embryonic development of the brain**
Left lateral view.

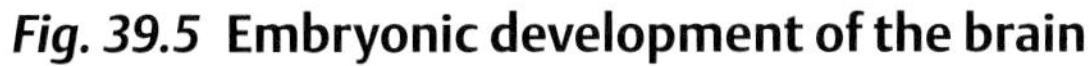

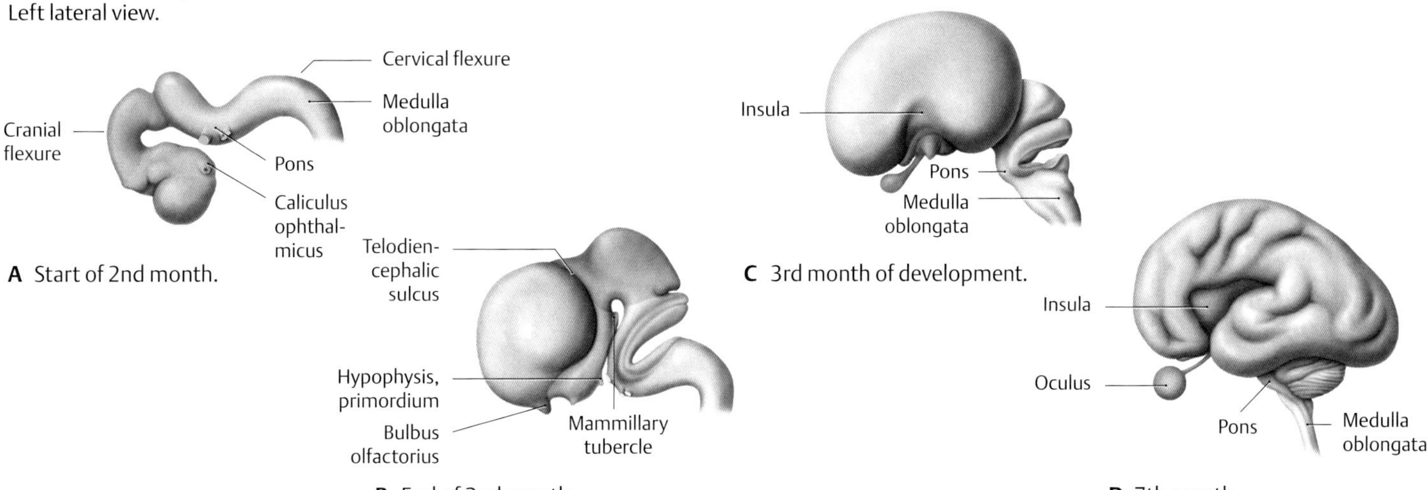
Cervical flexure
Medulla oblongata
Cranial flexure
Pons
Caliculus ophthalmicus
Telodiencephalic sulcus
Hypophysis, primordium
Bulbus olfactorius
Mammillary tubercle
Insula
Pons
Medulla oblongata
Insula
Oculus
Pons
Medulla oblongata

A Start of 2nd month.

B End of 2nd month.

C 3rd month of development.

D 7th month.

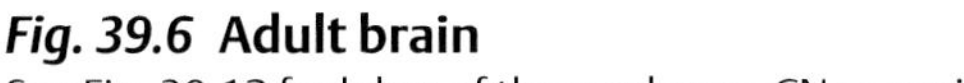

Fig. 39.6 **Adult brain**
See Fig. 39.12 for lobes of the cerebrum. CN = cranial nerve.

Gyrus precentralis
Sulcus centralis
Gyrus postcentralis
Lobus frontalis
Sulcus lateralis
Lobus temporalis
Pons
Medulla oblongata
Cerebellum
Lobus occipitalis
Lobus frontalis
Fissura longitudinalis cerebri
N. olfactorius (CN I)
N. opticus (CN II)
Hypophysis
Lobus temporalis
Pons
Medulla oblongata
Cerebellum
Medulla spinalis, pars cervicalis
Gyrus cinguli
Corpus callosum
Glandula pinealis
Hypothalamus
Hypophysis
Pons
Medulla oblongata
Lobus occipitalis
Cerebellum

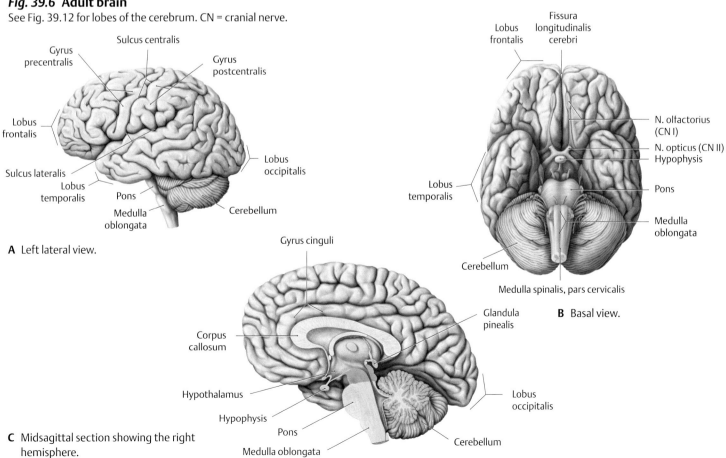

A Left lateral view.

B Basal view.

C Midsagittal section showing the right hemisphere.

Fig. 39.7 **Divisions of the telencephalon**
Coronal section, anterior view. The telencephalon is divided into cortex cerebri, substantia alba, and nuclei basales. The cortex cerebri is further divided into the allocortex and isocortex (neocortex).

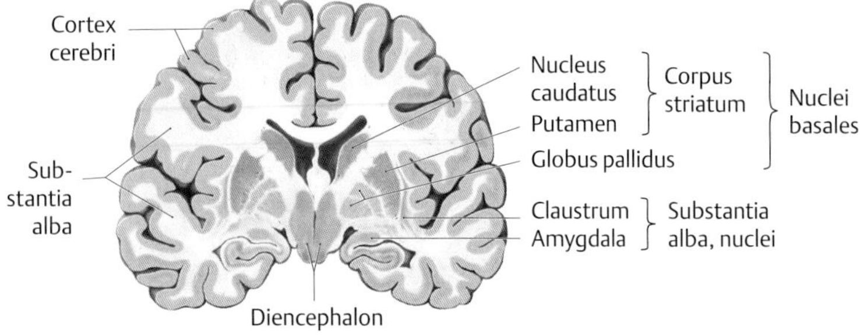
Cortex cerebri
Sub-stantia alba
Nucleus caudatus
Putamen
Corpus striatum
Nuclei basales
Globus pallidus
Claustrum
Amygdala
Substantia alba, nuclei
Diencephalon

Fig. 39.8 **Substantia alba**
A special preparation technique was used to show the fiber structure of the superficial layer of substantia alba.

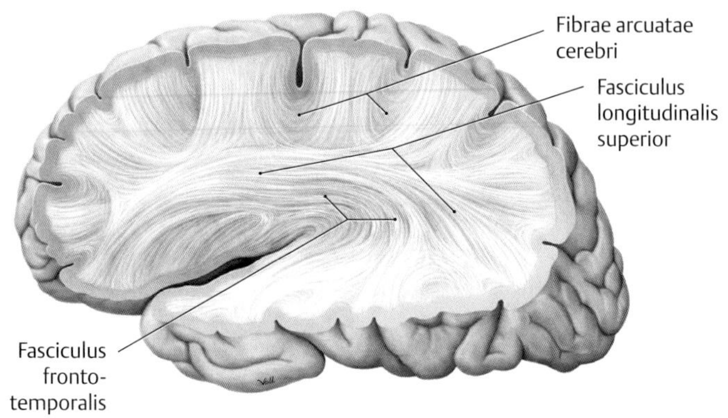
Fibrae arcuatae cerebri
Fasciculus longitudinalis superior
Fasciculus fronto-temporalis

A Lateral view of left hemisphere.

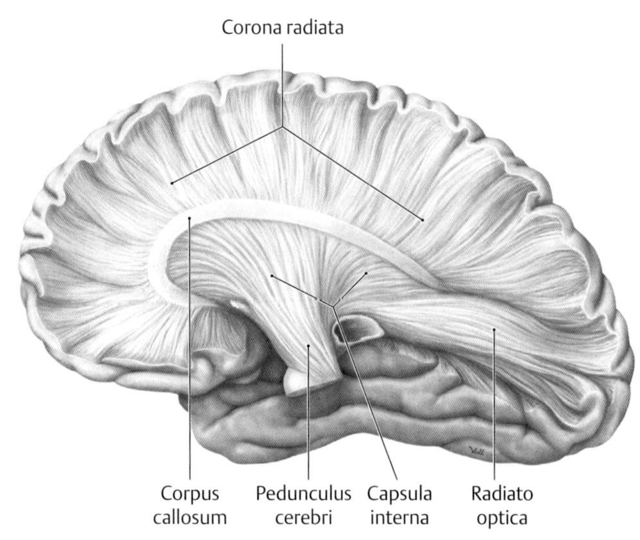
Corona radiata
Corpus callosum
Pedunculus cerebri
Capsula interna
Radiato optica

B Medial view of right hemisphere.

Fig. 39.9 **Nuclei basales**
Transverse section, superior view. The nuclei basales are an essential component of the motor system (see p. 615).

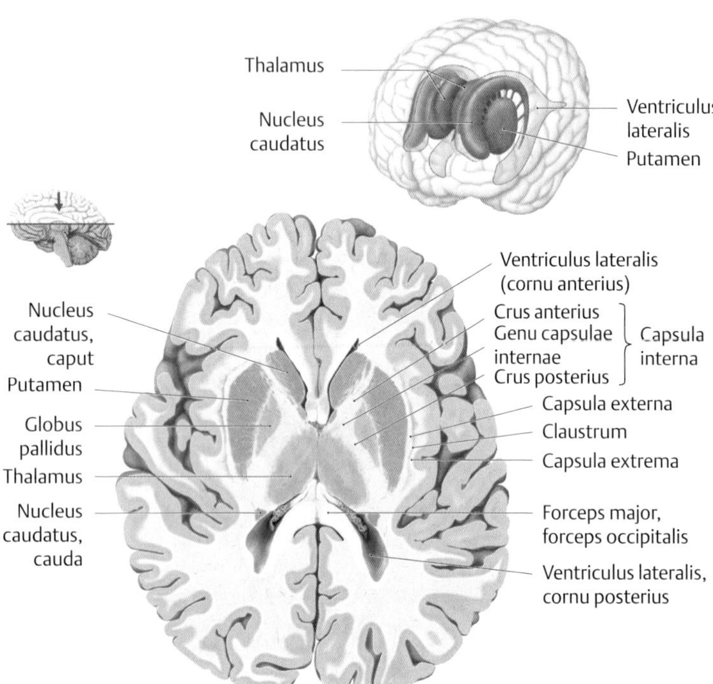
Thalamus
Nucleus caudatus
Ventriculus lateralis
Putamen
Ventriculus lateralis (cornu anterius)
Nucleus caudatus, caput
Putamen
Globus pallidus
Thalamus
Nucleus caudatus, cauda
Crus anterius
Genu capsulae internae
Crus posterius
Capsula interna
Capsula externa
Claustrum
Capsula extrema
Forceps major, forceps occipitalis
Ventriculus lateralis, cornu posterius

Fig. 39.10 **Allocortex**
The three-layered allocortex consists of the olfactory cortex (blue) and the hippocampus (pink).

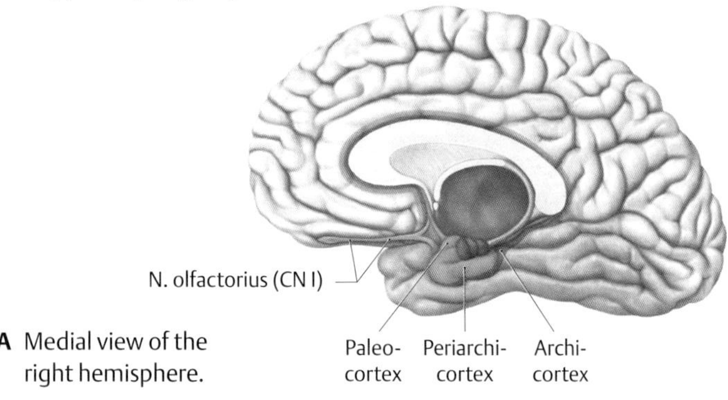
N. olfactorius (CN I)
Paleo-cortex
Periarchi-cortex
Archi-cortex

A Medial view of the right hemisphere.

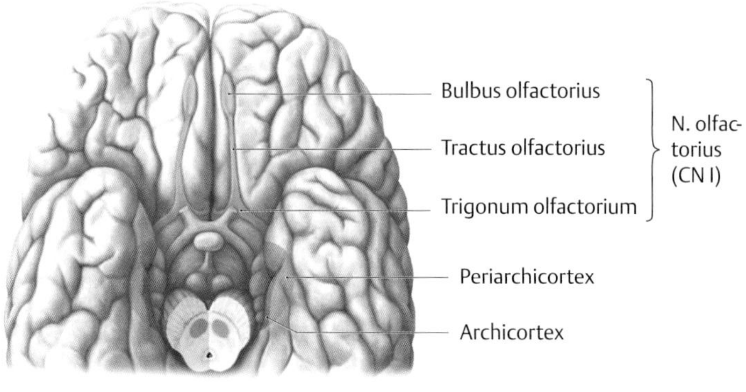
Bulbus olfactorius
Tractus olfactorius
Trigonum olfactorium
N. olfac-torius (CN I)
Periarchicortex
Archicortex

B Basal view.

Table 39.1 Development of the brain

	Primary vesicle	Region		Structure
Neural tube	Pros-encephalon (forebrain)	Telencephalon (cerebrum)		Cortex cerebri, substantia alba and nuclei basales
		Diencephalon		Epithalamus (glandula pinealis), thalamus, subthalamus, and hypothalamus
	Mesencephalon (midbrain)*			Tectum mesencephali, tegmentum, and pedunculi cerebri
	Rhombencephalon (hindbrain)	Metencephalon	Cerebellum	Cortex cerebelli, nuclei cerebelli, and pedunculi cerebri
			Pons*	Nuclei and fiber tracts
		Myelencephalon	Medulla oblongata*	

* The mesencephalon, pons, and medulla oblongata are collectively known as the brainstem.

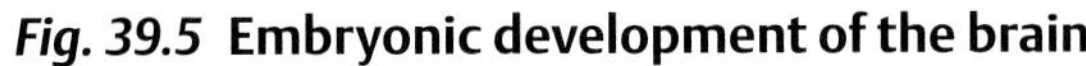

Fig. 39.5 Embryonic development of the brain

Left lateral view.

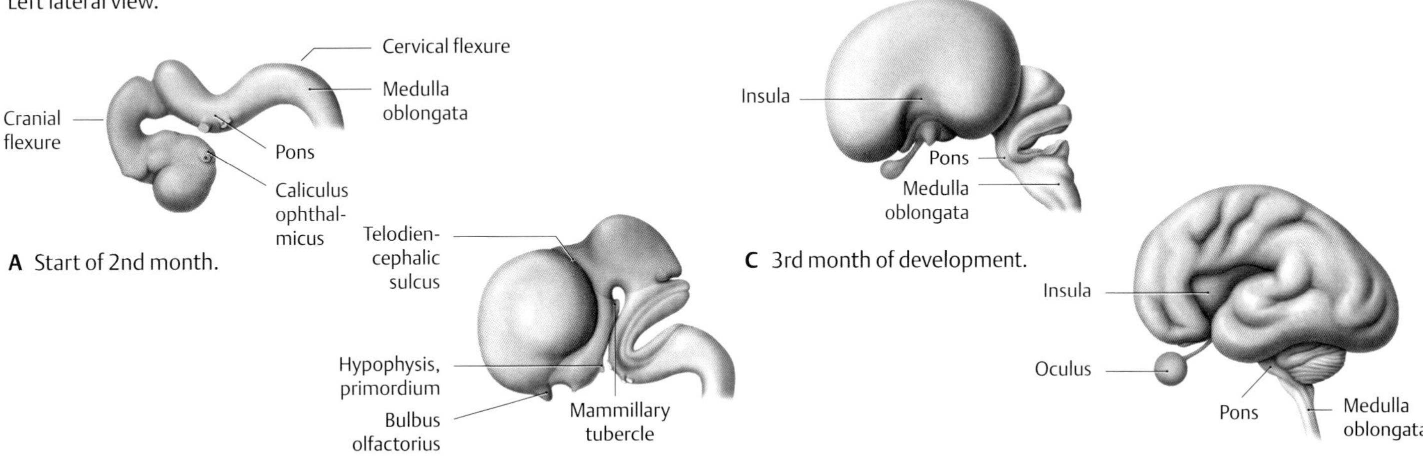
Cervical flexure
Medulla oblongata
Cranial flexure
Pons
Caliculus ophthalmicus
Telodiencephalic sulcus
Hypophysis, primordium
Bulbus olfactorius
Mammillary tubercle
Insula
Pons
Medulla oblongata
Insula
Oculus
Pons
Medulla oblongata

A Start of 2nd month.

B End of 2nd month.

C 3rd month of development.

D 7th month.

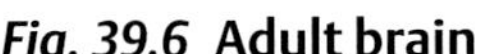

Fig. 39.6 Adult brain

See Fig. 39.12 for lobes of the cerebrum. CN = cranial nerve.

Sulcus centralis
Gyrus precentralis
Gyrus postcentralis
Lobus frontalis
Sulcus lateralis
Lobus temporalis
Lobus occipitalis
Pons
Medulla oblongata
Cerebellum

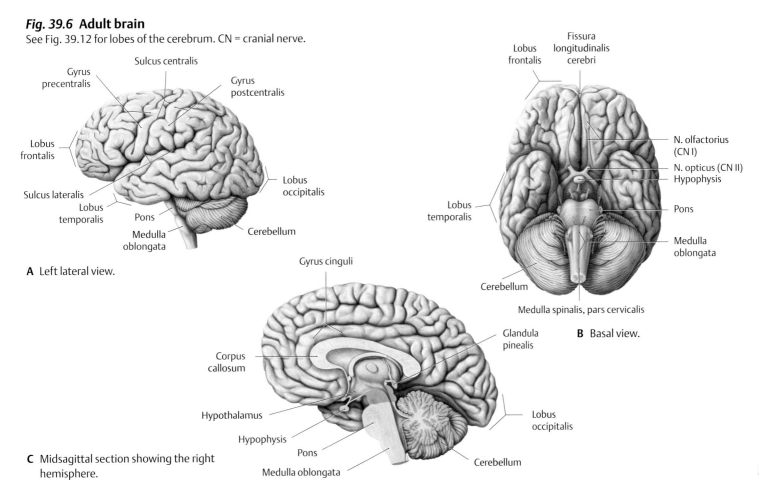

A Left lateral view.

Lobus frontalis
Fissura longitudinalis cerebri
N. olfactorius (CN I)
N. opticus (CN II)
Hypophysis
Lobus temporalis
Pons
Medulla oblongata
Cerebellum
Medulla spinalis, pars cervicalis

B Basal view.

Gyrus cinguli
Corpus callosum
Glandula pinealis
Hypothalamus
Hypophysis
Pons
Medulla oblongata
Lobus occipitalis
Cerebellum

C Midsagittal section showing the right hemisphere.

Telencephalon

Fig. 39.7 Divisions of the telencephalon

Coronal section, anterior view. The telencephalon is divided into cortex cerebri, substantia alba, and nuclei basales. The cortex cerebri is further divided into the allocortex and isocortex (neocortex).

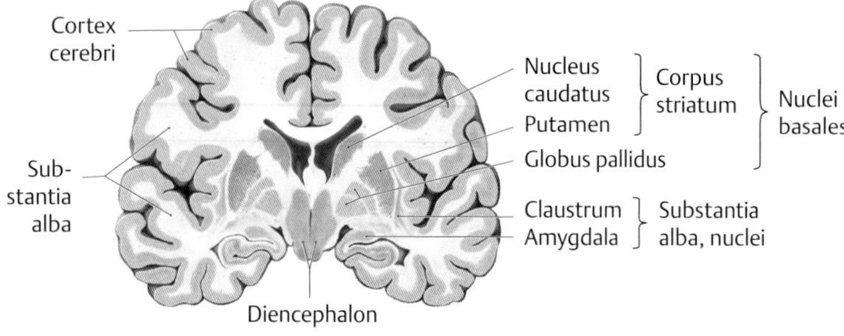
Cortex cerebri
Sub-stantia alba
Nucleus caudatus
Putamen
Corpus striatum
Nuclei basales
Globus pallidus
Claustrum
Amygdala
Substantia alba, nuclei
Diencephalon

Fig. 39.8 Substantia alba

A special preparation technique was used to show the fiber structure of the superficial layer of substantia alba.

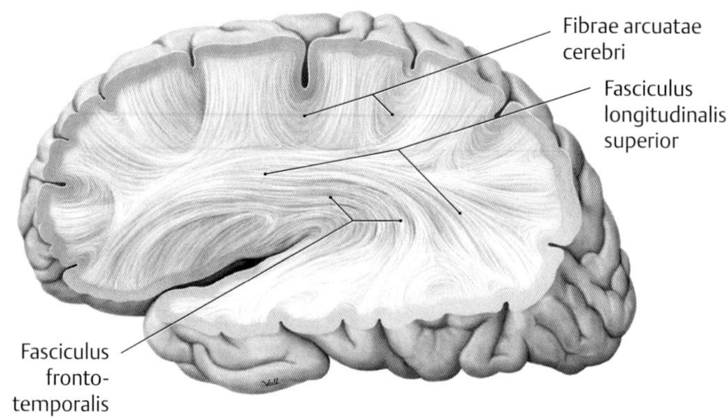
Fibrae arcuatae cerebri
Fasciculus longitudinalis superior
Fasciculus fronto-temporalis

A Lateral view of left hemisphere.

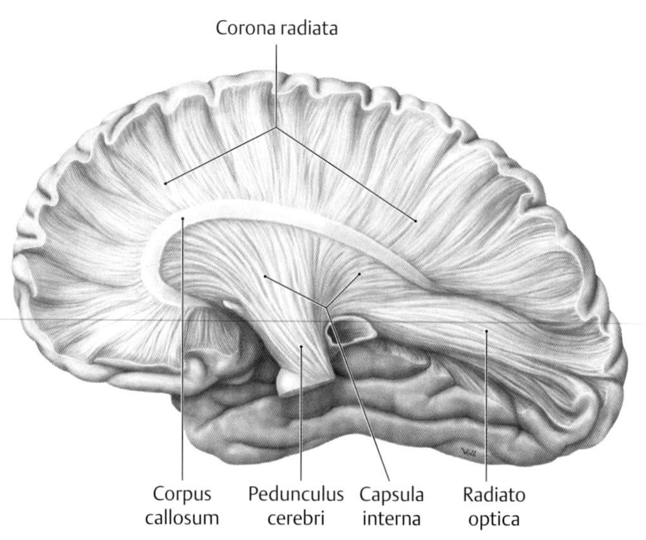
Corona radiata
Corpus callosum
Pedunculus cerebri
Capsula interna
Radiato optica

B Medial view of right hemisphere.

Fig. 39.9 Nuclei basales

Transverse section, superior view. The nuclei basales are an essential component of the motor system (see p. 615).

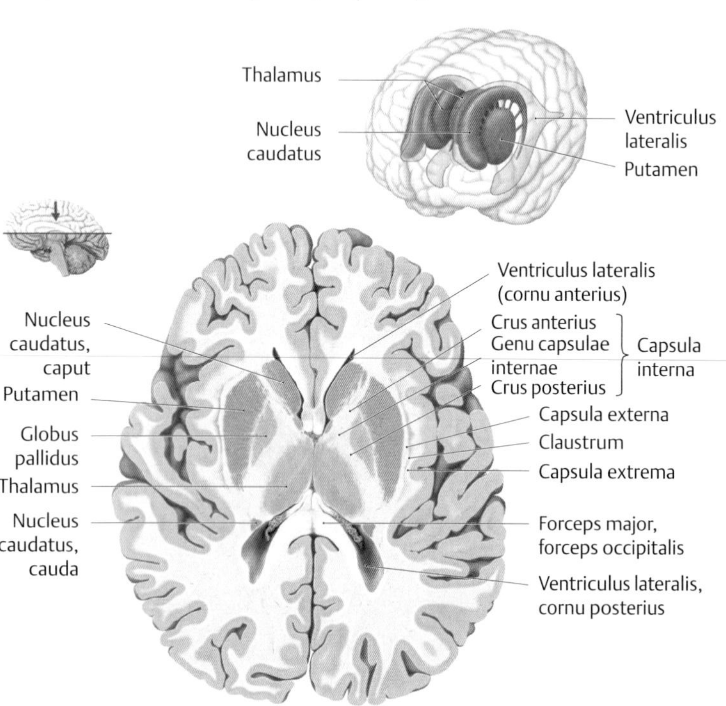
Thalamus
Nucleus caudatus
Ventriculus lateralis
Putamen
Nucleus caudatus, caput
Putamen
Globus pallidus
Thalamus
Nucleus caudatus, cauda
Ventriculus lateralis (cornu anterius)
Crus anterius
Genu capsulae internae
Crus posterius
Capsula interna
Capsula externa
Claustrum
Capsula extrema
Forceps major, forceps occipitalis
Ventriculus lateralis, cornu posterius

Fig. 39.10 Allocortex

The three-layered allocortex consists of the olfactory cortex (blue) and the hippocampus (pink).

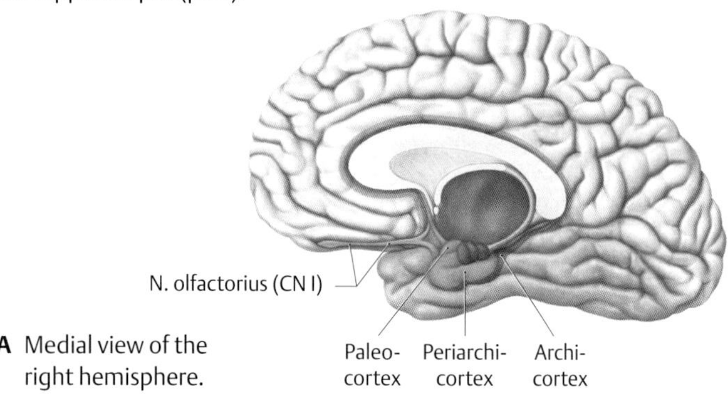
N. olfactorius (CN I)
Paleo-cortex
Periarchi-cortex
Archi-cortex

A Medial view of the right hemisphere.

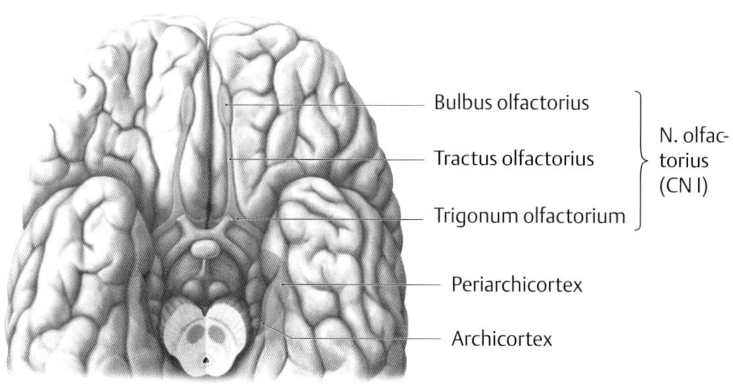
Bulbus olfactorius
Tractus olfactorius
Trigonum olfactorium
N. olfac-torius (CN I)
Periarchicortex
Archicortex

B Basal view.

Fig. 39.11 Isocortex: Columnar organization

Morphological considerations divide the isocortex into six horizontal layers; functional considerations divide it into cortical columns.

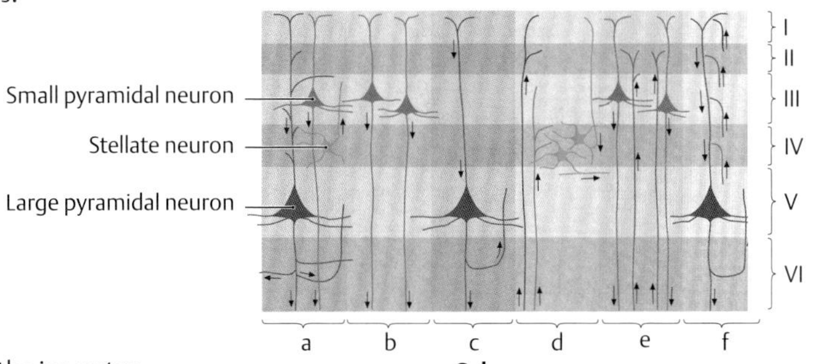

Cortical column
Pallium (neocortex)
Small pyramidal neuron
Stellate neuron
Large pyramidal neuron
I
II
III
IV
V
VI
a
b
c
d
e
f
Columns
Lamina molecularis (I)
Lamina granularis externa (II)
Lamina pyramidalis externa (III)
Lamina granularis interna (IV)
Lamina pyramidalis interna (V)
Lamina multiformis (VI)
Layers

A Histology of the isocortex.

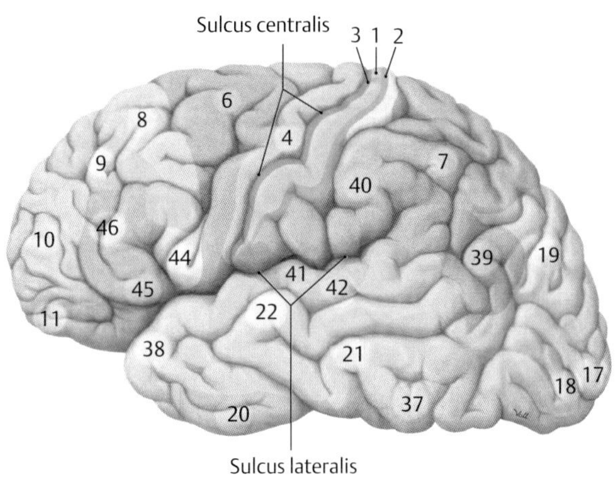

Sulcus centralis
3 1 2
6
8
4
9
7
40
10
46
44
41
39
19
42
45
22
11
38
21
18
17
37
20
Sulcus lateralis

B Brodmann (cortical) areas, lateral view of the left cerebral hemisphere.

Sulcus centralis
3 1 2
6
4
8
5
9
31
7
24
23
Sulcus parieto-occipitalis
10
33
32
19
30
Sulcus calcarinus
18
25
12
11
34
17
28
37
18
20
38
19

C Brodmann (cortical) areas, medial view of the right cerebral hemisphere.

Fig. 39.12 Lobes in the cerebral hemispheres

The isocortex also may be functionally divided into association areas (lobes).

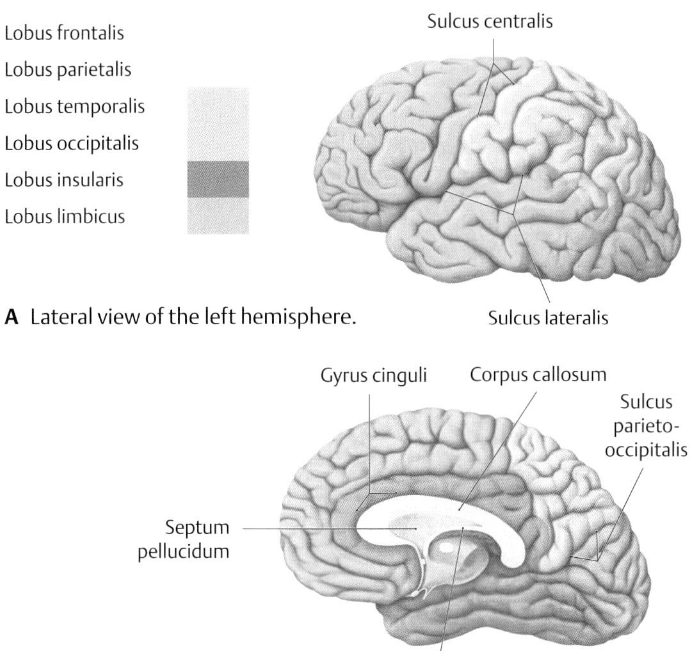

Lobus frontalis
Lobus parietalis
Lobus temporalis
Lobus occipitalis
Lobus insularis
Lobus limbicus
Sulcus centralis
Sulcus lateralis
Gyrus cinguli
Corpus callosum
Sulcus parieto-occipitalis
Septum pellucidum
Fornix

A Lateral view of the left hemisphere.

C Medial view of the right hemisphere.

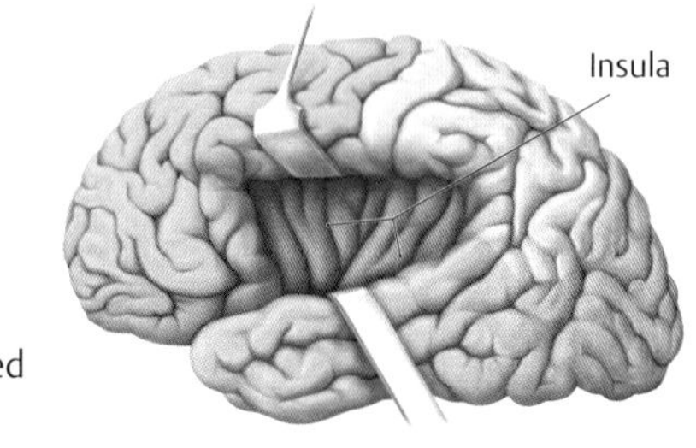

Insula

B Lateral view of the retracted left cerebral hemisphere.

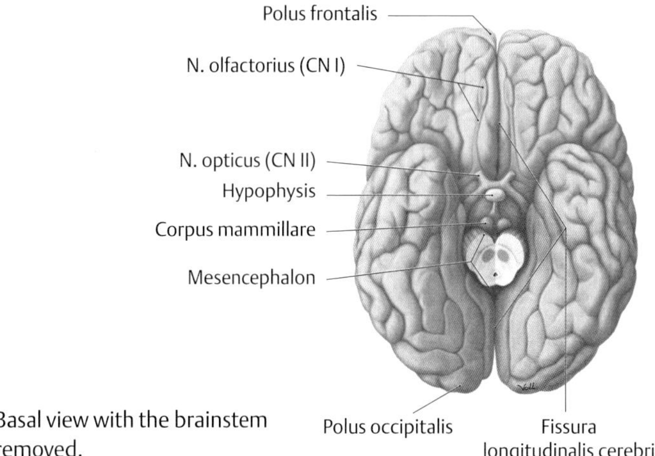

Polus frontalis
N. olfactorius (CN I)
N. opticus (CN II)
Hypophysis
Corpus mammillare
Mesencephalon
Polus occipitalis
Fissura longitudinalis cerebri

D Basal view with the brainstem removed.

Telencephalon & Diencephalon

Fig. 39.13 Hippocampal formation

The hippocampus, fornix, and amygdala are the major components of the limbic system (see p. 621).

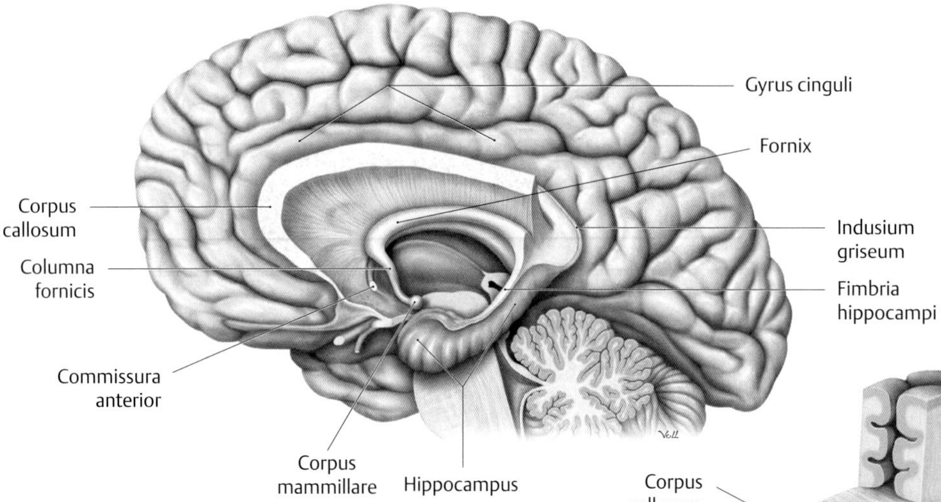

Gyrus cinguli
Fornix
Corpus callosum
Indusium griseum
Columna fornicis
Fimbria hippocampi
Commissura anterior
Corpus mammillare
Hippocampus

A Lateral view of the dissected left hemisphere.

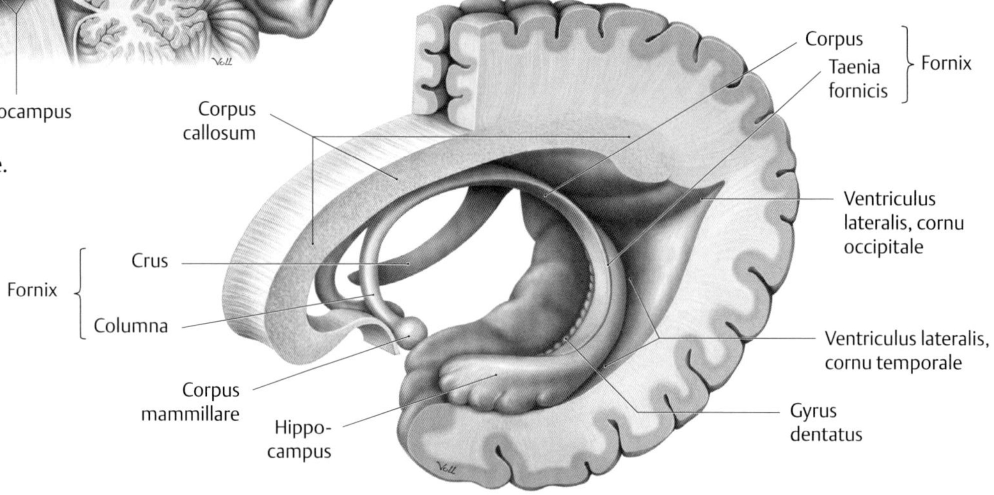

Corpus callosum
Corpus
Taenia fornicis
Fornix
Ventriculus lateralis, cornu occipitale
Fornix
Crus
Columna
Ventriculus lateralis, cornu temporale
Corpus mammillare
Hippocampus
Gyrus dentatus

B Left anterosuperior view.

Fig. 39.14 Diencephalon

Midsagittal section, medial view of the right hemisphere. The major components of the diencephalon are the thalamus, hypothalamus, and hypophysis (anterior lobe). See p. 598 for the extracted diencephalon.

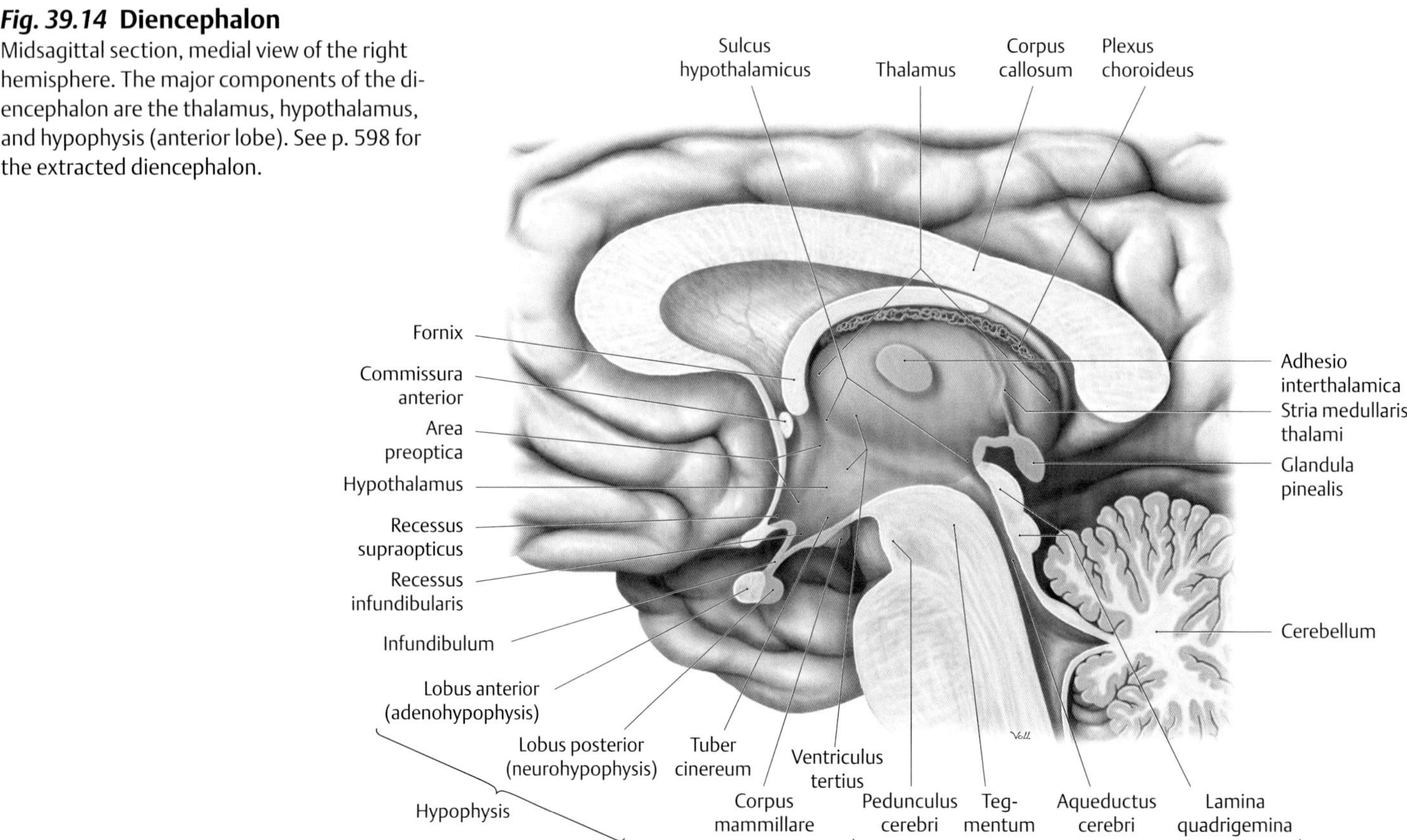
Sulcus hypothalamicus
Thalamus
Corpus callosum
Plexus choroideus
Fornix
Commissura anterior
Area preoptica
Hypothalamus
Recessus supraopticus
Recessus infundibularis
Infundibulum
Lobus anterior (adenohypophysis)
Lobus posterior (neurohypophysis)
Hypophysis
Tuber cinereum
Corpus mammillare
Ventriculus tertius
Pedunculus cerebri
Teg-mentum
Aqueductus cerebri
Lamina quadrigemina
Mesencephalon
Adhesio interthalamica
Stria medullaris thalami
Glandula pinealis
Cerebellum

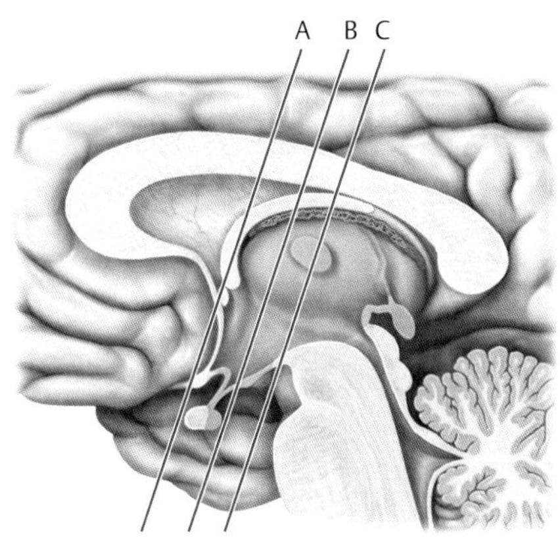
A
B
C

Table 39.2 Structures of the diencephalon

(P)	Recessus preopticus	
(OC)	Chiasma opticum	
(3V)	Ventriculus tertius	
(OT)	Tractus opticus	
(In)	Infundibulum	
(T)	Thalamus (with nuclei thalamici):	
	(R)	Nucleus reticularis
	(E)	Lamina medullaris externa
	(V)	Nuclei ventrolaterales
	(I)	Lamina medullaris interna
	(M)	Nuclei mediales
	(A)	Nuclei anteriores
	(P)	Nuclei paraventriculares
(S)	Nucleus subthalamicus	
(SN)*	Substantia nigra	
(MF)	Fasciculus mammillothalamicus	
(MB)	Corpus mammillaria	

*Actually a structure of the mesencephalon.

Table 39.3 Structures of the telencephalon

①	Corpus callosum
②	Septum pellucidum
③	Ventriculus lateralis
④	Fornix
⑤	Nucleus caudatus
⑥	Capsula interna
⑦	Putamen
⑧	Globus pallidus
⑨	Cavum septi pellucidi
⑩	Commissura anterior
⑪	Stria olfactoria lateralis
⑫	Plexus choroideus
⑬	Basal ganglia (nuclei basales)
⑭	Amygdala
⑮	Hippocampus

***Fig. 39.15* Telencephalon and diencephalon: Internal structure**
Coronal section.

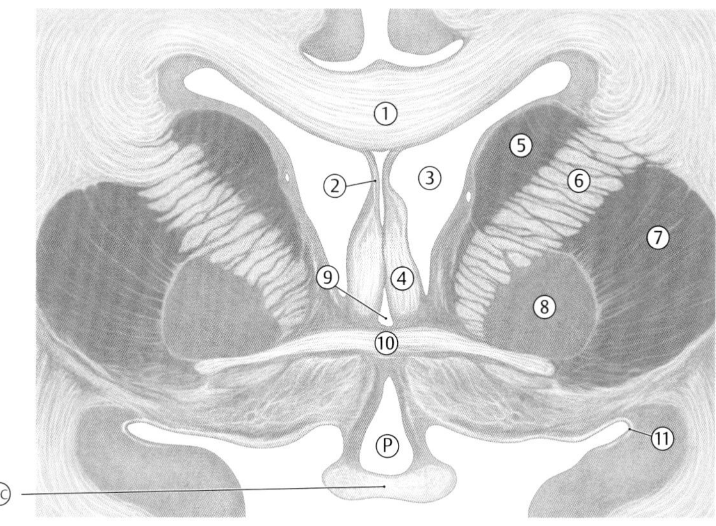
1
2
3
4
5
6
7
8
9
10
11
P
OC

A Level of chiasma opticum.

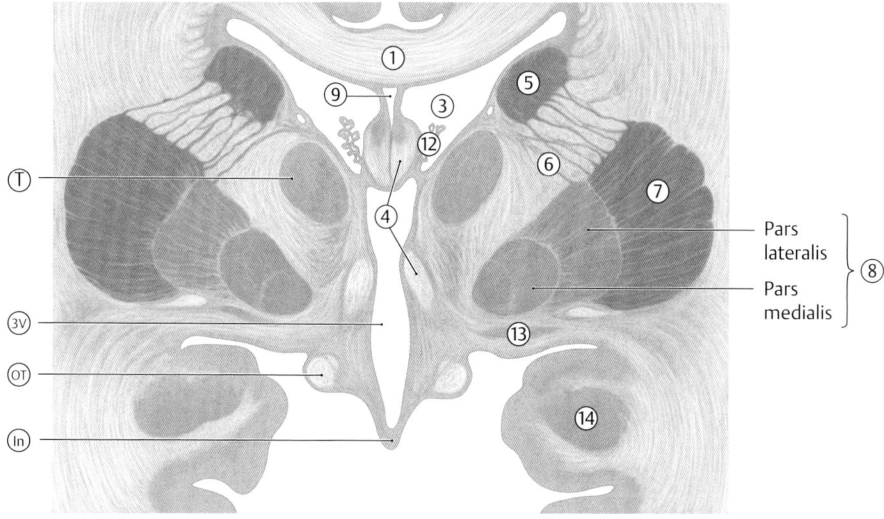
1
9
3
5
12
6
T
7
4
Pars lateralis
Pars medialis
8
3V
13
OT
14
In

B Level of the tuber cinereum.

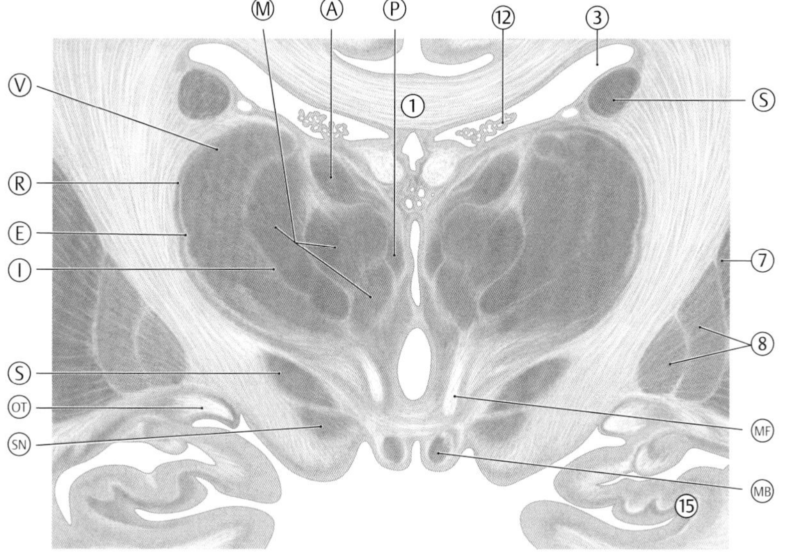
M
A
P
12
3
V
1
S
R
E
I
7
8
S
OT
MF
SN
MB
15

C Level of corpora mamillaria.

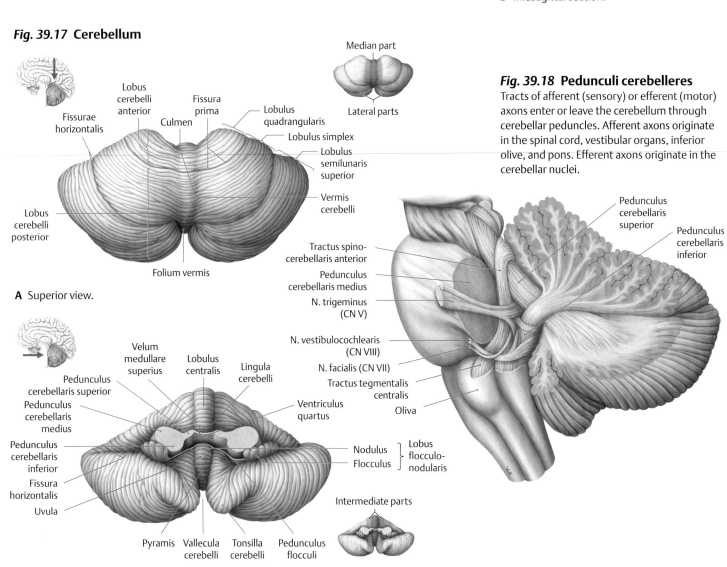

Fig. 39.16 Diencephalon, brainstem, and cerebellum
Left lateral view.

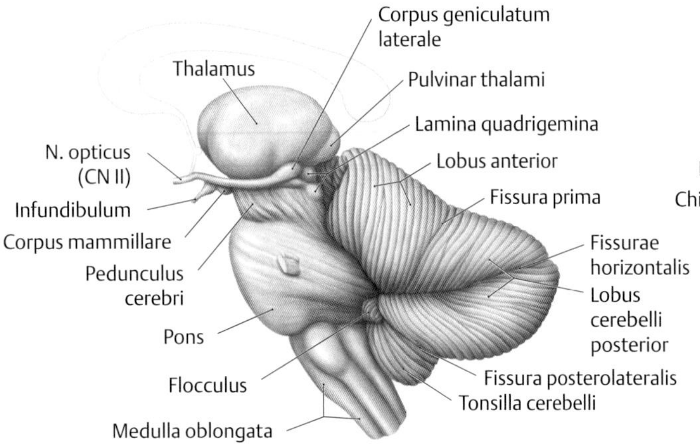

Corpus geniculatum laterale
Thalamus
Pulvinar thalami
Lamina quadrigemina
N. opticus (CN II)
Lobus anterior
Infundibulum
Fissura prima
Corpus mammillare
Fissurae horizontalis
Pedunculus cerebri
Lobus cerebelli posterior
Pons
Flocculus
Fissura posterolateralis
Tonsilla cerebelli
Medulla oblongata

A Isolated structures.

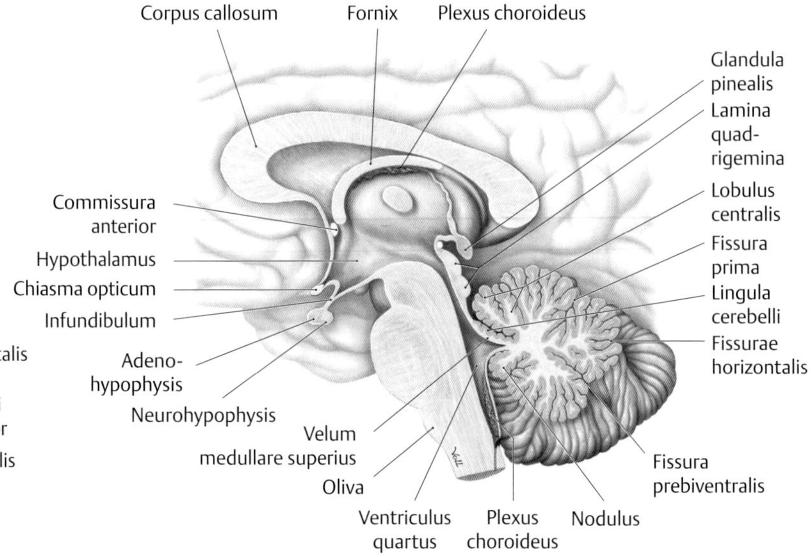

Corpus callosum
Fornix
Plexus choroideus
Glandula pinealis
Lamina quad-rigemina
Commissura anterior
Lobulus centralis
Hypothalamus
Fissura prima
Chiasma opticum
Lingula cerebelli
Infundibulum
Fissurae horizontalis
Adeno-hypophysis
Neurohypophysis
Velum medullare superius
Oliva
Fissura prebiventralis
Ventriculus quartus
Plexus choroideus
Nodulus

B Midsagittal section.

Fig. 39.17 Cerebellum

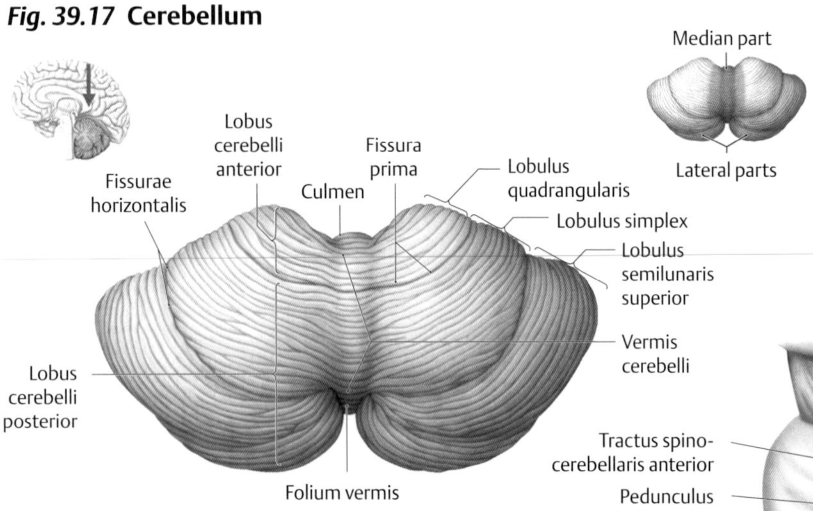

Median part
Lateral parts
Lobus cerebelli anterior
Fissura prima
Fissurae horizontalis
Culmen
Lobulus quadrangularis
Lobulus simplex
Lobulus semilunaris superior
Vermis cerebelli
Lobus cerebelli posterior
Folium vermis

A Superior view.

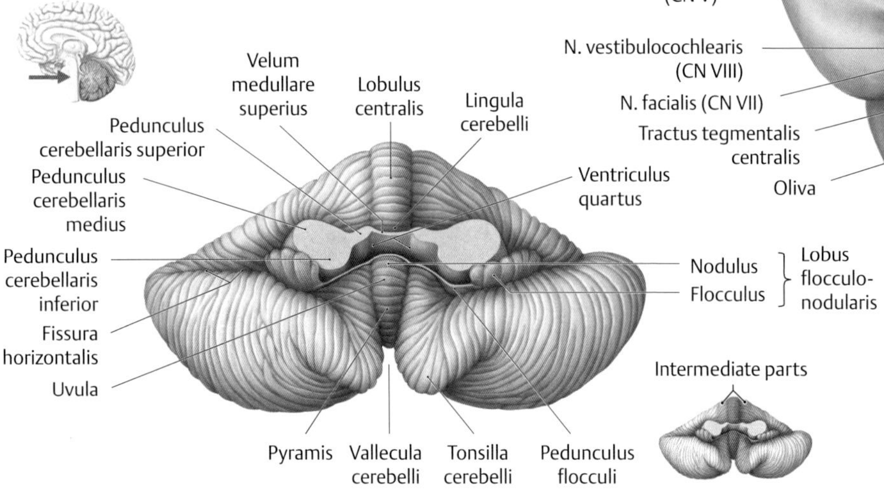

Velum medullare superius
Lobulus centralis
Lingula cerebelli
Pedunculus cerebellaris superior
Pedunculus cerebellaris medius
Ventriculus quartus
Pedunculus cerebellaris inferior
Nodulus
Flocculus
Lobus flocculo-nodularis
Fissura horizontalis
Uvula
Intermediate parts
Pyramis
Vallecula cerebelli
Tonsilla cerebelli
Pedunculus flocculi

B Anterior view.

Fig. 39.18 Pedunculi cerebelleres
Tracts of afferent (sensory) or efferent (motor) axons enter or leave the cerebellum through cerebellar peduncles. Afferent axons originate in the spinal cord, vestibular organs, inferior olive, and pons. Efferent axons originate in the cerebellar nuclei.

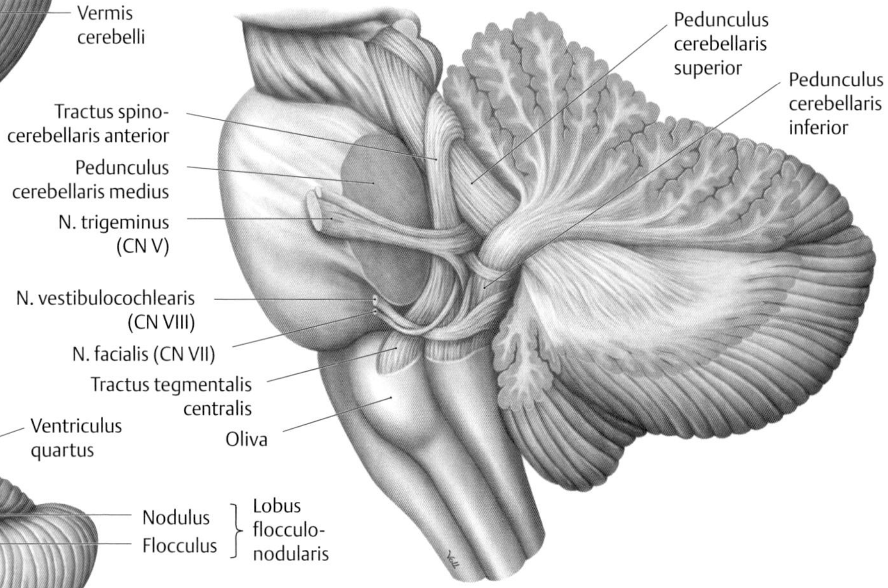

Pedunculus cerebellaris superior
Pedunculus cerebellaris inferior
Tractus spino-cerebellaris anterior
Pedunculus cerebellaris medius
N. trigeminus (CN V)
N. vestibulocochlearis (CN VIII)
N. facialis (CN VII)
Tractus tegmentalis centralis
Oliva

Fig. 39.19 **Brainstem**

The brainstem is the site of emergence and entry of the 10 pairs of true cranial nerves (CN III–XII). See p. 470 for an overview of the cranial nerves and their nuclei.

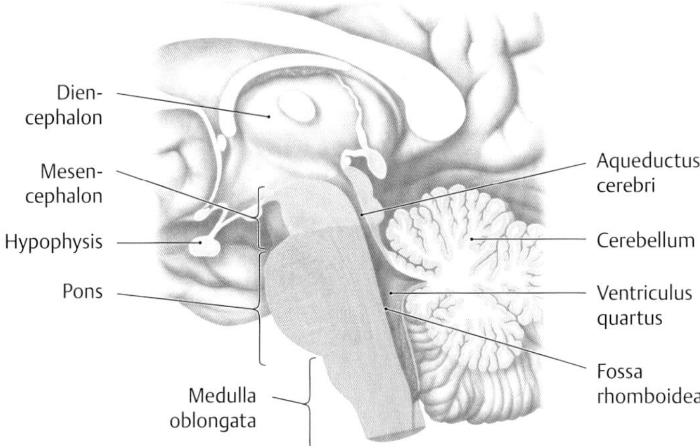
Dien-
cephalon
Mesen-
cephalon
Hypophysis
Pons
Medulla
oblongata
Aqueductus
cerebri
Cerebellum
Ventriculus
quartus
Fossa
rhomboidea

A Levels of the brainstem.

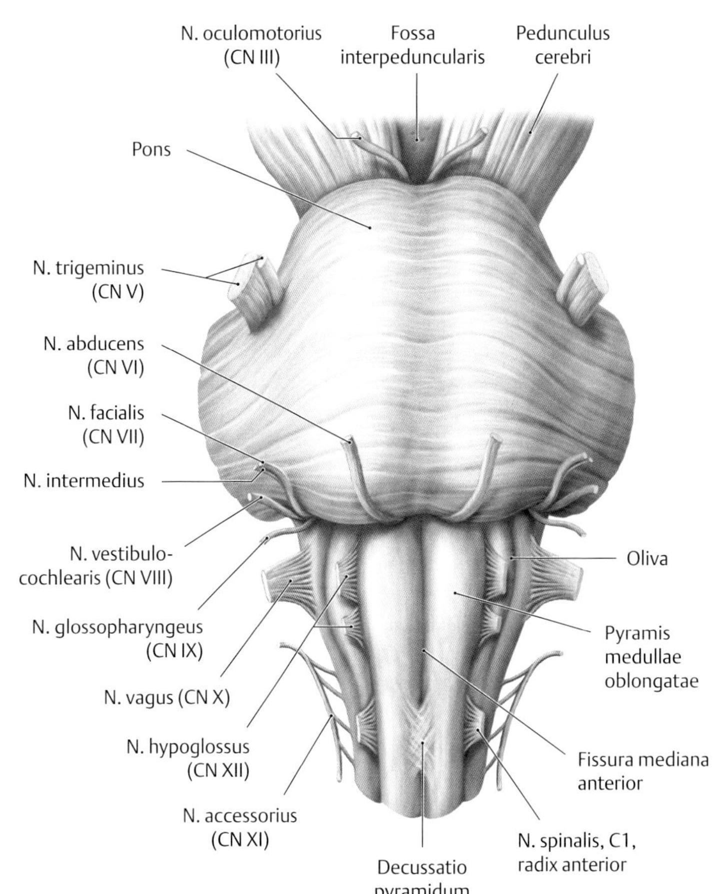
N. oculomotorius
(CN III)
Fossa
interpeduncularis
Pedunculus
cerebri
Pons
N. trigeminus
(CN V)
N. abducens
(CN VI)
N. facialis
(CN VII)
N. intermedius
N. vestibulo-
cochlearis (CN VIII)
N. glossopharyngeus
(CN IX)
N. vagus (CN X)
N. hypoglossus
(CN XII)
N. accessorius
(CN XI)
Decussatio
pyramidum
N. spinalis, C1,
radix anterior
Fissura mediana
anterior
Pyramis
medullae
oblongatae
Oliva

B Anterior view.

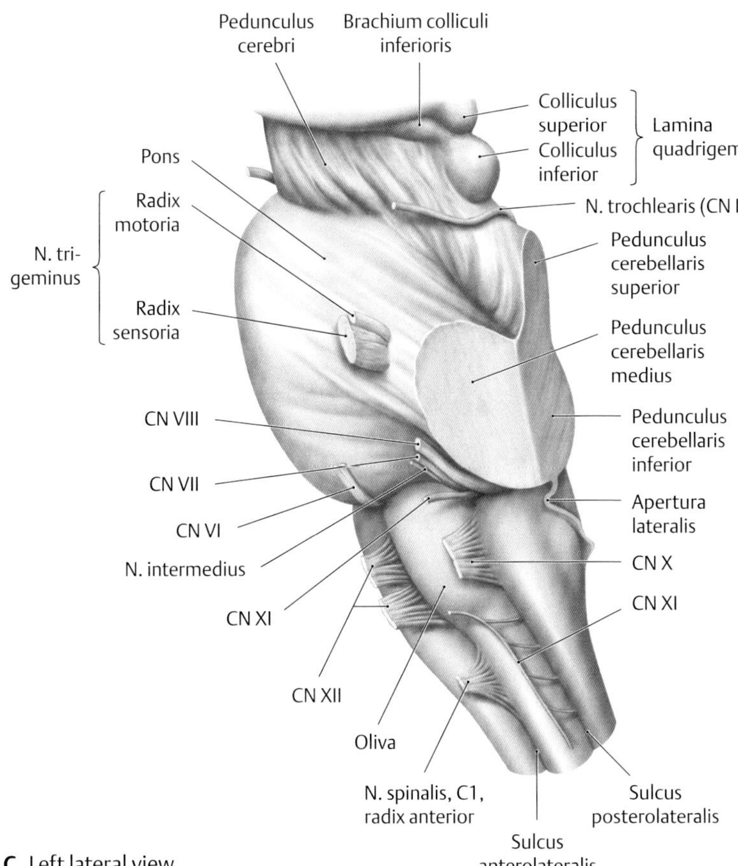
Pedunculus
cerebri
Brachium colliculi
inferioris
Colliculus
superior
Colliculus
inferior
Lamina
quadrigemina
Pons
N. tri-
geminus
Radix
motoria
Radix
sensoria
N. trochlearis (CN IV)
Pedunculus
cerebellaris
superior
Pedunculus
cerebellaris
medius
Pedunculus
cerebellaris
inferior
Apertura
lateralis
CN VIII
CN VII
CN VI
N. intermedius
CN XI
CN XII
Oliva
CN X
CN XI
N. spinalis, C1,
radix anterior
Sulcus
anterolateralis
Sulcus
posterolateralis

C Left lateral view.

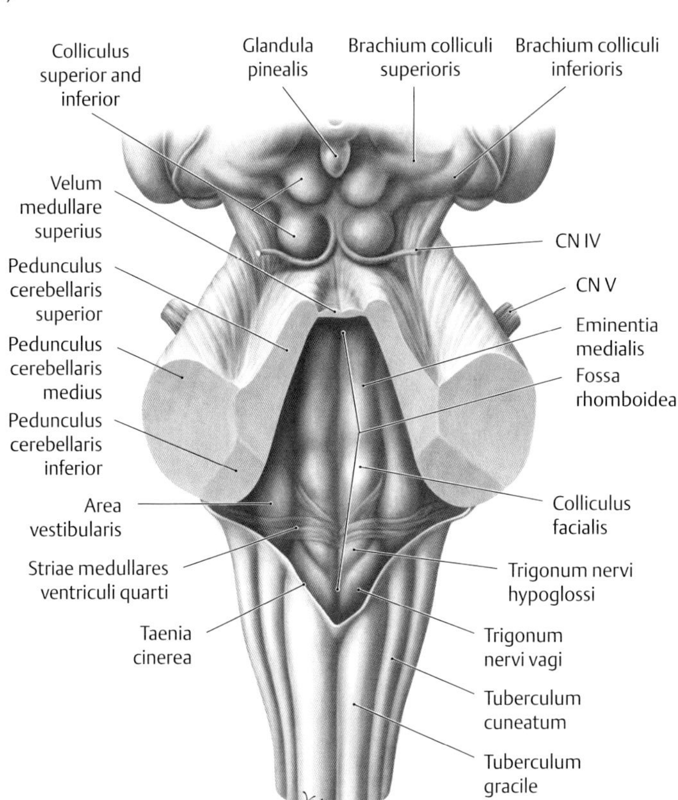
Colliculus
superior and
inferior
Glandula
pinealis
Brachium colliculi
superioris
Brachium colliculi
inferioris
Velum
medullare
superius
CN IV
CN V
Pedunculus
cerebellaris
superior
Pedunculus
cerebellaris
medius
Pedunculus
cerebellaris
inferior
Eminentia
medialis
Fossa
rhomboidea
Colliculus
facialis
Area
vestibularis
Striae medullares
ventriculi quarti
Trigonum nervi
hypoglossi
Taenia
cinerea
Trigonum
nervi vagi
Tuberculum
cuneatum
Tuberculum
gracile

D Posterior view.

Medulla Spinalis

Fig. 39.20 Medulla spinalis and segments

Medulla spinalis consists of 31 segments innervating a specific area in the trunk or limbs (see Fig. 39.22). Afferent (sensory) posterior rootlets and efferent (motor) anterior rootlets form the radix posterior and anterior, respectively. The two radicis fuse to form a mixed n. spinalis, which then divides into various branches.

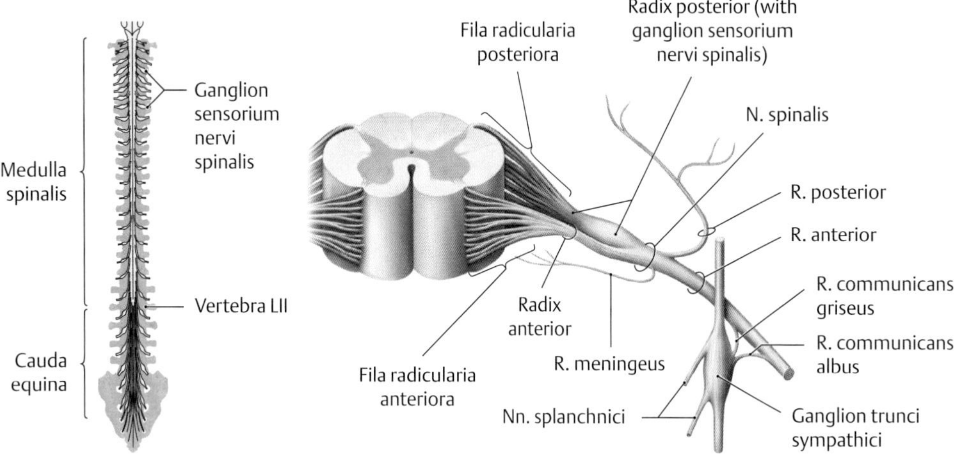

Ganglion sensorium nervi spinalis
Medulla spinalis
Vertebra LII
Cauda equina
Fila radicularia posteriora
Radix posterior (with ganglion sensorium nervi spinalis)
N. spinalis
R. posterior
R. anterior
R. communicans griseus
R. communicans albus
Ganglion trunci sympathici
Radix anterior
R. meningeus
Fila radicularia anteriora
Nn. splanchnici

A Spinal cord, posterior view.

B Spinal cord segment, anterior view.

Fig. 39.22 Segmental innervation of medulla spinalis lesions

Medulla spinalis is divided into four major regions: cervical, thoracic, lumbar, and sacral. Spinal cord segments are numbered by the exit points of their associated spinal nerves. (*Note:* This does not necessarily correlate numerically with the nearest skeletal element.)

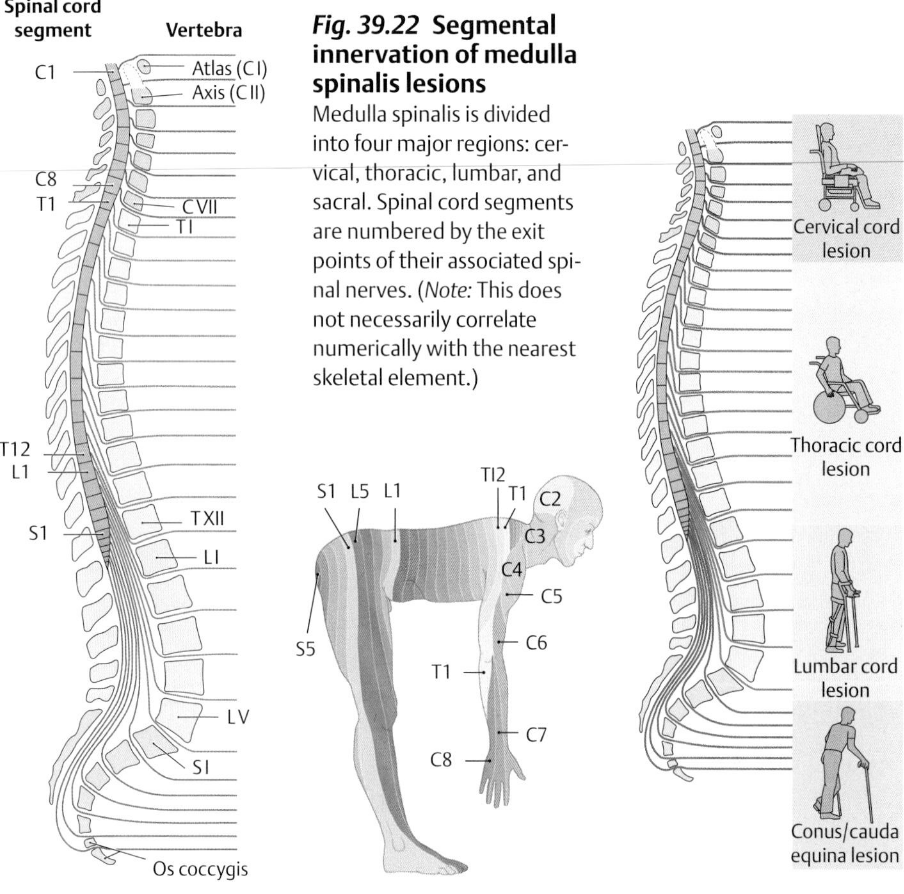

Spinal cord segment
Vertebra
C1
Atlas (CI)
Axis (CII)
C8
T1
CVII
TI
T12
L1
S1
TXII
LI
LV
SI
Os coccygis
S1 L5 L1
TI2
T1
C2
C3
C4
C5
C6
S5
T1
C7
C8
Cervical cord lesion
Thoracic cord lesion
Lumbar cord lesion
Conus/cauda equina lesion

A Spinal cord segments.

B Dermatomes. Each spinal cord segment innervates a particular skin area (dermatome).

C Spinal cord lesions.

Fig. 39.21 Medulla spinalis in situ

Posterior view with vertebral canal windowed.

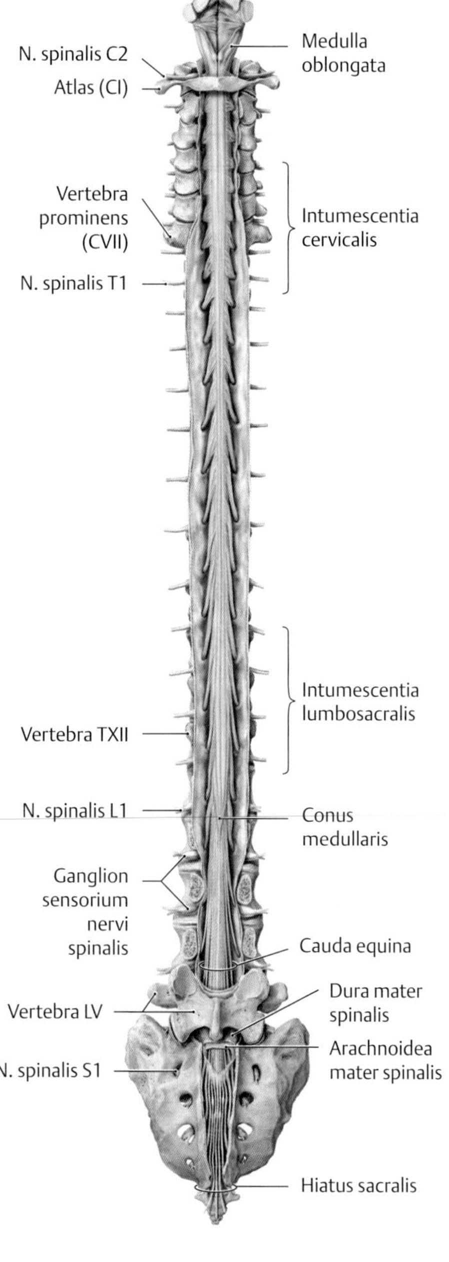

N. spinalis C2
Atlas (CI)
Medulla oblongata
Vertebra prominens (CVII)
Intumescentia cervicalis
N. spinalis T1
Intumescentia lumbosacralis
Vertebra TXII
N. spinalis L1
Conus medullaris
Ganglion sensorium nervi spinalis
Cauda equina
Vertebra LV
Dura mater spinalis
Arachnoidea mater spinalis
N. spinalis S1
Hiatus sacralis

Fig. 39.23 Spinal cord in situ: Transverse section

Superior view.

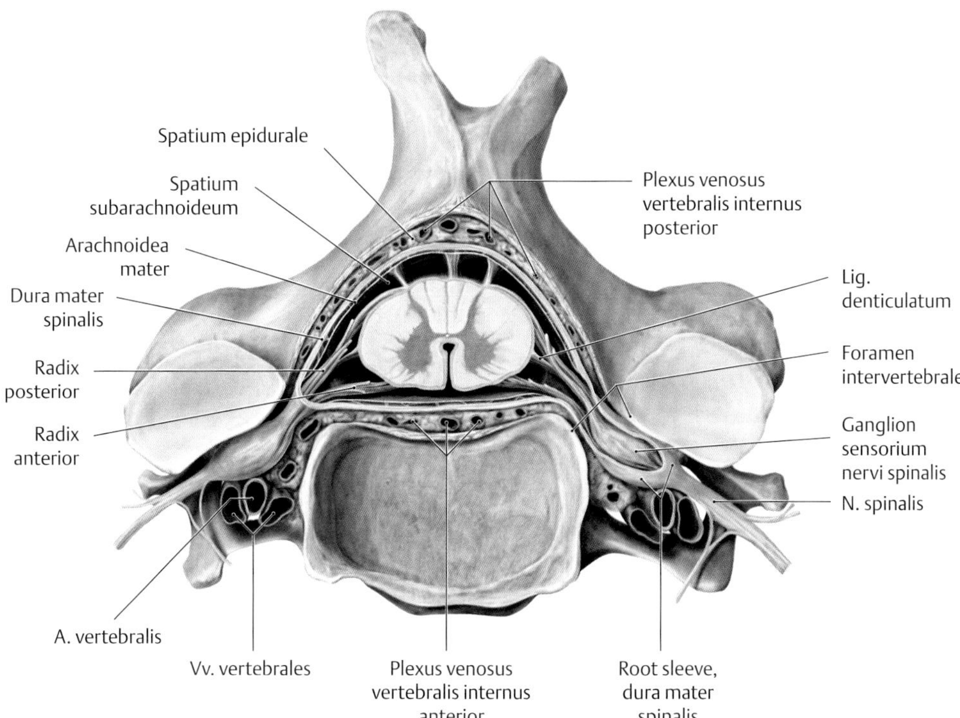

Spatium epidurale
Spatium subarachnoideum
Arachnoidea mater
Dura mater spinalis
Radix posterior
Radix anterior
A. vertebralis
Vv. vertebrales
Plexus venosus vertebralis internus anterior
Root sleeve, dura mater spinalis
N. spinalis
Ganglion sensorium nervi spinalis
Foramen intervertebrale
Lig. denticulatum
Plexus venosus vertebralis internus posterior

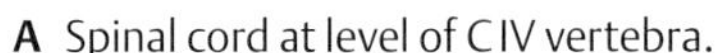

A Spinal cord at level of C IV vertebra.

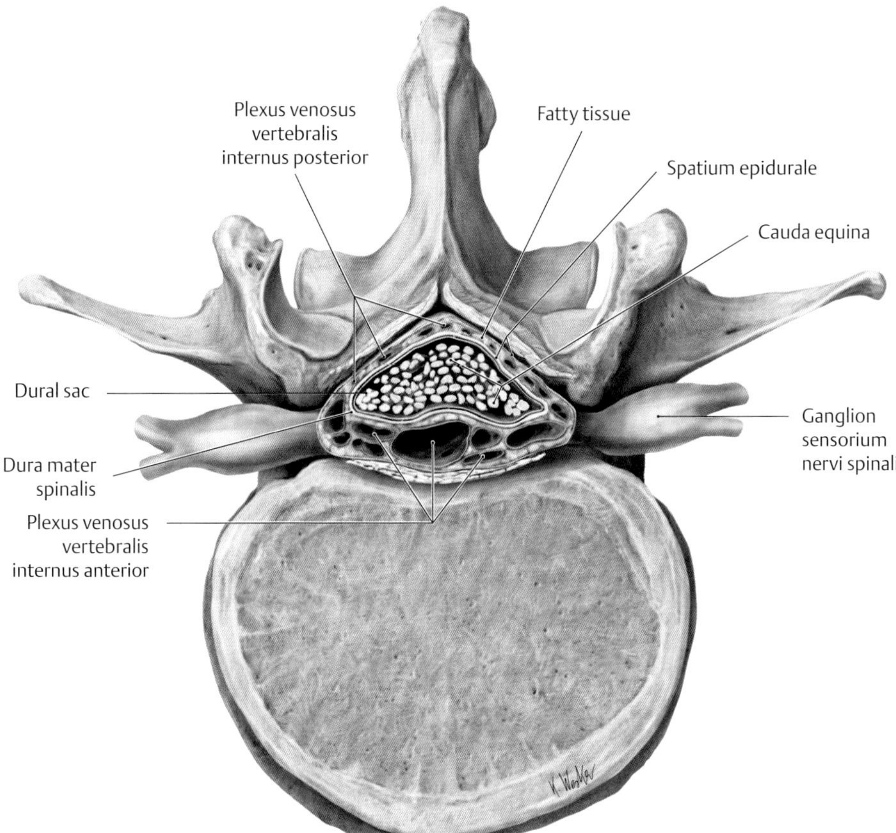

Plexus venosus vertebralis internus posterior
Fatty tissue
Spatium epidurale
Cauda equina
Dural sac
Dura mater spinalis
Plexus venosus vertebralis internus anterior
Ganglion sensorium nervi spinalis

B Cauda equina at level of L II vertebra.

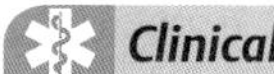

Clinical

Lumbar puncture

A needle introduced into the dural sac (lumbar cistern) generally slips past the spinal nerve roots without injuring the spinal cord. Cerebrospinal fluid (CSF) samples are therefore taken between the L III and L IV vertebrae (2), once the patient has leaned forward to separate the spinous processes of the lumbar spine.

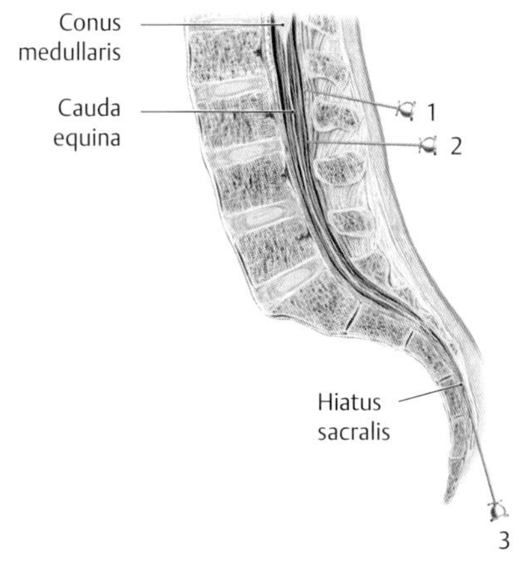

Conus medullaris
Cauda equina
1
2
Hiatus sacralis
3

Anesthesia

Lumbar anesthesia may be administered in a similar fashion (2). Epidural anesthesia is administered by placing a catheter in the epidural space without penetrating the dural sac (1). This may also be done by passing a needle through hiatus sacralis (3).

Fig. 39.24 Cauda equina

In adults, the spinal cord ends at approximately the level of L I. Below this, ventral and dorsal roots course through canalis vertebralis, uniting in the foramen intervertebrale to form the spinal nerve (see p. 36).

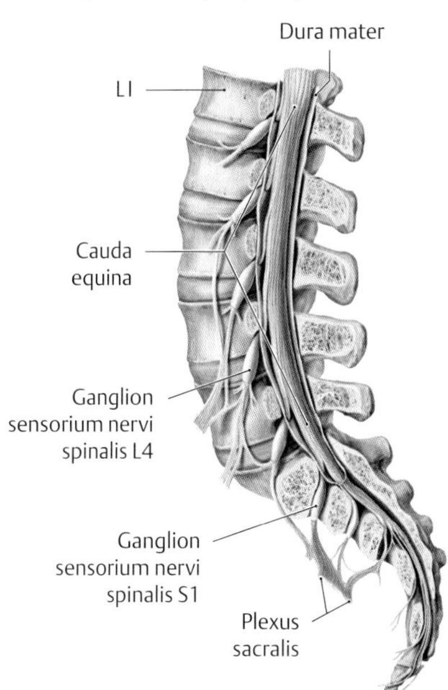

Dura mater
L I
Cauda equina
Ganglion sensorium nervi spinalis L4
Ganglion sensorium nervi spinalis S1
Plexus sacralis

Meninges

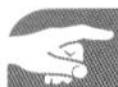

The brain and spinal cord are covered by membranes called meninges. The meninges are composed of three layers: dura mater (dura), arachnoidea mater, and pia mater.

The subarachnoid space, located between the arachnoid and pia, contains cerebrospinal fluid (CSF, see p. 604). See p. 601 for the coverings of the spinal cord.

Fig. 39.25 **Meninges**
See p. 606 for the veins of the brain.

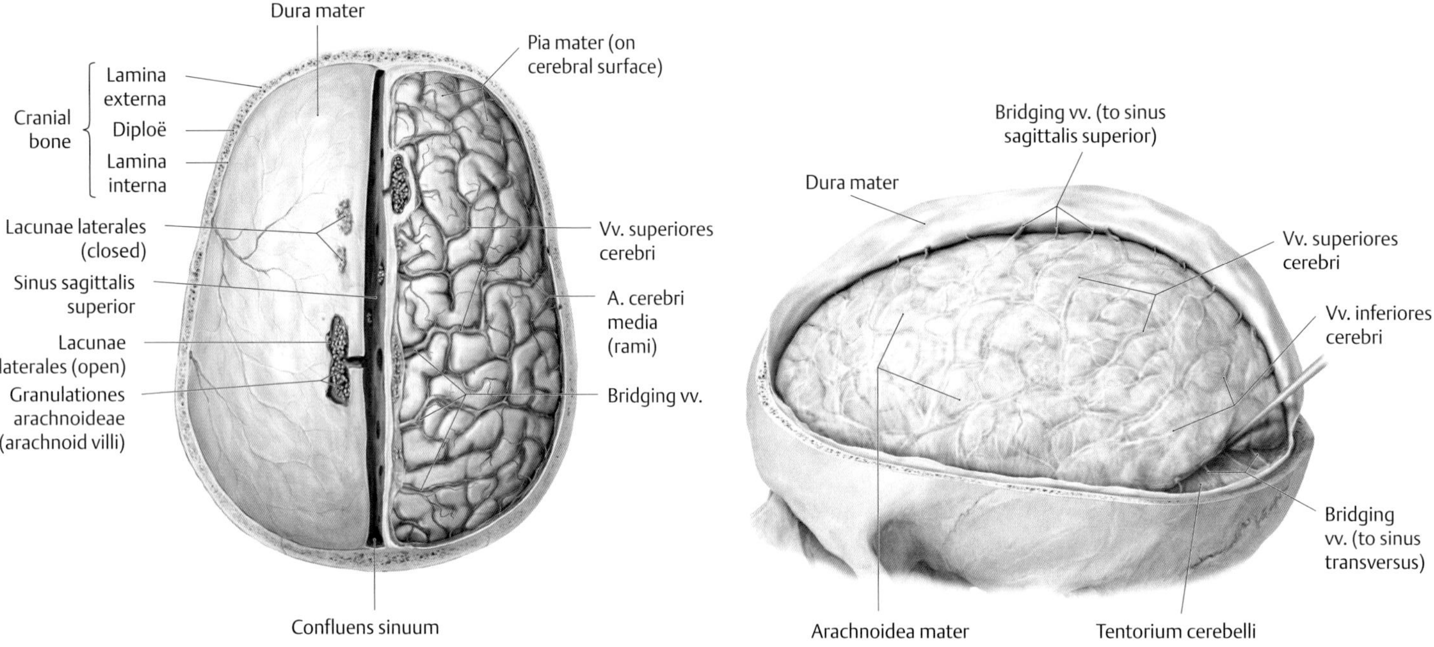
Dura mater
Pia mater (on cerebral surface)
Cranial bone
Lamina externa
Diploë
Lamina interna
Lacunae laterales (closed)
Sinus sagittalis superior
Lacunae laterales (open)
Granulationes arachnoideae (arachnoid villi)
Vv. superiores cerebri
A. cerebri media (rami)
Bridging vv.
Confluens sinuum
Bridging vv. (to sinus sagittalis superior)
Dura mater
Vv. superiores cerebri
Vv. inferiores cerebri
Bridging vv. (to sinus transversus)
Arachnoidea mater
Tentorium cerebelli

A Superior view. Left side: Dura mater (outer layer). Right side: Pia mater (inner layer). Granulationes arachnoidea (protrusions of the arachnoid) are sites for reabsorption of CSF.

B Arachnoidea mater, left anterior oblique view.

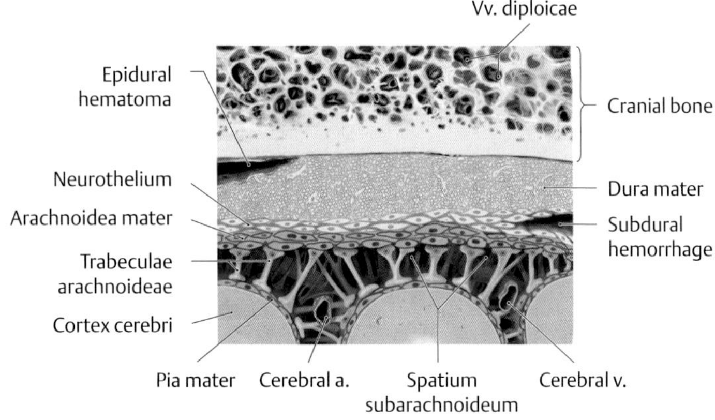
Vv. diploicae
Epidural hematoma
Cranial bone
Neurothelium
Dura mater
Arachnoidea mater
Subdural hemorrhage
Trabeculae arachnoideae
Cortex cerebri
Pia mater
Cerebral a.
Spatium subarachnoideum
Cerebral v.

C Layers of the meninges, coronal section, anterior view.

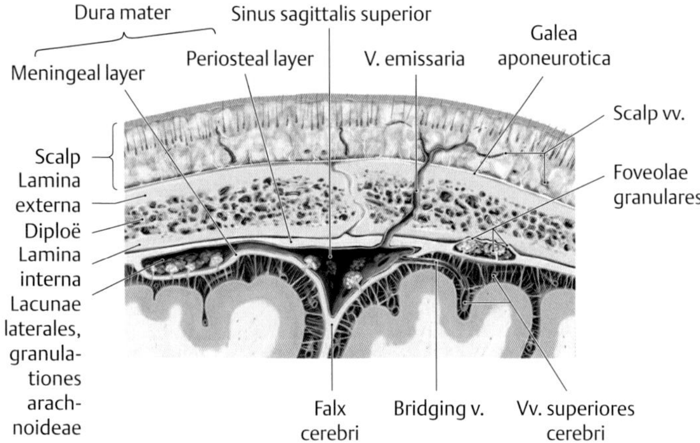
Dura mater
Sinus sagittalis superior
Galea aponeurotica
Meningeal layer
Periosteal layer
V. emissaria
Scalp vv.
Scalp
Lamina externa
Diploë
Lamina interna
Lacunae laterales, granulationes arachnoideae
Foveolae granulares
Falx cerebri
Bridging v.
Vv. superiores cerebri

D Dura mater and calvarium, coronal section, anterior view.

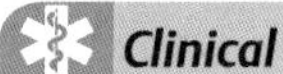

Clinical

Extracerebral hemorrhages

Bleeding between the bony calvarium and the soft tissue of the brain (extracerebral hemorrhage) exerts pressure on the brain. A rise of intracranial pressure may damage brain tissue both at the bleeding site and in more remote brain areas. Three types of intracranial hemorrhage are distinguished based on the relationship to the dura mater. See p. 608 for the arteries of the brain.

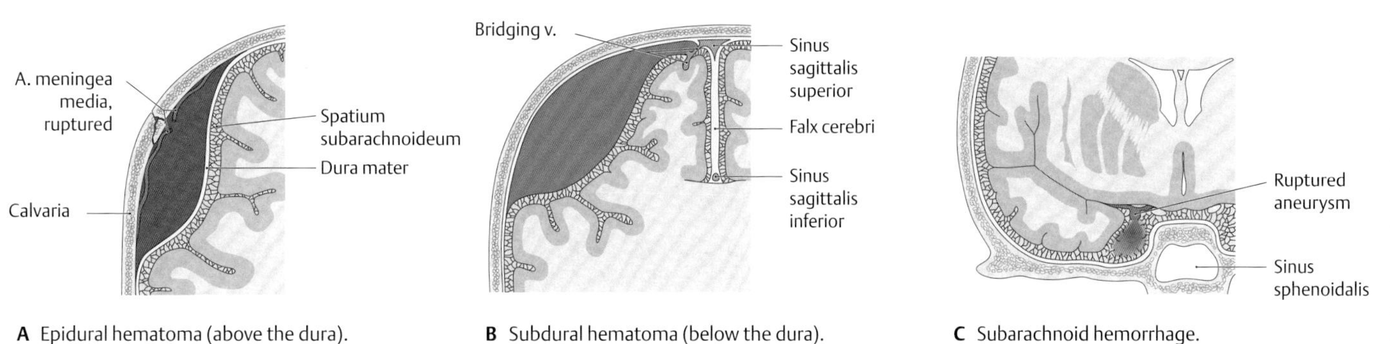

A. meningea media, ruptured
Spatium subarachnoideum
Dura mater
Calvaria
Bridging v.
Sinus sagittalis superior
Falx cerebri
Sinus sagittalis inferior
Ruptured aneurysm
Sinus sphenoidalis

A Epidural hematoma (above the dura).

B Subdural hematoma (below the dura).

C Subarachnoid hemorrhage.

Fig. 39.26 Dural septa

Left anterior oblique view. The major dural reflections are the falx cerebri, tentorium cerebelli, and falx cerebelli (not shown). The dural septa separate the regions of the brain from each other.

Incisura tentorii
Tentorium cerebelli
Bridging vv.
Falx cerebri
Diaphragma sellae
Crista galli
N. opticus
A. carotis interna

Fig. 39.27 Innervation of the dura mater

Superior view. *Removed:* Tentorium cerebelli (right side).

Lamina cribrosa
N. ethmoidalis anterior and posterior (r. meningeus)
CN V_1 and V_2 and V_3 (r. meningeus)
CN V_3 (r. meningeus)
Nn. cervicales 1 and 2 (r. meningeus)
CN X (r. meningeus)
CN V_1 and V_2 (r. tentorius)
Tentorium cerebelli

Fig. 39.28 Arteries of the dura mater

Midsagittal section, left lateral view. See p. 608 for the arteries of the brain.

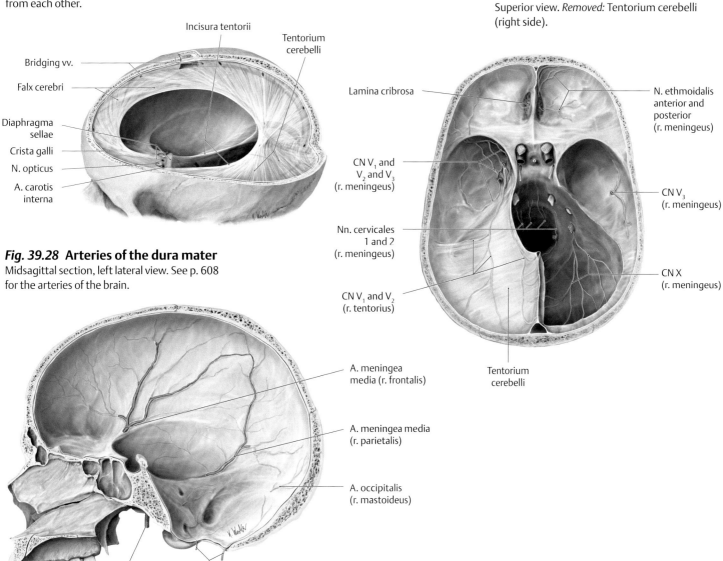

A. meningea media (r. frontalis)
A. meningea media (r. parietalis)
A. occipitalis (r. mastoideus)
A. meningea media (via foramen spinosum)
A. vertebralis (rami)

Fig. 39.29 **Circulation of liquor cerebrospinalis (cerebrospinal fluid, CSF)**
The brain and spinal cord are suspended in CSF. Produced in plexus choroideus, CSF occupies the spatium subarachnoideum and ventriculi of the brain.

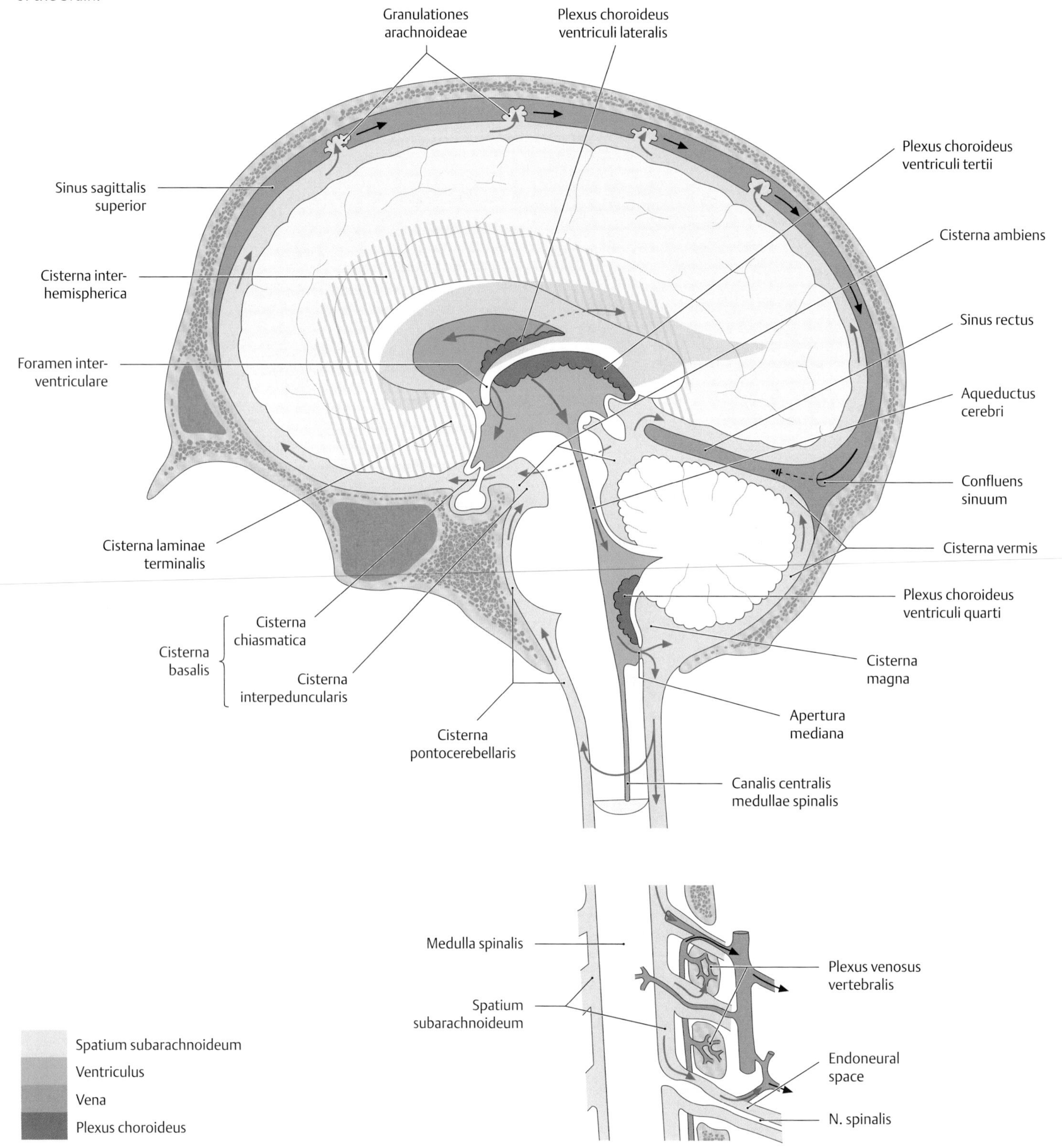
Granulationes arachnoideae
Plexus choroideus ventriculi lateralis
Plexus choroideus ventriculi tertii
Sinus sagittalis superior
Cisterna ambiens
Cisterna inter-hemispherica
Sinus rectus
Foramen inter-ventriculare
Aqueductus cerebri
Confluens sinuum
Cisterna laminae terminalis
Cisterna vermis
Plexus choroideus ventriculi quarti
Cisterna basalis
Cisterna chiasmatica
Cisterna interpeduncularis
Cisterna magna
Apertura mediana
Cisterna pontocerebellaris
Canalis centralis medullae spinalis
Medulla spinalis
Plexus venosus vertebralis
Spatium subarachnoideum
Endoneural space
N. spinalis
Spatium subarachnoideum
Ventriculus
Vena
Plexus choroideus

Fig. 39.30 Ventricular system

The ventricular system is a continuation of the central spinal canal into the brain. Cast specimens are used to demonstrate the connections between the four ventricular cavities.

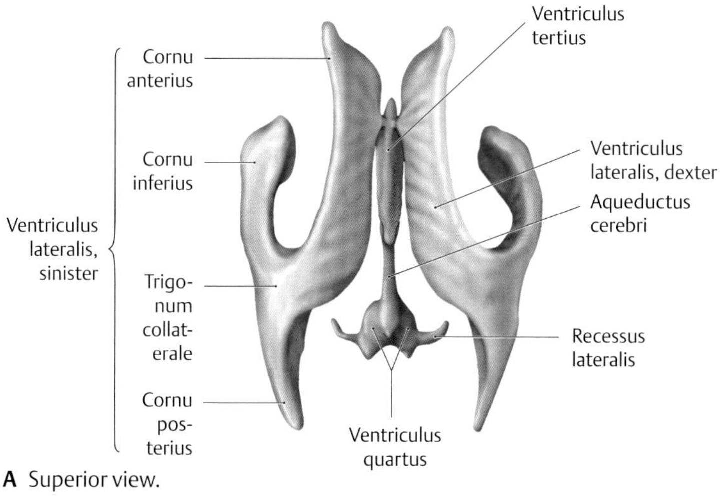

Ventriculus lateralis, sinister
Cornu anterius
Cornu inferius
Trigonum collaterale
Cornu posterius
Ventriculus tertius
Ventriculus lateralis, dexter
Aqueductus cerebri
Recessus lateralis
Ventriculus quartus

A Superior view.

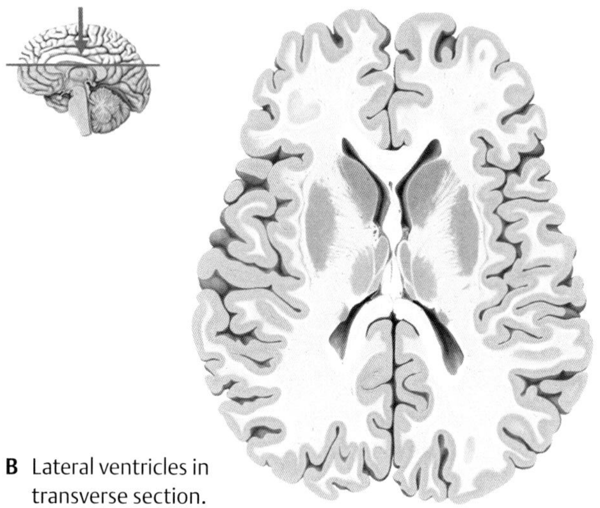

B Lateral ventricles in transverse section.

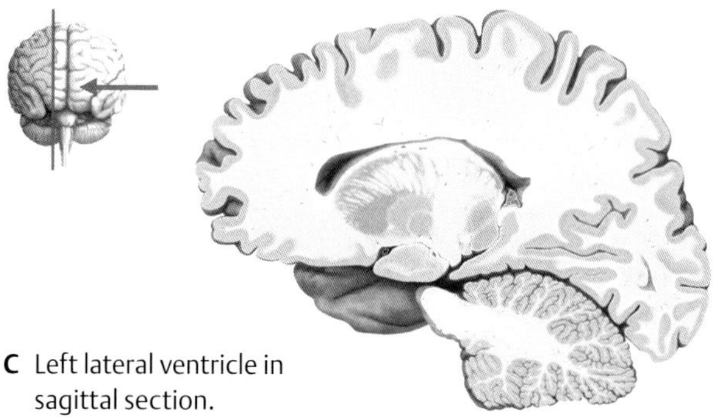

C Left lateral ventricle in sagittal section.

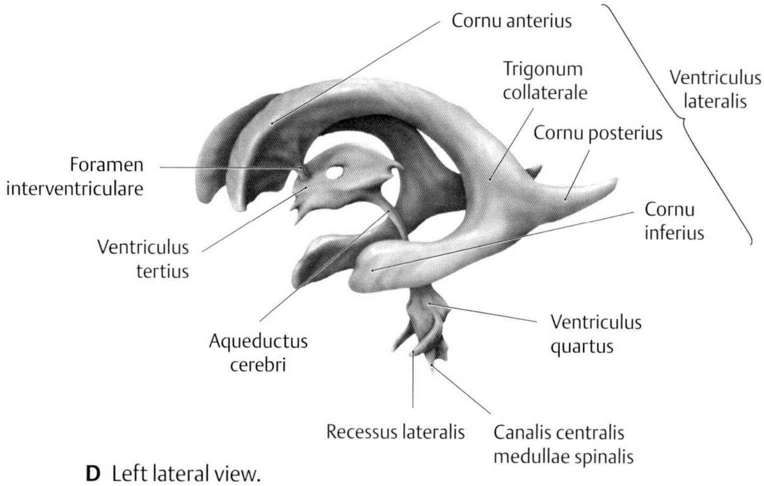

Cornu anterius
Trigonum collaterale
Ventriculus lateralis
Cornu posterius
Foramen interventriculare
Cornu inferius
Ventriculus tertius
Ventriculus quartus
Aqueductus cerebri
Recessus lateralis
Canalis centralis medullae spinalis

D Left lateral view.

Fig. 39.31 Ventricular system in situ

Left lateral view.

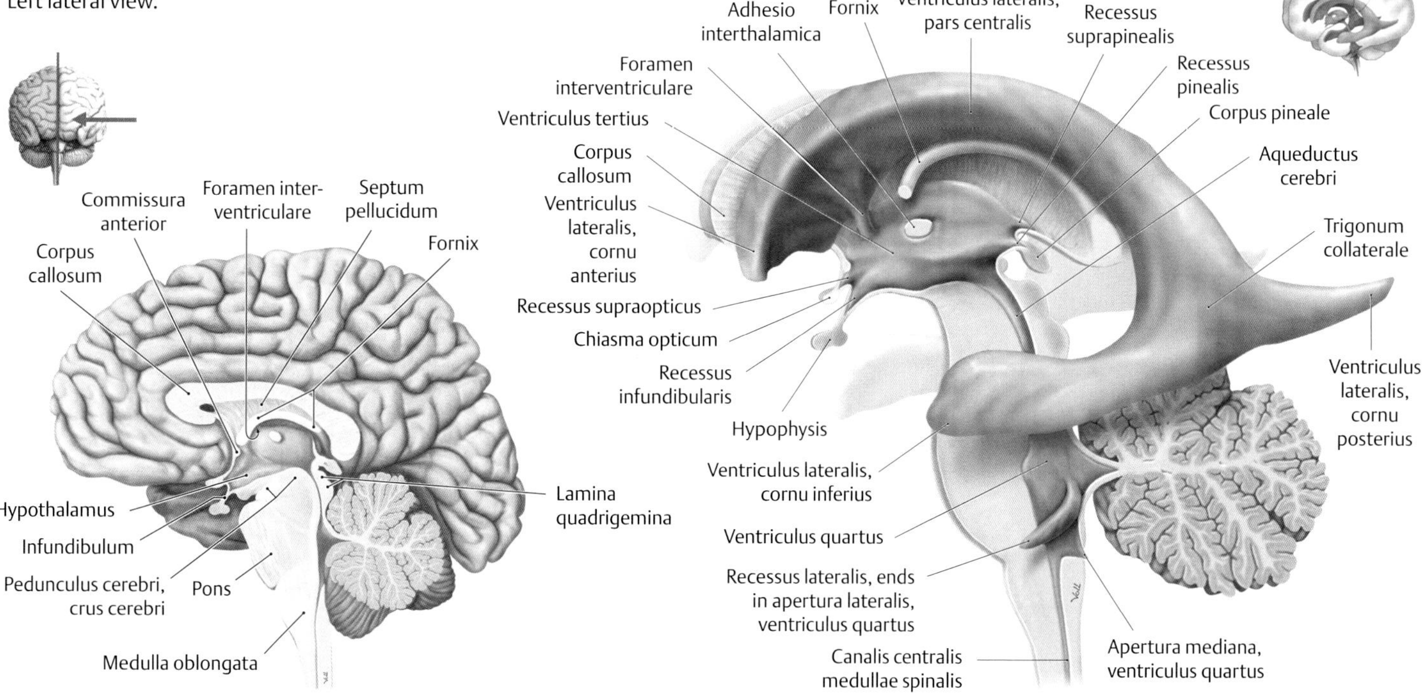
Commissura anterior
Foramen interventriculare
Septum pellucidum
Corpus callosum
Fornix
Hypothalamus
Infundibulum
Pedunculus cerebri, crus cerebri
Pons
Medulla oblongata
Lamina quadrigemina
Adhesio interthalamica
Fornix
Ventriculus lateralis, pars centralis
Recessus suprapinealis
Foramen interventriculare
Recessus pinealis
Ventriculus tertius
Corpus pineale
Corpus callosum
Aqueductus cerebri
Ventriculus lateralis, cornu anterius
Trigonum collaterale
Recessus supraopticus
Chiasma opticum
Recessus infundibularis
Ventriculus lateralis, cornu posterius
Hypophysis
Ventriculus lateralis, cornu inferius
Ventriculus quartus
Recessus lateralis, ends in apertura lateralis, ventriculus quartus
Canalis centralis medullae spinalis
Apertura mediana, ventriculus quartus

A 3rd and 4th ventricles in the midsagittal section.

B Ventricular system with neighboring structures.

Sinus Durae Matris & Veins of the Brain

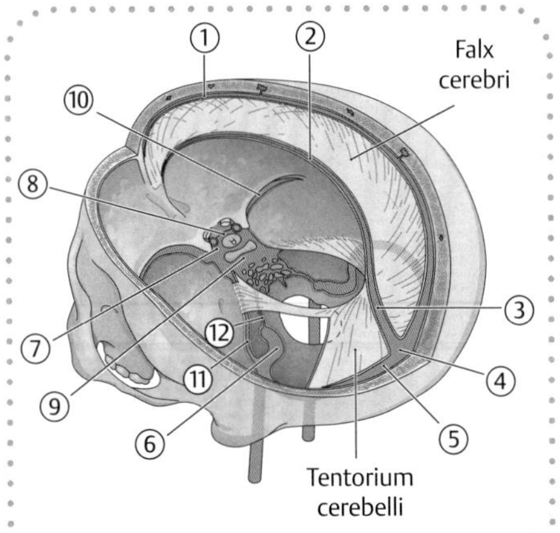

Falx cerebri
Tentorium cerebelli

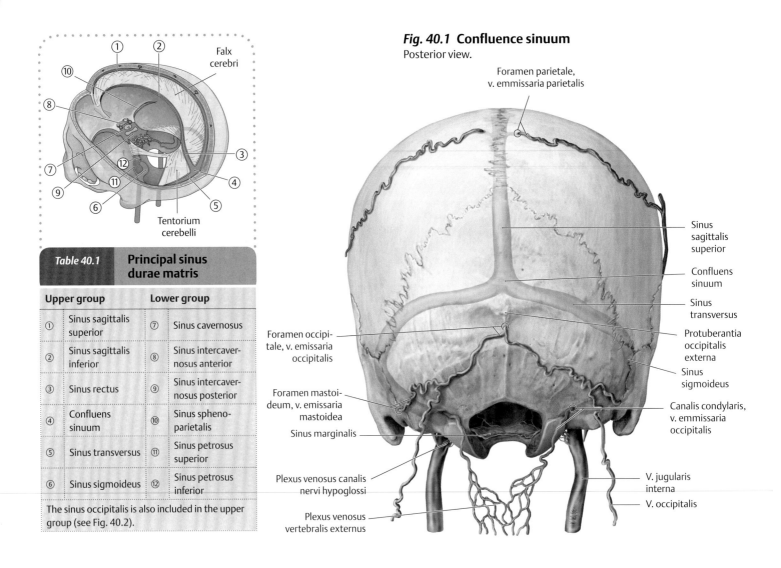

Table 40.1 Principal sinus durae matris

	Upper group		Lower group
①	Sinus sagittalis superior	⑦	Sinus cavernosus
②	Sinus sagittalis inferior	⑧	Sinus intercavernosus anterior
③	Sinus rectus	⑨	Sinus intercavernosus posterior
④	Confluens sinuum	⑩	Sinus sphenoparietalis
⑤	Sinus transversus	⑪	Sinus petrosus superior
⑥	Sinus sigmoideus	⑫	Sinus petrosus inferior

The sinus occipitalis is also included in the upper group (see Fig. 40.2).

***Fig. 40.1* Confluence sinuum**
Posterior view.

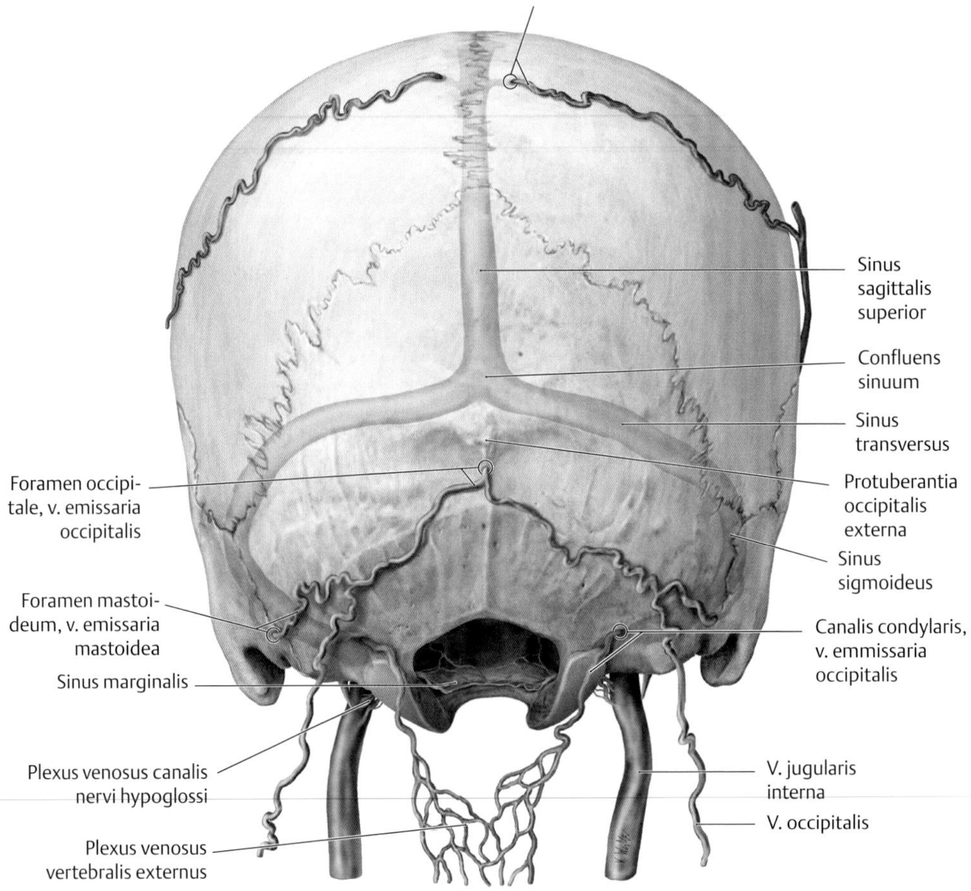

Foramen parietale, v. emmissaria parietalis
Sinus sagittalis superior
Confluens sinuum
Sinus transversus
Protuberantia occipitalis externa
Sinus sigmoideus
Canalis condylaris, v. emmissaria occipitalis
V. jugularis interna
V. occipitalis
Foramen occipitale, v. emissaria occipitalis
Foramen mastoideum, v. emissaria mastoidea
Sinus marginalis
Plexus venosus canalis nervi hypoglossi
Plexus venosus vertebralis externus

***Fig. 40.2* Vv. superficialis cerebri**

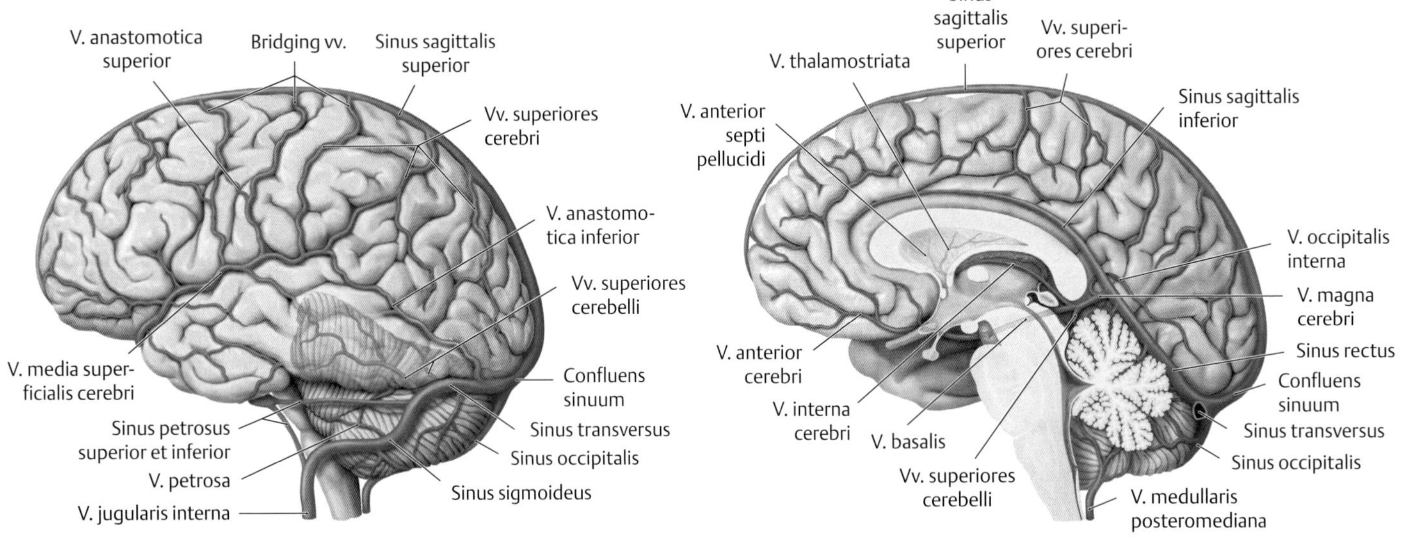
V. anastomotica superior
Bridging vv.
Sinus sagittalis superior
Vv. superiores cerebri
V. anastomotica inferior
Vv. superiores cerebelli
V. media superficialis cerebri
Confluens sinuum
Sinus petrosus superior et inferior
Sinus transversus
Sinus occipitalis
V. petrosa
Sinus sigmoideus
V. jugularis interna
Sinus sagittalis superior
Vv. superiores cerebri
V. thalamostriata
V. anterior septi pellucidi
Sinus sagittalis inferior
V. occipitalis interna
V. magna cerebri
Sinus rectus
V. anterior cerebri
Confluens sinuum
V. interna cerebri
Sinus transversus
V. basalis
Sinus occipitalis
Vv. superiores cerebelli
V. medullaris posteromediana

A Lateral view of the left hemisphere.

Fig. 40.3 **Basal cerebral venous system**
Basal view.

V. communicans anterior
V. inter-pedunculdaris
V. choroidea inferior
V. basalis
Confluens venosus posterior
V. media superficialis cerebri
V. anterior cerebri
V. media profunda cerebri
V. interna cerebri
V. magna cerebri

Fig. 40.4 **Veins of the brainstem**
Basal view.

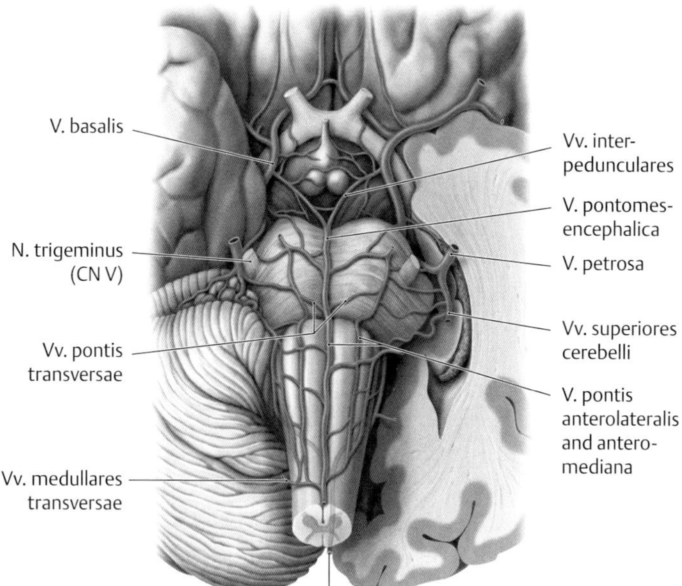

V. basalis
N. trigeminus (CN V)
Vv. pontis transversae
Vv. medullares transversae
V. medullaris posteromediana
Vv. inter-pedunculares
V. pontomes-encephalica
V. petrosa
Vv. superiores cerebelli
V. pontis anterolateralis and antero-mediana

Fig. 40.5 **Sinus durae matris in the skull base**
Superior view of the opened cranial cavity.
Removed: Tentorium cerebelli (right side).

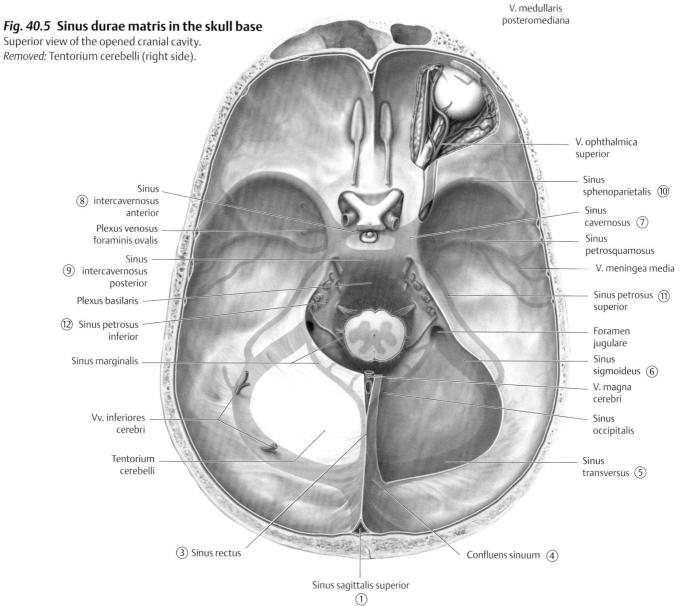

Sinus ⑧ intercavernosus anterior
Plexus venosus foraminis ovalis
Sinus ⑨ intercavernosus posterior
Plexus basilaris
⑫ Sinus petrosus inferior
Sinus marginalis
Vv. inferiores cerebri
Tentorium cerebelli
③ Sinus rectus
Sinus sagittalis superior ①
Confluens sinuum ④
V. ophthalmica superior
Sinus sphenoparietalis ⑩
Sinus cavernosus ⑦
Sinus petrosquamosus
V. meningea media
Sinus petrosus ⑪ superior
Foramen jugulare
Sinus sigmoideus ⑥
V. magna cerebri
Sinus occipitalis
Sinus transversus ⑤

Arteries of the Brain

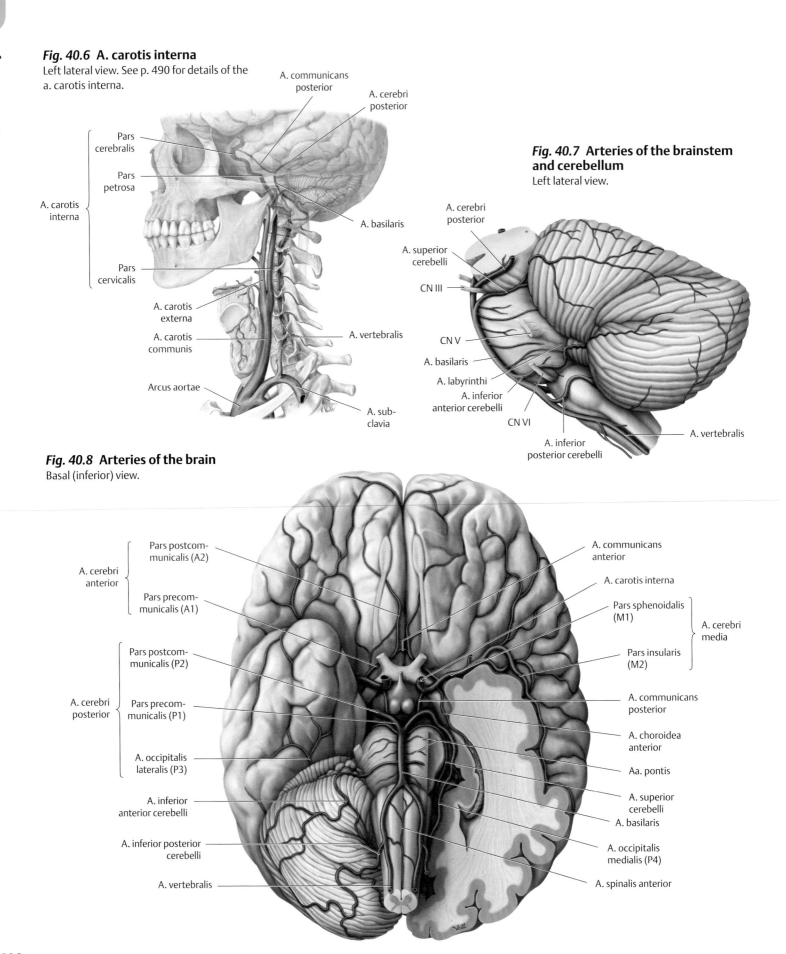

Fig. 40.6 A. carotis interna
Left lateral view. See p. 490 for details of the a. carotis interna.

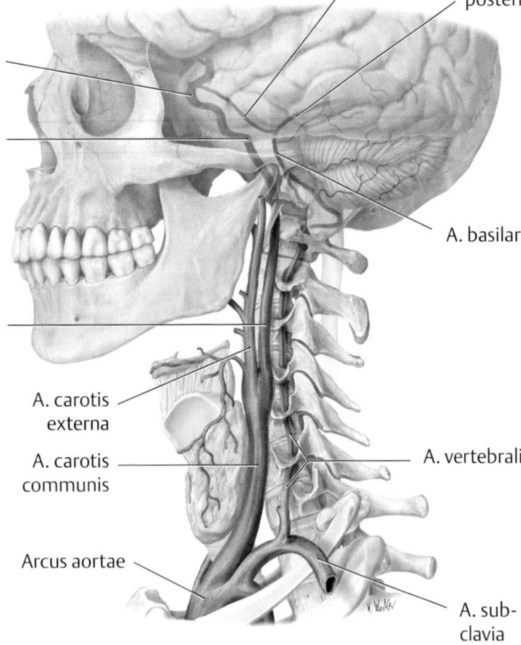

A. communicans posterior
A. cerebri posterior
Pars cerebralis
Pars petrosa
A. carotis interna
Pars cervicalis
A. basilaris
A. carotis externa
A. carotis communis
A. vertebralis
Arcus aortae
A. subclavia

Fig. 40.7 Arteries of the brainstem and cerebellum
Left lateral view.

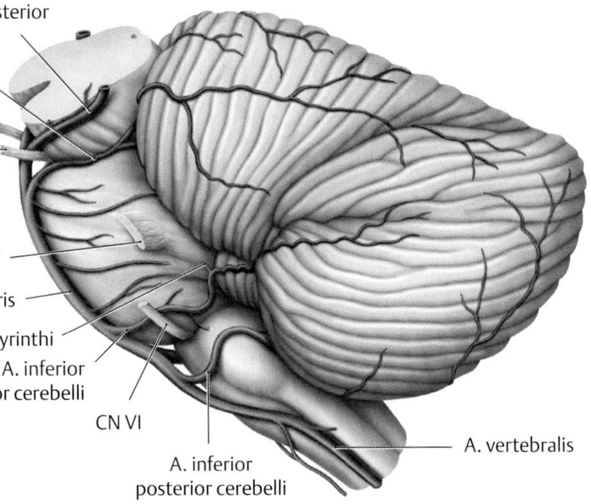

A. cerebri posterior
A. superior cerebelli
CN III
CN V
A. basilaris
A. labyrinthi
A. inferior anterior cerebelli
CN VI
A. inferior posterior cerebelli
A. vertebralis

Fig. 40.8 Arteries of the brain
Basal (inferior) view.

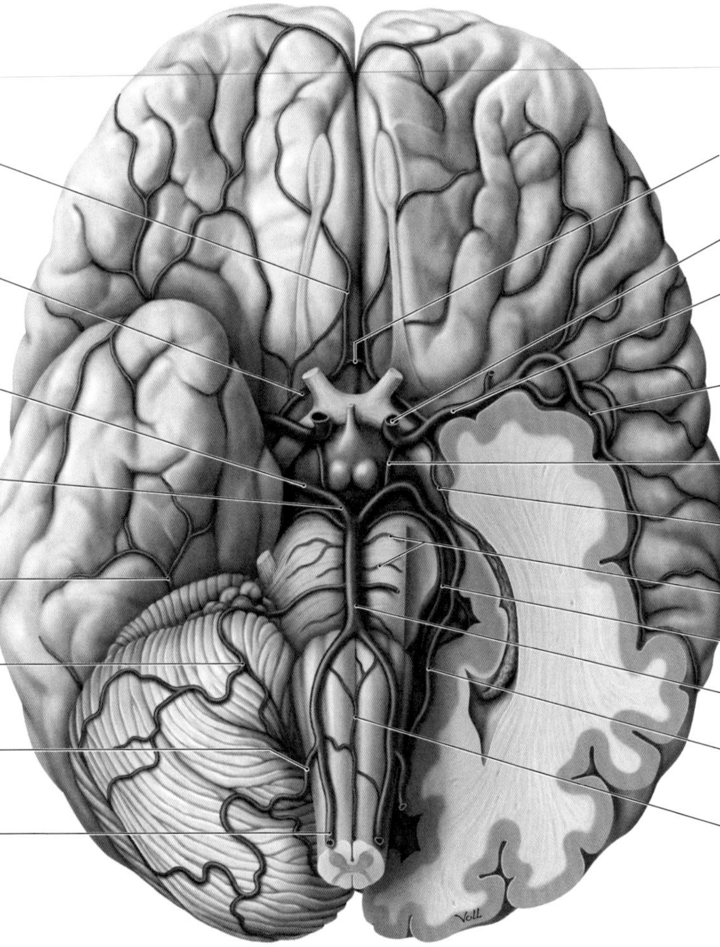

A. cerebri anterior
Pars postcommunicalis (A2)
Pars precommunicalis (A1)
A. cerebri posterior
Pars postcommunicalis (P2)
Pars precommunicalis (P1)
A. occipitalis lateralis (P3)
A. inferior anterior cerebelli
A. inferior posterior cerebelli
A. vertebralis
A. communicans anterior
A. carotis interna
A. cerebri media
Pars sphenoidalis (M1)
Pars insularis (M2)
A. communicans posterior
A. choroidea anterior
Aa. pontis
A. superior cerebelli
A. basilaris
A. occipitalis medialis (P4)
A. spinalis anterior

Fig. 40.9 Cerebral arteries

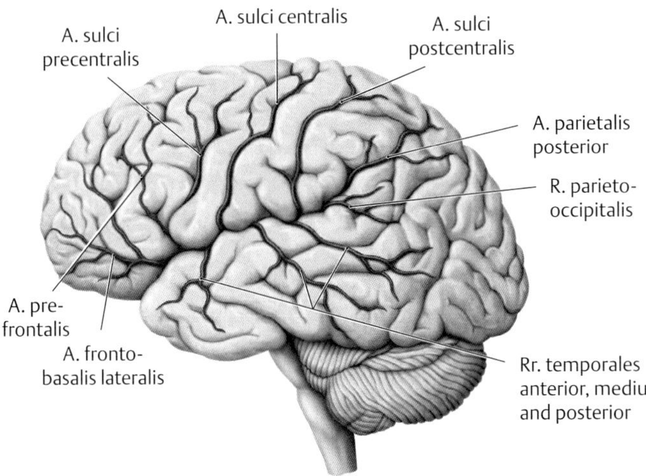
A. sulci precentralis
A. sulci centralis
A. sulci postcentralis
A. parietalis posterior
R. parieto-occipitalis
A. pre-frontalis
A. fronto-basalis lateralis
Rr. temporales anterior, medius and posterior

A A. cerebri media. Lateral view of the left hemisphere.

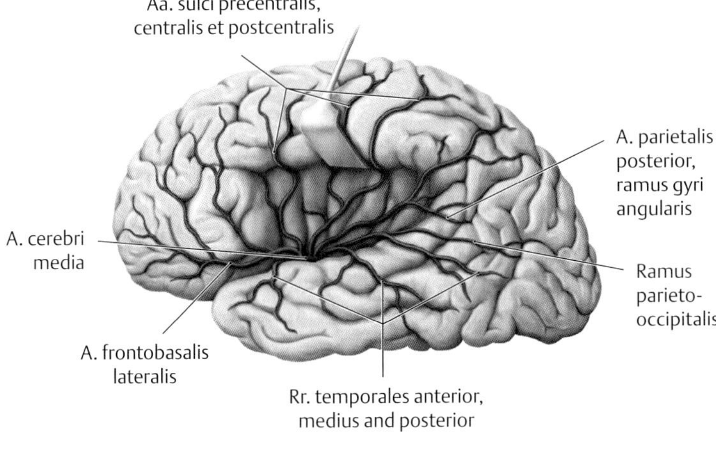
Aa. sulci precentralis, centralis et postcentralis
A. parietalis posterior, ramus gyri angularis
A. cerebri media
Ramus parieto-occipitalis
A. frontobasalis lateralis
Rr. temporales anterior, medius and posterior

B A. cerebri media. Left lateral view with the lateral sulcus retracted.

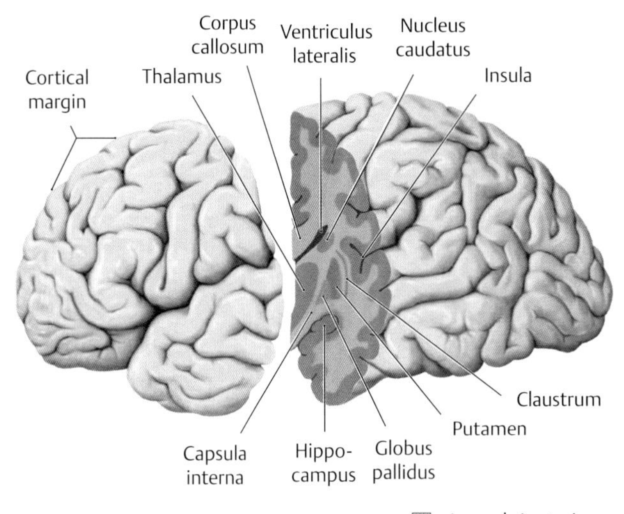
A. pericallosa
R. cingularis
Rr. para-centrales
A. calloso-marginalis
Rr. pre-cuneales
R. corporis callosi dorsalis
A. polaris frontalis
R. pari-etalis
A. cerebri anterior
A. occipitalis medialis (P4)
A. cerebri posterior
A. occipitalis lateralis (P3)
Rr. temporalis medii and posteriores

C Aa. cerebri anterior and posterior. Medial view of the right hemisphere.

Fig. 40.10 Cerebral arteries: Distribution areas
The central gray and white matter have a complex blood supply (yellow) that includes a. choroidea anterior.

Corpus callosum
Ventriculus lateralis
Nucleus caudatus
Cortical margin
Thalamus
Insula
Claustrum
Putamen
Capsula interna
Hippo-campus
Globus pallidus
A. cerebri anterior
A. cerebri media
A. cerebri posterior

A Lateral view of the left hemisphere.

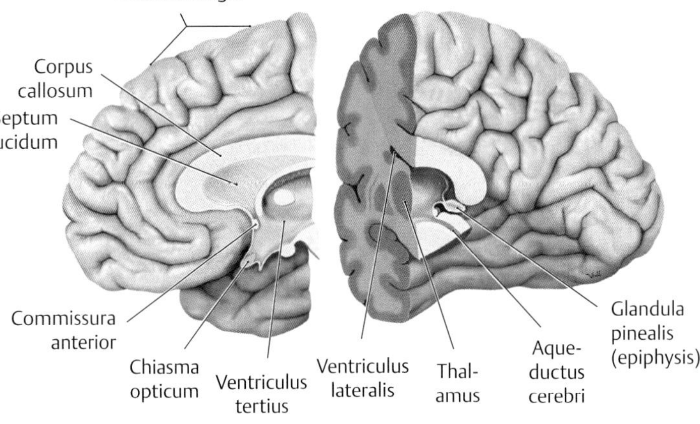
Cortical margin
Corpus callosum
Septum pellucidum
Commissura anterior
Chiasma opticum
Ventriculus tertius
Ventriculus lateralis
Thal-amus
Aque-ductus cerebri
Glandula pinealis (epiphysis)

B Medial view of the right hemisphere.

Arteries & Veins of Medulla Spinalis

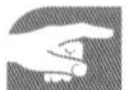

Like medulla spinalis itself, the arteries and veins of medulla spinalis consist of multiple horizontal systems (blood vessels of the spinal cord segments) that are integrated into a vertical system.

Fig. 40.11 Arteries of medulla spinalis

The unpaired anterior and paired posterior spinal arteries typically arise from the vertebral arteries. As they descend within canalis vertebralis, the spinal arteries are reinforced by anterior and posterior radicular arteries. Depending on the spinal level, these reinforcing branches may arise from the vertebral, ascending or deep cervical, posterior intercostal, lumbar, or lateral sacral arteries.

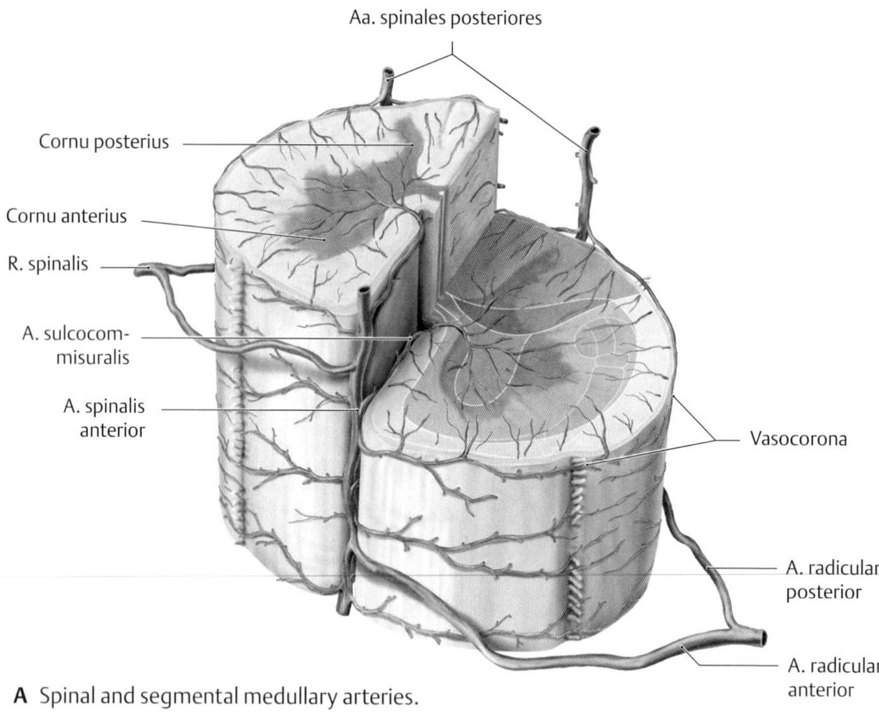
Aa. spinales posteriores
Cornu posterius
Cornu anterius
R. spinalis
A. sulcocommisuralis
A. spinalis anterior
Vasocorona
A. radicularis posterior
A. radicularis anterior

A Spinal and segmental medullary arteries.

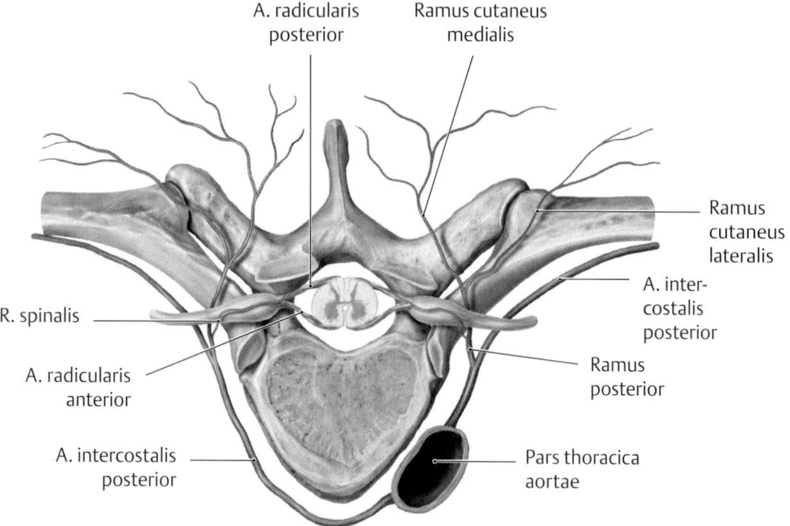
A. radicularis posterior
Ramus cutaneus medialis
Ramus cutaneus lateralis
A. intercostalis posterior
R. spinalis
A. radicularis anterior
Ramus posterior
A. intercostalis posterior
Pars thoracica aortae

B Origins of the radicular arteries. In the thorax, the segmental medullary arteries arise from the spinal branch of the posterior intercostal arteries (see p. 34).

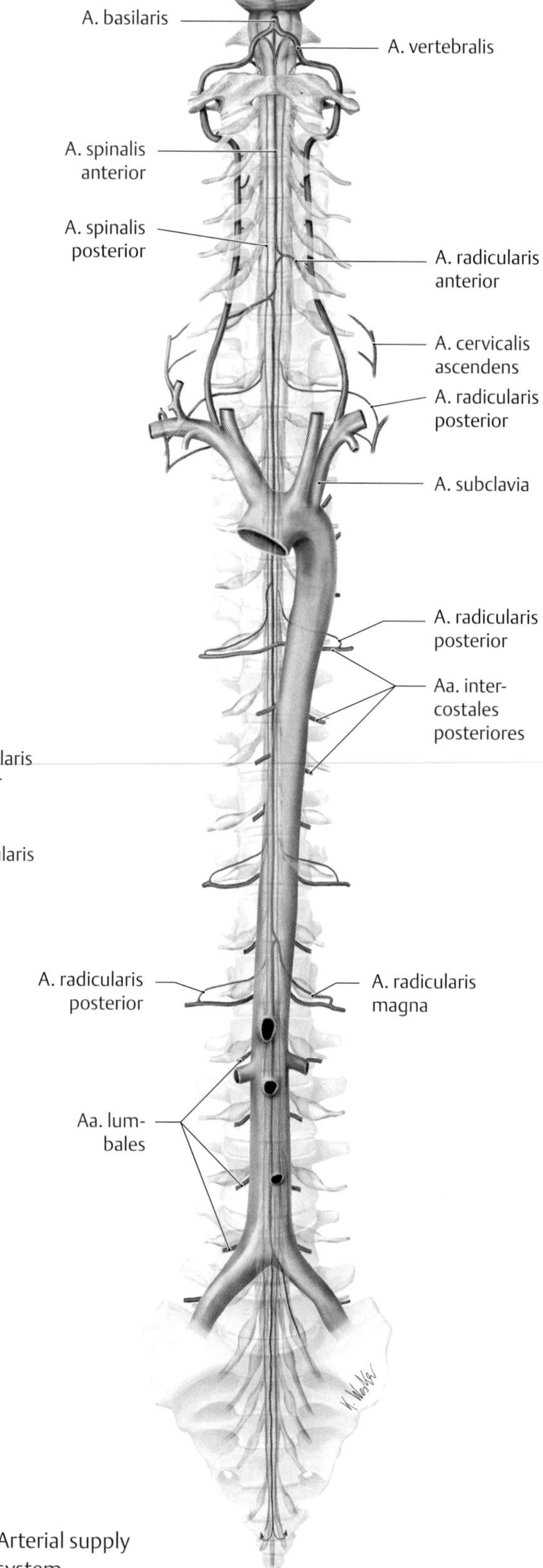
A. basilaris
A. vertebralis
A. spinalis anterior
A. spinalis posterior
A. radicularis anterior
A. cervicalis ascendens
A. radicularis posterior
A. subclavia
A. radicularis posterior
Aa. intercostales posteriores
A. radicularis posterior
A. radicularis magna
Aa. lumbales

C Arterial supply system.

Fig. 40.12 **Veins of medulla spinalis**

The interior of medulla spinalis drains via venous plexuses into vv. spinales anterior and posterior. The radicular and spinal veins connect the veins of the spinal cord with the plexus venosus vertebralis internus. The vv. intervertebrales and basivertebrales connect the internal and external venous plexuses, which drain into the azygos system.

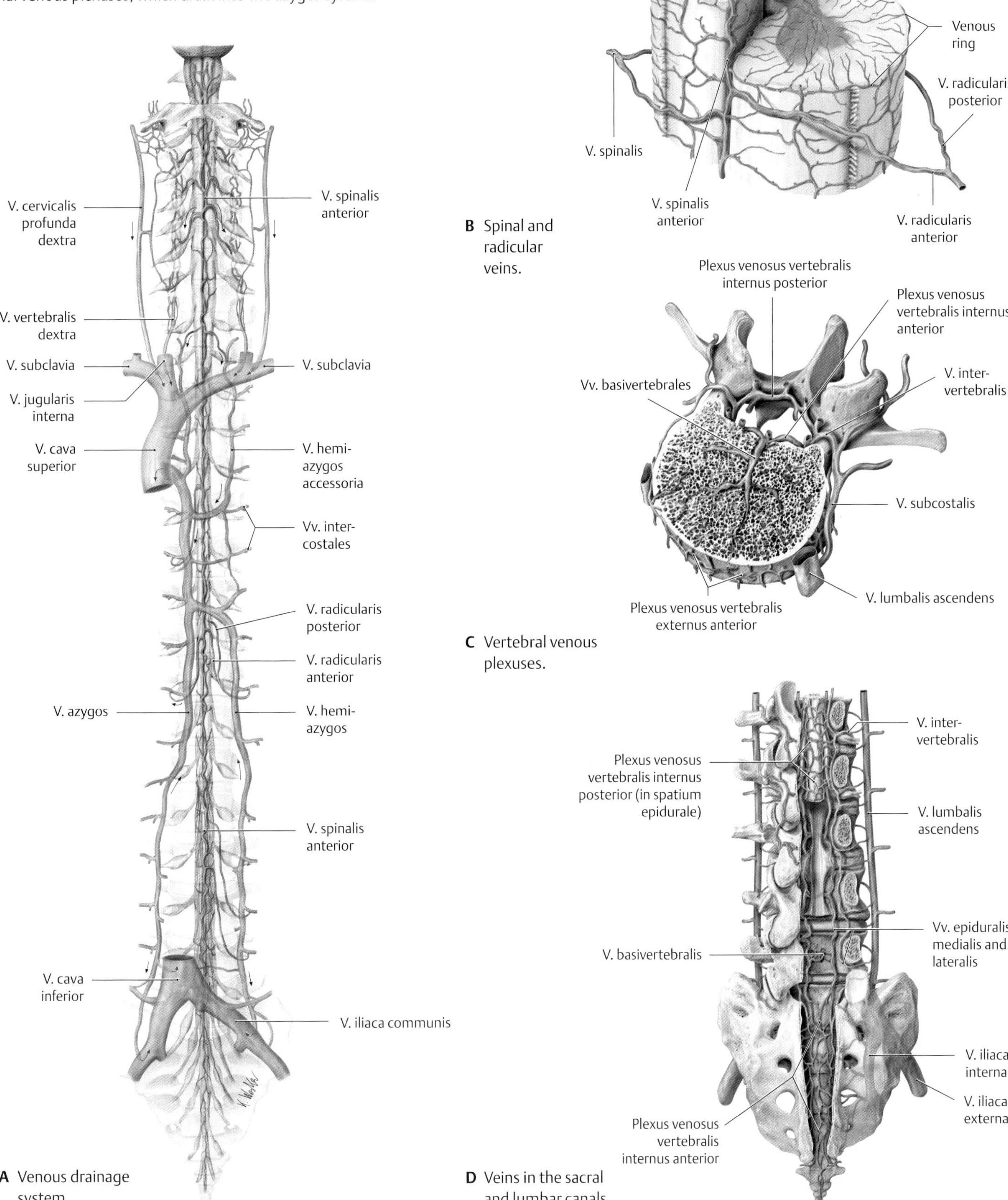
V. cervicalis profunda dextra
V. spinalis anterior
V. vertebralis dextra
V. subclavia
V. subclavia
V. jugularis interna
V. cava superior
V. hemi-azygos accessoria
Vv. inter-costales
V. radicularis posterior
V. radicularis anterior
V. azygos
V. hemi-azygos
V. spinalis anterior
V. cava inferior
V. iliaca communis
V. spinalis posterior
V. sulcalis
Venous ring
V. radicularis posterior
V. spinalis
V. spinalis anterior
V. radicularis anterior
Plexus venosus vertebralis internus posterior
Plexus venosus vertebralis internus anterior
Vv. basivertebrales
V. inter-vertebralis
V. subcostalis
V. lumbalis ascendens
Plexus venosus vertebralis externus anterior
V. inter-vertebralis
Plexus venosus vertebralis internus posterior (in spatium epidurale)
V. lumbalis ascendens
Vv. epiduralis medialis and lateralis
V. basivertebralis
V. iliaca interna
V. iliaca externa
Plexus venosus vertebralis internus anterior

A Venous drainage system.

B Spinal and radicular veins.

C Vertebral venous plexuses.

D Veins in the sacral and lumbar canals.

Circuitry

Fig. 41.1 Divisions of the nervous system

Direction of information flow divides nerve fibers into two types: afferent (sensory) fibers, which transmit impulses toward the central nervous system (CNS), and efferent (motor) fibers, which transmit impulses away. The nervous system may also be divided into a somatic and an autonomic part. The somatic nervous system mediates interaction with the environment, whereas the autonomic (visceral) nervous system coordinates the function of the internal organs.

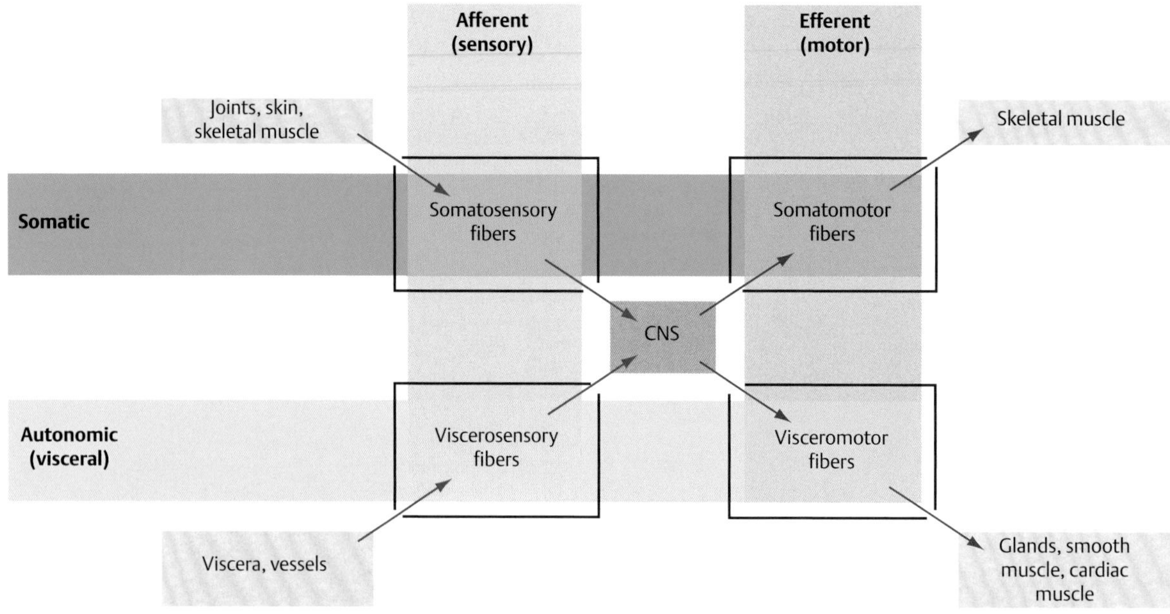
Afferent (sensory)
Efferent (motor)
Joints, skin, skeletal muscle
Skeletal muscle
Somatic
Somatosensory fibers
Somatomotor fibers
CNS
Autonomic (visceral)
Viscerosensory fibers
Visceromotor fibers
Viscera, vessels
Glands, smooth muscle, cardiac muscle

Fig. 41.2 Organization of substantia grisea

Left oblique anterosuperior view. Substantia grisea of the spinal cord is divided into three columns (horns). Afferent (blue) and efferent (red) neurons within these columns are clustered according to function.

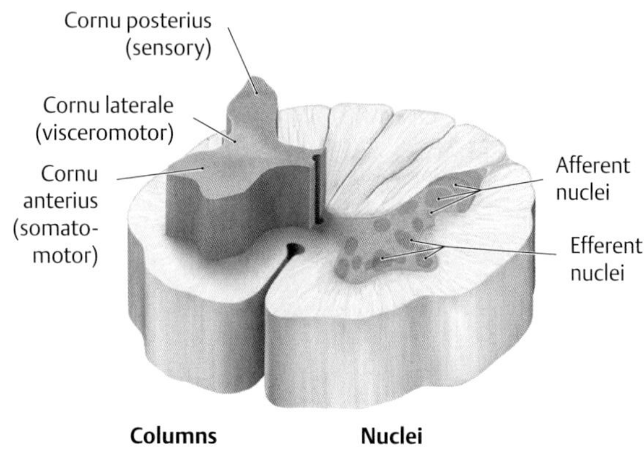
Cornu posterius (sensory)
Cornu laterale (visceromotor)
Cornu anterius (somato-motor)
Afferent nuclei
Efferent nuclei
Columns
Nuclei

Fig. 41.3 Muscle innervation

Indicator muscles are innervated by motor neurons in the anterior horn of one spinal cord segment. Most muscles (multisegmental muscles) receive innervation from a motor column, a vertical arrangement of motor nuclei spanning several segments.

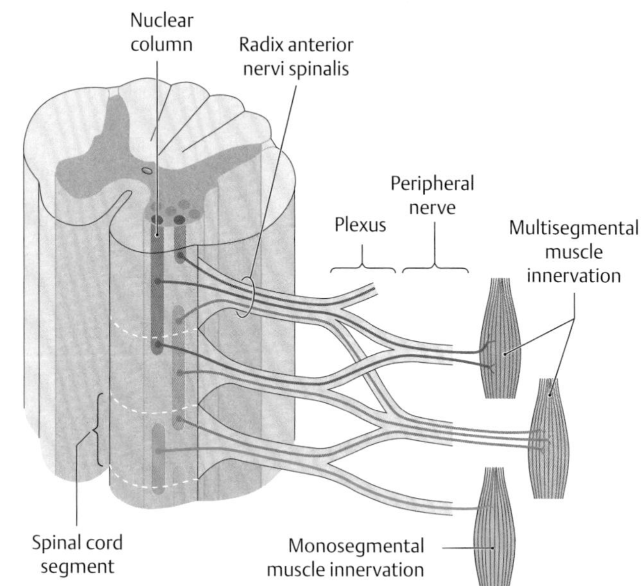
Nuclear column
Radix anterior nervi spinalis
Peripheral nerve
Plexus
Multisegmental muscle innervation
Spinal cord segment
Monosegmental muscle innervation

Fig. 41.4 Reflexes

Muscular function at the unconscious (reflex) level is controlled by substantia grisea of medulla spinalis.

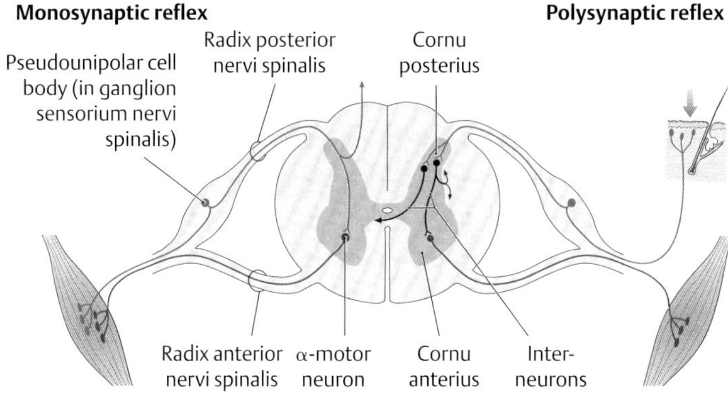

Monosynaptic reflex
Polysynaptic reflex
Radix posterior nervi spinalis
Cornu posterius
Pseudounipolar cell body (in ganglion sensorium nervi spinalis)
Radix anterior nervi spinalis
α-motor neuron
Cornu anterius
Inter-neurons

A Polysynaptic reflexes may be mediated by receptors inside of or remote from the muscle (i.e., skin); these receptors act via interneurons to stimulate muscle contraction.

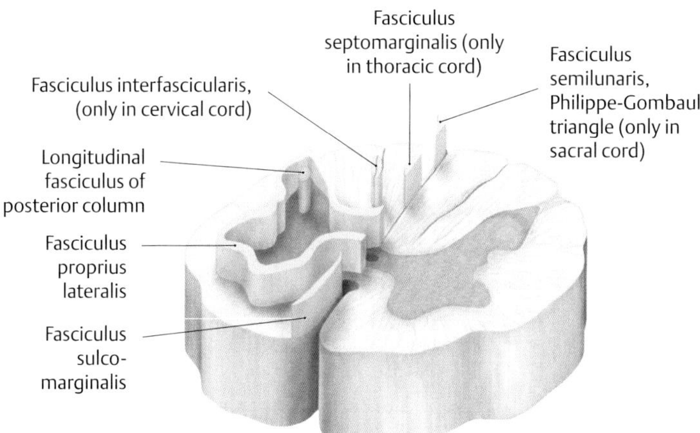

Fasciculus septomarginalis (only in thoracic cord)
Fasciculus interfascicularis, (only in cervical cord)
Fasciculus semilunaris, Philippe-Gombault triangle (only in sacral cord)
Longitudinal fasciculus of posterior column
Fasciculus proprius lateralis
Fasciculus sulco-marginalis

B Principal intrinsic fascicles of the spinal cord. The intrinsic fascicles are the conduction apparatus of the intrinsic circuits, allowing axons to ascend and descend to coordinate spinal reflexes for multisegmental muscles.

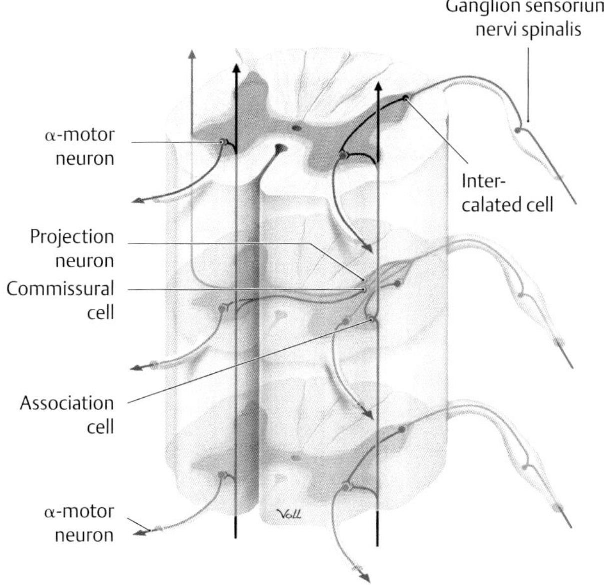

Ganglion sensorium nervi spinalis
α-motor neuron
Inter-calated cell
Projection neuron
Commissural cell
Association cell
α-motor neuron

C Intrinsic circuits of the spinal cord.

Fig. 41.5 Sensory and motor systems

The sensory system (see p. 614) and motor system (see p. 615) are so functionally interrelated they may be described as one (sensorimotor system).

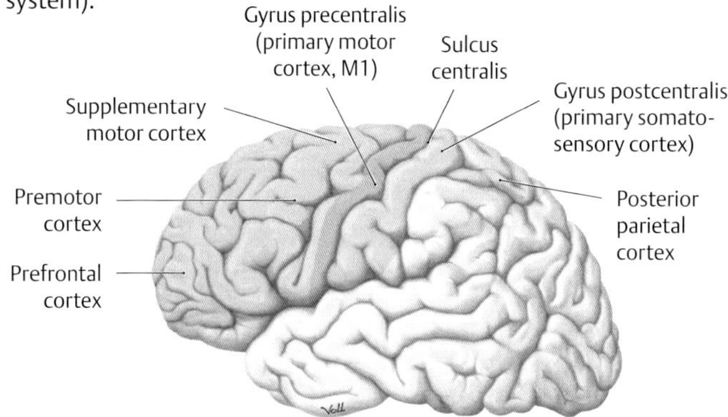

Gyrus precentralis (primary motor cortex, M1)
Sulcus centralis
Gyrus postcentralis (primary somato-sensory cortex)
Supplementary motor cortex
Premotor cortex
Posterior parietal cortex
Prefrontal cortex

A Cortical areas of the sensorimotor system. Lateral view of the left hemisphere.

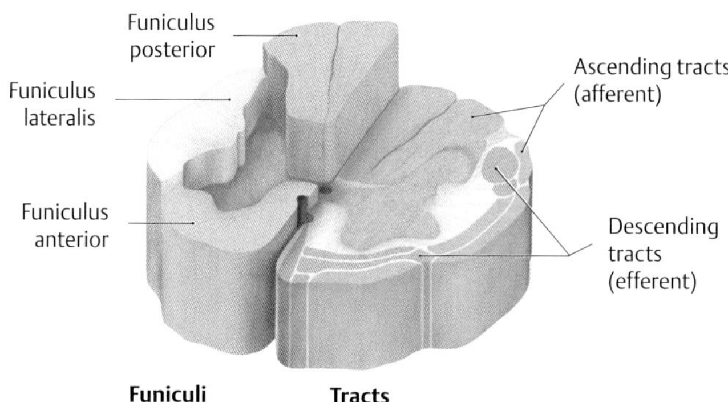

Funiculus posterior
Funiculus lateralis
Ascending tracts (afferent)
Funiculus anterior
Descending tracts (efferent)
Funiculi
Tracts

B White matter of the spinal cord. The white matter of the spinal cord contains ascending tracts (afferent, see p. 614) and descending tracts (efferent, see p. 615), which are the CNS equivalent of peripheral nerves.

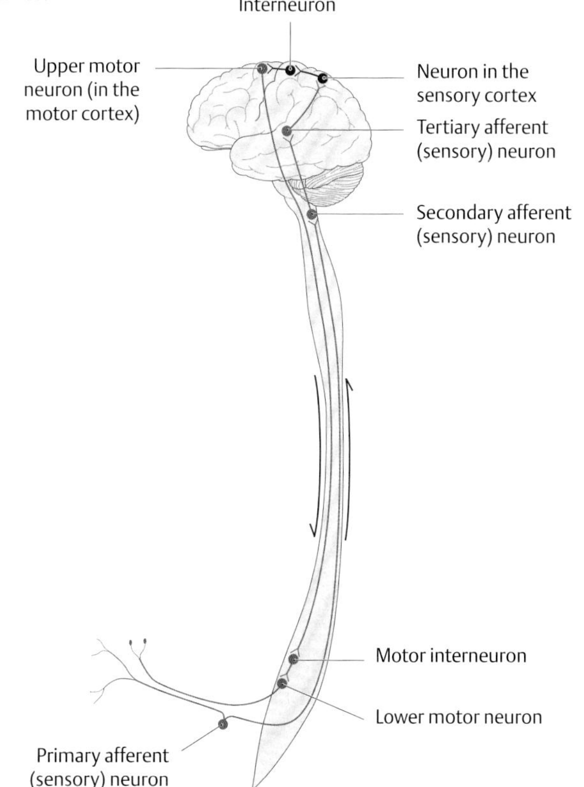

Interneuron
Upper motor neuron (in the motor cortex)
Neuron in the sensory cortex
Tertiary afferent (sensory) neuron
Secondary afferent (sensory) neuron
Motor interneuron
Lower motor neuron
Primary afferent (sensory) neuron

C Overview of sensorimotor integration.

Fig. 41.6 **Sensory pathways (ascending tracts)**

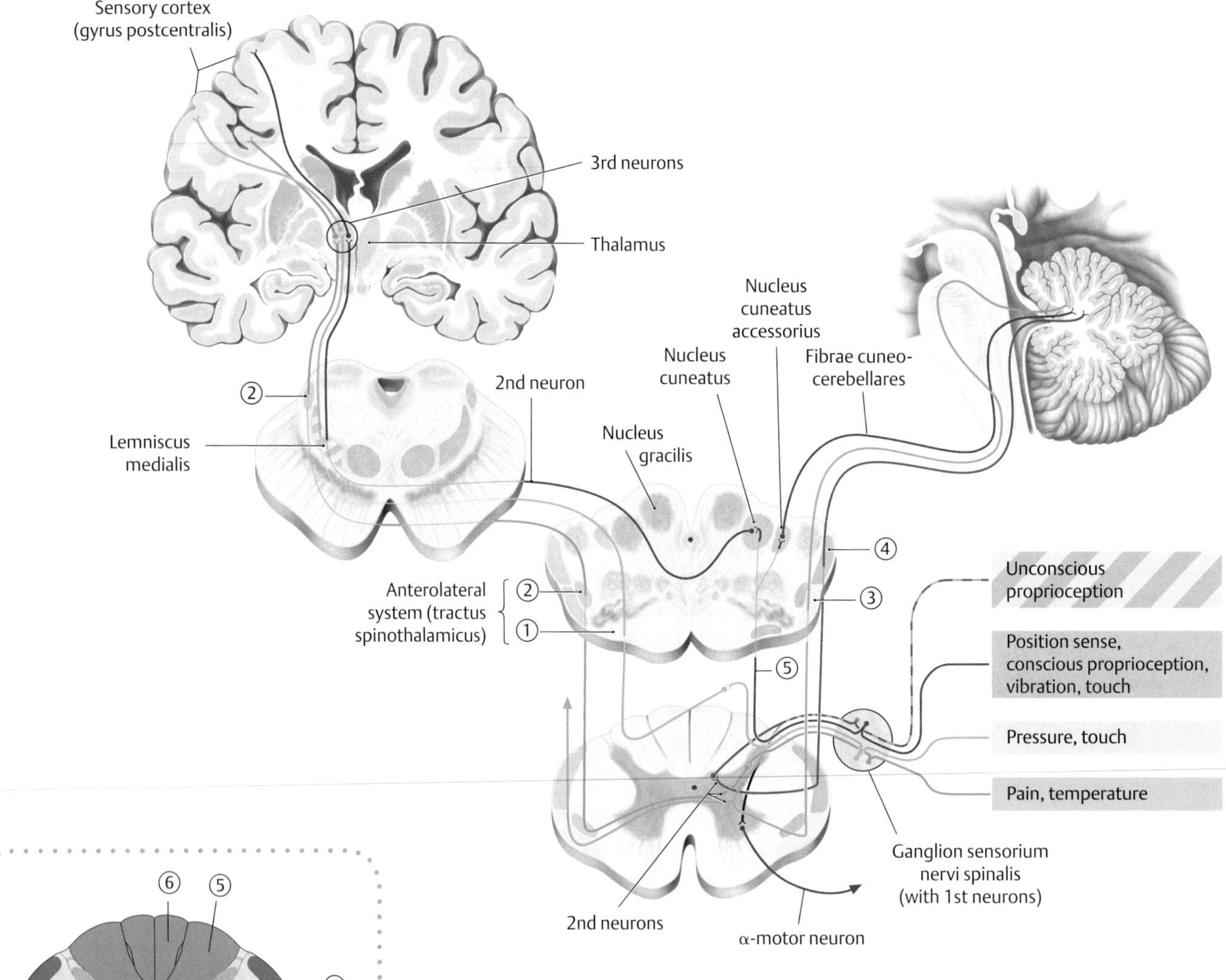
Sensory cortex (gyrus postcentralis)
3rd neurons
Thalamus
Nucleus cuneatus accessorius
Nucleus cuneatus
Fibrae cuneo-cerebellares
2nd neuron
②
Lemniscus medialis
Nucleus gracilis
④
Unconscious proprioception
Anterolateral system (tractus spinothalamicus)
②
①
③
⑤
Position sense, conscious proprioception, vibration, touch
Pressure, touch
Pain, temperature
Ganglion sensorium nervi spinalis (with 1st neurons)
2nd neurons
α-motor neuron
⑥
⑤
④
③
②
①

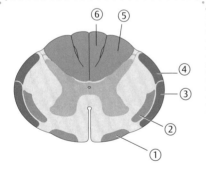

*The fasciculi cuneatus and gracilus convey information from the upper and lower limbs, respectively. At this level of medulla spinalis, only the fasciculus cuneatus is present.

Table 41.1 **Ascending tracts of the spinal cord**

	Tract	Location	Function		Neurons
①	Tractus spinothalamicus anterior	Funiculus anterior	Pathway for crude touch and pressure sensation		1st afferent neurons located in spinal ganglia; contain 2nd neurons and cross in commissura anterior
②	Tractus spinothalamicus lateralis	Funiculus lateralis and anterior	Pathway for pain, temperature, tickle, itch, and sexual sensation		
③	Tractus spinocerebellaris anterior	Funiculus lateralis	Pathway for unconscious coordination of motor activities (unconscious proprioception, automatic processes, e.g., jogging, riding a bike) to the cerebellum		Projection (2nd) neurons receive proprioceptive signals from 1st afferent fibers originating at the 1st neurons of spinal ganglia
④	Tractus spinocerebellaris posterior				
⑤	Fasciculus cuneatus	Funiculus posterior	Pathway for position sense (conscious proprioception) and fine cutaneous sensation (touch, vibration, fine pressure sense, two-point discrimination)	Conveys information from *upper* limb (not present below T3)	Cell bodies of 1st neuron located in spinal ganglion; pass uncrossed to the dorsal column nuclei
⑥	Fasciculus gracilis			Conveys information from *lower* limb	

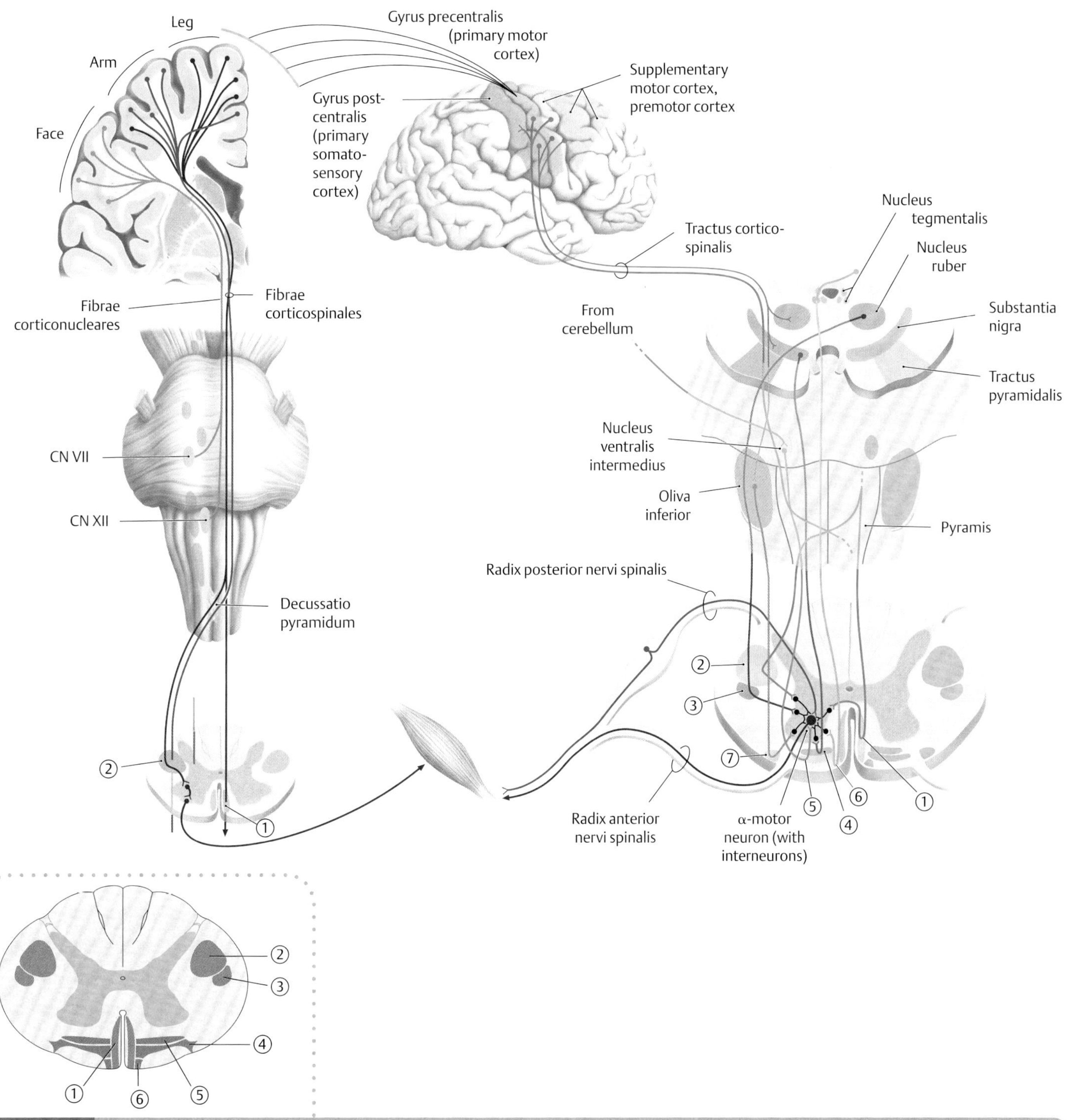

Leg
Arm
Face
Gyrus precentralis (primary motor cortex)
Gyrus post-centralis (primary somato-sensory cortex)
Supplementary motor cortex, premotor cortex
Fibrae corticonucleares
Fibrae corticospinales
CN VII
CN XII
Decussatio pyramidum
Tractus cortico-spinalis
Nucleus tegmentalis
Nucleus ruber
Substantia nigra
Tractus pyramidalis
From cerebellum
Nucleus ventralis intermedius
Oliva inferior
Pyramis
Radix posterior nervi spinalis
Radix anterior nervi spinalis
α-motor neuron (with interneurons)
①
②
③
④
⑤
⑥
⑦

***Fig. 41.7* Motor pathways (descending tracts)**

Table 41.2 Descending tracts of the spinal cord

Tract			Function	
Pyramidal tract	①	Tractus corticospinalis anterior	Most important pathway for voluntary motor function	Originates in the motor cortex *Corticonuclear* fibers to motor nuclei of cranial nerves *Corticospinal* fibers to motor cells in anterior horn of the spinal cord *Corticoreticular* fibers to nuclei of the reticular formation
	②	Tractus corticospinalis lateralis		
Descending pathways originating in the brainstem	③	Tractus rubrospinalis	Pathway for automatic and learned motor processes (e.g., walking, running, cycling)	
	④	Tractus reticulospinalis		
	⑤	Tractus vestibulospinalis		
	⑥	Tractus tectospinalis		
	⑦	Tractus olivospinalis		

Sensory Systems (I)

Table 41.3 Special sensory qualities (senses)

Sense	Cranial nerve		Ref.
Vision	N. opticus (CN II)		See p. 473
Balance	N. vestibulocochlearis (CN VIII)	N. vestibularis	See p. 480
Hearing		N. cochlearis	See p. 481
Taste	N. facialis (CN VII)		See p. 478
	N. glossopharyngeus (CN IX)		See p. 482
	N. vagus (CN X)		See p. 484
Smell	N. olfactorius (CN I)		See p. 472

Fig. 41.8 Visual system: Overview

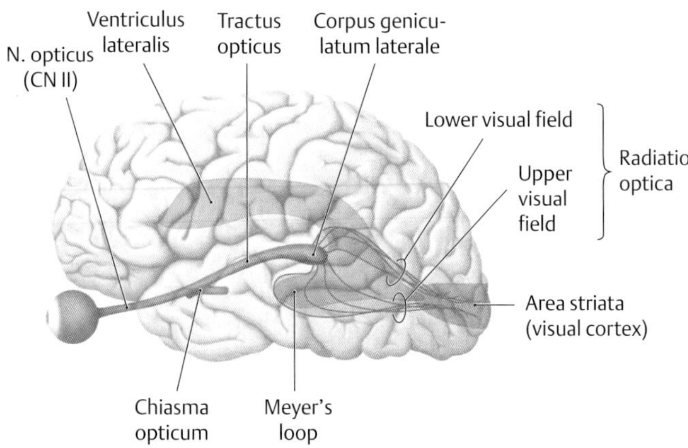

Ventriculus lateralis
Tractus opticus
Corpus geniculatum laterale
N. opticus (CN II)
Lower visual field
Upper visual field
Radiatio optica
Area striata (visual cortex)
Chiasma opticum
Meyer's loop

A Left lateral view.

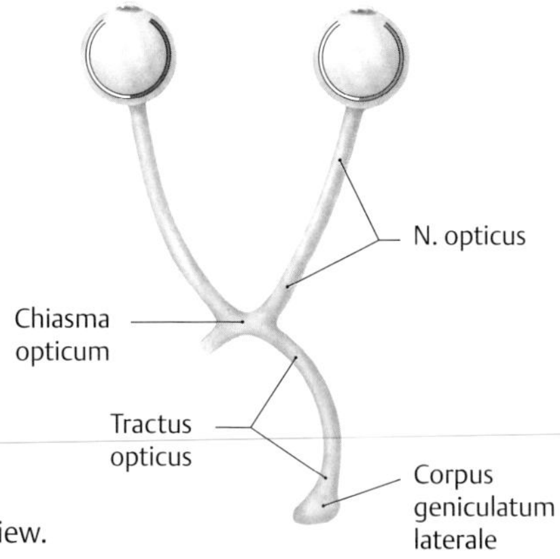

N. opticus
Chiasma opticum
Tractus opticus
Corpus geniculatum laterale

B Inferior view.

Fig. 41.9 Visual pathways

90% of optic nerve fibers terminate in corpus geniculatum laterale on neurons that project to the area striata (visual cortex). This forms the geniculate pathway, responsible for conscious visual perception. The remaining 10% travel along the medial root of the optic tract, forming the non-geniculate pathway. This pathway plays an important role in the unconscious regulation of vision-related processes and reflexes.

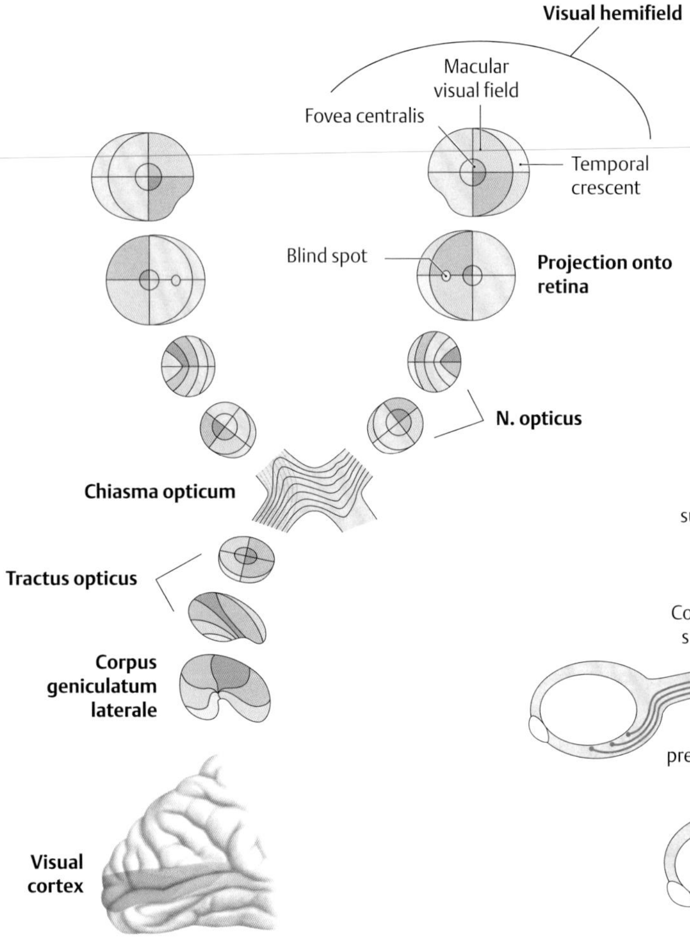

Visual hemifield
Macular visual field
Fovea centralis
Temporal crescent
Blind spot
Projection onto retina
N. opticus
Chiasma opticum
Tractus opticus
Corpus geniculatum laterale
Visual cortex

A Geniculate pathway. Left visual hemifield.

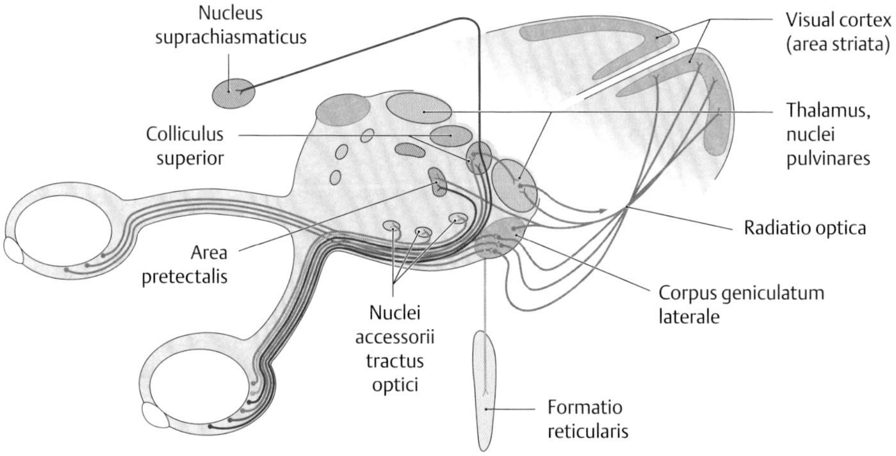

Nucleus suprachiasmaticus
Visual cortex (area striata)
Thalamus, nuclei pulvinares
Colliculus superior
Radiatio optica
Area pretectalis
Corpus geniculatum laterale
Nuclei accessorii tractus optici
Formatio reticularis

B Non-geniculate pathway.

Clinical

Lesions of the visual pathway

Visual field defects and lesion sites are here illustrated for the left visual pathway.

1 Unilateral lesion of n. opticus.
Blindness in affected eye

2 Lesion of chiasma opticum
Bitemporal hemianopia ("blinders")

3 Unilateral lesion of tractus opticus
Contralateral homonymous hemianopia

4 Unilateral lesion of radiatio optica in Meyer's loop (anterior temporal lobe)
Contralateral upper quadrantanopia ("pie-in-the-sky")

5 Unilateral lesion of radiatio optica, medial part
Contralateral lower quadrantanopia

6 Lesion of lobus occipitalis
Homonymous hemianopia

7 Lesion of polus occipitalis (cortical areas)
Homonymous hemianopic central scotoma

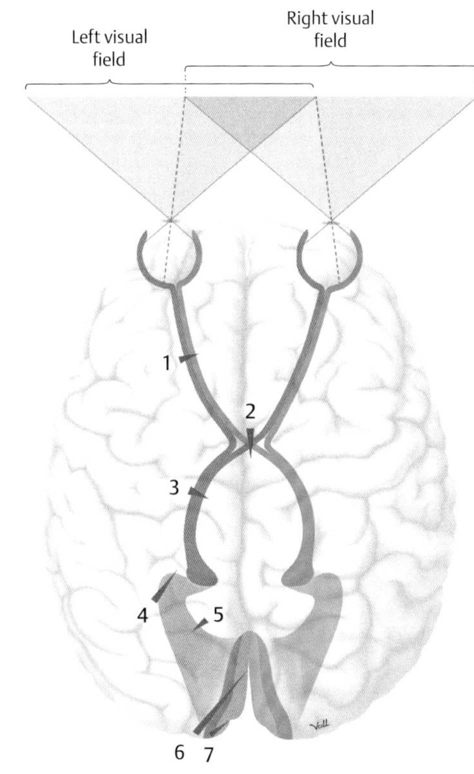
Left visual field
Right visual field
1
2
3
4
5
6
7

Fig. 41.10 Reflexes of the visual system

The reflexes of the visual system are mediated by the optic (afferent) and oculomotor (efferent) nerves.

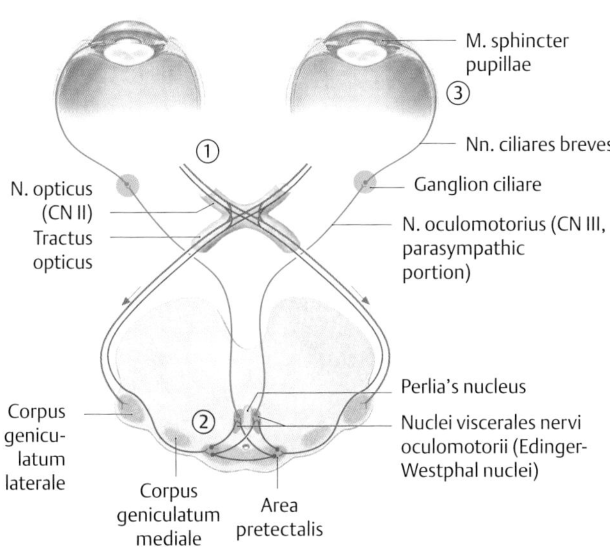
M. sphincter pupillae
③
①
Nn. ciliares breves
Ganglion ciliare
N. opticus (CN II)
Tractus opticus
N. oculomotorius (CN III, parasympathetic portion)
Perlia's nucleus
Corpus genicu-latum laterale
②
Nuclei viscerales nervi oculomotorii (Edinger-Westphal nuclei)
Corpus geniculatum mediale
Area pretectalis

A Pupillary light reflex.
① Incoming light is transmitted via the n. opticus.
② Large amounts of light are transmitted to the pretectal area, bypassing the geniculate pathway.
③ The neurons of the visceral oculomotor nucleus synapse on ganglion ciliare, which induces contraction of sphincter pupillae.

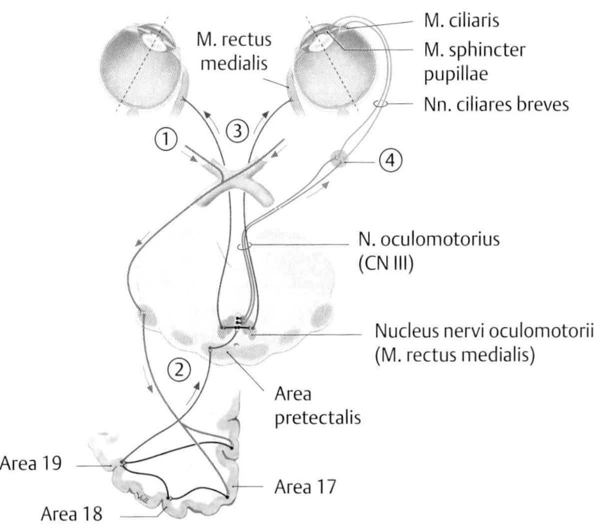
M. rectus medialis
M. ciliaris
M. sphincter pupillae
Nn. ciliares breves
①
③
④
N. oculomotorius (CN III)
Nucleus nervi oculomotorii (M. rectus medialis)
②
Area pretectalis
Area 19
Area 17
Area 18

B Pathways for convergence and accommodation.
① Light is received from an approaching object.
② Information is relayed via the primary (17) and secondary (19) visual cortices to the nuclei of n. oculomotorius.
③ Convergence: Constriction of the m. rectus medialis converges the visual axes of the eyes, keeping the approaching image on the fovea centralis, the point of maximum visual acuity.
④ Accommodation: The curvature of the lens is increased via contraction of the m. ciliaris. The m. sphincter pupillae also contracts.

Sensory Systems (II)

Fig. 41.11 **Balance**
Human balance is regulated by the visual, proprioceptive, and vestibular systems. All three systems send afferent fibers to the vestibular nuclei, which then distribute them to medulla spinalis (motor support), cerebellum (fine motor function), and brainstem (oculomotor function). Proprioception ("position sense") is the perception of limb position in space. *Note:* Efferents to the thalamus and cortex control spatial sense; efferents to the hypothalamus regulate vomiting in response to vertigo.

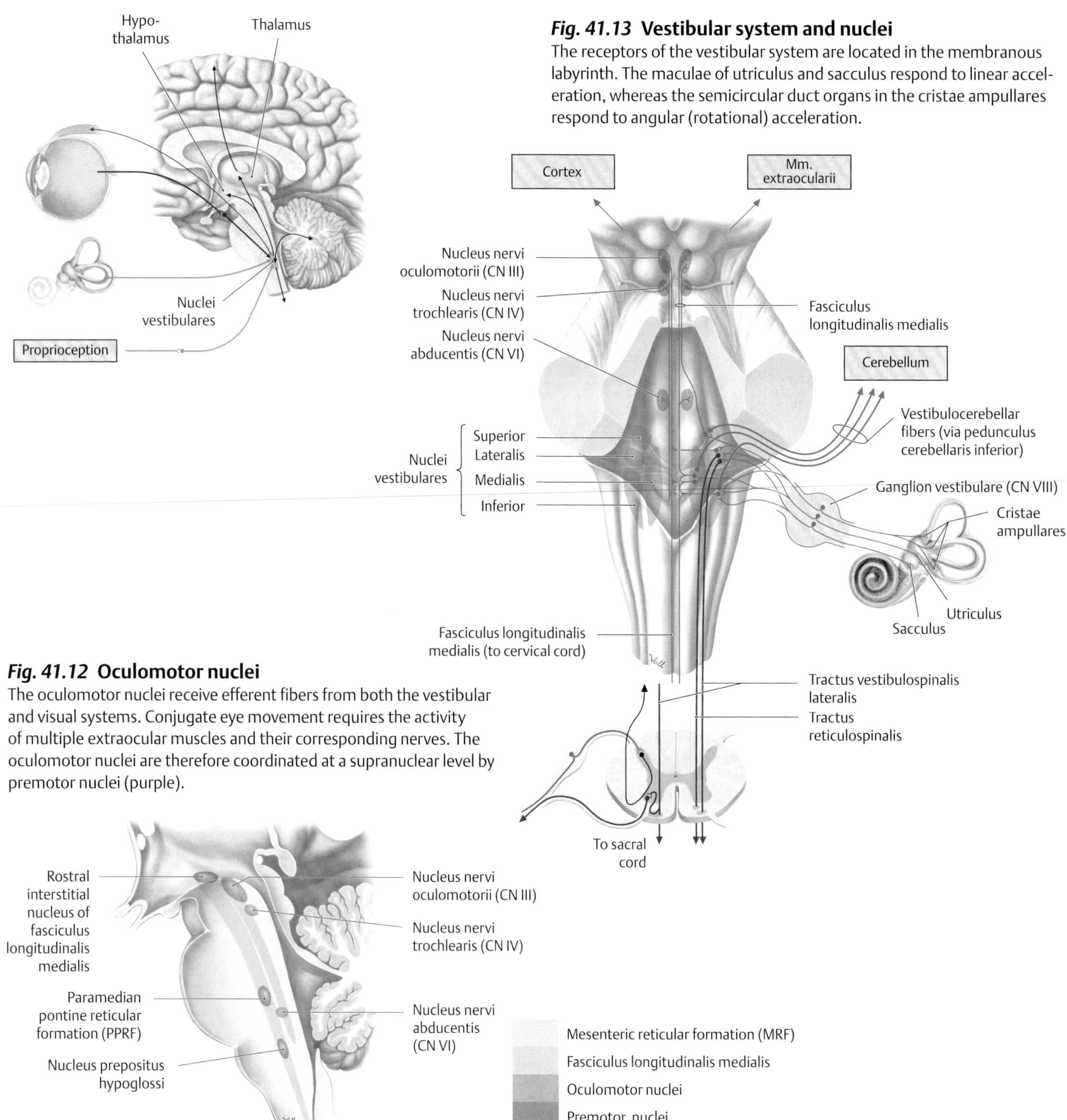

Hypo-
thalamus
Thalamus
Nuclei
vestibulares
Proprioception
Cortex
Mm.
extraocularii
Nucleus nervi
oculomotorii (CN III)
Nucleus nervi
trochlearis (CN IV)
Nucleus nervi
abducentis (CN VI)
Fasciculus
longitudinalis medialis
Cerebellum
Vestibulocerebellar
fibers (via pedunculus
cerebellaris inferior)
Nuclei
vestibulares
Superior
Lateralis
Medialis
Inferior
Ganglion vestibulare (CN VIII)
Cristae
ampullares
Utriculus
Sacculus
Fasciculus longitudinalis
medialis (to cervical cord)
Tractus vestibulospinalis
lateralis
Tractus
reticulospinalis
To sacral
cord
Rostral
interstitial
nucleus of
fasciculus
longitudinalis
medialis
Nucleus nervi
oculomotorii (CN III)
Nucleus nervi
trochlearis (CN IV)
Paramedian
pontine reticular
formation (PPRF)
Nucleus nervi
abducentis
(CN VI)
Nucleus prepositus
hypoglossi
Mesenteric reticular formation (MRF)
Fasciculus longitudinalis medialis
Oculomotor nuclei
Premotor nuclei

Fig. 41.13 **Vestibular system and nuclei**
The receptors of the vestibular system are located in the membranous labyrinth. The maculae of utriculus and sacculus respond to linear acceleration, whereas the semicircular duct organs in the cristae ampullares respond to angular (rotational) acceleration.

Fig. 41.12 **Oculomotor nuclei**
The oculomotor nuclei receive efferent fibers from both the vestibular and visual systems. Conjugate eye movement requires the activity of multiple extraocular muscles and their corresponding nerves. The oculomotor nuclei are therefore coordinated at a supranuclear level by premotor nuclei (purple).

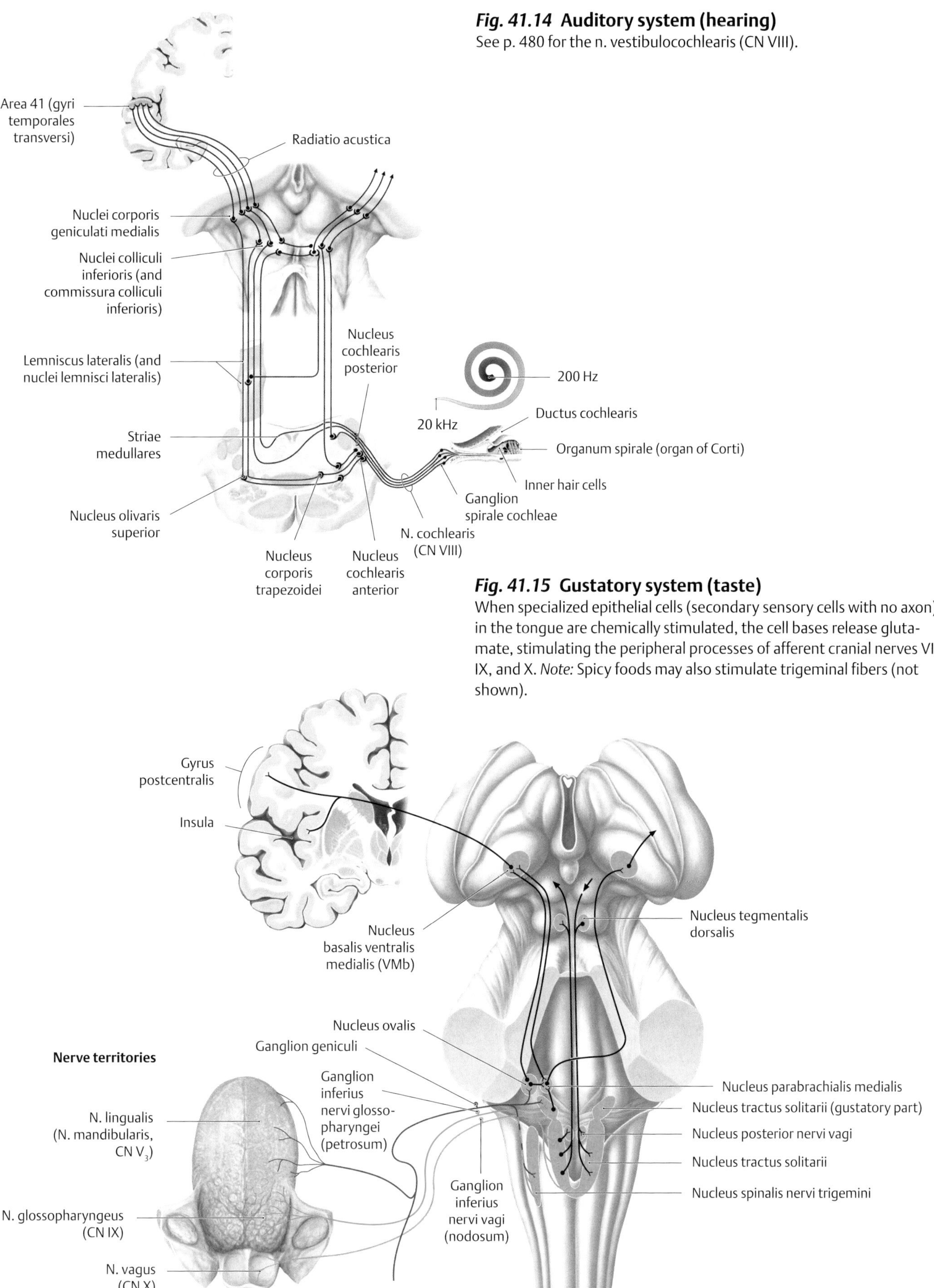
Area 41 (gyri temporales transversi)
Radiatio acustica
Nuclei corporis geniculati medialis
Nuclei colliculi inferioris (and commissura colliculi inferioris)
Lemniscus lateralis (and nuclei lemnisci lateralis)
Nucleus cochlearis posterior
200 Hz
20 kHz
Ductus cochlearis
Organum spirale (organ of Corti)
Inner hair cells
Striae medullares
Ganglion spirale cochleae
Nucleus olivaris superior
N. cochlearis (CN VIII)
Nucleus corporis trapezoidei
Nucleus cochlearis anterior
Gyrus postcentralis
Insula
Nucleus basalis ventralis medialis (VMb)
Nucleus tegmentalis dorsalis
Nucleus ovalis
Ganglion geniculi
Nerve territories
Ganglion inferius nervi glosso-pharyngei (petrosum)
Nucleus parabrachialis medialis
Nucleus tractus solitarii (gustatory part)
N. lingualis (N. mandibularis, CN V_3)
Nucleus posterior nervi vagi
Nucleus tractus solitarii
Nucleus spinalis nervi trigemini
Ganglion inferius nervi vagi (nodosum)
N. glossopharyngeus (CN IX)
N. vagus (CN X)

Fig. 41.14 **Auditory system (hearing)**
See p. 480 for the n. vestibulocochlearis (CN VIII).

Fig. 41.15 **Gustatory system (taste)**
When specialized epithelial cells (secondary sensory cells with no axon) in the tongue are chemically stimulated, the cell bases release glutamate, stimulating the peripheral processes of afferent cranial nerves VII, IX, and X. *Note:* Spicy foods may also stimulate trigeminal fibers (not shown).

Sensory Systems (III)

Fig. 41.16 Olfactory system (smell)

The olfactory system is the only sensory system not relayed in the thalamus before reaching the cortex (the prepiriform area is considered the primary olfactory cortex). The olfactory system is linked to other brain areas and can therefore evoke complex emotional and behavioral responses (mediated by the hypothalamus, thalamus, and limbic system): noxious smells induce nausea; appetizing smells evoke salivation.

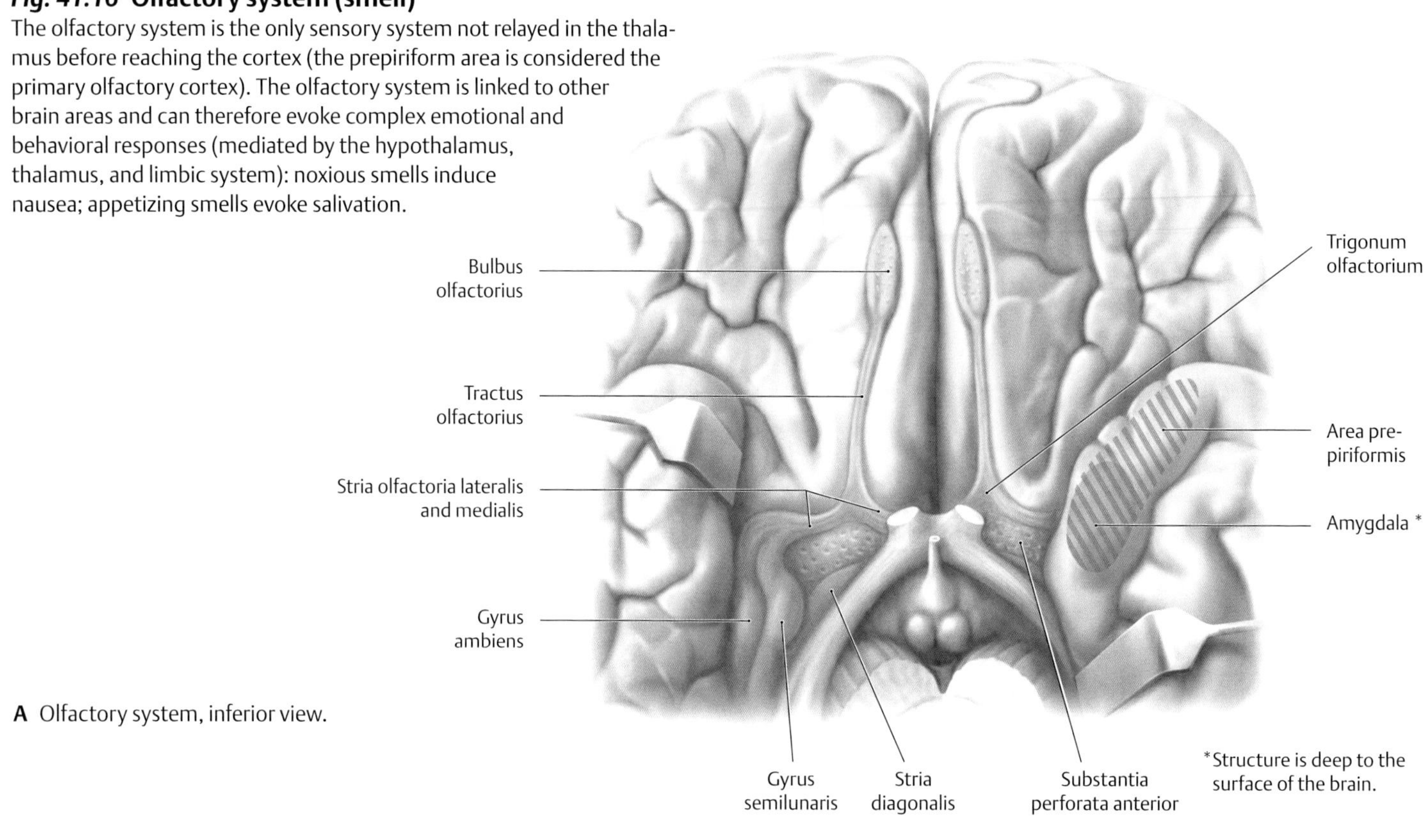
Bulbus olfactorius
Tractus olfactorius
Stria olfactoria lateralis and medialis
Gyrus ambiens
Trigonum olfactorium
Area pre-piriformis
Amygdala *
Gyrus semilunaris
Stria diagonalis
Substantia perforata anterior
*Structure is deep to the surface of the brain.

A Olfactory system, inferior view.

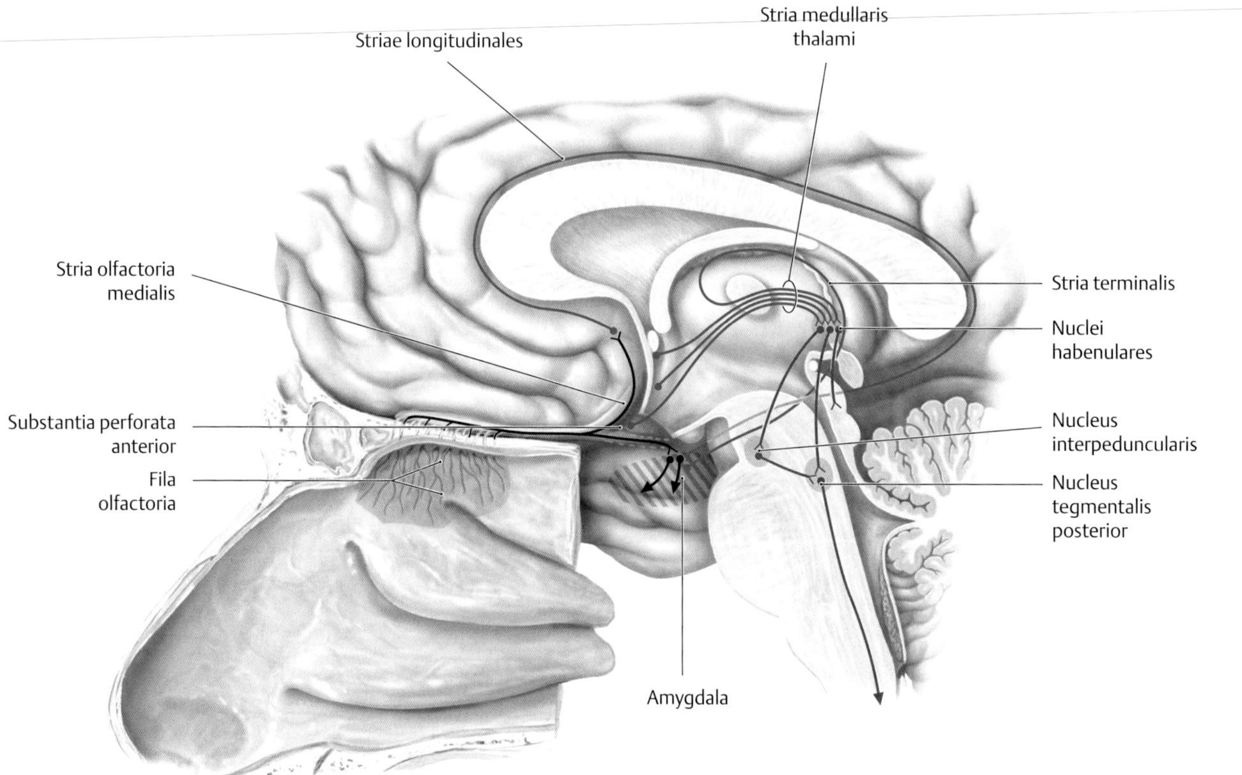
Striae longitudinales
Stria medullaris thalami
Stria olfactoria medialis
Substantia perforata anterior
Fila olfactoria
Amygdala
Stria terminalis
Nuclei habenulares
Nucleus interpeduncularis
Nucleus tegmentalis posterior

B Olfactory system with nuclei, left lateral view of midsagittal section.

The limbic system, which exchanges and integrates information between the telencephalon, diencephalon, and mesencephalon, regulates drive and affective behavior. It plays a crucial role in memory and learning.

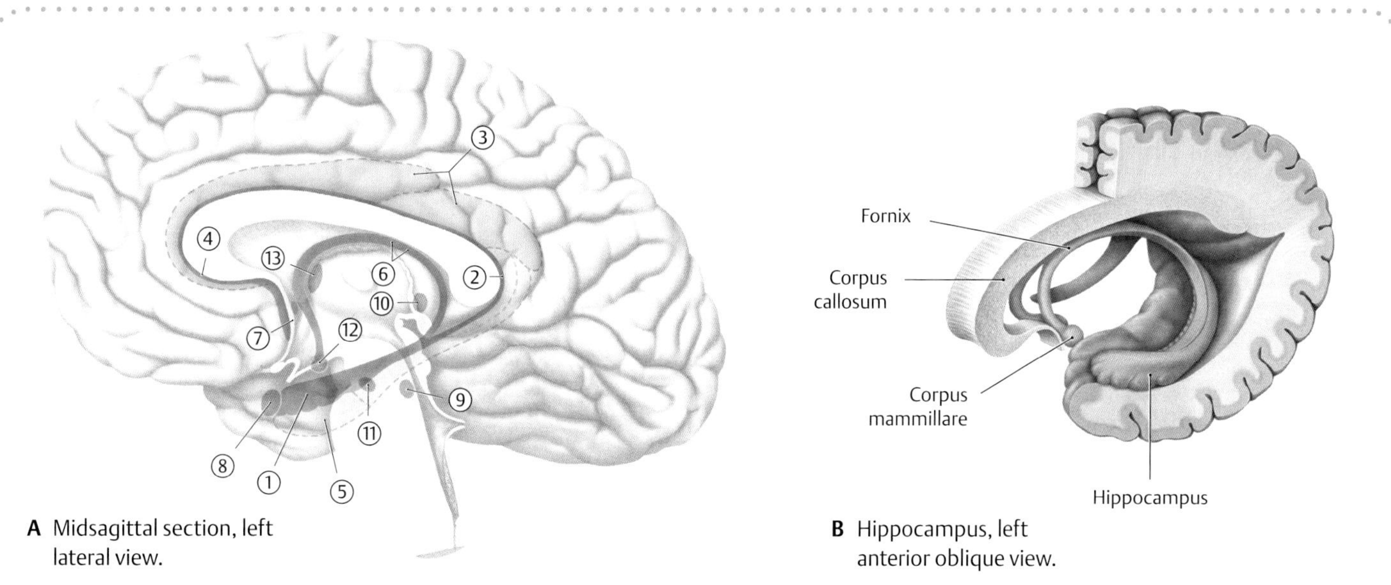

①
②
③
④
⑤
⑥
⑦
⑧
⑨
⑩
⑪
⑫
⑬
Fornix
Corpus callosum
Corpus mammillare
Hippocampus

A Midsagittal section, left lateral view.

B Hippocampus, left anterior oblique view.

Table 41.4 Structures of the limbic system

Outer arc		Inner arc*		Subcortical nuclei	
①	Gyrus parahippocampalis	⑤	Hippocampal formation (hippocampus, entorhinal area of gyrus parahippocampalis)	⑧	Amygdala
②	Indusium griseum	⑥	Fornix	⑨	Nuclei tegmentales dorsales
③	Area subcallosala (paraolfactory area)	⑦	Septal area (septum)	⑩	Nuclei habenulares
				⑪	Nucleus interpedunculares
④	Gyrus cinguli	Gyrus paraterminalis		⑫	Corpus mammillare
				⑬	Nuclei anteriores thalami

* The inner arc also contains the diagonal band of Broca (not shown).

Fig. 41.17 Limbic system nuclei

This neuronal circuit (Papez circuit) establishes a connection between information stored at the conscious and unconscious level.

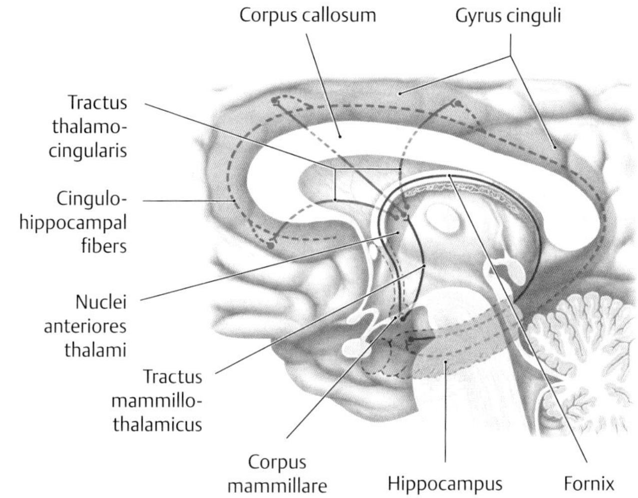

Corpus callosum
Gyrus cinguli
Tractus thalamo-cingularis
Cingulo-hippocampal fibers
Nuclei anteriores thalami
Tractus mammillo-thalamicus
Corpus mammillare
Hippocampus
Fornix

Fig. 41.18 Limbic regulation of the peripheral autonomic nervous system

The limbic system receives afferent feedback signals from its target organs. See p. 623 for the autonomic nervous system.

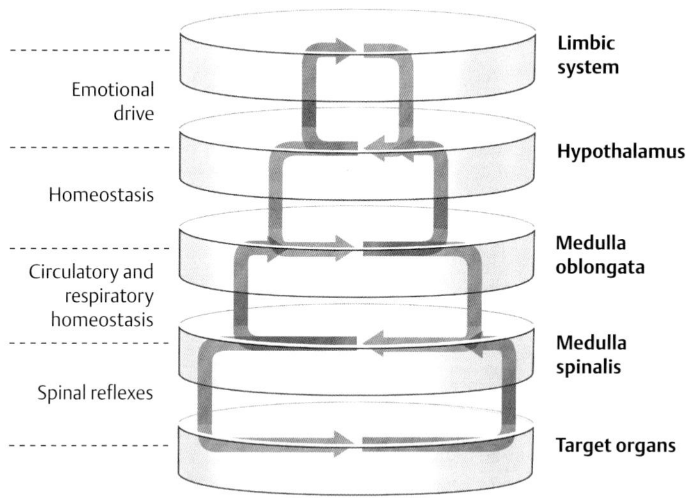

Emotional drive
Homeostasis
Circulatory and respiratory homeostasis
Spinal reflexes
Limbic system
Hypothalamus
Medulla oblongata
Medulla spinalis
Target organs

Autonomic Nervous System

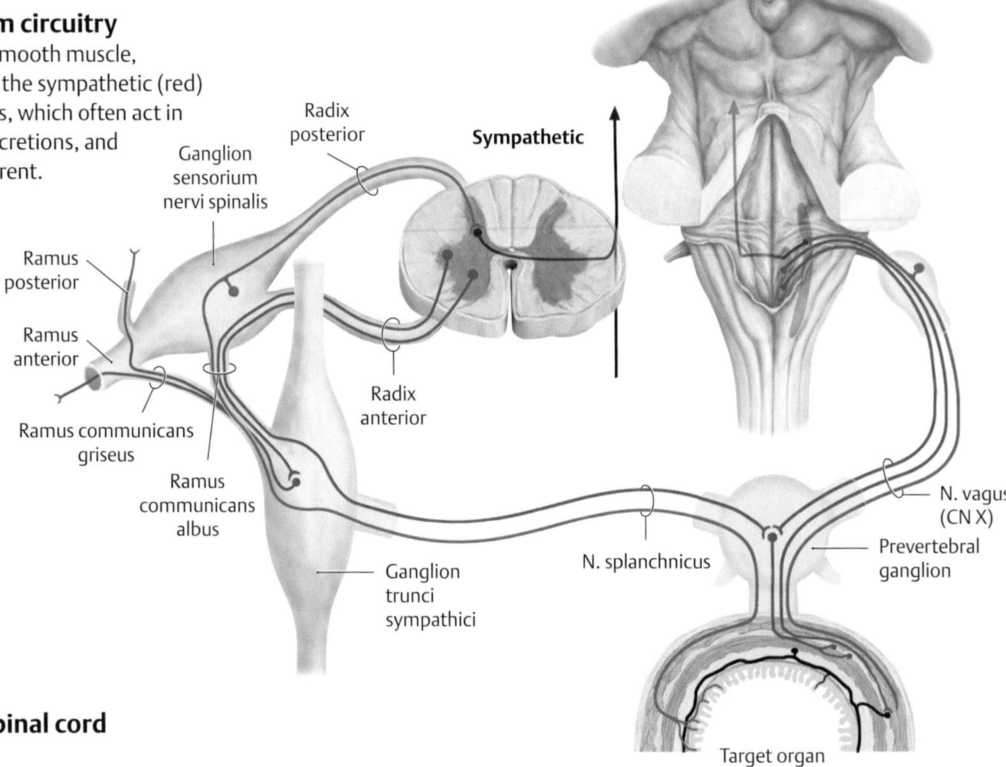

Parasympathetic
Sympathetic
Radix posterior
Ganglion sensorium nervi spinalis
Ramus posterior
Ramus anterior
Ramus communicans griseus
Ramus communicans albus
Radix anterior
Ganglion trunci sympathici
N. splanchnicus
N. vagus (CN X)
Prevertebral ganglion
Target organ

Fig. 42.1 Autonomic nervous system circuitry
The autonomic nervous system innervates smooth muscle, cardiac muscle, and glands. It is divided into the sympathetic (red) and parasympathetic (blue) nervous systems, which often act in antagonistic ways to regulate blood flow, secretions, and organ function. Green: Afferent. Purple: Efferent.

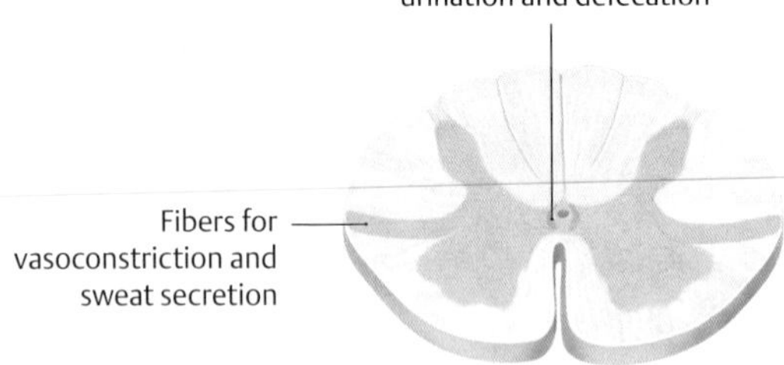

Fibers for genital function, urination and defecation
Fibers for vasoconstriction and sweat secretion

Fig. 42.2 Autonomic tracts in the spinal cord

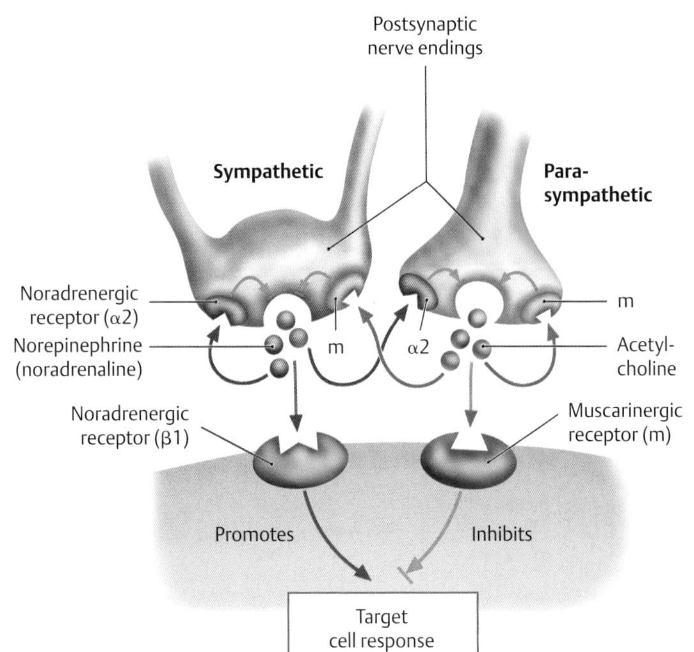

Postsynaptic nerve endings
Sympathetic
Para-sympathetic
Noradrenergic receptor (α2)
Norepinephrine (noradrenaline)
m
m
α2
Acetyl-choline
Noradrenergic receptor (β1)
Muscarinergic receptor (m)
Promotes
Inhibits
Target cell response

Fig. 42.3 Regulatory effects of the autonomic neurotransmitters

Fig. 42.4 Blood pressure regulation
Sympathetic fibers may release norepinephrine (noradrenaline), inducing the α1 receptor to mediate contraction of the vascular smooth muscle (thus increasing blood pressure). Circulating epinephrine (adrenaline) acts on the β2 receptors to induce vasodilation (decreasing blood pressure). *Note:* Parasympathetic fibers do not terminate on blood vessels.

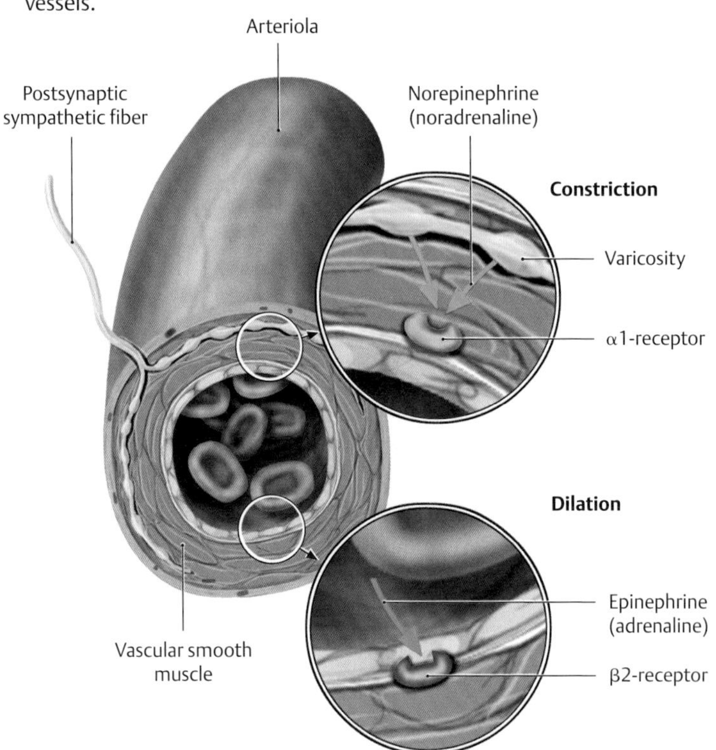

Arteriola
Postsynaptic sympathetic fiber
Norepinephrine (noradrenaline)
Constriction
Varicosity
α1-receptor
Dilation
Epinephrine (adrenaline)
β2-receptor
Vascular smooth muscle

Fig. 42.5 Autonomic nervous system

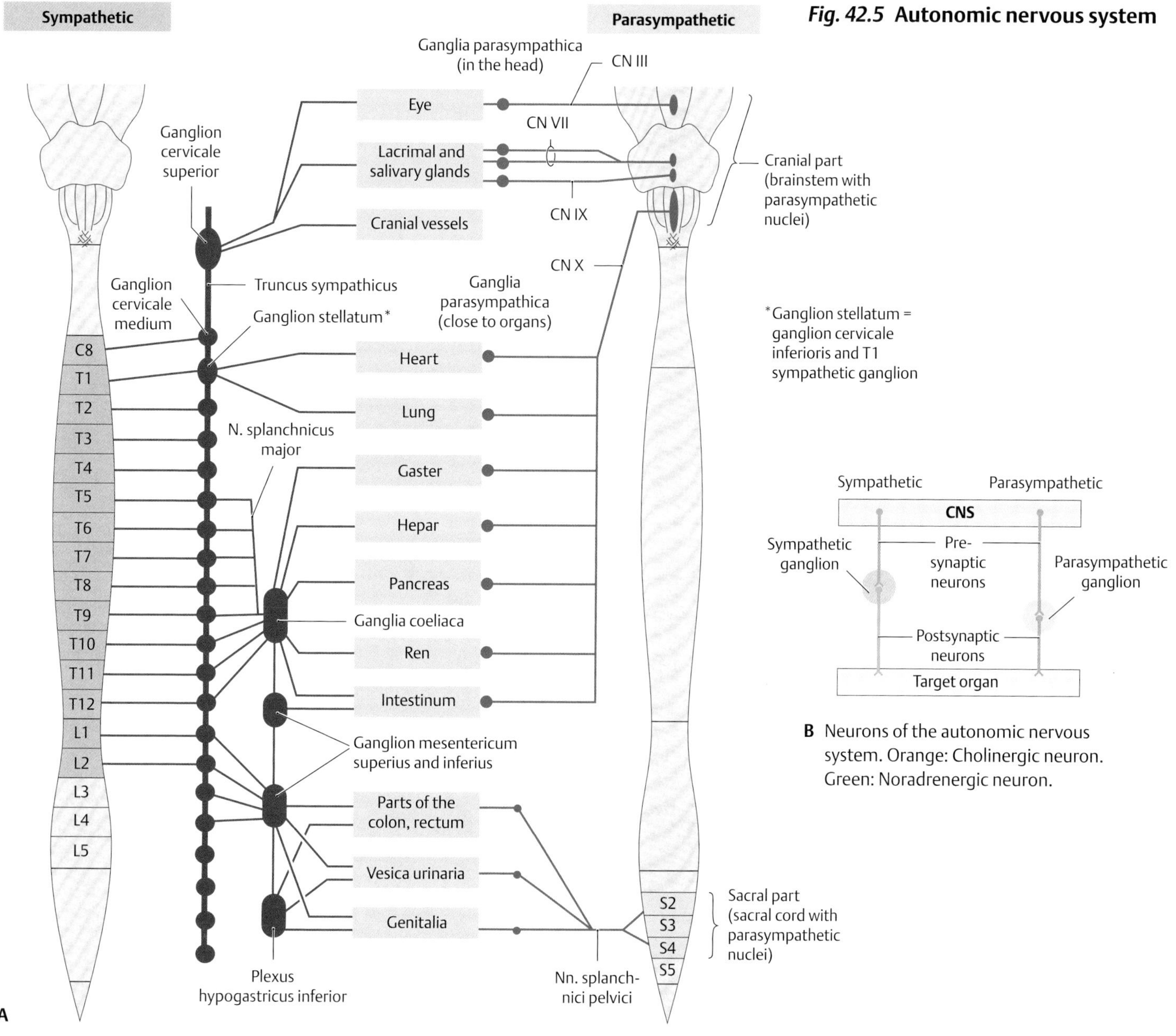
Sympathetic
Parasympathetic
Ganglia parasympathica (in the head)
CN III
Eye
CN VII
Lacrimal and salivary glands
Cranial vessels
CN IX
Ganglion cervicale superior
Cranial part (brainstem with parasympathetic nuclei)
CN X
Ganglion cervicale medium
Truncus sympathicus
Ganglion stellatum*
Ganglia parasympathica (close to organs)
C8
T1
T2
T3
T4
T5
T6
T7
T8
T9
T10
T11
T12
L1
L2
L3
L4
L5
Heart
Lung
N. splanchnicus major
Gaster
Hepar
Pancreas
Ganglia coeliaca
Ren
Intestinum
Ganglion mesentericum superius and inferius
Parts of the colon, rectum
Vesica urinaria
Genitalia
S2
S3
S4
S5
Sacral part (sacral cord with parasympathetic nuclei)
Plexus hypogastricus inferior
Nn. splanchnici pelvici
A
*Ganglion stellatum = ganglion cervicale inferioris and T1 sympathetic ganglion
Sympathetic
Parasympathetic
CNS
Sympathetic ganglion
Pre-synaptic neurons
Parasympathetic ganglion
Postsynaptic neurons
Target organ

B Neurons of the autonomic nervous system. Orange: Cholinergic neuron. Green: Noradrenergic neuron.

Table 42.1 Effects of the sympathetic and parasympathetic nervous systems

Organ (organ system)		Sympathetic NS effect	Parasympathetic NS effect
Gastro-intestinal tract	Tunica muscularis, stratum longitudinale and stratum circulare	Decreases motility	Increases motility
	Sphincter muscles	Contraction	Relaxation
	Glandulae intestinales	Decreases secretions	Increases secretions
Capsula splenica		Contraction	No effect
Hepar		Increases glycogenolysis/gluconeogenesis	
Pancreas	Endocrine pancreas	Decreases insulin secretion	
	Exocrine pancreas	Decreases secretion	Increases secretion
Vesica urinaria	M. detrusor vesicae	Relaxation	Contraction
	Functional bladder sphincter	Contraction	No effect
Glandula vesiculosa		Contraction (ejaculation)	
Vas deferens			
Uterus		Contraction or relaxation, depending on hormonal status	
Arteries		Vasoconstriction	Vasodilation of the arteries of the penis and clitoris (erection)

NS = nervous system. See also p. 244.

Appendix

Answers to Surface Anatomy Questions 626

Index 628

Answers to Surface Anatomy Questions

Back (pp. 40–41)

Q1: The superior boundaries of Michaelis' rhomboid run from processus spinosus of L IV to spina iliaca posterior superior. The rhomboid then follows the curve of crista iliaca to the anal cleft.

Q2: Angulus inferior scapulae is at the level of processus spinosus of T VII. Crista iliaca is at the level of processus spinosus of L IV. See p. 40 for palpable bony landmarks.

Thorax (pp. 120–121)

Q1: After careful inspection, undertake a systematic palpation of each breast. Palpate the tissue of each breast by quadrant in the following sequence: inferior lateral, inferior medial, superior medial, and superior lateral. Palpate the axilla to examine the axillary tail of breast tissue. The majority of lymph drainage from the breast is to nll. axillares. The nll. parasternales, which run along a. and v. thoracica interna, drain the medial portions of the breast. See p. 64 for the nll. axillares.

Q2: Valvae aortae and trunci pulmonales are best auscultated at the 2nd right and left intercostal spaces, respectively. Locate the 2nd intercostal spaces by finding the usually palpable angulus sterni (the junction between the manubrium and corpus of the sternum). The 2nd ribs attach to the sternum at the angulus sterni. The valva tricuspidalis (right atrioventricular valve) and valva mitralis (left atrioventricular valve) are best auscultated at the left 5th intercostal space. If the ribs are visible/palpable, the 5th rib can be found by counting up from below (the lowest rib at the midclavicular line is the 10th rib). See p. 87 for auscultation sites; see p. 120 for reference lines in the thorax.

Abdomen & Pelvis (pp. 248–249)

Q1: Use a vertical and a horizontal line through the umbilicus (at approximately the level of L IV) to divide the abdomen and pelvis into right and left upper and lower quadrants (see p. 142).

LUQ	Liver, stomach, colon transversum, small intestine, spleen, pancreas, duodenum, colon descendens, left kidney and glandula suprarenalis, left ureter.
RUQ	Liver, stomach, colon transversum, small intestine, gallbladder, pancreas, duodenum, colon ascendens, right kidney and glandula suprarenalis, right ureter.
LLQ	Small intestine, colon descendens, left ureter, urinary bladder, reproductive organs.
RLQ	Small intestine, colon ascendens (with cecum and appendix vermiform), right ureter, urinary bladder, reproductive organs.

Q2: *Direct* inguinal hernias are most common in middle-aged or older males and are believed to be caused by "wear and tear." They typically occupy the medial portion of canalis inguinalis (having exited the abdomen through the inguinal triangle). They may also exit via the superficial inguinal ring. Rarely, they enter the scrotum. *Indirect* hernias are seen in male children and young adults and are believed to have a congenital basis. They generally exit via the deep inguinal ring and thus may occupy the entire length of canalis inguinalis. They may also exit via the superficial inguinal ring, and occasionally enter the scrotum. See p. 135 for inguinal hernias.

Upper Limb (pp. 350–353)

Q1: The nn. cutanei antebrachii medialis and lateralis are both vulnerable during intravenous punctures in the fossa cubiti. The n. medianus is a direct branch from fasciculi medialis and lateralis of plexus brachialis; the lateral nerve is the cutaneous component of n. musculatocutaneus (fasciculus lateralis). See p. 339 for the cubital region.

Q2: With the elbow joint in flexion, the ulnar collateral ligament can be palpated using the olecranon, the epicondylus medialis and lateralis, and the processus coronoideus. The lig. collaterale radiale can be palpated using the epicondylus lateralis. See p. 284 for the collateral ligaments of the elbow.

Q3: In the wrist, the m. flexor carpi ulnaris tendon runs laterally to the a. and n. ulnaris until the canalis ulnaris. N. medianus is located between the palpable tendons of m. palmaris longus and m. flexor carpi radialis. A. radialis is slightly lateral to the m. flexor carpi radialis tendon. See p. 342 for the topography of the carpal region.

Q4: Tenderness at the base of the anatomic snuffbox suggests a fracture of os scaphoideum. See p. 347 for the anatomic snuffbox; see p. 299 for scaphoid fractures.

Lower Limb (pp. 450–451)

Q1: Caput femoris is located directly behind the a. femoralis. A. femoralis emerges below the midpoint of the ligamentum inguinale. See p. 436 for the inguinal region.

Q2: N. ischiadicus can be located as it exits foramen ischiadicum majus by identifying the midpoint between spina iliaca posterior superior and tuber ischiadicum. In the gluteal region (see pp. 438–439), n. ischiadicus passes just medial to the midpoint of a line connecting trochanter major of the femur and tuber ischiadicum. N. fibularis communis can be palpated on the lateral border of fossa poplitea as it courses along the medial border of the m. biceps femoris tendon (see p. 442). At the ankle, n. tibialis is located midway between the palpable medial malleolus and the calcaneal (Achilles') tendons (see p. 442).

Head & Neck (pp. 588–589)

Q1: A bolus of anesthetic injected approximately two thirds of the way up the posterior border of the m. sternocleidomastoideus would serve as a nerve block for the plexus cervicalis.

Q2: The confluence sinuum is found deep to the protuberantia occipitalis externa. See p. 608 for the sinus durae matris.

Q3: The regio cervicalis lateralis is bounded by the mm. sternocleidomastoideus and trapezius and clavicula. It contains the ramus externus of n. accessorius (CN XI) and plexus brachialis. See p. 576 for the triangles of the neck. See p. 582 for the contents of the regio cervicalis lateralis.

Q4: Trigonum caroticum is bounded by m. sternohyoideus, venter posterior of m. digastricus, and m. sternocleidomastoideus. It contains n. vagus (CN X). See p. 576 for the triangles of the neck. See p. 580 for the contents of trigonum caroticum.

Q5: Cartilago thyroidea (see p. 570) is commonly referred to as the "Adam's apple."

Index

Note: *Italicized* page numbers represent clinical applications. Tabular material is indicated by a "t" following the page number.

A

Abdomen, 124–249
  arteriae abdominales, 206–213
  female, 249
    aorta abdominalis, 208
  male, 249
  nervi lymphoidei aortici, 226, 226t
    abdomen parietale, 228
  organs of, 142, 142t, 143
  plexus autonomicus abdominales, 236, 236t
  surface anatomy of, 248–249
  transverse section, 156
  venae abdominales, 214–221
Abdominal wall
  internal surface anatomy of, 135
  musculi abdomini abdominal wall, 130–131, 138–139, 138t
  regio inguinalis and canalis inguinalis, 132–133, 133t
  vagina musculi recti abdominis, 134
Abducens, nervus (CN VI), 474, 474t
  injury to, effects of, 474t
  location, overview, 470
  origin, 471t
  palsy, *509*
Abduction/adduction axis of motion, 301
Abductor digiti minimi, musculus, 417, 417t
Abductor hallucis, musculus, 417, 417t
Abductor pollicis longus, musculus, 347
Accessorius, nervus (CN XI), 486, 486t
  basis cranii and, 464, 465
  injury to, effects of, 486t
  lesions of, 486
  location, overview, 470
  origin, 471t
Accessory sex glands, in male, 200
Accommodation, pathways for, 617
Acetabulum, 361
  ligamenta accetabuli, 364
  radiograph of, 125, 359
Acini, mammary, 63
Acromioclavicularis, articulatio, 252, 259
  injuries to, *259*
Acromioclavicularis, ligamentum
  articulatio glenohumerale and, 261
  rupture of, *259*
Acromium, 252–253
  in back surface anatomy, 40
"Acute abdomen," *143*
Adam's apple. *See* Thyroidea, cartilago
Adductors, musculi
  deep layer, 370–372, 377, 377t
  of sole of foot, 418–419, 418t
  superficial layer, 366–369, 376, 376t
Aditus, 553
Afferent axons, 471, 471t
Afferent (sensory) fibers, 612
Afferentes, nuclei, 471
Ala nasi, 520
Alaria, ligamenta, 17
Allocortex, 594
Alveoli, 111
Amygdala, 596–597, 597t
Anal triangle, in female perineal region, 136
Anastomosis
  arteria abdominalis, 207, 207t
  arteria carotis externa, 493
  arteria coronaria dextra et sinistra, 88
  arteriae intercostales, 56
  Galen's vein (vena magna cerebri), 575
  in right and left coronary arteries, *89*
  venous, of head and neck, 497t
"Anatomic snuffbox," 346, 352
Anconeus, musculus, 268, 270–271, 279, 279t
Anesthesia
  lumbar and epidural, *601*
  musculus sternocleidomastoideus and, 588
Angina pectoris, *89*
Angiotensin I/Angiotensin II, *209*
Angle-closure glaucoma, *518*
Angulus sterni, 46
  bifurcatio tracheae at, 110
  in thorax surface anatomy, 120
Angulus subpubicus, 127
Annulare, ligamentum, 284–285, 284t
  articulationes radioulnares and, 286
  radial head dislocation and, *287*
Anococcygealis, nervus
  in female perineum, 194
  in male perineum, 203
Ansa cervicalis, 37, 568
  roots of, 569
Antebrachii, nervus, 326, 326t
Anulus fibrosus
  in cardiac skeleton, 86
  discus invertebralis, 12
  disk herniation and, *13*
"Anvil" (incus), 532. *See also* Ossicular chain
Aorta, 56, 68, 206
  aorta abdominalis, 206, 206t
    anastomoses, 207, 207t
    in female abdomen, 208
  arteriae bronchiales and, 116
  arteria thoracica, 56, 56t, 68–69
    branches of, 69t
    dissection of, *69*
  in blood circulation, 82
Aortic dissection, *69*
Aortici nodi lymphoidei, 423
  male genitalia and, 234
  abdomini, 226, 226t
    parietales, of posterior abdominal wall, 228
  of pelvis, 227, 227t
  urinary organs and, 229
Apertura diaphragmatica, 53
Apex
  cordis, 92t
  pulmonis, 105
Apical segment opacity, 106
Apicales, ligamenta, 17
Aponeurosis
  lingualis, 548
  obliquus externus, 133, 133t, 134, 139
  obliquus internus, 130, 134, 139
  palmaris, 293, 306
    atrophy of, *306*
  plantaris, 411, 412
  transversus abdominis, 131, 139
  vagina musculi recti abdominis and, 134
Apparatura vestibulare, 536
  balance and, 618

Appendicitis, *143*
  Crohn's disease vs., *163*
Appendix, 164
Aqueous humor, glaucoma and, *518*
Arches
  palmar, 317, 345
  plantar, 410–411
Arcuate line, rectus sheath, 134
Arcus aorticus, in chest radiograph, 92
Arcus transversus, 410
Area septalis, limbic system and, 621, 621t
Area subcallosa, 621, 621t
Areola
  of female breast, 62
  in thorax surface anatomy, 121
Areolar glands, 62
Arm, 252–279. *See also* Forearm
  bones of, 252–253
  muscles of
    anterior, 264–267, 278, 278t
    posterior, 268–271, 279, 279t
  surface anatomy of, 350–351
  transverse sections of, 348–349
Arteriae. *See also individually named arteriae*
  of abdomen, 206–213
  of arcus tracheobronchiale, 116
  auricularis
    externa, 529
    interna, 537
    media, 534–535, 534t
  of back, 34
  of basis cranii, foramina for, 458
  of caput and neck, 490–495
  of cavitas nasalis, 524
  of cavitas thoracica, 66, 68–69
  cerebelli, 608
  of cerebellum, 608–609
  diaphragmaticae, 54, 55t
  dura mater, 603
  effects of autonomic nervous system on, 244t, 623t
  of esophagus, 99, 99t
  of eyeball, 517
  of genitalia
    female, 195, 225
    male, 202, 225
  of glandula thyroidea and glandula parathyroidea, 575
  of heart, 88–89
  of medulla spinalis, 610
  of membrum inferius, 420–421
  of membrum superius, 316–317
  of neck, 566
  of orbita, 506t, 510
  of palatum durum, 546
  of pelvis, 222–223, 222t
  of pulmo, 114–115, 115t, 118
  of rectum, 224
  of regio carpalis, 342
  of testis, 199, 199t
  of thoracic wall, 56, 56t
  of truncus encephali, 608
Arteriography, in stenosis arteria renalis, *209*
Articular processes, of vertebrae, 5, 5t
Articulatio genus, 382–391
  bursa periarticularis in, 385
  cavitas, 390–391
  ligaments of, 384–389, 384t
    cruciatum, 388–389
    ligamentum collaterale and patellare, 386
  meniscus in, 387
  radiographs of, 383, 391
Articulationes. *See also individually named articulationes*
  of cavitas oris. *See* Temporomandibularis, articulatio
  of columna vertebralis, 14–17
  of lower limb
    hip, 362–365
    knee, 382–391
    ankle, 404–407
    foot, 403–407
  of pelvic girdle, 124, 358
  of spine, 14–17
  of thoracic cage, 48–49
    articulatio costotransversalis, 49
    articulatio costovertebralis, 49
    articulatio sternocostalis, 49
    respiration and, 48
  of upper limb
    elbow, 282–285. *See also* Cubiti, articulatio
    shoulder, 258–261
    wrist and hand, 300–309
Arytenoidea, cartilago, 570
  vocal folds and, 571
Arytenoideus transversus, musculus, 572, 572t
Ascending lumbar veins, 214, 214t
Ascending tracts, 613, 614, 614t
ASD (atrial septal defect), *95*
Association areas, in cerebral hemispheres, 595
Asthma, *111*
Atherosclerosis
  arteria carotis, *491*
  disturbed coronary artery blood flow and, *89*
Atlantoaxiale, articulation, 16–17
Atlantooccipitale, articulatio, 16
Atlas (CI), 4, 6, 558
  in articulatio atlantoaxiale, 16
  in atlantooccipital joints, 16
  fracture of, 7
  ligamentum cruciforme of, 17
  tuberculum posterior of, 565
  processus transversus of, 565
Atria. *See* Atrium
Atrial septal defect (ASD), *95*
Atrioventricularis (AV), nodus, 90
Atrium (atria), 85
  blood circulation and, 82
  cardiac skeleton and, 86
  lymphatic drainage of, 100
Auditiva interna, arteria, 537
Auditory apparatus, 536
Auditory system, 619
Auricle, 529
Auriculares, musculi, 529
  in facial expression, 466, 466t
Auricularis, arteria
  anterior, 529
  posterior, 493, 493t, 529
    of auris media, 534, 534t
Auriculars, nervi, 37
Auris. *See also* Auricularis *entries*
  bones of, 526–527
  externa, 528–529. *See* Auricle
  interna, 536–537
  media, 530–535. *See* Middle ear
    arteries of, 534–535, 534t
    cavitas tympanica and, 530–531, 530t
    mastoid air cells and, *527*
    ossicular chain and membrana tympanica and, 532–533
  muscles of, 466, 466t
Auscultation, of cardiac valves, *87*
  sites for, 87t

Autonomic innervation. *See* Autonomic nervous system
Autonomic nervous system, 612, 621–622, 622t
abdominal and pelvic, 237, 244t
arcus tracheobronchiale and, 117
circuitry in, 621
esophagus and, 98
heart and, 91
intestines and, 240–241
intraperitoneal organs and, 245
plexuses, 236–237, 236t
thoracic, 74–75, 75t
urinary organs and, 246
Axilla, 336–337
nodi lymphatici of, 64t, 319
posterior shoulder and, 332
radial nerve compression in, *325*
tractus neurovasculares and, 333t
triangular and quadrangular spaces of, 333
walls of, 336, 336t
Axillaris, nervus, 324, 324t
injury to, *324*
Azygos system
in thoracic cavity, 70, 71, 71t
veins of medulla spinalis and, 611
Azygos, vena, 35

B

Back, 2–41
arteriae dorsales, 34
female, 41
male, 41
muscles of, 22–33
articulatio craniovertebralis and, 28, 28t
musculi prevertebrales, 29, 29t
overview, 22–23
short nuchal, 25, 28, 28t
nervi dorsales, 36, 36t
cutaneous innervation, 36t, 37
neurovasculature of, 34–39
ossa dorsales, 2–13
prominentiae ossae dorsales, 40
surface anatomy of, 40–41
venae dorsi, 35
Baker's cyst, *385*
Balance, 618
vestibular apparatus for, 536
Basis cranii, 458–459
and cavitas nasi, 520–521
and cavitas oris, 538–539
cerebral venous system of, 607
foramina of, 458
fossa pterygopalatina and, 505t
innervation of, 240
intestinum tenue, 160–163. *See also* Duodenum; Ileum; Jejunum
mesenterii of, 162
and orbita, 506–507
and os ethmoidale, 460
and os sphenoidale, 461
and os temporale, 526–527
referred pain from, *246*
sinus durae in, 607
Basivertebral veins, 611
Benign prostatic hyperplasia, *201*
Biceps brachii, musculus, 278, 278t
antebrachium anterior, 288–289
anterior shoulder and arm, 264–267
Biceps femoris, musculus, 370–373, 379, 379t
Biliary sphincter system, 172
Birth canal, episiotomy and, *193*
Bitemporal hemianopia, *617*
Bleeding
extracerebral hemorrhage, *603*
from nasopharynx, *495*
from nose, *525*
"Blinders," *617*
Blindness, *617*
Blood circulation, 82
Blood clots, *115*
Blood flow
disturbed, in arteriae coronariae, *89*
impeded, in neck, *567*
Blood pressure
autonomic regulation of, 622
fundus opticus examination in, *517*
Blood vessels. *See* Arteriae; Venae; *individually named vessels*
Bony prominences, palpable. *See* Palpable bony prominences
Brachialis, plexus, 320–321, 320t
in axilla topography, 337
fasciculus medialis and lateralis, 326, 326t
fasciculus posterior, 323, 323t
in axilla topography, 337
long (terminal) branches, 323t, 324–325
short branches, 323, 323t
long (terminal) branches, 326t, 327–329
nerves of, 320, 320t
short branches, 326, 326t
structure of, 321
supraclavicular branches, 322, 322t
Brachial region, topography of, 338
Brachii, musculi, 278, 278t
antebrachium anterior, 288–289
anterior shoulder and brachium, 266–267
posterior shoulder and brachium, 266–267
Brachii, nervus cutaneus, 326, 326t
Brachiocephalic lymph nodes, 100
Brachiocephalica, vena, 70, 71t
Brachiocephalicus, truncus, 68, 69t
Brachioradiales, musculi, 290–291, 294–295, 294t
Breast (female), 62–63
cancer of, *65*
lymphatic drainage in, 64
and sentinel node in breast cancer, *65*
in thorax surface anatomy, 121
Breast (male), in thorax surface anatomy, 121
Breast cancer, *65*
Brodmann (cortical) areas, 595
Bronchi, 110
foreign body in, *110*
Bronchial tree, 111
arteriae bronchiales and, 116
arteriae pulmonales and, 114
conditions associated with, *111*
lymphatic drainage of, 118
movements in respiration, 113
radiograph, 108
and trachea. *See* Tracheobronchiale tree
Bronchogram, posteroanterior, 108
Bronchopulmonary lymph nodes, 101, 118, 119
Bronchopulmonary segments, 108–109
Buccinator, musculus, 467, 467t
Bucket-handle tear, *387*
Bulbospongiosus, musculus
in female pelvis, 140, 140t, 154, 193
in male pelvis, 140, 140t, 143, 150, 154
Bulbourethralis, glandula, 200
primordium of, 205
Bulbus caroticus, calcified plaque in, *491*

Bursa(e)
  gastrocnemio-semimembranosus, *385*
  omentalis, 146–147, 146t
  periarticularis, 385
  subacromialis, 262–263
    cavitas glenoidalis and, 262
  subdeltoida, 262, 263

C

Caesarea, sectio, *127*
Calcaneocuboidea, articulatio, 403
Calcaneofibularis, ligamentum, 408t, 409
Calcaneus, 400–401
  facies articulationes and, 407
Calcification, in arteria carotis, *491*
Caloric testing, vertigo diagnosis and, *527*
Calvaria
  dura mater and, 602
  internal and external, 457
  structure of, 457
Canal of Schlemm, 518
  glaucoma and, *518*
Canales semicirculares, 528
  orientation and position for caloric testing, *527*
Canalis analis, 167, 167t
Canalis carpi, 343
  ligamenta of, 303
Canalis inguinalis, 133, 133t
Cancer. *See* Carcinoma
Capitatum, os, 300
  MR image of, 301
Capitis costae, articulatio, 49
Capitis, musculus longus, 564–565, 564t
Capituli radii, subluxation of, *287*
Capitullum, os, 256
Capsula articulatio genus, 385, 390
  attachments of, 390
  outpouching in, *385*
Capsula interna, 597, 597t
Caput. *See also specific regions, e.g.* Mouth, Nose, Orbita, Auris
  arteries of, 490–495
  bones of, 454–461
  muscles of, 462–469
  nerves of, 470–487
  neurovasculature, 488–505
  surface anatomy of, 588–589
  veins of, 496–497
Carcinoma
  of breast, *65*
  of colon, *165*
  gastric, *586*
  invasive ductal, *65*
  of prostata, *201*
Cardiac borders, 92, 92t
Cardiac conduction system, 90
Cardiac cycle, *90*
Cardiac murmur, *87*
Cardiac muscle contraction, 90
Cardiac skeleton, 86
Cardiac valves, 86–87
  auscultation of, *87*, 87t
  in ventricular diastole, 86
  in ventricular systole, 86
Cardiac veins, 88t
Cardinal directions of gaze, 508
Caroticotympanica, arteria, 534, 534t
Carotid sheath, fascia cervicalis profunda, 577, 577t
Carotis, arteria, 490–491. *See also* Carotis externa, arteria; Carotis interna, arteria
  atherosclerosis of, *491*
Carotis communis, arteria, 490–491. *See also* Carotis externa, arteria; Carotis interna, arteria
  aorta thoracica and, 68, 69t
  in blood circulation, 83
Carotis externa, arteria, 491, 491t
  anterior and medial branches, 492, 493t
  middle ear blood supply and, 534, 534t
  in neck, 566
  posterior branches, 493, 493t
  terminal branches, 494–495, 494t
Carotis interna, arteria, 490, 608
  course and branches of, 490
  middle ear blood supply and, 534, 534t
Carpal eminences, ulnar and radial, 303
Carpal region, topography of, 342. *See also* Canalis carpi; Canalis ulnaris
Carpal tunnel syndrome, *343*
Carpales, ossae, 252–253, 298–299, 298t
  fractures of, *299*
Carpometacarpale, articulatio, 300–301
  ligamenta of, 302
Carpus
  articulationes of, 300–301
  ligamenti of, 302–303
  ossae of, 298–299, 298t
  radiographs of, 299, 300
  and regio carpalis topography, 342–343
  surface anatomy of, 352–353
Cartilago
  arytenoideo, 570
  auricularis, 529
  corniculatio, 570
  costae, 44–45
  cricoidei, 570–571
  epiglottica, 570
  laryngea, 570
    musculi laryngei and, 572
  musculi thyroidei, 570–571
  triradiate, 125, 359
Cauda equina, 601
  in central and peripheral nervous systems, 592
Caudatus, nucleus, 597, 597t
Caval aortic lymph nodes. *See* Aortici nodi lymphoidei
Cavitas abdominis and pelvis, organs of, 142, 142t
Cavitas glenoidalis of scapula, 263
  radiograph of, 260
Cavitas nasi
  fossa pterygopalatina and, 505t
  neurovasculature of, 524–525
  ossae of, 520–521
  sinus paranasales of, 522–523
Cavitas oris, 538–557
  articulatio temporomandibularis and. *See* Temporomandibularis, articulatio
  dentes in, 542–543
  glandulae salvatorii in, 551
  lingua in, 548–549
  musculi of
    oral floor, 544, 545t, 547
    palatum molle, 545, 545t
    pharynx, 554–555
  nervus trigeminus in, 547
  ossae of, 538–539
  pars of, 550, 550t
  pharyngeal neurovasculature of, 556–557
  tonsillae and pharynx in, 552–553
  topography of, 550
Cavitas peritonealis, 144–145
  in female, 154
  in male, 143, 154
  organs of, 148
  posterior wall of, 149

Cavitas pleuralis
boundaries in, 102, 102t
bronchial tree in, 111
cavitas thoracis and, 66
lymphatic drainage of, 118–119
pleura parietalis, 102–103. *See also* Pleura parietalis
pleura visceralis, 102–103. *See* Pleura visceralis
in pneumothorax, *113*
pulmo, 105. *See also* Pulmo
skeleton thoracis and, 102
trachea in, 110
Cavitas subperitonealis, 154
Cavitas tympani, 530–531
arteriae of, 535
boundaries of, 530t
nervus glossopharyngeus in, 483
medial wall of, 481
ossicular chain in, 533
Cavum septum pellucidi, 597, 597t
Cecum, 164
Celiac lymph nodes, 231–232
of abdomen, 226, 226t, 230
parietal, of posterior abdominal wall, 228
Central nervous system (CNS), 592
Cerebellares, pedunculi, 598
Cerebellum, 598
arteries of, 608
Cerebral arteries, 609
Cerebral hemispheres, 595
Cerebral veins, 606–607
Cerebrospinal fluid (CSF), 604
extracting sample of, *601*
Cerebrum, 593, 593t
arteriae cerebri, 608–609
in central and peripheral nervous systems, 592
CSF and, 604
development of, 593, 593t
superficial veins of, 606
Cervical lymph nodes, 587, 587t
Cervical nerves, 464–465, 568t, 569
Cervical spine, 6–7, 558
injuries to, *7*
joints, 14–17
ligaments of, 16–19, 18t, 559
lordosis of, 2, *2*
nuchal muscles of, 24–25
palpable proc. spinosus at CVII, 4
structural elements, 5, 5t
Cervicale, trigonum, 589
Cervicales, regiones, 576, 576t
anterior topography, 578–579
lateral topography, 580–583
posterior topography, 584
trigonum caroticum in, 580
trigonum suboccipitale in, 585
Cervicalis, fascia
back muscles and, 23
deep, in neck, 577, 577t
Cervicalis, plexus, 568–569
skull base and, 465
Cervicalis, vertebrae (CIII-CVII). *See* Cervical spine
Cervicis, arteria transversa, in scapular region, 39
Cervicothoracic junction (CVII), 4
Cervix uteri, 151, 188–190
Chambers, cardiac, 85
lymphatic drainage of, 100
Chest. *See* Thorax (chest)
Chest radiographs, 92, 106
Chest tube insertion, *60*
Chiasma opticum, 473, 597, 597t, 616
lesion of, *617*
Childbirth, *127*
Choanae
of nose, 520, 521
of pharynx, 550, 552, 553
Choroideus, plexus, 597, 597t
CSF and, 604
Ciliare, corpus, 518–519
Ciliare, musculus, 518–519
Cingulum pelvicum
in abdomen and pelvis,124–127
membrum inferius, 358–359
Cingulus, gyrus, 621, 621t
Circulation, 82
fetal, 94–95. *See also* Newborn
Cisterna chyli, in abdominal lymphatic drainage
of intestinum, 232
of ren, 229
of pelvic organs, 235
of gaster, hepar, lien, pancreas, and duodenum, 231
Clavicula, 252–254
Clavicular notch, 44, 46
Clavipectoral triangle, 334
"Clawing" of hand, ulnar nerve damage and, *329*
Clitoris, 136, 151
function of, 186t
in urogenital system, 186
Cluneal nerves
in female perineum, 194
in male perineum, 203
CN, 470–471. *See* Cranial nerves; *individually named nerves*
CNS, 592–593. *See* Central nervous system (CNS)
Coccygeus, musculus, 140–141, 140t, 141
Coccygis, os, 10–11
as perineum boundary, 137
Cochlea, 536
ganglion spirale of, 481
Cochlearis, nervus. *See* Vestibulocochlearis, nervus (CN VIII)
Coeliaca, ganglion, 237–240
anterior abdominal organ innervation and, 238
small intestine innervation and, 240
urinary organ innervation and, 239
Coeliacus, plexus, 236, 236t
Coeliacus, truncus, 206–207, 206t
abdominal organs and, 210–211
Colic lymph nodes, 232
Colitis, *165*
Colitis ulcerosa, *165*
Collateral pathways, in portal system, 215
Collaterale radiale, ligamentum, 284–285, 284t
Collaterals, ligamentum, 388–389
in flexion and extension, 389
of hand, 302–305
of knee joint, 386
medial and lateral, of articulatio talocrurale, 408–409, 408t
Collecting ducts, embryonic derivatives of, 205t
Colles' fascia, of perineum, 136, 137, 154
Colles' fracture, in distal radius, *287*
Colli, musculus longus, 564–565, 564t
Colon, 164–165
carcinoma of, *165*
colon ascendens, 162, 164
colon descendens, 164
Colon sigmoideum, 164
Colon transversum, 144–147, 164
Colonoscopy, *165*
Columna vertebralis, 2–5. *See also* Spina
articulationes of, 14–17

overview, 14–15, 14t
regio craniovertebralis, 16–17
discus intervertebralis in, 12–13. *See* Intervertebralis, discus
elements of, 4–5
ligamenti of, 18–21, 559t
overview, 18, 18t
spina cervicalis, 19
spina thoracolumbalis, 20–21
ossae of, 2–13
Comminuted fracture, of humerus, *257*
Commissura anterior, 597, 597t
Common iliac lymph nodes, 226–229
female genitalia and, 235
male genitalia and, 234
Compartment syndrome, *445*
Conchae, of nose, 520, 521
Conduction system, cardiac, 90
Conjugate eye movements, 618
Conjunctiva, 514
Connecting vein, venous anastomoses and, 497t
Constrictions, esophageal, 96
Constrictor pharyngis superior, musculus, 554–555, 554t
Constrictors pharyngeales inferiors, musculi, 554–555, 554t
Constrictors pharyngeales medius, musculi, 554–555, 554t
Convergence, pathways for, 617
Coracoacromialis, arcus, 259, 261
subacromial space and, 262
Coracobrachialis, musculus, 264–267, 274, 274t
Coracoclaviculare, ligamentum, 259
articulatio glenohumerale and, 261
injury to, *259*
Coracoideus, articulatio, in thorax surface anatomy, 120
Cornea, 518
Corniculata, cartilago, 570
Coronaria, arteriae, 88–89, 88t
cardiac valves and, 86
disturbed blood flow in, *89*
Coronary stenosis, disturbed coronary artery blood flow and, *89*
Corpus callosum, 597, 597t
Corpus cavernosum, 200
Corpus geniculatum laterale, 616
Corpus mammillarius, 597, 597t
Corpus spongiosum, 200
Corti, organ of, 536
Costa cage, 44
articulationes of, 48–49
movement, 48
Costae, 44–47
in back surface anatomy, 40
and scapular extent, 255
size and shape variations in, 47
types of, 45
verae, 45
Costal angle, 44–45
Costal cartilage, 44–75
Costal groove, 47
Costal margins, in thoracic skeleton, 44
Costal tubercle, 44, 47
Costodiaphragmaticus, recess, 103
Costomediastinalis, recess, 103
Costotransversaria, articulatio, 49
Cortex cerebri, 594
allocortex of, 594
isocortex of, 595
Coxae, articulatio, 362–363
dislocation or dysplasia of, diagnosing, *363*
ligaments and capsule of, 364–365
Coxae, os, 358–359
in pelvic girdle, 124–125
Crani, fossa, 459
cranial nerves and, 511
fossa pterygopalatina and, 505t
Cranial nerves, 470–487. *See also individually named nerves*
brainstem and, 599
fibers of, classification, 471t
injury to,
nervus abducens, 474t
nervus accessorius, 486t
nervus facialis, 479t
nervus glossopharyngeus, 483t
nervus hypoglossus, 487t
nervus oculomotorius, 474t, 475
nervus trigeminus, 476t
nervus trochlearis, 474t
nervus vagus, 484t
nervus vestibulocochlearis, 480t
in meatus acousticus internus, 481
nuclei of, 471, 471t
in oral cavity innervation, 546
oral floor, 547
in orbit, 511
overview of, 470–471, 471t
in pharynx and pharyngeal space, 556–557
skull base foramina for, 458
Craniovertebral joints, 14t, 15–17. *See also* Atlantoaxiale, articulatio; Atlantooccipitale, articulatio
ligaments of, 16–17
muscles of, 28, 28t, 564–565, 564t
Cranium, 454–459, 454t
anterior, 455
basis cranii, 458–459
calvaria, 457
lateral, 454
musculi of, 462–469
origins and insertions, 464–465
neurovasculature of, 488–505
posterior, 456
surface anatomy of, 588–589
Cremaster, musculus, fascia and, 198, 199, 199t
Cricoarytenoideus, musculus, 572, 572t
Cricoidea, cartilago, 570, 571
Cricothyroideus, musculus, 572, 572t
Crista supraventricularis, 85
Crohn's disease, *163*
Cruciatum, ligamentum, 388–389
attachment sites, 387
in flexion and extension, 389
rupture of, *389*
Cruciforme, ligamentum
of atlas, 17
of fingers, 304
CSF. *See* Cerebrospinal fluid (CSF)
Cubiti, articulatio, 282
articulations in, 282–283
injuries to, assessing, *283*
ligaments of, 284–285, 284t
MR image of, 283
Cubiti, fossa
topography of, 339
veins of, 318
Cuboideum, os, 400–401
joints involving, articulation surfaces, 403
Cuneiform, os, 400–401
Cuneonaviculare, articulatio, 403
Cutaneus femoris lateralis, nervus, 426–427
plexus lumbosacralis, 424–425
Cutaneus femoris posterior, nervus, 430
in female perineum, 194

Cutaneus femoris posterior, nervus *(continued)*
in male perineum, 203
plexus lumbosacralis overview, 424–425
Cyst, synovial popliteal, *385*
Cystic lymph node, 231

D

Deciduous teeth, coding of, 543
Deep inguinal lymph nodes. *See* Inguinal lymph nodes
Deep segmental muscles, 32–33, 32t
Deferentiales, plexus, 243
Degenerative diseases, of spine, *9*
Delivery, episiotomy during, *193*
Deltoideum, ligamentum, 408
Deltoideus, musculus, 272, 272t
anterior shoulder and arm, 264–267
posterior shoulder and arm, 268–271, 332
in surface anatomy, 40, 120, 350–351
Deltopectoral groove, in thorax surface anatomy, 120
Dens axis (CII), 4, 6, 558
in articulatio atlantoaxiale, 16
dens fracture of, *7*
proc. spinosus of, 565
Dens caninus, 542
Dens incisivus, 542
Dens premolaris, 542
Dental panoramic tomogram, 543
Dentes, 542–543
in situ, 538–539
Dentes decidui, coding of, 543
Dentes permanentes, 542
coding of, 543
Dentition, DPT evaluation of, 543
Deoxygenated blood, in circulatory system, 82
arteriae pulmonales and, 116
Depressor anguli oris, musculus, 467, 467t
Dermatomes
of abdomen, 59
of back, 37
disk herniation and, *13*
of face, 488
of lower limb, 434–435
of medulla spinalis segments and, 600
of nuchal region, 568
of thoracic wall, 59
of upper limb, 330–331
Descending tracts, 613, 615, 615
Deviated septum nasi, *523*
Diabetes, fundus opticus examination in, *517*
Diaphragm leaflets, in chest radiograph, 92
Diaphragma
pelvis, 140–141, 140t
fascia of, anal canal and, 167
fascia thoracica, 52–53, 52t
liver attachment to, 170
neurovasculature of, 54–55, 55t
during respiration, 48
Diaphragma pelvis, musculi of, 140, 140t
in female, 136, 141, 152
in male, 137, 153
Diaphragmatica, facies, of heart, 84
Diencephalon, 596–598
internal structures of, 597, 597t
limbic system and, 621
nervus opticus and, 471t, 473
Diffusion distance, and respiratory compromise, *111*
Digastricus, musculus, 544, 545t, 562, 562t, 563
Digiti pedis. *See* Phalanges, of pes
Diplopia, *509*
Discus intervertebralis. *See* Intervertebralis, discus
Dislocation
articulatio cubiti, injury assessment and, *283*
of articulatio temporomandibularis, *541*
caput femoris, necrosis and, *421*
of hip, diagnosing, *363*
Dissection, aortic, *69*
Diverticula, *97*
duodenal, radiograph of, *161*
esophageal, *97*
Dorsalis scapuale, nervus, in plexus brachialis, 322, 322t
Double vision, *509*
DPT (dental panoramic tomogram), 543
Drainage, 226, 228
of gaster, hepar, lien, pancreas, and duodenum, 231
of intestines, 232
of kidneys, 229
lymphatic. *See* Lymphatic drainage of
pleural fluid, *60*
of pelvic organs, 235
"Drawer sign," ligamentum cruciatum rupture and, *389*
Duchenne's limp, *431*
Ductus
choledochus. *See* Bile duct(s)
ejaculatorius, 200
lactiferus, in female breast, 63
Müllerian, 205, 205t
nasolacrimalis, opening of, 522
thoracicus, lymphatic drainage and, 72–73
Wolffian, 205, 205t
Ductus arteriosus, 94–95
adult remnant of, 95t
Ductus choledochus, 172–173
endoscopy of, *161*
obstruction of, *173*
pancreatic. *See* Pancreatic bile ducts
Ductus deferens, 199–200
ampulla of, 143, 150, 200
effects of autonomic nervous system on, 244t, 623t
Ductus nasolacrimalis, 522
Ductus venosus, 94–95
adult remnant of, 95t
Duodenum, 160–161
lymph nodes and lymphatic drainage of, 231
and pancreas, 174
papillary region, endoscopy of, *161*
in retroperitoneum, 149
in situ, 146–147
truncus coeliacus and, 211
vena portae and, 218
wall of, biliary sphincter system in, 172
Dupuytren's contracture, *306*
Dura mater, 602
arteries of, 603
innervation of, 603
Dural septa, 602
Dysplasia, of hip, diagnosing, *363*

E

ECG (electrocardiogram), *90*
Ectopic (extrauterine) pregnancy, *143, 189*
Edema, pulmonary, *107*
Efferent axons, cranial nerves, 471, 471t

Efferent (motor) fibers, 612
Efferent nuclei, cranial nerves, 471
Einthoven limb leads, *90*
Einthoven triangle, *90*
Ejaculatorius, ductus, 200
Electrocardiogram (ECG), *90*
Electrodes, for ECG recordings, *90*
Embolism, pulmonary, *115*
Embryonic development
  of brain, 593, 593t
  of genital organs, 205, 205t
Encephali, truncus, 598–599
  arteries of, 608
  in brain development, 593t
  cranial nerves and, 470–471, 599. *See also* Cranial nerves; *individually named nerves*
    nervus accessorius, 486
    nervus opticus, 473
    nervus trigeminus, 476
  parasympathetic nervous system in thorax and, 75, 75t
  veins of, 607
Endoscopic retrograde cholangiopancreatography (ERCP), *161*
Endoscopy
  in Crohn's disease, *163*
  of papillary region of duodenum, *161*
  of stomach and antrum pylori, *159*
Epicolic lymph node, 232
Epicondylus(s)
  femoris, 356, 360–361, 450
  humeri, 253, 256–257, 350
Epididymis, 198
Epidural anesthesia, *601*
Epidural hematoma, *495, 603*
Epigaster, innervation of, 245
Epigastrica superior, arteria, 56
Epiglottica, cartilago, 570
Epiglottis, 571
Episiotomy, *193*
ERCP (endoscopic retrograde cholangiopancreatography), *161*
Erector muscles, of pelvic floor, 140, 140t
Erector spinae, musculus, 26, 30–31, 30t
  in back surface anatomy, 40
Esophagogastric junction, 97
Esophagus, 96–99
  lymphatic drainage of, 101
  neurovasculature of, 98–99, 99t
Ethmoidale, os, 460
  in paranasal sinuses, 523
Expiration, 112–113
  in pneumothorax, *113*
  rib cage movement in, 48
Extensor carpi radialis, musculus, 294–295, 294t
Extensor carpi ulnaris, musculus, 296–297, 296t
Extensor digitorum, musculus, of arm, 296–297, 296t
Extensor digitorum brevis, musculus, of foot, 416, 416t
Extensor digitorum longus, musculus, of foot, 397, 397t
Extensor hallucis brevis, musculus, 416, 416t
Extensor hallucis longus, musculus, 397, 397t
Extensor indicis, musculus, 296–297, 296t
Extensor pollicis, musculus, 296–297, 296t
  dorsum manus and, 347
External genitalia. *See also individual organs*
  development of, 204
  in female, 192–193
    blood vessels of, 195
    nerve supply, 194
    overview, 186, 186t
  in male, 187, 187t
External iliac lymph nodes
  female genitalia and, 235
  male genitalia and, 234
  parietal, of posterior abdominal wall, 228
  of pelvis, 227, 227t
Extra-articular fracture, of humerus, *257*
Extracerebral hemorrhages, *603*
Extracranial vein, venous anastomoses and, 497t
Extrahepatic bile ducts, 172, 173
Extraocular muscles, 508, 508t
  impaired coordination of, *509*
  innervation of, 509
    by oculomotor nerve, 475
Extraperitoneal organs, 142t
Extrapyramidal motor system, 615, 615t
  ganglion basale of, 594, 597, 597t
Extrauterine (ectopic) pregnancy, *143, 189*
Extrinsic muscles
  of back, 22, 30, 30t
    fascia thoracolumbalis and, 23
  lingualis, 548
  of neck, 560, 561, 561t
Eye, 516–519
Eye movements, conjugate, 618
Eyeball, 516
  blood vessels of, 517
Eyelids, 514

F

Face. *See also specific features of face, e.g.* Ossae, Nose, Orbita
  fractures of, *455*
  innervation of
    motor, 488
    sensory, 489
  muscles of, 462–469
    origins and insertions, 464–465
  neurovasculature of, 488–505
    fossa infratemporalis, 502–503
    fossa pterygopalatina, 504–505, 504t, 505t
    fossa temporale, 501
    parotid region, 500
    superficiale, 498–499
Facial expression, muscles of, 462–463
  actions of, 466–467, 466t–467t
  motor innervation of, 488
  origins and insertions, 464-465
Facialis, arteria, 492, 493t
Facialis, nervus (CN VII), 478–479, 479t
  auricle innervation by, 529
  glandula parotidea, 551
  gustatory system and, 619
  injury to, effects of, 479t
  location, overview, 470
  motor innervation of face, 464–465, 488
  muscles of facial expression and, 464–465
  in oral floor innervation, 547
  origin, 471t
  in os temporale, 478
Fallopian tube. *See* Tuba uterine
Falls
  articulatio acromioclaviculare damage and, *259*
  femur fractures and, *361*
  humerus fractures and, *257*
  radius fractures and, *287*
"False lumen," *69*
False pelvis, components of, 154
"False" pulsion diverticula, *97*
False ribs, 45

Far vision, light reflection by lens and, 519
Fascia
cervicalis. *See* Cervicalis, fascia
Colles', of perineum, 136, 137
fascia thoracolumbalis. *See* Thoracolumbalis, fascia
musculus cremaster testicularis and, 198, 199, 199t
penile, 150
transversalis, of canalis inguinalis, 133, 133t
visceralis. *See* Visceralis, fascia
Fasciculus cuneatus, 614, 614t
Fasciculus gracilis, 614, 614t
Fasciculus internus, of medulla spinalis, 613
Fasciculus longitudinalis medialis, 618
Fasciculus mammillothalamicus, 597, 597t
Fasciculus medialis longitudinalis, 618
Fasciculus, spinal intrinsic, 613
Fat pads, in articulatio cubiti injury assessment, *283*
Fauces (throat), 550, 550t
isthmus faucium of, 550, 553
muscles of, 555
Femoral hernia, *135*
Femoral ring, internal abdominal wall, 135
Femoral triangle, 440
Femoralis, nervus, 429
plexus lumbosacralis, overview, 424–425
Femoris, nervus cutaneus
lateralis, 426–427
plexus lumbosacralis overview, 424–425
posterior, 430, 430t
Femoropatellaris, articulatio, 383
Femur, 256–357, 360
anterior, topography of, 440
arteriae of, 421
fractures of, 361
head of, in hip joint, 361
musculi of
anterior, 366–369, 378, 378t
medial, 376–377
posterior, 370–373, 379, 379t
neurovasculature of, 448–449
posterior, topography of, 441
Fenestra vestibuli, ossicular chain and, 532, *533*
Fetal circulation, 94–95. *See also* Newborn
structures in, derivatives of, 95t
Fibrae somaticae
nervi craniales, 471, 471t
and referred pain, *246*
Fibrous pericardium, 80, 81
Fibrosus, anulus. *See* Anulus fibrosus
Fibula, 356–357, 380–381
fractures of, *381*
articulatio genu and, 382
Fibularis, nervus communis, 432
Fibularis, musculus, 392–393, 396, 396t
Fibularis tertius, musculus, 396, 397t
Fingers
bones of, 298–299, 298t
ligamenta digiti of, 304–305
longitudinal section of fingertip, 305
middle, lateral view of, 317
neurovascular structure of, 344
Fingertip, longitudinal section of, 305
Fissura horizontalis, of pulmo, 105
Fissura obliqua, of pulmo, 105
Fissures, pulmonary, 105
Flatfoot, 410
Flavum, ligamentum, 21
Flexion/extension motion
in articulatio genu
ligamentum cruciatum and collaterale, 389
menisci, 387
of articulatio metacarpophalangeale, 304
in hand and wrist, 301
suprapatellar pouch during flexion, 391
Flexor digiti minimi, musculus, 418–419, 418t
Flexor digitorum brevis, musculus, 417, 417t
Flexor digitorum longus, musculus, 399, 399t
Flexor hallucis brevis, musculus, 418–419, 418t
Flexor hallucis longus, musculus, 399, 399t
Flexor muscles
of anterior forearm, 288–289, 292–293, 292t
of posterior leg, 398–399, 398t, 399t
Flexorum, retinaculum
of manus, 342
of pes, 415
Floating ribs, 45
Fluid accumulation
abnormal pleural, drainage of, *60*
radiographic findings in lung, *107*
Foramen epiploica. *See* Foramen omentale (epiploic)
Foramen magnum, 458
Foramen (epiploicum) omentale, 147
boundaries of, 147t
Foramen ovale, 94–95
adult remnant of, 95t
open, *95*
Forearm, 280–297
arteries of, 317
bones of, 252–253, 280–281
muscles of, 294t, 295
anterior, 288–289, 292–293, 292t, 340
posterior, 290–291, 294–297, 294t, 296t, 341
radialis group, 294–295, 294t
neurovasculature, 340–341
transverse sections of, 348–349
veins of, 318
Forebrain, in brain development, 593t
Forefoot
arch of, 410
bones of, 400–401
Foregut, innervation of, 245
Forehead, muscles of, 466, 466t
Foreign bodies, ingested by children, *110*
Fornix, 597, 597t
in hippocampal formation, 596
limbic system and, 621, 621t
Fornix plantaris, 410
Fovea centralis, 519
Fractures
articulatio cubiti
injury assessment and, *283*
median nerve injury and, *328*
caput femoris, necrosis and, *421*
caput fibularis, *381*
distal radial, *287*
humerus, *257*
medulla spinalis, *7*
nervus facialis, *455*
nervus femoralis, *361*
os scaphoideum, *299*
Funiculi, spinal cord, 613, 614, 614t
Funiculus spermaticus, 132, 196
contents of, 196

G

Gait, waddling, *431*
Galen's anastomosis, 575
Gallstones, ultrasound of, *173*

Ganglia
aorticorenal. *See* Ganglion aorticorenale
autonomic plexuses of, 236, 236t
mesenteric. *See* Mesentericus inferius, plexus; Mesentericus superius, plexus
plexus basale, 594, 597, 597t
plexus coeliacus. *See* Coeliacus, plexus
plexus cochlearis, 481
plexus lumbalis, 237, 242
plexus pterygopalatinus, 505
plexus sacrale. *See* Sacralia, ganglia
plexus spinale, 601
plexus spirale, of cochlea, 481
in sympathetic nervous system. *See* Ganglion sympathicum
Ganglion aorticorenale
plexus autonomicus of, 236, 236t, 237
small intestine innervation and, 240
urinary organ innervation and, 239
Ganglion impar, 237
Ganglion mesentericum superior, 237
intestinum tenue innervation and, 240
urinary organ innervation and, 239
Ganglion sensorium nervi spinalis, 601
Ganglion spirale, vestibulare and cochleare, 481
Ganglion sympathicum, 237, 244
and postsynaptic neurons, 91
thoracic, 75, 75t
urinary organ innervation and, 239
Ganglion vestibulare, 481, 537
Gaster, 158–159. *See also* Gastric *entries*
bursa omentalis and, 146, 147
nodi lymphoidei and lymphatic drainage of, 230, 231
referred pain from, *246*
truncus coeliacus and, 210
vena portae and, 218
Gastric carcinoma, *586*
Gastric lymph nodes, 230, 231
Gastric ulcers, *159*
Gastricus, plexus, anterior abdominal organ innervation and, 238
Gastritis, *159*
Gastrocnemio-semimembranosus bursa, *385*
Gastrocnemius, musculus, 394–395, 398, 398t
Gastrocolicum, ligamentum, 146, 147
Gastrointestinal tract, effects of autonomic nervous system on, 244t, 623t
Gastro-omental lymph nodes, 230
Gaze, cardinal directions of, 508
Gemelli, musculi, 370–372, 374, 374t
Genioglossus, musculus, paralysis of, *549*
Geniohyoideus, musculus, 544, 545t, 548, 562, 562t, 563
Genitalia, 186–205. *See also individual organs*
development of, 204–205
in female, 188–195
autonomic innervation of, 247
autonomic plexus of, 236, 236t
blood vessels of, 225
coronal section, 191
embryonic derivatives, 205t
lymph nodes and lymphatic drainage of, 227, 235
neurovasculature, 194–195
overview, 186, 186t
in male, 196–203
autonomic innervation of, 247
autonomic plexus of, 236, 236t
blood vessels of, 225
embryonic derivatives, 205t
lymph nodes and lymphatic drainage of, 227, 234
neurovasculature, 202–203
overview, 187, 187t
Genitofemoralis, nervus, 426–427, 426t
in female perineum, 194
in male perineum, 203
plexus lumbosacralis, overview, 424–425
Genus articularis, musculus, 367, 378, 378t
Glands. *See individually named glands*
Glandular tissue, in female breast, 63
Glans clitoris, 136
Glans penis, 137
Glaucoma, *518*
Glenohumerale, articulatio, 256, 258
bony elements of, 260
capsula and ligamenta of, 261
cavitas in, 261. *See also* Cavitas glenoidalis of scapula
Globus pallidus, 597, 597t
Glossopharyngeus, nervus (CN IX), 482–483, 483t
auricula innervation by, 529
in cavitas tympani, 483
gustatory system and, 619
injury to, effects of, 483t
location, overview, 470
origin, 471t
skull base and, 465
visceral efferent fibers of, 483
Gluteal muscles, 374–375, 374t
in surface anatomy, 40, 451
in situ, 367–373
small, weakness in, *431*
Gluteal nerves, 424–425, 424t, 430t, 431
Glutealis inferior, arteria and vena, 222, 222t
Glutealis, regio, 366–373
anterior, 366–369
fasciae and cutaneous neurovasculature of, 438
and fossa ischioanalis fossa, 439
muscles of, 374–375, 374t
neurovasculature, 438–439, 441
posterior, 370–373
sensory innervation of, 430
Glutea superior, arteria and vena, 222, 222t
Goldberger lead, in ECG, *90*
Gonad primordium, 205, 205t
Gonads, referred pain from, *246*
Gracilis, musculus, 366–368, 376, 376t
Granulationes arachnoideae, in calvaria, 457
Great vessels, 66, 68–69
and heart in situ, 83
"Guarding," abdominal pain and, *143*
Gubernaculum, 205, 205t
ligamentum, 205, 205t
Gustatory system, 619

H

Hamatum, os, 300
MR image of, 301
"Hammer" (malleus), 532. *See also* Ossicular chain
"Hangman's" fracture, *7*
Hearing
auditory apparatus for, 536
ossicular chain in, *533*
Hearing loss, conductive, *533*
Heart, 82–93
auscultation of valves, 87t
and blood circulation, 82
pre- and postnatal, 94–95
chambers of, 85
conduction system, 90

Heart *(continued)*
  innervation of, 91
  lymphatic drainage of, 100
  normal, MR image of, 93
  radiographic appearance of, 92, 92t
  septal defects in, *95*
  in situ, 83
  surfaces of, 84
  transverse section (at T8), 93
  valves of. *See* Cardiac valves
Heart sounds, auscultation sites for, *87*, 87t
"Heartbeat," *90*
Helicobacter pylori, 159
Hematoma
  compartment syndrome and, *445*
  epidural, *495, 603*
  subdural, *603*
Hemianopia, *617*
Hemiazygos system, vena, 611
Hemorrhage. *See* Bleeding
Hepar, 168–171. *See also* Hepatic *entries*
  on abdominal MR image, 169
  attachment to diaphragma, 170
  effects of autonomic nervous system on, 244t, 623t
  lobes of, 171
  lymph nodes and lymphatic drainage of, 230–231
  referred pain from, *246*
  segments of, 170, 170t
  in situ, 146–147, 168
  surfaces of, 171
  truncus coeliacus and, 210
Hepatic lymph node, 230, 231
Hepatic metastasis, *215*
Hepatic vein(s), 82, 214, 214t
Hepaticus, ductus, 172, 173
Hepaticus, plexus
  anterior abdominal organ innervation and, 238
  small intestine innervation and, 240
Hepatoduodenale, ligamentum
  in bursa omentalis, 146
  duodenum and, 161
  in posterior peritoneal cavity, 149
  stomach and, 159
Hepatoesophageale, ligamentum, 159
Hepatogastrica, ligamentum, 158, 159
Hernia(s)/herniation
  discus intervertebralis, *13*
  inguinalis and femoralis, *135*
Hesselbach's triangle, 133, 135
Hilum, 105
  lymph drainage and. *See* Bronchopulmonary lymph nodes
  and perihilar radiolucency, 106
Hindfoot, bones of, 400–401
Hip muscles
  anterior, 366–369
  posterior, 370–373
Hippocampus, 594
  formation of, 596
  limbic system and, 621, 621t
  location of, 597, 597t
Histology
  of isocortex, 595
  of teeth, 542
Homonymous hemianopia, *617*
Humeroradiale, articulatio, 282, 284–285, 284t
Humeroulnar, articulatio, 283–285, 284t
Humerus, 256–257
  fractures of, *257*
  and musculus deltoideus, 272
  in upper limb, 252–253
Hyoideum, os, 539
  and larynx, 558
  muscle origins and insertions, 464
Hypertension
  fundus opticus examination in, *517*
  renal, *209*
Hypertrophy, prostatic, *201*
Hypogastricus. *See* Hypogastricus inferius, plexus; Hypogastricus superior, plexus
Hypogastricus inferius, plexus, 236, 236t
  large intestinal innervation and, 241
  pelvic innervation and, in female, 242
  urinary organ innervation and, 239
Hypogastricus superior, plexus, 236, 236t, 237
  intestinum crassum innervation and, 241
  pelvic innervation and
    in female, 242
    in male, 243
  urinary organ innervation and, 239
Hypoglossus, nervus (CN XII), 487, 487t
  damage to, *549*
  location, 470
  in oral floor innervation, 465, 547
  origin, 471t
  palsy, *549*
  in tongue innervation, 549
Hypoglossus, musculus, 544, 545t, 548
Hypopharyngeal (pharyngo-esophageal)
Hypophysis cerebri, 596
Hypothalamus, 596
Hypothenar muscles, 312–313, 312t

I

Ileitis terminalis (Crohn's disease), *162*
Ileocoecalis, valva, 164
Ileocolic lymph node(s), 232
Ileum, 162
  Crohn's disease and, *162*
  lymph nodes of, 232
Iliac crest (L4), 4, 124–127
  in back surface anatomy, 40
Iliac lymph nodes
  of abdomen, 226, 226t, 423
  female genitalia and, 235
  parietal, of posterior abdominal wall, 228
  male genitalia and, 234
  of pelvis, 227, 227t
Iliaca communis, arteria, 206, 206t, 208, 222–225, 222t
  arteria iliaca internal, branches of, 222, 222t
  in situ, 213, 216, 221
  ureters and, 180
Iliaca communis, vena, 214, 214t
Iliaca interna, arteria, branches of, 222, 222t
Iliacus muscles
  in abdominal wall, 138–139, 138t
  in hip and thigh, 366–369, 374–375, 374t
Iliacus, plexus
  male pelvic innervation and, 243
  urinary organ innervation and, 239
Iliocostalis muscles
  in back, 30, 30t, 31
  in neck, 560, 560t
Iliofemorale, ligamentum, 364–365
Iliohypogastricus, nervus, 426–427, 426t
  plexus lumbosacralis, overview, 424–425
Ilioinguinalis, nervus, 426–427, 426t
  in female perineum, 194
  in male perineum, 203
  plexus lumbosacralis, overview, 424–425
Iliolumbalis, arteria, 222, 222t

Iliopsoas, musculus, 366–368, 374–375, 374t
Ileum, 124–127, 358–359
Incisura
  clavicularis, 44, 46
  costalis, 46
  jugularis, of sternum, 44, 46
  scapularis,333, 333t
  suprajugularis, 120
Incus, 532. *See also* Ossicular chain
Indicator muscles, innervation of, 612
Indusium griseum, 621, 621t
Infection
  nasopharyngeal, *527*
  of sinus paranasalis, *523*
  of stomach, *159*
  of tonsilla pharyngea, *553*
Inflammation
  of large intestine, *165*
  of small intestine, *163*
Inflection points, line of gravity and, 3
Infracolic compartment, 144
Infrahyoideus, musculus, 560t, 562–563, 562t
  innervation of, 37, 569
Infraorbitalis, nervus, 547
Infraspinatus, musculus, 273, 273t
  posterior shoulder and arm and, 269
Infratemporalis, fossa, 502–503
  deep neurovasculature of, 503
  superficial neurovasculature of, 502
Infundibulum, 597, 597t
Inguinal hernia, *135*
Inguinal lymph nodes, superficial and deep, 423
  female genitalia and, 235
  male genitalia and, 234
  parietal, of posterior abdominal wall, 228
  in pelvis, 227, 227t
Inguinal ring(s), 130–133, 133t, 135
  dissection of, 133
  external, 437, 437t
  in pelvic surface anatomy, 248
Inguinale, ligamentum
  of canalis inguinalis, 133, 133t
  in surface anatomy, 249
Inguinalis, fossa
  lateralis, 131, 133–135, 133t
  medialis, 134–135
Inguinalis, regio, 132, 436
  sensory innervation of, 426
  structures of, 437, 437t
  superficial veins and lymph nodes of, 436
Innervation. *See also* Autonomic innervation; Parasympathetic innervation; Sympathetic innervation
  of abdominal organs, anterior, 238–239
  of auris, 529
  of back, 36, 36t
  of capsula articulatio temporomandibularis, 541
  of cavitas oris, 546–547
  of cavitas thoracis, 74–75, 75t
  diaphragma, 53–54
  of dura mater, 603
  of intestines, 240–241
  of lower limb, 434–435
  of membranous labyrinth, 537
  of muscles, 612. *See also under individual muscles*
  of musculi extraocularis, 509
    by nervus oculomotorius, 475
  of musculi pharyngeales, 485
  of orbita, 511
  of palm of hand, 345
  of pelvis, 242–243
  of regio nuchalis, 568–569, 568t
  segmental, medulla spinalis lesions and, 600
  of thoracic wall, 58–59
    muscles, 53
    peripheral sensory cutaneous, 58
  of tongue, 549
  of upper limb, 320, 320t
  of urinary organs, 239
Inspiration, 112–113
  in normal respiration vs. pneumothorax, *113*
  rib cage movement in, 48
Intercostal space, chest tube insertion via, *60*
Intercostales, arteriae, 56, 56t
Intercostales, musculi, 50–51, 50t
Intercostales, nervi, 36, 55
  in breast sensory innervation, 62
  course of, 59
Intercostalis, vena, 55
Intercostobrachialis, nervus, 326, 326t
Intermesentericus, plexus, 237
  large intestinal innervation and, 241
  pelvic innervation and, 242–243
  urinary organ innervation and, 239
Internal genitalia. *See also individual organs*
  development of, 205
  in female, 188–191
    overview, 186, 186t
  in male, 187, 187t
Internal organs
  abdominal, 158–179. *See also individually named organs*
    arteries of, 206–213
    innervation of, 236–241
    lymphatic drainage of, 228–233
    veins of, 214–221
  arteries of, 206–213, 222–225
  genital, 186–205. *See also* Genitalia
    arteries of, 222–225
    innervation of, 242–247
    lymphatic drainage of, 234–235
    veins of, 222–225
  lymphatic drainage of, 226–235
  pelvic, 180–205. *See also individually named organs*
    arteries of, 222–225
    innervation of, 242–247
    lymphatic drainage of, 227, 227t, 234–235
    veins of, 222–225
  referred pain from, *246*
  urinary, 176–185
    arteries of, 208–209
    innervation of, 246–247
    lymphatic drainage of, 229
    veins of, 214–215
  venae of, 214–225
Interossea cruris, membrana, 380
Interossei plantares, musculi, 418–419, 418t
Interosseus muscles
  atrophy of, nervus ulnaris damage and, *329*
  of hand, 314–315, 314t
  of sole of foot, 418–419, 418t
Interosseus talocalcaneus, ligamentum, 406–407
Interphalangealis, articulatio, 300
  ligaments of, 302
Interspinales, musculi, 32–33, 32t
Intertransversarii, musculi, 27, 32–33, 32t
Intertransversi, ligamentum, 21

Intervertebralis, discus, 12–13
posterolateral herniation, and spinal nerve compression, *13*
thoracic spine, 44
Intervertebral facet joints. *See* Zygapophysealis, articulatio
Intervertebralis, vena, 611
Intestines, 162–167
innervation of, 240–241
large, 164–167
lymph nodes and lymphatic drainage of, 232–233
small, 162–163
Intimal tear, *69*
Intra-articular fracture, of humerus, *257*
Intracranial pressure, fundus opticus examination and, *517*
Intraocular pressure, glaucoma and, *518*
Intraparotideus, plexus, 478
Intraperitoneal organs, 142t
autonomic innervation of, 245
Intraventricular septal defect (VSD), *95*
Intrinsic muscles
of back, 26–27, 30–33
deep, 32–33, 32t
fascia thoracolumbalis and, 23, 26
intermediate, 30–31, 30t
superficial, 30–31, 30t
basis cranii and, 464, 465
cervical spine, 24–25. *See also* nuchal muscles
Invasive ductal carcinoma, *65*
Investing layer, in fascia cervicalis profunda, 577, 577t
Iris, 518
Irrigation, of auditory canal, *527*
Ischiadicum, foramen, 439, 439t
Ischiadicus, nervus, 432–433, 432t, 433t
plexus lumbosacralis, overview, 424–425
plexus sacralis, overview, 430t
Ischioanalis, fossa, 154
regio glutealis and, 439
Ischiocavernosus, musculus
of female perineum, 193
of male perineum, 200
Ischiofemoralis, ligamentum, 364–365
Ischiopubis, ramus, as perineum boundary, 137
Ischii, os, 124–127, 358–359
Isocortex, 595

J

Jejunum, 162
lymph nodes of, 232
Joint capsules
of articulatio coxae, 364–365
of articulatio genu, 385, 390
outpouching in, *385*
articulatio glenohumerale, 261
articulatio temporomandibular, 463, 468
innervation of, 541
of elbow, 285
of fingers, 304
Jugular notch, 44
Jugularis, fossa, in thorax surface anatomy, 120
Jugularis, vena, 496, 496t
anterior, 496, 496t, 567
externa, 496, 496t, 567
impeded flow in, *567*
interna, 496, 496t, 567
ductus thoracicus drainage and, 72
Jugulosubclavialis junctions, articulatio, *586*
Juncturae columnae vertebralis faciei. *See* Zygapophyseales, articulationes
Juxtaintestinal lymph node, 232

K

Keratoconjunctivitis sicca, *515*
Kerckring, valves of, 160
Kiesselbach's area, nosebleeds and, *525*
Kyphosis, 2, *2*

L

Labia majora/labia minora, 136
function of, 186t
in urogenital system, 186
Labor, episiotomy during, *193*
Labyrinth, membranous, innervation of, 537
Lacrimal apparatus, 515
Lacrimal drainage, *515*
Lactiferus, ductus, 63
Lactiferus, sinus, 63
Lacunae musculorum, 437, 437t
Lacunae vasorum, 437, 437t
Lacunar lymph nodes, intermediate, 235
Lamina cribosa, constricted nervus opticus in, *518*
Lamina pretrachealis, of fascia cervicalis profunda, 577, 577t
Lamina prevertebralis, of fascia cervicalis profunda, 577, 577t
Landmarks, palpable. *See* Palpable bony prominences
Large intestine, 164–165. *See also* Colon; Rectum
diseases of, *165*
innervation of, 240
lymph nodes of, 233
radiographic appearance of, 165
referred pain from, *246*
Larynx, 570–573, 573t
cartilages of, 570, 589
muscles of, 572, 572t
innervation of, 485
neurovasculature of, 575
os hyoideum and, 558
vestibular and vocal folds of, 573
Latissimus dorsi, musculus, 277, 277t
anterior shoulder and arm, 264–267
in back surface anatomy, 40
posterior shoulder and arm, 268–271, 332
Le Fort fractures, *455*
Lead vectors, for ECG recording, *90*
Learning, limbic system and, 621
Leg, 380–399. *See also* Lower limb
arteries of, 421
bones of, 380–381. *See also* Fibula; Tibia
compartment syndrome in, *445*
compartments of, 444, 444t
muscles of, 396–399
anterior compartment, 392–393, 397, 397t
lateral compartment, 393, 396, 396t
posterior compartment, 398, 398t
neurovasculature of, 442–445
regio poplitealis, 443
veins of, 422
Lens, 518–519
Levator anguli oris, musculus, 467, 467t
Levator ani, musculus, 140–141, 140t
Levator labii inferioris, musculus, 467, 467t
Levator labii superioris alae nasi, musculus, 466, 466t
Levator labii superioris, musculus, 467, 467t
Levator scapulae, musculus, 276, 276t
Levator veli palatini, musculus, 545, 545t
Levatores costarum, musculi, 32–33, 32t

Lien, 174–175
location of, 146–147
nodi lymphoidei and lymphatic drainage of, 230, 231
truncus coeliacus and, 211
vena portae and, 219
Ligamenta. *See also individually named ligamenta, ligamentum*
of ankle, 406–407
of articulatio coxae, 364–365
of articulatio craniovertebralis, 16–17
of articulatio cubiti, 284–285, 284t
of articulatio genus, 384–385, 384t
collaterale, 386, 388–389
cruciatum, 388–389
patellaris, 386
of articulatio temporomandibularis, 540–541
of canalis inguinalis, 133, 133t
of columna vertebralis, 18–21, 559t
of digitus, 304–305
of hand and wrist, 302–303
of pelvis, 128–129
of pes, 408–409
articulatio subtalare, 406–407
articulatio talocruralis, 408–409, 408t
of scapula, 33t, 333
ossified, *255*
of shoulder, 258–259
articulatio glenohumerale and, 261
injury to, *259*
of spina cervicalis, 18–19, 18t, 559
of thoracolumbar spine, 20–21
Ligation, of arteria maxillaris, *495*
Light reflection, by lens, 519
Limbic system, 620, 621t
hippocampal formation and, 596
Limbs. *See* Lower limb; Upper limb; *individual limb parts*
Line of gravity
spine and, 3
whole-body, 357
Linea alba, 130, 131
rectus sheath and, 134
in surface anatomy, 120, 248
Linea semilunaris, 120, 248
Linea sternalis, cavitas pleuralis boundaries and, 102, 102t
Lingua, 548–549
as boundary of cavitas oris, 550
nervus hypoglossus injury and, 487t
nervus hypoglossus palsy of, *549*
Lingula, in lung architecture, 108t
Lingular pneumonia, *107*
Lingualis, arteria, 492, 493t
Lingualis, musculus, 465
Lobe opacity, in lung radiography, 106
Lobectomy, of lung, *109*
Lobus
of cerebral hemispheres, 595
of hepar, 171
of pulmo, 104, 105
removal, *109*
mammary, 63
Long bones, of upper limb, 252–253, 280–281
Longissimus dorsi, musculus
in back, 30–31, 30t
in neck, 560, 560t
Longitudinalis, arcus, 410–411
Longitudinalis, ligamentum
anterior
of cervical spine, 18–19, 18t
of thoracolumbar spine, 20
posterior
of articulatio craniovertebralis, 16
of cervical spine, 18–19, 18t
of thoracolumbar spine, 21
Lordosis, 2, *2*
Lower limb, 356–451. *See also* Ankle/ankle joint; Foot; Leg; Thigh
arteries of, 420–421
bones of, 356–357. *See also individually named bones*
lymphatic drainage of, 423
nerves of, superficial, 434–435
palpable bony prominences in, 357
surface anatomy of, 450–451
veins of, 422–423
perforating veins, 423
superficial, 434–435
Lucency, in lung radiography, 106
Lumbar anesthesia, *601*
Lumbar ganglia, 237, 242
Lumbar lymph nodes, 423
in abdomen, 226, 226t
parietal, of posterior abdominal wall, 228
urinary organs and, 229
Lumbalis, plexus, 424t, 425–427, 426t
muscles innervated by, 426t, 427
nervus femoralis of, 429, 429t
nervus obturatorius of, 428, 428t
Lumbar puncture, *601*
Lumbar spine, 9
articulatio zygapophyseales of, 14
disk herniation in, *13*
lordosis of, 2, *2*
osteoporotic, radiograph of, *9*
palpable proc. spinosus at L4, 4
structure, 5, 5t
Lumbalis, vertebra (L1–L5). *See* Lumbar spine
Lumbosacralis, plexus, 424–425, 424t. *See also* Lumbalis, plexus; Sacralis, plexus; *individually named nerves*
Lumbrical muscles
of foot, 418–419, 418t
of hand, 314–315, 314t
Lunate, 300
MR image of, 301
Lung(s), 104–109. *See also* Pulmonary *entries*
blood supply to, 114–115, 115t, 118
boundaries in, 102, 102t
bronchopulmonary segment of, 108–109
in chest radiograph, 92
diseases of, *107*
lobes of, 105
lymphatic drainage of, 118
metastasis in, *215*
in pleural cavities, 102, 102t
radiographic appearance of, 106
resection of, *109*
in respiration, 112–113
segmental architecture of, 108, 108t
structure, 105
Lung volume, respiratory changes in, 112
Lymph
drainage of. *See* Lymphatic drainage
formation of, 118
Lymph nodes
of abdomen, 226, 226t
parietal, of posterior abdominal wall, 228
urinary organs, 229
axillary, levels of, 64t
cavitas thoracia, 100
cervical
superficial and deep, 587, 587t
tumor metastasis via, *586*

Lymph nodes *(continued)*
  of ileum, 232
  of intestines, 231–232
  of jejunum, 232
  in lower limb, 423
    regio poplitealis of leg, 443
  mediastinal, 100–101
  metastasis to, *586*
  in neck, superficial and deep cervical, 587, 587t
  paraesophageal, 101
  paratracheal, 101
  of pelvis, 227, 227t
  phrenic, superior and inferior, 100
  supraclavicular, gastric carcinoma
  thoracic, 73
  truncus brachiocephalicus, 100
  truncus bronchopulmonalis, 101, 118, 119
  in upper limb, 319
Lymphatic drainage
  of abdomen, 226, 226t
  of esophagus, 101
  in female breast, 64
    and sentinel node in breast cancer, *65*
  of heart, 100
  of internal organs, 231
  of lower limb, 423
  of manus 319
  of mediastinum, 100–101
  of neck, 586
  of pelvis, 227, 227t
  of pleural cavity, 118–119
  of ren, 229
  in thoracic cavity, 72–73
    pathways, 73
    by quadrant, 73
    trunks, 72
  of upper limb, 319
Lymphatic system, 72–73
  ductus thoracicus in, 72, 73
  thymus in, 80
  tumor metastasis via, *65*
Lymphomas, systemic, *586*

M

MA (midaxillary line), 102, 102t
Malleus, 532. *See also* Ossicular chain
Mammariae, lobi, 63
Mammary ridges, 62
Mammography, normal vs. abnormal, *65*
Mandibula, 539
  muscles of mastication and, 463, 468–469, 468t, 469t
    origins and insertions, 464
  teeth, 542
Mandibularis, nervus (CN V_3), in fossa infratemporalis, 503
Manubrium. *See* Sternum
Manus, 298–315
  arteries of, 317
  bones of, 252–253, 298–299, 298t
  carpal region, 342–343
  "clawing" of, nervus ulnaris damage and, *329*
  dorsum, 346–347
  joints of, 300–301
  ligaments of, 302–303
  lymphatic drainage of, 319
  muscles of, 306–315
    dorsal, 310–311
    hypothenar, 312–313, 312t
    metacarpal, 314–315, 314t
    middle and deep layers, 308–309
    superficial and middle layers, 306–307
    thenar, 312–313, 312t
  palm, topography of, 344–345
  pronation and supination of, articulatio radioulnaris and, 286
  surface anatomy of, 352–353
  tendons
    carpus and digitus, 306
    dorsal, 310, 310t
  veins of, 318
Masseter, musculus, 463, 468, 468t
Mastication, musculi, 463–464, 468–469
  motor innervation of, 488
Masticatory muscle sling, 469, 469t
Mastoid lymph nodes, 587, 587t
Mastoideus, processus, *527*
Maxilla, 538
  sinuses maxillae, DPT evaluation, 543
  teeth of, 542
  tuberositas of, fossa pterygopalatina and, 504t
Maxillaria, arteria, 494t, 495
  branches of, 504, 504t
    terminal, of middle ear, 534, 534t
  ligation of, *495*
Maxillomandibular, os, DPT evaluation of, 543
MC. *See* Midclavicular line (MC)
Meatus accusticus
  externus, 528
    curvatura of, *528*
  internus, cranial nerves and, 481, 537
  irrigation of, *527*
Meatus, nasal structures and, 522
Median sacral vein, 214, 214t
Medianus, nervus, 326t, 328, 328t
  injury to, *328*
  muscles innervated by, 328t
  sensory distribution, 328
"Mediastinal flutter," *113*
Mediastinum, 76–101
  anterius, contents of, 76t
  cavitas thoracica and, 66
  contents of, 76t, 77
  divisions of, 76
    cavitas thoracica and, 67
  esophagus in, 96–99. *See also* Esophagus
  heart, 82–87. *See also* Heart
  mediastinum inferius
    contents of, 76t
    heart in, 82–83
    structures of, 78–79
  lymphatic drainage of, 100–101
  medius, contents of, 76t
  overview of, 76–77
  in pneumothorax, *113*
  posterius, contents of, 76t
  structures of, 78–79
  superius
    contents of, 76t
    structures of, 78–79
    thymus in, 80
Medulla oblongata, 593, 539t
  nervus accessorius and, 486
  nervus glossopharyngeus (CN VIX) and, 482
  nervus hypoglossus and, 487
  nervus vagus and, 484
  nervus vestibulocochlearis (CN VIII) and, 480
Medulla spinalis, 600–601
  arteriae of, 34, 610
  autonomic tracts in, 622
  in central and peripheral nervous systems, 592
  CSF and, 604
  sympathetic nervous system in thorax and, 75, 75t

tracti ascendens of, 613–614, 614t
tracti descendens of, 613, 615, 615t
venae of, 35, 611
Medullaris segmentalis, arteria, 610
Membrana arachnoidea, 602
Membrana synovialis, in articulatio coxae, 364
Membrana tympanica, 528, 532
arteriae of, 534
in otoscopy, *529*
sound waves and, *533*
Membranous labyrinth, 537
vestibular stem receptors and, 618
Membrum superius, 252–353. *See also* Axilla; Antebrachii; Brachii; Carpus; Manus; Shoulder; *individually named bones*
arteriae of, 316–317
lymphatic drainage of, 319
musculi of, 272–279
innervation by plexus brachialis, 320, 320t
nervi of, 330–331
ossae of, 252–257, 280–281
palpable bony prominences in, 253
posterior shoulder and axilla and, 332–333
regio brachialis of, 338
regio cubitalis of, 339
shoulder, 332–335
surface anatomy of, 350–351
venae of, 318
superficial, 330
Memory, limbic system and, 621
Meningea, arteria
of auris media, 534, 534t
in calvaria, 457
injury to, 495
Meningea media, arteria, injury to, *495*
Meninges, 602–603
Meningitis, *527*
Menisci, 387
injury to, *387*
Mentalis, musculus, 467, 467t
Mesencephalon
in brain development, 593t
components of, 596
and formatio reticularis, 618
limbic system and, 621
nervus oculomotorius and nervus trochlearis and, 471t, 474, 474t
Mesenteric lymph nodes, 232
in abdomen, 226, 226t, 231, 232
female genitalia and, 235
inferior, 226–227, 232
intermediate, 232
male genitalia and, 234
parietal, of posterior abdominal wall, 228
in pelvis, 227, 227t
Mesenterica inferior,
arteria, 206–207, 206t, 213
ganglion, 237
large intestinal innervation and, 241
urinary organ innervation and, 239
vena, 221
Mesenterica superior
arteria, 206–207, 206t, 212
arterial anastomoses and, 207
vena, 215, 220
Mesenterici superiors, nodi lymphoidei, 232
in abdomen, 226, 226t, 231, 232
parietal, of posterior abdominal wall, 228
in pelvis, 227, 227t
Mesentericus, plexus. *See* Mesentericus inferius, plexus; Mesenteric superior, plexus
female internal genitalia and, 188
of peritoneal cavity, 145, 148
peritoneum and, 142, 142t
of small intestine, 162
of stomach, 159
Mesentericus inferius, plexus, 236, 236t
large intestinal innervation and, 241
pelvic innervation, 242–243
Mesentericus superior, plexus, 236, 236t
anterior abdominal organ innervation and, 238
intestinum tenue innervation and, 240
Mesometrium, 188
Mesosalpinx, 188
Mesovarium, 188
Metacarpale
articulatio, 300
ligamentum, 302
ossae, 252–253, 298–299, 298t
third, transverse section of, 305
Metacarpales, musculi, 314–315, 314t
Metacarpophalangeallis, articulatio, 300
extension and flexion of, 304
ligaments of, 302
MR image of, 301
Metastasis. *See* Tumor metastasis
Metatarsale, ossa, 400–401
Metatarsophalangealis, articulatio, 403
Metatarsus
arch of, 410
bones of, 400–401
Meyer's loop, 473
Michaelis' rhomboid, 41
Midaxillary line (MA), 102, 102t
Midclavicular line (MC), 121
pleural cavity boundaries and, 102, 102t
Midgut, innervation of, 245
Molar teeth, 542
Monosynaptic reflex, 613
Mons pubis, 136, 186t
Motility, ocular, 508
Motion
of articulatio genus, in flexion and extension
ligamentum cruciatum and ligamentum collaterale, 389
menisci, 387
axes of, hand and wrist, 301
pelvic stability and, 358
Motor system, 613
extrapyramidal. *See* Extrapyramidal motor system
pathways in, 613, 615, 615t
Mouth, muscles of, 467, 467t
"Mouth breathing," *553*
Mucosa
lateral nasal wall, 525
lingualis, 548
pharyngealis, 553
septum nasi, 524
Müllerian duct, 205, 205t
Musculus multifidus, 32–33, 32t
Multiple sclerosis, *517*
Multisegmental muscles
innervation of, 612
spinal reflexes and, 613
Muscle edema, compartment syndrome and, *445*
Muscle sling, masticatory, 469, 469t
Muscle weakness, Musculus gluteus minimus, *431*
Musculi. *See also individual musculi*
of abdominal wall, 130–131, 138–139, 138t
surface anatomy of, 248

Musculi *(continued)*
- of antebrachium
  - anterior, 288–289
  - posterior, 290–291
- of arm
  - anterior, 264–267, 278, 278t
  - posterior, 268–271, 279, 279t
  - surface anatomy of, 350–351
- of auricle, 529
- of back, 22–33. *See also* Back, muscles of
  - surface anatomy of, 40–41
- of ear, 466, 466t
  - external, 529
- erectile, in female, 193
- of facial expression, 462–463, 466–467
  - origins and insertions, 464–465
- of hip, 374–375, 374t
  - anterior, 366–369
  - posterior, 370–373
- innervation of, 612. *See also under individual musculi*
- of larynx, 572, 572t
- of leg
  - anterior, 392–393, 397, 397t
  - lateral, 393, 396, 396t
  - posterior, 394–395, 398, 398t
- of lingua, 548
- of lower limb. *See individual regions, e.g.* of region glutealis, of leg, of thigh, of pes
- of manus
  - hypothenar muscles, 312–313, 312t
  - metacarpus, 314–315, 314t
  - middle and deep layers, 308–309
  - superficial and middle layers, 306–307
  - surface anatomy of, 352–353
  - thenar muscles, 312–313, 312t
- of mastication, 468–469, 468t, 469t
  - location, 463
  - origins and insertions, 464–465
- of neck, 560–565
  - classification, 560t
  - deep, 564–565, 564t
  - infrahyoidale, 561t, 562–563, 562t
  - nuchal, 560, 560t
  - superficial, 560, 561, 561t
  - suprahyoidale, 561t, 562–563, 562t
- of oral cavity
  - as boundary of cavitas oris, 550
  - oral floor, 544, 545t
  - palatum molle, 545, 545t
- of os, 467, 467t
- of pelvic floor, 140, 140t
  - in female, 136, 141, 152
  - in male, 137, 153
- of pes
  - of sole, 412–413, 417–419, 417t, 418t
  - of dorsum, 414–416, 416t
- of region glutealis, 374–375, 374t
  - anterior, 366–369
  - posterior, 370–373
- of shoulder, 264–271. *See also* Shoulder, muscles of
- of skull and face, 462–469
  - forehead, nasi, and auris, 466, 466t
  - origins and insertions, 464–465
  - os, 467, 467t
- of stomach, layers, 158
- of thigh
  - anterior, 366–369, 378, 378t
  - medial group, 376–377, 376t, 377t
  - posterior, 370–373, 379, 379t
- thoracic wall, 50–51, 50t. *See also* Diaphragma
- of thorax, 120
- of upper limb, 350–351
  - innervation by plexus brachialis, 320, 320t

Muscularis externa
- of canalis analis, 167
- of duodenum, 160

Muscularis extrema, 158
Musculocutaneus, nervus, 326t, 327
- muscles innervated by, 327, 327t
- sensory distribution, 327

Musculophrenica, arteria, 55, 55t, 56t, 56
Myelination, 592
Mylohyoideus, musculus, 544, 545t, 562, 562t, 563
Myocardial infarction, types of, *89*

N

Nares, 520
Nasalis, musculi, 466, 466t
Nasalis pharyngis, pars, 520
- infection in, *527*

Nasopharyngeal bleeding, *495*
Nausea, 620
Navicularis, os, 400–401
- articulationes involving, facies articularis, 403

Near vision, light reflection by lens and, 519
Neck (Cervix). *See also* Larynx; Nuchae *entries*
- arteriae of, 490–495, 566
  - impeded flow in, *567*
- bony structures of, 558
- boundaries of, 558
- chronic pain in, *15*
- glandulae in. *See* Parathyroidea, glandula; Thyroidea, glandula
- lamina profunda of, 577, 577t
- musculi of, 560–565
  - classification, 560t
  - infrahyoidei, 561t, 562–563, 562t
  - nuchae, 560, 560t
  - profunda, 564–565, 564t
  - superficialis, 560, 561, 561t
  - suprahyoidei, 561t, 562–563, 562t
- nervus vagus branches in, 485
- regions of, 576, 576t. *See also* Regio cervicalis
- sensory innervation of, 489, 568t, 569
- surface anatomy of, 588–589
- vas lymphaticum of, 586–587
- venae of, 496–497, 567
  - principalis superficialis, 496t
  - profunda, 497

Necrosis, avascular, os scaphoideum fractures and, *299*
Nerve cells. *See* Neurons
Nerve compression
- in crus, *445*
- nervus radialis *325*
- nervus spinalis, *13, 15*
- nervus suprascapularis, *255*

Nervi. *See also individually named nervi*
- of auris internum, 537
- of back, 36, 36t
- of cavitas nasi, 525
- of cavitas thoracis, 66, 74–75
- craniales, 470–471. *See* Craniales, nervi; *individually named nervi*
- in fossa pterygopalatina, 505
- of male perineum and genitalia, 203
- of membrum inferius, superficialis, 434–435
- of membrum superius, superficialis, 330–331
- orbita and, 506t
- of palatum durum, 546
- plexus. *See* Autonomic plexus; Plexus (nervi)

of plexus brachialis, 320–321
of plexus lumbosacralis, 424–425, 424t
of regio carpalis, 342
of regio nuchalis, 37
Nervous system, divisions of, 612
Neural tube, development of, 593t
Neurocranium, 454t
Neuronal circuit, in systema limbica, 621
Neurons
in autonomic nervous system, 622
components of, 592
Neurotransmitters, 592
regulatory effects of, 622
Neurovasculature
of auris internum, 537
of back, 34–39
of caput and facies, 488–505
of cavitas nasi, 524–525
of cavitas oris, 546
palatum durum, 546
oral floor, 547
of crus, 442–445
anterior, 445
lateral, 444
regio poplitea, 443
posterior, 442, 447
of diaphragma, 54–55, 55t
of digiti, 344
of esophagus, 98–99
of facies
fossa infratemporalis, 502–503
fossa pterygopalatina, 504–505, 504t, 505t
fossa temporalis, 501
regio parotidea, 500
superficialis, 498–499
of femur, 448–449
anterior, 440
posterior, 441
of genitalia
female, 194–195
male, 202–203
of glandula parathyroidea, 575
of glandula thyroidea, 575
of larynx, 575
of lingua, 549
of orbita, 510–511, 512, 513
fossa pterygopalatina and, 505t
structural openings, 506t
of palma manus, 344–355
of pes, 445–447
of perineum
in female, 195
in male, 203
of pharynx, 556–557
of regio nuchalis, 38
of thoracic wall, 60–61
of tracheobronchial tree, 116–117
Newborn
circulation in, 95
kyphotic curvatura spinalis in, *2*
septum nasii defects in, *95*
Nodus sinuatrialis, 90
and postsynaptic neurons, 91
Non-geniculate pathway, 616
Nose, 520–525
musculi of, 466, 466t
os ethmoidale of, 460
skeleton of, 520
structural openings into, 522, 522t
Nosebleeds, *525*
Nuchalis, fascia, 23
Nuchae, ligamentum, 18t, 19
of articulatio craniovertebrales, 16
Nuchalis, musculi, 24–25. *See also* Intrinsic musculi
basis cranii and, 464, 465
classification of, 560, 560t
Nuchalis, regio
innervation of, 568–569, 568t
nervi of, 37
neurovasculature of, 38
surface anatomy of, 588–589
vascular supply to, 34
Nuclei
abducens, 474
accessorius, 486
facialis, 478
glossopharyngeus, 482
hypoglossus, 487
nervi cranialis, 471
occulomotorius, 474
premotor, 618
systema limbicus, 621
systema vestibularis and, 618
trigeminus, 476
trochlearis, 474
vagus, 484
vestibulocochlearis, 480
Nuclei basale, of telencephalon, 594, 597, 597t
Nucleus pulposus, 12
disk herniation and, *13*
Nucleus subthalamicus, 597, 597t
"Nursemaid's elbow," *287*

O

Obliquus capitis, musculus, 28, 28t, 564–565, 564t
Obliquus externus, musculus, 138–139, 138t
in abdominal wall, 130–131
of canalis inguinalis, aponeurosis of, 133, 133t
rectus sheath and, 134
in surface anatomy, 40, 248
Obliquus internus, musculus, 138–139, 138t
in abdominal wall, 130–131
aponeurosis, 130
of canalis inguinalis, 133, 133t
rectus sheath and, 134
Obliquus oculi, musculus, 508, 508t
Obstetrical procedure, *193*
Obturatoria, arteria and venae, 222, 222t
Obturatorii, nodi lymphoidei, 235, 587, 587t
Obturatorius externus, musculus, 366–368, 377, 377t
Obturatorius internus, musculus
in coxa and femur, 370, 374, 374t, 375
in pelvic wall, 140, 140t
Obturatorius, nervus, 424–426, 424t, 426, 426t
motor and sensory rami, 428–429, 428t, 429t
sensory distribution, 428
Occipitalis, arteria, 493, 493t
Occipitalis, lobus, 595
lesions of, *617*
Occipitalis, nervus, 37
Occipitofrontalis, musculus, 466, 466t
Occiput, venae of, 497
Ocular motility, 508
Oculomotorius, nervus (CN III), 474–475
balance and, 618
injury to, effects of, 474t, 475
location, overview, 470
origin, 471t
palsy, 474, *509*
reflexes of visual system, 617

Oesophageales, plexus, 98
Olfactorius, bulbus, 472
Olfactorius, cortex, 594
Olfactorius, nervus, (CN I), 472
  location, overview, 470
  origin, 471t
  in smell, 620
Olfactory system, 620
Omentum
  bursa of. *See* Lesser sac (bursa omentalis)
  major, 144–145
  minus, 159
Omohyoideus, musculus, 562–563, 562t
Opacity, in pulmonal radiography, 106
Open-angle glaucoma, *518*
Ophthalmica, arteria, 517
Ophthalmicae, venae, 517
Opponens digiti minimi, musculus, 418–419, 418t
Opticus, fundus, *517*
Opticus, nervus (CN II), 473
  constricted, glaucom and, *518*
  lesion of, *617*
  location, overview, 470
  origin, 471t
  reflexes of visual system, 617
Opticus, tractus, 597, 597t
  lesion of, *617*
Opticus, axis, bulbus oculi and, 516
Oral floor, muscli of, 544, 545t
  as boundary of cavitas oris, 550
  innervation of, 547
Orbicularis oculi, musculus, 466, 466t
Orbicularis oris, musculus, 467, 467t
Orbita, 506–515
  apparatus lacrimalis and, 515
  axis of
    bulbus oculi and, 516
    nervus oculomotorius palsy and, *509*
  bulbus oculi and, 516
  fossa pterygopalatina and, 505t
  innervation of, 511
  musculi of, 508–509, 508t
  nervi craniales in, 511
  neurovasculature of, 510–513
    contents, 513
    passage through orbita, 512
    structural openings, 506t
  palpebrae and conjunctiva and, 514
  structures surrounding, 507t
  topography of, 514
Organ blockage, *143*
Organ contact areas
  hepar, 170
  ren, 176
Organ of cortex, 536
Organs
  internal, 158–185. *See* Internal organs
  reproductive, 186–205. *See* Genitalia
  urinary, 176–185. *See* Urinary organs
Ossae. *See also individually named ossae*
  of antebrachium, 280–281
  of auris, 526–527
  of back, 2–11
  of brachium, 256–257
  of caput, 454–461
  of carpus, 298–299
  of cavitas nasii, 520–521
    sinus paranasii and, 523
  of cavitas oralis, 538–539
    articulatio temporomandibularis and, 540
  of cingulum pelviucm, 124–127, 358–359
  of columna vertebralis, 2–13
  of femur, 360–361
  of manus, 298–299
  of membrum inferius, 356–357
  of membrum superior, 252–257
  of neck, 558
  of orbita, 506–507
  of pes, 400–401
  of shoulder, 254–257
  of sinus paranasii, 523
  of sura, 380–381
  of thorax, 44–47
  of vertebra, 2–11
Ossicula auditus. *See* Ossicular chain
Ossicular chain, 532–533
  arteriae of, 534
  ossae of, 532
  in hearing, *533*
Ossiculorum auditus, musculi. *See* Ossicular chain
Ossification, of ligamentum transversum superior of scapula, *255*
Osteomeatal unit, 522
Osteophytes, nervus spinalis compression and, *15*
Osteoporose, *9*
  femoral fractures and, *361*
Otoscope, insertion of, *529*
Ovar, 188–189
  ligamentum suspensorium of, 151
  in pelvis, 151
  in systema urogenitales, 186
Ovarian primordium, 205
Ovarica, venae, 214, 214t
Ovaricus, plexus, 236–237, 236t, 242
  intestinum tenue innervation and, 240
Oxygenated blood, in circulatory system, 82
  venae pulmonales and, 82

P

Pacemaker. *See* Nodus sinuatrialis (SA)
Pain
  acute abdominal, *143*
  chronic neck, *15*
  referred, from internal organs, *246*
Palatinum, os, 538
  fossa pterygopalatina and, 504t
Palatoglossus, musculus, 545t, 548
  innervation of, 549
Palatopharyngeus, musculus, 545t, 555
Palatum
  durum, as paries superior of cavitas oris, 538
  fossa pterygopalatina and, 505t
  molle, musculi of, 545, 545t
Palatum durum, 538–539
  neurovasculature of, 546
  as cavitas oris boundary, 550
Palatum molle
  as cavitas oris boundary, 550
  musculi of, 545–555, 545t
Palma of manus, 344–345
  surface anatomy of, 353
Palmaris longus, musculus, 288, 292, 292t
Palpable bony prominences
  in abdomen and pelvis, 248
  in back, 40
  of caput and neck, 588–589
  in manus and carpus, 352–353
  in membrum inferius, 357, 450–451
  in membrum superius, 253, 350–351
  processi spinosi
    vertebra lumbales (L IV), 4, 9
    as spinal landmarks, 4
    12th vertebra thoracis (T XII), 4, 8
    vertebra prominens (C VII), 4, 6
  in thorax, 120

Palsy. *See also* Paralysis
  nervus abducens, *509*
  nervus oculomotorius, 474, *509*
  nervus trochlearis, *509*
Pancreas, 174–175
  effects of autonomic nervous system on, 244t, 623t
  location of, 146
  nodi lymphatici and lymphatic drainage of, 230–231
  referred pain from, *246*
  truncus coeliacus and, 211
  vena porta and, 219
Pancreaticocholedochus, ductus
  pancreas and, 174
  vesica fellea and, 172, 173
Pancreaticoduodenales, nodi lymphoidei, 231
Pancreaticus, plexus, anterior abdominal organ innervation and, 238
Pancreatitis, cholelithiasis and, *173*
Papez circuit, 621
Papilla mammaria, 62, 63
  accessoriae, 62
  in thorax surface anatomy, 121
Papillae, lingual, 548
Paracolici, nodi lymphoidei, 232
Paraoesophageales, nodi lymphoidei, 101
Parahippocampales, gyrus, 621, 621t
Paralysis. *See also* Palsy
  facial, 479t
  of musculi extra- and intraoculares, 474
  of musculus genioglossus, *549*
  nervus hypoglossus injury and, 487t
  sternocleidomastoideus, 486
  trapezius, 486
Parasternales, nodi lymphoidei, 64
  tumor spread and, *65*
Parasympathetic innervation. *See* Systema nervosa parasympathica
Parathyroidea, glandula, 574
  neurovasculature of, 575
Paratracheales, nodi lymphoidei, 101
Paravertebrales, linea (PV), 102, 102t
Parietales, fascia, pelvic, 154
Parietales, musculi, pelvic wall, 140, 140t, 141
Peritoneum, 144
Peritoneum parietale
  of canalis inguinalis, 133, 133t
  vagina musculi recti abdominis and, 134
Parotidei, nodi lymphoidei, 587, 587t
Parotideomasseterica, regio, topography of, 500
Parotis, glandula, 551
Patella, 383
  articulation with femur, 382
Patellae, ligamenti, 386
Pectineus, musculus, 366–368, 376, 376t
Pectorales, nervi, 326, 326t
Pectoralis major, musculus, 274, 274t
  anterior shoulder and brachium, 264–267
  nodi lymphoidei axillares and, 64
  in thorax surface anatomy, 120
Pectoralis minor, musculus, 275, 275t
  anterior shoulder and brachium and, 265
  nodi lymphoidei axillares and, 319
Peduncula, cerebellares, 598
Pelvica, ganglia, autonomic plexuses of, 236, 236t
Pelvis
  arteriae of, 222–225
  autonomic plexuses of, 236, 236t
  divisions of, 154t
  female, 126–127, 127t, 249
    arteriae and venae of, 222, 222t, 223
    in childbirth, *127*
    contents of, 151
    coronal section, 155
    features of, 127, 127t
    innervation of, 242
    measurements, 129
    nodi lymphoidei of, 235
    peritoneal relationships in, 152
    transverse section, 157
    ureter in, 181
    urethra in, 185
    vesica urinaria in, 183
  floor of. *See* Diaphragma pelvis
  ligamenti of, 128–129
  male, 126–127, 127t, 249
    arteriae and venae of, 222, 222t, 223
    contents of, 150
    coronal section, 155
    features of, 127, 127t
    innervation of, 243
    nodi lymphoidei of, 234
    peritoneal relationships in, 153
    transverse section, 157
    ureter in, 181
    urethra in, 185
    vesica urinaria in, 182
  musculi of
    diaphragma pelvis, 140, 140t, 141
    diaphragma pelvis. *See under* Diaphragma pelvis
    pelvic wall, 140, 140t, 141
  musculus gluteus minimus and, *431*
  nodi lymphoidei and lymphatic drainage of, 227, 227t, 234–235
  organs of, 142, 142t
  and regio urogenitalis, 154
  surface anatomy of, 248–249
  venae of, 222–225
Pelvis renalis and calices, embryonic derivatives of, 205t
Penis, 137, 196–197
  ligamentum suspensorium of, 150
  neurovasculature of, 202
  urethra and, 185
Peptic ulcus, *143*
Peribronchial network, for lymph drainage, 118
Pericardiaphrenica, arteria, 55, 55t
Pericardium, 80–81
  and mediastinal lymph drainage, 100
Pericardium serosum, parietalis and visceralis, 81
  cardiac surfaces and, 84
Perihilaris, regio, radiolucency of, 106
Perimenopausal women, lacrimal drainage in, *515*
Perinea, raphe, 137
Perineum
  boundaries of, 137
  divisions of, 154t
  in female, 136
    diaphragma pelvis and, 136
    neurovasculature, 195
  in male, 137
    diaphragma pelvis and, 137
    neurovasculature, 203
Peripheral pulmo, lymphatic drainage of, 118
Peritoneum
  and mesenterium, 142, 142t
  parietal
    of canalis inguinalis, 133, 133t
    vagina musculi recti abdominis and, 134
Pes, 400–419
  arches of, 410–411
  arteriae pedis, 420

Pes *(continued)*
- articulatio pedes of, 402–407
  - articulatio subtalare, 404–407
  - articulatio talocruralis, 404–405
  - facies articulationes distales and proximales, 403
- force distribution, 410
- ligaments of, 408–409
  - in articulatio subtalaris, 406–407
  - in articulatio talocruralis, 408–409, 408t
- muscles of, 412–419
  - deep intrinsic, 414
  - intrinsic dorsal, 416, 416t
- nervus tibialis in, 433
- neurovasculature of, 445–447
- ossa pedes, 400–401
- posterior compartment of, medial view, 443
- stabilizers of, 410–411
- veins of, 422

Pes cavus, 410

Pes planus, 410

Pes rectus, 410

Pes transversoplanus, 410

Petrosus, nervus, ganglion pterygopalatinum and, 505

Peyer plaques, 162

Phalanges
- of manus, 252–253, 298–299, 298t
- of pes, 400–401

Pharyngea ascendens, arteria, 492, 493t
- of auris media, 534, 534t

Pharyngis, musculi, 554–555, 554t
- innervation of, 485
- neurovasculature of, 556
- basis cranii and, 465

Pharynx, 550, 550t, 553–557
- auris media communication with, 530
- faucial isthmus of, 550, 553
- mucosa of, 553
- musculi of, 554–555
- neurovasculature of, 556–557
- paries superior of, 552

Philippe-Gombault triangle, 613

Phombencephalon, in brain development, 593t

Phrenica, arteria, 55, 55t

Phrenica inferior, vena, 214, 214t

Phrenici, nodi lymphoidei, 100
- inferior, 100
  - in abdomen, 226, 226t, 228
  - parietal, of posterior abdominal wall, 228
  - urinary organs and, 229
- superior, 100

Phrenicus, nervus, in diaphragmatic innervation, 54–55

Phrenica, vena, 55

Phrenicocolicum, ligamentum, 147, 161

Pia mater, 602

Piriformis, musculus
- in coxa and femur, 366–368, 374–375, 374t
- in pelvic wall, 140–141, 140t

Pisiforme, os, 300

Pituitaria, glandula, 596

Placenta, in prenatal circulation, 94

Planes
- subcostales, 121
- transumbilicales, 248

Planta of pes
- arteriae of, 420
- musculi of
  - deep intrinsic, 418–419, 418t
  - intrinsic, 412–413
  - superficial intrinsic, 417, 417t
- venae of, 422

Plantaris, musculus, 394–395, 398, 398t

Platysma, 463, 467t
- in neck, 561t

Pleura parietales, 103
- cavitas pleuralis boundaries and, 102t
- injury to, pneumothorax and, *113*
- parts of, 103

Plexus (nervi)
- autonomic. *See* Autonomic plexus
- brachialis, 320–321. *See also* Brachialis, plexus
- cervicalis. *See* Cervicalis, plexus
- choroideus. *See* Choroideus, plexus
- coeliacus, 236, 236t
- deferentialis, 243
- esophageus, 98
- gastrici, 238
- hepaticus. *See* Hepaticus, plexus
- hypogastricus. *See* Hypogastricus inferior, plexus; Hypogastricus superior, plexus
- iliacus. *See* Iliacus, plexus
- intermesentericus. *See* Intermesentericus, plexus
- of lien. *See* Lienalis, plexus
- lumbosacralis, 424–425, 424t. *See also* Lumbalis, plexus; Sacralis, plexus; *individually named nervi*
- mesentericus. *See* Mesentericus inferior, plexus; Mesentericus superior, plexus
- ovaricus. *See* Ovaricus, plexus
- pancreaticus, 238
- parotideus, 478
- of prostata. *See* Prostaticus, plexus
- of rectum. *See* Rectalis, plexus
- of ren. *See* Renalis, plexus
- suprarenalis. *See* Suprarenalis, plexus
- of testes. *See* Testicularis, plexus
- uretericus. *See* Uretericus, plexus
- uterovaginalis, 242
- vesicalis. *See* Vesicalis, plexus

Plexus (venosus)
- vertebralis, 57, 611
  - externa and interna, 35
- vesicalis, 222, 222t

Plexus autonomicus. *See* Autonomic nervous sytem

Plica vestibularis, 573

Plica vocalis, 573
- cartilago arytenoidea and, 571

Pneumatization, of sinus paransales, 522

Pneumonektomie, *109*

Pneumonie, lingualis, *107*

Pneumothorax, *113*

PNS. *See* Peripheral nervous system (PNS)

Polysynaptic reflex, 613

Polythelia, 62

Pons, 598–599
- development, 593, 593t
- nervi craniales and, 470, 471t
- nervus abducens (CN VI) and, 474
- nervus facialis (CN VII) and, 478–479, 479t
- nervus trigeminus (CN V) and, 476

Poplitea, fossa, Baker's cyst in, *385*

Poplitei, nodi lymphoidei, 423, 443

Popliteus, musculus, 394–395, 399, 399t

Portae, vena, 215, 218–219

Portal circulation, 82

Portosystemic collaterals, 215

"Position sense," 618
Postnatal circulation, 95
Postsynaptic neurons
in autonomic innervation of heart, 91
of esophagus, 98
Postsynaptic potentials, 592
Preaortici, nodi lymphoidei
in abdomen, 226, 226t
in pelvis, 227, 227t
urinary organs and, 229
Precaecales, nodi lymphoidei, 232
Pregnancy, extrauterine (ectopic), *143, 189*
Prenatal circulation, 94
Presynaptic neurons
in autonomic innervation of heart, 91
and esophagus, 98
Prevertebrales, musculi
in back, 29, 29t
basis cranii and, 465
in neck, 560t, 564–565, 564t
Procerus, musculus, 466, 466t
Promontorii, nodi lymphoidei
female genitalia and, 235
male genitalia and, 234
urinary organs and, 229
Pronation, of articulatio radioulnaris, 286–287
Pronator quadratus, musculus, 292–293, 292t
antebrachium anterior, 288–289
antebrachium posterior, 290–291
Pronator teres, musculus, 288–289, 292, 292t
Proprioception, 618
Prosencephalon, in encephalon development, 593t
Prostata, 200–201
primordium of, 205
in situ, 143, 150
Prostate-specific antigen (PSA), *201*
Prostatic carcinoma, *201*
Prostatic hypertrophy, *201*
Prostaticus, plexus, 243
urinary organ innervation and, 239
Proximal articulatio radioulnaris, 282, 284–285, 284t
PSA (prostate-specific antigen), *201*
Pseudopolyps, in early-stage colitis, 165
Psoas, musculus
in abdominal wall, 138–139, 138t
in coxa and femur, 366–369, 374–375, 374t
Pterygoideus, musculus, lateral and medial, 469, 469t
Pterygopalatina, fossa, 504–505, 504t, 505t
Pubis, ramus, 124–127
of diaphragma pelvis, 136
in female pelvis, 151
in male pelvis, 150
Pubis, os, 124–127, 358–359
Pubofemorale, ligamentum, 364–365
Puborectalis, musculus, 166
Pudenda interna, arteria and vena, 222, 222t
Pudendus, nervus, 424–425, 424t
in female perineum, 194
in male perineum, 203
Pulmonales, arteriae, 114–115, 115t, 118
Pulmonary arteriogram, arterial and venous phases in, 115
Pulmonary circulation, 82
Pulmonary edema, *107*
Pulmonary embolism, *115*
Pulmonary emphysema, *107*
Pulmonales, lobuli, venae pulmonales and, 114
Pulmonales, venae, 114–115, 115t, 118
blood circulation and, 82
Pupil size, 519
Pupillary light reflex, 617
Putamen, 597, 597t
PV (Linea paravertebralis), 102, 102t
Pyramidalis, musculus, 138–139, 138t
Pyramidalis, tractus, 615, 615t

Q

Quadrantanopia, *617*
Quadratus femoris, musculus, 370–372, 374, 374t
Quadratus lumborum, musculus, 27, 138–139, 138t
Quadratus plantae, musculus, 418–419, 418t
Quadriceps femoris, musculus, 366–368, 378, 378t
in surface anatomy, 248

R

Radial tear, *387*
Radialis, arteria, 317
Radialis group, musculus
antebrachium anterior, 288–289, 292, 292t
antebrachium posterior, 290–291, 294, 294t
Radialis, nervus, 325, 325t
compression of, *325*
damage to, humeral fracture and, *257*
musculi innervated by, 325, 325t
sensory distribution, 325
Radiatio optica, 473
lesions of, *617*
Radiculares, venae, 611
Radiocarpalis, articulatio, 300
Radiolabeling, in breast cancer assessment, *65*
Radiolucency, in pulmo, 106
Radioulnaris, articulatio
distal, 287, 300
proximal, 282, 284–285, 284t, 287
supination and pronation of, 286
Radioulnaris distalis rotation, articulatio, 287
Radius, 280–281
at carpus, 298, 299
fracture, *287*
in membrum superius, 252–253
Ramus (rami). *See also* Ramus communicans griseus
anterior
nervus lumbalis and, 242–243
nervus sacralis and, 237, 239, 242
in back innervation, 36, 36t
ischiopubic, as perineum boundary, 137
of nervus cervicalis, 464–465, 568t
pubic, 136
in regio nuchalis innervation, 37, 568t
in thoracic wall innervation, 59
Ramus communicans griseus nervi spinalis, 237
pelvic innervation and
in female, 242
in male, 243
Rays, in the pes, 410
Recessus praeopticus, 597, 597t
Recessus sphenoethmoidalis, 522

Rectales superiors, nodi lymphoidei, 232
Rectalis, arteria and venae, media and inferior, 222, 222t
Rectalis, plexus, 242–243
  urinary organ innervation and, 239
Rectum, 166–167, 167t
  lymphatic drainage of, 227
  vas sanguineum of, 224
Rectus abdominis, musculus, 138–139, 138t
  in abdominal wall, 131
  in surface anatomy, 248
Rectus capitis, musculus, 564–565, 564t
  posterior, 28, 28t, 564–565, 564t
Rectus femoris, musculus, 366–369, 373, 378, 378t
Rectus oculi, musculus, 508, 508t
Reference lines, cavitas pleuralis boundaries and, 102, 102t
Referred pain, from internal organs, *246*
Reflexes
  musculi, 613
  of visual system, 617
Ren, 176–179. *See also* Renal *entries*
  effects of autonomic nervous system on, 244t, 623t
  lymphatic drainage of, 229
  organ contact areas with, 176
  referred pain from, *246*
  in retroperitoneum, 149, 177
  structure, 178–179
Renal bed, ren in, 176
Renal hypertension, *209*
Renalis, arteria, 209
  stenose of, *209*
Renalis, plexus, 236–237, 236t
  intestinum tenue innervation and, 240
  urinary organ innervation and, 239
Renalis, vena, 217
  tributaries of, 214
  as tributaries of vena cava inferior, 214, 214t
Reproductive organs, 186–205. *See also* Genitalia; *individual organs*
  overview of, 186–187, 186t, 187t
Respiration, 112–113
  costa cage movement in, 48
Respiratory compromise, conditions causing, *111*
Retinaculum (retinacula), 415
Retinaculum extensorum
  of manus, 310
  of pedis, 415
Retroaortici, nodi lymphoidei, 226, 226t
  parietal, of posterior abdominal wall, 228
Retroauricularis, nodi lymphoidei, 587, 587t
Retroperitoneum
  ren and glandula suprarenalis in, 177
  structures of, 149, 149t
Retropylorici, nodi lymphoidei, 231
Rhombencephalon, in encephalon development, 593t
Rhomboideus, musculus, 276, 276t
Rima glottidis, effects of musculi laryngis action on, 572t
Rima palpebrarum, musculi of, 466, 466t
Rings, fibrous, in cardiac skeleton, 86
Risorius, musculus, 462, 467t
Rotation, of articulatio radioulnaris distalis, 287
Rotator cuff, musculi of, 273, 273t
Rotators, musculi, 32, 32t, 33
Rotundum, ligamentum, 151
Rupture, of ligamentum cruicatum, *389*

S

SA. *See* Nodus sinuatrialis
Sacralia, foramina, nervus spinalis rami in, 36
Sacralia, ganglia, 237
  urinary organ innervation and, 239
Sacralis, arteria and vena, lateralis, 222, 222t
Sacralis, hiatus, epidural anesthesia and, *601*
Sacralis, nervus, 430
Sacralis, nodi lymphoidei
  female genitalia and, 235
  male genitalia and, 234
  parietal, of posterior abdominal wall, 228
  of pelvis, 227, 227t
Sacralis, plexus, 237, 430–433, 432t, 433t, 601
  musculi innervated by, 430t
  pelvic innervation and, 242
  plexus lumbosacralis, overview, 424–425, 424t
Sacroiliaca, articulatio, ligamenti of, 129
Sacrotuberale, ligamentum, as perineum boundary, 137
Sacrum, os, 10–11
  features, 5, 5t
  kyphosis of, 2, *2*
  and os coccygis, 10–11
  radiograph of, 10–11
  in surface anatomy, 40, 451
  vascular supply to, 34
"Sail sign," in articulatio cubiti injury assessment, *283*
Salivary glands, 551
Salivation, 620
Salpingopharyngeus, musculus, 555
Sartorius, musculus, 366–368, 378, 378t
  in surface anatomy, 248
Scaleni, musculus
  in neck, 560t, 564–565, 564t
    innervation of, 569
  in thoracic wall, 50–51, 50t
Scalenus anterior, musculus
  in neck, 560t, 564–565, 564t
    innervation of, 569
  in thoracic wall, 50–51, 50t
Scalenus medius, musculus
  innervation of, 569
  in neck, 560t, 564–565, 564t
  in thoracic wall, 50–51, 50t
Scalenus posterior, musculus
  in neck, 560t, 564–565, 564t
    innervation of, 569
  in thoracic wall, 50–51, 50t
Scaphoideum, os, 298–299
  fractures of, *299*
  MR image of, 301
  tuberculi of, 299, 303
Scapula, 252–253, 255
  ligamenti of, 33t, 333
  neurovascular tracts of, 333t
  ossified ligamentum transversum of, *255*
Scapulae, angulus inferior (TVII), 4, 40
Scapulae, foramen, *255*
Scapular arcade, 317
Scapulothoracicum, articulatio, 258
Scotoma, *617*
Scrotum, 196–199
  neurovasculature of, 202
  in perineum, 137
  cutis of, 198–199, 199t

Segmentation of pulmo, 108
architecture, 108t
bronchopulmonary, 109
Segmentectomy (wedge resection), *109*
Semimembranosus, musculus, 370–372, 379, 379t
Semipronation, of articulatio radioulnaris, 287
Semispinales, musculus
in back, 32–33, 32t, 268–269
in neck, 560, 560t
Semitendinosus, musculus, 370–371, 379, 379t
Senses, 616–621
balance, 618
hearing, 619
sensory system and, 616, 616t
sight, 616–617
smell, 620
taste, 619
Sensorimotor system, 613
integration in, 613
Sensory systems, 613, 616–621
auditory, 619
balance, 618
gustatory, 619
olfactory, 620
pathways in, 613, 614, 614t
special qualities of, 616t
visual, 616–617. *See also* Visual system
Sentinel node, *586*
in breast cancer, *65*
Septal defects, *95*
Septoplasty, *523*
Septum
intraventriculare, 87
nasi. *See* Septum nasi
scroti, 143, 150
Septum nasi, 520
deviated, *523*
mucosa and neurovasculature of, 524, 525
Septum pellucidum, 597, 597t
Septum scrotalis, 143, 150
Septum ventriculare defect (VSD), *95*
Serous layers, of cavita pleuralis, 103
Serratus anterior, musculus, 266–267, 269, 275, 275t
in thorax surface anatomy, 120
Serratus posterior, musculus, 26, 30–31, 30t
in membrum inferior, 269
"Shadows" in pulmo radiography, 106, *107*
Short musculi nuchales, 25, 28, 28t, 560t, 564, 564t, 565
Shoulder
anterior, 334–335
musculi of, 264–267, 274–275
neurovascular contents, 334–335
articulationes of
glenohumeralis. *See* Glenohumeralis, articulatio
overview, 258–259
musculi of
anterior, 264–267, 274–275
musculus deltoideus and rotator cuff, 272–273, 273t
posterior, 256–277, 268–271
ossae of, 252–253
posterior
and axilla, 332–333
musculi of, 268–271, 276–277
neurovascular tracts and, 333t
radiograph of, 260
Shoulder girdle, 258. *See also* Clavicula; Scapula
Sinus durae matris, 606–607, 606t
venous, 457
Sinus(es)
lactiferi, 63
maxillaris, DPT evaluation of, 543
os ethmoidale and, 460
paranasales, 522–523
Sinus nasales et paranasales, 522–523
Sinus paranasales, 522–523
bony structures of, 523
infection of, *523*
MR image of, 523
pneumatization of, 522
Sinus sigmoideus, plexus venosus vertebralis and, 35
Sinus urogenitalis, 205, 205t
Sinus venosus, anastomoses and, 497t
Sinusitis, *523*
Skeleton
cardiac, 86
thoracic, 44
Smell, 620
Soleus, musculus, 394–395, 398, 398t
Somatic nervous system, 612
Somatosensory innervation, of lingua, 549
Sound waves, ossicular chain and, *533*
Spatium pharyngeum, 556
Spatium pleuralis, chest tube insertion into, *60*
Spatium quadrangulare of axilla, 333, 333t
Spatium retropubicum
in female, 152
in male, 150, 153
Spatium subacromialis, 262
Spatium subglotticum 573t
Spatium supraglotticum, 573t
Spatium transglotticum, 573t
Spatium triangulare, of axilla, 333, 333t
Spermatica, fascia, externa and interna, 198–199, 199t
Sphenoidale, os, 460
fossa pterygopalatina and, 504t
Sphenopalatina, arteria, bleeding from, *495*
Sphincter
ani externus, 167
biliary system, 172
at esophagogastric junction, 97
musculi, 140, 140t
Sphincter ani externus, musculus, 167
Spina iliaca, 124–127
in surface anatomy, 40, 120, 248
Spina. *See also* Spina cervicalis; Spina lumbalis; Sacrum, os; Spina thoracica
cervical, 6–7
curvaturae of, 2, *2*
development of, *2*
lumbar, 9
normal anatomical position of, 3
palpable landmarks in. *See under* Palpable bony prominences
plexus venosus vertebralis and, 35
sacral, 10–11
thoracic, 8, 44
Spina sacralis. *See* Sacrum, os
Spina scapulae (TIII), 4
in back surface anatomy, 40
Spinales, musculi, 30, 30t, 31
Spinales, nervi
branches of, 36–37, 36t
compression of
osteophytes and, *15*
posterolateral disk herniation and, *13*
in oral floor innervation, 547
in thoracic wall innervation, 59
processus uncinatus proximity to, *15*
Spinales, venae, 611
Spinalis, arteria, 610

Spinocerebellaris, tractus, 614, 614t
Spinothalamicus, tractus, 614, 614t
Spinosus, processus
of axis, 565
palpable. *See under* Palpable bony prominences
in spina cervicalis, 44
thoracic, 44, 45
of vertebra, 5, 5t
Splayfoot, 410
Splenicus, plexus
anterior abdominal organ innervation and, 238
Intestinum tenue innervation and, 240
Splenii, musculi, 30–31, 30t
in back, 26
in neck, 560, 560t
Spondylolisthesis, traumatic, *7*
stapes, 532. *See also* Ossicular chain
conductive hearing loss and, *533*
Stenosis, of arteria renalis, *209*
Sternoclavicularis, articulatio, 252, 259
Sternocleidomastoidea, regio, 576, 576t
Sternocleidomastoideus, musculus, 560–561, 561t
anesthesia injection and, 588
insertion on basis cranii, 464–465
paralysis of, 486
in surface anatomy, 120, 588–589
Sternocostal joints, 49
Sternocostalis, facies (anterior), of heart, 84
Sternohyoideus, musculus, 562–563, 562t
Sternothyroideus, musculus, 562–563, 562t
Sternum, 44, 46
articulatione sternoclaviculare and, 259
and heart in situ, 82–83
"Stirrup." *See* Stapes
Stria olfactoria, lateralis, 597, 597t
Styloglossus, musculus, 548
Stylohyoideus, musculus, 544, 545t, 562–563, 562t
Stylomastoidea, arteria, 534, 534t
Stylopharyngeus, musculus, 555
Subarachnoid hemorrhage, *603*
Subclavia, arteria
aorta thoracica and, 68, 69t
blood circulation and, 83
in neck, 566
rami of, 317
thoracic wall, 56, 56t
Subclavia, vena, 72
Subclaviculares, nervus, 62
Subclavius, musculus, 275, 275t
Subcostales, musculus, 50–51, 50t
Subdural hematoma, *603*
Sublingualis, glandula, 551
Subluxation, of caput radii, *287*
Submandibulares, nodi lymphoidei, 587, 587t
Submandibularis, glandula, 551
Submentales, nodi lymphoidei, 587, 587t
Suboccipital nerve, 37
Suboccipitalis, musculus
in back, 28, 28t
in neck, 560t, 564–565, 564t
suboccipital triangle and, 585
Subpleural network, for lymph drainage, 118
Subpylorici, nodi lymphoidei, 230, 231
Subscapulares, musculus, 273, 273t
anterior shoulder and brachium, 265–267
Subscapulares, nervus, in plexus brachialis, 323, 323t
Substantia alba
in central nervous system, 592
of medulla spinalis, 613
in telencephalon, 594
Substantia grisea
in central nervous system, 592
reflex control and, 613
of medulla spinalis, organization of, 612
Substantia nigra, 597, 597t
Subtalaris, articulatio, 404–405
Sulcus terminalis, 548
Superficiales, musculi. *See* Extrinsic musculi
Superficiales, venae
of back, 39
of caput and neck, 496
of membrum inferior, 434–435
of membrum superior, 330–331
of thoracic wall, 57
Supination, of articulatio radioulnaris, 286, 287
Supinator, musculus, 296, 296t
antebrachium anterior, 288–289
antebrachium posterior, 290–291
Supraclaviculares, nodi lymphoidei, gastric carcinoma metastasis to, *586*
Supracolic compartment, 144
Suprahyoidei, musculi, 464, 544, 545t, 560t, 562–563, 562t
Suprapatellar pouch, during flexion, 391
Suprapylorici, nodi lymphoidei, 230, 231
Suprarenales, venae, 214, 214t
Suprarenalis, glandula, 176, 178
effects of autonomic nervous system on, 244t, 623t
Suprarenalis, plexus, 236, 236t, 237
urinary organ innervation and, 239
Suprascapulares, nervus
compression of, *255*
in plexus brachialis, 322, 322t
Supraspinatus, musculus, 273, 273t
anterior shoulder and brachium, 266–267
bursa subacromialis and, 262
posterior shoulder and brachium, 269, 332
Supraspinatus, tendina, 263
in rotator cuff tear, *273*
Supravesicalis, fossa, 135
Surface anatomy
of back, 40–41
of brachium, 350–351
of caput, 588–589
of carpus, 352–353
of manus, 352–353
of membrum inferius, 450–451
of membrum superius, 350–351
of neck, 588–589
of pelvis, 248–249
of thorax, 120–121
Surfactant production, respiratory compromise and, *111*
Sympathetic innervation
of abdomen and pelvis, effects of, 244t
of esophagus, 98
of heart, 91
of tracheobronchial tree, 98
Sympathetic nervous system, 623
in abdomen and pelvis, 244
effects of, 244t
autonomic plexuses and, 237
effects of, 623t
genitalia and, 247
in thorax, 75, 75t
urinary organs and, 246
Symphysis, pubica, 248
Symphysis pubica, 124–127
diaphragma pelvis musculi and, 141
in female pelvis, 151
in male pelvis, 150
as perineal boundary, 137

Synaptic organization, in autonomic nervous system, 622
Syndesmosis, tibiofibulare, 380, 409
  fibular fracture and, *381*
Syndesmotic ligamenti, of articulatio talocruralis, 408–409, 408t
Synovial popliteal cyst, *385*
Systema nervosa parasympathica, 623
  in abdomen and pelvis, 244
    effects of, 244t
  effects of, 623t
  esophagus and, 98
  genitalia and, 247
  heart and, 91
  in thorax, 75t
  tracheobronchial tree, 98
  urinary organs and, 246
Systema nervosum periphericum (PNS)
  components of, 592
  components of limbic regulation of, 621

T

Talocalcanea, articulatio, 406
Talocalcaneonavicularis, articulatio, 406
Talocruralis, articulatio, 402, 404–405
  ligamenta of, 408–409, 408t
  tendon sheaths and retinacula of, 415
  tibiofibular syndesmosis and, 380
Talofibulare, ligamentum, 408t, 409
Talometatarsale, articulatio, 403
Talonavicularis, articulatio, 403
Talus, 407
Tarsus
  arcus of, 410
  ossae of, 400–401
Taste, 619
Taste innervation, 549
TDLU, 63, 65. *See* Terminal duct lobular unit (TDLU)
Tears, to menisci, *387*
Telencephalon, 594–595
  in encephalon development, 593t
  formatio hippocampalis and, 596
  internal structures of, 597, 597t
  limbic system and, 621
  nervus olfactorius and, 471t, 472
Temporale, os, 526–527
  nervus facialis in, 478
  nervus vestibulocochlearis in, 481
  structures in, *527*
Temporalis, fossa, topography of, 501
Temporalis, musculus, 468, 468t
Temporalis superficialis, arteria, 494, 494t
Temporomandibularis, articulatio, 540–541
  capsula, 463, 468
    innervation of, 541
  dislocation of, *541*
Tendinae
  of digiti, 304–305
  of dorsum manus, 347
  palpable, of carpus, 352
  supraspinatus. *See* Supraspinatus, *tendina*
Tension pneumothorax, *113*
Tensor fasciae latae, musculus, 374, 374t
  anterior femur, 366–367
Tensor veli palatini, musculus, 545, 545t
Teres major, musculus, 277, 277t
  anterior shoulder and brachium, 264–267
  in back surface anatomy, 40
  posterior shoulder and brachium, 268–271, 332
Teres minor, musculus, 273, 273t
  in back surface anatomy, 40
  posterior shoulder and brachium, 268–271
Terminal duct lobular unit (TDLU), 63
  in breast cancer, *65*
Testicular primordium, 205
Testiculares, venae, 214, 214t
Testicularis, plexus, 236, 236t, 237
  intestinum tenue innervation and, 240
  urinary organ innervation and, 239
Testis, 198–199, 199t
  descendus of, 204
  vas sanguineum of, 199, 199t
Thalamus, 596–597, 597t
  spatial sense and, 618
Thenaris, musculi, 312–313, 312t
Thoracic volume, respiratory changes in, 112
Thoracic wall, 44–65
  arteriae and venae of, 56–57, 56t
  articulationes of, 48–49
  female mamma, 62–65. *See also* Mamma (female)
  innervation of, 58–59
  movement of, 48
  musculi of, 50–51, 50t. *See also* Diaphragma
  neurovasculature of, 60–61
Thoracica, arteria, 56
Thoracica interna, vena, 70, 71t
Thoracica, segmenta (costa VI pair), 45
  elements of, 45t
  structure of, 45
Thoracica, spina, 5, 5t, 8
  articulationes zygapophysiales of, 14
  kyphosis of, 2, *2*
  palpable processus spinosus at TXII, 4
  typical (TVI) structure of, 8
Thoracicae, vertebrae (TI–TXII). *See* Thoracica, spina
Thoracicus, ductus, lymphatic drainage and, 72–73
Thoracicus, nervus, longus, 322, 322t
Thoracis, cavitas, 66–75
  arteriae, 66, 68–69
  divisions of, 66
  innervation of, 74–75
  lymphatics of, 72–73
  mediastinum divisions in, 67
  nodi lymphoidei, 100
  sectional CT views of, 67
  structures of, 66t
  venae, 66, 70–71
Thoracoacromialis, arteria, 56, 56t
Thoracodorsalis, nervus, 323, 323t
Thoracolumbalis, fascia, 23
  lamina superficialis 26
  in surface anatomy, 40
Thoracolumbales, ligamenti, 20–21
Thorax (chest), 66–75. *See also* Thoracis, cavitas
  arteria medullaris segmentalis and, 610
  bony prominences of, 120
  cavitas pleuralis in, 102–119. *See also* Cavitas(tis) pleuralis
  female, 121
    male vs., 44
  lymphatic pathways in, 73
  male, 121
    vs. female, 44
  mediastinum in, 76–101. *See also* Mediastinum
  musculi of, 120
  surface anatomy of, 120–121
  wall of, 44–65. *See also* Thoracic wall
Thromboembolus, *115*
Thymus, 80
Thyroarytenoideus, musculus, 572, 572t
Thyrohyoideus, musculus, 562–563, 562t

Thyroidea, arteria, superior, 492, 493t
Thyroidea, cartilago, 570–571
  in caput and neck surface anatomy, 589
  in thorax surface anatomy, 120
Thyroidea, glandula, 574
  neurovasculature of, 575
Tibia, 356–357, 380–381
Tibial plateau, 382, 387
Tibialis anterior, musculus, 397, 397t
  anterior compartment, 392–393
Tibialis, nervus, communis, 433, 433t
Tibialis posterior, musculus, 399, 399t
  posterior compartment, 394–395
Tibiofibulares, ligamenti, 408t, 409
Tissue, erectile, in female, 193
Tonsilla palatina, 552
  infections of, *553*
Tonsilla pharyngea, 552
  infections of, *553*
Tonsillae, 552
  infections of, *553*
Trachea, 110
Tracheobronchial tree, 116–117
Tractus, medulla spinalis
  ascendens, 613–614, 614t
  descendens, 613, 615, 615t
Transversalis, fascia, 133, 133t
Transversum superior, ligamentum
  articulatio glenohumeralis and, 261
  of scapula, ossified, *255*
Tranversi, processi
  of atlas, 565
  in spina thoracica, 44, 45
  vertebral, 5, 5t
Transversospinalis, musculus, 32–33, 32t
Transversus abdominis, musculus, 130–131, 138–139, 138t
  of canalis inguinalis, 133, 133t
  vagina musculi recti abdominis and, 134
Transversus thoracis, musculus, 50–51, 50t
Trapezium, os, 300
  MR image of, 301
  tuberculi of, 299, 303
Trapezius, musculus, 276, 276t
  anterior shoulder and brachium, 264–267
  in back surface anatomy, 40
  in neck and, 560–561, 561t
  origins and insertions, 464–465
  paralysis of, 486
  posterior shoulder and brachium, 268–271, 332
Trapezoideum, os, 300
  MR image of, 301
Triceps brachii, musculus, 279, 279t
  axilla and, 333, 333t
  in back surface anatomy, 40
  posterior antebrachium, 290–291
  posterior shoulder and brachium, 268–271
Triceps surae, musculus, 398, 398t
  posterior compartment, 394–395
Trigeminus, nervus (CN V), 476–477
  in cavitas oris, 547
  injury to, effects of, 476t
  location, overview, 470
  mandibular division (CN V_3), 476–477, 476t
    in fossa infratemporalis, 503
    musculi masticatorii and, 464, 468, 488
  maxillary division (CN V_2), 476–477, 476t
    fossa pterygopalatina and, 505
  nervus auricularis innervation by, 529
  ophthalmic division (CN V_1), 476–477, 476t
  origin, 471t
  sensory rami of, 489
Trigoni
  in cardiac skeleton, 86
  hypoglossal, 487
  olfactory, 472
Trigonum caroticum, 580, 589
Trigonum sacralis in back surface anatomy, 41
Trigonum suboccipitalis, 585
Triquetrum, os, 300
  MR image of, 301
Triradiatus, cartilago, 125, 359
Trochanter major, in back surface anatomy, 40
Trochlea humeri, 256–257
Trochlearis, nervus (CN IV), 474
  injury to, effects of, 474t
  location, overview, 470
  origin, 471t
  palsy, *509*
"True" traction diverticula, *97*
Tuba auditiva, 530
  infection in, *527*
  musculi of, 555
Tuba (fallopi) uterina, 188–189
  function of, 186t
  pelvis and, 151
  in urogenital system, 186
Tubal (extrauterine) pregnancy, *143, 189*
Tuberculi
  of atlas, 565
  costalis. *See* Costae, tuberculum
  of os scaphoideum, 303
  of os trapezium, 303
  pubic, 248, 362
  in spina cervicalis, 558
Tuberculosis, *107*
Tuberositas ischii, 124–127
  in back surface anatomy, 40
  as perineum boundary, 137
Tuberositas minus, in thoracic surface anatomy, 120
Tuberositas, in surface anatomy
  of back, 40
  of thorax, 120
Tubuli seminiferi, 199
Tumor metastasis
  in breast cancer, *65*
  to nodi lymphoidei cervicales, *586*
  portal venous system and, *215*
Tunica albuginea, 198–199
Tunica dartos, 196, 198–199, 199t
Tunica vaginalis, 196
  lamina parietalis and visceralis, 198–199, 199t
Twelfth costa (TXII), palpable processus spinosus at, 4, 8
Tympanica superior, arteria, 534, 534t

U

Ulcera
  gastric, *159*
  peptic, *143*
Ulna, 280–281
  at carpus, 298, 299
  in membrum superius, 252–253
Ulnar tunnel, 343
Ulnare, ligamentum collaterale, 284–285, 284t
Ulnaris, arteria, 317
Ulnaris, nervus, 326t, 329
  damage to, *329*
  musculi innervated by, 329t

in regio carpalis, 342
sensory distribution, 329
Ulnaris palsy, nervus, *329*
Umbilicales, plicae, 135
Umbilicalis, arteria, 222, 222t
adult remnant of, 95t
postnatal, 95
in prenatal circulation, 94
Umbilicalis, medulla, postnatal, 95
Umbilicalis, vena, 94–95
adult remnant of, 95t
Umbilicus, 130–131
in prenatal circulation, 94
in thorax surface anatomy, 21, 120
Uncinatus, processus, 15
articulatio uncovertebralis and, 14, 14t, 15
nervus spinalis and arteria vertebralis proximity to, *15*
in spina cervicalis, 558
Uncovertebralis, articulatio, 14–15, 14t
Ureter, 180–181
embryonic derivatives of, 205t
accessory sex glands and, 200
Uretericus, plexus, 237
pelvic innervation and
in female, 242
in male, 243
urinary organ innervation and, 239
Urethra, 184–185, 200
embryonic derivatives of, 205t
lymphatic drainage of, 227
Urinaria, vesica, 182–185
effects of autonomic nervous system on, 244t, 623t
embryonic derivatives of, 205t
in female, 183–185
lymphatic drainage of, 227
in male, 182, 184–185
accessory sex glands and, 200
referred pain from, *246*
Urinary organs, 176–185
autonomic innervation of, 246
effects of autonomic nervous system on, 244t, 623t
nodi lymphoidei of, 228
Urogenital system, 186–187
embryonic structures, derivatives of, 205t
Urogenitalis, regio, 154
in female regio perinealis, 136
Uterovaginalis, plexus, 242
Uterus, 188–189
effects of autonomic nervous system on, 244t, 623t
function of, 186t
in pelvis, 151
in urogenital system, 186
Uvula, 550, 552–553
Uvulae, musculus, 545, 545t

V

Vagina, 190–191, 136, 151
function of, 186t
location of, 136, 151
in urogenital system, 186
vestibulum vaginae of, and glandulae vestibulares, 192
Vagina musculi recti abdominis, abdominal wall and, 134
Vaginae tendinae carpales, of dorsum of manus, 310, 310t
Vaginae tendinum
carpal and digital, 306
communication between, *307*
of tarsus, 415
Vagus, nervus (CN X), 470, 471t, 484–485, 484t
basis cranii and, 465
course and rami of, 485
esophageal innervation and, 98
gustatory system and, 619
injury to, effects of, 484t
in lingua innervation, 549
nervus auricularis innervation by, 529
in parasympathetic nervous system in thorax, 75, 75t
Valva aortae, 86, 87
auscultation site for, *87,* 87t
Valva of Kerckring, 160
Valva pneumothorax, *113*
Valva semilunares, during ventricular diastole, 86
Valva trunci pulmonalis, 86–87
auscultation site for, *87,* 87t
Valvae atrioventriculares, 86–87
auscultation sites for, *87,* 87t
Valvular heart disease, heart sounds and, *87,* 87t
Vasculature. *See* Arteriae; Neurovasculature; Venae; *individually named arteries and veins*
Vasti, musculi, 366–369, 378, 378t
Vena cava inferior, 70–71, 214–216
azygos system and, 70–71
in blood circulation, 82
in prenatal circulation, 94
tributaries of, 214, 214t
Vena cava superior, 70–71, 71t
in blood circulation, 82
impeded flow in, *567*
in prenatal circulation, 94
thoracic tributaries of, 71t
Vena jugularis. *See* Jugularis, vena
Venae. *See also individually named venae*
of abdomen, 214–221
of auris interna, 537
of back, 35
of basis cranii, 607
foramina for, 458
of brainstem, 607
of bulbus oculi, 517
of caput and neck, 496–497
of cavitas thoracica, 66, 70–71
of diaphragma, 54, 55t
of encephalon, 606
of esophagus, 99, 99t
of genitalia
female, 195, 225
male, 202, 225
of glandula thyroidea and parathyroidea, 575
of heart, 88–89
of medulla spinalis, 611
of membrum inferius, 422
superficialis, 434–435
venae perforantes, 423
of membrum superius, 318
venae superficiales, 330
of neck, 567
of orbita, 510
orbita and, 506t
of pelvis, 222–225, 222t
of pulmo, 114–115, 115t, 118
of rectum, 224
of testis, 199, 199t
of thoracic wall, 57
of tracheobronchial tree, 117
Venipuncture, *318*
Ventricular system, in encephalon, 605
in situ, 605
Ventriculus lateralis, 597, 597t, 605

Ventriculus (encephalon), 597, 597t
  and CSF circulation, 604
  system of, 605
Ventriculus (heart), 85–86
  arteria pulmonalis and, 114
  arteriae coronariae distribution and, 89
  blood circulation and, 82
  lymphatic drainage of, 100
Vertebra prominens (C7), 6, 558
  in back surface anatomy, 40
  ligamentum nuchae and, 19
Vertebrae, 2, 5, 5t
  cervicales, 6–7. *See* Spina cervicalis
  lumbales, 9. *See* Spina lumbalis
  sacrales, 10–11. *See Os* sacrum
  thoracicae, 8. *See* Spina thoracica
Vertebrae, arcus
  articulationes of, 14–15, 14t. *See also* Zygapophyseales, articulationes
  ligamenti of, 18, 559t
Vertebrae, corpus, 5, 5t
  articulationes of, 14, 14t, 15. *See also* Uncovertebrales, articulationes; Zygapophyseales, articulationes
  ligamenti of, 559t
  thoracic, 44, 45
  ventral slippage of, *7*
Vertebrae, ligamenti, 18–19, 18t
Vertebrae sacrales (SI–SIV). *See* Sacrum, os
Vertebrale, foramen, 5, 5t
  plexus venosus vertebralis and, 35
Vertebralis, arteria, processus uncinatus proximity to, *15*
Vertebralis, plexus venosus, 57, 611
Vesica biliaris, 172–173
  location of, 147
  referred pain from, *246*
  truncus coeliacus and, 210
Vesica seminales, 200, 243
  effects of autonomic nervous system on, 244t, 623t
Vesica urinea. *See* Urinary bladder
Vesicalis, arteria and venae, 222, 222t
Vesicalis, plexus, pelvic innervation and
  in female, 242
  in male, 243
  urinary organ innervation and, 239
Vesicalis, plexus venosus, 222, 222t
Vestibular system, 618
Vestibulare, glandulae, major and minor, 186
  function of, 186t
  primordium of, 205
  in urogenital system, 186
  and vestibulum vaginae, 192
Vestibularis, nervus. *See* Vestibulocochlearis, nervus (CN VIII)
Vestibulocochlearis, nervus (CN VIII), 480, 480t, 537
  auditory system and, 619
  in auris interna, 537
  injury to, effects of, 480t
  location, overview, 470
  origin, 471t
  in os temporale, 481
Vestibulum oris, 550, 550t
Visceralis, fascia(e)
  cervicalis profunda, 577, 577t
  in female pelvis, 151, 152
  in male pelvis, 150, 153
  pelvic, 154
Visceralis, fibrae
  nervi craniales, 471, 471t
    efferent, of nervus glossopharyngeus, 483
  and referred pain, *246*
Visceral nervous system. *See* Autonomic nervous system
Visceralis, pleura, 103
  lymphatic drainage of, 118
Viscerocranium, 454t
Vision, light reflection by lens and, 519
Visual axis, nervus oculomotorius palsy and, *509*
Visual cortex, 616
Visual field defects, *617*
Visual perception, 616
Visual system, 616–617, 616t
  lesions of, *617*
Vocalis, musculus, 572, 572t
VSD (septum ventriculare defect), *95*
Vulva, 186t

W

Waldeyer's ring, 552, 552t
Waves, in ECG recording, *90*
Weakness, of musculus gluteus minimus, *431*
Wedge resection (segmentectomy), *109*
"Whiplash" injury, *7*
Wilson lead, in ECG, *90*
Wolffian duct, 205, 205t

X

Xiphoideus, processus, 44, 46, 120
  diaphragma and, 52
  thoracic wall musculi and, 51

Z

"Z" line, 97
Zenker's diverticula, *97*
Zona orbicularis, 364
Zonulares, fibrae, 518
  light reflection by lens and, 519
Zygapophyseales, articulationes, 14, 14t
  innervation of, 36
  in spina cervicalis, 558
Zygomaticus, musculus, 467, 467t